TOXICOLOGY
OF
PESTICIDES

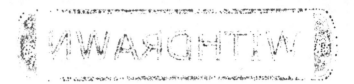

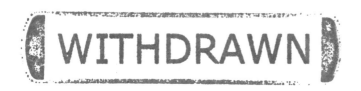

TOXICOLOGY OF PESTICIDES

Wayland J. Hayes, Jr., M.D., Ph.D.

Professor of Biochemistry
Center in Environmental Toxicology, Department of Biochemistry
Vanderbilt University School of Medicine
Nashville, Tenn.

Formerly Chief Toxicologist,
Pesticides Program, National Communicable Disease Center
U.S. Public Health Service

The Williams & Wilkins Company/*Baltimore*

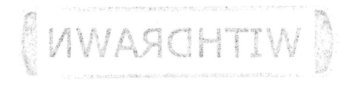

Made in the United States of America

Library of Congress Cataloging in Publication Data

Hayes, Wayland J   1917–
    Toxicology of pesticides.
    1. Pesticides—Toxicology.   I.   Title.
[DNLM: 1.   Pesticides—Poisoning.   WA24O H418t]
RA1270.P4H38   615.9′02   74-17329
ISBN 0-683-03897-4

The writing of this book was partially supported by Public Health Service
Grant No. ES-00267

Composed and printed at the
Waverly Press, Inc.
Mt. Royal and Guilford Aves.
Baltimore, Md. 21202, U.S.A.

TO

Philip Theophrastus Bombast von Hohenheim

called

PARACELSUS

who said

**Was ist das nit gifft ist? alle ding sind
gifft vnd nichts ohn gifft/Allein die dosis macht
das ein ding kein gift ist.***

or in more
familiar language

Dosage Alone Determines Poisoning

* Reproduction by permission of the National Library of Medicine from their copy
of Paracelsus' *Drey Bücher* printed in Cologne by the Heirs of Arnold Byrckmann in
1564.

PREFACE

The past two decades have been marked by public concern over the effects of pesticides on human health and on the environment. Examples of this concern may be found in numerous conferences and in the reports of several official committees. In its evaluation of the balance between benefit and risk in the use of pesticides, one of these committees, chaired by Senator Abraham Ribicoff, concluded that: "... the quantity and quality of empirical information as to both the benefits and risks of chemical pesticides available to scientists and administrators in Government agencies, academic institutions, and private industry were far more extensive than was generally recognized." This conclusion was accurate, and yet years after the report there was no single source to which a person could go for a description of the basic principles of toxicology and information about pesticides that would permit a rational decision about safety.

Widespread use of my *Clinical Handbook on Economic Poisons*, both in its English and its Spanish editions, encouraged me to undertake a book of much broader scope. Like the *Handbook*, the present volume is directed partly to the practicing physician who must advise his patients about the safe use of pesticides and always be ready, if an emergency occurs, to diagnose and treat poisoning. Like the *Handbook*, this volume will also be of use to county agents, health officers, legal experts, manufacturers, formulators, and applicators of pesticides.

Unlike the *Handbook*, this volume is con-cerned less with individual compounds, but rather deals with the principles, the general conditions of exposure, the observed effects of this exposure on human health, the problems of diagnosis and treatment, the means of preventing injury, and brief outlines of the impact of pesticides on domestic animals and wildlife. The book is written in the hope of showing how the modern, quantitative science of toxicology can help to achieve a rational approach to environmental chemicals.

Many misunderstandings regarding pesticides could be avoided if the persons involved were familiar with dosage-response relationships, which constitute the most important single principle in toxicology. It is for this reason that the book is dedicated to Paracelsus, whose famous statement about the importance of dosage in determining poisoning was published at least as early as 1564. The importance of dosage cannot be appreciated fully except in association with a quantitative study of all factors bearing on toxicity. It is possible to measure the contribution each of the more important factors usually makes to variation in toxicity and to point out the contribution it can make in exceptional circumstances. In contrast with the limited importance of other factors, the dosage of any compound always is decisive in determining its effect. Therefore, wherever possible, clinicians should be provided with information on tolerated doses or blood levels of pesticides, as well as information on doses or blood levels that have produced illness and larger ones that have produced death. Differences in exposure can explain how a compound that is dangerous to workers may be safe for the general population or *vice versa*. In a similar way, the completely different habits of different species may explain why one will receive a large or even fatal dosage in the same general environment in which other species, including man, receive only trivial exposure. Thus, quantitative toxicology permits both the clinician and the ecologist to reach a correct diagnosis.

An effort to describe or even to outline the aspects of toxicology that relate to pesticides indicates to what extent toxicology is intertwined with other disciplines. Toxicology is now far different from the classical combination of clinical and forensic medicine with analytical chemistry that constituted toxicology for more than a century and that the general public still identifies with the subject.

Most effort in toxicology now is devoted to safety evaluation. Forensic medicine is no less important than in the past, but far more toxicologists today are concerned with laws that regulate the safe use of chemicals than are involved with laws regarding detection of poisoning and the punishment of poisoners.

The pesticide problem is not merely one concerning the chemical industry and professional farmers, foresters, and applicators, or one concerning only those who wish to protect wildlife, or those responsible for control of malaria and other vector-borne diseases of man and his livestock. Rather, the pesticide problem concerns every person who wants food at a reasonable price and who wants his home free of vermin. The problem can be solved only on the basis of sound toxicological principles. Knowledge of these principles permits agreement and a cooperative approach on the part of persons professionally responsible for protection of our food, our health, and our wildlife, respectively. Ignorance of these principles limits some other persons to a partisan approach that may be dangerous to the common good.

This book will accomplish one of its important objectives if it suggests the scope of modern toxicology and indicates to those interested in one or another aspect of the pesticide problem how toxicology can and must contribute to a scientific evaluation of pesticides and other chemicals and thus to their judicious use. Of course, basic toxicological principles that apply to pesticides apply to other compounds. In fact, it may come as a surprise how many materials first employed as pesticides have been used as drugs and *vice versa*.

The redefinition and expansion of toxicology is not static. New segments are being added. Old concepts continually are being reexamined. The change is so rapid that even some toxicologists are not aware of it all. For example, one part of modern toxicology is concerned with poisons elaborated by a wide variety of plants and animals and with the defenses that other organisms have evolved for their protection against these poisons. By elucidating these interactions, toxicology contributes to the understanding of biology and ecology. This understanding, in turn, may have practical implications for the recurring problem of resistance of organisms to compounds of both biological and synthetic origin. It is also possible that study of the wide range of poisons produced by other organisms may reveal one or more new compounds useful as pesticides or drugs.

Another objective of this book is to point out needs in toxicology. The greatest single theoretical and practical need is for a thorough exploration of the statistical and biochemical aspects of the effects of small dosages. This is discussed in connection with thresholds of beneficial and harmful actions and their chemical bases, the beneficial effects of small dosages, and mathematical models for dosage-response relationships. Other important but more restricted needs vary all the way from that for a dependable test for hypersensitivity to a specific chemical to the need for an objective way to evaluate various ecological factors known to influence populations. The test for hypersensitivity would improve the care of individual patients. The ecological evaluation would improve our insight into the fate of the falcon and the plight of the pelican. Many other deficiencies in our knowledge are mentioned in connection with discussion of relevant information already available.

I am indebted to several scientists and publishers for permission to reproduce copyrighted material, and this is duly recorded in connection with the specific tables and figures. Chapter 5 of this book is an updated and expanded version of my essay published in 1968 as part of *Modern Trends in Toxicology*. I am thankful to Butterworth & Company Ltd. for permission to reuse much of the original writing. I am grateful also to the Royal Society who generously allowed me to use selected parts of my paper on "Toxicity of Pesticides to Man: Risks from Present Levels," published earlier in the Proceedings of the Society.

I am grateful to my colleagues, all of whom have been supportive and in many instances very helpful. Dr. John Barnes reviewed the outline at an early stage and helped to determine the subjects covered and their arrangement. Dr. William F. Durham reviewed the entire book. Dr. George Decker reviewed the section on the benefits of pesticides to agriculture. Dr. Robert A. Neal reviewed the section on qualitative metabolism, and Dr. John Robinson reviewed the part on the dynamics of storage. The late Dr. Rudolph Radeleff reviewed the chapter on domestic animals. Dr. Lucille and William Stickel reviewed the chapter on wildlife in an unusually detailed and constructive way. Dr. Harry Hays and Dr. William Upholt supplied information on regulatory matters. Dr. M. Vandekar and Dr. John Copplestone furnished valuable information on international aspects of pesticides, including their contribution to improved health and economic development through control of malaria and other vector-borne diseases. Dr. Henry M. Kissman and Mr. Bruno M. Vasta reviewed Appendix I and supplied the CAS Register Numbers contained in it. Mrs. Claudia Lewis helped with references. Mrs. Lynn Wilson and Miss Karin Brewer edited the manuscript, read proof, and prepared much of the index. Mrs. Carol Blythe, Mrs. Joanne Liddle, and Miss Lynn Holt typed the manuscript. In spite of the important assistance given by my friends, they must not be blamed for omissions and mistakes that inevitably persist. I hope that a wider range of friends will now draw these defects to my attention.

Wayland J. Hayes, Jr.

CONTENTS

Chapter 1.
INTRODUCTION **1**

1.1 Definition of Toxicology   1
1.2 Scope of Toxicology   1
  1.2.1 The Major Subdivision of Toxi-
     cology   2
     1.2.1.1 Toxicological Aspects of
        Legal Medicine   2
     1.2.1.2 Toxicological Aspects of
        Occupational Health   4
     1.2.1.3 Relation of Toxicology to
        Experimental Pathology . .   5
     1.2.1.4 Clinical and Veterinary
        Toxicology   5
     1.2.1.5 Evaluation of Safety   5
     1.2.1.6 Environmental Toxicology.   6
  1.2.2 Training of Toxicologists   8
  1.2.3 Societies Related to Toxicol-
     ogy   8
1.3 Definition of Pesticides   9
1.4 Benefits from Pesticides   9
  1.4.1 Health and Comfort   10
     1.4.1.1 Kinds of Diseases Con-
        trolled   10
     1.4.1.2 Benefits from Disease
        Control   10
  1.4.2 Agriculture and Forestry   15
     1.4.2.1 Losses Caused by Pests . .   15
     1.4.2.2 Utilization of Farm Land in
        the United States of Amer-
        ica   16
     1.4.2.3 Crop Production per Unit
        Area   17

     1.4.2.4 Factors Permitting Main-
        tenance of Food Supply . . .   17
     1.4.2.5 Agricultural Benefits from
        Pesticides   18
  1.4.3 Protection of Stored Products .   19
1.5 Production and Use of Pesticides .   **20**
  1.5.1 Production of Pesticides   20
     1.5.1.1 Introduction of Pesticides .   20
     1.5.1.2 USA Production   21
     1.5.1.3 World Production   22
     1.5.1.4 USA Imports and Exports .   22
  1.5.2 Economic Value of Pesticides .   23
     1.5.2.1 Cost of Pesticides   23
     1.5.2.2 Wholesale Cost of Imports
        and Exports   24
  1.5.3 Use of Pesticides   24
     1.5.3.1 Tonnage Used   24
     1.5.3.2 Number of Compounds
        and Products   24
  1.5.4 Methods of Application   26
**1.6 Pesticide Problems and Their Solu-
  tions** **27**
  1.6.1 Nature of Pesticide Problems .   27
  1.6.2 Proposed Solutions   27
     1.6.2.1 The Economic Approach .   28
     1.6.2.2 Empirical Approaches to
        Pesticide Problems   28
1.7 Standard References on Pesticides .   **29**
  1.7.1 Nomenclature   29
  1.7.2 General Information   31
1.8 Conventions Used in This Book . . .   **33**

xi

Chapter 2.
GENERAL PRINCIPLES: DOSAGE AND OTHER FACTORS
INFLUENCING TOXICITY 37

2.1 Kinds of Toxicity 37
  2.1.1 Nature of Injury 37
  2.1.2 Duration of Injury 37
    2.1.2.1 Factors in the Chronicity of Injury 37
    2.1.2.2 Reversibility 38
2.2 Quantitation of Dosage-Response Relationships 39
  2.2.1 The ED 50 or LD 50 39
    2.2.1.1 The 1-Dose ED 50 or LD 50 39
    2.2.1.2 The 90-Dose ED 50 or LD 50 43
    2.2.1.3 Kinds of Phenomena Showing a Cumulative Log-Normal Form in Their Dosage-Response Relationships .. 45
  2.2.2 The Chronicity Index 45
  2.2.3 Time Relationships 46
    2.2.3.1 The ET 50 or LT 50 47
    2.2.3.2 The Logtime-Logdosage Curve 48
  2.2.4 Problem of Measuring Effect of Dispersed Toxicants 52
    2.2.4.1 The EC 50 and LC 50 53
  2.2.5 Measurement of Graded Responses 53
  2.2.6 Dosage at the Tissue Level ... 53
  2.2.7 Statistical Considerations 53
    2.2.7.1 Number of Subjects 53
    2.2.7.2 Randomization of Subjects 55
    2.2.7.3 Selection of Dosage Levels 55
    2.2.7.4 Effects of Small Dosages .. 55
    2.2.7.5 The Geometric Mean 62
    2.2.7.6 Reproducibility of Results. 63
    2.2.7.7 Abnormal Values in Control Groups 64
2.3 Dosage-Response Relationships in Different Kinds of Toxicity or Change 64
  2.3.1 Toxicity (*Sensu Stricto*) 64
  2.3.2 Neurotoxicity 64
  2.3.3 Teratogenesis 64
  2.3.4 Carcinogenesis 64
  2.3.5 Mutagenesis 65
  2.3.6 Hypersensitivity and Allergy .. 65
  2.3.7 Metabolism and Storage 65
  2.3.8 Induction of Enzymes 65
2.4 Factors Influencing Toxicity of Any Kind 67

  2.4.1 Compound 68
    2.4.1.1 Primary Compounds 68
    2.4.1.2 Derived Compounds 69
  2.4.2 Dosage 69
  2.4.3 Schedule of Dosage 69
  2.4.4 Duration of Dosage 70
  2.4.5 Route of Exposure 71
  2.4.6 Interaction of Compounds 72
    2.4.6.1 Kinds of Interaction 72
    2.4.6.2 Mechanisms of Interaction 75
  2.4.7 Species and Strain Differences 75
    2.4.7.1 Differences between Parasites and Hosts 75
    2.4.7.2 Differences between Vertebrates 76
  2.4.8 Individual Differences 78
  2.4.9 Sex and Other Endocrines 80
    2.4.9.1 Sex 80
    2.4.9.2 Other Endocrines 81
  2.4.10 Age 81
  2.4.11 Nutrition 82
    2.4.11.1 General Nutritional Condition 82
    2.4.11.2 Effects of Protein 82
    2.4.11.3 Miscellaneous Nutritional Effects 83
  2.4.12 Isolation and Crowding 84
    2.4.12.1 Effects of Isolation and Aggregation 84
    2.4.12.2 Effect of Crowding 85
  2.4.13 Other Social or Psychological Factors 85
  2.4.14 Disease 85
  2.4.15 Temperature 87
  2.4.16 Pressure and Altitude 88
  2.4.17 Light and Other Radiation ... 88
    2.4.17.1 Direct Biological Effects of Radiation 89
    2.4.17.2 Photosensitization 89
  2.4.18 Circadian and Other Rhythms. 91
    2.4.18.1 Circadian Rhythms in Mammals 96
  2.4.19 Other Factors Influencing Toxicity 97
    2.4.19.1 Seasonal Differences 97
    2.4.19.2 Relative Humidity 97
    2.4.19.3 Aquatic Factors 97
  2.4.20 Discussion of Factors Influencing Toxicity 98

Chapter 3.
GENERAL PRINCIPLES: METABOLISM 107

3.1 Qualitative Aspects of Metabolism 107
  3.1.1 Possibility of "External Metabolism" 107
  3.1.2 Biotransformation 107
    3.1.2.1 Known Reactions 107
    3.1.2.2 Enzymatic Basis of Biotransformation 108
    3.1.2.3 Relation of Enzymes to Toxicity 117
  3.1.3 Species, Strain, Individual, and Genetic Factors in Metabolism 118
    3.1.3.1 Species Differences in Metabolism 118
    3.1.3.2 Individual and Strain Differences in Metabolism . . . 118
    3.1.3.3 Genetic Factors 127
  3.1.4 Toxicity of Metabolites 129
3.2 Quantitative Aspects of Metabolism 129
  3.2.1 Factors Influencing the Transfer and Availability of Chemicals in the Body 129
    3.2.1.1 Properties of Membranes . 130
    3.2.1.2 Ionization 130
    3.2.1.3 Protein Binding 131
    3.2.1.4 Passive and Specialized Transfer 132
  3.2.2 Absorption 133
    3.2.2.1 Indirect Measurement of Absorption 134
    3.2.2.2 Direct Measurement of Absorption 134

    3.2.2.3 Gastrointestinal Absorption 135
    3.2.2.4 Respiratory Absorption . . 136
    3.2.2.5 Dermal Absorption 140
    3.2.2.6 Absorption by Other Routes 150
  3.2.3 Dynamics of Distribution and Storage 150
    3.2.3.1 Distribution after a Single Dose 151
    3.2.3.2 Storage in Relation to Repeated Intake 154
    3.2.3.3 Factors Other than Dosage and Time that Affect Storage 161
    3.2.3.4 Storage in Relation to Toxicity 166
    3.2.3.5 Storage in Relation to the Ecosystem 167
  3.2.4 Excretion 168
    3.2.4.1 Respiratory Excretion 168
    3.2.4.2 Biliary and Fecal Excretion 168
    3.2.4.3 Urinary Excretion and Its Relation to Other Forms of Excretion 169
    3.2.4.4 Excretion in Milk 170
    3.2.4.5 Factors Changing The Rate of Excretion 170
  3.2.5 Balance Studies 171
3.3 Methods of Studying Metabolism . 172
  3.3.1 Tracers 172
  3.3.2 New Chemical Techniques 172
  3.3.3 Metabolic Pool Technique 172

Chapter 4.
GENERAL PRINCIPLES: NATURE OF INJURIES AND TESTS FOR THEM 182

4.1 Mode of Action 182
  4.1.1 Nonspecific Actions 183
    4.1.1.1 Corrosive Action 183
    4.1.1.2 Ferguson's Principle 183
  4.1.2 Specific Action 184
    4.1.2.1 Enzymes 184
    4.1.2.2 Critical Molecules 185
    4.1.2.3 Membranes 186
4.2 Effects on Cells and Tissues 187
  4.2.1 Cells 187
    4.2.1.1 Spindle Poisoning 187
    4.2.1.2 Mutagenesis 188
    4.2.1.3 Carcinogenesis 190
  4.2.2 Cardiovascular System 194
    4.2.2.1 Blood and Lymph Vessels 194

  4.2.3 Respiratory System 194
    4.2.3.1 Lungs 194
  4.2.4 Gastrointestinal System and Intermediary Metabolism 195
    4.2.4.1 Liver 195
  4.2.5 Urinary System 195
    4.2.5.1 Kidneys 195
  4.2.6 Muscles, Supportive Tissues, and Skin 196
    4.2.6.1 Mesothelial Layers 196
  4.2.7 Nervous System and Sense Organs 196
    4.2.7.1 Central Nervous System . . 196
    4.2.7.2 Peripheral Nervous System 197
    4.2.7.3 Eye 197

4.2.8 Endocrine Glands 197
  4.2.8.1 Pancreas 197
  4.2.8.2 Thyroid 197
4.2.9 Reproductive System 197
  4.2.9.1 Testis 197
4.2.10 Embryo and Fetus 197
  4.2.10.1 Teratogenesis 197
  4.2.10.2 Teratogenesis in Man ... 201
4.3 Some Techniques for Measuring Different Kinds of Injury 201
  4.3.1 Biochemical and Biophysical Investigations 203
  4.3.2 Toxicological Studies on Isolated Cells 203
  4.3.3 Tests of Mutagenesis 204
    4.3.3.1 Background of Tests of Mutagenesis 204
    4.3.3.2 Outline of Tests 204

    4.3.3.3 Toxicological Aspects of Tests of Mutagenesis 206
  4.3.4 Tests of Carcinogenesis 207
  4.3.5 Tests of Effects Specific to Certain Organs or Systems 207
    4.3.5.1 Pharmacological Tests ... 207
    4.3.5.2 Tests of Respiratory Toxicity 208
    4.3.5.3 Tests of Dermal Toxicity, Irritation, and Sensitization 208
    4.3.5.4 Tests of Irritation of the Eye 214
    4.3.5.5 Tests of Behavior 214
    4.3.5.6 Tests of Reproduction 215
    4.3.5.7 Techniques for Study of Teratogenesis 217
    4.3.5.8 Tests of Oral Toxicity 217

Chapter 5.
STUDIES IN MAN **225**

5.1 Cases 226
5.2 Medical Use 226
5.3 Use Experience 226
5.4 Volunteers 228
  5.4.1 Introduction 228
    5.4.1.1 Kinds of Studies 228
  5.4.2 Legal Considerations 235
    5.4.2.1 Codes of Practice 235
    5.4.2.2 Regulation of Clinical Research and Investigations .. 236
    5.4.2.3 A Law Permitting Tests in Man 236
    5.4.2.4 Legal and Other Requirements for Tests in Man ... 237
    5.4.2.5 Court Action 238
    5.4.2.6 Consent 239
  5.4.3 Design of Studies 240
    5.4.3.1 Selection of Parameters .. 240
    5.4.3.2 Selection of Dosage 241
    5.4.3.3 Choice of Volunteers 241
    5.4.3.4 Studies of Workers 243
    5.4.3.5 Protocol and Conduct of the Study 243
    5.4.3.6 Protection of the Volunteer 246
    5.4.3.7 Protection of the Investigator 247
  5.4.4 Motivation of Volunteers 248
  5.4.5 Conclusion 248

5.5 Measurement of Exposure Under Practical Conditions 249
  5.5.1 Measurement of Respiratory Exposure 249
    5.5.1.1 Estimation of Respiratory Exposure from Air Concentration 250
    5.5.1.2 Estimation of Respiratory Exposure from Trapping Toxicant in Inhaled Air ... 251
  5.5.2 Measurement of Dermal Exposure 252
    5.5.2.1 Estimation of Dermal Exposure from Air Concentration 252
    5.5.2.2 Estimation of Dermal Exposure from Absorbent Samplers 253
    5.5.2.3 Estimation of Dermal Exposure from Washing 253
    5.5.2.4 Conventions for Measuring Dermal Exposure 254
  5.5.3 Measurement of Oral Exposure 255
  5.5.4 Problems of Measuring Contributions from Different Routes of Exposure 256
    5.5.4.1 Smyth Technique 256
    5.5.4.2 Differential Protection Technique 256

Chapter 6.
RECOGNIZED AND POSSIBLE EXPOSURE TO PESTICIDES **265**

6.1 Residues in Food 265
  6.1.1 Residues in Animal Products .. 266
    6.1.1.1 Observed Residues 266

    6.1.1.2 Factors Influencing Residues in Animal Products .. 267
  6.1.2 Residues in Vegetable Prod-

ucts 267
6.1.2.1 Observed Residues 267
6.1.2.2 Factors Influencing Residues on Plants and Plant Products 269
6.1.3 Residues in Water 274
6.1.3.1 Residues in Potential Drinking Water 274
6.1.3.2 Residues in Other Water and Sediments 274
6.1.4 Removal of Residues from Food and Water 275
6.1.4.1 Removal of Residues from Food 275
6.1.4.2 Removal of Residues from Water 276
6.1.5 Residues in Total Diet 276
6.1.5.1 Regular Diet 276
6.1.5.2 Special Diet 281
6.2 Residues in air 282
6.2.1 Observed Residues in Community Air 282
6.2.2 Drift and Related Matters 283
6.2.2.1 Local Drift 283
6.2.2.2 Worldwide Drift 284
6.2.2.3 Factors Influencing Residues in Community Air ... 285

6.2.3 Exposure of Workers 288
6.2.3.1 Respiratory and Dermal Exposures of Workers 288
6.2.3.2 Oral Exposure of Workers . 294
6.3 Residues in soil 294
6.3.1 Observed Residues in Soil 295
6.3.1.1 Residues Following Application to Crops 295
6.3.1.2 Residues Following Direct Application to Soil 297
6.3.2 Physical and Chemical Changes of Pesticides in the Soil 298
6.3.2.1 Nature of Changes 298
6.3.2.2 Factors Influencing Residues in Soil 298
6.3.2.3 Distribution of Residues in the Mud Walls of Houses .. 303
6.4 Importance of Residues in Different Media 304
6.4.1 Importance to Man 304
6.4.2 Importance to Other Organisms 305
6.4.2.1 Domestic Animals 305
6.4.2.2 Wildlife 306
6.5 Degradation of Poisons in Nature 306

Chapter 7.
RECOGNIZED AND POSSIBLE EFFECTS OF PESTICIDES IN MAN 311

7.1 Incidence of Poisoning 311
7.1.1 Poisoning Generally 311
7.1.1.1 Mortality 311
7.1.1.2 Morbidity 313
7.1.2 Poisoning by Pesticides 316
7.1.2.1 Compounds that Have Caused Poisoning 316
7.1.2.2 Endemic Mortality 316
7.1.2.3 Endemic Morbidity 320
7.1.2.4 Epidemics of Poisoning by Pesticides 322
7.1.2.5 Experience of Special Groups 325
7.1.3 Record of Different Countries . 333
7.1.4 Factors in Poisoning 334
7.1.4.1 Compound 334
7.1.4.2 Dosage 335
7.1.4.3 Route of Exposure 335
7.1.4.4 Interaction of Compounds . 336
7.1.4.5 Race and Ethnic Group ... 336
7.1.4.6 Sex 336
7.1.4.7 Age and Competency 336
7.1.4.8 Accessibility 337
7.1.4.9 Containers and Labeling .. 338
7.1.4.10 Occupation 339
7.2 Incidence of Storage or Excretion . 339

7.2.1 Storage of Certain Chlorinated Hydrocarbon Pesticides 340
7.2.1.1 Storage in Bone 340
7.2.1.2 Storage in Fat 340
7.2.1.3 Storage in Blood 346
7.2.1.4 Storage in Organs 349
7.2.1.5 Storage in the Fetus 349
7.2.2 Excretion of Certain Chlorinated Hydrocarbon Pesticides . 349
7.2.2.1 Excretion in Milk 349
7.2.2.2 Excretion in Urine 352
7.2.2.3 Excretion in Feces 352
7.2.2.4 Excretion in Expired Air .. 353
7.2.3 Storage and Excretion of Other Pesticides 353
7.2.4 Factors Involved in Storage and Excretion 355
7.2.4.1 Identity of Factors 355
7.2.4.2 Evaluation of Factors Influencing Storage of Pesticides in Man 361
7.3 Other Effects of Pesticides 362
7.4 Possible Effects of Pesticides 363
7.4.1 Marginal Effects 363
7.4.2 Speculative Effects 366
7.5 Criteria of Safety 367

Chapter 8.
DIAGNOSIS AND TREATMENT OF POISONING **379**

8.1 Diagnosis **379**
  8.1.1 Chemical Epidemiology 379
    8.1.1.1 Retrospective Study 381
    8.1.1.2 Prospective Study 381
  8.1.2 History of Exposure 382
  8.1.3 Clinical Findings 382
  8.1.4 Laboratory Findings 383
    8.1.4.1 Diagnostic Tests 383
    8.1.4.2 Supportive Tests 391
8.2 Treatment **391**
  8.2.1 Removal of Poison 391
    8.2.1.1 Emesis 393
    8.2.1.2 Gastric Aspiration and Lavage 395
    8.2.1.3 Evacuation of the Gut . . . 397
    8.2.1.4 Removal of External Poison 398
    8.2.1.5 Removal to Fresh Air 399
  8.2.2 Supportive Treatment 399
    8.2.2.1 Maintenance of Airway and Artificial Respiration 399

    8.2.2.2 Oxygen Therapy 401
    8.2.2.3 Infusions and Transfusions 402
    8.2.2.4 Sedatives 403
    8.2.2.5 Stimulants 404
    8.2.2.6 Antiemetics 405
    8.2.2.7 Steroids 406
    8.2.2.8 Antibiotics 406
    8.2.2.9 Nursing Care 406
  8.2.3 Antidotes 407
    8.2.3.1 Detoxifying or Neutralizing Antidotes 407
    8.2.3.2 Pharmacological Antidotes . 409
    8.2.3.3 Oximes 410
    8.2.3.4 Chelating Agents 417
    8.2.3.5 Antidotes for Poisoning by Cyanide 421
    8.2.3.6 Oxygen 422
    8.2.3.7 Calcium 423
    8.2.3.8 Vitamin K 423

Chapter 9.
PREVENTION OF INJURY BY PESTICIDES **429**

9.1 Regulations **429**
  9.1.1 Regulation of Labeling 430
    9.1.1.1 Labeling in the United States of America 430
    9.1.1.2 Labeling in Great Britain . . 432
    9.1.1.3 International Proposals for Labeling 433
    9.1.1.4 Graphic Warning Labels . . 433
  9.1.2 Regulation of Transport and Storage 434
    9.1.2.1 Regulation of Transport in the United States of America 434
    9.1.2.2 International Regulation of Transportation 436
    9.1.2.3 Regulation of Storage 436
  9.1.3 Regulation of Use 436
    9.1.3.1 Regulation of Importation or Sale 436
    9.1.3.2 Regulation of Application . 436
    9.1.3.3 Licensing of Operators . . . 437
    9.1.3.4 Regulation of Working Conditions 438
    9.1.3.5 Inspection 438
  9.1.4 Regulation of Residues 439
    9.1.4.1 The Bases for Safety Factors 439
    9.1.4.2 Acceptable Daily Intake . . 442
    9.1.4.3 Tolerances 442
    9.1.4.4 Water Standards 446
    9.1.4.5 Threshold Limit Values or

        Maximal Allowable Concentrations 446
    9.1.4.6 Other Standards 452
    9.1.4.7 Toxicity Rating or Class . . 453
  9.1.5 Cost of Regulations 453
  9.1.6 Liability 455
9.2 Choice of Compound and Formulation **455**
  9.2.1 Choice of Compound 455
  9.2.2 Choice of Formulation 456
    9.2.2.1 Liquid and Paste Formulations 456
    9.2.2.2 Dry Formulations 457
    9.2.2.3 Protective Additives 458
9.3 Protective Practices and Devices . **458**
  9.3.1 Protective Practices 458
    9.3.1.1 Avoidance of Exposure . . . 458
    9.3.1.2 Removal of Contamination 458
    9.3.1.3 Working in Pairs 459
    9.3.1.4 Storage for Safety 459
    9.3.1.5 Disposal of Empty Containers 460
    9.3.1.6 Disposal of Unwanted Pesticide 461
    9.3.1.7 Environmental Surveillance 462
    9.3.1.8 Medical Surveillance 463
  9.3.2 Protective Devices 464
    9.3.2.1 Industrial Protective Equipment 464
    9.3.2.2 Personal Respiratory Pro-

tection 464
9.3.2.3 Protective Clothing 468
9.3.2.4 Other Prophylactic Devices 469
**9.4 Education and Cooperative Com-
munity Relations** **470**
9.4.1 Education 470
9.4.1.1 Training of Workers 470

9.4.1.2 Training of the Public 471
9.4.2 Community Relations 472
9.4.2.1 Interdepartmental Committees and Bilateral
Agreements 473
**9.5 Alternative Methods of Pest Con-
trol** **474**

Chapter 10.
EFFECTS ON DOMESTIC ANIMALS 478

10.1 Incidence of Poisoning **478**
10.1.1 Poisoning Generally 478
10.1.2 Poisoning by Pesticides 479
10.1.2.1 Endemic Mortality and
Morbidity 479
10.1.2.2 Epidemics of Poisoning by
Pesticides 479

**10.2 Incidence of Storage and Excre-
tion** **481**
**10.3 Other Possible Effects of Pesti-
cides** **481**
10.4 Factors in Poisoning **481**

Chapter 11.
EFFECTS ON WILDLIFE 483

11.1 Toxicology **483**
11.1.1 Inherent Susceptibility of
Wildlife to Pesticides 483
11.1.2 Storage of Pesticides in Wildlife 483
11.1.2.1 Compounds Found in
Wildlife 484
11.1.2.2 Monitoring of Pesticides . 484
11.1.2.3 Geographical Distribution
of Pesticides 484
**11.2 Ecological Factors in Pest Con-
trol** **485**
11.2.1 Pest and Their Natural Control 485
11.2.1.1 The Nature of Pests 485
11.2.1.2 Natural Control 486
11.2.2 Biotic Simplification, a Cause
of Pest Problems 486
11.2.2.1 Faunal Imbalance 487
11.2.2.2 Emergent Pests 487
11.2.2.3 Evaluation of Biotic Simplification as a Cause of
Pest Problems 488
11.2.3 Food Chains 488
11.2.3.1 Secondary Poisoning 488
11.2.3.2 Biological Magnification . 489
11.2.3.3 Bases for Population De-

clines Among Certain
Falcons and Fish-Eating
Birds 492
11.2.3.4 Evaluation of Biological
Magnification 502
11.2.4 The Nature of Pest Control .. 503
11.3 Injury to Wildlife **503**
11.3.1 Injury in Relation to Kind of
Treatment 504
11.3.1.1 Application to Water ... 504
11.3.1.2 Application to Non-Agricultural Land 505
11.3.1.3 Application to Agricultural Land 507
11.3.1.4 Accidental Contamination 507
11.3.2 Overall Evaluation of Injury . 508
11.4 Control of Wildlife **509**
11.5 Limitation of Injury to Wildlife .. **510**
11.5.1 Ecological Methods 510
11.5.2 Modified Use of Pesticides .. 510
11.5.2.1 Choice of Compound 510
11.5.2.2 Limitation of Dosage 511
11.5.2.3 Limitation of Area of Application 511
11.5.2.4 Timing of Application .. 512
11.5.3 Alternative Methods 512

Appendix I.
Chemical Names and CAS Registry Numbers of Pesticide Compounds
Mentioned in This Volume Arranged by Group **517**

Appendix II.
Some Units of Measure Used in This Book **534**

Appendix III.
Conversion Table for the Units of Measure Frequently Used in Connection
with the Toxicology of Pesticides **535**

Appendix IV.
Approximate Dosages (mg/kg/day) of a Compound for Certain Animals on
Diets Containing It at Different Concentrations that Do Not Influence Food
Intake **536**

Index **537**

1

INTRODUCTION

1.1 Definition of Toxicology

Toxicology is the qualitative and especially the quantitative study of the injurious effects of chemical and physical agents, as observed in alterations of structure and response in living systems; it includes the application of the findings of these studies to the evaluation of safety and to the prevention of injury to man and all useful forms of life.

Toxicology is concerned with untoward effects, but the toxicologist must base his judgments on a broad understanding of medicine. He must know the range of normal in order to identify correctly the abnormal. He must consider intended use in judging what is "adverse."

The dosage-response relationship is of such importance that it must be considered a part of the definition of toxicology. In fact it is mainly this principle that is signified by the word "quantitative" in the definition above. The principle was first stated by Paracelsus in his "Third Defense" of treatments he recommended, especially the use of mercury for treating syphilis. Since he was defending the harmlessness of his remedies, he stated the rule in a negative sense emphasizing that the *dosis* alone makes a thing not poison (see Dedication of this book). In what is thought to be the first complete Latin translation of the works of Paracelsus (1603), the passage in question appears on page 122 of the Second Book as follows: *"Dosis sola facit, vt venenum non fit."* Apparently this version was later shortened and made positive by dropping three words. In any event, one commonly sees the aphorism in the form *"Dosis sola facit ve-*

nenum." The English version in the Dedication expresses the sense of modern toxicology.

1.2 Scope of Toxicology

Modern toxicology contributes to clinical medicine, legal medicine, occupational medicine and hygiene, veterinary medicine, experimental pathology, and safety evaluation. Each of these disciplines would be incomplete without the subject matter and point of view that distinguish toxicology. However, the importance of toxicology in these professions and disciplines varies greatly. Since the abandonment of Lister's form of asepsis, the surgeon has little concern for toxicology, but the pediatrician may be involved for several hours per week. The person responsible for safety evaluation devotes essentially 100% of his professional time to toxicology.

There is no aspect of toxicology that does not overlap other disciplines. Legal medicine involves not only toxicology but also law and pathology; it is largely concerned with evidence regarding causes of death, especially unnatural causes. Occupational health involves both medical and engineering aspects of toxicology, but of course it encompasses the proper lighting of workplaces, the problem of the working mother, and a host of other environmental relationships entirely separate from toxicology. Experimental pathology is, as the name implies, concerned mainly with pathology, but toxins often are used as tools to create morphological changes for study. The evaluation of safety of chemical compounds is the aspect of toxicology that overlaps other disci-

1

plines least, yet even here one must make constant use of pharmacology, biochemistry, analytical chemistry, pathology, and statistics.

1.2.1 The Major Subdivision of Toxicology

Table 1-1 lists books that constitute landmarks in toxicology. Some of them, concerned with a particular application of toxicology, are

discussed in the following sections. Others, concerned more with principles than with application, are discussed in Sections 1.1, 3.1.4, and 4.1.2.

1.2.1.1 Toxicological Aspects of Legal Medicine. In prehistoric times, people probably were familiar with the injurious effects of certain plants and minerals at least as soon as

Table 1-1

Books that Constitute Landmarks in Toxicology

Author	Title	Date of publication first edition	later editions[a]	Contribution
Abano, Pietro d' 1250-1315?	De venenis	1472	Eng. trans. 1924	one of the earliest of the important treatises on poisons
Ellenbog, Ulrich 1440-1499	Von den gifftigen besen Tempffen und Reuchen	1524[b]	Eng. trans. 1932	description of occupational poisoning by lead and mercury
Agricola, Georgius 1494-1555	De re metallica	1556	1621 1657 Eng. trans. 1919, 1950	description of pulmonary disease in miners
Paracelsus, 1493-1541	Von der Bergsucht oder Bergkranckheiten drey Bücher	1567		attributed pulmonary and other diseases to metal dusts and fumes
Ramazzini, Bernardino 1633-1714	De morbis artificium diatriba	1700	2nd 1703 Eng. trans. 1705, 1746	first comprehensive treatise on occupational diseases
Fontana Felice 1730-1805	Traité sur le vénin de la vipère sur les poisons américains, sur le laurier-cerise, et quelques autres poisons végétaux; on y a joint des observations sur la structure primitive du corps animal, différentes expériences sur la reproduction des nerfs et la description d'un nouveau canal de l'oeil	1781	Eng. trans. 1787 1795	descriptions of poisons and of antidotes
Delille, R. and Magendie, François 1783-1855	Des effets de l'Upas Tienté sur l'économie animal	1809		animal studies of arrow poisons
Orfila, Matthieu Joseph Bonaventure 1787-1853	Traité des poisons tirés des règnes minéral, végétal et animal ou toxicologie générale considérée sous les rapports de la pathologie et de la médecine légale	1814- 1815	2nd 1818 5th 1852 Eng. trans 1817	first treatment of toxicology as a separate discipline
Orfila, M.J.B.	Eléments de chimie médicale	1817	4th 1828 8th 1851	first treatise on chemical analysis in toxicology
Orfila, M.J.B.	Leçons de médecine légale	1821- 1823	2nd 1828 4th 1848	first treatise on legal medicine, especially forensic toxicology
Orfila, M.J.B.	Secours à donner aux personnes empoisonnées ou asphyxiées, suivis des moyens propres à reconnaître les poisons et les vins frelatés et à destinguer la mort réelle de la mort apparente	1818	2nd 1821 3rd 1825 Eng. trans. 1818, 1819 1926	a popular condensation of the Traité des poisons

Table 1-1 (continued)

Author	Title	Date of publication		Contribution
		first edition	later editions[a]	
Chevallier, Jean-Baptiste-Alphonse 1793-1879	Dictionnaires des altérations et falsifications des substances alimentaires médicamenteuses et commerciales, avec l'indication des moyens de les reconnaître	1850	2nd 1854-55 3rd 1857-58	comprehensive treatise on the adulteration of foods, drugs, and commercial substances and briefer essays on many aspects of public health, including the health of workers exposed to lead, arsenic, and phosphorus
Bernard, Claude 1813-1878	Leçons sur les effets des substances toxiques et médicamenteuses	1857		introduction of experimental pathology
Lehmann Karl Bernhard 1858-1940	Die Methoden der praktischen Hygiene; Anleitung zuer Untersuchung und Benrtheilung der Aufgaben des täglichen Lebens; für Aertze, Chemiker und Juristen	1890	2nd 1901 Eng. trans. 1893	chemical and bacteriologic methods, examination of air, soil, and water for contaminants, and many other matters bearing on hygienic control
Kobert, Edward Rudolph 1854-1918	Lehrbuch der Intoxikationen	1893	Eng. trans.1897 1902-1906 (2 vols. 2nd ed.)	outstanding text, emphasis on forensic medicine
Lewin, Louis 1850-1929	Lehrbuch der Toxikologie[c]	1885	2nd 1897 4th 1929	valuable text
Lewin, L.	Die Gifte in der Weltgeschichte	1920		an account of poisons in world history
Peters, Rudolph A. 1889-	Biochemical Lesion and Lethal Synthesis	1963		elaboration of two basic concepts of toxicology

a. Editions and English translations. Translations are referenced separately only if they are discussed in the text.
b. Written in 1473 but not published until 1524.
c. Title as first published in 1885. Gifte und Vergiftungen is the title of the fourth edition, published in 1929.

they became aware of the therapeutic action of some of them. Certainly poisions were mentioned in written records as early as any that describe beneficial drugs. Hemlock (coniine), aconite, hyocyames, hellebore, opium, lead, antimony, and copper were mentioned in the Ebers Papyrus, thought to have been written about 1550 BC, but based on considerably earlier sources (Ebers, 1875; Bryan, 1931).

The earliest recognized poisons were capable of causing severe injury and of being used for murder or official executions. Socrates was killed with hemlock (*Conium maculatum*) as described by Plato (Church, 1896). Thus, knowledge of poisons was associated very early with one or another aspect of law. A very thorough description of the place of poisons in world history may be found in a book by Lewin (1920).

Noteworthy individual contributions to medicolegal toxicology appeared from time to time, as outlined in Table 1-1. However, it was not until the first quarter of the 19th Century that there was reason to recognize toxicology as a distinct discipline separable from pharmacology on the one hand and general clinical medicine on the other. This birth of toxicology as a separate discipline was accomplished by Bonaventura Orfila through publication of his first book in 1814 and 1815. This book, and three subsequent ones, each went through several editions and received widespread attention. Long before the end of his life in 1853, Orfila was recognized internationally as the founder of toxicology (Anonymous, 1853).

The first book, as indicated by its title (see Table 1-1), dealt with toxicology largely from the standpoint of clinical findings, pathology, and legal medicine. The unique contribution of the book was that it brought together previously scattered information in such a way that both its unity and utility were apparent. The book was translated promptly into several languages. English versions appeared within a few years not only in England but in the United States of America. An excellent translation, abridged chiefly by reducing the number of case histories but comprising over 500 pages, was published in Philadelphia (Nancrede, 1817). In the following year, Orfila himself issued (as his third book) a far more drastic abridgement to which, however, he added some items not in the original work.

The second book by Orfila (1817) emphasized the chemistry of poisons. He advocated positive analytical findings as a prerequisite for diagnosis of poisoning, and he developed a number of analytical procedures. Thus, several important aspects of the subject were recognizable as soon as toxicology itself was established as a separate discipline. In fact, for a long time the association of analytical chemistry and legal medicine constituted almost the whole of toxicology, and persons, especially chemists, who did this kind of work were the only recognized toxicologists.

Orfila did not neglect the strictly clinical aspects of toxicology. His third book, published in 1818, was concerned with the recognition and treatment of poisoning. Orfila realized the ineffectiveness of many remedies, including theriaca, consisting of a mixture of drugs. Following experiments, he recommended treatment such as artificial respiration, and a few antidotes such as white of egg, milk, common salt, vinegar, lemon juice, soap, gallnuts, and calcined magnesia. It may be seen that his antidotes included material to adsorb or expel poisons or to neutralize acids or alkalis. This clinical book was essentially a condensation of the longer treatise first published 4 years earlier. It was this abridged version more than the basic one that was translated into various languages, including English. Several translations appeared in the United States of America (Price, 1818; Black, 1819; Stevenson, 1826).

Orfila's fourth book (1821–1823) concerned legal medicine. Even the first edition was a substantial work, the two volumes consisting of 737 and 503 pages, respectively.

Whereas a sophisticated understanding of the dosage-response relationship was not achieved until the 20th Century (see Section 2.2.1.1), a general appreciation of its importance appeared early. Orfila (1814–1815) even attempted to study in dogs the mode of action of repeated small doses. Although he found this work difficult and not completely satisfactory, he concluded: "We have remarked, however, that the disease produced by poison given in small doses, presented the greatest analogy with that which followed the introduction of a larger quantity; the same observations were made on the lesions of textures [pathological lesions]." In spite of this generality, Orfila also recorded that consumption of small quantities of spurred rye (ergot) produces nervous symptoms, whereas consumption of a great deal at one time or consumption of small amounts for a long time produces gangrene. Undoubtedly a very important reason that the early writers gave little attention to the dosage-response relationship was their preoccupation with practical matters. As Orfila (1814–1815) stated in the preface to his first book, his concern was with "the effects of poisonous substances when administered in doses capable of producing serious accidents."

In Orfila's time, appreciation of the importance of dosage was based almost entirely on clinical observation, whether of man or animals. For about a century after toxicology was recognized as a separate discipline, it required the best chemistry could offer to detect a poison in the vomitus, excreta, or tissues of a victim. It was only with the development of modern analytical methods that toxicologists were forced to make a distinction between harmless and harmful levels of a wide range of inorganic and synthetic chemicals in human tissues and excreta. It is now becoming necessary to make a similar distinction between harmless and harmful changes in enzymes and other body functions that are altered by chemical and physical agents.

Orfila guided the early development of toxicology in the United States of America not only through translations of his books but also through the influence of his concepts on American authors (Coley, 1832) and on other authors whose books were republished in America (Christison, 1845).

1.2.1.2 Toxicological Aspects of Occupational Health. The origins of occupational toxicology were largely separate from those of legal medicine. As outlined in Table 1-1, there were some important early publications on occupational toxicology. However, because of the relative simplicity of early chemical industry and the prevalence of a laissez-faire attitude, occupational toxicology as it now exists is a product of the 20th Century.

Today, occupational toxicology is a complex, interdisciplinary field, requiring both physicians and engineers. Physical methods of medical examination retain their value but are supplemented by an ever growing list of valuable clinical laboratory tests. Engineers and other industrial hygienists monitor the exposure of workers, and through proper plant design, ventilation, and perhaps personal protective devices, guard against excessive exposure to a wide range of chemicals. Both the industrial physician and the industrial hygienist require a clear understanding of the dosage-response relationship. Chemical industry would be impractical if workers could tolerate no exposure whatever, and this industry now would be socially unacceptable if the chemical tolerance of workers were exceeded except in connection with rare and unavoidable accidents.

1.2.1.3 Relation of Toxicology to Experimental Pathology.

Working along lines suggested by Claude Bernard (1857), those interested in experimental pathology frequently utilize chemicals to produce characteristic lesions of basic interest to pathologists or physiologists. Chemicals can produce pathological changes that are no less astonishing for their specificity in relation to individual compounds than for their variety in relation to the tissues or functions that are changed by at least one compound.

Chemicals may be used to alter chromosomes or other structures within cells or their effects may be grossly visible in one or more tissues. Chemicals may affect different stages of the organism from the zygote through old age. This fact is the basis of further specialization. For example, much of teratology is experimental pathology in relation to the embryo and fetus. Some diseases may be produced or at least approximated through the use of chemicals—for example, the production of diabetes mellitus in rats by alloxan. Other examples are given in Chapter 4.

Even though the emphasis of experimental pathology is on lesions rather than on the agents that produce them, the discipline obviously makes an important contribution to toxicology.

1.2.1.4 Clinical and Veterinary Toxicology.

Clinical and veterinary problems must have been among the first aspects of toxicology to attract attention, but they were not an object of early specialization. Often it was only when poisoning aroused suspicion of foul play that it attracted the attention of a specialist. Most patients suffering from accidental poisoning were attended by a general practitioner. The situation was similar in veterinary medicine, except that this entire branch of medicine developed much more recently.

Although most cases of poisoning are still attended by physicians who are relatively unspecialized in toxicology, the clinician now can obtain information more promptly and efficiently than in the past because of poison control centers. Furthermore, some physicians now specialize in the care of patients poisoned by drugs and other chemicals. The American Academy of Clinical Toxicology has been formed to advance this aspect of the field.

Modern veterinary toxicology is well developed in its clinical and safety evaluation aspects. There is relatively little development of veterinary legal medicine, foul play being a human prerogative.

1.2.1.5 Evaluation of Safety.

More money and work are now expended on evaluation of safety than on all other aspects of toxicology combined. There has been no lessening of the importance of the toxicological features of patient care, legal medicine, occupational health, or experimental pathology. The concept of pretesting developed gradually. Drugs were among the first materials so tested. The first animal experiments were not required by law and were not very thorough by modern standards. Today, elaborate tests are required by law (21 USC 321 *et seq.*).

Industrial management has long recognized the necessity of learning the hazards of compounds in order to protect the men who make or formulate them. However, the rapid development of chemical industry, including the pesticide industry, and a concurrent increase in protective regulations (see Section 9.1) have led to a tremendous increase in testing to determine the safety of each compound before it is permitted to be sold or to be used for a particular purpose. Among the material now regulated and tested are the detergents, bleaches, glues, and other chemicals commonly used in the household.

The evaluation of safety is a continuing process for drugs and industrial chemicals, including pesticides. After a compound is released for a particular use, the possibility exists that side effects will be observed in patients, formulators, applicators, or others whose exposure is greater than that of most people. If a new use for the compound is discovered, then new studies may have to be carried out in animals in order to evaluate safety under the new conditions. Finally, a marked change in emphasis on a particular kind of injury (eg, emphasis on teratology following the epidemic caused by thalidomide) or merely the development of a new test may call for reevaluation of some compounds, including those in safe use for many years.

No matter what the outcome of tests may be, either before or after a compound is introduced for use, the toxic effects must be balanced against the benefits offered by the compound or by the process in which it is involved. No material is harmless. All are fatal at some dosage. The probability that any person will receive a harmful dose depends at least as much on how the material is used as on its inherent toxicity. Furthermore, it long has been accepted that greater hazard may be permitted in connection with drugs to combat life-threatening diseases than can be permitted in connection with drugs to allay minor discomfort.

In connection with industrial chemicals, the considerations are more purely economic. It is agreed that any compound can be made and formulated safely provided that enough precautions are taken (eg, special ventilation, completely automated closed system, and the like). However, if the cost of necessary precautions exceeds the economic value of the compound, its manufacture is doomed.

The extensive investigations that continue to be carried out in connection with air pollution and water pollution can be considered a part of safety evaluation. In this connection, few if any compounds are studied prior to their "introduction into use." By definition, most "pollutants" are accomplished facts. However, continuing research is needed on the toxicology of wastes discharged into air and water in order to distinguish the dangerous from the annoying. Certainly, marked reduction of pollution is justified on esthetic grounds. Waste can be lessened by the technological equivalent of tidiness or good housekeeping, often with little expense and sometimes at a saving. However, it is only on the basis of thorough laboratory and epidemiological study that a rational judgment can be made regarding the balance between cost and benefit in those situations where progressive improvement in waste control can be accomplished only by an exponential increase in the expense.

Some of the same considerations of cost eventually must be faced in connection with testing compounds before use, just as it is in connection with testing wastes after they have been released. This aspect of the cost of pesticides is discussed in Section 9.1.5.

Advances in biochemistry, analytical chemistry, electrophysiology, and electron microscopy have permitted the development of more sensitive and accurate toxicological tests. On the other hand, the need to establish practical assurance of the safety of chemicals has been a stimulus for specialized applications of chemistry, physiology, and pathology, and sometimes for fundamental advances in these fields.

However, the requirements for safety evaluation have never been more rigorously enforced or broadly interpreted than in connection with pesticides. Some of the details are offered in Section 9.1.

Safety evaluation is no longer restricted to drugs, industrial chemicals, pollutants, and other materials recognized as poisonous for one or more species. It is coming to be recognized that the need for safety evaluation extends to materials that were formerly taken for

granted. This is especially true in connection with the normal or essentially inevitable constituents of food. Examples of normal constituents are the cyclopropanoid fatty acids found in some important vegetable oils used as food. Examples of essentially inevitable constituents are the aflatoxin and other fungal toxins. The importance of these compounds for man remains uncertain. However, in some experimental situations, the cyclopropanoid fatty acids are powerful cocarcinogens, and aflatoxin B_1 is the most powerful carcinogen known. Many other examples are given in *Toxicants Occurring Naturally in Foods* (National Academy of Sciences, 1966a) and *Toxic Constituents in Plant Foodstuffs* (Liener, 1969). Antinutritive substances as well as toxic compounds are found in food (Gontzea and Sutzescu, 1968).

1.2.1.6 Environmental Toxicology.

The term *environmental toxicology* is relatively new, and its exact usage is not established fully. The term ought to be reserved for all applications of toxicology to organisms other than man and his domestic animals. Defined in this way, environmental toxicology has had three main lines of development: toxinology, ecological toxicology, and wildlife toxicology.

Confusion arises when one of the expressions, "environmental toxicology" or "environmental pharmacology," is sometimes used to designate evaluations made in the interest of man but dealing with compounds in the "environment." This unfortunate usage seems more opportunistic than scientific. It attempts to gain attention through current interest in the "environment" but it raises indefensible distinctions between different parts of man's surroundings. For example, this ill advised usage lends itself to such unproductive debates as whether contamination of river water is more "environmental" than contamination of workroom air.

Toxinology. It is easy to understand that the first toxicants produced by living organisms to be noticed and studied were those dangerous to man. Interest in poisonous plants and in the venom of snakes, spiders, bees, wasps, etc., probably is more ancient than any other aspect of toxicology. Certainly, this interest was a part of the mainstream of early clinical and medicolegal toxicology. More recently, poisons produced by living organisms have become the subject of biochemical and other detailed investigation characteristic of modern safety evaluation. This is particularly true of the bacterial and fungal toxins, which have caused dramatic outbreaks of acute poisoning in man and useful animals, and some of which are the proven cause of chronic illness in animals and the suspected cause of similar effects in man.

When poisons produced by living organisms were studied chemically it became evident that some of plant origin (mainly alkaloids) were stable, while others of plant, animal, or bacterial origin were unstable, proteinaceous, and often capable of giving rise to specific tolerance in man and other mammals. These labile poisons were called "toxins" or "toxines" and the protective materials produced by mammals were called "antitoxins." The meaning of "antitoxin" remains intact. The meaning of "toxin" has been eroded by common use of the word as a synonym for "poison" or "toxicant." The specialized meaning persists in the derivative, "toxinology," which is the study of toxins in the restricted sense. The reason that both words now find limited use is that the chemical distinction they were meant to signify is now of limited use. Modern toxicology generally requires finer chemical distinctions. There is, however, some etymological reason also to discard the specialized usage of "toxin," for there is no reason to suppose that the ancient Greek arrow poison was unstable or proteinaceous. The word "venom", derived from the Latin word, *venenum* (and perhaps ultimately from a love potion of Venus), clearly designates the poisonous matter produced by snakes, scorpions, bees, and others. Implicit in the meaning of "venom" is that the material is produced by a healthy organism for its own use.

Ecological Toxicology.   Ecological toxicology is the study of all toxicants produced by living organisms and of the ecological relationships made possible by these poisons. This discipline is, then, much broader than toxinology. Whereas some of the compounds by which organisms of one species influence those of another include the most toxic compounds known, many are of low toxicity to mammals. In fact, a large number of these secondary chemicals occur in our ordinary food, especially our vegetable food (for references see Section 1.2.1.5.)

Regardless of their exact degree of toxicity, these chemicals that modulate interactions between species have been called "allelochemics" and the class of interactions are termed "allelochemic" (Whittaker, 1970a, 1970b). The compounds are distinguished by their function from hormones, which modulate interactions between organs or tissues, and pheromones, which modulate interactions between individuals of the same species.

In a masterful review, Whittaker and Feeny (1971) have shown how protista, bacteria, fungi, higher plants, and animals have made use of chemicals for their adaptive advantage,

only to have their prey, enemies, or competitors develop countermeasures, for example the ability to detoxify the compounds adequately or to use them as cues. Thus, the same compounds may come to have adaptive value to both kinds of species, as is true of the mustard oils and their glycosides that deter many insects that otherwise would feed on members of the *Cruciferae* but have been exploited as attractants by cabbage butterflies and some other enemies of these plants.

Concerning the importance of allelochemics in ecology, the reviewers stated: "In all communities chemical interrelations are important aspects of the adaptation of species to one another; in some communities chemical relations seem to be the principal basis of species niche differentiation and community organization. Ecologists consider that ecosystems are given functional unity by the transfer of energy, inorganic nutrients, and foods between environment and organisms. To these two classes of materials in community transfer, inorganic nutrients and foods, should be added the third, allelochemics. An intricate pattern of exchanges of materials of all three classes relates the organisms of a community to the environment and to one another. If the inorganic and organic nutrients provide the essential fabric of this pattern, the allelochemics provide much of the color and detail of its design."

In this broad context, man's use of poisons and his defenses against them can be viewed as an extension of processes found in many forms of life. This is true whether one considers primitive arrow poisons or the most modern synthetic toxicants designed for maximal effectiveness and safety, including biodegradability.

The origins of ecological toxicology lie in general biology, especially ecology. Some of the facts that contribute to this new science are old, but the integrating concepts in their modern chemical forms are new. Both classical toxicology and modern safety evaluation, while based on general biology, are most directly related to human and veterinary medicine and pharmacology. In view of their different origins, it is remarkable that environmental toxicology and the remainder of the discipline have so much in common. Actually, the most beautiful examples of the conformity of a dosage to its purpose may be found among the solitary wasps. Some of these wasps sting selected species of insects or spiders in such a way that the victim is not killed but permanently paralyzed so that in due course it may serve as food for a wasp's larvae. Compared to these wasps, the Borgias were amateurs.

Environmental toxicologists are beginning to make refined measurements of the dosage-response relationships by which the chemical control of ecological processes is regulated. The value of these measurements confirms the unity of toxicological principles.

Some of the techniques developed for safety evaluation may prove valuable in experimental approaches to environmental toxicology. Conversely, ecological toxicology can broaden the outlook of many toxicologists by emphasizing the applicability of toxicological principles to all living things. It is clear that organisms frequently have been successful in developing defense against chemical attack as well as against infection. No pesticide, whether chemical or living, will prove completely and permanently effective. The battle that has been going on since life began must continue between man and the pests that attack him or his property. Undoubtedly there is much to be learned from finding out how the battle has gone for the last million years.

Wildlife Toxicology. Wildlife toxicology involves study of the effects of toxicants of any origin on wildlife, in exactly the same sense that veterinary toxicology is related to domestic animals. Wildlife toxicology has achieved high scientific standards in safety evaluation. In one sense, the problems of this evaluation for a given kind of wildlife are relatively simple, because the organism itself can be studied, and there usually is no need for extrapolation from one species to another, even in connection with destructive tests. However, the subdiscipline faces two important technical difficulties: (a) the problem of the great range of organisms, in the interest of which safety evaluations ought to be carried out; and (b) the problem of raising or otherwise obtaining an adequate supply of some species and of treating them as experimental animals.

Because wildlife toxicology is concerned with safety evaluation, it might have been discussed as a major subdivision of the foregoing section. However, because the fish, birds, and mammals thought of as wildlife form such an important part of our environment and since studies related to them contribute so much of what is known about the ecological effects of chemicals in the environment, it seems best to list the subject as one apsect of environmental toxicology.

Chapter 11 consists of a brief discussion of wildlife toxicology insofar as it involves pesticides.

1.2.2 Training of Toxicologists

According to one interpretation, toxicology is what toxicologists do. What they do is, to some degree, an extension of their training. Table 1-2 shows the training and duties, and Table 1-3 shows the affiliations of the charter members of the Society of Toxicology as recorded in *American Men of Science.* It may be seen that about one-third of these toxicologists were trained as pharmacologists, about one-fifth as physicians, almost one-fifth as biochemists, and the remainder in a wide variety of disciplines. Only a few were originally trained as toxicologists.

European toxicologists, at least those concerned with drug toxicity, have a different distribution of training, and in fact the distribution varies greatly from one country to another. Based on 226 questionnaries completed by members of the European Society of Drug Toxicity, Tripod and Stamm (1969) reported that the basic training of just over half of these toxicologists was medicine whereas between 9 and 14% were trained in chemistry, pharmacy, veterinary medicine, and natural sciences, respectively. Almost 20% of the men were trained in a combination of two of these disciplines and over 10% were trained in three of them. A very high percentage had some supplementary training in one or more disciplines in addition to the one or more in which they were fully qualified. The report does not specify the ages at which European toxicologists have completed their basic training. It does state regarding the training of future toxicologists: ". . . the would-be toxicologist can expect to have to undergo a programme of specialized training every bit as prolonged and as costly as those currently required for any other branch of scientific specialisation, including particularly medicine."

Toxicology now depends on the teamwork of men and women trained in different disciplines. This situation is likely to continue. Training in toxicology probably will be required to an increasing degree to provide beginners with the special orientation that present leaders in the field have acquired through experience. However, a need will remain in toxicology for persons with the most thorough training and continuing experience in human and veterinary medicine, pharmacology, analytical chemistry, biochemistry, pathology, statistics, and a number of other separate disciplines.

1.2.3 Societies Related to Toxicology

A number of societies, including the American Society for Pharmacology and Experimental Therapeutics, the American Chemical Society, the New York Academy of Sciences, and the American Medical Association, have fos-

Table 1-2

Training and Duties of 183 Charter Members
of the Society of Toxicology

Discipline	Training	Duties
medicine	21.3%	0 %
veterinary medicine	5.5	1.6
pharmacology	34.4	33.9
chemistry	6.0	1.6
biochemistry	18.5	10.3
toxicology	1.6	17.0
others	20.8[a]	37.7[b]
total	108.1%	102.1%

a. Pathology, biology, physiology, etc.

b. Chiefly administration.

Table 1-3

Affiliation of Charter Members of
the Society of Toxicology

Affiliation	Percentage
industry	46.7
university	25.4
government	17.9
private institutes	10.0
total	100.0

tered an interest in toxicology. However, although toxicology has been recognized as a discipline since the early 19th Century, societies devoted exclusively to the discipline were begun only recently. The Society of Toxicology was organized in 1961. It was the intention of the founders that the Society of Toxicology would be international, and members now come from at least 16 countries. However, all meetings so far have been in the United States of America. The only deterrent to becoming truly international is the expense of travel. Under the circumstances, it is not astonishing that national or regional groups are appearing. These include the Canadian Association for Research in Toxicology and the Sociedad Venezolana de Toxicologia. A Swedish discussion group in toxicology has been organized.

Other societies indicate by their names as well as by their activities an interest in different aspects of toxicology or of disciplines closely associated with it. These societies include: the American Academy of Clinical Toxicology, the American College of Veterinary Toxicology, the American Conference of Governmental Industrial Hygienists, the American Industrial Hygiene Association, the American Society for Experimental Pathology, the Environmental Mutagen Society, the European Association of Poison Control Centres, the European Society for the Study of Drug Toxicity, the International Society of Toxinology, the National Association of Coroners, and the Weed Society of America.

1.3 Definition of Pesticides

Pesticides are defined under the Federal Environmental Pesticide Control Act as including: ". . . (1) any substance or mixture of substances intended for preventing, destroying, repelling, or mitigating any pest [insect, rodent, nematode, fungus, weed, other forms of terrestrial or aquatic plant or animal life or viruses, bacteria, or other micro-organisms, except viruses, bacteria, or other micro-organisms on or in living man or other animals, which the Administrator declares to be a pest] and (2) any substance or mixture of substances intended for use as a plant regulator, defoliant or desiccant."

1.4 Benefits from Pesticides

A full understanding of toxicology must involve knowledge of the benefits arising from chemicals or from physical forces whose real or potentially injurious effects toxicologists study and attempt to prevent. Only a few compounds are of such basic interest that their toxicological study is merited in the absence of real or prospective use. The tremendous diagnostic and therapeutic value of drugs justifies their use, and in turn requires a detailed study of their side effects. Only the economic value and use of most industrial chemicals justifies a study of their toxicology. The same is true of pesticides. Their important contributions to our health and economy guarantee their continued use as a class, and require the most complete knowledge of their toxicology we can achieve and the avoidance of their hazards.

The contributions of pesticides to health and

economy are closely interrelated. They contribute directly to our health through control of certain vector-borne diseases; they contribute directly to the economy through increased production of food and fiber and through the protection of many materials during storage. However, improved health has sometimes permitted a more prosperous and stable economy. In some countries, greater and more dependable production of food has eliminated famine and thus contributed as much to health as to the economy.

1.4.1 Health and Comfort

Simmons (1959) reviewed the contribution of pesticides to the control of human diseases spread by arthropods and other vectors. His compendium was detailed and based on 668 references.

Unfortunately, no new but equally comprehensive account has appeared to bring the whole picture up to date. However, malaira remains the most important endemic and epidemic vector-borne disease, and several excellent reviews of its control have been published (Soper et al., 1961; Bruce-Chwatt and Haworth, 1965; and World Health Organization, 1967).

1.4.1.1 Kinds of Diseases Controlled. Outbreaks of malaria, louse-borne typhus, plague, and urban yellow fever, four of the most important epidemic diseases of history, have been controlled by DDT. Simmons (1959) listed over 20 other diseases that have been controlled to some degree by this compound, including filariasis, dengue, various virus encephalitides, louse-borne relapsing fever, trench fever, murine typhus, shigellosis, amebiasis, leishmaniasis, bartonellosis, onchocerciasis, sandfly fever, trypanosomiasis, yaws, infectious conjunctivitis, cholera, Chagas disease, scrub typhus, scabies, rickettsialpox, tick-borne relapsing fever, Rocky Mountain spotted fever, and tularemia. Now one may add various hemorrhagic fevers and Kyasanur forest disease to the list.

Other pesticides have made some contribution, but the chlorinated hydrocarbon insecticides, especially DDT, have been of greatest importance in the control of insect-borne diseases of man. A variety of compounds ranging from DDT to pyrethrum have contributed greatly to human comfort through control of household insects, which, although not known to carry disease, are an annoyance.

Systematic use of rodenticides helps to prevent the transmission of diseases acquired by man from rats and other rodents. However,

any effort to kill rats in the face of an epidemic of plague may lead to increased spread of the disease, because infected fleas leave the dead rats and may attack man. In the face of epidemics, DDT has proved valuable by killing fleas before they could leave the rats or have a chance to contact man. In fact, it was not until DDT was used that an epidemic of plague was ever stopped.

Not only are human diseases spread by insects, ticks, and rats, but a few require snails as intermediate hosts. The most important of these is schistosomiasis, a major endemic disease in some parts of the world. The three forms of schistosomiasis may be controlled to some degree by molluscicides.

1.4.1.2 Benefits from Disease Control. Control of a particular disease may have not only a direct clinical benefit but also a secondary effect in reducing other, entirely unrelated diseases. It can have direct economic benefits such as reduction of medical costs and loss of time at work. It may have indirect economic benefits such as increased agricultural and economic potential. Finally, control of disease may be of tremendous military importance.

These different kinds of benefits are illustrated in the following paragraphs devoted to malaria.

Military Importance of Malaria. It is fair to say that the military importance of malaria is so vast it never has been described or evaluated fully. One must be satisfied with a few examples.

Melville (1910) has recalled the Walcheren Expedition in the Netherlands (1809) in which the British forces were overcome by malaria within a month of disembarkation. In the French campaign in Madagascar in 1895 there were 13 deaths in action and over 4,000 deaths "due almost entirely to malaria fevers and their sequelae." Of the British campaign in West Africa in 1864, Melville said: "It can scarely be called a war, as an enemy was never seen, or a grain of powder expended; our troops were defeated by disease, much of which was preventable."

During World War I, the British, French, and German armies in Macedonia were immobilized by malaria for 3 years. The answer of one French general to an order to attack was: "Regret that my army is in the hospital with malaria." During 1916 to 1918 when the average British strength was only 124,000, there were 162,512 admissions to hospital for malaria but only a total of 23,762 killed, wounded, taken prisoner, or missing. Over 2 million man-days were lost to the British Army in Macedonia in 1918 alone (Mac-Donald, 1923).

The malaria picture was completely changed during World War II through the use of DDT and other preventive measures. Within the continental United States, hospital admission rates for malaria in the US Army reached 14 per 1,000 average strength during the summers of 1917, 1919, and 1920 but during World War II did not reach 5 per 1,000. In fact, the maximal summer rate was systematically reduced from a little over 4 per 1,000 in 1941 to less than 1 per 1,000 in 1944. In 1943 the attack rate for malaria in the US Army worldwide was 25.45 per 1,000 average strength. DDT was first added to US Army supply lists in May, 1943. The attack rates in 1944 and 1945 were 21.58 and 16.95 per 1,000. The corresponding rates of death due to malaria were 1.64, 1.14, and 1.01 per 100,000 average strength in 1943, 1944, and 1945, respectively (Coates et al., 1963).

The worldwide rates offer little idea of the problem faced in some advanced sections. In 1944 the attack rates just exceeded 200 per 1,000 average strength in the Base Section of the India-Burma Theater, but reached over 400 in the Intermediate Section and 1,000 in the Advance Section. The rate was greatly reduced (<50) in all sections during the last 10 months of 1945. The malaria pressure was even greater in some areas. For example, in Guadalcanal, rates for entire divisions rose as high as 3,700 per 1,000 and in some groups exceeded 14,000 (Coates et al. 1963).

History of Malaria. Of all communicable diseases, malaria has had greatest effect on society in most tropical and subtropical countries. In the past, it was a serious problem in the United States of America as far north as Illinois, an area few would consider subtropical.

During the first half of this century, it is estimated that some 300 million people in the world suffered from malaria each year, and of these over 3 million died of it. The potential of the disease was illustrated by the 1934–1935 epidemic in Ceylon. Morbidity was greater than 50% of the entire population, and 80,000 people—1.4% of the population—died. A major outbreak occurred as recently as 1958 when an estimated 200,000 people died of malaria in Ethiopia. Even now it is estimated that between 200,000 and 500,000 infants and young children in tropical Africa die each year from the direct effects of malaria (Bruce-Chwatt and Haworth, 1965).

Malaria is such a debilitating disease that it has a marked influence on lowering resistance to other diseases, not merely in a long-run sense, but in day-to-day battles (Newman, 1965). Although it is difficult to estimate the extent of indirect injury done by any disease, this was possible for malaria in Ceylon. Control efforts not only reduced mortality from malaria but reduced general mortality also. It was concluded that the total deaths due to malaria were of the order of 5 times the number of deaths actually ascribed to the disease. It was recognized that some deaths were incorrectly ascribed to malaria but it was felt that this error was more than overbalanced by the opposite mistake. In portions of Ceylon where the spleen index was high, malaria control led to a marked increase in the crude rate of population growth. Where the spleen index was low, malaria control had little effect on population growth. In British Guiana, malaria control had little influence on the general trend of population growth but it did almost eliminate the wide annual variation (Newman, 1965).

Before the development of DDT, many attempts were made to control malaria by drainage, drugs, and larvicides. There were a few stunning victories, notably the one that permitted building of the Panama Canal (1904–1914). Dr. William C. Gorgas (1915) reduced the number of canal workers hospitalized for malaria from 821 per 1,000 in 1906 to 76 per 1,000 7 years later. Gorgas and his team were credited with saving 39,500,000 man-days of illness and preventing 71,000 deaths. Even such a victory involved limited populations, a level of control that would be unacceptable today, and expense that could be met only under unusual circumstances such as the building of a canal.

The use of residual insecticides beginning in the 1940's revolutionized the concept of control and led to the possibility of eradication. It has been known for many years that female anopheline mosquitoes are necessary for transmission of the disease, and that after taking a blood meal they usually rest on a nearby indoor surface for several hours while the blood digests and the eggs mature. Each female mosquito requires a blood meal every 2 or 3 days, but the malaria parasite requires at least 10 days in the mosquito to reach a stage that can infect man. It followed that any mosquito feeding in a house with all the inside surfaces sprayed with an effective residual insecticide would come into contact with toxic surfaces on several occasions and would die before it could pass on the infection. Thus, house spraying with DDT and to a lesser extent with BHC became the major tool in malaria control. For the first time it became possible not only to reduce illness caused by malaria, but to interrupt its transmission. Fig. 1-1 exemplifies how the initiation of a DDT spray program led to a reduction of mosquitoes indoors and, thus, to a reduction of cases of malaria.

The concept of national malaria eradication dates back at least to 1916 (Hoffman, 1916), a period when its achievement would have been technically difficult, but its importance for the economy as well as for health was fully appreciated. The ending of transmission of malaria and the elimination of the reservoir of infective cases in the United States of America and in large areas of Venezuela and Guyana was recognized as eradication of malaria in those areas and led to the concept of continent-wide malaria eradication. This objective was enunciated at the Thirteenth Pan American Sanitary Conference in 1950 and more forcefully by the Fourteenth Pan American Sanitary Conference in Santiago in October, 1954. In 1955, the Eighth World Health Assembly in Mexico City recommended eradication rather than control as an international objective. This objective was defined and elaborated by the Sixth Report of the WHO Expert Committee on Malaria (World Health Organization, 1957).

The contribution of many persons and institutions to developing the concept of malaria eradication has been reviewed in detail (Soper et al., 1961).

Protection from Malaria. Today malaria eradication is an accomplished fact for 619 million people who live in areas once malarious. Where eradication has been achieved it has stood the test of time. An additional 334 million people live in areas where transmission of the parasite is no longer a major problem. These 953 million people now constitute over one-fourth of the population of the world, and their protection is an accomplishment without parallel (World Health Organization, 1967).

Unfortunately, there is another side to the coin. There are 638 million people living in areas where transmission of malaria still continues. At the end of 1965, the population in malarious areas where eradication programs have not yet started numbered 362 million. Of these, 190 million were in the African Region of WHO. Progress has been uneven. The European, South East Asian, and American Regions account for 95% of people benefitting from the later phases of eradication programs. In the African Region the proportion of people living in areas in the later phases of eradication is under 3% of the total population in malarious areas. The situation is intermediate

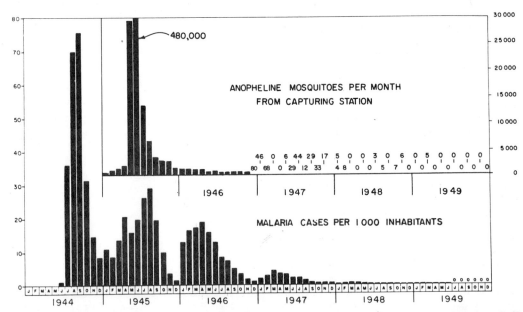

Fig. 1-1. Number of anopheline mosquitoes per month from capturing stations in Latina Province, Italy, and number of malaria cases per 1,000 inhabitants of the same province following spraying with DDT from June, 1945, onward. Modified from Simmons (1959) and reproduced by permission of Birkäuser Verlag, Basel.

in the Eastern Mediterranean Region and the Western Pacific Region. The difficulties, which depend on administrative and other causes as well as technical complications, were discussed at length in the Thirteenth Report of the WHO Expert Committee on Malaria (World Health Organization, 1967). Suffice it to say here that the main technical dificulties involve resistance of mosquitoes to insecticides and the fact that some strains of anopheline mosquitoes often bite and rest outdoors and are, therefore, little affected by indoor spraying. Other technical difficulties involve resistance of malaria parasites to drugs and factors related to human ecology, including population movements, outdoor sleeping, types of dwellings unsuitable for the use of residual insecticides, and interferences with the residual insecticide deposit.

These difficulties, especially the resistance of insects to certain insecticides, led to a need to develop other effective compounds. A long-range program has been initiated by the World Health Organization to discover and test these compounds. Already there has been some practical success (World Health Organization, 1969).

In a few areas, for example, some in Venezuela, malaria eradication has failed only because of a combination of severe technical difficulties. However, with the exception of the areas just mentioned, failure to eradicate malaria usually has occurred only in areas that are retarded economically, administratively, or in other ways. These problems may be attributed partly to ill health, to which malaria contributes a considerable part. With the attainment of eradication elsewhere, the gap is widening. Malaria eradication is considered the key to the solution of Africa's major problems in education, agriculture, industry, and transportation, and of its other diseases and poverty. While malaria is important in many other parts of the world, in Africa the solution of this problem is fundamental to all progress (Soper *et al.*, 1961). Furthermore, the persistence of malaria anywhere represents a potential threat to people in all the formerly malarious areas of the world. It is in the common interest to promote global eradication (World Health Organization, 1967).

Economic Benefits. No study of the economic effects of malaria control has been reported for most programs. Although some of the few economic studies that have been made involved programs that were incomplete and difficult, all of them have indicated a net profit.

The economic impact of a few early programs, especially those in Afghanistan, several areas of India, Ceylon, Belgian Congo, Southern Rhodesia, and the Transvaal, were reviewed by Simmons (1959). Observed benefits included reductions in illness, hospitalization, and absenteeism from work; increases in agricultural production (sometimes to the extent of 400%); increases in land values; reclamation of new land; increases in bank clearings and other business activity; and establishment of industries.

Perhaps the most complete report of the economic benefits of malaria control is that of Livadas and Athanassatos (1963) concerning Greece. A control program mapped by Livadas was blocked by World War II. After the war, the plan was revised and implemented to take advantage of DDT, which had become available. The campaign, based exclusively on annual house spraying, began in 1946 before the transmission season. Even during the first year, there was a sharp drop in the incidence of malaria, and by the end of 1949 transmission had practically ceased. Early in 1951, a sudden shortage of insecticide made it necessary to discontinue routine spraying in a part of the country. Active epidemiological surveillance was continued in the hope of maintaining the advantages gained insofar as possible. Actually, there was no significant recurrence of disease even though as recently as 1972 it had not yet been eradicated.

The direct economic profit from malaria control in Greece was calculated on the basis of reduction of: (*a*) time lost from work (6 days per year for recognized cases in persons of productive age); (*b*) expense for drugs; (*c*) expense for medical care; (*d*) economic loss related to mortality caused directly by malaria; and (*e*) loss from mortality caused indirectly by malaria. The annual losses associated with these several causes were estimated as follows: (*a*) US $12,000,000; (*b*) $1,000,000; (*c*) $2,500,000; (*d*) $7,500,000; (*e*) $3,000,000; or a total of $26,000,000 each year. By contrast, the cost of the program did not exceed $1,500,000 annually. The difference between cost and savings may have been greater, for the savings were estimated in a most conservative way. One may hesitate to place a monetary value on a human life, but few would consider the amount of $1,500 used by the authors as excessive!

Livadas and Athanassatos (1963) pointed out the difficulty of measuring the indirect economic benefits of malaria control, since there were many factors contributing to the improvements in agriculture, manufacturing, commerce, and other elements of the gross national product. However, they emphasized that many of the improvements would have been impossible if the country had still been subject to malaria. This relationship was especially clear in connection with increased tourism and rice production. Information from the paper under discussion is reproduced in Tables 1-4 and 1-5. It is interesting to observe the lag that occurred in agricultural production. Although malaria was suppressed in 1946, it was not until about 1949 that there was a distinct improvement in the rate of production per hectare under cultivation. There followed a period of steady improvement through about 1953 when an almost steady state was reached, changed only by some further increase in production per hectare about 1957. The end result was doubling of wheat production, quadrupling of cotton production, and an increase of 15 times in the production of rice. This experience probably exemplifies a general truth: it requires several years to gain the full advantage of disease control.

Although agricultural production reached a plateau in Greece about 1953, manufacturing, wholesale and retail trade, transportation and communication, and other elements of the gross national product continued to increase (Table 1-5). Tourism was one important contribution to the economy that would have been impossible without malaria control. In fact, until DDT was put to use in 1946 the situation had not improved greatly since Sir Ronald Ross, who in 1898 discovered the transmission of malaria in birds, wrote of his visit to Greece in 1906 as follows: "One also might expect to find numerous suitable hostels for tourists in a country where every hill or brook has been made sacred through its literature, art and history and which ought to be visited every year by thousands of foreigners from all parts of the world. At present in all these great valleys you only see scenes of desolation, bare hills, deserted tracts of land, and a poor and scanty population" (Ross, 1906).

In India, the number of malaria cases dropped from 100,000,000 annually in 1933–1935 before control to 150,000 in 1966. During the same period, the loss to the economy was reduced from $1,300,000,000 annually to $2,-000,000 annually. Between 1952 and 1966, the

Table 1-4

Area and Production of Wheat, Rice and Cotton in Greece 1935-1938 and 1948-1960. Area is Expressed in Thousands of Hectares and Production in Thousands of Metric Tons

From Livadas and Athanassatos (1963).

Calendar year	Wheat		Cotton		Rice	
	area	production	area	production	area	production
1935-1938	850	768	62	44	2	4
1948	843	800	45	35	4	9
1949	763	839	57	48	8	21
1950	867	850	77	79	10	32
1951	954	930	87	89	19	56
1952	965	1,050	82	77	21	75
1953	1,045	1,400	89	95	17	66
1954	1,045	1,219	109	128	21	86
1955	1,040	1,337	166	189	18	61
1956	1,062	1,245	160	154	11	43
1957	1,088	1,720	156	191	14	60
1958	1,111	1,786	162	187	17	66
1959	1,163	1,767	131	170	18	67
1960	1,142	1,666	165	184	14	55

Table 1-5

Gross Domestic Products of Greece: 1955-1961
Expressed in Millions of Drachmae (30 dr. = 1 dollar U. S.)

From Livadas and Athanassatos (1963).

Branch	1955	1956	1957	1958	1959	1960	1961
agriculture forestry-fishing	20,093	22,768	25,022	23,731	23,833	23,700	28,400
manufacturing	10,521	12,134	12,984	14,186	14,519	15,859	17,174
wholesale and retail trade	6,658	8,030	8,411	8,828	9,230	9,469	10,475
transportation and communication	4,567	5,106	5,351	5,579	6,044	6,666	7,292
public administration and deference	4,091	5,137	5,158	5,673	6,173	6,674	7,163
all others	12,375	14,462	15,671	17,265	18,851	21,169	23,293
gross domestic product	58,305	67,627	72,197	75,234	78,650	83,537	93,797

number of man-days of productive labor of people between the ages of 15 and 50 saved was estimated at 179,500,000 days. The total cost of the eradication campaign in India up to now has been only $200,000,000 annually, much less than the original annual loss to the economy (World Health Organization, 1968).

Malaria, apparently brought to Sardinia by the Carthaginians, made the island essentially worthless to the Romans, who invaded it in 238 BC. There was no real relief until malaria was eradicated. Levi (1968) wrote a fascinating account of the change under the title "Sardinia Reborn." Cicero and many lesser men warned against travel to Sardinia. Now it has become a thriving agricultural and industrial area, and a haven for tourists.

1.4.2 Agriculture and Forestry

Pesticides are only one of a series of factors that have permitted maintenance of our supply of food and agricultural fiber in spite of a continued increase of the population and some decrease of the area suitable for farming. The factors that have permitted maintenance of our supply of food and fiber are listed and discussed in Section 1.4.2.4, but they can be understood only in connection with information on (a) losses caused by pests; (b) the changing pattern of land use; and (c) certain increases of crop production per unit area.

1.4.2.1 Losses Caused by Pests. Food and fiber are subject to damage by pests during every stage of their production, transportation, and storage. It is difficult to estimate this damage, and improved, standardized methods are needed (Chiarappa et al., 1972). One problem is that measurement may be impossible until control of losses reveals the true potential for production (see Section 1.4.2.5). Only a few examples of losses can be given here.

It was reported by the Minnesota Agricultural Extension Service (1964) that weeds caused average losses of 22 to 44% of production of soybeans, corn, small grain, flax, and forage as compared to weed-free or weed-controlled fields of the same crops. Other examples of damage by weeds are given by two studies represented by Fig. 1-2. In these studies, the spaces between rows were kept clean by ordinary cultivation. The only weeds (giant foxtails) allowed to remain were in the rows themselves. As may be seen, a large number of weeds caused a reduction of about 25% in the production of both corn and soybeans. However, a small number of weeds did a disproportionate amount of damage. Only about three weeds per meter of row reduced production by about 5%.

During the decade 1951–1960, it is estimated that plant diseases cost the United States of America $4,250 million, plus an additional $250 million expended on disease control programs. These costs do not include

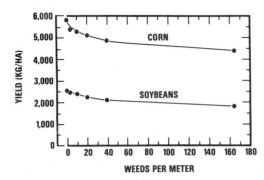

Fig. 1-2. Effect of weeds on the production of corn and soybeans. Spaces between the rows were kept clean by ordinary cultivation. From data of Illinois Agricultural Extension Service (1961).

losses of food and other agricultural products in the market or in the hands of the consumer. In general, it is thought that losses caused by fungi amounted to 10% of gross agricultural production (National Academy of Sciences, 1968a).

It is estimated that, in developed countries in the temperate zone, weeds waste 10 to 15% of the total value of agricultural and forest products. The burden is about equally divided between the expense of chemical and other measures to control weeds and actual losses in yield and quality. Losses from weeds are greatest in tropical countries. In some instances, weed control may triple the yield of tropical rice (National Academy of Sciences, 1968b).

The available estimates of losses caused by insects concern only major pests that cause damage repeatedly. During the period 1951–1960, these major pests caused an estimated annual loss of $6,800 million in the United States of America alone. Although this figure does not include sporadic losses or losses from minor pests, it does include relevant damage to rangeland, turf, ornamental plants, forests, forest products, stored products, livestock, poultry, and honeybees as well as crops. Crops differ in their susceptibility to insects, during both production and storage. Estimates of the proportion lost during production during the period 1951–1960 were: 15% for alfalfa intended for hay, 12% for corn, 13% for apples, 19% for cotton, 6% for oranges, 4% for rice, and 3% for soybeans. During the same period losses during storage were 5.5% for corn and 3% for wheat (National Academy of Sciences, 1969). Put another way, the annual losses to agriculture caused by insects are about 10 times what farmers spend for pesticides (see Section 1.5.2.1) indicating that only the most severe, concentrated injuries are being com-

bated. Of course, the losses are not equally distributed. Losses to agriculture as a whole are a burden; losses to the individual farmer may be a disaster.

By far the most complete study of worldwide crop losses caused by insects, fungi, and weeds is that of Cramer (1967). It was concluded: the total loss caused by pests to crops is in the order of $75,000 million annually or about 35% from the potential production. To the total loss, insects contribute 13.8%; fungi, 11.6%; weeds, 9.5%; and other pests, the remaining 0.1%. The losses are not evenly distributed. For example, those caused by insects amount to 5% of potential production in Europe, 7% in Oceania, 9% in North and Central America, 10% in South America, USSR, and the People's Republic of China, 13% in Africa, and 21% in those parts of Asia not already mentioned. These differences are due in part to climatic and other ecological factors, but they also reflect the extent to which control measures are established in the different regions. The largest loss is that of cereals, especially rice, but all classes of food and fiber are involved.

1.4.2.2 Utilization of Farm Land in the United States of America. The main elements of the utilization of farm land in the United States of America are summarized in Fig. 1-3. The curves show the uninterrupted increase of population, the early increase and eventual decline in the area of farms and croplands, and the way in which this decrease in area has been compensated for by increased crop production per unit area. The area used for crops reached its maximum in 1930. The area devoted to farming reached its maximum in 1950 with 468,871,660 hectares. This area constituted 60.9% of the total land area available in the 48 contiguous states. The proportion of land in farms now stands at only 48.7%, partly because of some decrease in farm acreage in the contiguous states but mostly because the vast area of Alaska is now counted in the total land area. Some of the land now in use is marginal for crops. It would not be agriculturally or economically feasible to convert a significant amount of rangeland or forest to the production of crops.

The increased production per unit area and the increased number of persons that an average farmer now can feed are both evidence for the improved efficiency of crop production that has compensated for the fact that the area of crop land declined since 1930 while the population rose steadily. If it were not for this improved efficiency, the relative cost of our food would be greater. A larger proportion of the population would have to be occupied in

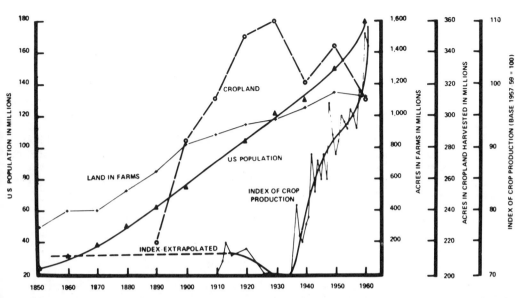

Fig. 1-3. A graphic presentation of data on the acreage of land in farms, the acreage in cultivated crops, and the general index of crop production per acre to illustrate their possible relationship to increases in the human population of the United States of America. Modified from Decker (1966) and reproduced by permission of the American Medical Association.

the production of food and fiber. The basis of our economy would be undermined by this displacement of people to agriculture. This economic damage probably would occur sooner than damage to health through malnutrition.

1.4.2.3 Crop Production per Unit Area.
Many people are unaware of progress that has been made in increasing the yield of staple foods. Others are unaware that each crop and each ecological area presents separate problems and that once a gain is achieved it often can be maintained only at the cost of continuing interdisciplinary research. An important reason for the achievement of the advanced countries compared to the developing nations is their greater success in increasing the productivity of their staple foods. The entire problem has been discussed in masterly fashion by Sprague (1967), and the following examples of increased productivity are drawn from his paper.

The average production of rice in Japan, which formerly was approximately 1,800 kg/ha, reached about 4,000 kg/ha in 1963. The average production of corn (maize) in the United States of America, which was 1,418 kg/ha in 1933, reached 4,243 kg/ha in 1963. Corresponding values for production of wheat in Mexico were 750 kg/ha in 1945 and 2,600 kg/ha in 1964.

It is an inescapable fact that substantial increases have been made by a number of

countries in their rate of production of staple foods. If those changes had not occurred, the world population problem would be even more severe than it is now. Any significant worsening of production would lead to disaster.

1.4.2.4 Factors Permitting Maintenance of Food Supply.
No one factor is responsible for maintenance of productivity of a single crop—much less our total food supply. Factors known to contribute include: (a) mechanization of farming, (b) improved varieties of plants and animals; (c) fertilizers for crops and feed adjuvants for domestic animals and birds; (d) monoculture (the growing of a crop in extensive fields and frequently in adjacent fields so that an entire region is devoted largely to a single crop to which that region is adapted); (e) pesticides for protection of plants and animals, and drugs and vaccines for protection of livestock; and (f) other methods of pest control.

These factors are always interdependent to some degree and sometimes to an astonishing degree. Laymen rarely appreciate that a strain improved for one area may be poorly adapted for another area.

Some persons suppose that fertilizer is a panacea for poor agricultural production. The fact is that any important benefit from the use of additional fertilizer may depend on development of a strain adapted to the area and capable of utilizing the supplement (Sprague, 1967).

Potential benefit from the use of improved strains that are adapted to an area may not be realized unless other factors are brought into play to hold the advantage that has been won. Hybrid corn can be grown in greater density than the best strains commonly available during the 1930's. However, the full benefit is not realized unless weeds are controlled and damage from insects is minimized (Sprague, 1967). In many situations, chemical control of pests is the only practical approach. However, the advantage gained may be lost through variation in a single factor, and chemical control is not always possible. In 1970 a new strain of the southern corn leaf blight, *Helminthosporium maydis,* suddenly spread from Texas and Florida in the South to Minnesota and Wisconsin in the North and destroyed what was first estimated as 10% of the crop (Gruchow, 1970) but was finally estimated as 15%. Although infestation could be prevented by the fungicide zineb, its use was not economically feasible for field corn.

Another example of interaction involves monoculture which permits efficient use of land especially adapted to a particular crop. Full development of agricultural mechanization for land preparation, planting, weed control, and harvesting with all its benefits depends on the use of monocultures. However, monocultures favor the development of insect pests and plant diseases. Thus, increased use of pesticides is often one condition for any increase in production beyond that achieved through peasant agriculture.

1.4.2.5 Agricultural Benefits from Pesticides. Agricultural benefits from pesticides are of two kinds. It is often easy to demonstrate benefit to the individual farmer. It is often difficult to determine the separate contributions of pesticides (among the many interrelated factors discussed in the preceding section) toward the total regional or national production of an important crop.

Profit to the Farmer. Use of pesticides may increase net profit by (a) providing a more economical way of weeding or thinning, (b) increasing quality, (c) increasing yield, and (d) reducing loss during storage and transport to market. Pesticides have an important insurance function by stabilizing production.

Farmers are unimpressed by the fact that the total monetary value of a crop in an area may be similar in good and bad years, because the price tends to vary inversely with supply. However, it requires no great insight on the part of a farmer to realize he will make no money if it is *his* crop that is destroyed. His profit will be small if his cows give little milk

because they are harassed by flies. Farmers easily understand the competitive character of their business. Persons who object to the use of pesticides express not only the truth but a deep conviction when they point out that blemishes on fruit are often skin-deep and that worms in fruit are not harmful to health. However, the orchardist knows that his fruit will be sold in competition with that of other producers. If nice looking fruit is placed beside defective fruit in a supermarket, the better product will sell in spite of a price differential. There just are not enough people who prefer wormy apples to make them profitable.

An illustration of personal gain and also of the interaction of factors that influence crop production may be found in a publication of the National Research Council (1962). At a time when the wholesale price of tomatoes was $12 per ton for US No. 2 fruit but $23 per ton for US No. 1 fruit, a farmer could gross $128 per acre (approximately the cost of production) if he neither fertilized nor sprayed. Fertilizing tended to increase production while spraying had the added effect of improving the quality of fruit. Fertilizing alone increased the farmer's gross income by $136 (196%); spraying alone raised it by $96 (75%); but a combination of the two increased his gross income by $336 (262%).

Another way to express the benefit of pesticides to the individual farmer is to estimate the monetary value of increased production resulting under practical conditions from a given investment in pesticides and their application. It has been estimated that in the United States of America agriculture can produce an average of $4 of additional product for each dollar spent on pesticides (Headley, 1968). In England, the estimate was five units of new income for each unit of expenditure (Strickland, 1970). Obviously, these estimates apply to the profit realized from adequate, judicious use of pesticides as compared to no use whatever. If the rate of application were increased progressively, the profit margin would decline and disappear.

Benefit to Society. The fact that pesticides increase the production and improve the competitive position of the individual farmer is indirect evidence for the contribution of these compounds to society in general.

A different sort of evidence is provided by Fig. 1-4, which shows the average rate of production of corn (maize) in Illinois between 1900 and 1962. It may be seen that the introduction of the first hybrid corn, which began about 1935 and was nearly complete by 1940 (period 1) produced a sharp, limited increase in

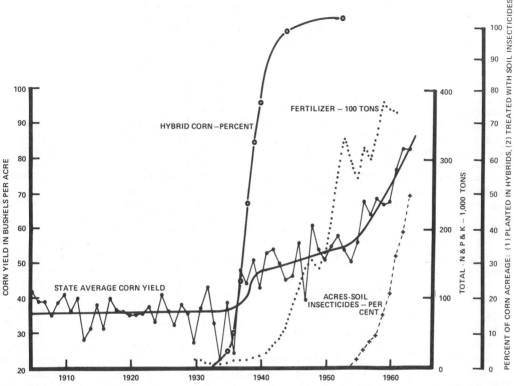

Fig. 1-4. A comparison of the increased use of hybrid seed, fertilizer, and pesticidal chemicals with rising corn yields in Illinois, 1900–1962. Modified from Decker (1966) and reproduced by permission of the American Medical Association.

production. The increase in the use of fertilizer between 1940 and 1953 (period 2) led to a further gradual advance in production. Even though the use of fertilizer was essentially stable for about 5 years after 1953 (period 3) the production of corn increased rapidly during this period in response to the introduction and rapidly increasing use of soil insecticides. Thus, it was possible to recognize the separate contributions of pesticides even though multiple factors were involved in the overall increase in the yield of corn.

When DDT was introduced, there was an unprecedented increase in the production of those crops on which it was used, and the increase corresponded to the degree of its use (Decker, 1966). Crops such as cotton, peanuts, and potatoes, on which pesticides are used most extensively, showed gains ranging from 68 to 119%. The production of alfalfa seed increased from 300 to 600% in states where the crop was treated intensively with insecticides, but remained essentially stable in states where the crop is raised for hay and, therefore, receives little treatment with insecticides.

Decker has pointed out that, if the United

States of America were to revert to production methods and levels that prevailed in 1930, an increase of 76,488,300 ha of cropland and 272,767,800 ha of farmland would be required to feed the population. The land is simply not available.

1.4.3 Protection of Stored Products

No single agency is responsible for the protection of stored products in the sense that ministries of health and agriculture are responsible for disease control and crop protection. One result is that, whereas information is minimal on the benefits of pesticides to health and to agricultural production, information is even more fragmentary on the benefits of pesticides to the protection of stored products. However, one has only to think of a few examples of the damage of various grain insects to food, the damage of moths to wool, or the damage of termites to wood to realize how much destruction would occur if some control were not exercised. In primitive societies, loss of food has led to starvation. In some tropical areas, it still is assumed that houses will be rebuilt every few years because decay and the ravages of termites have made them unsound. By use of preservatives, wood may be protected even if it must be left in the open. Thus, most utility poles, railroad ties, and dock pilings are impregnated. It has been estimated that this use of chemicals saves as much wood in the United States of America alone each year as would be produced annually by a forest the size of the state of New Hampshire.

Losses that occur during storage are caused mainly by insects, mites, rodents, and fungi, all of which are susceptible to chemical control, at least under some circumstances.

It has been estimated that at least 10% of harvested food crops—enough to feed 200 million people without additional land or cultivation—are lost during storage. In the tropics, the loss is mainly in the quantity of food stored. In temperate climates, the loss is mainly of quality and acceptability (Parkin, 1967).

1.5 Production and Use of Pesticides

The production and use of pesticides is a reflection of their value to one or more segments of society. On the other hand, any hazard each of them may present is proportional to the amount of it used. Thus, information on production and use constitutes one important factor determining both benefit and hazard.

A valuable source of information on production, consumption, importation, and exportation of pesticides is a book by Arrington (1956). It gives data for the United States of America for the period 1945 to 1955 and briefer information for over 60 other countries in North and South America, Europe, Asia, Africa, and Oceania.

1.5.1 Production of Pesticides

1.5.1.1 Introduction of Pesticides.
Pesticides have been used to a limited degree since ancient times. The Ebers Papyrus, written about 1550 BC, lists preparations to expel fleas from a house (Bryan, 1931). Homer relates how Odysseus burned sulfur ". . . to purge the hall and the house and the court" (*Odyssey XXII*, 492–494). By 900 AD, the Chinese were using arsenic to control garden insects. In 1669, the earliest known record of arsenic as an insecticide in the Western world mentioned its use with honey as an ant bait. Use of tobacco as a contact insecticide was mentioned later in the same century. A very small number of materials were added during the 18th Century. Even during the early 19th Century, only a few compounds were available, and their use was not general. Beginning about

1870, the number of conpounds available for use increased gradually. Equipment for applying pesticides to crops began to be developed about the same time. The equipment shown in Fig. 1-5 seems quaint by present standards, but it serves to remind us that mechanized chemical pest control is older than most of us can remember.

The rate at which important insecticides, fungicides, and herbicides were introduced is shown in Fig. 1-6. The dates of introduction of compounds through 1946 are taken from Shepard (1951) and based on sources cited by him. The year of introduction of each compound that came into use after 1947 is taken as the year of its first registration under the Federal Insecticide, Fungicide, and Rodenticide Act (FIFRA). Information on some of these compounds was supplied by a personal communication from the late Mr. Justus Ward, who for many years was responsible for administering that Act. More recent information has been supplied by the manufacturers.

It is clear from Fig. 1-6 that the introductions of insecticides, fungicides, and herbicides have followed separate courses, although admittedly many compounds in each of these groups were introduced in the period from about 1942 through 1965. Use of registration under FIFRA would tend to overemphasize the first enforcement of the Act as a critical period in the introduction of pesticides. However, the graph indicates that no such influence was evident; accelerated introduction of insecticides and fungicides began before the Act was passed and introduction of these compounds and herbicides continued with little or no change for years thereafter.

A recognizable acceleration in the rate of introduction of insecticides began in 1877. There was a further increase in rate beginning in 1924 and a still further increase beginning in 1946. Some important insecticides were discovered during World War II, but these discoveries had far less to do with the war *per se* than is commonly supposed. In fact, the rate of introduction beginning in 1946 continued at least as late as 1963 and decreased only very slightly from then until 1971, the last year of record.

The increased introduction of fungicides dates from 1943 and that of herbicides from 1947, both much later than the first two phases of increase of insecticides.

There was some reduction in the rate of introduction of new pesticide compounds about 1965. The fact that the changes were not simultaneous for insecticides, fungicides, and herbicides suggests that the factor involved may be different for each of these classes of

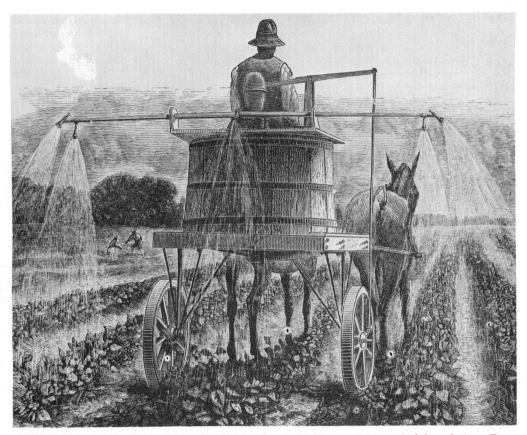

Fig. 1-5. The Johnson Wheeled Sprinkler patented in 1873 for spraying arsenical formulations. From Riley (1885).

pesticides or that the relative importance of multiple factors may be different for each. No prediction of future introductions of new compounds in the USA seems possible. There certainly are some compounds of great promise now unregistered, and research and development of pesticides continued to increase at least through 1970. It seems likely that some countries will introduce the new compounds into use.

1.5.1.2 USA Production.   Production data on synthetic organic chemicals are published by the United States Tariff Commission. The Commission presents statistics in as great detail as is possible without revealing the operations of individual producers. Statistics for an individual chemical or group of chemicals are not given unless there are three or more producers, no one or two of which may be predominant. Moreover, even when there are three or more producers, statistics are not given if there is any possibility that their publication would violate the statutory provisions relating to unlawful disclosure of information accepted in confidence by the Commission.

This means there is no official record for many compounds that are interesting from the standpoint of toxicology. It means that information on many other materials is incomplete. However, for certain compounds, the record is essentially complete and very impressive.

Fig. 1-7 shows the production of DDT and synthetic organic pesticides in the United States of America. Values for production and estimates for future production of "all insecticides" and "all pesticides" were published formerly. However, chemicals used as grain fumigants, as well as many of the inorganic materials used as pesticides (eg, sulfur, copper sulfate, and sodium chlorate), have other important uses unrelated to pest control. The amount of these materials used for pest control is known only approximately, if at all. Thus, the only dependable values are for synthetic compounds used as pesticides only.

Although the production of synthetic pesticides increased greatly and rather steadily over the years, some important compounds or groups of compounds reached a relatively steady state of production, or were almost

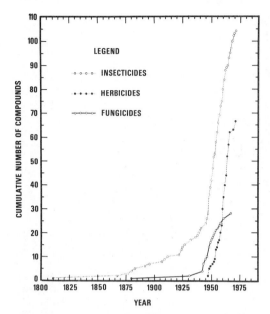

Fig. 1-6. Dates of introduction of some important pesticides. The date of introduction of each compound in use before 1948 was taken mainly from Shepard (1951). The date of first registration under the Federal Insecticide, Fungicide, and Rodenticide Act of 1947 was taken as the time of introduction for each compound first used in 1948 or later. Information on registration was supplied by the manufacturers. No account has been taken in the graph of the fact that some of the compounds gradually were replaced by others and thus became relatively unimportant.

supplanted by newer materials. This is illustrated by Fig. 1-8. The arsenicals were largely replaced by DDT and BHC. Production of BHC was curtailed when it became evident that it imparted an undesirable flavor to some crops. Production of DDT in the United States of America continued to increase until about 1963. However, from about 1953 onward the increased production was sustained mainly by exports. As discussed in Section 1.5.3.1, the annual use of DDT in this country increased only slightly between 1953 and 1959 and then decreased gradually.

1.5.1.3 World Production. No systematic study apparently has been made of world production of pesticides. The nearest approach was an investigation by Arrington (1956), but that was confined largely to imports and exports. The fact that Japan, the Netherlands, the United Kingdom, and West Germany were leading exporters of pesticides and that Australia, Belgium, Denmark, Italy, Yugoslavia, and Switzerland were important exporters in

1954 proves that they were important producers also. Undoubtedly they met most of their own internal needs, but this may have been true of some countries that exported little or no pesticidal material. Arrington's report contained no information on the Soviet Union, probably an important producer of pesticides.

Countries that were important in pesticide production in 1954 remain important, but production has also increased in a number of other countries.

1.5.1.4 USA Imports and Exports. The United States of America is both an importer and exporter of pesticides. This may seem strange but is largely explained by the fact that the materials imported generally are different from those exported. Necessity to import a compound may result from (a) lack of natural resources or appropriate climate, or (b) commercial considerations. The USA imports arsenic from countries where it is abundant and imports pyrethrum and rotenone from the tropical countries where they are grown. The USA imports certain synthetic organic pesticides because the foreign companies that hold the patents prefer to realize the profit resulting from manufacture rather than the lesser profit that might be obtained through royalties. In other instances, a rapid increase in demand for a locally manufactured compound can be met more economically by importation than by building new manufacturing facilities.

Exports of pesticides from the USA consist almost entirely of synthetic organic compounds. Of these exports in 1970, insecticides comprised 54%, herbicides 28%, fungicides 11%, fumigants 2.5%, rodenticides 0.1%, and

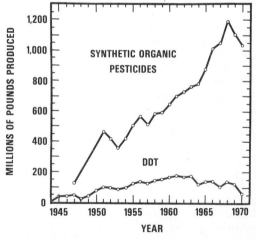

Fig. 1-7. United States production of DDT and synthetic organic pesticides. Based on data from US Tariff Commission.

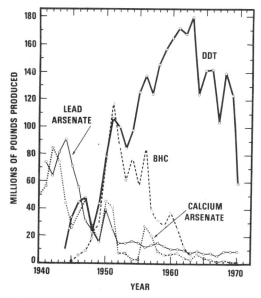

Fig. 1-8. United States production of two arsenical insecticides and two synthetic insecticides. Based on data from US Tariff Commission.

others less than 5%. The organophosphorus insecticides comprised 18% of the total pesticides exported, DDT 6.5%, and other chlorinated hydrocarbon insecticides 9.4%.

1.5.2 Economic Value of Pesticides

From a toxicological standpoint, it is more valuable to know the weight of pesticides produced (Section 1.5.1.2) than to know their cost. The tonnage of a specific product produced in 1 year is directly comparable with the tonnage of the same material produced in another year. The prices are not directly comparable because of changes in the value of money and because the basis of reporting may be different. Even so, there is considerable interest in the price. Certain basically economic considerations, including monetary profit to the individual farmer, are discussed in Section 1.4.2.5. It remains to review the monetary value of the entire market created by the needs of farmers and others.

1.5.2.1 Cost of Pesticides.

Wholesale Cost. Release of official statistics regarding the cost of pesticides at the producer's level is subject to the same limitation as release of information on production (see Section 1.5.1.2). Information on all classes of pesticides is incomplete. It is most nearly complete for synthetic organic compounds; therefore, these materials are emphasized in this account.

With the exception of 1957 and 1969, the wholesale value of synthetic organic pesticides in the United States of America increased each year from 1954 through 1970. In 1957 the reduction in total value was a combined effect of reduced production and reduced average unit cost. In 1969, the reduction in total value was entirely the result of reduced production; the average unit cost actually increased 6.7%. The total wholesale value of synthetic organic pesticides produced in the United States of America increased from about $157,599,000 in 1954 to $1,072,115,000 in 1970. The value of these same materials actually sold within the country or exported increased from $102,145,000 to $870,314,000 during the same period.

The increase in wholesale cost involved at least three factors: increased production, monetary inflation, and the gradual substitution of more expensive compounds for less expensive ones. A combination of the last two factors is reflected in the average, wholesale, unit price. With the exception of 1957, this index increased each year from 1954 through 1969. Specifically, it increased from $0.376 per pound in 1954 to $0.951 per pound in 1969. Inflation did not influence the cost of all compounds equally. In fact, the cost of DDT declined from a rate of $0.230 per pound during 1959 and 1960 to a low of $0.166 per pound in 1964 and only $0.179 in 1967. However, a variety of factors led to an increase to $0.220 in 1971.

Retail Cost to Farmers. Apparently the only part of the retail pesticide market that has been subjected to detailed analysis is the agricultural one. Even here, the latest year for which the figures are available is 1966 (Blake *et al.*, 1970). In 1966, farmers in the United States of America paid $560.8 million for pesticides, not including the cost of application. Of this amount, $505.8 million went for crop pests, $29.5 million for livestock pests, and $25.5 million for all other pests. This latter figure was broken down as follows: $6.0 million for seed treatments and stored crops, $5.3 million for seedbeds and transplants, $2.0 million for other noncropland uses, $0.2 million for treatment of buildings, and just under $12.0 million for rodent control.

Herbicides cost farmers $243.2 million, or 48% of the total pesticide expenditure for crops. Insecticides for crops cost farmers $194.6 million, more than 38% of the total for crops. Fungicides cost $32.9 million, or nearly 7% of the total.

Weed control for corn, cotton, and soybeans accounted for almost 70% of the expenditures for herbicides. Insecticides for corn and cotton together were 50% of insect control expenses.

Disease control in producing fruit, including citrus, accounted for 65% of total expenditures for fungicides.

Only 14% of planted cropland in 1966 was treated with some type of pesticide material, at an average cost of $3.98 per acre. However, over 90% of land planted in Irish potatoes, tobacco, apples, and citrus was treated. Annual costs for pesticides varied from $0.45 per acre for some grains to $54.80 per acre for apples. Because of the extent of the crops and their relatively high requirements for pesticides, the highest expenditures for individual crops were for corn ($135 million) and cotton ($94 million).

Farms with gross sales of $40,000 or more comprised less than 5% of all farms but accounted for 46% ($257 million) of all expenditures for pesticides. Farms with gross sales of less than $10,000 comprised about 70% of farms but accounted for only 17% of all expenditures for pesticides.

1.5.2.2 Wholesale Cost of Imports and Exports. The reasons that pesticides are imported as well as exported are discussed in Section 1.5.1.4.

In the United States of America, the total monetary value of exported pesticides has exceeded the value of imported ones by factors varying from 22 to 44 during the last 5 years reported. However, the average unit cost of imports ($0.753 to $1.114 per pound) was uniformly higher than the unit cost of exports ($0.436 to $0.512 per pound) during the same period. The differential undoubtedly reflects the high cost of pyrethrum.

Both imports and exports have increased but the rate of increase has been greatest for imports, at least for the last 5 years reported. It is premature to say that this represents a real trend. The available records on imports cover only a few years and the values are highly variable. Even the unit cost for imports shows twice as much variation during the last 5 years as does the unit cost of exports.

Although the total value of pesticide exports has varied considerably from year to year, the trend has been remarkably consistent since 1952, or perhaps earlier; doubling has occurred approximately every 8 years. Prior to 1952 the rate of increase may have been more rapid (doubling about every 5 years) if the statistics for 1945 are really comparable. In any event, exports of pesticides were valued at $18 million in 1945; in 1951 and 1952 they averaged $55 million, and from this level they increased to over $220 million in 1970.

1.5.3 Use of Pesticides

1.5.3.1 Tonnage Used. For a country that both imports and exports pesticides, it is difficult to determine the amount really used. Information on the use of pesticides in the United States of America is even more limited than information on their production. DDT is an example of a compound that increased in production for a number of years after its use in the USA had reached a steady state. Table 1-6 shows the amount of several pesticides used in the United States of America. Comparison of the data for lead arsenate, calcium arsenate, BHC, and DDT suggests that the trend for use and the trend for production often are similar. However, the two trends may be opposite if exports constitute a high proportion of sales. This was true of DDT for many years. By 1953, the annual use of DDT already had reached 62,500,000 pounds in the United States of America. It increased about 25% to reach its highest value for any year (78,682,000 pounds) in 1959. From 1959 onward, the domestic use of DDT decreased gradually to about one-third that amount in 1970 and then dropped to essentially zero in 1973. If the trend evident from 1959 through 1970 had continued without interruption, use of DDT in the USA would have reached zero in 1975.

Use of pesticides is subject to more irregular and rapid variation in a state or other limited area than in a country. For example, in contrast to the pattern of use in the country as a whole, the use of DDT in Arizona increased by a factor of 4.6 from 1965 to 1967 and then fell back below the original level by the following year (Roan *et al.*, 1969). The changes in use reflect changes in regulations and economics and, generally most important, in weather (a major determinant of pest abundance) (Roan *et al.*, 1969).

1.5.3.2 Number of Compounds and Products.

Number of Compounds Used. The 4th edition of the *Pesticide Index* (Frear, 1969a) lists approximately 1,475 separate compounds as well as synonyms for many of them. Since the Index was published, some new compounds have been introduced experimentally or even commercially. It is difficult to say how many of these compounds are important either for some specialized use or even for more extensive uses requiring many tons of product each year. Fig. 1-6 is based on 199 compounds of undoubted importance. All pesticide products registered by the US Department of Agriculture in 1967 were based on only 368 basic chemicals (Mulhern, 1967), and a few of them were of little importance. Considering the introduction of new compounds, and the existence of some variation in the choice of compounds by different countries, 350 would seem to be a good

Table 1-6

Pesticide Consumption in the United States of America, 1953-1970

(Figures shown in thousands of pounds. [a])

Year	Compound						
	Aldrin-toxaphene group	BHC (gamma basis)	DDT	2,4-D (acid basis)	2,4,5-T (acid basis)	Calcium arsenate	Lead arsenate
1953	34,050	7,300	62,500	23,449	4,438	7,000	16,000
1954	35,420	8,500	45,117	23,841	2,761	3,190	16,000
1955	54,400	7,138	61,800	23,889	2,359	3,911	13,269
1956	61,570	9,450	75,000	24,000	4,260	23,000	11,500
1957	52,500	6,600	71,000	20,500	1,800	18,250	12,000
1958	78,834	5,500	66,700	21,300	3,800	9,000	12,897
1959	73,331	4,276	78,682	34,102	5,508	--	10,618
1960	75,766	5,111	70,146	31,131	5,859	7,314	11,173
1961	78,260	4,577	64,068	31,067	5,444	4,874	8,967
1962	82,125	2,204	67,245	35,903	8,102	4,541	7,957
1963	79,275	1,299	61,165	33,199	7,179	3,960	6,954
1964	83,161	--	50,542	43,986	8,912	3,611	7,951
1965	80,568	--	52,986	50,535	7,244	3,474	8,090
1966	86,646	--	46,672	63,903	17,080	2,942	6,944
1967	86,289	--	40,257	46,955	13,381	2,329	6,152
1968	38,710	--	32,753	43,404	13,304	1,992	4,747
1969	89,721	--	30,256	49,526	3,218	2,117	7,721
1970	62,282	--	25,457	46,942	4,871	2,900	5,860

a. Data from U.S. Tariff Commission

estimate for the total number of compounds of real importance.

Number of Products Used. No information is available on the number of products for sale before the Federal Insecticide, Fungicide, and Rodenticide Act went into effect in 1947. Beginning at that time, existing commercial products were registered as quickly as their labeling could be brought into conformity with the Act. Many new products were introduced, most of them based on very recently developed compounds. It was a time of tremendous increase in the variety of pesticides and especially of their formulations. Furthermore, the increase in products appeared even greater than it was because, for a variety of reasons, minor changes were made in many formula-

tions, and each change or set of simultaneous changes in a single product required a separate labeling action. Understandably, the US Department of Agriculture kept a record of each action, but unfortunately lacked any mechanism during the early years to know how many products had been dropped from the market. The cumulative number of approved labels increased in an essentially straight line fashion from about 10,000 in 1949 to about 90,000 in 1958 (Ward, 1958) and continued to increase at the same rate to a level of 134,193 in 1963 (Shepard, 1963). However, these cumulative figures were never realistic estimates of the total number of products available for sale at any one time. In addition to the thousands of products deleted for commercial reasons, the registrations of thousands of others were canceled because of official limitation of the use of arsenic, DDT, and other compounds.

It is estimated that the largest number of pesticidal products commercially available in the United States of America was about 60,000 during the mid-1960's. By 1969, the number had fallen to about 45,000. In 1972 it was about 34,000 and still decreasing (Hays, 1972).

The decline in the number of commercially available products was reflected by editions of the *Pesticide Handbook,* which lists important agricultural preparations, but few household preparations. The number of products listed gradually increased to about 8,000 in 1969 and then decreased to approximately 7,000 in 1972 (Frear, 1969b, 1972). If the ratios of these values to the estimated total number of products available in 1969 and 1972 are meaningful, it indicates that coverage by the Handbook continued to improve even though the number of entries decreased.

No matter what the number of commercial products registered for sale at any one time, there is considerable overlapping or duplication of formulations. It is estimated that there are only about 3,000 basically different formulations of pesticides, and for the last 20 years their number has been far more constant than the number of separately registered products.

1.5.4 Methods of Application

Not only have the number of pesticides and their tonnage increased, but the number and variety of their uses and the methods of their application have increased also. Crops are treated that formerly were left unprotected. There is extensive use of planes as well as ground equipment. Fig. 1-9 shows the trend of the number of acres of cropland in California treated by aircraft. The expansion of suburbs has been associated with increased use of pesticides by amateurs for lawns or small flower or vegetable gardens. However, an increasing proportion of treatments are made by pest control applicators or custom applicators. Such professional service now is used commonly for lawns and golf courses, as well as for buildings, ships, and crops.

New formulations have been developed. For example, water-wettable powders, an outgrowth of wettable sulfur and wettable lime sulfur powders, were improved technically during the 1950's; they now constitute the most important single kind of formulation for control of both agricultural pests and disease vectors. Another change of formulation involves concentration. There has been a trend toward the application of more concentrated

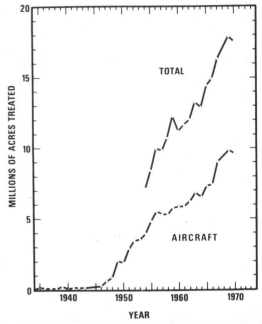

Fig. 1-9. Area of land in California treated with pesticides. Based on data from California Department of Agriculture Annual Reports.

sprays in lower volume in order to achieve the same or somewhat smaller dosage per unit area. This practice may reduce the amount of expensive solvent required for a given task. An aircraft can treat more area per load using ultra-low-volume spray. The physical properties of undiluted technical malathion are peculiarly adapted to ultra-low-volume application. The paper (Skoog *et al.,* 1965) describing the use of malathion in this way in 1963, apparently for the first time, also gives a history of the early development of the technique with other compounds and, in this connection, cites papers as early as 1946.

In addition to the advantages already enumerated, malathion applied to plants in ultra-low-volume produces longer lasting surface residues than less concentrated formulations applied at the same dosage of active material (Nolan, 1967; Awad *et al.,* 1967; Saini and Dorough, 1970). This fact is explained in some degree by the greater penetration into leaves of malathion formulated with an emulsifier (Awad et al., 1967). However, ultra-low-volume residues last longer on glass plates as well as on leaves (Saini and Dorough, 1970), so that differences of evaporation determined by differences in the physical form of the residue must be important. Although it has been suggested that plant enzymes degrade ultra-low-volume residues less rapidly, evidence for this effect is questionable (Awad *et al.*, 1967). Regardless of the factors involved, the net effect is that control can be achieved with less malathion per unit area if it is applied as an ultra-low-volume spray.

1.6 Pesticide Problems and Their Solutions

1.6.1 Nature of Pesticide Problems

The use of any biologically active compound poses potential problems of toxicity. Persons most likely to be affected are those with direct contact, including those who manufacture, formulate, or use the compound. However, if the material is used in or around the home, many more people potentially are affected. If the compound is used in any stage of food production, then residues of it or of its derivatives may persist in food when it is eaten; thus, the entire population may be exposed to traces of the material. Finally, domestic and useful wild animals also may be affected, depending on the way in which the compound is used and its persistence after use.

What is commonly referred to as "the pesticide problem" is more than the sum of real and potential injuries from pesticides. To a large degree, it is the result of disagreement among people about the need for pest control, about what environmental features deserve serious concern, about what pesticides ought to do, and about what side effects from them are tolerable. An instructive discussion of the matter and what realistically might be done about it, is that by Beirne (1967).

It is the duty of the toxicologist to identify and evaluate the problems and, on the basis of scientific study, to prevent injury and to develop methods of treating illness if it occurs. More specifically, it is the duty of toxicologists to study each new compound early in its development, so that it may be permitted only for safe uses and under safe conditions. The preliminary study ought to identify the nature and degree of potential injury and methods for avoiding such injury. The early study also may develop methods of treating illness if it occurs. Once a compound, whether old or new, is in use, toxicologists have a duty to monitor its effects, especially on those most heavily exposed. Finally, toxicologists must investigate any claims of injury and fairly evaluate them.

1.6.2 Proposed Solutions

Two things must be pointed out at the beginning. First, if toxicologists did their work perfectly from the beginning, and if it were always possible to release for use only compounds with essentially no effect on any organism except the target pest, there would be no problem and no need for a solution. Unfortunately, our knowledge of testing is imperfect. Furthermore, it is and will continue to be impossible to test all the species that may eventually prove to be affected to a significant degree. Practical means have not yet been devised for ensuring even that information on the susceptibility of people will be gathered with the efficiency and speed that modern techniques permit. Perhaps even more important, in the absence of a truly satisfactory way to control a particular pest at a particular time, a compound may be used where the danger is known clearly not only to toxicologists but to the applicators or other workers. This is not a situation peculiar to pesticides. The problem extends to drugs and other chemical and to mechanical devices, including automobiles. Statistically, private automobiles are not as safe as public transportation, but in many situations no practical alternative exists. The same is true of pesticides, particularly some of the more toxic ones.

Second, it must be realized that the majority of pesticidal compounds offer little or no threat to human health or to the environment under practical conditions of use. Only a minority of compounds have given trouble when used according to label directions. On the other hand, no compound, whether pesticide or not, is harmless if sufficiently misused. On the average, the duty of the toxicologist has been discharged well in recent years.

There remains the challenge to develop toxicological tests that are more efficient (and hopefully more economical) in evaluating real hazards, both old and recently discovered. As an example of an important recent advance in testing for a danger that became apparent largely in the last decade, one may mention the model ecosystem developed by Metcalf for the purpose of detecting compounds that undergo biological magnification (see Sections 3.2.3.2 and 11.2.3.2). There also remains the continuing challenge to toxicologists to cooperate with physicians, educators, industrial hygienists, and regulatory officials in promoting the safe use not only of pesticides but of drugs, household chemicals, industrial compounds, and other substances.

In fact, an important aspect of the problem of testing either effectiveness or toxicity is the difficulty of getting good communication between persons in the laboratory and those who carry out large scale tests and eventually use the product under field conditions. The WHO program for testing pesticides discussed in

Section 7.1.2.5 is an example of communication at its best.

1.6.2.1 The Economic Approach. It has been suggested by Headley and Lewis (1967) that public policy with regard to the use of pesticides ought to be based on the cost and the returns associated with such use. To this end, they offered what they called a conceptual decision framework for the formulation of policy in their belief that "the so-called pesticide problem is largely and inescapably economic in nature." Basically, the proposal is to express direct and indirect benefits and direct and indirect costs in a single unit, namely dollars, and to determine policy on the basis of a balance between benefit and cost. Nothing could be simpler.

Increased sales value of a crop is an example of a direct benefit. Increased sales value of a neighbor's crop (through drift of pesticide to the neighbor's field and reduction of the number of pests capable of migrating to the neighbor's field) would be an example of an indirect benefit. (Actually, indirect benefits are poorly documented in agriculture but they may be important in public health; there are many examples of the control of other diseases by programs for control of malaria.) The cost of pesticide and of labor to apply it plus the prorated cost of equipment for the application constitute the cost of application. The cost of pesticide presumably covers the prorated cost of developing the compound. The cost of any accidents, whether to people or to crops or livestock, constitutes the indirect cost to the farmer. The cost of any damage to the environment, as well as the prorated cost of regulation and monitoring, constitute the indirect (or external) cost to society, including the farmer.

Unfortunately, many real situations are not adequately covered by the model proposed by Headley and Lewis (1967) and represented by their second figure. Benefits often do not increase indefinitely as the amount of pesticide applied increases. Excessive application may, for example, produce phytotoxicity and decrease production. Granted that those indirect costs of pesticides resulting from injury to nontarget organisms would be a sigmoid function (if the increase in pesticide input is linear), there is no reason to suppose that the curve passes through the origin. Furthermore, there is no reason there should be a greater than linear increase corresponding to a linear increase in pesticide use. As a matter of fact, the increase in direct cost would be somewhat less than linear because of a relative reduction in the cost for labor and equipment.

Finally, there may be real difficulty in measuring the benefits and costs in a particular situation. This is especially true, as Headley and Lewis admit, where it becomes necessary to fix a monetary value on human life.

1.6.2.2 Empirical Approaches to Pesticide Problems. A number of editorials and reviews have discussed the pest control problem. In most instances the suggestions for solution of the problem have been nonspecific or they have placed an emphasis on alternative methods of control that is not justified by practical experience.

It must be recognized that when pesticide problems have arisen that could be evaluated accurately in economic terms, they have been solved promptly. For example, when the chlorophenoxy herbicides were first developed, there were a number of instances in which sensitive crops such as cotton were injured by drift from an application intended for other crops such as rice. Claims were brought in court and the value of the destroyed cotton or other crops was adjudicated. Such losses could not be allowed to continue. Farmers became acquainted with the problem and regulations were established to minimize drift. Furthermore, it was soon realized that most, if not all, of these mishaps were associated with use of highly volatile compounds. Manufacture of these compounds was stopped. Following these changes, injury to crops from drift of chlorophenoxy herbicides has become rare.

Reasonable agreement also has been reached on other questions where a direct comparison is possible, no matter what the unit of measure. For example, it is easy to justify the control of malaria and other vector-borne diseases even though it is a matter of record that some of the compounds (eg, dieldrin) used for this purpose have caused illness among the spraymen. The number of human lives saved by these programs is much greater than the number of persons injured by pesticides, whether used for disease control or some other purpose. Under these circumstances, one cannot oppose the use of pesticides for malaria control without being suspected of advocating malaria as a means of population control in developing nations in the tropics.

In many countries, society has adjusted to a considerable degree to a low level of accidental injury to people by pesticides, just as they have adjusted to the more numerous injuries caused by accidental ingestion of drugs. Fortunately, it has been possible through education to reduce the frequency of such injury.

In other countries, the actual or potential rate of injury has been judged too high. A number of developing countries have prohibited the sale or use of one or more highly toxic compounds. Such decisions are based mainly on considerations of safety but may be conditioned by a lack of need for the compound.

The pesticide problems that have given greatest difficulty are those in which no valid matching of benefits and indirect costs is possible. No real way has been found to compare the benefit from improvement of a particular crop with injury to one or more species of wildlife. Quite aside from the interests of the individual farmer or forester, there is no way to compare the economic benefits to society resulting from abundant food and fiber with the mainly esthetic injury to society resulting from damage to birds. This problem, too, may be adjudicated eventually. Unfortunately, the trial tends to be one in which the plaintiff and the defendant speak separate languages, each different from that of the judge. In the meantime, there is a danger that the majority of the public, being ignorant of the basic principles of toxicology and unfamiliar with the farmer's problems, will, through their elected representatives, compromise their own food supply.

Toxicologists cannot solve such problems alone. However, it would be constructive if it were more widely recognized that scientists can reach complete agreement about the safety of a pesticide for man and its danger for another desirable species, for example a form of wildlife.

In the meantime, some environmentalists have been so critical of the chemical industry and so eager to have technology limited by government action that realization of their proposals under a system of free enterprise may not have been envisioned. However, based on actual performance, there seems little reason to believe that a strong centralized and planned economy has any notable advantages over other economic systems in preventing environmental disruption (Goldman, 1970). The fact is that a perfect solution of pest control is not known. Realistic efforts to solve individual pest problems must take into account people who produce food and those who eat.

Realistic efforts to strike a balance between the benefits and the subtle, indirect costs of pesticides must take all humanity into account. As Mrs. Indira Gandhi (1972) said, ". . . How can we speak to those who live in villages and in slums about keeping the oceans, the rivers and the air clean when their own lives are contaminated at the source? The environment cannot be improved in conditions of poverty. Nor can poverty be eradicated without the use of science and technology."

1.7 Standard References on Pesticides

1.7.1 Nomenclature

When compounds are first considered as pesticides, they are designated by chemical name and seldom in any other way, except perhaps a code number assigned to them for the purpose of record keeping by the public agency or commercial company carrying out the investigation. When a particular compound begins to attract attention outside the laboratory in which it was first studied, it often continues to be known by its code number. A considerable literature may be built up in which the code number is the working designation. Thus, the rodenticide, monosodium fluoroacetate, introduced in the early 1940's, is still known as "compound 1080" or merely as "1080." If the material justifies its early promise, it almost always will be assigned at least one proprietary name by the sponsoring company. If more than one use is known, more than one proprietary name may be assigned. Proprietary names are those owned by a company and used to designate their products. Such names are referred to frequently but inaccurately as "trade names." Actually, according to trademark law, a trade name is synonymous with the company name.

Unfortunately, most chemical names are too complicated to be remembered easily, especially by those who are not chemists. Furthermore, there are serious objections to using a proprietary name as a scientific term. Such use invites confusion, partly because definition of these words is controlled only by the companies that own them, and partly because important compounds may come to have several proprietary names. The multiple names may come from the same or different companies. A company may use different proprietary names to designate different grades or uses of its compound. For example, one company has sold fenthion as Endex® for indoor use, as Baytex® for many outdoor uses, and as Queletox® for control of birds. This is a reasonable procedure that, among other benefits, undoubtedly helps to prevent a salesman or a buyer from getting the wrong formulation for his purpose. The fact remains, however, that use of proprietary names can lead to confusion in scientific discussion and literature.

Nonproprietary names are spoken of as "common names," "coined names," and "generic names," and these terms may be considered interchangeable. Such a term becomes an "approved name" if it is issued by an authoritative private or governmental agency, and it becomes an "official name" if issued by a governmental agency under authority of a law specifically authorizing the establishment of names. The 1972 amendments of the Federal Insecticide, Fungicide, and Rodenticide Act authorize the Administrator to determine and establish suitable names to be used in the ingredient statement of labels for pesticides.

Need for Nonproprietary Names. An approved nonproprietary name makes a compound identifiable. To this extent, the name clarifies regulatory procedures regarding the compound and the frequently numerous commercial products containing it. Finally, nonproprietary names serve to protect proprietary names and trademarks, which often have great commercial value. The federal law concerning the granting of trademarks provides that a proprietary name may fall into the public domain if the public adopts it as a common name. The trademark rights to the word "aspirin" were lost in the United States of America in this way.

The need for nonproprietary names is evident, but their acquisition presents many problems. Before considering these problems, it would be helpful to review the solution reached in connection with drugs.

Nonproprietary Names for Drugs. Alessandri and Jerome (1970) provided a history of nonproprietary names for drugs, a detailed discussion of the underlying problems, and valuable description of the conventions now observed in promulgating these names. In the United States of America, nonproprietary names for drugs now are selected by the United States Adopted Name Council (USAN Council). Names so adopted are designated USAN. The Council has five members and three sponsors (the American Medical Association, the United States Pharmacopeia, and the American Pharmaceutical Association). Each sponsor appoints one member. A fourth member-at-large must be approved by all three sponsors, and a fifth member is appointed by the Food and Drug Administration. Under federal law, the Commissioner of the Food and Drug Administration (acting for the Secretary of Health, Education, and Welfare) has authority to designate an official name for any drug. According to present agreement, the Food and Drug Administration accepts those names unanimously approved by the USAN Council but reserves the right to select an official name in those instances in which the Council cannot reach unanimous agreement. A name becomes official when published in the *Federal Register*.

Of course other countries have their own systems for the approval of names. International cooperation in the selection of nonpro-

prietary names of drugs is carried out under the auspices of the World Health Organization. A word is first listed as a proposed international nonproprietary name (pINN) and later as a recommended international nonproprietary name (recINN).

The methods for establishing approved nonproprietary names in the United States of America and in the international community are more advanced for drugs than for pesticides. Those interested in the nomenclature of pesticides could learn much from those responsible for naming drugs.

Problems Involving Nonproprietary Names. It would be ideal if all reports of the effectiveness, toxicity, and other properties of each pesticide were made in terms of its unique nonproprietary name. Realization of such an ideal situation would require not only that each nonproprietary name be adopted very early in the development of the corresponding pesticide but that the same name would be adopted in every country. This would require prompt, international action—a most difficult combination to achieve, especially in view of the fact that each name must be suitable in each country in which it is used. The nonproprietary name must not duplicate or be easily confused with other names (including proprietary names) of other pesticides or of drugs or industrial chemicals, or even of other things or ideas.

Certainly, most progress will be made if all persons concerned with any aspect of pesticides recognize the problems involved with nonproprietary names and work for their solution. Such problems include: (*a*) real difficulty of avoiding duplicate or otherwise unsuitable names; (*b*) shortsighted unwillingness of some companies to release their proprietary names for use as nonproprietary names; (*c*) thinly disguised commercialism of some agencies entrusted with establishment of nonproprietary names; (*d*) rigid requirement of certain languages that names end with a particular letter or combination of letters. At least in the past, another difficulty has involved: (*e*) improper use of a nonproprietary name to designate a mixture rather than a single, characteristic compound. All technical grade pesticides are mixtures, but it only leads to confusion to give these mixtures nonproprietary names. It is shortsighted even for the manufacturer, because improvements in manufacturing technique often lead to a progressive increase in the concentration of the intended active ingredient in the technical product. In this book, regardless of its original meaning, each nonproprietary name is used to designate a compound—not a mixture. When required for clarity, the nonproprietary name is used with a suitable modifier to show that the technical mixture or an isomer or some other form is meant.

CAS Registry Number. Chemical Abstracts Service has developed a series of "registry numbers" for individual compounds. This number may become the most useful single synonym for each compound. Of course, there is no possibility or intension that registry numbers would replace approved nonproprietary names. Numbers are not adapted for human memory, but they are ideal for computers. The CAS registry number is unique for a particular compound; isomers receive separate numbers. The CAS registry number may be used through the Chemical Abstracts Service for establishing the equivalence or lack of correspondence of other code numbers, nonproprietary names, proprietary names, and chemical names, and as a key to computer searches of the chemical literature.

Sources of Information on Nomenclature. Pesticides have been and are named by a number of public, professional, and other groups. Coined names in the strict sense were first given to insecticides by the Interdepartmental Committee on Pest Control (ICPC) composed of representatives of the United States Departments of Agriculture; Defense; Interior; and Health, Education, and Welfare. Subsequently, arrangements were made for the American Standards Association (ASA) [later the American National Standards Institute, Inc. (ANSI)] to take responsibility for naming pesticides. A list of the pesticides named by the Institute is available in their catalog (American National Standards Institute, 1972) and a brochure on each compound is available for purchase. Unlike other groups of pesticides, most herbicides are named in North America by the Weed Society of America (WSA) (1967), the approved forms being specified in their *Herbicide Handbook.* Some other groups issue lists of acceptable names even though they do not name compounds themselves. These include the Entomological Society of America (Kenaga and Allison, 1969) and the US Department of Agriculture (Caswell, 1967).

British common names for pesticides are set by the British Standards Institution (BSI) (1961).

Pesticide names found in Russian technical literature have been published in the Latin as well as the Cyrillic alphabet along with their English equivalents (Busbey, 1961). Additional information on equivalent Russian and English names may be found by comparing the Russian and English editions of the valuable book on the chemistry of pesticides by Melnikov (1971).

Considerable international agreement on nonproprietary names for pesticides has been reached through the International Organization for Standardization (ISO), of which the various national standards organizations are members.

The most valuable single published source of information on nomenclature of pesticides is Frear's *Pesticide Index* first published in 1961. The most recent edition (Frear, 1969a) lists over 1,400 compounds and a larger number of synonyms. Other sources of information on various aspects of pesticides including their nomenclature are bulletins or journal articles by the Association of American Pesticide Control Officials (1966), and by Martin (1964).

The most important source of information on proprietary names of pesticides is Frear's *Pesticide Handbook.* The 24th annual edition (Frear, 1972) listed approximately 7,000 products.

1.7.2 General Information

Books. Books dealing with some special aspects of the toxicology of pesticides are referred to in this book in the chapter dealing with the same subject. However, several valuable references must be mentioned here, either because their subject matter is very general, or because they provide background information essential to an understanding of toxicology of pesticides even though they are not concerned directly with it.

A good reference on legal medicine is entitled *Legal Medicine: Pathology and Toxicology* (Gonzales *et al.*, 1954).

The leading reference on toxicological aspects of occupational health is *Industrial Hygiene and Toxicology* (Patty, 1958 *et seq.*).

Evaluation of safety is represented by a number of books dealing with techniques, especially techniques suitable for drugs. Important ones are cited in Chapters 2, 3, and 4. The book *Air Pollution: A Comprehensive Treatise* (Stern, 1962) should be consulted by anyone interested in this aspect of safety evaluation.

The best introduction to the problems created by pests and to the full range of biological and chemical methods available for their control is a series of six volumes published by the National Academy of Sciences (1968–1970). Each of the first five volumes was prepared by a committee of experts on a particular class of pests, namely, microorganisms that cause plant diseases, weeds, insect pests, plant-parasitic nematodes, and vertebrate pests. The sixth volume was prepared by a committee expert on the effects of pesticides on fruit and vegetable physiology. Emphasis in all of the books is on basic ecology and physiology. Particular attention is given to problems that lack satisfactory solution.

A book with more emphasis on alternative methods of pest control and a realistic evaluation of these methods was published a little later by the National Academy of Sciences (1972).

An excellent introduction to problems and methods of insect control is *Insect Control by Chemicals* (Brown, 1951). It contains information not only on the compounds themselves but on their pharmacology in insects, equipment for applying insecticides from the ground and from the air, phytotoxicity, and an unusually perceptive early appraisal of the effect of insecticides on the environment. Another useful book that is somewhat similar but gives more emphasis to individual compounds and to human toxicology is *Toxicologie des Produits Phytopharmaceutiques* (Fabre and Truhaut, 1954).

Books that emphasize the chemistry of pesticides and/or their action against pests are *Chemicals for Pest Control* (Hartley and West, 1969), *Organic Insecticides—Their Chemistry and Mode of Action* (Metcalf, 1955), and *The Chemistry and Action of Pesticides* (Shephard, 1951). The latter book is notable for the historical insight and the information on production it offers. The most recent and most generally useful book is the *Pesticide Manual* by Martin (1972).

Books dealing with methods of chemical analysis of pesticides include: *Analytical Methods for Pesticides, Plant Growth Regulators, and Food Additives* (Zweig, 1963; 1964a; 1964b; 1964c; 1967; 1972); *Handbook of Analytical Toxicology* (Sunshine, 1969); and *Analysis of Pesticide Residues in Human and Environmental Samples* (Thompson, 1971).

Proceedings. Among the proceedings of various symposia and hearings, the following must be mentioned: *Agricultural Control Chemicals* (American Chemical Society, 1950); *Plant Protection Conference, 1956* (Plant Protection Ltd., 1957); *New Approaches to Pest Control and Eradication* (American Chemical Society, 1963); the Ribicoff Report, *Pesticides and Public Policy* (US Senate, 1966) and the record of hearings on which it was based (US Senate, 1964); *Natural Pest Control Agents* (American Chemical Society, 1966a); *Organic Pesticides in the Environment* (American Chemical Society, 1966b); *Scientific Aspects of Pest Control* (National Academy of Sciences, 1966b); *Biological Effects of Pesticides in Mammalian Systems* (New York Academy of Sciences, 1969); *Chemical Fallout: Current Research on Persistent Pesticides* (Miller and Berg, 1969); *Report of the Secretary's Commission on Pesticides and Their Relationship to Environmental Health* (US Department of HEW, 1969). These proceedings contain some valuable reviews and offer pictures of the state of the art at the time they were issued. Some of these proceedings, especially those issued by the American Chemical Society, contain reports of original research as well as reviews and position papers.

Reviews. Reviews about toxicology and often about pesticides are published in *Residue Reviews, Essays in Toxicology, Critical Reviews in Toxicology,* and less frequently in *Pharmacological Reviews* and *Annual Review of Pharmacology.*

Primary Journals. Original papers on toxicology are published in a wide range of journals, and those on pesticides are no exception. Because of demonstrated relevance, over 1,100 journals of all sorts are scanned systematically for articles abstracted in Pesticides Abstracts, formerly called Health Aspects of Pesticides Abstract Bulletin. Of these, the great majority are scientific journals; a few are trade or news bulletins. Of course many articles on the toxicology of pesticides appear in a relatively small number of journals including: Acta Pharmacologica et Toxicologica, American Industrial Hygiene Association Journal, Archiv fur Toxikologie, Archives of Contamination and Toxicology, Archives of Environmental Health, Archives Internationales de Pharmacodynamie et de Therapie, Biochemical Pharmacology, British Journal of Industrial Medicine, Bulletin of Environmental Contamination and Toxicology, Bulletin of the World Health Organization, Canadian Journal of Physiology and Pharmacology, Canadian Medical Association Journal, Clinical Toxicology, European Journal of Pharmacology, European Journal of Toxicology, Experimentia Farmakologii i Toksikologiia, Food and Cosmetics Toxicology, Industrial Medicine and Surgery, Journal of Agriculture and Food Chemistry, Journal of Environmental Health, Journal of Occupational Medicine, Journal of Pharmacology and Experimental Therapeutics, Life Sciences, Nature, Pesticide Biochemistry and Physiology, Pesticides Monitoring Journal, Pesticide Science, Science, Toxicology and Applied Pharmacology, Xenobiotica, and Zeitschrift fur Naturforschung.

Secondary Journals. Original reports, reviews, and discussions on the toxicology of pesticides are indexed with varying emphasis and completeness of coverage by Index Medicus, Chemical Abstracts, Biological Abstracts, Biosciences Information Service, Toxicity Bibliography, Excerpta Medica (Sections 30 and 35), Pollution Abstracts, and Abstracts on Health Effects of Environmental Pollutants.

The only major journal dealing exclusively with the toxicology of pesticides is Pesticides Abstracts, published by the Environmental Protection Agency and issued by the United States Government Printing Office. It is of great value in itself and an invaluable means of access to the original literature.

Computer Service. The most recent development in the retrieval of references and abstracts involves the use of computers. Such a service, called TOXLINE, is now available from the National Library of Medicine through its Toxicology Information Program. Particular attention is given to pesticides. The system employs the same computer as that used for MEDLINE. It permits on-line, interactive retrieval of toxicological information through a nationwide communication network. Users with access to terminals in medical schools and in some other large laboratories can use key words and index terms to search both the titles and the abstracts of over 250,000 journal articles in toxicology and related fields from 1965 to the present. Off-line printouts may be obtained if desired.

Persons with or without access to a computer terminal also may purchase literature searches from the Toxicology Information Response Center of the Oak Ridge National Laboratory. This service depends largely, but not entirely, on TOXLINE.

1.8 Conventions Used in This Book

Nomenclature. Insofar as possible, pesticides are designated in this book by their nonproprietary names (see Section 1.7.1). For a few chemically simple compounds, the chemical name is also the common name. When there is no common name but a compound is known generally by a trade name, then the trade name is employed. Complicated chemical names have been used to designate compounds only where there is no other choice. Appendix I lists the names selected and the chemical identity of each.

Units. Metric units are used in this book in most instances. An important exception is that statistics on the production, use, and cost of pesticides are given in the units in which they are supplied by official sources. Another exception involves some figures reproduced from earlier publications.

To facilitate comparisons in toxicology, a single unit has been selected to express each concept of measurement; these units are shown in Appendix II. This policy has made it necessary to convert many values from the units, whether metric or otherwise, in which they were stated originally. Appendix III is a conversion table especially for the help of persons who prefer some other set of units and wish to continue their use.

References. References to scientific books and papers are given in the usual way at the end of each chapter. It is customary to give references to laws, regulations, and legal notices in very concise, highly stylized form entirely different from that of scientific references. Therefore, legal citations are given in full in the text and not repeated at the end of the chapter in which they appear.

REFERENCES

Abano, P. (1472). *De venenis.* J. Wurster and F. van Siebenburgen, Mantua, 364 pp. Translated into English by H. M. Brown (1924), Ann. Med. Hist.

Agricola, G. (1556). *De re metallica.* H. Frobenium and N. Episcopivm, Basilae, 538 pp. Translated into English by H. C. Hoover and L. H. Hoover (1950) Dover Publications, Inc., New York.

Alessandri, M. C., and Jerome, J. B. (1970). Drug nomenclature—United States adopted names. In: *Remington's Pharmaceutical Sciences,* Ed. 14, pp. 509–516. Mack Publishing Company, Easton, Pa.

American Chemical Society (1950). *Agricultural Control Chemicals.* Adv. Chem. Ser. 1. American Chemical Society, Washington, DC.

American Chemical Society (1963). *New Approaches to Pest Control and Eradication.* Adv. Chem. Ser. 41. American Chemical Society, Washington, DC.

American Chemical Society (1966a). *Natural Pest Control Agents.* Adv. Chem. Ser. 53. American Chemical Society, Washington, DC.

American Chemical Society (1966b). *Organic Pesticides in the Environment.* Adv. Chem. Ser. 60. American Chemical Society, Washington, DC.

American National Standards Institute (1972). *Catalog,* Section K–62. American National Standards Institute, New York.

Anonymous (1853). Biographical sketch of the late M. Orfila. **Lancet, 1:326–327.**

Arrington, L. G. (1956). *World Survey of Pest Control Products.* US Government Printing Office, Washington, DC.

Association of American Pesticide Control Officials, Inc. (1966). *Pesticide Chemicals Official Compendium.* AAPCO, Inc.

Awad, T. M., Wilson, S. B., and Brazzel, J. R. (1967). Effect of environmental and biological factors on persistence of malathion applied as ultra-low-volume or emulsifiable concentrate to cotton plants. J. Agric. Food Chem., 15:1009–1013.

Beirne, B. P. (1967). *Pest Management.* Leonard Hill, London.

Bernard, C. (1857). *Leçons sur les Effets des Substances Toxiques et Médicamenteuses.* J. B. Baillière et Fils, Paris.

Black, R. H. (1819). *Directions for the Treatment of Persons who have taken Poison, and those in a State of Apparent Death; Together with the Means of Detecting Poisons and Adulterations in Wine; also, of Distinguishing Real from Apparent Death.* Translated from the French of M. P. Orfila. 1st Amer. Ed. N. G. Maxwell, Baltimore.

Blake, H. T., Andrilenas, P. A., Jenkins, R. P., Eichers, T. R., and Fox, A. S. (1970). *Farmer's Pesticide Expenditures in 1966.* Agricultural Economic Rept. 192, US Department of Agriculture, Washington, DC.

British Standards Institution (1961). *Recommended Common Names for Pesticides.* British Standards House, London.

British Standards Institution (1965). *Recommended Common Names for Pesticides.* British Standards House, London.

Brown, A. W. A. (1951). *Insect Control by Chemicals.* John Wiley & Sons, Inc., New York.

Bruce-Chwatt, L. J., and Haworth, J. (1965). Malaria eradication: Its present status. Isr. J. Med. Sci., 1:284–289.

Bryan, C. P. (1931). *The Papyrus Ebers,* Translated from the German version. D. Appleton and Company, New York.

Busbey, R. L. (1961). Pesticide names found in U.S.S.R. technical literature. J. Econ. Entomol. 54:254–257.

Caswell, R. L. (1967). *Acceptable Common Names and Chemical Names for the Ingredient Statement on Economic Poison (Pesticide and Plant Growth Regulator) Labels.* US Department of Agriculture, Washington, DC.

Chevallier, J.-B.-A. (1850). *Dictionnaires des Altérations et Falsifications des Substances Alimentaires Médicamenteuses et Commerciales, avec l'Indication des Moyens de les Reconnaître* Vols. 1 and 2, 479 and 580 pp. Bechetjeune, Paris.

Chiarappa, L., Chiang. H. C., and Smith, R. F. (1972). Plant pests and diseases: Assessment of crop losses. Science, 176:769–773.

Christison, R. (1845). *A Treatise on Poisons in Relation to Medical Jurisprudence, Physiology, and the Practice of Physic.* E. Barrington and G. D. Haswell, Philadelphia.

Church, E. J. (1896). *The Trial and Death of Socrates.* Macmillan, London.

Coates, J. B., Jr., Hoff, E. C., and Hoff, P. M. (1963). *Preventive Medicine in World War II.* Vol. 6, *Communicable Diseases—Malaria.* US Government Printing Office, Washington, DC.

Coley, H. (1832). *A Treatise on Medical Jurisprudence. Part I. Comprising the Consideration of Poisons and Asphyxia.* William Stodart, New York.

Cramer, H. H. (1967). Plant protection and world crop production. Pflanzenschutz-Nachr. 1:1–524.

Decker, G. C. (1966). Chemicals in the production of food. In: *Proc. Western Hemisphere Nutrition Congress.* American Medical Association, Chicago, pp. 127–135.

Delille, R., and Magendie, F. (1809). Des effets de l'Upas Tienté sur l'économie animal. Nouv. Bull. Sci. par la Soc. Phil. Paris, 1:368–371.

Ebers, G. (1875). *Papyros Ebers Das Hermetische Buch über die Arzeneimittel der alten Agypter in hieratischer schrift.* W. Engelmann, Leipzig.

Ellenbog, U. (1524). *Von den giftigen besen Tempffen und Reuchen.* M. Ramminger, Augsburg. Translated into English by Cyril Bernard (1932), Lancet, 1:270–271.

Fabre, R., and Truhaut, R. (1954). *Toxicologie des Produits Phytopharmaceutiques.* Soc. d'Edit. d'Enseignement Supérieur, Paris.

Fontana, F. (1781). *Traité sur le Venin de la Vipère, sur les Poisons Américains, sur le Laurier-Cerise, et quelques autres Poisons Végétaux; On y a Joint des Observations sur la Structure Primitive du Corps Animal, Différentes Expériences sur la Reproduction des Nerfs et la Description d'un Nouveau Canal de L'oeil,* Vols. 1 and 2, 328 and 373 pp. Florence. Translated into English by Joseph Skinner (1787), J. Murray, London.

Frear, D. E. H (ed.) (1969a). *Pesticide Index,* Ed. 4. College Science Publishers, State College, Pa.

Frear, D. E. H. (ed.) (1969b). *Pesticide Handbook—Entoma,* Ed. 21. College Science Publishers, State College, Pa.

Frear, D. E. H. (ed.) (1972). *Pesticide Handbook—Entoma,* Ed. 24. College Science Pubishers, State College, Pa.

Gandhi, I. (1972). Address to the United Nations Conference on the Human Environment held at Stockholm, June 5–16, 1972.

Goldman, M. I. (1970). The convergence of environmental disruption. Science, 170: 38–42.

Gontzea, I., and Sutzescu, P. (1968). *Natural Antinutritive Substances in Foodstuffs and Forages.* S. Karger, New York.

Gonzales, T. A., Vance, M., Helpern, M., and Umberger, C. J. (1954). *Legal Medicine: Pathology and Toxicology,* Ed. 2. Appleton-Century-Crofts, New York.

Gorgas, W. C. (1915). *Sanitation in Panama.* D. Appleton and Company, New York.

Gruchow, N. (1970). Corn blight threatens crop. Science, 169:961.

Hartley, G. S., and West, T. F. (1969). *Chemicals for Pest Control.* Pergamon Press, Inc., New York.

Hays, H. (1972). Personal communication.

Headley, J. C. (1968). Estimating the productivity of agricultural pesticides. Am. J. Agric. Econ., 50:13.

Headley, J. C., and Lewis, J. N. (1967). *The Pesticide Problem: An Economic Approach to Public Policy.* Johns Hopkins Press, Baltimore.

Hoffman, F. L. (1916). A plea for National Committee on the eradication of malaria. South. Med. J., 9:413–420.

Illinois Agricultural Extension Service (1961) Circular 828.

Kenaga, E. E., and Allison, W. E. (1969). Commercial and experimental organic insecticides (1969 revision). Bull. Entomol. Soc. Am., 15:85–148.

Kobert, E. R. (1902–1906). *Lehrbuch der Intoxikationen,* Vols. 1 and 2. F. Enke, Stuttgart. An English translation by L. H. Friedburg (1897) was published in a related compendium, *Practical Toxicology for Physicians and Students,* W. R. Jenkins, New York.

Lehmann, K. B. (1890). *Die Methoden der praktischen Hygiene; Anleitung zuer Untersuchung und Benrtheilung der Aufgaben des täglichen Lebens; für Aertze, Chemiker und Juristen.* J. F. Bergmann, Wiesbaden, 594 pp. Translated into English by W. Crookes (1893). Kegan Paul, London.

Levi, G. (1968). Sardinia reborn. World Health, pp. 12–25.

Lewin, L. (1885). *Lerbuch der Toxicologie.* Urban and Schwarzenberg, Wien.

Lewin, L. (1920). *Die Gifte in der Weltgeschichte.* Springer, Berlin.

Lewin, L. (1929). *Gifte und Vergiftungen,* Ed. 4. Auflage, Stilke, Berlin.

Liener, I. E. (1969). *Toxic Constituents in Plant Foodstuffs.* Academic Press, Inc., New York.

Livadas, G., and Athanassatos, D. (1963). The economic benefits of malaria eradication in Greece. Riv. Malarial, 42:177–187.

MacDonald, A. G. (1923). Prevention of malaria. In: *History of the Great War Based on Official Documents. Medical Services, Hygiene of the War,* edited by W. G. Macpherson, W. H. Horrocks, and W. O. Beveridge, Vol. 2, pp. 189–238. H.M.S.O., London.

Martin, H. (1964). *Guide to the Chemicals Used in Crop Protection.* Canada Dept. Agri. Publ. 1093.

Martin, H. (1972). *Pesticide Manual.* Basic information on the chemicals used as active components of pesticides, Ed. 3. British Crop Protection Council.

Melnikov, N. N. (1971). Chemistry of pesticides. Residue Rev. *36*:1–480. (The English translation is based on a version of the 1968 Russian edition as revised by the author in 1970.)

Melville, C. H. (1910). The prevention of malaria in war. In: *The Prevention of Malaria,* Ed. 2, edited by R. Ross, pp. 577–599. John Murray, London.

Metcalf, R. L. (1955). *Organic Insecticides—Their Chemistry and Mode of Action.* Interscience Publishers, Inc., New York.

Miller, M. W., and Berg, G. G. (1969). *Chemical Fallout.* Charles C Thomas, Springfield, Ill.

Minnesota Agricultural Extension Service (1964). Special Report 13.

Mulhern, F. J. (1967). *Hearings before a Subcommittee of the Committee on Appropriations, House of Representatives, Ninetieth Congress, First Session: Department of Agriculture and Related Agencies Appropriations for 1968.* Part 2. US Government Printing Office, Washington, D.C.

Nancrede, J. G. (1817). *A General System of Toxicology: Or, A Treatise on Poisons.* Abridged and partly translated from the French of M. P. Orfila. M. Carey and Son, Philadelphia.

National Academy of Sciences (1966a). *Toxicants Occurring Naturally in Foods.* Publ. 1354, Washington, DC.

National Academy of Sciences (1966b). *Scientific Aspects of Pest Control.* Publ. 1402, Washington, DC.

National Academy of Sciences (1968a). *Principles of Plant and Animal Pest Control.* Vol. 1, *Plant Disease Development and Control.* Publ. 1596, Washington, DC.

National Academy of Sciences (1968b). *Principles of Plant and Animal Pest Control.* Vol. 2, *Weed Control.* Publ. 1597, Washington, DC.

National Academy of Sciences (1968c). *Principles of Plant and Animal Pest Control.* Vol. 4, *Control of Plant-Parasitic Nematodes.* Publ. 1696, Washington, DC.

National Academy of Sciences (1968d). *Principles of Plant and Animal Pest Control.* Vol. 6, *Effects of Pesticides on Fruit and Vegetable Physiology.* Publ. 1698, Washington, DC.

National Academy of Sciences (1969). *Principles of Plant and Animal Pest Control.* Vol. 3, *Insect-Pest Management and Control.* Publ. 1695, Washington, DC.

National Academy of Sciences (1970). *Principles of Plant and Animal Pest Control.* Vol. 5, *Vertebrate Pests: Problems and Control.* Publ. 1697, Washington, DC.

National Academy of Sciences (1972). *Pest Control: Strategies for the Future.* Washington, D.C.

National Research Council (1962). *New Developments and Problems in the Use of Pesticides.* Publ. 1082, Washington, DC.

Newman, P. (1965). *Malaria Eradication and Population Growth—with Special Reference to Ceylon and British Guiana.* Bureau of Public Health Economics Research Series No. 10, University of Michigan, Ann Arbor.

New York Academy of Sciences (1969). *Biological Effects of Pesticides in Mammalian Systems.* New York.

Nolan, K. G. (1967). American Cynamid Co., Princeton, NJ. Private communication, to T. M. Awad, S. B. Vinson, and J. R. Brazzel.

Orfila, M. J. B. (1814–1815). *Traité des Poisons Tirés des Règnes Minéral, v"gétal et Animal ou Toxicologie Genérale Considérée sous les Rapports de la Pathologie et de la Médecine Légale.* Crochard, Paris. Translation into English by Nancrede is listed separately in this bibliography.

Orfila, M. J. B. (1817). *Eléments de Chimie Médicale,* Vols. 1 and 2, pp. 575 and 610. Crochard, Paris.

Orfila, M. J. B. (1818). *Secours à donner aux Personnes Empoisonnées ou Asphyxiées.* Feugueray, Paris. Translations into English by Black, Price, and Stevenson are listed separately in this bibliography.

Orfila, M. J. B. (1821–1823). *Leçons de médecine légale,* Vols. 1 and 2, pp. 503 and 737. Bechetjeune, Paris.

Paracelsus. (1564). *Philosophiae ad Athenienses Drey Bucher.* Erhen A. Bryrckmanni, Coln.

Paracelsus. (1567). *Von der Bergsucht oder Bergkranckheiten drey Bücher.* S. Mayer, Dilingen. English translation may be found in Temkin, C. L., Rosen, G., Zilboorg, and Sigerist, H. E. (1941). *Four Treatises of Theophras-*

tus von Hohenheim called Paracelsus, Johns Hopkins Press, Baltimore.

Paracelsus. (1603). *Operum Medico-Chimicorum sive Paradoxorum,* Tomus Genuinus Secundus. Collegio Musarum Palthenianarum, Francofurto.

Parkin, E. A. (1967). Food and health—the value of pest control. Proc. Second Brit. Pest Control Conf., 2nd Session, pp. 5–8.

Patty, F. A. (ed.) (1958 et seq.). *Industrial Hygiene and Toxicology,* Ed. 2 (revised), Vols. 1. and 2. Interscience Publishers, Inc., New York.

Peters, R. (1963). *Biochemical Lesions and Lethal Synthesis.* Pergamon Press, Oxford.

Plant Protection Ltd. (1957). *Plant Protection Conference 1956.* Butterworths, London.

Price, W. (1818). *A Popular Treatise on the Remedies to be Employed in Cases of Poisoning and Apparent Death Including the Means of Detecting Poisons, of Distinguishing Real from Apparent Death and of Ascertaining the Adulteration of Wines.* Translated from the French of M. P. Orfila, pp. 1–170, Solomon W. Conrad, Philadelphia.

Ramazzini, B. (1700). *De Morbis Artificium Diatriba,* A. Capponi, Mutince, 360 pp. Translated into English by Hoffman (1746), London.

Riley, C. V. (1885). *Fourth Report of the United States Entomological Commission.* US Government Printing Office, Washington, DC.

Roan, C. C., Morgan, D. P., Kreader, C. H., and Moore, L. (1969). Pesticide use in Arizona as shown by sales. Progressive Agric. Ariz., 21:14–15.

Ross, R. (1906). *Report to the Liverpool School of Tropical Medicine.* Athens. Cited by Lividas, G., and Anthanassatos, D. (1963). The economic benefits of malaria eradication in Greece. Riv. Malariol, 42:177–187.

Saini, M. L., and Dorough, H. W. (1970). Persistence of malathion and methyl parathion when applied as ultralow-volume and emulsifiable concentrate sprays. J. Econ. Entomol., 63:405–408.

Shepard, H. H. (1951). *The Chemistry and Action of Insecticides,* Ed. 1 McGraw-Hill, New York.

Shepard, H. H. (1963). Personal communication, October 2.

Simmons, S. W. (1959). The use of DDT insecticides in human medicine. In: *DDT, The Insecticide Dichlorodiphenyltrichloroethane and its Significance,* edited by P. Muller, pp. 251–502, Birkhaüser Verlag, Basel.

Skoog, F. E., Cowan, F. T., and Messenger, K. (1965). Ultra-low-volume aerial spraying of dieldrin and malathion for rangeland grasshopper control. J. Econ. Entomol., 58:559–565.

Soper, F. L., Andrews, J. A., Bode, K. F., Coatney, G. R., Earle, W. C., Keeny, S. M., Knipling. E. F., Logan, J. A., Metcalf, R. L., Quarterman, K. D., Russell, P. F., and Williams, L. L. (1961). Report and recommendations on malaria: A Summary. Am. J. Trop. Med. Hyg., 10:451–502.

Sprague, F. G. (1967). Agricultural production in the developing countries. Science, 157:774–778.

Stern, A. C. (ed.) (1962). *Air Pollution: A Comprehensive Treatise,* Vols. 1 and 2. Academic Press, Inc., New York.

Stevenson, J. G. (1826). *A Practical Treatise on Poisons and Asphyxies Adapted to General Use. Followed by Directions for the Treatment of Burns, and for the Distinction of Real from Apparent Death.* Translated from the French of M. P. Orfila. Hilliard, Gray, Little, and Wilkins, Boston.

Strickland, A. H. (1970). Economic principles of management. In: *Concepts of Pest Management.* Proceedings of a conference held at North Carolina State University, Raleigh.

Sunshine, I. (ed.) (1969). *Handbook of Analytical Toxicology.* The Chemical Rubber Publishing Company, Cleveland.

Thompson, J. F. (ed.) (1971). *Analysis of Pesticide Residues in Human and Environmental Samples.* Perrine Primate Research Laboratories, Perrine, Fla.

Tripod, J., and Stamm. W. (1969). What are toxicologists? Proc. Eur. Soc. Study Drug Toxicity, 10:122–138.

United States Department of Health, Education, and Welfare (1969). *Report of the Secretary's Commission on Pesticides and Their Relationships to Environmental Health.* US Government Printing Office, Washington, DC.

United States Senate (1964). Hearings before the Subcommittee on Reorganization and International Organizations of the Committee on Government Operations, United States Senate. Parts 1–10, including Appendices I–V to Part 1. US Government Printing Office, Washington, DC.

United States Seante (1966). *Pesyicides and Public Policy.* Report of the Committee on Government Operations, United States Senate, made by its Subcommittee on Reorganization and International Organizations. Rept. No. 1379. US Government Printing Office, Washington, DC.

Ward, J. C. (1958). Use pesticides with care. Pest Control, 26:14–16.

Weed Society of America (1967). *Herbicide Handbook,* Ed. 1. W. F. Humphrey Press, Inc., Geneva, NY.

Whittaker, R. H. (1970a). In: *Chemical Ecology,* edited by E. Sondheimer and J. B. Simeone. Academic Press, Inc., New York.

Whittaker, R. H. (1970b). *Communities and Ecosystems.* Macmillan, New York.

Whittaker, R. H., and Feeny, P. P. (1971). Allelochemics: Chemical interactions between species. Science, 171:757–770.

World Health Organization (1957). WHO Expert Committee on Malaria, Sixth Report. WHO Tech. Rep. Ser. No. 123.

World Health Organization (1967). WHO Expert Committee on Malaria, Thirteenth Report. WHO Tech. Rep. Ser. No. 357.

World Health Organization (1968). Malaria—Economic facts. World Health, April, pp. 10–11.

World Health Organization (1969). Evaluating and testing new insecticides. WHO Chron., 23:530–531.

Zweig, G. (ed.) (1963). *Analytical Methods for Pesticides and Plant Growth Regulators.* Vol. 1, *Principles, Methods, and General Applications.* Academic Press, Inc., New York.

Zweig, G. (ed.) (1964a). *Analytical Methods for Pesticides and Plant Growth Regulators.* Vol. 2, *Insecticides.* Academic Press, Inc., New York.

Zweig, G. (ed.) (1964b). *Analytical Methods for Pesticides and Plant Growth Regulators.* Vol. 3, *Fungicides, Nematocides and Soil Fumigants, Rodenticides, and Food and Feed Additives.* Academic Press, Inc., New York.

Zweig, G. (ed.) (1964c). *Analytical Methods for Pesticides and Plant Growth Regulators.* Vol. 4, *Herbicides.* Academic Press, Inc., New York.

Zweig, G. (ed.) (1967). *Analytical Methods for Pesticides and Plant Growth Regulators.* Vol. 5, *Additional Principles and Methods of Analysis.* Academic Press, Inc., New York.

Zweig, G. (ed.) (1972). *Analytical Methods for Pesticides and Plant Growth Regulators.* Vol. 6, *Gas Chromatographic Analyses.* Academic Press, Inc., New York.

2

GENERAL PRINCIPLES: DOSAGE AND OTHER FACTORS INFLUENCING TOXICITY

This and the following three chapters are intended as an introduction to the toxicology of pesticides and an evaluation of methods for their study. These chapters are not meant as a set of guides for testing a particular compound intended for a particular purpose. Of course, the importance of such guides is recognized, and some of them are listed in appropriate sections of the four chapters. Besides offering suggestions about where details on technique may be found, an effort is made to identify (a) parameters in need of special study, and (b) the variety and limitations of present approaches to such study. Under the circumstances, it has seemed best to organize the discussion of techniques conceptually and not in the usual, operational way according to actue and chronic tests, dermal toxicity, and the like. Briefly, the statistical and other methods for studying toxic reactions in intact animals are discussed in this chapter. Methods for studying absorption, distribution, metabolism, storage, storage loss, and excretion, are considered in Chapter 3. Techniques for measuring different kinds of injury and injury in different tissues are outlined in Chapter 4, and methods for measuring exposure and quantitative metabolism in people under occupational and other practical conditions are discussed in Chapter 5.

2.1 Kinds of Toxicity

Toxicity may be classified according to the nature or the duration of the injury involved.

2.1.1 Nature of Injury

The kinds of injury or change that may be produced by chemicals and are known to be of practical importance in certain circumstances are: acute and chronic toxicity in the restricted sense, neurotoxicity, teratogenesis, carcinogenesis, hypersensitivity, metabolism and storage, and induction of enzymes. The dosage-response relations in these different kinds of toxicity or change are described in Section 2.3. Methods for studying the different kinds of toxicity are described in Section 4.3.

2.1.2 Duration of Injury

2.1.2.1 Factors in the Chronicity of Injury. At least three major, independent factors (compound, dosage, and duration of dosing) and a separately measurable, dependent factor (storage) are involved in what is often lumped with misleading simplicity under the term "chronic toxicity."

Some compounds are inherently likely to produce chronic effects, which is largely the same as saying that their effects are highly irreversible. In some instances, a single dose sufficient to produce any immediate effect or perhaps no detectable immediate effect eventually leads to chronic illness.

It is important to realize that there is no necessary relationship between the number of doses and the chronicity of illness. Of course, if a material capable of producing chronic effects is administered repeatedly, the chance that chronic effects will occur is increased, and the chance that only actue poisoning will occur is decreased. However, both acute and chronic effects can occur as part of a single illness. Among the materials that can produce chronic illness by a single dose are thallium and arsenic (Moeschlin, 1965), triorthocresyl phosphate (Smith *et al.*, 1930), or certain carcinogens (Bryan and Shimkin, 1943; Schoental and Magee, 1957; Magee and Barnes, 1962; Carnaghan, 1967). Undoubtedly some other materials such as lead often would cause both acute and chronic effects if there commonly were occasion to absorb a sufficiently large single dose of them.

Other compounds such as potassium cyanide have so far produced only acute illness. In other words, with cyanide the illness is similar whether it follows a single large dose or many somewhat smaller doses. If recovery occurs, it progresses at a rate determined by the severity of illness rather than by the number of doses received. The production of persisting effects is not characteristic of cyanide, although such effects may follow tissue anoxia of whatever cause.

Some compounds are intermediate to the examples cited in regard to the chronicity of their effects. Chronic poisoning cannot be produced by one drink of alcohol, but persistent excessive drinking can lead to chronic organic damage. There is considerable evidence that prolonged excessive intake of sodium in the form of table salt produces chronic hypertension (Meneely, 1966). In these instances, the easy reversibility of the injury finally is overcome by prolonged high dosage.

Much confusion would be avoided if the expression "chronic poisoning" were restricted to chronic disease produced by a chemical or by the chemical changes secondary to radiation or other physical agent. Since chronic disease may be caused by a single dose and acute poisoning may follow repeated exposure, the duration of exposure ought to be specified separately.

Chronic illness (whether secondary to poisoning, infection, malnutrition, metabolic disorder, circulatory malfunction, neoplasia, genetic defect, or some unknown cause) is characterized not only by long duration but by certain pathological features, especially scarring and atrophy.

It is sometimes implied that chronic illness is necessarily obscure and difficult to diagnose. This simply is not true. Most of the poisoning produced by the alkyl mercury fungicides is both chronic and tragically obvious. Difficulty in diagnosis is more likely to be associated with very mild, transient illness or with failure to suspect the possibility of poisoning than with any particular set of clinical characteristics.

2.1.2.2 Reversibility. The matter of reversibility is subject to several qualifications. Even when a chemical lesion is rapidly and completely reversible, as in the case of thiamine deficiency in its early stages, severe poisoning may lead to irreversible complications. Secondly, many compounds have two or more actions, which may differ in reversibility. Finally, the mode of action of many toxicants is unknown. It is therefore important to determine whether animals actually poisoned by a particular toxicant are capable of complete recovery or whether they are left with some residual functional or structural injury. As discussed in the preceding section, it is characteristic of some compounds that they produce chronic illness (sometimes after a single dose), while others produce illness only while dosage is maintained at a sufficiently high level. Section 2.2.2 presents a quantitative method for recording the tendency of each chemical to produce cumulative *effects* following repeated dosing, and Section 3.2.3.2 discusses the related but separable phenomenon of cumulative *storage* of compounds or their metabolites.

The effects of many toxicants, including many pesticides, are fully reversible, but since a number of factors may be involved the possibility of recovery must be tested directly for each compound. Unfortunately, little use is made of the technique of keeping the survivors of the higher doses of ordinary 1-dose LD 50 tests for long periods without further dosing in order to observe possible latent effects. This technique is far from new. It has had some use in Great Britain in the systematic testing of pesticides. In fact, the procedure is recommended explicitly in the Pesticides Safety Precautions Scheme Agreed between Government Departments and Industry, issued by the Pesticides Branch of the Ministry of Agriculture, Fisheries and Food (Great Britain, 1966). The method is simple and capable of revealing the ultimate in irreversibility. It is especially suitable for discovering what Barnes (1968) has called "hit-and-run" poisons. As already mentioned, a single dose of several natural and synthetic compounds has been shown capable of causing cancer and other chronic injury when administered orally or by other routes.

On the contrary, the possible reversibility of lesions produced by repeated doses is often neglected also. Thus, one could cite examples in which certain morphological changes of the liver have been called cancer without evidence of invasion or metastasis and without any effort to find whether the changes would regress if dosing were discontinued. Such neglect represents not only poor toxicology but irresponsibility.

2.2 Quantitation of Dosage-Response Relationships

Scientific study of the effects of chemical or physical agents on living organisms requires measurement. A distinction is made as to whether each measurement involves an agent alone (dose) or an agent in relation to an organism (dosage). A 1.0-mg dose of a compound is identical no matter whether it is administered to a 20-g mouse or a 5,000-kg elephant but the dosages are vastly different, being 50 mg/kg for the mouse and 0.002 mg/kg for the elephant. The susceptibility of different species or even different individuals can be compared precisely only if their body weight is taken into account.

This does not mean that large animals always require a higher dose than small ones of the same species to manifest the same effect. The tendency in this direction may be obscured by individual variation, particularly since large animals frequently are older or better nourished than small ones and may differ in other ways also. Even so, the significance of individual differences of whatever origin can be studied most effectively if dosage rather than dose is considered.

The word dosage is properly applied to any rate or ratio involving a dose. Thus the expressions milligram per kilogram and milligram per square centimeter both designate a dosage. Dosages often involve the dimension of time (eg, milligram per kilogram per day) but the meaning is not restricted to this relationship.

The acute or 1-dose ED 50 defined below and generally expressed in terms of milligrams of material per kilogram of body weight is the universally accepted, primary way of expressing acute effects of solids and liquids that are swallowed, contaminate the skin, or are administered subcutaneously, intravenously, or by other parenteral routes. An LD 50 is a special case of the ED 50 in which the effect measured is death. The numerical form of these ED 50 or LD 50 values permits useful comparisons between the acute effects of different compounds or of the same compound administered by different routes. There is no generally accepted, comparable way to express

the effects of repeated dosing, but use of the 90-dose ED 50 (or LD 50) and the chronicity index both may help to express the results of repeated dosing.

The use of ED 50 and LD 50 values—whether for 1 dose or 90 doses—is the ideal way to express toxicity because they are direct measures of the dosage received by the test organism. However, there is no direct or easy way to measure the dosage of a gas received by animals that breathe air or to measure the dosage of a solution or suspension by fish or other organisms that live in water and obtain their oxygen from it. Under these circumstances, the investigator often must be satisfied with a statistical estimate of the time required for a given concentration to produce a specified effect or with an estimate of the concentration required to produce a specified effect in a fixed time.

No matter what the physical form of the chemical or the habits of the test species, there is obvious interest in determining the largest dosage or concentration that produces no observable effect or no significant observable effect. This is the largest safe dosage for the test organism under the conditions of the test. Such a "no effect" level is often used as a basis for estimating a lower value considered safe under more varied conditions, including the exposure of another species, especially man (see Sections 2.2.7.4 and 9.1.4.1).

Finally, dosages may be compared in terms of tissue levels no matter what the physical form of the compound, the habits of the species, the route of absorption, or the duration of dosing.

The dosage-response relationship is the most fundamental single principle in toxicology. It extends to all kinds of injurious effects (see Section 2.3), and it implies the existence of a threshold dosage for each compound below which, under defined conditions, no harmful effect is produced (see Section 2.2.7.4).

2.2.1 The ED 50 or LD 50

2.2.1.1 The 1-Dose ED 50 or LD 50. An ED 50 is a statistical estimate of the dosage of a material that would produce a specified effect in 50% of a very large population of a text species under stated conditions, for example a single oral dose of an aqueous solution given to male rats. Of course it would be impractical to use hundreds or even thousands of animals to make such a test, and, even if this were done, it would be unlikely that the investigator would hit upon the dosage to produce the effect in exactly half of the animals. That is why the parameter must be estimated statistically. In practice, test animals are divided into groups of moderate size—frequently about 10 per group. Each group is given one of a series of geometrically increasing dosages selected in such a way that the smallest dosage will produce the intended effect in only a small proportion of the group receiving it, while the largest dosage produces the same effect in the majority of animals receiving it. The result for each group is expressed as the percentage of animals showing the effect under study. By one technique or another, the percentage effect for each group is converted to a probit and related to the logarithm of the dosage that produced it. Any effect measured in this way must be recorded as an all-or-none response. However, phenomena that show continuous variation may be treated on an all-or-none basis merely by selecting an arbitrary limit. For example, systolic blood pressure may vary widely but could be made the basis of an ED 50 by counting all animals whose pressure exceeded 150 mm Hg.

Form of the ED 50 or LD 50 Curve. Several matters regarding determination of ED 50 and LD 50 values are illustrated by Fig. 2-1 based on LD 50 studies of DDT. All parts of the graph represent the results of tests in which groups of rats were given various dosages of the compound. In part A, the dosage for each group has been plotted on plain graph paper against the percentage of mortality. The observed points fall along a broad S-shaped pattern. The fundamental statistical principles illustrated by part A first were defined clearly by Trevan (1927). Specifically, he pointed out that there was no such thing as a minimal lethal dosage or minimal effective dosage as, according to Trevan, was then conceived, namely, a dosage that would be just sufficient to produce the effect in all animals of a given species. He noted that the variability of individuals in a population led to the characteristic S-shaped curve and that there seemed to be less variability at the 50% level of response. Trevan proposed the equivalent terms, "median lethal dose" and "LD 50," both in their presently accepted meaning. He also suggested that dosages that kill other proportions of large groups of animals be designated by analogous symbols, for example "LD 25" and "LD 75" for dosages that kill 25 and 75%, respectively. In Trevan's paper in the Proceedings of the Royal Society, the symbols were printed with a space between the letter "D" and the appropriate number. This style has been adopted for this book, partly because it is authentic and partly because it is completely clear when it becomes necessary in theoretical discussions to refer to fractions of a percent, as in "LD 0.01."

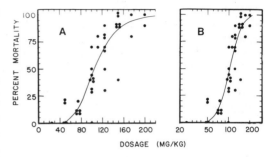

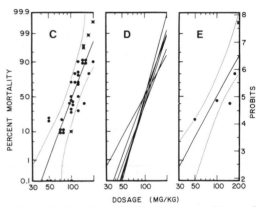

Fig. 2-1. Mortality of white rats caused by oral doses of DDT. Each point represents one group of animals, usually 10. A, percentage mortality in six separate tests plotted against dosage. B, the same data with percentage plotted against logarithm of dosage. C, the same data with percentage mortality expressed as probits plotted against logarithm of dosage; the 19/20 confidence limits are shown by dotted lines on either side of the dosage-response curve. D, dosage-response curves for each of the six separate tests. E, the dosage-response curve that differed most from the others, showing its relatively wide confidence limits.

The LD 50 can be read from the curve even in its S-shaped form on plain paper. Thus, in part A, the level for 50% mortality intersects the curve at a dosage of about 113 mg/kg.

It may be noted parenthetically that the middle portion of the sigmoid curve—say in the region of 20 to 80% response—often is indistinguishable from a straight line. The fact that a simple straight line relationship between dosage and percentage response adequately describes some sets of data must not obscure the fact that more complete data determine a sigmoid curve on plain paper.

Part B of Fig. 2-1 represents the same data as those shown in part A, but dosage is now shown on a logarithmic scale rather than on a simple arithmetic scale. The S-shaped pattern persists, but the curve approaches a straight line. Part C of the graph represents the same data plotted with an additional conversion. Here, the logarithm of dosage is plotted against percentage mortality expressed as probits. The correspondence between percentage and probits is shown by the scales on the left and right of the lower portion of the graph. As may be seen, the points are scattered about a straight line when the full (logprobit) conversion is made. The logarithmic conversion apparently was introduced first by Krogh and Hemmingsen (1928), but it was the subject of numerous publications cited by Gaddum (1933) in the classical paper in which he introduced the full conversion essentially in the form still used today. Actually, Gaddum employed normal equivalent deviations rather than probits, which are commonly used today. However, a probit is merely a normal equivalent deviation to which 5.0 has been added for convenience to eliminate negative values. The paper by Gaddum was shortly followed by three by Bliss (1934a; 1934b; 1935a), and these four papers on the statistical relationship between dosage and response are still basic today. The facts regarding probit analysis were summarized in a masterful way by Finney (1952) in a book first published in 1947 and revised in 1952. A more general treatment of the principles of biological assay is that of Emmens (1948).

It remains to state that the slender sigmoid curve we have discussed constitutes (insofar as data permit one to judge) a cumulative lognormal curve. Conversion of the percentage response to normal equivalent derivatives or probits is merely a statistical device for converting the sigmoid curve into a straight line. Although Gaddum (1933) employed the logarithmic conversion as well as the normal equivalent deviation conversion for use in toxicity measurements, it apparently was not until 1945 that he introduced the word "lognormal" to describe the situation in which log x is normally distributed. In the same paper, Gaddum (1945) emphasized that the distribution of values for many parameters in nature is not statistically normal. This means only that the distribution frequently does not conform to any of the family of curves commonly called "normal" or "Gaussian" after Karl Friedrich Gauss who first popularized this particular pattern of variation. Use of the word "normal" in this connection has no bearing on physical or biological normalcy. In fact, Gaddum pointed out that if the distribution of the volume of particles is normal the distribution of their diameters will, of necessity, not be normal.

Gaddum stressed the importance of converting measurements in such a way that the results may be subjected to statistical evaluation. In addition to logarithmic conversion of each variable for this purpose, he suggested that a positive or negative constant might be added to each variable prior to its logarithmic conversion.

The logprobit conversion has great value for purposes of description and statistical analysis. However, in spite of its great practical value, the basic assumption that the relationship of variables is perfectly lognormal cannot be considered proved, because the upper and lower extremities of the curve have not been studied experimentally. This detail is discussed in Section 2.2.7.4 under the heading, The Logprobit Model and Quantitative Study of the Effects of Small Dosages.

The ED 50, ED 1, ED 99, and Corresponding LD Values. Returning to part C of Fig. 2-1, it may be seen that the level of 50% mortality intersects the curve at a dosage of 113 mg/kg, and this is the oral LD 50 for DDT as indicated by the observed data. In a similar way, the 1% mortality level intersects the curve at a dosage of 52 mg/kg, which, therefore, is the LD 1. Mortality of 99% is not shown on the graph but would fall at a dosage of 223 mg/kg, which is the LD 99.

Confidence Limits and Reproducibility. The degree of scatter of the observed values may be evaluated by calculation and expressed as confidence limits. These limits are shown by dotted lines on both sides of the solid line in part C of the graph. These particular confidence limits indicate the area or range within which the dosage-response line may be expected to fall in 19 of 20 samples taken at random from the same population. It may be seen that a series of such curves will correspond closely with one another at the 50% mortality level but will agree less well as the mortality approaches either 0 or 100%. This is a graphic representation of the fact first noted by Trevan (1927) that the LD 50 may be estimated more accurately than corresponding statistics for greater or lesser effect (eg, LD 99 or LD 1). Exactly the same is true of ED 50 values and corresponding ED 99 and ED 1 values.

The points represented in parts A, B, and C of Fig. 2-1 represent the results of six separate tests made in six different years for the purpose of determining whether there was any change, genetic or otherwise, in the susceptibility of the particular colony of rats to acute poisoning by DDT. Part D of the graph shows the dosage-response lines determined in connection with the six separate tests. The lines correspond very closely at the 50% mortality level but diverge somewhat in connection with higher or lower mortality rates. Actually, all of the lines are in good agreement, indicating that there was no detectable change in the colony concerning susceptibility to DDT. In fact, the dependability of this kind of test is well recognized. Weil *et al.* (1966) reported that they had done 1-dose oral LD 50's on 26 chemicals annually for 11 or 12 years each to determine the reproducibility of the test and the dependability of commercial production of the chemicals. The resultant median lethal doses were relatively unaffected by the different annual samples of each chemical, by changes in the stock of rats, by the degree of dilution of the toxicants, or by change in the personnel performing the tests. Only one variable, the weight of the rat, appeared to have a significant effect on the values obtained.

Slope and Its Relation to Confidence Limits. Part E of Fig. 2-1 shows the data and resulting curves for a single LD 50 determination, namely the particular test that differed most from the average of the six tests. It may be seen that the slope of the line is greater than the slopes of the other LD 50 lines (shown in part D). This increase in slope is a graphic representation of the greater variability of the data on which this particular determination was based. The greater variability of the data is also reflected by the fact that the dotted curves (representing confidence limits) stand further away from the solid line than the corresponding curves do in part C of the graph.

Procedures for Determining ED 50 and LD 50 Values. Parts C and E of Fig. 2-1 represent actual determinations of LD 50 values using the graphic method proposed by Litchfield and Wilcoxon (1949) who also supplied details of the method for calculating the 19/20 confidence limits. There are a number of nongraphic methods for determining ED 50 or LD 50 values including the method of Bliss (1935a; 1935b; 1938). The nongraphic methods have in common the fact that percentage values must be transformed by means of an appropriate table or calculation. A wide variety of methods has been reviewed by McIntosh (1961) who concluded that the differences among results within the 15 to 85% response range are negligible. Thus the selection of the method to use depends largely on personal choice.

Repeated determinations of an ED 50 or LD 50 for a particular compound under the same conditions should give not only statistically indistinguishable values but also statistically indistinguishable slopes of the dosage-response curves. Of course different compounds may give different values and different slopes for the dosage-response curves as shown in Fig. 2-2. The curves may be related in such a way that the ED 50 (or LD 50) values are statistically distinguishable but other values such as the ED 1 (or LD 1) are not distinguishable. Fig. 2-2 offers an example. The LD 50 values for dieldrin and toxaphene are different but the LD 1 values for these compounds are statistically indistinguishable.

Tests Using Small Numbers of Animals. The conventional procedures for determining ED 50 or LD 50 values require the use of approximately 50 to 100 animals. The use of this many rats or mice may be practical, even though somewhat expensive. The use of a similar number of dogs or monkeys often is entirely impractical. To meet this problem a number of methods have been developed that permit the use of a small number of animals per group to determine approximate ED 50 or LD 50 values (Gaddum, 1933; Deichmann and LeBlanc, 1943; Weil, 1952; Smyth *et al.*, 1962).

Volume of Each Dose. If the results of toxicological tests are to be compared, it is wise to keep all conditions as nearly uniform

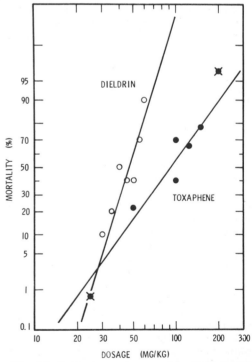

Fig. 2-2. Dosage-response curves for dieldrin and toxaphene given orally to white rats. Points adjusted according to the method of Litchfield and Wilcoxon (1949) are distinguished by a superimposed ×.

as possible. One variable that should be standardized is the volume of solution or suspension in which compounds are administered. It has been found practical to give most oral doses at the rate of 0.005 ml per gram of body weight and to give dermal applications at the rate of 0.0016 ml per gram of body weight. Differences in dosage are determined by changing the concentration. The value of 0.0016 ml/g was chosen for dermal application because it represents a plausible exposure of about 100 ml for a man and also gives even numbers for dosage associated with many formulations actually used in the field. Thus, at this rate of application, the dose for a 70-kg man would be 112 ml—a not unlikely degree of contamination as the result of spillage. Formulations of 0.312, 0.625, 1.25, 2.5, 5, and 10% produce dosages of 5, 10, 20, 40, 80, and 160 mg/kg, respectively, when applied at the rate of 0.0016 milliliter per gram of body weight.

2.2.1.2 The 90-Dose ED 50 or LD 50. It has been suggested, more or less empirically, that subacute tests should occupy up to one-tenth of the lifespan of the experimental animals (commonly considered to be about 90 days for the rat and 1 year for the dog) (FAO/WHO, 1958).

Boyd (1961) accepted the concept of one-tenth of the lifespan, but considered it to be 100 days in the rat. However, the important thing is not the choice or definition of a particular fraction of the lifespan but the selection of a testing interval that is as short as practicable and yet will give meaningful information about the effect of absorbing the toxicant during an entire lifetime. Secondarily, it would be desirable to have a standard test so that results from different laboratories would be reported in the same terms.

Apparently Boyd and Boyd (1962) were the first to report subacute toxicity in the form of an LD 50. The compound was administered intramusculary for as long as 100 days. In connection wth oral doses it was proposed (Boyd and Selby, 1962) that the compound under test be administered by stomach tube for 100 days. The test differed in some technical requirements from the 90-dose test described below. In spite of this, the two tests are fundamentally similar, and the results of one are largely interchangeable with those of the other.

Several years after he had proposed the 100-day test, Boyd (1968) pointed out that, for the compounds he studied, the test could be reduced to about 70 days with little or no loss of important information.

Weil and McCollister (1963) showed that the results of 90-day studies not only in rats but even in dogs were similar to corresponding lifetime studies in these species for a wide range of compounds.

Hayes (1967b) pointed out that a 30-day test in the rat would be adequate for some compounds (eg, potassium cyanide). However, a review of data on certain chemosterilants showed that, although 30 doses were entirely inadequate to reveal the potential injury caused by repeated doses of any of them, 90 doses gave for most of them essentially the same results as those of tests lasting twice as long. Thus, although a test involving less than 90 doses would be adequate to reveal the effect of long-term exposure to many compounds, a 90-dose test is more generally valid for predicting lifetime effects. In fact, even a 90-dose schedule is inadequate to define the long-term toxicity of some compounds such as hempa (hexamethyl phosphoric triamide); however, it was clearly evident after 90 or even somewhat fewer days that animals being dosed with hempa were still dying and that the exposure would have to be prolonged in order to assess the toxicity properly. Thus, 90 doses were selected as standard for quantitative study of the effects of repeated doses, partly because 90-dose tests were already widely accepted for other purposes and in spite of the limitations just mentioned.

The 90-dose ED 50 (or 90-dose LD 50) is statistically comparable to a 1-dose ED 50 (or 1-dose LD 50). In both, percent effect expressed as probits is related to dosage expressed as logarithms.

The results of a 1-dose and a 90-dose LD 50 study of warfarin are shown in Fig. 2-3. It may be seen that the curves are similar in slope although the dosages that proved critical differ by a factor of about 20. Table 2-1 shows the LD 50 values and related statistics for warfarin.

Determination of the 90-Dose ED 50 or LD 50. In calculating the conventional 1-dose LD 50 no account is taken of time, although, of course, animals given a single dose do not respond to it simultaneously. The 90-dose ED 50 is managed in a similar way; the animals are held long enough after the last dose to be sure all reactions have been counted. The two procedures differ, since in the 1-dose test all animals in a group receive the same dosage, but in the 90-dose test animals in the same group may receive different total dosages because some may survive longer than others. This difference does not invalidate a comparison of the results of the two tests.

In determining the acute oral ED 50, the compound is usually administered by stomach tube. In determining the oral 90-dose ED 50 the compound is administered as a mixture in

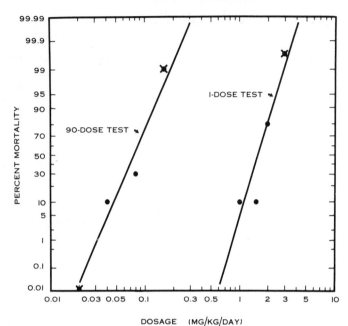

Fig. 2-3. One-dose and 90-dose oral dosage-response curves for warfarin. Points adjusted according to the method of Litchfield and Wilcoxon (1949) are distinguished by a superimposed ×. From Hayes (1967a) by permission of Academic Press, Inc., New York.

Table 2-1

Toxicity of Warfarin to Male Rats

From Hayes (1967b) by permission of Academic Press.

	1-dose	90-dose
no. rats tested	50	110
survival time (days)	5-10	3-43 [a]
LD 50 [b]	1.6	0.077
19/20 confidence limits [b]	1.4-1.9	0.055-0.108
lowest dose to kill [b]	1.0	0.04 [c]
LD 1 [b]	0.84	0.032

a. The true range may be 3-25 days; warfarin was probably not the cause of death in the rat that died after eating the compound for 43 days.

b. Expressed as mg/kg for 1-dose test or mg/kg/day for 90-dose test.

c. This death probably was not caused by warfarin. The smallest dosage to cause a death clearly related to warfarin was 0.08 mg/kg/day.

the diet. This difference in technique of oral administration introduces a second kind of difference (applying to this route only) between the two kinds of oral ED 50 value, but it has two advantages: convenience and realism. Obviously it is more convenient to maintain an animal on a special diet for 90 days than to dose the animal by stomach tube for the same period. Except in connection with drugs, which are administered in discrete doses, it is also more realistic to administer repeated doses in the diet rather than by stomach tube. If people receive relatively regular repeated doses of an environmental compound, the intake is usually distributed throughout a considerable portion of most days as the result of either occupational or dietary exposure. On the contrary, if acute poisoning occurs in man, it is usually the result of a single massive exposure due to a splash or other spillage associated with occupation, or the ingestion of a relatively concentrated material due to accident or suicide. Furthermore, if a number of compounds are administered by any particular route in such a way that the absorption of a single dose of each is concentrated in as short a period as possible, but the absorption of repeated doses of each is distributed as evenly as is practical over each day, then any difference in cumulative effect of the compounds will be demonstrated to greatest advantage.

Thus, to determine the oral 90-dose ED 50 (or LD 50) of a compound, appropriate concentrations in ground chow are fed to groups of animals for 90 days. All survivors are then fed uncontaminated feed for a minimum of 2 weeks, and, if any of them are still affected, they must be observed for as long as necessary until they have died or recovered. The dosage (expressed as milligrams per kilogram per day) is calculated from measured food consumption (Hayes, 1967b).

2.2.1.3 Kinds of Phenomena Showing a Cumulative Lognormal Form in Their Dosage-Response Relationships.

As reviewed in the foregoing sections, the pharmacological and lethal effects of compounds on intact organisms have the form of cumulative lognormal curves which can be plotted as straight lines following probit conversion. In biology, the lognormal curve rarely is used except in measuring the responses of intact organisms. However, similar curves are obtained when the concentration of a compound is plotted against its effect on an isolated piece of animal tissue or against the inhibition it causes in the activity of an enzyme. The dissociation curves of oxyhemoglobin also have a similar form (Gaddum, 1937). The fact that this form of dosage-response relationship is found in connection with tissues, enzymes, and macromolecules indicates its fundamental nature.

In fact, when the initial concentration (or dosage) of one kind of molecule (eg, a toxicant) is plotted against the percentage of these molecules reacted with another kind of molecule (eg, an enzyme or macromolecule) present in excess, the resulting graphs are statistically indistinguishable from straight lines within the range of 10 to 90% reaction. At the extremes, that is below 10% and above 90%, deviation from linearity is observed. Such effects can be modeled using simple expressions derived from the law of mass action or, more appropriately, expressions derived from a consideration of cooperative ligand binding (eg, the Hill equation). The concept of a threshold can be incorporated into either model. However, a truly realistic model must include kinetic consideration of the rate of inactivation of the poison and the repair of the biochemical lesion. Certainly, this realistic modeling would be complex. However, it might be useful in defining the quantitative aspects of remaining problems. Of course, it is already known that small concentrations of a toxicant may be withstood by the intact organism because it can tolerate some inactivation of enzymes and macromolecules and because critical molecules are replaced in the course of normal repair. Known examples of a chemical basis for thresholds in dosage-response relationships are discussed in Section 2.2.7.4.

2.2.2 The Chronicity Index

It is evident that regardless of the method chosen for its expression, the ratio between the 1-dose and multiple-dose LD 50 values of a compound constitutes a measure of its cumulative effect. For a long time, it has been customary to convey some idea of how well animals withstand repeated doses of a compound by reporting what fraction of the acute LD 50 they can tolerate daily. Boyd *et al.* (1966) refined this procedure by suggesting that the comparison be made at the LD 50 levels for both the acute and the subacute tests. Specifically, he proposed that a one-tenth lifespan (0.1L) "chronic/acute LD $_{50(0.1L)}$ index" (C/A LD $_{50(0.1L)}$ index) be calculated by expressing the multiple dose LD 50 as a percentage of the acute LD 50. (Both kinds of LD 50 values involved stomach tube administration, but the acute dose was given to fasted rats while the repeated daily doses were given to nonfasted animals.) The C/A index for sodium chloride was found to be 72, indicating that 100 daily doses of table salt each at a rate 72% of the acute LD 50 would kill half of a very large population of rats.

The term "chronicity factor," introduced independently by Hayes (1967b), is expressed as quotient rather than a percentage. However, this "factor" is really an index, and ought to be designated as such in the future. Excluding differences in the procedures for measuring the LD 50 values, the chronicity index for a compound is the reciprocal of its C/A LD $_{50(0.1L)}$

index expressed as a fraction instead of as a percentage; that is:

$$\text{chronicity index} = \frac{100}{\text{C/A LD}_{50(0.1L)} \text{ index}}$$

For example, the C/A LD $_{50(0.1L)}$ index for sodium chloride (71.7) would correspond to a chronicity index of 1.395.

Since each chronicity index is a ratio, these indices may be used to compare the tendency of different compounds to have cumulative effects without reference to their absolute toxicities. This index is determined on the basis of observed effect. No distinction is made between effects that depend in part on cumulation of the toxicant (eg, lead) and those that do not (eg, alcohol).

The chronicity index for each compound is obtained by dividing its 1-dose LD 50 (expressed as milligrams per kilogram) by its 90-dose LD 50 (expressed as milligrams per kilogram per day). The resulting number is large (2.0 or more) for compounds that are relatively cumulative in their effects and small (less than 2.0) for compounds that show little cumulative effect. The index of 2.0 is recognized as an arbitrary dividing point, but it appears plausible from the limited data available. In any event, if a compound were absolutely cumulative (in the sense that 1/90th of the 1-dose LD 50 was exactly the 90-dose LD 50), the chronicity index would be 90. A chronicity index of 1.0 associated with oral intake indicates that daily ingestion of the 1-dose LD 50 mixed into the regular diet leads to death of half of a very large population so exposed for 90 days.

Table 2-2 summarizes the 1-dose and 90-dose LD 50 values and also the chronicity indices for warfarin and several other compounds. The marked cumulative effect of warfarin and the chemosterilants; the small magnitude of such an effect of table salt, caffeine, and some organic phosphorus compounds, and the essential lack of cumulative effect of potassium cyanide are recorded. The 90-dose LD 50 of warfarin was only about 1/20 of the 1-dose LD 50, indicating a chronicity index of about 20 for that compound. It required daily ingestion of approximately a 1-dose LD 50 of several organic phosphorus insecticides to kill half of the test animals in 90 days, indicating a chronicity index of approximately 1 in each instance. Rats tolerated daily 25 1-dose LD 50's of potassium cyanide mixed with their regular food with no mortality, indicating a chronicity factor of less than 0.04. This tolerance for organic phosphorus compounds and cyanide undoubtedly indicates the ability of the body, and especially the liver, to detoxify

moderate dosages of these materials provided there is time in which to accomplish the task. The chronicity index permits comparison of the effects of different classes of compounds and it may permit comparison of the effects of different compounds of the same class. Whether these smaller intraclass distinctions are really significant or whether they are outweighed by differences caused by species or other factors must be determined by future experience. It is certainly to be hoped that increasing use will be made of 90-dose LD 50 and ED 50 values and of the chronicity index in order that the study of long-term toxicity may be made more quantitative.

The chronicity index is a measure of cumulative *effect*. As discussed in Section 3.2.3.2, a concentration index has been proposed as a measure of cumulative *storage*. As discussed at greater length in Section 3.2.3.2, the effect of a compound cannot be less than that determined by its storage in the body, especially its presence (storage) in sensitive tissues. In this sense, a compound that has a high concentration index will tend to have a high chronicity index. However, some compounds are highly cumulative in their effects even though they show a minimal tendency to storage. Thus, the two indices do not vary in a parallel fashion.

It is generally agreed that what has been called biological magnification is the basis for the injury caused by DDT and a few other compounds to certain large, predatory forms of wildlife. Biological magnification occurs in situations in which a compound shows a high concentration index in each successive species in a food chain. The problem of measuring the tendency of different compounds to exhibit biological magnification is discussed in Sections 3.2.3.2 and 11.2.3.2.

2.2.3 Time Relationships

The report of essentially every toxicity test should include information on the time relationships of the effects observed. It is important whether a single dose produces its effect soon after dosing or only after hours or days and whether the effect is brief or prolonged. From a practical standpoint, it is important to know whether a patient, who is only mildly sick an hour after overexposure to a toxicant, is really "over the worst of it" or likely to slip at any moment into a critical condition. From a theoretical standpoint, rapid onset of illness following dosage of experimental animals at or below the LD 50 level suggests that the toxicant is absorbed rapidly and acts directly. Rapid recovery following dosing at a substantial rate suggests that the toxicant is excreted or detoxified rapidly. On the other hand, slow

Table 2-2
Absolute and Relative, Acute and Subacute Oral Toxicity
of Certain Pesticides and Drugs.
From Hayes (1967b), except as noted, by permission of Academic Press.

Compound	Species	Sex	1-dose LD 50 (mg/kg)	90-dose LD 50 (mg/kg/day)	Chronicity index
mirex	rat	F	365	6.0	60.8
dieldrin	rat	M	102	8.2	12.8
DDT	rat	M	250	46.0	5.4
warfarin	rat	M	1.6	0.077	20.8
metepa	rat	M	136	7.5	18.1
apholate	rat	M	98	17	5.8
paraquat	rat	F	110	20.5	5.4
atropine	rabbit	M	588[a]	78[a]	7.5
benzylpenicillin	rat	M	6,700[b]	4,140[b]	1.6
sodium chloride	rat	M	3,750[c]	2,690[d]	1.4
caffeine	rat	F	192[e]	150[f]	1.3
dichlorvos	rat	F	56	>70	<0.80
parathion	rat	F	3.6	{ 3.5 / 3.1	{ 1.03 / 1.16
azinphosmethyl	rat	F	11.0	10.5	1.05
EPN	rat	F	7.7	12.0	0.64
potassium cyanide	rat	M	10	>250[g]	<0.04

a.   Boyd and Boyd, 1962 (100 intramuscular dose test).

b.   Boyd and Selby, 1962 (100-dose test).

c.   Boyd and Shanas, 1963.

d.   Boyd et al., 1966 (100-dose test).

e.   Boyd, 1959.

f.   Boyd et al., 1965 (100-dose test).

g.   No mortality occurred at 250 mg/kg/day, the highest dosage administered.

onset of illness following dosing at almost any level suggests that the toxicant is absorbed slowly or must be metabolized before it can act. Prolonged illness following dosage at or below the LD 50 level usually suggests that detoxification and excretion of the toxicant are inefficient, but sometimes means that the toxicant produces some anatomical or biochemical lesion that recovers slowly or not at all.

Time relationships in toxicity often can be expressed best by recording the range and mean of time required to produce an observed effect. However, a more elaborate statistical treatment sometimes is indicated. An ET 50 or LT 50 gives a more precise estimate of time to be anticipated in repeated tests than can be expressed by a simple average. The logtime-logdosage curve has considerable theoretical interest and, in some instances, may be used to predict the proper dosages to be used in long-term studies.

2.2.3.1 The ET 50 or LT 50. An ET 50 is a statistical estimate of the interval or time from dosage to a specific all-or-none response of 50% of the organisms in a very large population subjected to a toxicant under specified conditions. As used here, an all-or-none effect may be a specified level of a quantitative response, for example, time of appearance of first tumor or time at which the systolic blood pressure reaches 150 mm Hg. An LT 50 is a special case of an ET 50 in which the effect reported is death. ET 50 and LT 50 values are determined by relating the cumulative percentage effect (expressed as probits) to the logarithm of time required to produce the effect. In practice, the calculation (Bliss, 1937) or graphic solution

(Litchfield, 1949) is carried out in a manner essentially identical to those used for ED 50 and LD 50 values.

There is one striking difference in the form of these statistics for dosage and time. In considering dosage *per se,* the time of response is ignored completely. A series of tests involving several dosage levels of a compound results in a single dosage-response curve. On the other hand, in considering time of response, dosage cannot be ignored, and a series of tests involving several dosage levels results in a series of separate curves of different slope. A sufficiently low dosage of any compound will generate a curve coinciding with the baseline, indicating that no animals were affected. The critical range will generate a series of curves such that both the slope and the magnitude of the ET 50 are inversely proportional to dosage. In general, progressive increase of the dosage beyond that necessary to affect all animals will cause progressively less and less change in the slope and position of the ET 50 curves. However, in some instances, progressive increase in dosage beyond that necessary to kill all animals will cause a relatively sudden shift of the very high-dosage ET 50 curves to the left accompanied by an unpredictable change in their slopes. Such a change indicates that a different mode of action has come into play. Any dosage above that necessary to kill all organisms in a population is a "supralethal" dosage, but the term is used most often in connection with dosages that involve some difference in mode of action. Examples may be found most commonly in the toxicology of compounds of which the ordinary effects are delayed. Such compounds are discussed further in Section 2.2.3.2.

Except for the phenomenon of changed mode of action, the points discussed in the last paragraph are illustrated by Fig. 2-4 which shows LT 50 curves resulting from different dosage levels of warfarin administered in connection with a 90-dose LD 50 study. (Similar LT 50 curves were obtained in connection with a 1-dose LD 50 study.) It may be seen from Fig. 2-4 that, in practice, the progression of curves from right to left is not always completely orderly. The curves at the right tend to be horizontal or incomplete (indicated by dashed lines) because only a portion of the animals in these groups die. The curves at the left tend to approach the vertical, but there is some irregularity, caused no doubt by individual differences and the fact that only a limited number of animals are used in each group. The data on which Fig. 2-4 was based were used in a different form in connection with the corresponding dosage levels in Fig. 2-6. A comparison of the two figures shows the value of the

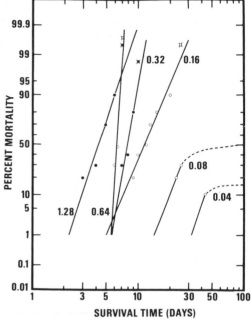

Fig. 2-4. LT 50 curves for male Sherman strain white rats administered repeated dosages of warfarin ranging from 0.04 to 1.28 mg/kg/day, respectively. Points adjusted according to the method of Litchfield and Wilcoxon (1949) are distinguished by a superimposed ×.

two kinds of graphs for illustrating different aspects of the same results.

2.2.3.2 The Logtime-Logdosage Curve. Compounds may show one or more of the following interrelations between dosage and time to response, no matter whether there are one or more doses: (*a*) a uniform delay between the first dose and the response; (*b*) a prolongation of the interval that is inversely related to dosage; and (*c*) a complete absence of detectable effect at low dosages and, therefore, an interval that exceeds the period of observation (which may be the lifetime of the subjects).

As is well known, there is a lag in the appearance of a detectable effect of some compounds. In other words, there is an inherent delay in their action, which is not accounted for by the time necessary for their absorption and distribution to the target organ. The inherent delay is not fully overcome by substituting larger doses or by using intravenous injection. Examples are offered by: (*a*) carcinogens, for which an induction period is apparently always required; (*b*) certain organic phosphorus compounds that produce paralysis in man or the chicken, but only following a delay of about 10 days; and (*c*) the coumarin-derived anticoagulants, which inhibit prothrombin formation but have no clinical effect until the existing supply of prothrombin becomes depleted. In these instances, the toxicants have little or no initial effect unless the dosage is massive. Some other compounds, notably alkylating agents (Hayes, 1964), produce delayed effects but generally produce some illness promptly after a dose at or even below the LD 50 level.

A compound cannot produce a delayed effect unless it or its metabolites or a direct or indirect pharmacological action persists until the effect appears. This persistence of a compound or its action is the very stuff of which cumulative effects are made. On the contrary, the coumarin-derived anticoagulants exhibit the delay but do not produce a truly chronic disease.

Although the necessary delay in the onset of the effect of some compounds is well known, it has not been customary to represent it graphically. By contrast, curves relating the increasing interval from the first and sometimes only dose until the appearance of a selected effect were used at least as early as 1937 and were based on data published as early as 1908 (Clark, 1937). Clark showed that, for a certain range of dosages characteristic of each test system, there often is a straight line relationship when the logarithm of time to response is plotted against the logarithm of dosage producing the response. Both the graphic and the mathematical features of the relationship were thoroughly investigated by Bliss (1940). Fig. 2-5 indicates the form of a typical curve. Recognition of the relationship apparently has not been general, with the result that it·has been rediscovered from time to time.

It is a general principle of toxicology that any compound may be tolerated without injury provided the dosage is sufficiently small. It has not been customary to represent this relationship graphically. As discussed below, such representation is desirable, for it reveals what may be basic differences in the behavior of different compounds.

Form of the Complete Logtime-Logdosage Curve. Summarizing the last several paragraphs, it is evident that a complete logtime-logdosage curve would have three segments: (1) a first segment representing the minimal time necessary to produce an effect even with dosages larger than the minimal one required; (2) a second segment to represent the increasing times necessary to produce an effect with successively smaller dosages; and finally (3) a third segment indicating a dosage a little below which the effect is not produced, no matter for how long dosing may be continued. Such a curve based on a study of warfarin is shown in Fig. 2-6. The three segments are well shown. The second segment was established by dos-

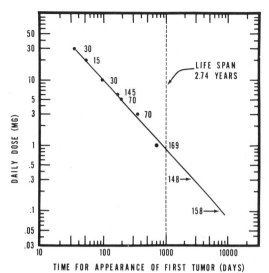

Fig. 2-5. Responses of rats to graded daily doses of 4-dimethylaminoazobenzene (4-DAB) administered orally. No liver tumor was obtained with the two lower doses employed, indicated by arrows. The number associated with each point or arrow refers to the number of animals tested at that dosage. From data of Druckrey (1959).

ages of 0.16, 0.32, 0.64, and 1.28 mg/kg/day, and in each instance the time necessary for half of the animals to die was 10 days or less. (The points in Fig. 2-6 represent geometric means as explained in the legend. LT 50 values could have been used and would have given essentially identical results. The choice was based on convenience, especially in connection with groups in which only a few animals died.)

As may be seen, the third segment in Fig. 2-6 has been drawn out horizontally at the level of the 90-dose LD 50 value for warfarin as determined by the original, detailed form of the 90-dose curve in Fig. 2-3. The corresponding LD 10, LD 1, LD 0.1, and LD 0.01 have been indicated also. Since the lowest dosage tested (0.02 mg/kg/day) lies between what were calculated to be the LD 0.1 and LD 0.01 levels, there is little wonder no effect was observed among a group of only 10 animals.

It appears that a few compounds (eg, warfarin, Fig. 2-6) exhibit all three segments of the theoretical curve, some (eg, 4-DAB, Fig. 2-5) exhibit the first and second segments only, and most compounds exhibit the second and third segments only. Perhaps some compounds exhibit the second segment only, but no illustration is at hand. It is impossible to make a more exact statement at this stage because there has been so little study of comparative, quantitative toxicology. In fact, it is not established that all compounds exhibit a typical

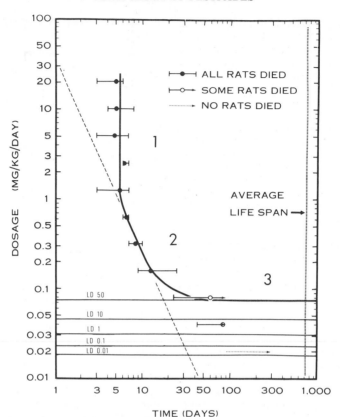

Fig. 2-6. Relationship between dosage of warfarin and time of death in rats. A short vertical line indicates the time of death of the first animal in a group to die, and a solid point indicates the geometric mean time to death for a group in which all the animals died. In those groups in which some animals did not die, their survival is indicated by an arrow, and the best estimated geometric time to death is indicated by an open circle. The tip of each arrowhead indicates the end of the dosage period. Since it could not be assumed without proof that the survivors would live a normal life span, it was empirically assumed for purposes of calculation that the survivors died on the last day of the test. Thus, the true position of these estimated values always lies to the right of the open circle. Note that no rats died when dosed for 300 days at a rate of 0.02 mg/kg/day. The graph also shows the 90-dose LD 50 and some other dosage-response values for 90 doses of warfarin. Slightly modified from Hayes (1967a) by permission of Academic Press.

second segment of the theoretical curve, although this appears likely. Curved second segments shown by some authors (Clark, 1937) may, in fact, represent a transition between second and third segments.

The presence of a delayed reaction following large dosages does not exclude the possibility that small dosages of the same compound may be tolerated. Fig. 2-6 offers an illustration of this kind of tolerance in rats fed warfarin. Another example is offered by the works of Siegel *et al.* (1965) who showed that a mixture of tricresyl and other triaryl phosphates, which produced paralysis of chickens and rabbits after only about 20 days of high-level exposure, was tolerated by both species for as long as 90 days when given at lower dosage levels. Of course, it is easy to demonstrate tolerance for small dosages of most compounds, albeit

they do not elicit a significant latent period when absorbed at high dosage levels.

In all instances studied so far, carcinogenesis is associated with lack of a third segment in the logtime-logdosage curve. In connection with toxicity generally, lack of this segment is exceptional. The presence of the third segment strongly implies the existence of a threshold at a level only a little less than the level of the segment itself. It is not certain how the absence of a third segment ought to be interpreted, but there is no evidence to exclude the possibility that a threshold exists here also, that is at a dosage level just below that required to produce tumors in animals that survive as long as any of their species. Regardless of the logtime-logdosage response, the existence of a threshold should be demonstrated chemically, as discussed in Section 2.2.7.4.

Use of the Logtime-Logdosage Curve for Prediction. Aside from its basic interest for toxicology, the logtime-logdosage curve may be used in connection with a brief test to predict appropriate dosage to use in long-term studies. Reference to Fig. 2-5 shows that only about 90 days of testing of 4-DAB in rats at dosages of 10, 18, and 32 mg/rat/day would have been sufficient to predict that a dosage of about 0.9 mg/rat/day produces an effect within the lifetime of that species. On the contrary, use of the same technique in connection with warfarin (Fig. 2-6) predicted a limiting value which, however, did not correspond closely with the value actually observed in a long-term experiment. By extrapolation of the second segment of the curve (as shown in part by the dashed line in Fig. 2-6), one would predict that a dosage of approximately 0.002 mg/kg/day would kill half of a sufficiently large group of similar animals within 90 days. This prediction for warfarin is seriously inaccurate when compared to the 90-dose LD 50 of 0.077 mg/kg/day based on all the dosage levels tested, including a dosage of 0.020 mg/kg/day, which was tolerated for 300 days without any mortality.

The fact that the value predicted may be only limiting and may not correspond closely with observed long-term toxicity does not make the test useless. The test does have the advantage of relative brevity. It is better to know a limiting value than to have no valid guide whatever for choosing dosages for long-term study.

The logtime-logdosage curve also may be used in the bioassay of bacterial and other toxins. What may have been the first effort along this line (Boroff and Fitzgerald, 1958) confirmed the straight-line, loglog relationship demonstrated earlier for other substances and showed that by the intravenous injection of relatively large doses a test could be completed in less than 2 hours instead of the 4 days required for the conventional test for toxins. It was shown later that by using dilutions that had been tested by the conventional way, it was possible to construct a standard curve relating the log of the mean survival time in minutes to the log of concentration or log of the number of lethal doses per unit volume, thus providing a prompt measurement expressed in the desired unit (Boroff and Fleck, 1966).

Haber's Rule. Apparently the only statement Haber made of what has come to be called his rule is contained in a footnote to the last of a series of five lectures this chemist made during the period 1920–1923 (Haber, 1924). The particular lecture involved was on the history of gas warfare, and all the toxicological considerations were in this context. This means, among other things, that only brief exposures were considered. At that time, no chemical was known that would not drift away or be diluted to a harmless concentration soon after its release. The complete footnote (quoted by permission of Springer-Verlag) may be translated as follows:

"A simple and practical measure for toxicity can be obtained that suffices for all practical purposes. For each war gas, the amount (*C*) present in one cubic meter of air is expressed in milligrams and multiplied by the time (t) in minutes necessary for the experimental animal inhaling this air to obtain a lethal effect. The smaller this product (*C* × *t*) is, the greater is the toxicity of the war gas. A few values obtained during the war are given in the table. More detailed information can be found in the medical literature. The values were all obtained by using cats as experimental animals. The chemicals are listed according to the order of their introduction as war gases.

Substances	First used by	$C \times t$
ethylbromoacetate	France	3000 and less
chloracetone	France	3000
xylylbromide	Germany	6000
chlorine	Germany	7500
perchlormethyl mercaptan	France	3000 and less
hydrocyanic acid*	France	1000
phosgene	France	450
methylchloroformate	Germany	500

*The value of (*C* × *t*) for hydrogen cyanide depends on its concentration. The value given refers to the concentration of 1/2% obtainable in the field. The values are much higher with smaller concentrations."

It may be noted that the footnote implies but does not state what is now called Haber's rule for equitoxic doses, especially fatal doses, namely:

$$Ct = K$$

where *C* is concentration, *t* is time, and *K* is a constant characteristic of a particular compound.

Actually the concept was not original with Haber. Apparently it was stated first by Warren (1900) in connection with his studies of the effect of different concentrations of sodium chloride on *Daphnia magna*. Warren stated the relation as:

$$T(X - 8) = \text{constant}$$

where *T* = time of killing, and *X* = strength of

salt solution. The value, 8, was an observed constant, being the concentration below which the relationship did not hold and survival of the animals was influenced little or not at all by the salt. Thus, Warren recognized that the relationship was true only within certain limits of time and concentration. It is clear from his note on hydrocyanic acid that Haber, too, was fully aware of the limitation of the constant relationship.

Bliss (1940) reviewed some earlier papers on the subject and presented an elaborate mathematical analysis of the relationship between exposure time and concentration.

Restatement of Haber's Rule. Further study has emphasized the limited applicability of the rule. Recognition of this limitation has led to a restatement of the relationship as follows:

$$\frac{[(CVm) - De]\,tR}{w} = D$$

where:

D = dosage (mg/kg) received during time, t

C = concentration of toxicant (mg/m³)

Vm = minute volume rate of respiration (m³/min)

De = detoxification rate (mg/min)

t = time (min) of exposure

w = body weight (kg)

R = retention coefficient expressed as a decimal fraction.

This equation shows that a sufficiently high rate of detoxification would negate prolonged exposure to a sufficiently low concentration. It thus expresses quantitatively the limitation on the rule when applied to easily detoxified materials like hydrocyanic acid. It will be seen that in this equation dosage (D) is not necessarily a constant for all combinations of concentration and time that produce the same effect, since the detoxification rate and perhaps the retention coefficient may vary with dosage.

Relation of Haber's Rule to the Logtime-Logdosage Curve. If one considers the relationship, $Ct = K$, which constitutes Haber's rule, it is clear that it represents a special case of the second segment of the logtime-logdosage curve (the dosage being expressed, of course, as concentration). When plotted on loglog paper, all solutions of the equation lie on a straight line passing through two points, namely:

$$C = 1, t = K$$
and 　　　　$C = K, t = 1.$

Furthermore, on the same set of coordinates, all solutions of all other equations of the same

form will lie parallel to the first but pass through K_1, K_2, etc, instead of K. The slope of these lines is algebraically the same, and it is 45° on ordinary loglog paper.

Some logtime-logdosage curves based on observed data have a slope statistically indistinguishable from that determined by Haber's rule. Fig. 2-5 is an example. However, other real curves show greater or lesser slope (Clark, 1937; Bliss, 1940; Druckrey, 1943, 1967; Scholz, 1965). Examination of Fig. 2-6 shows that the second segment slopes downward more steeply than 45°. In other words, within the range of dosage from 1.28 down to 0.16 mg/kg/day, the smaller dosages are progressively more effective than would be predicted by Haber's rule. That is, progressively less total dosage is required as shown in Table 2-3. The significance of slopes greater than or less than 45° is not clear; in fact, both have been observed for warfarin under different conditions. In any event, there is no relationship between the slope of the second segment of the curve and the occurrence of a third segment.

2.2.4 Problem of Measuring Effect of Dispersed Toxicants

Although it is desirable to express dosage in terms of weight of toxicant per weight of organism, this is difficult if the dose is absorbed from air by the lungs or tracheae of land animals or from water by the gills of aquatic animals. Under these circumstances, it may be convenient and even necessary to consider toxicity in terms of concentration of the toxicant in the medium. If there is continuous exposure to constant concentrations, the data are expressed in the form of EC 50 values as explained below. If time is also a variable, the time results may be presented in terms of a logtime-logdosage curve as discussed in connection with Haber's rule.

When possible, dosage in terms of milligrams per kilogram should be calculated from the concentration of toxicant, the respiratory

Table 2-3

Dosage Relationship for the Second Segment of the Curve in Figure 2-6

Daily dosage (mg/kg)	Total dosage (mg/kg)
1.28	7.17
.64	4.28
.32	2.69
.16	2.03

volume, and the proportion of toxicant retained. The result of this calculation offers one important way of comparing toxicity by the respiratory route with that by other routes. Another approach is to measure plasma or other tissue levels of toxicant following exposure by different routes (see Section 2.2.6).

2.2.4.1 The EC 50 and LC 50. An EC 50 is a statistical estimate of the concentration of a toxicant in the ambient medium necessary to produce a particular effect in 50% of a very large population under specified conditions. An LC 50 is a special case of the EC 50 in which the effect recorded is death. EC 50 and LC 50 values are determined in a similar way to ED 50 and LD 50 values, ie, probits representing the percentages of animals showing a response in a series of tests are related to the logarithms of the concentrations that produced the responses. EC 1 and EC 99 values may be determined and confidence limits of the various estimates may be calculated. ET 50 and LT 50 values may be calculated on the basis of concentration instead of dosage.

2.2.5 Measurement of Graded Responses

What has been said so far about quantitation of dosage-response relationships was concerned with all-or-none effects or effects that can be treated in this way. However, many responses of organisms are graded in character and need to be so reported. Such reports may take many forms including tables and line and bar graphs and represent the whole gamut of pharmacological effects. In some instances, the data may be treated mathematically. Some examples are given in the section on storage (3.2.3). However, graded responses do not lend themselves to neat quantitative tabulation such as may be applied, for example, to the LD 50 values of a series of compounds.

2.2.6 Dosage at the Tissue Level

A simple but profound change in pharmacology began in the 1940's when increased emphasis was placed on the importance of tissue levels of drugs. It had long been known that chemicals act at a cellular level, and the change in emphasis was conditioned largely by the rapidly increasing ability to carry out the necessary measurements. In any event, a series of such measurements made it possible to relate the effectiveness of many drugs to their minimal plasma levels or, to be more exact, to minimal plasma levels of free compound. This critical index of the concentration available to cells made it possible to devise rational, nontoxic uses of several compounds that previously had been too slowly effective or too toxic

to be practical. The factors that can be involved in determining the plasma levels of free compounds have been reviewed by Brodie (1967) and by the National Academy of Sciences (1969).

Some factors other than dosage that control the concentration of foreign compounds available at the tissue level are discussed in Chapter 3. It seems inevitable that the toxicity of pesticides would be far better understood if the influence of these factors on pesticides were explored much more fully.

2.2.7 Statistical Considerations

There are several good reference books on statistics applicable to problems in toxicology. These include volumes by Pearson and Hartley (1958), Mainland (1963), Steel and Torrie (1960), and Snedecor (1967). Useful statistical tables may be found in books by Beyer (1966) and Fisher and Yates (1963).

This section is not intended as a substitute for the references just cited, and such books must be consulted by anyone interested in the mathematical details. This section does discuss some broad guidelines regarding: (a) how many subjects are required for ordinary tests; (b) randomization of subjects; (c) selection of dosage levels; and (d) special considerations associated with the effects of small dosages.

2.2.7.1 Number of Subjects. As discussed in Section 2.2.1.1 and illustrated graphically in Fig 2-1, the accuracy of statistical measurement can be increased by running more tests under the same conditions.

Number of Independent Units. Table 2-4 shows the difference that must appear between two equal groups to be significant at a level of $P = 0.05$, using groups of 50, 40, 30, 20, and 10 subjects, respectively. The simplest situation is that in which the effect under study does not occur in the controls. Inspection of the table shows that when no controls are affected, there still must be 5 reactors (50%) among a group of 10 experimental subjects in order to achieve assurance that the difference between the two groups has not occurred by chance. If the groups are larger a smaller proportion of reactors is required. Thus, with groups of 50 subjects each, only 6 reactors (12%) are needed in the experimental group to indicate a statistical significance of difference when no controls react. Put another way, groups of 50 subjects each will be required to demonstrate dependably an effect that occurs in 12% of a very large population even when there are no reactors among the controls. Larger groups are required if events that occur at a lower frequency are to be demonstrated.

Table 2-4

Differences Between Two Groups Necessary for Significance (P = 0.05)

From National Academy of Sciences (1960) by permission of the Academy.

50 animals per group		40 animals per group		30 animals per group		20 animals per group		10 animals per group	
Percentage incidence		Percentage incidence		Percentage incidence		Percentage incidence		Percentage incidence	
Least affected	Most affected	Least affected	Most affected	Least affected	Most affected	Least affected	Most affected	Least affected	Most affected
0	12	0	15	0	20	0	30	0	50
4	16	5	20	3 1/3	26 2/3	5	35	10	70
10	26	10	27 1/2	10	36 2/3	10	45	20	80
20	38	20	42 1/2	20	46 2/3	20	55	30	90
30	50	30	52 1/2	30	56 2/3	30	65	40	100
40	60	40	62 1/2	40	66 2/3	40	75	50	100
50	70	50	72 1/2	50	76 2/3	50	85	60	--
60	80	60	82 1/2	60	86 2/3	60	90	70	--
70	88	70	90	70	93 1/3	70	100	80	--
80	94	80	95	80	100	80	--	90	--
90	--	90	--	90	--	90	--		

The second and succeeding lines of Table 2-4 are concerned with the situation in which there are reactors among the control group. If one group has a certain percentage of reactors, the other group must have a specified larger percentage in order for the difference to be significant. Thus, at least 50 animals per group would be necessary in order to give reasonable assurance that 26% incidence in one group and 10% incidence in the other group are in reality different.

Table 2-4 is intended to illustrate the principles just outlined. A more complete table suitable for guiding experimental work was provided by Mainland (1963).

Needless to say, even a mild clinical effect of a compound would be intolerable if it occurred in 1% of the general population who encounter traces of the material. If the effect were at all serious, an incidence of 1% among workers would be intolerable also.

The solution of the problem from the standpoint of ordinary testing is to keep the limitations of precision in mind and to design experiments and select dosages in such a way that there will be one or more groups in which the parameter of interest approaches an incidence of 100%, while the incidence in the control is held very low. Interpretation of the results must be based not only on statistical consideration, but also on judgment regarding the severity and reversibility of the effect under discussion, and the relevance of the test as a whole to the human situation.

Identity of Sampling Units. As critically reviewed by Weil (1970), it is an error to count individual subjects as statistical experimental units when these subjects are not randomly selected. For example, in studies of reproduction or teratogenesis, mothers (or litters) and not the number of offspring are the proper basis for statistical analysis. It is misleading to report the number of malformed young produced; instead, one may report the number of litters showing any malformation or, more precisely, the proportion of malformed young per litter. The reason, of course, is that the fate of any particular offspring is conditioned by the physiology of its mother and by the dosage she received. Counting young rather than litters counts the same thing over and over. This tends to exaggerate the statistical significance of the results and may lead to the conclusion that observed differences are significant when they easily might occur by chance.

The same precaution must be observed in connection with studies of carcinogenicity started with newborn or infant animals.

Other types of unjustified grouping for statistical analysis are the combination of dosage groups, sexes, or strains without testing the data statistically and finding that a particular combination is justified.

2.2.7.2 Randomization of Subjects. There is a possibility that error will be introduced into experiments through nonrandom selection of subjects, whether animals or people. For example, in selecting animals from a holding cage, there is a chance that the quieter ones will be taken first and the livelier ones caught later. If they are placed in groups as they are caught, there will be a tendency for successive groups to be more active, and the degree of activity may represent a basic physiological difference. The remedy is to give the animals temporary numbers as they are caught and then assign them to groups according to a table of random numbers. Such tables frequently are included in books of statistical tables. After the animals have been divided into groups, each one may be given a permanent identification number in serial order.

What has just been said about randomization concerns populations that either are considered homogeneous or exhibit variation impractical to control. Of course, recognized variation may be made the object of controlled experimentation. For example, if differences involving sex are to be studied, the males and females must be segregated, after which subjects of each sex may be assigned randomly to appropriate groups. Since populations may lack homogeneity in many obvious ways, it may be desirable to select subjects carefully in order to avoid introducing unwanted but controllable variables. For example, it is often desirable to limit a series of tests to animals of a preselected age or weight.

In working with a limited supply of subjects, it may be better to ignore strict randomicity in order to distribute some obvious variables among the different experimental groups. For example, if 30 men of widely different ages are to be placed in three dosage groups, it may be desirable to place their names on cards, arrange the cards in order by year and date of birth, and then deal the cards into three groups in the order: 1, 2, 3, 3, 2, 1, 1, 2, etc. Although such a distribution is not random, it will eliminate bias. After a test has been run in this way, the data may be examined to see whether recognized variables affected the result. The results for each group may be plotted by age, or a coefficient of correlation may be calculated to see whether the outcome was significantly influenced by this variable. The results for one race may be compared to those for another, and other variables may be considered in turn.

2.2.7.3 Selection of Dosage Levels. Since the effects of chemicals expressed as probits usually form a straight line when plotted against the logarithm of dosage, it is best to choose a series of dosage levels that form a geometric progression. A factor of 2.0 (log interval of 0.3) is often used. More detailed information will be obtained if a smaller factor such as 1.26 (log interval of 0.1) is used, especially in the region of the ED 50. Conversely, less (but sometimes sufficient) information can be obtained by testing dosage levels separated by a factor of 4 or more.

Selection of the general range of dosages to be studied is simply a matter of judgment supplemented by cautious trial. A number of methods for efficient use of small numbers of animals for determining ED 50 and LD 50 values are referenced in Section 2.2.1.1. Use of the logtime-logdosage curve for predicting the proper dosage range for tests involving repeated doses is discussed in Section 2.2.3.2.

2.2.7.4 Effects of Small Dosages. Safety evaluation is much concerned with the effects of dosages just below and just above the threshold of observable effect, that is with the *no significant effect level* and *lowest effect level* in practical experiments. After a consideration of these practical matters, the following paragraphs go on to discuss what is known about the existence of thresholds and the beneficial effects of small dosages. These theoretical matters have clear implications for the probable outcome of the quantitative study of the effects of dosages so small that extremely large groups of subjects are required for their meaningful investigation. Because of its difficulty and expense, this kind of quantitative study has never been carried out, but such study would have tremendous theoretical and practical importance. The strictly toxicological study ought to be coordinated with biochemical investigations that could offer a reason for the statistical findings, no matter what they may be.

The No Significant Effect Level. The concept of "no effect" is one of the most commonly employed in safety evluation. The "no effect level" is the maximal or near maximal dosage level at which no difference from untreated or vehicle-treated controls is detected. It is not a level so far below any effective one as to be insignificant. Although the term "no effect" often is applied in connection with a dietary concentration, it is always in the context of the dosage administered. Although the term could be employed in connection with one or a few doses, it is employed mainly in connection with long-term tests. Use of the expression implies an organized study and careful observation—not the casual result of a test with some other purpose. Any study designed to reveal a dosage producing no effect should contain, in addition to a control group receiving no toxicant, one or more groups of subjects given larger dosages fully expected to produce measurable effects of the compound. Since such tests are almost always prolonged, particular attention must be given to the number of subjects assigned to each group so that the number available at the end of the study will be adequate to reach a statistically significant result (see Section 2.2.7.1).

There are several reasons for placing the expression, "no effect" in quotation marks. First, many studies reveal effects that are obvious, reproducible, and highly significant from a statistical standpoint but of questionable biological significance. Depending on circumstances, an example might be partial inhibition of an easily regenerated enzyme. There is no substitute for judgment in toxicology. Second, as discussed in one of the following sections, the effects of small dosages of toxic compounds may be beneficial and thus qualitatively different from the effects of larger dosages. Third, failure to detect any effect by an elaborate scheme of testing does not exclude the possibility that an effect would have been detected if some other scheme had been used. Rapid progress has been made recently in chemical detection of toxicants or their metabolites. Analytical chemists have already achieved such skill that they easily measure biologically unimportant traces of several pesticides. Biochemists and physiologists are not far behind.

For these reasons, it is generally recognized that what is needed is a "no significant effect" or "no adverse effect" level, that is, a level that causes no detectable injurious effect. There is no complete substitute for long-term tests, but increasing attention must be given to evaluating the biological significance of observed effects that involve no demonstrable injury to health. A toxicologist may do as much harm by unnecessarily condemning a compound as by failing to detect and to prevent a real toxic hazard.

The Lowest Effect Level as a Practical Toxicological Measurement. As already mentioned, it usually is impractical to use such a large number of subjects per group that the possibility of a rare (<1%) but highly undesirable effect, such as neurotoxicity or carcinogenesis, can be excluded in the lower dosage range. This problem is not of such importance as may appear at first because the frequency of an effect can be increased by increasing the dosage—just one reason for using injurious

dosages in long-term studies. Thus, the existence of a highly undesirable effect of a particular compound can be taken into account in the selection of a safety factor. A more serious objection from a purely scientific standpoint is the imprecision of finding the highest "no significant effect" level. From a statistical point of view, it would be preferable to employ for safety evaluation the lowest effect level, that is, the smallest one at which a meaningful, injurious effect or even a relevant, harmless effect is detected. This implies: (a) that the "no significant effect" is determined in order to put a limit on what is meant by the smallest effect level; but (b) the more objective, positive finding is used for safety evaluation; and (c) the nature of any injurious effect observed will be taken into account in choosing a safety factor.

The matter of safety factors based either on the "no significant effect" dosage level or on effective dosage levels is discussed in Section 9.1.4.1

Threshold Levels as Biological Facts. The practical difficulty in establishing a "no effect" level for a particular compound using a manageable number of experimental animals and the more complex problem of extrapolating a safe level for man must not be permitted to obscure the fact that thresholds do exist. The toxicologist faced with a single limited experiment would be wise to recall the impossibility of proving a negative. The logician faced with a complete lack of supporting evidence would be wise not to press pure logic too far and conclude that no threshold exists so that even a single molecule may represent a hazard. As pointed out by Friedman (1973), the question of the existence of a threshold is a problem of biology, not of mathematics or of probability. In not a single instance has the absence of a threshold been demonstrated. On the contrary, concentrations are known at which compounds with the highest biological activity are inactive.

For example, as described by Friedman (1973), limitation of vitamin A intake to 10% of the minimal required dosage leads to severe deficiency disease and yet it constitutes a dosage of 3.6×10^{15} molecules per kilogram of body weight or a concentration of 6×10^{-9} M in the body. In a similar way, ineffective levels of vitamin D and vitamin B_{12} (where the daily requirements are only 10 μg/day and 1 μg/day, respectively) are 4×10^{-11} M and 1×10^{-12} M. By conservative estimates, postmenopausal women and adult men have 1.5×10^{12} molecules of estradiol per kilogram of body weight or the equivalent of 2.6×10^{-12} M.

For tetrachlorodibenzdioxin, reported to

have an LD 50 value of 0.0006 mg/kg in guinea pigs, a harmless dose would still produce a concentration of 1.9×10^{-10} M in guinea pigs. For botulinum toxin, where talk of activity in terms of molecules has long been common, an amount of toxin that would produce absolutely no effect in mice would represent a dosage of 4.2×10^7 molecules per kilogram or a concentration in the mouse of 7×10^{-17} M, assuming a molecular weight of 900,000.

Values of the same orders of magnitude apply to some carcinogens. An ineffective amount of aflatoxin in the rat determines a dosage of 9.6×10^{12} molecules per kilogram and a concentration of 1.6×10^{-11} M. However, many strong carcinogens are less potent. For 1,2,5,6-dibenzanthracene, methylcholanthrene, and 3,4-benzpyrene administered by different routes, the ineffective concentration in the body ranges from 1×10^{-8} to 1×10^{-1} M.

Of course, the limiting level is even higher for compounds that are not inherently very active. For example, an ineffective amount of Aramite® as a carcinogen involves a concentration of 3×10^{-1} M.

Hutchinson (1964) and later Dinman (1972) suggested that 10^4 molecules per cell is the limiting concentration for biological activity, whether pharmacological or injurious. As pointed out by Friedman (1973), there are about 6×10^{13} cells in a 70-kg human body, from which it follows that the suggested limiting level for activity is 8.6×10^{15} molecules per kilogram or about 1×10^{-8} M. The demonstrated no effect levels for vitamin D, vitamin B_{12}, and estradiol (10^{-11} to 10^{-12}M) are so low that the corresponding thresholds may be somewhat lower than the limiting level of 1×10^{-8} just discussed. The same reasoning applies to the thresholds of toxic action of tetrachlorodibenzdioxin and botulinum toxin and the threshold of carcinogenic action of aflatoxin. Further evidence that the limiting concentration for the activity of a few highly active compounds is less than 10^{-8} M is the report that certain pheromones have thresholds of the order of 1×10^{-12} M. Of course, these values do not prove that the limiting concentration is ever less than 10^{-8} M in susceptible cells, since some compounds, such as botulinum toxin, have an extremely high affinity for the cells on which they act, and their distribution in the body at critical dosage may be very uneven.

However, exactly what concentration is limiting is far less important than the fact that thresholds do exist even for the most active compounds. No one doubts that the existence of deficiency conditions proves that minimal or threshold concentrations of vitamins, hormones, and other beneficial compounds are required for proper action. There is no chemical or other scientific reason to suppose that there is an inherent difference in the dosage-response relation of injurious compounds.

Beneficial Effects of Small Dosages. Schulz (1888) may have been the first to observe stimulation from very low concentrations of poisons. He investigated the effect of mercuric chloride, iodine, bromine, arsenous acid, chromic acid, formic acid, and salicylic acid on yeast and concluded that, when sufficiently diluted, all of them can increase the vitality of yeast over a longer or shorter period of time. Only a few years later the bacteriologist, Hueppe (1896), stated the rule that has come to bear his name: "Every substance that kills and destroys protoplasm in certain concentrations, inhibits development in lower concentrations, but acts as a stimulus and increases the potential of life at even lower concentrations beyond a point of neutrality." In stating this principle, Hueppe mentioned certain apparent exceptions. He also acknowledged the independent discovery of the rule by Arndt and Schulz.

A special, universally accepted instance of the beneficial effects of small dosages involves the reactions of plants to what are now called essential trace elements. A plant cannot live if even a single one of these metals or metaloids is completely absent from the medium in which the plant is grown, but an excess of any one or them is injurious. This is the law of optimal nutritive concentration. Recognition of it must be credited to Gabriel Bertrand even though he may never have stated it concisely in publication. The relationship of beneficial and harmful effects of trace elements was implied in the discussion that followed his presentation on "complementary nutrients" at the Fifth International Congress of Applied Chemistry held in 1903 in Berlin (Bertrand, 1903). Personal communications from his son, Dr. Didier Bertrand, and one of his students, Dr. Rene Truhaut, establish that Gabriel Bertrand presented the law of optimal nutritive concentration in his courses at the Sorbonne from 1908 through 1930. Later, Didier Bertrand (1962a, 1962b, 1969) generalized the law and expressed it in mathematical form.

As reviewed by Townsend and Luckey (1960) and in a very different way by Smyth (1967), evidence has continued to accumulate that small dosages of many compounds are beneficial even though larger dosages of the same compounds are injurious. Townsend and Luckey tabulated many examples from the pharmacological literature. Smyth offered several original examples of benefits from small doses of toxicants. The benefit may be substantial and include increased rate of growth, greater fertility, and prolonged lifespan. The phenomenon of benefit from small dosages may extend to cell cultures and involve pesticides such as dimethoate, disulfoton, and malathion (Gabliks *et al.,* 1967).

In the course of its repeated rediscovery, the phenomenon or variants of it have received different names. Thus the noun "hormesis" and the adjective "hormetic" were proposed for the stimulatory action of a subinhibitory amount of a toxicant (Southam and Ehrlich, 1943). The term "hormoligosis" (from the Greek, *hormao,* I rouse or set in motion, and *oligos,* small) was proposed (Luckey, 1956) to indicate the more general process by which a small amount of anything, regardless of its toxicity, produces stimulation. The same author used the term "hormoligant" to indicate something that stimulates when given in a small amount. The term "sufficient challenge" introduced by Smyth (1967) refers to the entire range of phenomena and emphasizes the need of the organism for some measure of stress, whether it be a small amount of poison, a small amount of radiation, or early, immunizing infection. In fact, he points out that he took the term from Toynbee's concept of "sufficient but not overpowering challenge" in connection with human history.

There is a tendency to take for granted the beneficial effects of small amounts of certain classes of compounds, which we call drugs, nutrients, or growth promoters, and to ignore completely the beneficial effects of small amounts of other materials, some of which we call poisons. The difference depends largely on our supposed understanding of their actions.

Since antiquity, the use of therapeutic drugs has seemed reasonable to people. Thus we "understand" the benefits from this one class of materials that are clearly toxic. A nutritional mechanism for the stimulation produced by low concentrations of certain toxic substances offers another basis for understanding. A number of minerals, vitamins, amino acids, and fatty acids are known to be essential to animals. The fact that excessive intake of some of them, notably several of the metals and vitamins A and D, has led to cases of human poisoning has not detracted from acceptance of their benefit. The discovery of the induction of processing enzymes, especially the mixed function oxidases of the liver, has added a third means of understanding the benefit of small amounts of some drugs, pesticides, and other chemicals. Finally, the effectiveness of growth promoting feed additives is understood in a somewhat different sense. There is little or no reason to think that the effectiveness of arsanilic acid and various antibiotic feed additives depends on any nutritive value. Their mode of action when given in the usual, homeopathic dosages remains unknown, but their ability to make chickens, pigs, and calves grow faster is inescapable. Here "understanding" is in terms of commercial success.

There is a tendency to ignore the beneficial effects of small doses of toxic compounds unless they are understood in terms of therapeutic action, nutritional requirement, growth promotion, or perhaps enzyme induction. In the latter case, there is some ambivalence and tendency to view adaptive change as evidence of injury. A few scientists have courage to see in the induction of enzymes an evidence of adaptation at the molecular level. Toxicologists should combat all bias. The existence of a phenomenon does not depend on our understanding of it. Statistically established evidence of benefit from small dosages ought to be viewed just as objectively as statistically established evidence of injury from larger dosages. This statement is not meant to underestimate the importance of increasing our basic understanding; it is a plea to explore widely and to face facts when they are found.

Many compounds have two or more modes of action, which reach expression at different, though perhaps overlapping, dosage levels. Possession of more than one mode of action certainly opens the possibility that low dosages of a compound will be beneficial rather than merely harmless. However, both benefit and harm may be associated with a single mode of action. Most of the side effects of drugs are excessive expressions of their therapeutic actions and the result of overdosage.

It is a general principle that excessive dosages of beneficial compounds are always toxic. It may be that the converse is also true, for the possibility cannot be excluded that sufficiently small dosages of toxic compounds are always beneficial in some living system; each apparent exception may be merely the result of failure to test a particular material under appropriate conditions.

The Logprobit Model and Quantitative Study of the Effects of Small Dosages. It is implied by the logprobit curve for dosage-response that an effect occurring in a low proportion of a population—say on the average of 1 in 10,000—is merely the result of a smaller dosage than those that would produce the same effect in a high proportion of the same population. The number of subjects necessary to measure the effect of a truly small dosage is very great unless this effect is qualitatively different from that produced by a large dosage.

If a small dosage produces a beneficial effect compared to the control, it may be possible to establish this fact with no more experimental subjects than are required to show that a larger dosage is harmful, and the presence of a positive benefit may exclude the possibility of a hypothetical injury from the same dosage. This principle is illustrated by facts regarding selenium, a trace element essential to life. Using groups of only eight animals each, Siami (1971) showed clearly that rats fed a dietary supplement of 1 ppm selenium grew better than rats fed the same regular commercial rat feed which contained only 0.15 ppm of the element. Rats receiving a supplement of 2 ppm also grew better than the controls but not so well as those receiving the 1-ppm supplement. Rats receiving a 3-ppm supplement showed definite toxicity, including liver cirrhosis, and those receiving 5 ppm of selenium died in only 5 weeks. Thus, the presence of a positive benefit at 2 ppm excludes, within the limits of the experiment, the possibility of injury from this exposure even though 3 ppm were distinctly injurious.

If the effects of different dosages are qualitatively identical and if it requires groups of 10 subjects to identify with acceptable precision the dosage that causes an event on the average once in every two chances (ED 50), then it would require groups of 500 subjects to find with the same precision the dosage that on the average causes an event once in 100 chances (ED 1). For an event affecting 1 in 10,000 (ED 0.01), groups of 50,000 subjects each would be required. Such large groups of subjects are required to measure the effects of small dosages directly that this measurement is entirely impractical in connection with routine toxicological testing. In fact, such studies have not been done.

Reasons for not doing statistical studies of small dosages include: (a) their great expense; (b) the technical difficulty of preventing or even recognizing effects caused by uncontrolled variables; and (c) the fact that tests employing a reasonable number of animals per group give results of practical value entirely suitable for determining safe levels of human exposure. The safety factor (whether in the form of a fraction of the "no significant effect" level or the "lowest effect" level or in the form of standard deviations [see Section 9.1.4.1]) removes the acceptable dosage one or two orders of magnitude from the lowest dosage tested experimentally and, therefore, far from the area of danger.

The main reason for doing thorough, direct,

statistical studies of the effects of small dosages is that we do not know the answers. For practical purposes, we can compensate for our ignorance by using safety factors that exceed the degree of uncertainty involved. However, there might be practical as well as theoretical value in exploring with precision the effects of small dosages. Sound information would reveal the limits of variability and thus indicate more accurately what safety factors really are needed—a practical result, greatly to be desired.

The straight line, logprobit, dosage-response curve was developed on the basis of observed facts, but, in addition, it involves the theoretical assumption that response to dosage follows a lognormal distribution. The logprobit model fits the observed facts and greatly facilitates their orderly study and presentation (see Section 2.2.1). However, there is no way to be sure that the model fits the facts in an area where almost no measurements have been made.

Hypothetically, the logprobit curve could deviate from a straight line either upward or downward in the low dosage region. Any true deviation would indicate that the distribution for a complete range of dosage levels is not lognormal under the conditions tested. A deviation in the low dosage level would not indicate that the distribution for dosages near the ED 50 level is not essentially lognormal, for the conditions relative to this level and to low dosages may be qualitatively different.

The direction of deviation would depend on the nature of the physiological factor responsible for nonnormal distribution. If there is no threshold for the effect under study so that no dosage, no matter how small, is totally without the effect measured, then the line must deviate upward and approach a horizontal direction in such a way that it will pass through absolute zero located an infinite number of logarithmic cycles to the left. There is no example to illustrate this condition, but it must be considered from the standpoint of logic. If a statistically valid example were found, it would indicate either an unsuspected variable in the experiment or the existence of a yet undiscovered principle of toxicological action.

If the threshold for the effect under study does not lie in the lognormal distribution but at a dosage higher than predicted by this distribution, then the logprobit line must deviate downward and approach a vertical direction. There are literally thousands of possible examples of this situation. As often as not the lower part of a logprobit curve is made up of points "adjusted" from zero values. The adjustment is made in the faith that a lognormal distribution is involved, even though some of the observed zero values are based on large enough groups of subjects to be statistically likely to give values higher than zero. Of course a number of examples will have to be tested at low dosage levels and with very large groups of subjects before a conclusion about the existence and eventually the frequency of non-lognormal distribution may be reached. If this kind of non-lognormal distribution were demonstrated, the statistical model would have to be adjusted, but no new principle of toxicological action would be indicated. The mechanism would have to be learned in each instance, but possibilities are known. For example, the downward flexure of the curve might correspond to the transition between low dosages metabolized easily by one pathway and higher dosages that overload the normal pathway and involve other pathways also.

It appears likely that, if the kind of deviation from lognormal distribution under discussion exists, it is related more often to the ability of an enzyme to cope successfully with low dosage levels than it is related to beneficial effects. Unlike the situation with selenium mentioned earlier, beneficial dosages of many essential elements are one or more orders of magnitude smaller than the smallest dosage observed to be injurious.

Fig. 2-7 illustrates the matters that have just been discussed. The figure shows the proportion of different groups of mice that developed tumors at the site of injection of a single subcutaneous dose of 20-methylcholanthrene as reported by Bryan and Shimkin (1943). It may be seen that the observed values in the area of the ED 50 correspond well to the expected lognormal distribution. The adjusted values for low dosage levels also correspond well, for they have been made to do so. However, each of these adjusted values for low dosages (shown by "×") is derived from an observed value of zero. In Fig. 2-7, the straight line required by the observed values in the area of the ED 50 has been extended at each end as required by a lognormal distribution of all values. However, in the low dosage area, an upward flexure of the curve has been inserted (dotted line) to illustrate a "no threshold" relationship, and a downward flexure has been inserted (dashed line) to illustrate the opposite deviation from a lognormal distribution.

Similar reasoning could be applied to the upper portion of the curve, but it would be of no real interest from the standpoint of safety evaluation.

Other Models of Dosage-Response Relationship. Other ways for describing dosage-response relationships include the logit and 1-hit models. They give results very similar to those

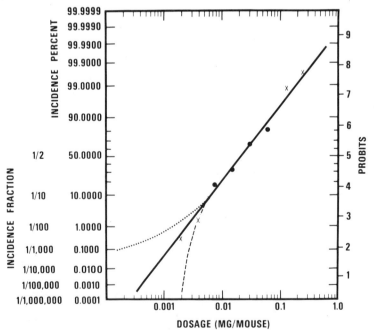

Fig. 2-7. Incidence of tumors in mice following a single subcutaneous dose of 20-methylcholanthrene; (●) observed values, (×) values adjusted from 0 or 100% by the method of Litchfield and Wilcoxon (1949). Hypothetical deviations from the straight line logprobit relationship are shown by a dotted and a dashed line as discussed in the text. Data from Bryan and Shimkin (1943).

for the logprobit method of analysis at the ED 50 level and even in some instances at the ED 16 level. However, the logit and 1-hit models predict effects of low dosages quite different from those predicted by the logprobit model. The tails of the distributions differ widely even though the central portions are similar (Mantel, 1963). Thus, the degree of reduction of the dosage that produces tumors in 1% of subjects necessary to achieve virtual safety (defined as the production of only one tumor in 100 million subjects), differs widely for the three models, namely: 1/100, for the logprobit model; 1/100,000, for the logistic model; and 1/1,000,000, for the 1-hit model (Mantel and Bryan, 1961). In other words, the curves for these other models deviate upward and to the left as compared to the straight-line logprobit relationship.

The objective studies of the effects of small dosages discussed in the foregoing section would test all three models simultaneously. It is not necessary to test extremely low dosages but only to learn whether the observed points deviate from the logprobit relationship and, if so, in what direction. For example, in Fig. 2-7 and for groups of 1,000 each, the estimated number of mice developing tumors following a dosage of 0.0039 mg per mouse would be 50 for no threshold, 35 for lognormal distribution, and 18 if a threshold is involved. After a dosage of 0.00195 mg per mouse, the estimates would be 20, 5, and 0.001 (ie, zero) mice, respectively. Certainly it ought to be possible to distinguish values of these magnitudes with only a relatively few replications of an experiment.

Chemical Basis of Thresholds in Dosage-Response Relationships. A great deal is known about the biotransformation of foreign compounds and also about the effects of toxic substances on the otherwise normal metabolism of the body. This knowledge, discussed in Chapters 3 and 4, explains many toxic actions and dosage-response relationships. However, the biochemical basis of the effects of small dosages is poorly explored, just as their dosage-response relationships are poorly studied.

It is clear in a general way that thresholds involve dosage but are not necessarily directly proportional to it, and that they are conditioned by the ability of the body to repair some injuries. Sufficiently small doses are without detectable effect. The effects of somewhat larger doses may be harmless in themselves and completely repaired before the next dose is received. This relationship is well illustrated by the action of inhibitors on enzymes, when administered at rates that do not cause illness. What is not clear is the identity and relative

importance of mechanisms that do not correspond directly with differences in dosage and, in this sense, may be regarded as qualitative differences. It is often speculated that small doses are biotransformed by "normal" pathways without taxing them, but that larger doses saturate these pathways, flood others, and thus interfere with endogenous metabolism. Unfortunately, details frequently are lacking, but there are notable exceptions, some of which are discussed in the following paragraphs.

Capacity for biotransformation may explain the presence of a threshold. Furthermore, biotransformation may be one mechanism of repair as is illustrated by the classical example of cyanide poisoning. Prompt metabolism of the cyanide ion to the much less toxic thiocyanate ion serves to prevent a combination of cyanide with cytochrome oxidase (the biochemical lesion in this instance). However, if the lesion already has formed, metabolism of cyanide to thiocyanate helps to establish a gradient that favors release of cyanide from combination with cytochrome oxidase and in this way promotes repair of the biochemical lesion. The tremendous efficiency of the metabolism of small doses of cyanide to thiocyanate explains why we are able to withstand the small amounts of cyanide we receive daily from food and other sources. However, above a certain threshold, cyanide is dangerous. In this instance, the limiting factor is not the capacity of the enzyme, rhodanese, but the immediate availability of sulfur to form thiocyanate. Moderate doses of cyanide cannot be metabolized efficiently because the sulfur compounds ordinarily used for this purpose are limited in availability. That this limitation of sulfur is, in fact, the reason for the threshold above which cyanide becomes dangerous is demonstrated by the fact that the threshold is moved upward if a suitable source of sulfur is furnished. The difference can be measured best not in terms of the threshold itself, but in terms of the LD 50. It was shown by Way *et al.* (1966) that the LD 50 of potassium cyanide can be shifted from 9 to 33 mg/kg merely by supplying sodium thiosulfate.

Glyoxylate is significantly more toxic than ethylene glycol, of which it is a metabolite, and it probably is largely responsible for the toxicity of the parent compound. When the dosage of glyoxylate to monkeys was reduced from 500 to 60 mg/kg, the proportion excreted unchanged was reduced from a maximum of 59% to a maximum of 1.5% and the proportion metabolized to carbon dioxide increased. Thus the kidney, which is specifically susceptible to injury by ethylene glycol and glyoxylate, is protected to a disproportionate degree by the metabolism of low dosages as compared to the metabolism of high dosages (McChesney et al., 1972).

Liver glutathione (GSH) has a relation to the toxicity of bromobenzene somewhat analogous to that of available sulfur to the toxicity of cyanide. There is a close relationship between the covalent binding of halogenated benzenes and their ability to cause necrosis of the liver. However, covalent binding of bromobenzene metabolites to mouse liver protein remains low until a critical dosage of 1.20 to 2.15 mmoles/kg is reached. At dosages of 2.15 and 4.06 mmoles/kg (which produces minimal and extensive toxicity, respectively) the rate of covalent binding is not only high, but is over twice what would be predicted by extrapolation of the rates for lower, nontoxic dosages (Reid and Krishna, 1973). Bromobenzene, or especially its epoxide, depletes liver glutathione in the process of forming a mercapturic acid. Little covalent binding of bromobenzene metabolites occurs while the supply of GSH is adequate and mercapturic acid is being formed, but considerable covalent binding occurs when 90% of the liver GSH is lost and little mercapturic acid can be formed (Jollow et al., 1974). Anything that reduces liver GSH (even though harmless in itself) makes the liver more susceptible to injury by bromobenzene. Finally, as outlined in Section 3.1.4, bromobenzene is capable of metabolism by different pathways and the protection is at least partially independent of GSH availability. Thus the metabolism of bromobenzene is complex, but the available facts all help to explain its disproportionate increase in toxicity above a threshold.

As reviewed by Gillette (1973), the toxicity of acetaminophen shows a disproportionate increase above a threshold and this relationship depends at least in part on the availability of liver GSH.

Another example involves the onset of toxicity at dosage levels that exceed the metabolic capacity of the liver. Golberg (1967) found that 2,4,6-tri-tert.-butylphenol at a dosage of 0.5 mg/kg/day for 6 days induced hepatic processing enzymes, and their efficiency was such that the concentration of the compound in the liver was indistinguishable after dosages of 10, 25, and 50 mg/kg/day. However, a dosage of 75 mg/kg/day produced an approximately eight-fold increase in average liver storage, and it was only at this threshold dosage range of 50 to 75 mg/kg/day that toxicity as indicated by histopathological changes in the liver first appeared. In a study of a series of substituted phenols, it was found that liver processing

enzymes invariably were induced by dosages lower than those required to alter the activity of liver microsomal phosphatases or to produce histopathological change (Golberg et al., 1967).

Stokinger (1953) reviewed evidence that the tissue distributions of beryllium, silver, iron, and iodine differ—sometimes greatly—according to dosage. His interest was focused on the serious errors that may be introduced by extrapolating the results of the storage of small, tracer doses to the storage of therapeutic or even toxic doses. Although his interest was in tissue distribution rather than toxicity per se, he noted that one might expect to find a different pattern of toxic manifestations solely because of the different amounts of the toxic agents in various organ sites. As mechanisms governing the distribution of the elements listed, Stokinger suggested: (a) dose-dependent formation of colloidal hydroxides such as those of beryllium, which are then phagocytized by cells of the reticuloendothelial system; (b) formation of complexes with serum proteins or other colloids (eg, complexes of silver), which are then phagocytized; and (c) complex physiological regulation such as those of iodine and iron.

As discussed above, nonlinear, dose-dependent differences in the toxicity of foreign organic compounds, unlike those of the elements, are likely to depend on other mechanisms, namely: (d) biotransformation; and (e) biorepair. There may be other mechanisms also, for the subject has been studied inadequately.

It is pointed out above that the only beneficial effects of small dosages of toxic substances that now are accepted generally are those that are "understood." There is something to be said for this uncompromising demand for intellectual justification. In any event, it is clear that the concept of threshold and the observed beneficial effects of small dosages will be more readily accepted if their biochemical basis is elucidated more completely. Studies of dosage-related biochemistry ought to go hand in hand with statistical studies of the clinical effects of small dosages.

2.2.7.5 The Geometric Mean. Francis Galton (1879) pointed out that, in many vital phenomena, equal intervals of effect are produced by logarithmic intervals of stimulus. He used as a specific example Fechner's law, which in its simplest form states that sensation is proportional to the log of stimulus. Galton emphasized that, for such phenomena, the true mean is the geometric one. In the geometric series, 1, 2, 4, 8, 16, 32, etc., the geometric mean of 4 and 16 is 8 (ie, 4:8::8:16) and not 10 (ie, not [4 + 16]/2). Use of the geometric mean where appropriate avoids the consequences of assuming that errors in excess or in deficiency of the truth are equally probable. To show how absurd or misleading this assumption can be, Galton recalled that, since there are giants more than twice as tall as the mean height of their race, the assumption "implies the possibility of the existence of dwarfs whose stature is less than nothing at all."

By his brief, rational paper, Galton introduced a more technical mathematical study by Donald McAlister (1879) entitled "The Law of the Geometric Mean." This law has not received the attention or use it deserves. It is appropriate for calculating the average storage of a compound in a population or the average time of death in a series of animals all dosed in the same way. On the other hand, few of the published arithmetic means are so much in error that they ought to be discarded. As Galton (1879) noted, the difference between the arithmetic and the geometric mean is small if the range of the values averaged is narrow.

2.2.7.6 Reproducibility of Results. Ideally, the results of any particular measurement ought to be reproducible in the same laboratory or from one laboratory to another. This becomes especially important when the numerical results may be used as guides for diagnosis and therapy, or when any results may be used to determine whether a compound does or does not satisfy legal criteria (for example, criteria of registration, residue tolerances, or whatever). However, results can be meaningful and important even when it is impossible to standardize the conditions to the point that control values are statistically identical from one trial to another.

An astonishing proportion of biological and biochemical studies are recognized as valuable contributions if the results for each experimental group show a clearcut relation to the results for the corresponding control in the same experiment. Of course, no study can be considered confirmed until the *relationships* demonstrated in the initial experiment have been redemonstrated in the same laboratory or, even better, in different laboratories.

Whereas all scientific procedures are examined from the standpoint of reproducibility within an experiment, only a few toxicological methods have been examined thoroughly for reproducibility in a broader sense. In these studies, it seldom has been possible to identify all of the causes of variation. In animal experiments, some of the variables discussed in Section 2.4 may be detected (Weil and Wright, 1967).

Probably the most important single factor in determining reproducibility is the objectivity of the endpoint. In a study of the oral LD 50, where the endpoint is clearcut, different protocols in use in well established laboratories produced results that differed so little that choice of one or the other would not change the interpretation of the relative hazard of any particular compound. Specifically, the highest and lowest LD 50 values for each of 10 compounds as determined in eight laboratories by various protocols differed by factors ranging from 1.30 to 5.48. The degree of variation was less, but not statistically less, when each laboratory used a reference protocol and a reference stock of rats (as compared with (a) reference protocol and rats commonly used in the laboratory, or (b) both protocol and rats commonly used in the laboratory) (Weil and Wright, 1967).

Far greater differences were found in a study of intralaboratory and interlaboratory variability in the results of eye and skin irritation tests, where the endpoints are subjective. Although other factors were involved, it was concluded that the main factor contributing to variability was difficulty in reading the reactions. Although numerical factors of difference (between highest and lowest values) could not be assigned, some of the differences obviously were very great. The majority of laboratories performed the tests competently and reproducibly; however, others were far afield. Some materials were rated the most irritating by some laboratories and rated the least irritating by others. Some of the laboratories that were most out of line were industrial and some were governmental. Therefore, restricting testing to any one type of laboratory would not solve the problem. In fact, it was concluded that the tests, which have been in general use for 20 years, are not now dependable ways of classifying a material as an irritant or a nonirritant. It was suggested that modification of the tests themselves would not be helpful but that careful reeducation of those who perform the tests would be required if any improvement is to be made (Weil and Scala, 1971). The Council of the Society of Toxicology supported this emphasis on training and a lack of emphasis on rigid standardization of protocols (Hayes, 1971).

One factor that may contribute to the failure of a laboratory to agree with the majority of others in a particular test is unfamiliarity with it. In a study of the reproducibility of measurements of blood lead, it was noted that some of the laboratories ordinarily had occasion to use the test only a few times per year (Keppler *et al.*, 1970). Here is not only one explanation for poor performance but an indication that the study may not have reflected the accuracy of experienced laboratories. Reeducation would be most efficient if it could be provided when needed, that is, just before an infrequently used test is required. However, if only a few tests are to be run, it probably would be more efficient to refer them to another laboratory than to arrange training.

2.2.7.7 Abnormal Values in Control Groups. It sometimes occurs that statistically significant difference between an experimental group and its control depends on an abnormality of the control and not on any deviation in the experimental group. This is an important reason why, in order to be indicative of deleterious effect, changes must be produced that are dosage-related and illustrate a trend away from the norm for the population under study (Weil and Carpenter, 1969).

2.3 Dosage-Response Relationships in Different Kinds of Toxicity or Change

2.3.1 Toxicity (Sensu Stricto)

All people with toxicological or medical training are aware that toxicity in the restricted sense corresponds to dosage for any particular compound. However, use of the various procedures described in Section 2.2 for measuring dosage-response relationships is restricted all too often to this limited kind of toxicity.

The less common or less familiar a phenomenon is, the more likely that its relationship to an actual or supposed etiology will be viewed qualitatively rather than quantitatively. Phenomena often viewed in this way include neurotoxicity, teratogenesis, carcinogenesis, mutagenesis, hypersensitivity, and storage, as well as adaptive response of microsomal enzymes.

2.3.2 Neurotoxicity

By neurotoxicity is meant the delayed but persistent paralysis caused by certain organic phosphorus compounds. The classical example is "jake leg" paralysis caused by triorthocresyl phosphate. Most studies of neurotoxicity have attempted to learn which molecular configurations are capable of producing the phenomenon and which are not. When active compounds were investigated quantitatively, it was found that a sufficiently low dosage was tolerated, and progressively larger dosages increased the frequency and severity, and often reduced the latency of neurotoxicity (Davies *et al.*, 1960; Aldridge and Barnes, 1961; Cavanagh *et al.*, 1961; Siegel *et al.*, 1965).

2.3.3 Teratogenesis

Although most research in teratogenesis has been centered on the nature of the phenome-

non itself and the biological factors which influence it, a few quantitative studies have been made, and they illustrate that for any given compound and experimental situation there is a dependable relationship between dosage and effect (Wilson, 1964; Murphy, 1965). It has been pointed out that there is no way to exclude that any given compound may be teratogenic to some species under certain conditions (Bough *et al.*, 1963; Karnofsky, 1965).

Steep dosage-response curves for teratogenic action such as those shown in Fig. 2-8 are not uncommon and, in fact, appear to be the rule. Agents can be tolerated in low dosage without any recognizable effect on development or viability, but most of them that have detectable teratogenicity rather quickly become lethal to all embryos at higher dosages. Between these ranges of normality and lethality, there exists a narrow zone of dosages in which variable numbers of embryos survive with varying degrees of teratogenic involvement. A sharp rise of the dosage-response curve is also characteristic of the teratogenic action of x-radiation (Wilson, 1964).

Further details regarding dosage-response relationships in teratogenesis are given in Section 4.2.10.1.

2.3.4 Carcinogenesis

Strong carcinogens demonstrate a striking dosage-response relationship whether expressed on the usual basis of incidence versus dosage (Figs. 2-7 and 2-9) or on the basis of logtime versus logdosage (Fig. 2-5). Thorough

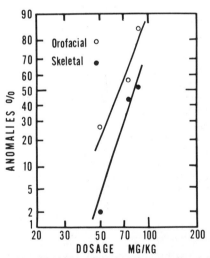

Fig. 2-8. Incidence of orofacial anomalies (○) and skeletal anomalies (●) in fetal mice whose mothers received different dosages of diphenylhydantoin by intraperitoneal injection on gestation days 11, 12, and 13. Data from Harbison and Becker (1970).

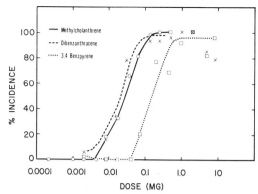

Fig. 2-9. Responses of mice to graded single doses of each of three polycyclic aromatic hydrocarbon carcinogens dissolved in tricaprylin and injected subcutaneously. Approximately 20 animals per dose of each compound. From National Academy of Sciences (1960) by permission of the Academy.

reviews of the matter have been written by Druckrey (1967) and by Shabad (1971). However, so much research on carcinogenesis has been centered on the phenomenon itself and so little attention has been given to quantitation of the actions of chemicals that even some experts in the field seem unfamiliar with the fact that chemical carcinogenesis follows clear-cut dosage-response relationships.

There is no doubt that only a small dosage of certain compounds is necessary to increase the incidence of cancer in susceptible animals. For example, as shown in Table 2-5 (p. 68), the ED 50 for carcinogenesis following a single subcutaneous injection of three of the classical laboratory carcinogens in mice ranges from 0.76 to 4.6 mg/kg. The naturally occurring carcinogen, aflatoxin, also is effective when administered subcutaneously at a total dosage of about 1.8 mg/kg (Dickens et al., 1966) but its danger by the oral route is more important. Dietary intake of aflatoxin B_1 during only 2 weeks at a total dosage of about 2.6 mg/kg produces carcinoma in male rats and a lower daily intake for a longer period also produces cancer when the total dosage is less than 0.5 mg/kg (Wogan and Newberne, 1967).

Unfortunately, little or no attention has been given to the dosage-response relationships of weak carcinogens.

Problems of the quantitative study of the effects of small dosages discussed in Section 2.2.7.4 are relevant to carcinogens as well as other toxicants. In fact, Fig. 2-7 is based on a study of 20-methylcholanthrene, and Fig. 2-9 is based on three carcinogens.

There is evidence, sometimes of a very tenuous nature, that some pesticides are tumorigens if not carcinogens (see Section 4.2.1.3).

2.3.5 Mutagenesis

Nearly all studies of chemical mutagenesis have been concerned with identifying mechanisms of action or with learning whether selected chemicals can or cannot cause some mutagenic effect in the system under study. Little attention has been paid to dosage-response relationships. However, such a relationship apparently has always been found when looked for. Examples from his own work and that of others on the induction of phage were given by Heinemann (1971). Dominant lethal mutations produced in insects and mammals by many alkylating agents and some other compounds regularly show dosage-response relationships. The toxicity of some of these compounds considered for use as insect chemosterilants has been reviewed (Hayes, 1968).

2.3.6 Hypersensitivity and Allergy

The extreme sensitivity of some people is illustrated by the fact that anaphylactic reactions to penicillin have been produced during skin testing with as little as 10 units of it (Mayer et al., 1953).

The fact that some people are "allergic" and others are either not allergic or at least highly resistant tends to obscure the fact that the various forms of hypersensitivity are dosage-related within a homogeneous population. Individuals who suffer from allergy often find that a reduction of dosage will lead to clinical improvement. For example, people who are sensitive to pollen often get some relief by closing most of the air inlets of their homes and placing filters on the remaining ones, even though this procedure does not eliminate their exposure to pollen but merely reduces it. Under experimental conditions in which the susceptibility of animals was made uniform by passive transfer, the onset of anaphylaxis was directly related to the dose of antigen (Pruzansky et al., 1959). Human leukocytes isolated from ragweed-sensitive donors release histamine at rates determined by the concentrations of purified antigen derived from the pollen (Lichtenstein and Osler, 1964). Other forms of hypersensitivity may be dose-related also. For example, blood dyscrasias, especially aplastic anemia, are a recognized hazard of the otherwise valuable drug chloramphenicol. Hodgkinson (1954) showed that these dangerous side effects occurred predominantly in cases in which the drug had been administered at a rate significantly higher than usual.

The fact that even hypersensitivity often is dosage-related emphasizes the importance of searching for suspected but undemonstrated dangers of a particular compound among peo-

ple whose exposure is most intensive and prolonged.

2.3.7 Metabolism and Storage

People trained in the biological sciences are
generally familiar with the fact that absorbed
compounds tend to reach a steady state of
storage, and that for each compound the storage at equilibrium corresponds to dosage. People not trained in the biological sciences are
usually unfamiliar with these facts and suppose that compounds are of two distinct sorts,
those that are stored and those that are not.
They suppose that compounds that are stored
at all continue to accumulate indefinitely with
no tendency to reach a steady state in which
the amount lost each day is equal to the
amount absorbed. It may seem odd to mention
this folklore in a book such as this, but the
views of the public must be taken into account
in any long-term effort to achieve popular
understanding of industrial chemicals in general and pesticides in particular.

The relationships between equilibrium storage and daily dosage for DDT in man, rat,
rhesus monkey, dog, and turkey are shown in
Fig. 2-10. It is clear that equilibrium storage
corresponds to daily dosage in all species studied. However, the details of this relationship
differ according to species and, at least in the
rat, according to sex and dosage level. Specifically, storage is the same in male and female
rats up to a dosage of about 0.02 mg/kg/day,
but above this level storage is greater in

females. Although species differences are to be
expected, the pattern reported for the dog is
remarkably different from the patterns for
other species and ought to be reexplored, especially at lower dosage levels.

The relation of dosage to the dynamics of
storage is considered in Section 3.2.3.2. The
relation of dosage to storage in man is illustrated in Section 7.2.4.1.

2.3.8 Induction of Enzymes

One of the most exciting developments in
recent years concerns the microsomal enzymes
(see Section 3.1). They help to explain a number of otherwise obscure facts in toxicology. It
is generally admitted that their net effect is
adaptive, although some persons fear that
stimulation of enzymes by one chemical will
lead to greater injury to the organism when
faced with some other challenge. Biologists
tend to believe firmly in adaptation, but they
are often skeptical about specific examples.
Regardless of the final toxicological evaluation
of the process of induction, it is clear from
work already complete that they are orderly
relationships between dosage and response for
compounds that stimulate microsomal enzymes. In fact, one of the very early papers by
Conney et al. (1956) demonstrated very clear
dosage-response relationships for demethylase
and DAB-reductase following injection of 3-
methylcholanthrene. The same paper demonstrated a similarly clear relationship for inhibition by ethionine.

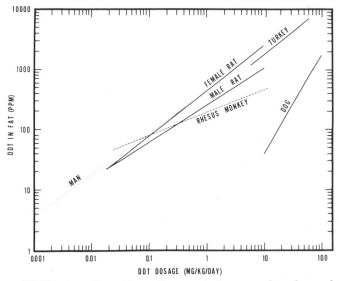

Fig. 2-10. Storage of DDT in the adipose tissue of man, rat, rhesus monkey, dog, and turkey. The curves
have not been extrapolated beyond the dosage levels studied. The curves are based on human data
referenced in connection with Fig. 7–7 and a reevaluation of animal data referenced by Hayes (1959).

Apparently the first such studies of pesticides as inducers of microsomal enzymes were those of Hart and his colleagues regarding chlordane and DDT. No obvious dosage-response relationships were found either with single or multiple doses of chlordane (Hart *et al.*, 1963). Some indication of a dosage-response relationship was evident from tabular values for DDT, but the relationship apparently was not discussed (Hart and Fouts, 1963), or discussed only briefly (Hart and Fouts, 1965) in connection with these early studies. It was Kinoshita *et al.* (1966) who first demonstrated clearly a dosage-related effect of DDT and toxaphene on enzyme induction. The result has been confirmed in connection with DDT (Gillett, 1968; Hoffman *et al.*, 1970) and other compounds (Hoffman *et al.*, 1968; Gielen and Nebert, 1971).

Sufficiently small dosages produce no detectable effect on enzyme activity. There is considerable evidence that the threshold dosage for enzyme induction corresponds to the upper limit of intake that can be metabolized by the unstimulated liver (Hoffman *et al.*, 1970).

The threshold dosage of DDT for induction of various microsomal enzymes in the rat has been estimated at about 0.05 mg/kg/day (ie, a dietary level of 1 ppm) (Kinoshita *et al.*, 1966) or 0.5 mg/kg/day (Schwabe and Wendling, 1967). Datta and Nelson (1968) found that a dietary level of 4 ppm (about 0.2 mg/kg/day) induced enzymes. Gillett (1968) found that the threshold is 0.125 mg/kg/day. Street *et al.* (1969) estimated the threshold at 0.05 mg/kg/day. The different estimates are not necessarily inconsistent, since they depend on different test systems. In any event, the lowest estimate (0.05 mg/kg/day) is only 0.2 times that known to be effective in man (Laws *et al.*, 1967; Poland *et al.*, 1970) whereas it is 50 times greater than the average dietary intake of all DDT-related materials by a 16- to 19-year-old man, that is, 0.0009 mg/kg/day (Duggan, 1968).

The enzyme-inducing dosage of DDT (0.5 mg/kg/day) used by Schwabe and Wendling (1967) led in 14 days to a storage level of 10 ppm in the adipose tissue of rats. The dosage of about 0.2 mg/kg/day used by Datta and Nelson produced in 20 weeks a storage of 39 and 76 ppm in the adipose tissue of males and females, respectively. Twelve weeks after dietary feeding of DDT was stopped, the storage levels of DDT-related materials had fallen to 11 and 21 ppm, respectively, compared to 6 and 9 ppm, respectively, in the controls. The rats previously fed DDT still showed some induction of liver enzymes 12 weeks after dosing was stopped. Neither the rats reported by Schwabe and Wendling nor those reported by Datta and Nelson were in a steady state of DDT storage when their values were between 10 and 21 ppm. It is therefore open to serious question whether these storage values are at all comparable to those found in people in the general population.

2.4 Factors Influencing Toxicity of Any Kind

Although dosage is the main factor determining whether a particular chemical will or will not produce a given effect, there are other factors that influence response. Factors of a biological nature include route of exposure, species and individual differences, sex, age, nutrition, and disease. Physicochemical factors include temperature and other environmental variables and, of course, the schedule and duration of dosage and the formulation in which the chemical is administered. There is no theoretical and frequently little practical limit to the range of dosage that may be explored experimentally, and there is frequently little practical limit to the range of human dosage that may be encountered at least occasionally. Thus, at one end of the spectrum it may be possible to find unexposed populations and at the other end of the spectrum to find an occasional person who is killed by accidental ingestion of a single large dose. Compared to dosage, the other factors that influence response to a particular chemical have been subject to less quantitative study. However, some have been studied, and it can be said, for example, that, on the average, pesticides are a little over 4 times more toxic by the oral route than by the dermal route. Factors other than dosage are important only in special circumstances. Thus, altitude (atmospheric pressure) is unimportant for toxicology in the parts of the world where most people live, but becomes progressively more important in connection with some compounds as altitude increases from about 5,000 feet and progressively greater strain is placed on cardiorespiratory function. There are certain factors that are almost universally relevant in toxicology and may affect man, while other factors (such as the details of caging) apply directly to animal experiments only.

The response of liver microsomal enzymes to dosage was mentioned in a preceding section (2.3.8). Differences in these enzymes or in their ability to be induced explain many differences in susceptibility to poisoning associated with interaction of compounds, differences in species, sex, age, and perhaps other factors. These enzymes are discussed in more detail in Section 3.1.2.2.

In addition to differences in metabolizing enzymes, changes in membranes, ionization, protein binding, and bile flow (discussed in Section 3.2.1) in some instances may explain observed interactions of compounds or differences of susceptibility to poisons associated with age, diet, and the like.

2.4.1 Compound

2.4.1.1 Primary Compounds. Compounds show a tremendous range of inherent toxicity. Pesticides constitute only a small proportion of all industrial chemicals, but even pesticides show a wide range of toxicity. For example, the oral toxicity of tetraethylpyrophosphate is approximately 588 times greater than that of pyrethrum extract. However, it must not be

supposed that the difference depends on the fact that one of the compounds is synthetic and the other of plant origin. The difference is sometimes in the opposite direction. Nicotine, a plant product, is about 103 times more toxic than difenphos, a synthetic organic phosphorus compound. The most toxic materials known are produced by living organisms. The nearer blood the nearer bloody!

Table 2-5 illustrates the range of toxicity produced by one or a few doses of selected pesticides and some other materials. There is, of course, some tendency for compounds of similar chemical nature to resemble one another in toxicity. However, the resemblance is more likely to be qualitative rather than quantitative. Thus, the organic phosphorus com-

Table 2-5
Toxicity of One Dose of Selected Materials;
Doses are Oral Unless Indicated

Material and route	Species	Sex	Dosage (mg/kg)	Effect	Reference
botulinal toxin A					
α-fraction (IV)	mouse	-	0.000,000,27	LD 50	Dasgupta et al., 1966
unfractionated (IP)	"	-	0.000,001,4	LD 50	Lamanna & Carr, 1967
same (PO)	"	-	0.001,4	LD 50	Lamanna & Carr, 1967
same (PO)	man	-	<0.000,014	LD	Schantz & Sugiyama, 1974
O-ethyl-methyl-S-phosphorylthio-choline iodide (IP)	"	-	0.03	LD 50	Holmstedt, 1959
N,N'-di-n-butylphos-phorodiamine fluoride (IM)	chicken	F	2.0	LD 50	Davies et al., 1966
same (IM)	"	F	0.05	para[a]	Davies et al., 1966
dibenzanthracene (SC)	mouse	M	0.76	ED 50[b]	Bryan & Shimkin, 1943
methylcholanthrene(SC)	"	M	0.96	ED 50[b]	Bryan & Shimkin, 1943
benzpyrene (SC)	"	M	4.6	ED 50[b]	Bryan & Shimkin, 1943
aldicarb	rat	M	0.8	LD 50	Gaines, 1969
tetraethylpyro-phosphate	"	M	0.8	LD 50	Gaines, 1969
parathion	"	M	13	LD 50	Gaines, 1960
endrin	"	M	17.8	LD 50	Gaines, 1960
arsenic trioxide	"	M	72	LD 50	Gaines, 1968
nicotine sulfate	"	F	83	LD 50	Gaines, 1960
DDT	"	M	113	LD 50	Gaines, 1960
pyrethrum	"	M	470	LD 50	Gaines, 1968
acetylsalicyclic acid	"	-	1,360	LD 50	Eagle & Carlson, 1950
malathion	"	M	1,375	LD 50	Gaines, 1960
sodium chloride	"	M	3,550	LD 50	Gaines, 1968
difenphos	"	M	8,600	LD 50	Gaines et al., 1967

a. para = paralysis   b. carcinogenesis

pounds all produce a similar clinical picture, but difenphos does so only at a dosage over 10,000 times greater than that required by tepp. In the last analysis, the toxicity of each compound must be judged on its own merits.

Compounds also show variation in inherent toxicity when given repeatedly. Butler (1965) reported that aflatoxin, a poison elaborated in food by certain fungi, produces cancer in rats when given at a dosage of only 0.01 mg/day, while the synthetics dimethylnitrosamine and butter yellow require dosages of 0.75 and 9.0 mg/day, respectively, to produce the same effect.

The fact that some compounds are inherently likely to produce chronic illness whereas others produce acute poisoning only, regardless of the duration of intake, was discussed in Section 2.1.2 but must be reemphasized here.

2.4.1.2 Derived Compounds. Not only do compounds differ in their inherent toxicity, but they differ in the ease with which they undergo chemical change. Some pesticides may decompose during storage. Others change when their residues are exposed to ultraviolet light, plant enzymes, or soil microorganisms. Thus, one or more derivatives, in addition to the original compound, may be absorbed by men or animals exposed in one of several ways, including exposure by eating food treated earlier by a pesticide. Of course, nearly all compounds (whether viewed as primary or derivative) are metabolized following absorption by man or animals. No two compounds are exactly alike. Each derivative and metabolite will differ chemically and toxicologically in some degree from its precursor.

There is no rule regarding the relative toxicity of compounds and their nonmetabolic derivatives. Metabolism tends to render compounds more water-soluble and less toxic, but there are exceptions. Peters coined the term "lethal synthesis" in 1951 for biotransformation of a compound to a significantly more toxic product (see Section 3.1.4).

Full understanding of the toxicology of each pesticide can be acquired only through recognition and study of its derivatives as well as the primary compound. Such study may reveal that the toxicity of a compound depends on a lethal synthesis. This discovery may or may not suggest the possibility of some preventive or therapeutic measure. However, in no event will discovery of the details change the inherent toxicity of the primary compound. Contrary to what some lay persons seem to think, parathion is no more—or less—toxic since the discovery that its toxicity depends largely on its conversion to paraoxon.

2.4.2 Dosage

Control of dosage is the basis of all safety in the use of chemicals. This rule applies not only to compounds of relatively high toxicity but also to compounds of low toxicity including those necessary to life. Babies have been killed by putting salt in their formula in place of sugar (Finberg *et al.*, 1963), and it is said that the ancient Chinese carried out executions using water as a toxicant. On the other hand, all of us tolerate traces of arsenic, lead, and mercury (Monier-Williams, 1949), which are naturally occurring elements widely distributed in food and water. They are found in marine fish and in undeveloped areas where they have no use in industry or as pesticides.

A sufficiently large dosage of an ordinarily harmless material is fatal. On the other hand a sufficiently small dosage of the most virulent poison is without effect. For every compound, dosage can make the difference between health and death; in this sense the importance of this factor is infinite.

Although age, nutrition, and perhaps other factors, may be independent determinants of toxicity in animals of the same strain and sex (see Sections 2.4.10 and 2.4.11), it is astonishing how infrequently the effective dosage for small and large (mainly juvenile and mature) animals of the same strain can be distinguished statistically. This conclusion is consistent with the results of a study of botulinum toxin (Lamanna and Hart, 1968), certainly the most thorough investigation of the relation between body size and effective dosage. Even though the extreme affinity of botulinum toxin for its receptor is unique, it still follows that strain and species differences, which involve many compounds and often are substantial, cannot be explained by differences of size *per se*. Similarly the striking difference of the susceptibility of young and old rats to antu cannot be explained by their size. Dosage-response relationships that are truly different are emphasized, not hidden, when expressed in terms of body weight.

2.4.3 Schedule of Dosage

It is common knowledge among toxicologists that the schedule of dosage may have an important influence on the quantitative results. Usually anything that permits greater detoxification or excretion of a toxin tends to reduce the injury it produces. An oral dose given on an empty stomach is absorbed over a briefer period than the same dose administered when the stomach is at least partly full. Ingestion of a certain daily dosage mixed in the diet often is less injurious than the same dosage of the same compound administered daily by stomach tube. The compound reaches a lower maximal concentration in blood and other tissues when the same dosage is distributed throughout the day rather than being concentrated in a brief period. The microsomal enzymes, excretion, and other defenses may be able to cope indefinitely with a low concentration of compound but may not be capable of handling peak levels.

Similar reasoning applies to schedules that permit rest periods as compared to those that do not. Truly continuous exposure is usually more damaging than intermittent exposure at the same daily rate. An example may be cited for lead (Kehoe, 1961). It must be noted, however, that the distinction between continuous and intermittent exposure is blurred somewhat for a compound stored like lead.

An even more dramatic example involves carbon tetrachloride studied in connection with the possible continuous exposure of men in submarine vessels or stations. It was found that intermittent exposure (8 hours day, 5 days week) to carbon tetrachloride at a concentration of 515 mg/m^3 killed a small proportion of experimental animals and caused injury, especially to the liver, of many of those that survived for 6 weeks. About the same degree of injury was produced by continuous exposure at a concentration of only 61 mg/m^3, and this occurred within about the first 6 weeks (Prendergast et al., 1967). Thus, under these conditions, continuous exposure was about 8 times more dangerous dose-for-dose than intermittent exposure similar in schedule to much occupational exposure.

The cited work by Prendergast and his colleagues and earlier related work by the same and other groups of investigators offer some indication that a considerably smaller dosage of each of a number of compounds is required to cause injury if exposure is continuous rather than intermittent. Unfortunately, many of the investigations are reported in such a way that a meaningful comparison is impossible. Since many people are exposed to air pollution, some of them continuously, it seems tragic not to compare the effects of continuous and intermittent exposure at equal intervals of time since initial exposure. This is particularly true because the equipment and procedure for continuous exposure is specialized and costly. As long as tests are to be done, little difficulty or expense would be added by gathering and presenting comparable data. Certainly the number of persons now exposed continuously to ordinary air pollution is vast compared to the number who will enter the closed atmos-

pheres of spacecraft or submarine vessels or stations in the foreseeable future.

The general rule that rest periods and avoidance of peak blood levels tend to be protective usually applies best to compounds that are easily detoxified and excreted, and least to compounds against which the defenses of the body are inherently poor, with the result that the compounds or their effects are relatively cumulative. The cumulation may occur over relatively long periods as, for example, with lead, or over short periods as, for example, with carbon monoxide. In the former case, the cumulation frequently involves months. In the latter case, the cumulative effect may involve hours or days but is not prominent in connection with longer periods. All of us inhale some carbon monoxide, and those who smoke tobacco inhale more than nonsmokers (Hanson and Hastings, 1993). Some garage workers encounter a level of exposure that is marginal in respect to injury. Higher levels of exposure involve progressively more hazard with the result that in some countries carbon monoxide kills more people than any other single compound.

In some instances (Saffiotti and Shubik, 1956; Waud et al., 1958), repeated small doses produce greater effect than a smaller number of larger ones even though the total dosage resulting from the larger number of applications is less. This relationship would appear to violate a dosage-response relationship. The explanation may involve a failure of one or a few doses to reach the target tissue. Prolonged action may be required when there is an inherent delay between the initial dose and first observed effect regardless of whether this effect follows one or more doses. The apparently inverted dosage-response may involve a purely pharmacological effect such as the depletion of tissue norepinephrine by reserpine (Waud et al., 1958) or it may involve toxic effects as discussed in a different way in Section 2.2.3.2.

The modifying effect of schedule and a number of other factors must be taken into account in any consideration of dosage. Tests to establish safe levels should involve the dosage schedule, route, and other conditions people are expected to encounter. When these modifying factors are taken into account, the paramount importance of dosage becomes even more evident.

2.4.4 Duration of Dosage

Weil and McCollister (1963) investigated the degree of toxicity revealed by short-term and long-term tests in rats. For 22 compounds, the ratios of the dosages producing the minimal effect observed in short-term and in 2-year feeding tests varied from 0.5 to 20.0 and averaged 2.9. Ratios greater than 1.0 indicated the degree of apparent increase in toxicity associated with long-term testing. Ratios less than 1.0 may have indicated adaptation, experimental variation, or both. It was possible to compare the maximal dosages of 33 compounds producing no effect; these ratios ranged from 0.5 to 12.0 and averaged 2.3.

Some methods for measuring the effects of duration of dosage are discussed in Sections 2.2.1.2, 2.2.2, and 2.2.3.2.

Similar studies were continued by Weil *et al.* (1969) and expressed in somewhat different terms. The comparisons involved 20 compounds including 11 pesticides. The LD 50 values were determined and the compounds were fed to rats for 7 and 90 days, respectively. The results were compared to those in 2-year studies done earlier. The LD 50 values offered a poor indication of the results of repeated dosing. However, the results of long-term exposure could be predicted in an efficient way from the results of exposure lasting only 7 days. Using subscripts to indicate the number of days of exposure, it was found that the relationships for predicting the lowest dosage large enough to produce a minimal effect (MiE) were those shown in Table 2-6.

2.4.5 Route of Exposure

The route by which a compound is absorbed helps to determine not only the ease of absorption, but also, in some instances, the ease of metabolism. Compounds are usually more toxic by the oral than by the dermal route, and this was true of 64 of 67 compounds studied by Gaines (1960, 1969) and analyzed in this regard by Hayes (1967a). However, there were three exceptions, that is three compounds more toxic by the dermal route. Considering all 67 pounds, the factor of difference by which oral toxicity exceeded dermal toxicity ranged from 0.2 to 21 and averaged 4.2.

The lesser toxicity of one of the compounds (isolan) by the oral route was markedly influenced by metabolism. Five of six rats survived infusion of isolan into an intestinal vein for an hour at a rate that led to death within 18 to 35 minutes in six comparable animals infused via the femoral vein (Gaines *et al.,* 1966). Thus, a single pass through the liver is sufficient to make the difference between life and death in connection with isolan, and this phenomenon helps to explain the high dermal, and low oral toxicity of the compound.

Gaines (1969) found that about one-third of the pesticides he tested had such a low or variable dermal toxicity that no LD 50 could be determined. Thus the true average difference beween oral and dermal toxicity is greater than that calculated for compounds for which definite dermal as well as oral LD 50 values can be measured. Furthermore, relatively low dermal toxicity may be characteristic of an even higher proportion of compounds generally than is true of pesticides.

For practical reasons, respiratory toxicity is studied and reported in terms of concentration of chemical and duration of exposure. Values obtained in this way cannot be converted easily to dosage in terms of body weight, and direct comparison with toxicity by other routes is not usually possible. Some notion of the respiratory toxicity of a compound may be inferred from its intravenous toxicity (DuBois and Geiling, 1959). However, the method is of limited value partly because gases and aerosols are absorbed by the respiratory tract to different degrees depending on the compound and the particle size.

Table 2-6

Ratios for Predicting the Results of Long-Term Feeding
from the Results of Short-Term Feeding

Slightly modified from Weil et al. (1969) by permission of Academic Press.

Value	Ratios for predicting result of	
	90-day feeding study	2-year feeding study
median value	$MiE_7/3.0$	$MiE_{90}/1.8$ or $MiE_7/5.4$
95th percentile	$MiE_7/6.2$	$MiE_{90}/5.7$ or $MiE_7/35.3$

2.4.6 Interaction of Compounds

In a broad sense, it is probable that all compounds in the body interact, directly or otherwise. Most of the interactions are so complex, obscure, or trivial that they remain unidentified. However, some foreign chemicals have distinct interactions in the body, and in some instances the mechanisms of these interactions have been identified.

2.4.6.1 Kinds of Interaction. The effects of different foreign chemicals may: (*a*) mutually interfere with one another; (*b*) be simply additive; or (*c*) potentiate one another. The essentially additive relation is most common. Both exceptional conditions—mutual antagonism and potentiation—may be of practical and theoretical importance. From a practical standpoint, interference (antagonism) between two compounds may cancel the benefit or antidote the injury expected from one of them. Potentiation may increase benefit or harm depending on circumstances. From a theoretical standpoint, study of either antagonism or potentiation often leads to a better understanding of the mechanisms of action of the compounds involved.

Methods of Measuring Interaction. It has been pointed out that, for statistical reasons, it is possible to estimate the dosage responsible for an ED 50 more accurately than the dosage responsible for some greater or lesser effect. It is for this reason that in studying the interaction of two or more compounds, they are often administered in equal fractions of their respective ED 50 values. If two compounds are compared, the dosages should be a geometric series based on one-half; for three compounds, the dosage should be a geometric series based on one-third, and so on. Thus, if the effects of two compounds are exactly additive, administration of half an ED 50 of compound A and half an ED 50 of compound B should result in exactly one ED 50 for the mixture. This relationship may be written as an equation: (1/2 ED 50 A + 1/2 ED 50 B) × 1.0 = 1 ED 50 M. If the compounds are antagonistic by a factor of 2, the relationship may be written: (1 ED 50 A + 1 ED 50 B) × 0.5 = 1 ED 50 M. If the effects of the compounds potentiate one another by a factor of 4, the relationship may be written (1/8 ED 50 A + 1/8 ED 50 B) × 4.0 = 1 ED 50 M. Written in this way the multiplicand indicates the ratio between the observed and the expected ED 50 for the mixture and expresses the degree and kind of interaction. Thus, 1.0 indicates an exactly additive relation, progressively smaller fractions indicate progressively greater antagonism, and numbers progressively greater than 1.0 indicate progressively

greater potentiation. Actually, the error of measurement is such that fractions or numbers differing from 1.0 by no more than a factor of 2 or 3 cannot be distinguished from the simple additive relationship.

In some instances, it is desirable to study the interaction of two compounds at many dosage ratios. The results of such tests may be recorded in a diagram such as that shown in Fig. 2-11. This kind of diagram apparently was introduced in 1926 through a paper devoted to theoretical and mathematical considerations (Loewe and Muischnek, 1926) and another dealing with the antagonism between barbital and aminopyrine (Kaer and Loewe, 1926). Loewe and Muischnek (1926) introduced the term "isobole" (from the Greek *isos* equal and *bolos* a blow or stroke) to designate a line passing through points of equal action or injury, eg, a series of ED 50 values resulting from administering two compounds in different ratios. In Fig. 2-11, the dotted line indicates all possible comparisons at equal ratios of the two ED 50 values. The three points on the diagram indicate the same relationships of dosage as those presented by the three equations in the preceding paragraph. The solid straight line is the isobole of exactly additive action at all dosage ratios. All lines (including the one shown) lying to the right and above this straight solid line represent some degree of antagonism. All lines (including the one shown) lying below and to the left of the straight solid one represent some degree of potentiation. Real curves are not always symmetrical.

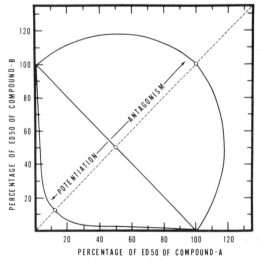

Fig. 2-11. Isoboles of ED 50 values of compounds A and B, illustrating additive, antagonistic, and potentiative interactions. See text.

A number of other theoretical relations or special cases in addition to additive, antagonistic, and potentiative have been mentioned but whether they exist in nature or can be meaningfully distinguished by the type of diagram shown in Fig. 2-11 is not clear. Examples include a combination of antagonism and synergism between the same pair of compounds at different dosage ratios, sensitization, and desensitization.

The axes of the diagram need not be measured off in percentage but may indicate dosage directly as shown in Fig. 2-12, which records the toxic (therapeutic) effect of pyrimethamine and sulfadiazine, administered both singly and together in various proportions, to combat malaria organisms infecting chicks.

Systematic Study of Interaction. Only a few studies have been made of the possible interactions of compounds in such a way that the results can be compared meaningfully. One such study was that of Keplinger and Deichmann (1967). It involved over 100 combinations of eight chlorinated hydrocarbon insecticides, six organic phosphorus insecticides, and one carbamate insecticide in sets of two and three compounds in rats and mice. The results were expressed as the quotient of the ratio of the expected to the observed LD 50 values. The largest quotient obtained was only 2.26, indicating a very small or even questionable potentiation between chlordane and methoxychlor in mice. The smallest quotient obtained was 0.36, indicating a minor degree of antagonism between aldrin and trithion in rats. The

data for combinations of three compounds did not reveal any effects of toxicity that could not have been predicted from the combination of two compounds.

In a 2-year rat-feeding study using a combination of six pesticides (DDT, aldrin, pyrethrin, piperonyl butoxide, malathion, and 2,4-D) and eight food additives at use levels or higher, significant alteration of toxicity in comparison with the toxicity of individual substances was not found (Fitzhugh, 1966).

For industrial chemicals as well as for pesticides, the most common joint action is a simple additive one (Smyth *et al.,* 1969).

Antagonism. Although, as just stated, some instances of interference are encountered in general surveys of interaction, the examples are usually small in magnitude and unexplained. The best examples, both from a practical and theoretical standpoint, involve antidotes, which are discussed under Section 8.2.3.

A rapid change in the degree of antagonism may be of more clinical significance than antagonism *per se.* For example, Cucinell and his colleagues (1966) reported a fatal hemorrhage in a patient who had received chloral hydrate and bishydroxycoumarin in combination without ill effect. However, when medication with chloral hydrate was stopped but bishydroxycoumarin was continued, the prothrombin time increased and hemorrhage occurred. It was later shown that chloral hydrate stimulates the metabolism of this anticoagulant. The danger lies in too rapid withdrawal of the inducer without an appropriate reduction in

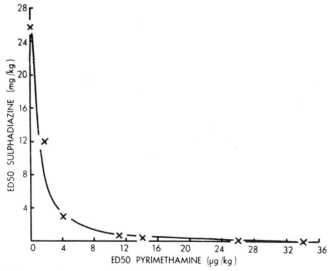

Fig. 2-12. ED 50's (dosages reducing parasitemia to 50% of the mean parasitemia of untreated controls) of pyrimethamine and sulfadiazine, administered both singly and together in various proportions to chicks infected with malaria. Each ED 50 was determined graphically from a dosage-response curve. Redrawn from Rollo (1955) by permission of the British Journal of Pharmacology.

the dose of anticoagulant. The same danger does not exist in connection with inducers that are stored to a significant degree in the tissues because, even if their administration is discontinued, their action decreases very gradually corresponding to their slow elimination.

Potentiation. A few examples of clinically important potentiation are known to involve pesticides. Many chlorinated hydrocarbon solvents and fumigants, notably carbon tetrachloride, are much more likely to injure the liver if alcohol is consumed about the same time. In a totally different way, the dithiocarbamate fungicides, which are closely related to Antabuse, interfere with the metabolism of alcohol so that it becomes more toxic.

True potentiation is a comparatively rare phenomenon except in connection with certain organic phosphorus insecticides and at least some classes of teratogens. The reason for the interaction of organic phosphorus compounds is that many of them inhibit aliesterases responsible for the efficient detoxification of some other members of the same class (Su *et al.*, 1971). This is the mechanism that explains the potentiation of the toxicity of malathion by EPN when the dosage of both is substantial (Murphy and DuBois, 1957). However, if the dosage of the two compounds is sufficiently small, there is enough enzyme to detoxify both of them, and the phenomenon of potentiation is not manifest. Rider *et al.* (1959) have shown that people can tolerate 3 mg/day of EPN plus 16 mg/day of malathion or 6 mg/day of EPN plus 8 mg/day of malathion for prolonged periods without significant depression of red cell or plasma cholinesterase. The combination of 6 mg/day of EPN plus 16 mg/day of malathion (Rider *et al.*, 1959) or 16 and 5 mg/man/day, respectively (Moeller and Rider, 1962a), did produce asymptomatic depression of both enzymes, but the effect was only additive. No potentiation was noted. The highest dosage of malathion alone tolerated without even slight inhibition of cholinesterase is 16 mg/man/day (Moeller and Rider, 1962a), whereas that for EPN is 6 mg/kg/day (Rider *et al.*, 1959). Thus, potentiation among this class of compounds may be important for overexposed workers but not for people who eat ordinary residues.

Other mechanisms of interaction are outlined in Section 2.4.6.2.

In a study of the interaction of six recognized teratogens, it was found that all pairs showed appreciable potentiation of teratogenic action provided the dosage of each was above a level producing at least a 1% effect. In several instances, potentiation occurred even when one or more materials were given at subthreshold dosage. No such consistent pattern of interaction was observed as regards intrauterine death (Wilson, 1964).

It seems likely that the mechanism of cocarcinogenesis will not be explained until neoplasia itself is explained. However, in what may have been the only quantitative study of this kind of potentiation, a dosage-response relationship was found not only for 9,10-dimethyl-1,2-benzanthracene but also for it in combination with the carcinogen croton oil (Graffi, 1953).

Whether potentiation will be of any practical importance depends on its degree and on the chance a person or useful animal may have of adequate and essentially simultaneous exposures to two potentiating compounds. Potentiation as high as 4- or 5-fold, such as that seen with some organic phosphorus insecticides, is of limited toxicological importance. The chance that a person or useful animal will encounter both members of a potentiating pair is smaller than the chance of encountering either one separately. This is especially true because, to be effective, the two compounds must be absorbed at about the same time and at dosages not very different from those that would be dangerous if only a single compound were absorbed. Traces are not effective.

Potentiation may be of critical importance in isolated instances, but it is virtually impossible to predict them, partly because there may be no apparent—and, therefore, predictive—pharmacological relationship between the two compounds involved and also because the mechanism of their interaction (Section 2.4.6.2) may not be known before the fact. An exception involves the organic phosphorus insecticides. DuBois *et al.* (1968) developed a quantitative procedure for measuring the potency of these compounds to inhibit aliesterases and amidases that are critical to their detoxification. DuBois (1972) has suggested that the use of this procedure constitutes a practical method of determining the dietary levels that might potentiate the toxicity of pharmacologically active compounds normally detoxified by esterases.

A factor of more than 100 times was found for potentiation between malathion and triorthocresylphosphate (Murphy *et al.*, 1959). Although triorthocresylphosphate is an organic phosphorus compound it is not a pesticide. Potentiating compounds need not belong to the same chemical class. An example is the potentiation of the toxicity of parathion by chlorophenothiazine (Gaines, 1962). Furthermore, the chance of encountering two compounds at about the same time is not always random. Striking exceptions are compounds used in related procedures, including drugs taken concurrently or used to treat intoxication. The reason for singling out drugs is that many are taken at dosages that equal or exceed the daily dosages of pesticides absorbed by the most exposed workers. Of course, the exact opposite of potentiation is expected when exposure to a toxicant and its antidote are associated either for prophylaxis or treatment. However, less thoroughly studied combinations of toxicants and drugs might prove to be potentiating, particularly if the drug is taken at about the same time that the toxicant has been absorbed in sufficient dosage to produce illness. In this situation, even a moderate degree of potentiation might prove critical.

It is important that the clinician be aware of the possibility of interaction and that appropriate studies be made in all cases in which poisoning appears to have occurred but in which the degree of known exposure seems inadequate to account for the observed effects.

2.4.6.2 Mechanisms of Interaction.

Compounds interact in the body by a wide range of mechanisms including chelation, alteration of ionization, alteration of protein binding, and the inhibition, reactivation, or induction of enzymes. Original access to the body may be altered by some of these same mechanisms or by solvents, by ion-exchange resins or adsorptive colloids, or by a change of the intestinal flora. The final pharmacological or toxicological effect of one or more interactions usually cannot be predicted except by careful study of a pair of compounds. The mechanisms involved in interaction of compounds are described at greater length in other sections as noted in the following brief summary.

The possible complexity of interactions must be emphasized. For example, calcium disodium edetate (EDTA) is useful for removing lead from the body (Section 8.2.3.4), but treatment that is too intense or prolonged or the use of certain other chelating agents can cause injury by disturbing the distribution of essential trace metals in the tissues. In their net effects, charcoal (Section 8.2.3.1) and ion-exchange resins are similar to chelating agents.

Section 3.2.1.2 describes the tremendous differences in transport that can be made by differences in ionization within tolerated limits of pH.

The discussion of protein binding (Section 3.2.1.3) includes an illustration of competition for binding sites as the basis for the interaction of two compounds.

The action of several pesticides depends on the inhibition of enzymes. The success of several antidotes depends on their ability to reactivate these inhibited enzymes. Thus EDTA, BAL, and other chelating agents (Section

8.2.3.4) may restore enzymes blocked by heavy metals. Oximes such as 2-PAM (Section 8.2.3.3) may restore enzymes blocked by organic phosphorus compounds. Combined use of nitrites and sodium thiosulfate releases cytochrome oxidase blocked by cyanide (Section 8.2.3.5).

The matter of enzyme induction is described in Section 3.1.2.2. When the same substrate and enzyme are involved, inhibition and induction have opposite pharmacological effects. Thus, inhibition of liver S-desulfurase by SKF 525-A or by feeding a protein-free diet antagonizes the action of azinphosmethyl. Conversely, induction of the same enzyme by 3-methylcholanthrene or 3,4-benzpyrene potentiates the action of the insecticide (Murphy and DuBois, 1958). Under different circumstances (especially the involvement of an enzyme of opposite pharmacological action) the effect of inhibition and induction may be reversed. For example, inhibition of liver aliesterase by EPN, TOCP, or a number of other compounds potentiates the action of malathion (Murphy *et al.*, 1959; Murphy and Cheever, 1968).

No doubt other mechanisms of interaction could be identified.

Effect of Formulation. The toxicity of a compound may be modified by differences in formulation. Solvents are especially important in this connection, but wetting agents and other ancillary compounds may be involved. When these chemicals promote or retard the toxicity of a pesticide, it is usually through promotion or retardation of absorption. The facilitating action may involve injury to a barrier, especially in the skin (see Section 3.2.2.5). Increase in absorption may also involve a solvent that, by its own ready absorption, helps to carry the toxicant along as discussed in the same section and illustrated in Table 3-9.

Importance of Environmental Chemicals. The source of a compound that influences the toxicological or pharmacological action of a recognized compound is not always obvious. A striking example is the alteration of drug metabolism in rats and mice by cedarwood bedding in their cages (Ferguson, 1966; Vesell, 1967; Wade *et al.*, 1968). Another example is the change in reaction to molybdenum caused by the traces of zinc derived from galvanized cages (see Section 2.4.11.3). An example from human experience of a toxic interaction that was at first obscure is that between exposures to asbestos dust and cigarette smoke.

2.4.7 Species and Strain Differences

2.4.7.1 Differences between Parasites and

Hosts. There is a tendency to ignore as objects of scientific interest and wonder the differences in the susceptibility of pests and of organisms we hope to protect. This attitude may be justified if the difference is based more on difference in exposure than on inherent susceptibility. The difference cannot be ignored when it involves "systemics," that is, pesticides used as drugs to combat parasites on or in their host. Examples of systemics for mammals include crufomate, trichlorfon, dichlorvos, ronnel, and coumaphos. Some of these compounds were originally developed to destroy botflies that pass their larval stages in the tissues of cattle, the mucous membranes or nasal sinuses of sheep, or the stomach and anterior small intestines of horses. Ronnel is used as a systemic treatment for fleas and the action of dichlorvos on fleas may be partially systemic. During the early studies, it was found that control extended to some but not all species of nematodes, including some in the tissues rather than the intestinal lumen. Trichlorfon has been used to treat helminthiasis, including ankylostomiasis, ascariasis, trichuriasis, and creeping eruption in man (Cerf *et al.*, 1962). The expected pharmacological effects of the drug did appear as side effects but these effects were no more severe or frequent than those of other anthelminthics. Trichlorfon was also tried by others to treat schistosomiasis but later work showed it to be essentially ineffective.

The control of botfly larvae and fleas is certainly due to the anticholinesterase and other antiesterase action of the drugs and no other mode of action is known against the susceptible nematodes. The fact that the compounds can be effective against parasites in the tissues without injuring the host is striking evidence of very great difference in susceptibility to absorbed drug. The mechanism of the difference is poorly understood but probably depends on the greater susceptibility of the esterases of the parasite and the greater metabolic power of the microsomal enzymes of the host.

(It may be noted that systemics for plants are compounds capable of being absorbed by one part of the plant and then translocated to another part so that the plant becomes pesticidal. Absorption is usually by the roots but may be by the leaves or other plant organs.)

2.4.7.2 Differences between Vertebrates. As a general rule, small species of warm blooded animals eat more food than large ones in relation to their body weight. Therefore, if both kinds receive the same contaminated diet, the small species will receive a larger dosage of toxicant. The relationship is illustrated in Appendix IV.

However, the most notable examples of species differences do not depend on differences in food intake but are inherent. Sometimes the inherent difference may be explained in terms of metabolic or genetic differences as discussed in Section 3.1.3. Very large differences in susceptibility are more likely among species belonging to different phyla but may occur among species of the same class. Norbormide is associated with a wide range of susceptibility among mammalian species. The LD 50 for albino Norway rats is 4.3 mg/kg, while dogs, cats, monkeys, sheep, chickens, and turkeys are unaffected by single doses at the rate of 1000 mg/kg (Roszkowski *et al.*, 1964; Roszkowski, 1965). Thus, the factor of difference for these species for norbormide is greater than 230. Even the wild strain of Norway rat is less susceptible (LD 50, 12 mg/kg). Another example of marked species susceptibility involves ducks and diazinon (see Section 10.4).

Apparently the largest difference in species susceptibility that has been measured involves the teratogenic effects of thalidomide. Human embryos have been deformed by as little as 0.5 to 1.0 mg/kg taken daily by the mother for several days. At the other extreme, no injury to cat embryos was produced by a maternal dosage of 500 mg/kg/day, indicating a difference of more than 1,000-fold. In fact, all other species studied require a dosage greater than that which is teratogenic in some women. The rabbit responds rather uniformly to dosages of 30 to 50 mg/kg/day, whereas many strains of rats fail to respond to 4,000 mg/kg/day even though a dosage of 50 mg/kg/day is teratogenic in a few strains (Kalter, 1965).

Some differences between species may be of such degree as to be essentially qualitative. Examples include the propensity of ducks to develop cataracts of the lens in response to dinitro compounds, or that of hens and man to develop delayed but permanent paralysis in response to triorthocresylphosphate and some other organic phosphorus compounds. Although these are unusual situations, they emphasize how different from one another species can be.

Examination of Table 2-7 shows that for many pesticides the factor of difference in susceptibility of the mouse, guinea pig, rabbit, and dog ranges from 0.2 to 11.8 and averages close to 1.0 as compared to the susceptibility of the male rat. The fact that the species difference is usually small is confirmed by comparisons based on the kind of test that may be applied to both people and experimental ani-

Table 2-7

Relative Susceptibility of Different Species to Pesticides
Based on Oral LD 50 Values (Gaines, 1960; FAO-WHO, 1965;
Lehman, 1965) and Using the Male Rat as Standard.
From Hayes (1967a) by permission of the Royal Society, London.

Compound	Susceptibility factor [a]			
	mouse	guinea-pig	rabbit	dog
chlorobenzilate	1.4	--	--	--
DDT	0.3 - 0.8	0.3	0.3 - 0.5	--
methoxychlor [b]	2.7 - 3.8	--	--	--
lindane	1.0	0.7 - 0.9	0.4 - 1.5	--
aldrin	0.9 - 1.2	1.2 - 1.6	0.5 - 1.1	0.4 - 0.8
chlordane	0.8	--	1.1 - 3.4	--
dieldrin	1.2	0.9 - 1.0	0.9 - 1.0	0.7 - 0.8
endrin	--	0.5 - 2.7 [c]	1.8 - 6.2	--
heptachlor	0.6 - 1.5	0.8 - 0.9	--	--
azinphosmethyl	1.6	0.2	--	--
Chlorthion (R)	0.7	--	--	--
diazinon	0.9 - 1.4	0.3	0.8	--
dimethoate	3.0 - 5.4	0.5 - 0.9	--	--
dioxathion	--	--	--	1.1 - 11.8
malathion	1.6 - 1.9	--	--	--
methyl parathion	0.4	--	--	--
mevinphos	0.9 - 1.6	--	--	--
oxydemetonmethyl	1.0 - 2.5	0.3 - 0.6	--	--
parathion	0.2 - 5.0	1.6 - 3.2	0.5 - 3.0	--
phosphamidon	1.3	--	--	--

a.   A factor of less than 1.0 indicates less susceptibility than that of the
      male rat; a factor greater than 1.0 indicates greater susceptibility.

b.   Both sexes.

c.   Approximate.

mals, or on information obtained in connection with accidents to man. Such comparisons of the susceptibility of man and animals are shown in Tables 2-8 and 2-9. Inspection of the tables indicates, for example, that man is more susceptible than the rat to lindane, about equally susceptible as the female rat to parathion, and distinctly less susceptible to warfarin than rats of either sex. Although in many instances in which a direct comparison is possible there is no marked difference, the difference appears to be about 100-fold for a few compounds and over 1,000-fold for thalidomide. Furthermore, the tables by necessity involve phenomena that can be studied in laboratory animals. Much of the reason for making tests in man is the existence of hypersensitivity, subjective responses, and other phenomena that do not lend themselves to study in animals.

Certain animals do lend themselves to testing for a limited number of specific forms of toxicity. Thus, hens are used to screen for possible neurotoxicity of organic phosphorus compounds, not only because they are highly susceptible to this injury, but because this susceptibility seems to resemble that of man. In a similar way, ducks are used to test the tendency of dinitro compounds to cause cataract. Additional (but often less clearcut) examples are given in Chapter 4. Section 4.3 lists useful references on laboratory animals.

The ideal scheme would be to have a species of experimental animal resembling man so closely in susceptibility to poisons that any differences would be unimportant. Unfortunately, no such animal has been identified or is likely to exist. Monkeys and apes have been suggested. They are valuable for special purposes, but there is no convincing evidence that their average value is greater than that of any other laboratory animal. In some instances they are distinctly inferior to other animals. For example, when fed DDT, the rhesus monkey metabolizes little or no DDE, although both rats and man form this compound readily (Durham et al., 1963).

Variation between species must be considered every time a new compound that has been properly tested in animals is used for the first time. It is frequently suggested that the tests be made in a large number of species. If the results in the different animals are similar, it is likely that human response to the compound will not be greatly different. If, however, there is a wide variation in the response of different

Table 2-8

Comparison of the Susceptibility of Man and Other Animals to Certain
Pesticides. All doses are single and oral unless otherwise noted.
From Hayes (1967a) by permission of the Royal Society, London.

Compound	Species	Dosage (mg/kg)								References
		Largest without clinical effect	Smallest with clinical effect	Median clinical CD 50	Smallest with serious effect	Largest non-fatal	Smallest fatal	LD 50	Uniformly fatal	
DDT	man	--	6	10	16[a]	285[b]	--	--	--	Garrett, 1947; Hsieh, 1954; Neal et al., 1946; Velbinger, 1947; Hayes, 1959
	rat, F	--	--	--	75	150	100	118	200	Gaines[c]
	rat, M	25	--	--	50	175	50	113	200	Gaines[c]
lindane	man	--	0.4[d]	0.4[d]	0.5[a]	--	--	--	--	Graeve and Herrnring, 1951
	rat, F	--	--	--	--	125	75	91	--	Gaines[c]
	rat, M	--	--	--	50	125	75	87	200	Gaines[c]
	calf	2.5	--	--	5	--	--	--	--	Radeleff et al., 1955
chlordane	man	--	--	--	32[a,b]	--	--	--	--	Dadey and Kammer, 1953
	man	--	--	--	--	--	29-57	--	--	Hayes, 1963
	infant	--	--	--	10[a]	--	--	--	--	Lensky and Evans, 1952
	rat, F	100	200	--	300	550	350	430	600	Gaines[c]
	rat, M	--	--	--	250	400	250	335	450	Gaines[c]
dieldrin	man	--	--	--	10	--	--	--	--	Princi, 1952
	rat, M,F	--	--	--	30	60	30	46	--	Gaines[c]
endrin	man	--	--	--	0.2	--	--	--	--	Davies and Lewis, 1956
	rat, F	--	--	--	6	10	6	7.5	--	Gaines[c]
	rat, M	--	--	--	10	25	10	17.8	30	Gaines[c]
dichlorvos	man	--	--	--	51	--	--	--	--	Hayes, 1963
	rat, F	--	--	--	--	100	37	56	125	Gaines[c]
	rat, M	--	--	--	--	125	75	80	150	Gaines[c]
	cow	--	--	--	27	--	--	--	--	Tracy et al., 1960
	horse	--	--	--	25	--	--	--	--	Jackson et al., 1960
diazinon	man	--	--	--	2.2[e]	--	--	--	--	Hayes, 1963
	man	--	--	--	--	250	--	--	--	Bockel, 1957
	rat, M	--	--	--	200	300	200	250	350	Gaines[c]
	calf	--	--	--	1	--	10	--	--	Radeleff et al., 1955
malathion	man	--	--	--	--	200	71	--	--	Walters, 1957; Paul, 1960
	rat, F	--	--	--	750	1,250	750	1,000	1,500	Gaines[c]
	rat, M	500	--	--	1,000	1,750	1,000	1,375	2,000	Gaines[c]
	sheep	150	100	--	100	300	150	--	--	Radeleff et al., 1955
parathion	man	--	--	--	--	6.4	2.0	--	13	Goldblatt, 1950; Hayes, 1963
	child	--	--	--	--	--	0.1	--	--	Kanagaratnam et al., 1960
	rat, F	--	--	--	1	4.5	3.0	3.6	5	Gaines[c]
	rat, M	5.0	--	--	10	20	10	13.0	30	Gaines[c]
	calf	--	--	--	0.5	--	1.5	--	--	Radeleff et al., 1955
	sheep	50	--	--	--	75	20	--	--	Radeleff et al., 1955
	steer	25	--	--	--	--	--	--	--	Radeleff et al., 1955
tepp	man	--	0.05	--	3.5	--	--	--	--	Grob and Harvey, 1949; Grob et al., 1950
	rat, M	--	--	--	--	--	1.0	1.05	--	Gaines[c]

a. Convulsions.
b. Part of dose vomited.
c. Based partly on published papers (Gaines, 1960; 1969) and partly on the original data from which the papers were drawn.
d. 3 times a day for 3 days; highly dispersed formulation.
e. Dermal.

species, then conservatism forces us to suppose, until there is direct evidence to the contrary, that man may be at least as sensitive as the most susceptible species.

No matter what the pattern of response in experimental animals, the ultimate test must be in man. It is best that such tests be carried out under circumstances permitting scientific observations (see Chapter 5).

2.4.8 Individual Differences

Individual differences are apparent in every toxicological test including those carried out on people. Study of a paper by Gaines (1969), in which he reports the acute oral toxicity of pesticides, shows that for 69 compounds the LD 50 value for male rats ranged from 1.20 to 7.14 times greater than the corresponding LD

1 value. The average factor of difference was 2.42. The corresponding factors of difference for the dermal toxicity of 42 pesticides were 1.37 to 14.93 with an average of 3.00. In other words, judged in this way individual variation although very real is usually relatively small. In studies of storage and excretion, the greatest individual average excretion of malathion-

Table 2-9

Comparison of the Susceptibility of Man and Other Animals to Repeated Doses of Certain Pesticides. All doses are oral unless otherwise noted.

From Hayes (1967a) by permission of the Royal Society, London.

Compound	Species	Dosage (mg/kg/day)	Duration (days)	Results	References
DDT	man	0.5	>600	increased storage; no clinical effect	Hayes et al., 1956
	rat, M, F	0.24	161	histopathological changes of the liver	Laug et al., 1950
methoxychlor	man	2	56	no effect	Stein et al., 1965
	rat, M, F	4.87	750	no effect level	Lehman, 1965
demeton	man	0.05	24	15% reduction of plasma ChE only	Moeller & Rider, 1962b
	rat, F	0.05	112	no significant depression of ChE	Barnes & Denz, 1954
	rat, F	0.14	112	30% inhibition of ChE	Barnes & Denz, 1954
	rat, F	0.24	66	60% reduction of plasma and 40% reduction of RBC ChE	Gaines, unpub. results
	dog, M, F	0.025	168	no significant depression of ChE	Frawley & Fuyat, 1957
	dog, M, F	0.047	168	significant depression of ChE	Frawley & Fuyat, 1957
dimofox	man	0.002	70	no effect on ChE	Edson, 1964
	man	0.0034	70	25% reduction of whole blood ChE	Edson, 1964
	rat, F	0.024	28	about 50% inhibition of RBC ChE; no effect on plasma ChE	Edson, 1964
	rat, F	0.095	28	75% reduction of RBC ChE; 25% reduction of plasma ChE	Edson, 1964
	rat, F	0.475	28	almost complete inhibition of RBC ChE 75% reduction of plasma ChE	Edson, 1964
dioxathion	man	0.05	59	no inhibition of RBC and plasma ChE	Frawley et al., 1963
	man	0.1	28	slight inhibition of plasma ChE; no effect on RBC ChE	Frawley et al., 1963
	rat, M, F	0.22	91	no significant effect on ChE	Frawley et al., 1963
	rat, M, F	0.78	91	significant reduction of RBC and plasma ChE	Frawley et al., 1963
	dog, M, F	0.25	12	marked effect on plasma ChE; no effect on RBC ChE	Frawley et al., 1963
	dog, M, F	0.8	12	marked effect on plasma ChE; no effect on RBC ChE	Frawley et al., 1963
malathion	man	0.34	56	maximal reduction of 25% plasma and RBC ChE	Moeller Rider 1962a
	rat, F	3.2	90	29% reduction in RBC and no reduction of plasma ChE on 30th day; recovery by 90th day	Gaines, unpub. results
	rat, M	4.5	730	10 to 30% inhibition of plasma and RBC ChE	Hazelton & Holland, 1953
methyl parathion	man	0.1	24	15% reduction of plasma ChE only	Moeller & Rider, 1962b
	dog, M, F	0.94	84	significant depression of plasma and RBC ChE	Williams et al., 1959
parathion	man	0.1	42	33% reduction of whole blood ChE; 16% inhibition of RBC ChE; 37% inhibition of plasma ChE	Edson, 1964
	rat, F	0.07	90	no effect	Gaines, unpub. results
	rat, F	0.26	84	80% reduction of RBC ChE; slight inhibition of plasma ChE	Edson, 1964
	rat, F	0.35	90	37% reduction of plasma and 44% reduction of RBC ChE	Gaines, unpub. results
	dog	0.047	168	60% inhibition of plasma ChE	Frawley and Fuyat, 1957
	pig	4.0	49	80% inhibition of RBC ChE; no inhibition of plasma ChE	Edson, 1964
schradan	man	0.014	44	25% reduction of blood ChE	Edson, 1964
	man	0.06	60	77% inhibition of RBC ChE; 50% inhibition of plasma ChE	Edson, 1964
	rat, M, F	0.045	112	substantial reduction of ChE; no effect on plasma ChE	Edson, 1964
	rat, M	0.22	14-85	complete inhibition of RBC ChE	Edson, 1964
	pig, F	0.1	102	55% inhibition of RBC ChE; slight reduction of plasma ChE	Edson, 1964

Table 2-9 Continued

Compound	Species	Dosage (mg/kg/day)	Duration (days)	Results	References
arsenic trioxide	man	0.44	?	frequent mild poisoning	Sollmann, 1957
	sheep	10	---	tolerated without symptoms	Reeves, 1925
	horse	4.7	---	tolerated without symptoms	Reeves, 1925
warfarin	man	0.14	indef.	maintenance therapeutic dose	Friedman, 1959
	man	0.29-1.45	15	hemorrhage in 12 people (4 to 70 y) followed by recovery	Lange & Terveer, 1954
	man	1.7	6	hemorrhage in 22 y man followed by recovery	Holmes & Love, 1952
	man	0.83-2.06	15	fatal to boy (19 y) and girl (3 y)	Lange & Terveer, 1954
	rat, M, F	0.08	40	killed 5 of 10	Hayes & Gaines, 1959
	rat, M, F	0.39	15	killed all of 10 rats	Hayes & Gaines, 1959
2,4-D	man	14-37	18	tolerated	Seabury, 1963
	man	66	1	coma, hyporeflexia; incontinence	Seabury, 1963
	rat, F	15	112	tolerated	Hill & Carlisle, 1947
	dog	9	84	tolerated	Drill & Hiratzka, 1953

derived material differed from the smallest individual average excretion at the same dosage by factors of only 2.2 to 8.7 for different groups of people (Hayes *et al.*, 1960). Thus, the degree of difference was relatively constant in tests carried out at different dosage levels or at different times. A similar observation was made regarding the storage of DDT and the excretion of DDA in man. In separate tests, the maximal storage of DDT was 1.3 to 5.9 times the minimal storage at the same dosage level. For a single dosage group, the maximal rate of excretion of DDA by one man in any one day was 18.0 times greater than his own minimal rate, and the difference between the lowest minimum and highest maximum within the group was 21.5 times (Hayes *et al.*, 1971). In all of these tests the relative constancy of one individual as compared with another was noted.

Although individual differences may be understood in statistical terms, physiological understanding of it is lacking almost entirely. Of course, if a population is sufficiently heterozygous, the differences between individuals may depend on their genetic diversity. However, individual differences persist to some degree in a homozygous population. This is illustrated by the failure of the LD 50 values of four pesticides in a particular population of mice to change in the course of 12 or more generations even though each succeeding generation was bred from mice that had survived an LD 50 dose (Guthrie *et al.*, 1971).

2.4.9 Sex and Other Endocrines

2.4.9.1 Sex. Chiefly because of its convenience, the rat is used more than any other species for studies in toxicology. The rat also has the apparent distinction of showing more variation between the sexes in its response to

chemicals than any other species. This fact may have led to more concern than is justified regarding possible differences in the susceptibility of men and women to chemicals. In any event, calculations from data provided by Gaines (1960, 1969) for the oral toxicity of 69 pesticides showed that the difference in the oral LD 50 for male and female rats ranged from 0.21 (indicating greater susceptibility of the female) to 4.62 (indicating greater susceptibility of the male), and averaged 0.94. The corresponding factors for the dermal toxicity of 37 pesticides were 0.11 to 2.93 with an average of 0.81 (Hayes, 1967a). The differences in the susceptibility of male and female rats are associated to a large degree with differences in their liver microsomal enzymes (see Section 3.1.2.2).

In contrast to the situation in rats and to a lesser degree in other rodents, significant differences between the sexes of other species in their susceptibility to poisons usually have not been reported. Such differences were looked for but not found in relation to the storage of DDT in monkeys (Ortega *et al.*, 1956; Durham *et al.*, 1963). As discussed in Section 7.2.4.1, such differences among men and women are small or lacking entirely. Small, reported differences in the storage of chlorinated hydrocarbon insecticides in men and women are discussed in Section 7.2.4.1.

Pregnancy. Susceptibility to a particular compound may be either greater, less, or identical in pregnant females than in nonpregnant ones in the same strain and age. For example, pregnancy exaggerates the danger of anticoagulants but reduces the danger of paraquat. In some instances, such as susceptibility to anticoagulants, the reason for difference is clear. In most instances the reason is obscure.

In a systematic study of 19 drugs, given by

different routes, pregnant mice were more susceptible than nonpregnant ones by factors ranging from 0.74 to 14.55 and averaging 1.90—or only 1.27 if one excludes the single high value (Beliles, 1972).

2.4.9.2 Other Endocrines. There is considerable evidence that the pituitary adrenal axis may be influenced by photoperiodicity and in turn may influence susceptibility to toxicants (see Section 2.4.17).

2.4.10 Age

Children and young animals are often more susceptible than adults to poisons in food. The most common reason is that children and other young animals eat more than adults in proportion to their weight. Thus, when given the same contaminated food, young animals receive a higher dosage of toxicant. The relationship for rats is shown in Fig. 2-13. Although the figure is based on DDT, it applies equally well to any compound that does not cause a reduction of food intake.

However, other factors may be involved. It is now well known that a number of drugs are poorly metabolized by infants, particularly prematures (Fouts and Adamson, 1959). Although it is seldom possible to quantitate the difference, it is clear that a dosage of some drugs easily tolerated by human adults may lead to severe illness or even death in very young children.

Calves and sometimes lambs are markedly more susceptible than adult cattle or sheep to sprays or dips of chlordane, dieldrin, and lindane (Radeleff, 1964).

Systematic study of drugs (Hoppe *et al.*, 1965; Yeary and Benish, 1965) and pesticides (Brodeur and DuBois, 1963; Lu *et al.*, 1965) indicates that newborn animals are generally more susceptible than adults of the same species regardless of route of administration. However, the difference may be small and there are some exceptions in which the newborn are actually less susceptible than adults (Brodeur and DuBois, 1963; Hoppe *et al.*, 1965). As reviewed by Durham (1969), the difference, no matter what its direction, can often be explained in terms of the recognized activity of microsomal enzymes in activating or deactivating the chemical in question. Other factors that may be of importance are renal function and membrane permeability. Fortunately, compounds of similar pharmacological action tend to show similar differences in their toxicity to young and adult animals (Yeary and Benish, 1965). In studying drugs, Yeary and Benish found that newborn rats were 0.6 to 10.0 times more susceptible than adults. Hoppe *et al.* (1965) found a similar range of 0.7 to 6.2. Goldenthal (1971) studied a much larger number of drugs and a few other compounds (290 in all) and reported a much wider range of factors of difference: <0.02 to 750. However, by omitting only one low factor and eight high ones, the range was narrowed to 0.1 to 20. The geometric mean of all of the factors (no exceptions) was 2.78.

In their studies of 15 organic phosphorus

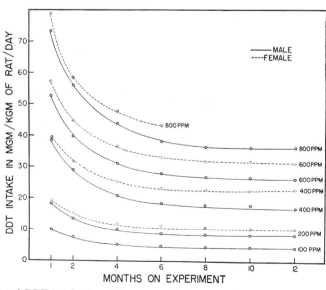

Fig. 2-13. Calculated DDT intake in milligrams per kilogram of body weight in rats receiving various levels of DDT in the diet. From Fitzhugh and Nelson (1947) by permission of The Williams & Wilkins Co., Baltimore.

insecticides or defoliants, Brodeur and DuBois (1963) found that weanling male rats were 0.2 to 4.1 times more susceptible than adults with a mean of 1.8. DDT is less toxic to infant rats than to adults (see Section 7.2.2.1).

2.4.11 Nutrition

2.4.11.1 General Nutritional Condition. Apparently only extremes of general nutrition have produced observable alterations in the toxicity of pesticides. As reviewed elsewhere (Hayes, 1959), various mammals and even fish are relatively resistant to poisoning by DDT if they are fat rather than thin. The same result has been produced with dieldrin under experimental conditions (Barnes and Heath, 1964). Other factors may be involved, but certainly distribution of the insecticide to adipose tissue tends to reduce the concentration of the insecticide at the site of action and thus protects the organism.

Paired feedings may be used to distinguish those effects of a toxicant secondary to reduced intake of food.

Effect of Starvation. If DDT is stored in body fat in sufficient concentration, rapid mobilization of the fat through starvation may lead to poisoning (Fitzhugh and Nelson, 1947). There is an increase in the concentration of poison in the small amount of fat remaining and, by the same token, in all tissues of the body (Dale *et al.*, 1962). During mobilization of DDT, excretion is increased by a factor of about 1.4, but the increase is insufficient to prevent poisoning in some rats. It was pointed out by Dale and associates that starvation is unlikely to precipitate poisoning by DDT in man because even people with heavy occupational exposure to the compound do not store enough of it to produce the effect and because the metabolism of man is inherently slower than that of the rat so that man cannot starve so fast.

Some other chlorinated hydrocarbon insecticides are excreted more efficiently than DDT. For example, Heath and Vandekar (1964) found that the average excretion of dieldrin in rats was relatively rapid (5%/day), and that it was more than doubled following a few days of starvation. Therefore, it is not astonishing that it was not possible to precipitate dieldrin poisoning in rats by starving them after they had been fed for 7 to 18 months at dietary levels up to 15 ppm (Treon and Cleveland, 1955).

The toxicological effects of weight loss associated with infection may be indistinguishable from those associated with starvation (see Section 2.4.14).

2.4.11.2 Effects of Protein.

Quantity of Dietary Protein. In addition to the action involving storage just discussed, nutrition may influence toxicity through metabolism promoted by the liver microsomal enzymes. Murphy and DuBois (1958) showed that male rats maintained on a protein-free diet for 4 weeks had only 24% as much microsomal enzyme activity as normal rats. Also, the liver enzymes of rats which did not receive protein could not be induced by compounds that orinarily stimulate these enzymes.

There is great variation in the influence of protein malnutrition on susceptibility to acute poisoning by different compounds. This variation may depend on: (*a*) the net effect of biotransformation, whether detoxication or toxication; (*b*) differences in the relative contribution of biotransformation to toxicity; (*c*) the ability of some compounds to cause anorexia or other disruption of nutrition; and (*d*) perhaps other mechanisms.

As an example of difference in the net effect of biotransformation, it may be recalled that the toxicity of aflatoxin, which is detoxified by the liver, is increased by protein deficiency, whereas the toxicity of carbon tetrachloride, which is rendered toxic by metabolism, is decreased greatly by protein deficiency (McLean and McLean, 1969).

The LD 50 of DDT and the associated clinicopathological effects showed only slight variation among rats previously maintained for 4 weeks on ordinary laboratory feed, and others fed a synthetic diet containing either normal protein (27% casein) or deficient protein (8% casein) (Boyd and De Castro, 1968). Even after a diet containing 0.0% protein, the toxicity of DDT was increased only 4-fold (Boyd and Krijnen, 1969b). By extreme contrast, the acute toxicity of captan was increased 2,100-fold in rats maintained without protein as compared to those fed normal protein (Krijnen and Boyd, 1970). The results for DDT, captan, and a number of other pesticides are summarized in Table 2-10. It may be seen that even a very great increase in protein is without important effect on susceptibility to pesticides. The same is true of a reduction of protein to only one-third of normal. However, when protein restriction is severe and especially when it is complete, susceptibility to some pesticides is increased dramatically. It must be recalled that rats that have been maintained without protein for 28 days from weaning weigh about 30% less than they did when placed on the diet. Two-thirds of such rats die in the first 3 days after their food is withdrawn even though

Table 2-10

Estimates of the Increase in the Acute Toxicity
of Certain Pesticides in Albino Rats as Related
to the Concentration of Protein in Their Diet,
during 28 Days from Weaning until Dosing.

From Boyd et al. (1970) by permission of the American Medical Society.

Agent	Percent in diet					Reference
	0.0	3.5	9.0	26.0	81.0	
captan	2,100.0	26.3	1.2	1.0	2.4	Krijnen & Boyd, 1970
carbaryl	8.6	6.5	1.1	1.0	1.0	Boyd & Krijnen, 1969a
CIPC	8.7	4.0	1.7	1.0	--	Boyd & Carsky, 1969
diazinon	7.4	1.9	1.8	1.0	2.0	Boyd et al., 1969
DDT	4.0	2.9	1.5	1.0	3.7	Boyd & Krijnen, 1969b
endosulfan	20.0	4.3	1.8	1.0	1.0	Boyd et al., 1970
lindane	12.3	1.9	1.0	1.0	1.8	Boyd et al., 1969
monuron	11.5	3.0	1.8	1.0	--	Boyd & Dobos, 1969
toxaphene	--	3.7	--	1.0	--	Boyd & Taylor, 1971

no chemical is administered. It is little wonder that their susceptibility to compounds that cause anorexia is striking.

Other compounds that have been studied in relation to protein deprivation include Banol®, parathion, and chlordane (Casterline and Williams, 1969), and dieldrin (Lee *et al.*, 1964).

In a thorough review of diet and toxicity, McLean and McLean (1969) emphasized the opposite effects of protein deficiency on the toxicity of compounds that are detoxicated and those that are toxicated by biotransformation (see Section 3.1.4), especially in those instances where the site of biotransformation is also the site of toxic injury. The reviewers also pointed out that reversal of one aspect of deficiency (such as the induction of microsomal enzymes by a foreign compound or by a component of natural diets in animals with borderline protein deficiency) may reverse the entire effect of diet on toxicity. Although there is evidence that malnourished people are unduly susceptible to infection, there is no clear evidence that the cell's general ability to withstand change and trauma is altered by malnutrition. The relation of nutrition to toxicity must be determined separately for each compound, and, under practical conditions, other factors must be taken into account.

Quality of Dietary Protein. The acute oral toxicity of heptachlor was found to be 1.6 to 2.1 times greater in rats pair-fed casein than in those fed on gluten, regardless of whether protein constituted 10 or 18% of the diet. The difference was less or even reversed when the casein diet was fed *ad lib.* and weight gain was greater (Webb and Miranda, 1973). Gluten is an incomplete protein that reduces food intake and permits only an abnormally small increase in body weight of rats that consume it *ad lib.* as their only source of protein. It seems likely that the lower toxicity of heptachlor in rats fed gluten depends on limited conversion of the compound to heptachlor epoxide as a result of limited activity of the microsomal enzymes of the liver. On the other hand, the even greater protection offered by normal intake of high quality protein may result from the presence of normal fat deposits and the sequestering of both heptachlor and its epoxide in the fat.

2.4.11.3 Miscellaneous Nutritional Effects. Deficiency of any essential trace element is injurious in itself. However, a borderline deficiency may predispose to injury by a toxicant. Furthermore, there may be an interaction in the metabolism of trace elements whether essential or not. For example, Brinkman and Miller (1961) found that rats fed molybdenum gained less weight and had lower hemoglobin levels if they were kept in galvanized cages instead of stainless steel cages. Similar effects were produced by increasing the zinc content of the diet of rats fed molybdenum and kept in stainless steel cages.

2.4.12 Isolation and Crowding

Either isolation or crowding may influence the behavior, biochemistry, and morphology of animals. Rodents have been most studied in this regard but it seems unlikely that nonrodents are immune. Although very few drugs have been studied in this way, enough work has been done to show that either isolation or crowding has a dramatic effect on the susceptibility of some strains to certain drugs, but little or no effect on their susceptibility to others.

Animals are caged separately in most tests of toxicity. This practice facilitates observation of each animal and permits measurement of individual food intake and collection of individual samples of excreta for analysis. It has been suggested (Hatch *et al.*, 1963) that the results of tests on isolated rats do not reflect the functioning of normal animals. It is true that many wild rodents tend to live in small groups and that common laboratory rodents will cluster if permitted to do so. Consideration of isolation and crowding might be crucial in the study of a rodenticide from the standpoint of rodent control. The ultimate objective of most toxicity testing is the safety of man, not that of rodents. However, in all tests of toxicity, there is a clear need to keep in mind the possible effects of isolation and crowding. Differences in the handling of animals may lead to marked differences in the results of tests in different laboratories, or in the same laboratory at different times.

2.4.12.1 Effects of Isolation and Aggregation.

Physiological Effects of Isolation. The effects of isolation may depend on sex, strain, and duration of isolation (Wiberg and Grice, 1965). When these factors are held constant, the effects may vary depending on the past history of each animal in regard to grouping (Thiessen, 1963). In other words, isolation changed the susceptibility of animals to crowding. Isolated mice had relatively heavier testes and showed much less locomotion in a standard test than mice held in groups of five each. However, when previously isolated mice were placed in groups of 10 each, they showed increased fighting, diminution of testis weight, and a higher level of locomotor activity than mice that had been in groups of five before being placed in groups of 10.

According to a review by Hatch *et al.* (1963), isolation of rats or mice for 10 days or less may produce lowered resistance to stress, lower food consumption and weight gain, and smaller adrenals, as compared to animals held in groups of two or more. Isolation longer than a month may produce the opposite effects, including greater food consumption and a tendency toward larger adrenals. In addition, lower weights of the thyroid, thymus, spleen, and ovary, an increase in oxygen consumption, and absolute leukopenia and eosinopenia have been observed. Other changes have been reported less commonly. The authors interpreted their own findings and those of others as indicating that isolation produces an endocrinopathy probably involving the adrenal cortex.

The effects of isolation are reversible when previously isolated rodents are grouped (Balazs *et al.*, 1962).

Effects of Isolation on Susceptibility to Chemicals. Isolation may have a marked effect on the reaction of rodents to some chemicals. In other instances, isolation may change the threshold of susceptibility but have little effect at the LD 50 level (Wiberg and Grice, 1965). A very dramatic effect of isolation and its duration on susceptibility to a drug is shown in Fig. 2-14. Not shown by the figure is the fact that rats conditioned by isolation for 3 months remained highly susceptible to isoprenaline even after they had been regrouped for a week (Balazs *et al.*, 1962).

Perhaps it is the conditioning produced by isolation rather than isolation itself which is of greatest or most frequent importance in influencing the action of chemicals. It was shown very early (Gunn and Gurd, 1940) that α-amphetamine is more toxic for aggregated than for isolated mice, and this result has been confirmed many times. Recently, it has been shown that this effect is very much more striking if the mice are isolated for an extended period before dosing and grouping. Thus, although the susceptibility of pre-

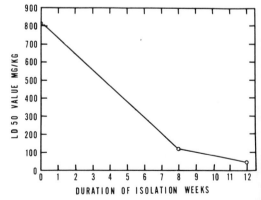

Fig. 2-14. Effect of isolation on susceptibility of rats to isoproterenol. Based on data from Hatch *et al.*, 1963.

grouped mice was increased by grouping as compared to isolation immediately after dosing (these mice died in an average of 53 minutes when grouped, but isolated ones survived 69 minutes), the susceptibility of preisolated mice was increased drastically by grouping but was also inherently greater (these mice died in an average of 14 minutes when grouped and even isolated ones suvived only 51 minutes) (Welch and Welch, 1966).

At least in connection with stimulants of the central nervous system, the effects of aggregation may be due to hyperpyrexia associated with increased motor activity resulting from greater response to external stimuli (Peterson and Hardinge, 1967).

It is impossible to discuss here the varied and complex differences in brain and adrenal catecholamines that have been shown to depend on group density. Enough has been said, however, to emphasize the importance of carrying out toxicological experiments under standardized conditions or of varying the conditions knowingly.

2.4.12.2 Effect of Crowding. Crowding is not merely the absence of isolation but a deviation from the norm in the opposite direction. It can cause striking clinical injury and social disintegration, at least in some species. The phenomenon has been studied mostly in relation to population control. In a review of this aspect, Christian and Davis (1964) concluded that excess population density leads to increased aggressiveness and other forms of competition and thus (through an endocrine feedback mechanism involving pituitary-adrenocortical activity and inhibition of reproduction), to regulation and limitation of population growth. This mechanism has been demonstrated for some rodents, lagomorphs, and deer, and it may apply to other mammals. According to this concept, other factors such as disease, predation, and weather limit populations occasionally, but the feedback mechanism remains as a safety device to prevent destruction of the environment and consequent extinction.

A tranquilizer can reduce aggression in a population and raise the limit at which the growth curve reaches equilibrium. After three populations of house mice had become crowded and aggression and reproduction had leveled off, chlorpromazine was added to the diet of two of the populations at a concentration of 750 ppm. Although this concentration of chlorpromazine slightly reduced the reproduction of individual pairs of mice tested separately, it decreased aggression and increased breeding success of the crowded mice. Population growth was renewed while the drug was being administered. When chlorpromazine was removed from one of the treated populations, the rate of aggression increased and the number of mice declined. The third population, which served as a control, declined slightly but probably not significantly while the other two increased under the influence of chlorpromazine (Vessey, 1967).

Although crowding (in the sense used in population dynamics) is not likely to occur in a toxicology laboratory, population density undoubtedly has a bearing on the practical use of rodenticides and other poisons to control pests.

2.4.13 Other Social or Psychological Factors

Anything that disturbs an animal may influence its physiological reactions and thus possibly change its reactions to foreign chemicals. In some instances, disturbance may have several components and it may be difficult to determine their relative importance. For example, each visit of the investigator or attendant to the animal room involves auditory, visual, olfactory, and sometimes tactile stimuli animals can detect. Their responses may be unconditioned or conditioned by previous experience.

The mere placing of an animal in a cage that differs in shape, area, material, or bedding may influence behavior. Changing the shape of a cage may cause mice to produce wet feces and would interfere with the testing of diuretics or purgatives (d'Arcy, 1962). Chance (1947) reported that by using larger cages he could reduce to about half the toxicity of amphetamine and ephedrine to individually caged mice. Other effects of caging were reviewed by Chance and Mackintosh (1962).

Audiogenic seizures are a dramatic, specialized response of some species to certain frequencies and intensities of noise. Approximately 36% of normal Sherman strain rats had seizures in response to intense noise from an electric bell, but the response rose to about 80% in rats receiving dieldrin at a dietary rate of 25 ppm. Although a number of compounds have been studied in this regard, the relationship between response and the tone, intensity, and pulse frequency of sound apparently have received little attention.

2.4.14 Disease

Few studies have been made of the relationship between the toxicity of chemicals and the occurrence of disease of other cause. A few exceptions are clearly recognized; for example, silicosis predisposes to tuberculosis. A dosage-response relationship appears to hold, for there is no evidence that inhalation of silica insufficient to cause silicosis has any effect on the occurrence of tuberculosis.

In one instance, a laboratory using pathogen-free rats consistently found higher LD 50 values for a series of test compounds than did other laboratories using normal rats of the same strain in a prearranged study (Weil and Wright, 1967).

In an unpublished study it was found that tube feeding of rats with larvae of *Trichinella spiralis* at the rate of 20 larvae per gram of body weight produced a marked, temporary decrease in food intake and a corresponding loss of body weight of about 60 g. The loss occurred over a period of 10 days in rats receiving no other treatment, but continued at a much slower rate for another 6 days in rats that previously had received DDT at a dietary level of 200 ppm (8.5 mg/kg/day for males and 10.5 mg/kg/day for females) for 359 days before infestation with larvae. Biopsy 10 days after infestation showed that the concentration of DDT in body fat had increased from an earlier biopsy average of $1,319 \pm 163$ (S.E.) ppm to $3,105 \pm 1,071$ ppm as a result of fat mobilization and a partial failure of metabolism and excretion to keep pace with the DDT so mobilized. The surviving rats had recovered fully 38 days later; at that time the DDT concentration in their fat was only 874 ± 10 ppm, because they had increased their fat stores into which the remaining DDT and that accumulated from continuing dietary intake were distributed. The reduction of food intake and the resulting loss of body weight produced by severe, nonfatal trichinosis were adequate to account for the initial increase in the concentration of DDT-derived material, and the subsequent recovery of weight was adequate to account for the final decrease in the concentration of this material stored in the fat of rats with the gastrointestinal phase of this disease. Thus, all of the observed changes could be explained in terms of body weight just as was true in connection with simple food deprivation (see Section 2.4.11.1).

A different and less understood kind of interaction is that in which chemicals appear to reduce resistance to infection or to increase the virulence of an infecting organism. Inasmuch as some compounds are antibiotic, it is logical that others may be probiotic. However, although some antibiotic reactions have been studied in great detail and are well understood, no careful study has been made of any probiotic interaction. The antibiotic reactions show dosage-response relationships, and the compounds tend to be specific for groups of microorganisms, and sometimes for species or even strains. These same characteristics are likely to characterize any genuine probiotic reactions. Examples of probiosis have been reported, but more investigation is needed to establish their validity, and very much more work is required to learn whether they are of practical importance and, if so, under what conditions. Although the implications of some individual reports of probiosis seem to have been exaggerated, the broadest theoretical implications have been neglected. In the absence of systematic study, it is impossible to exclude the possibility that probiosis is equally as important as antibiosis. That would certainly be true if chemical carcinogenesis turned out to be a form of probiosis rather than an action on the host—a relationship strongly suggested by the work of Price *et al.* (1972).

Reports of probiosis involve polychlorinated biphenyls and duck hepatitis virus in ducks (Friend and Trainer, 1970a); p,p'-DDT or dieldrin, respectively, and the same virus in ducks (Friend and Trainer, 1970b); and lead nitrate and *Salmonella typhimurium* in mice (Hemphill *et al.*, 1971).

One report (Wassermann *et al.*, 1969) suggests that any change in response to infection may be complex but may involve the immunological system. Rats given a 200-ppm aqueous suspension of DDT of unstated stability as their only source of water for 35 days not only had heavier livers but slightly heavier adrenals and lighter spleens. The DDT-treated animals showed a rise of serum albumin and some globulin fractions but a decrease of other globulin fractions. Although DDT alone caused a slight increase in the size of the adrenal, it tended to inhibit the greater increase produced by surgery. Whereas the average titer of antibodies to ovalbumin in rats receiving DDT was slightly less than that in controls injected with ovalbumin in the same way, the range of titers in different animals in the same group was so great that the result was difficult to evaluate.

It has not always been possible to confirm reports of a relationship between disease resistance and the intake of a chemical. For example, it has been reported that change in the phagocytic activity of white blood cells is an indication of early intoxication by DDT (Kun'ev, 1965). To test this report, DDT was given to male rats by stomach tube at a rate of 0.25 mg/kg/day for 31 days. Blood taken at intervals from 10 of these rats and from 10 controls was incubated with *Staphylococcus epidermidis*. The proportion of white cells ingesting bacteria and the average number of bacteria ingested per cell were measured. The same measurements were made at intervals on white blood cells from 15 dosed and 15 control rats after they had received bacteria by intracardiac injection. There was no statistical difference in phagocytic activity between the dosed and control rats in either the *in vitro* or the *in vivo* study (Kaliser, 1968).

2.4.15 Temperature

The interaction of temperature and the effects of foreign chemicals is complex, but it must be taken into account in the design and interpretation of experiments. Such interaction is most likely to occur in connection with compounds that influence temperature control or metabolic rate, but is not confined to compounds known to have one of these actions. Disturbances in temperature control are more likely to be important in small animals (such as rats and mice) or young animals, simply because their control of body temperature is imperfect at best. No matter what the size of the animals, the investigator should record both the ambient temperature and the body temperature in any study involving temperature as a variable. In some instances, skin temperature or the temperature of the extremities should be recorded because it may be critical but distinctly different from the body or visceral temperature.

For most compounds, minimal toxicity occurs at some temperature between room temperature and thermal neutrality, ie, the temperature at which the animal consumes least oxygen while at rest. In such instances, toxicity increases at temperatures both below or above this point, so that a graph of mortality or other measure of toxicity against ambient temperature is U-shaped. Examples include antu (Meyer and Karel, 1948), parathion (Baetjer and Smith, 1956), warfarin, strychnine, and several common solvents (Keplinger *et al.*, 1959). Other examples include two important antidotes, BAL (McDonald, 1948) and atropine (Keplinger *et al.*, 1959). Apparently no compound is known in which the opposite relationship exists, ie, maximal toxicity at some intermediate temperature with lesser toxicity at both lower and higher temperatures.

A smaller number of compounds demonstrate a more or less continuous increase in toxicity corresponding to increasing ambient temperature. In this instance, the graph of toxicity against temperature may be thought of as the right-hand branch of a U-shaped curve. It is often an open question whether the remainder of the curve would be demonstrated if sufficiently lower temperatures were investi-

gated. In any event, continuously increasing toxicity with increasing temperature has been found for dinitrophenol (Fuhrman *et al.*, 1943; Keplinger *et al.*, 1959) and for picrotoxin (Chen *et al.*, 1943).

A very few compounds may be more toxic at lower temperatures so that the graph of toxicity against temperature may be considered the left-hand branch of a U-shaped curve. Whether higher temperatures would complete the curve is often unknown. According to Bogdanovic (1961) picrotoxin is an example but, as already noted, Chen *et al.* (1943) found the opposite in a very careful study.

At least for some compounds that affect body temperature, there are critical ambient temperatures above which compounds cause a rise of body temperature and below which they cause a fall. Different compounds often have different critical temperatures in the same species (Shemano and Nickerson, 1958, 1959). If the change in body temperature is sufficient it may be a major cause of death. Even in the absence of a drug, an ambient temperature of 38°C is lethal to about 50% of mice in 3 hours at a relative humidity of 20% (Adolph, 1947). Rats fed malathion at a dietary rate of 4,000 ppm died sooner than controls when both were clipped and exposed to an ambient temperature of 1.5° C, but only after their body temperature had fallen to 18° C, which is half of normal (Marton *et al.*, 1962). As Keplinger *et al.* (1959) pointed out, it may be difficult to decide whether the stress of heat or cold renders an animal more susceptible to a compound or whether the compound renders it more susceptible to heat or cold. In fact, cold causes tetanus and hyperresponsiveness of the spinal cord similar in some respects to those caused by strychnine and some other compounds (Koizumi, 1955; Brooks *et al.*, 1955).

Many studies of the interaction of temperature and toxicity are carried out in nonacclimated animals. This was true of most of the studies cited in this section. As shown in a paper by Johnson *et al.* (1963) and the associated discussion, acclimatization may alter or even reverse the effect of either heat or cold. For example, Craig pointed out in the discussion that the toxicity of DFP, sarin, and atropine to rats and mice was increased by exposure to cold only if the animals were unacclimatized. This means that the conditions of each study must be stated clearly. It does not mean that investigations of unacclimatized animals are unimportant. People may encounter foreign chemicals at ambient temperatures to which they are not accustomed. The use of hypothermy in medicine is the most dramatic, but perhaps not the most important example.

Temperature can affect absorption, distribution, and action. As measured by excretion of paranitrophenol, parathion is absorbed more rapidly from human skin at higher ambient temperatures (Funckes *et al.*, 1963; Wolfe *et al.*, 1970). The maximal average increase in absorption is apparently in the order of 5 times but may be increased by a factor greater than 10 for the first few hours of exposure (Funckes *et al.*, 1963).

Some differences in action at different temperatures may be explained on the basis of dosage at the tissue level, as is true of chlorpromazine (Berti and Cima, 1954). However, this is not always true. For example, the central nervous system depressant norpipanone is about 3 times more toxic to mice at 29° C than at 18° C ambient temperature (Herr *et al.*, 1953). Although the difference is explained, at least in part, by the fact that following identical doses the concentration of the compound in the brain is about 40% greater at the higher temperature, there may be an inherent difference in the reactivity of the tissue. A higher dosage (96 mg/kg) and a resulting higher concentration in the brain (30 ppm) were required to produce the same effect (LD 50) at 18° C than the dosage (33 mg/kg) and brain level (6.7 ppm) required at 29° C (Herr *et al.*, 1954). Another example involves the action of DDT on the isolated frog heart. Hoffman and Lendle (1948) found that in December at a low room temperature a concentration of 300 ppm was required to produce the same effect that could be produced by 1 ppm or even 0.1 ppm in June at a temperature of at least 22° C.

The same compound may produce qualitatively different effects at different temperatures. Fatal doses of chlorpromazine given to mice at an ambient temperature of 38° C cause violent convulsions, but at 13° C they cause prolonged central depression (Berti and Cima, 1955).

The quantitative differences in toxicity associated with temperature are often small but are sometimes dramatic. Cold increased the toxicity of reserpine to unacclimatized mice by 1,200 times (LD 50 0.015 mg/kg at 20° C as compared to 18.84 mg/kg at 30° C) (Johnson *et al.*, 1963). Cold increased the susceptibility of rats to isoprenaline by factors of about 1,000 in males and 10,000 in females (Balazs *et al.*, 1962).

2.4.16 Pressure and Altitude

Pressure resulting from altitude may be a factor in the toxicity of any compound, especially one that influences cardiorespiratory function. An example involves the greater toxicities of red quill and digitalis at high altitudes as compared to the altitude of most communities (Ward *et al.*, 1940). Strychnine is also more toxic at high altitudes (Moore and Ward, 1935). On the other hand, a difference in pressure does not always determine a difference in toxicity. Of practical interest is the finding that dichlorvos, at exposure levels far in excess of those proposed for the disinsection of aircraft, exhibited no toxicity to people at 2,438 m, a cabin altitude seldom exceeded in normal airline operations of pressurized aircraft (Smith *et al.*, 1972).

New problems of toxicology have arisen since submarines and spacecraft may remain out of contact with the atmosphere of the earth for long periods. Maintenance of a small closed atmosphere offers a possibility for the accumulation of various gases and vapors that dissipate rapidly in ordinary situations. The toxicity of anything in the small space may be influenced by the fact that the pressure may not be that to which we are accustomed. Elaborate equipment for study of these problems was first described by Thomas (1965).

2.4.17 Light and Other Radiation

Although this section is concerned with the biological effects of light on toxicity, it should be recalled that some compounds undergo chemical change when exposed to radiation. Some of these changes have been demonstrated in pesticides and others may occur. Reactions in the upper atmosphere are considered important in degrading a variety of airborne compounds (see Section 6.2.2.1).

Some pesticides known to be susceptible to photodynamic action include: *p,p'*-DDT (Roburn, 1963), *p,p'*-DDE (Roburn, 1963), *p,p'*-DDD (Roburn, 1963), aldrin (Roburn, 1963), dieldrin (Roburn, 1963; Robinson *et al.*, 1966), and endrin (Roburn, 1963). It has not been proved that these purely physicochemical changes are of any practical importance in the toxicology of any pesticide. There is some evidence that poisoning of crop workers may result from residues of paraoxon in fields treated with parathion (Milby *et al.*, 1964). Conversion of parathion to paraoxon and other derivatives has been demonstrated in the laboratory (Payton, 1953; Frawley *et al.*, 1958). However, it is not clear what factors favor the production and persistence of enough paraoxon in the field to produce poisoning.

An old but still useful review of photodynamic action and diseases caused by light is that of Blum (1941).

2.4.17.1 Direct Biological Effects of Radiation.

Ionizing Radiation. The biological effects produced by x-rays and other ionizing radiation have been studied extensively. A description of these effects is beyond the scope of this book, even though gamma rays from radioactive cobalt were used to sterilize screw-worm flies in order to eradicate this destructive species in the southeastern United States of America.

A useful review of the biological effects of ionizing radiation is that of Schwan and Piersol (1954, 1955).

Ultraviolet Radiation. In addition to the direct photochemical action mentioned at the beginning of this section, ultraviolet radiation with a wavelength in the range 0.29 to 0.32 μm is responsible for sunburn. Ultraviolet light also produces "farmer's skin," an increased incidence of skin cancer, and the conversion of 7-dehydrocholesterol or a similar precursor in the skin to vitamin D. These effects and the action of sunlight generally were reviewed in detail by Blum (1945).

Visible Radiation. Differences in the intensity and wavelength of light within the visible range may influence the production of a variety of physiological effects, which may interact with the effects of toxic substances or even become manifest only in the presence of such substances. Kueter and Ott (1964) reported acceleration of the appearance of carcinoma, increased aggressiveness, and reversal of the sex ratio as effects of artificial light from various commonly used sources.

Photoperiodicity. Photoperiodicity of visible light determines or synchronizes circadian rhythms and, in combination with changes in temperature, is responsible for seasonal changes in physiology. See Sections 2.4.15 and 2.4.18.

2.4.17.2 Photosensitization.

Some chemicals make cells more susceptible to the action of light, especially ultraviolet light. Effects have been reported to result from wavelengths ranging from 0.29 to 0.50 μm (Daniels, 1965). Most compounds with this property are fluorescent (Blum, 1941). Although photosensitization usually affects the skin of vertebrates, other tissues are not immune. For example, the perfused turtle heart was arrested by a porphyrin preparation when exposed to light, but not in the dark. The reaction was not caused by a diffusible toxin. A second heart perfused in the dark with the perfusate from the first heart was not affected (Rask and Howell, 1928). Actions on other vertebrate tissues as well as free-living cells, viruses, and proteins including enzymes have been demonstrated (Blum, 1941).

One of the outstanding characteristics of photodynamic processes is that they occur only in the presence of molecular oxygen. However, photodynamic uptake of oxygen differs strikingly from normal oxidative metabolism in regard to respiratory quotient and sensitivity to heat and chemical inhibitors (Blum, 1941).

Whereas chemical photosensitization generally is activated by ultraviolet light, visible light may be active also, at least in some organisms. For example, while paramecia are not injured or sensitized to heat by visible light of high intensity, they readily are killed by this light in the presence of photodynamic dyes, and they are sensitized to heat by sublethal dosages of light. Cells so sensitized are killed when subjected to otherwise harmless temperatures. If the light and heat are applied in the reverse order, no ill effects are observed (Giese and Crossman, 1946).

In most instances, the biochemical basis of photosensitization is not understood, but it certainly can involve basic components of protoplasm. Deoxyribonucleic acid suspensions become less vicous when irradiated *in vitro* in the presence of eosin, methylene blue, 1,2-benzanthracene, or 20-methylcholanthrene. It is thought that the reaction involves depolymerization (Koffler and Markert, 1951).

Photosensitization has been caused in one species or another by a wide range of compounds. In addition to the prophyrins discussed below, the following materials have caused some degree of photosensitization in man: methylene blue, many phenothiazine compounds, many furocoumarin compounds, anthracene and acridine derivatives, 5-methoxypsoralem (the active principal of oil of bergamot used in perfumes) and related materials from other plants, griseofulvin, demethylchlortetracycline and some other antibiotics, sulfonamids and their derivatives, including some oral hypoglycemic agents, bithionol, hexachlorophene, and other miscellaneous drugs. It may be noted that many of these compounds consist of three aromatic or heterocyclic rings in a linear configuration. Substitution with sulfur or nitrogen may lead to an increase in photosensitizing capacity (Daniels, 1965).

A number of pesticides have chemical structures suggesting they might act as photosensitizers, and this property has been observed in connection with oxythioquinox, phenothiazine, and griseofulvin.

Porphyria. Porphyrins are probably the cause of more frequent and more serious photosensitization in man than all other materials combined. However, photosensitization does not occur in all cases in which the concentration of porphyrins in the blood and excreta is increased. It is important to review porphyria—any disturbance of porphyrin metabolism—because the chemical most effective for disturbing this metabolism is a pesticide, hexachlorobenzene. Recent detailed reviews are those by De Matteis (1967), Schmid (1966), and Jaffé (1968).

Porphyria may be an inborn error of metabolism, or it may be the result of injury by a foreign chemical, an infectious disease, or a vitamin deficiency in a genetically normal organism. Between these two extremes are situations in which it is difficult to evaluate the importance of genetic deficiency on the one hand and exogenous injury on the other. It is certain that persons who suffer from latent acute intermittent porphyria may bring on an acute attack by barbiturates, alcohol, and apronal. However, porphyria was produced in rabbits by sulfonethylmethane in 1895 (Stokvis, 1895) and more recently by 2-isopropyl-4-pentenoyl urea (Schmid and Schwartz, 1952). The reviews cited above list a number of other chemicals, including chlordane, lindane, and some other chlorinated hydrocarbon insecticides, that produce porphyria in animals or produce excess porphyrins in liver cell cultures. The porphyrins produced in excess are all type III isomers (Granick and Levere, 1964). Some increase in the concentration of porphyrins in the blood and urine accompanies lead poisoning in man so frequently that one is forced to conclude that lead causes a direct injury to some aspect of porphyrin metabolism and does not merely trigger the effect in the genetically susceptible. The same is true of abnormal porphyrin metabolism in persons with infectious hepatitis, poliomyelitis, pellagra, and pernicious anemia. Finally, at least one case is known in which porphyria was the result of a hepatic tumor and disappeared when the tumor was successfully removed (Tio, 1956; Tio et al., 1957). This situation suggests that the tumor cells differed genetically from those of the surrounding liver.

Table 2–11 shows the identity of compounds that occur in excess in the blood, tissues, and excreta in porphyria, whether of genetic or toxic origin. The main conditions characterized by abnormal concentrations of these compounds are listed. As may be seen from the structural formulae at the top of the table, porphin consists of a great ring composed of four pyrrole rings. Although porphin does not occur in living organisms, a large number of vitally important compounds may be considered as derivatives of porphin through methyl,

vinyl, acetic acid, and propionic acid substitutions for hydrogen. The table shows the chemical relation of some of the most frequently occurring, abnormal porphyrins as well as the normal porphyrins leading to heme and hemoglobin, but fails to show their close relation with cytochrome and chlorophyll.

Present understanding of the origin and interrelation of these materials is shown in Fig. 2–15. Some of the reactions shown in the figure occur mainly in the liver, while others, especially those directly involving the formulation of heme, occur in the bone marrow. It follows that injury or genetic defect of either or both of these organs may cause porphyria. Congenital porphyria, erythropoietic protoporphyria, and porphyria caused by lead involve the bone marrow; most other porphyrias involve the liver. Griseofulvin and 3,5-dimethoxycarbonyl–1,4–dihydrocollidine (DDC) affect both bone marrow and liver.

Some forms of porphyria are listed in Table 2–12. It may be seen that the different conditions can be distinguished clinically, chemically, and genetically. Each one, at least in theory, is characterized by a particular spectrum of concentrations of δ-aminolevulinic acid (δ-ALA) and/or porphyrins in urine, feces, serum, and red cells. The conditions produced in genetically normal people by some chemicals resemble the hereditary conditions, but only imperfectly. Different chemicals tend to produce different derangements of porphyrin metabolism.

As reviewed by Granick and Levere (1964) and others, there is considerable evidence that some porphyria is the result of increased production of δ-ALA synthetase, which depends on DNA–mediated synthesis of RNA. Increases of the enzyme and of the production of porphyria by chemicals are prevented by puromycin, actinomycin D, and other inhibitors of protein and RNA synthesis. The synthesis of δ-ALA synthetase is normally regulated by heme. If the concentration of inducing drugs is not too high, increased porphyrin production in liver cell culture can be prevented by the addition of heme (Granick, 1966). Thus, clinical disease may be caused by various chemicals that induce δ-ALA synthetase or by some defect of the normal regulatory mechanism by which heme represses formation of the enzyme. The hereditary porphyrias apparently differ from most heritable diseases because they depend on increased synthesis of a specific enzyme (δ-ALA synthetase) rather than on decreased activity of an enzyme, as is usually the case (Granick, 1965; 1966). However, more recent evidence indicates that in persons with acute intermittent porphyria the excessive synthesis is caused by induction by certain steroid metabolites that are produced in excess because these persons have a hereditary deficiency of activity of the enzyme(s) steroid Δ^4-5 α-reductase (Kappas *et al.*, 1972). In rats, some chemically induced porphyria is prevented by prior treatment with phenobarbital; presumably the inducer is detoxicated by drug-metabolizing enzymes of the liver (Kaufman *et al.*, 1970). A useful review of porphyrin metabolism is that of Pindyck *et al.* (1971).

Exogenous toxins that produce porphyria apparently are of two sorts: (*a*) those that lead to excessive δ-ALA synthetase (Meyer and Marver, 1971) and are, therefore, models of some spontaneous porphyrias, and (*b*) those, such as lead, that inhibit δ-ALA dehyrase (Hernberg *et al.*, 1970; Haeger-Arosen *et al.*, 1971; Gajdos and Gajdos-Török, 1971). Both enzyme changes have the same effect: the presence at one site or another of an excessive amount of δ-ALA and consequent disruption of heme synthesis. Howwever, if production of δ-ALA is judged by its excretion, normal variation must be kept in mind. Thus, urinary δ-ALA is principally a function of urine osmolality when the urinary level of lead is below 0.024 ppm, and principally a function of lead exposure when the urinary level of lead is above 0.146 ppm (Barnes *et al.*, 1972).

Although heme is considered the normal regulator of δ-ALA synthetase, it is not effective in most experimental situations. A few other materials either reduce porphyrin production or form relatively harmless complexes with abnormal porphyrins. Gajdos and Gajdos-Török (1961) showed that adenosine-5-monophosphate was beneficial to rats poisoned by hexachlorobenzene. Treatment caused a reduction in the concentration of certain porphyrins in liver, kidney, lung, and urine. The authors emphasized that further research would be required to establish the reason for the benefit. However, they placed little emphasis in the fact just mentioned and favored a hypothesis similar to that of Labbe (1967) discussed below.

Copper forms very stable, nonfluorescent complexes with porphyrins. Intravenous or intramuscular injections of 4 to 20 mg of cupric chloride into rats made porphyric by hexachlorobenzene at a dietary level of 2,000 ppm for 8 to 10 weeks led to very rapid loss of fluorescence in urine, skin, liver, and other viscera. Howerver, these parenteral doses were poorly tolerated. Cutaneous sensitivity to long wavelength ultraviolet light appeared diminished in porphyric rats consuming water containing 0.15% cupric sulfate. The apparent excretion of coproporphyrin and uroporphyrin in the urine of these rats was much reduced. These results probably were due to the quenching of fluorescence by copper and not to any effect on the production or metabolism of porphyrin. The hepatotoxicity of copper indicates great caution in even exploring copper as an antidote, but the results of the experiment suggest the possibility that some other quenching substance might be of value (Photinopoulos and Lorincz, 1965).

It was demonstrated many years ago that a porphyrin affects isolated cells only in the presence of light (Hausmann, 1908). When porphyrin is injected into healthy animals exposed to light, it causes marked cutaneous irritation, illness, and in some instances death, although the same dosage is harmless to animals kept in the dark (Hausmann, 1911, 1914; Rask and Howell, 1928). The intravenous dosage used in these *in vivo* studies ranged from 50 mg/kg to more than 100 mg/kg. Evidence was presented that this porphyrin combines slowly with one or more substances in the tissues whether in the light or in the dark. It is the action of light on this combination that produces injurious effects. Irradiation of the porphyrin before injection is without effect. It is not yet clear why some abnormalties of porphyrin metabolism cause sensitivity to light, or acute illness, or both, while others do not. It may be that the difference is caused by differences in the concentration of porphyrin complexes in those tissues exposed to light, but appropriate measurements have not been made. It may be that these conditions are the result of particular ratios as well as particular concentrations of porphyrins, In any event, sensitivity to light cannot be explained simply by the presence of a critical concentration of any single porphyrin in urine or any other single kind of specimen commonly used for measurement. Labbe (1967) has suggested that porphyrinogenesis may be secondary in importance, and inhibition of mitochondrial terminal electron transport and energy generation may be the primary biochemical lesion, but this, too, is speculation and the problem remains unsolved.

2.4.18 Circadian and Other Rhythms

A wide range of biological rhythms and their basis have been reviewed at length (Sollberger, 1965).

The word "circadian," from Latin *circa* (about) and *dies* (a day), refers to the rhythmic repetition of certain phenomena in living organisms at about the same time each day.

Table 2-11

Identity of δ-Aminolevulinic Acid, Porphobilinogen, Protoporphyrin, Heme, and Various
Other Porphyrins with Notes on their Occurrence in Health and Disease

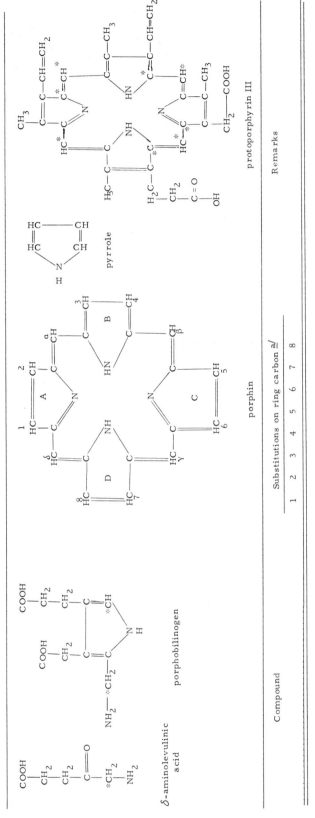

δ-aminolevulinic acid

porphobilinogen

pyrrole

porphin

protoporphyrin III

Compound	Substitutions on ring carbon [a]								Remarks
	1	2	3	4	5	6	7	8	
δ-aminolevulinic acid (ALA)									found in normal urine; greatly increased in acute porphyria; moderately increased in lead poisoning but not increased in hexachlorobenzene-induced porphyria
porphobilinogen (PBG)									trace in normal urine, greatly increased in acute porphyria and in protocoproporphyria, but not in other porphyrias

92

Compound	Substitutions on ring carbon [a]								Remarks
	1	2	3	4	5	6	7	8	
uroporphyrin I	A	P	A	P	A	P	A	P	found only in traces in normal urine; greatly increased in urine -- and also present in bones and teeth -- in most cases of congenital porphyria but rarely in urine in acute porphyria
uroporphyrin III	A	P	A	P	A	P	P	A	not found in normal urine; found in most cases of acute porphyria and hexachlorobenzene-induced porphyria
corproporphyrin I	M	P	M	P	M	P	M	P	found in normal urine, bile, and feces; increased in urine in infectious hepatitis; increased in feces in pernicious anemia and hemolytic jaundice; increased in urine and feces in most cases of congenital porphyria but rarely in acute porphyria
corproporphyrin III	M	P	M	P	M	P	P	M	found in normal urine; increased in urine of persons with poliomyelitis, those treated with salvarsan, and those poisoned by lead and hexachlorobenzene; increased in urine in most cases of acute porphyria but rarely in congenital porphyria; greatly increased in feces in HCB porphyria
protoporphyrin III (PP) [b]	M	V	M	V	M	P	P	M	found in urine in pellagra and in feces in HCB porphyria
heme [b]	M	V	M	V	M	P	P	M	

* Carbon atoms derived from the α-carbon of glycine and, therefore, the δ-carbon of ALA; the remaining 26 carbons of heme are derived from intermediates of the tricarboxylic acid cycle.

a. Substitutions: M = methyl ($-CH_3$); V = vinyl ($-CH=CH_2$); A = acetic acid ($-CH_2-COOH$); P = proprionic acid ($-CH_2-CH_2-COOH$).

b. Protoporphyrin III + Fe^{++} = heme; heme + globin = hemaglobin.

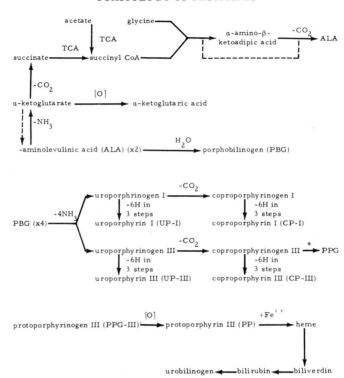

Fig. 2-15. Origin and interrelation of heme and other porphyrins. Uroporphyrinogen I forms uroporphyrin I and coproporphyrin I but not protoporphyrinogen or heme. TCA indicates the tricarboxylic acid cycle and the asterisk indicates oxidative decarboxylation.

Table 2-12

Concentration of δ-Aminolevulinic Acid (ALA), Porphobilinogen (PBG), Uroporphyrin (UP), Coproporphyrin (CP), and Protoporphyrin (PP), in Urine, Feces, Serum, and Red Blood Cells in Normal Persons and Those with Different Types of Porphyria. In some instances, only the degree of increase can be shown.

Type of porphyria	Compound[a]	Urine (ppm)	Dry feces (ppm)	Serum (ppm)	RBC (ppm)	Sensitivity to light	Acute illness	Hereditary pattern	Decade onset
normal	ALA	2 (0.03-10.2)							
	PBG	1-1.5							
	UP-I	0.015-0.03							
	CP-I	0.1-0.3	0.03-0.04		0.01-0.02				
	PP		0.1		0.1-0.6				
congenital erythropoietic porphyria, congenital photosensitive porphyria, Günther's disease	ALA	N		-		marked leading to blisters, scars, hypertrichosis	none, but splenomegaly and hemolytic anemia frequent; bones and teeth may be stained	homozygous autosomal recessive	1
	PBG	N							
	UP-I	~100[b]	~2,000	+	+++				
	CP-I	~10[b]	~130,000	+	++				
	PP		(+)	±	(+)				
erythropoietic protoporphyria	ALA	N		N		some; no blisters or scars	none, but occasional hemolytic anemia	heterozygous autosomal dominant	1
	PBG	N							
	UP-III	N	N	-	N				
	CP-III	N-0.5	20-80	-	(+)				
	PP		20-100	(+)	+++				
pyrroloporphyria, acute intermittent porphyria, Swedish porphyria, porphyria acuta intermitans (PAI) latent	ALA	~20		(+)		none	none[c]		
	PBG	~20							
	UP-III	++[b]							
	CP-III	+[b]		+				heterozygous autosomal dominant	2-4
	PP			+	N				
manifest	ALA	20-180		+		none	marked during attacks[d]		
	PBG	30-300							
	UP-III	+++[b]							
	CP-III	++	+						
	PP		+		N				

Table 2-12 Continued

Type of porphyria	Compound[a]	Urine (ppm)	Dry feces (ppm)	Serum (ppm)	RBC (ppm)	Sensitivity to light	Acute illness	Hereditary pattern	Decade onset
protocopro-porphyria, South African porphyria, mixed or varigate porphyria — latent	ALA	4.3		N		none	none	heterozygous autosomal dominant	2
	PBG	1.7							
	UP-III	0.24							
	CP-III	0.6	~400						
	PP		~650						
manifest	ALA	8-219		+		some to light but more to trauma	some, especially after drugs		
	PBG	20-200							
	UP-III	+++ [b]							
	CP-III	++	500-900						
	PP		800-1400		-				
delayed cutaneous porphyria, porphyria cutanea tarda (PCT), pyrroloporphyria — latent	ALA	N		N		none	none	familial; mechanism unknown	3-5
	PBG	N							
	UP	++							
	CP	(+)	+++						
	PP		++	N					
manifest	ALA	(+)		-		marked	none		
	PBG	N							
	UP	+++							
	CP	++	++						
	PP			+	+				
lead-induced porphyria	ALA	+++		++		none		none [e]	any
	PBG	N							
	UP-III	N							
	CP-III	+++	N						
	PP								
hexachlorobenzene-induced porphyria	ALA	0.5-2.3		-		marked blisters, scars, hypertrichosis, osteoporosis	hepatomegaly but few abdominal or neurological symptoms	none [e]	any, but mostly children
	PBG	0.3-0.7							
	UP-III	2.4-28.0 [b]							
	CP-III	0.1-4.7	18-222						
	PP		38-50		N				

(+) to ++ = increased.   N = normal.   - = Information not available.   ~ = About

a. The predominant isomer is indicated where known.

b. Chiefly made in vitro from PBG

c. May be precipitated by barbiturates, sulfonamids, griseofulvin, and estrogens.

d. Abdominal colic; sometimes oliguria, azotemia, hypertension, peripheral and central neuropathy, psychosis, and even coma, paralysis, and respiratory failure.

e. Not hereditary, but small doses of these and other chemicals may trigger an attack in genetically susceptible persons.

Of course, some circadian rhythms have been common knowledge for centuries. Some animals are nocturnal and others are diurnal. One might suppose that this difference in activity pattern depended merely on species differences regarding direct response to light. Experimentation has revealed that the situation is often not so simple. The activity pattern may persist, with or without modification, when an animal is placed in continuous darkness or continuous light. Even when experimentally imposed conditions of light change the pattern, the regulation may be temporary and the natural rhythm may eventually exert itself. For example, although Siegel (1961) found that the diurnal feeding pattern of rats disappeared in 6 to 10 days in rats transferred to continuous light, Wiepkema (1966) found that mice reared for two generations in continuous light showed a marked circadian rhythm in their feeding.

The persistence of circadian rhythm is the absence of any known external clue to the passage of time is one kind of evidence that has led to the hypothesis of the "physiological clock." Although the anatomical location and mode of action of such a clock is unknown, there is convincing evidence that some circadian rhythms are endogenous. Both endogenous and exogenous circadian rhythms are adjusted and regulated by photoperiod.

Under natural conditions, photoperiodicity depends on the movement of the earth. Rotation of the earth produces the succession of day and night. Revolution of the earth around the sun produces the seasons. In the temperate and arctic zones, the days are longer in summer and shorter in winter. Furthermore, the difference in the length of daylight at these seasons increases progressively from the equator to the poles. Consequently, during spring and fall, the rate of change in the relative length of light and darkness is greatest at the poles and least near the equator. The ability of organisms to use photoperiodic cycles as clues to impending seasonal change implies that they possess the ability to distinguish between long and short lengths of daylight. This ability is one factor in the complex adaptation of organisms to their environment.

The complicated and varied effects of photoperiodicity on organisms have been abundantly demonstrated by experiments designed for the purpose. There is a danger that the possible importance of photoperiodicity will be forgotten in experiments designed for other reasons. Many modern animal rooms have only artificial lighting, but the lighting cycle and the adaptation of the animals to it frequently are not mentioned in descriptions of methods used in toxicological studies.

It appears that the effects of circadian rhythms and photoperiodicity in invertebrates, especially insects, have been studied more thoroughly than those effects in mammals. Valuable reviews of the physiology and ecology of photoperiodism in insects are those of Beck (1963) and Danilevskii (1965). It is impossible to go into the matter in detail here. It is pertinent to record that one or more species of insects or mites show definite diurnal variation in their susceptibility to some pesticides, including dichlorvos (Polcik et al., 1964), methyl parathion (Cole and Adkisson, 1964), DDT (Beck, 1963), and potassium cyanide (Beck, 1963).

Probably some of the information on invertebrates would be of value in connection with studies in mammals. However this may be, it is already clear that circadian rhythms are important in a number of physiological functions of mammals, including their susceptibility to some poisons.

2.4.18.1 Circadian Rhythms in Mammals. In mammals, as in insects, endocrine functions may be influenced directly or otherwise by light, and may involve circadian rhythms. For example, hepatic tryptophan pyrrolase and its circulating substrate, whole blood tryptophan, have a circadian rhythm in mice that is practically eliminated by adrenalectomy (Rapoport et al., 1966). However, not all liver enzymes are so much influenced by adrenalectomy. Civen et al. (1967) showed that the rhythmicity of tyrosine α-ketoglutarate transaminase (TKT) is little altered after adrenalectomy.

The same authors (Civen et al., 1967) noted that TKT is rapidly induced by various agents but that phenylalanine-pyruvate transaminase (PPT) is not induced during the same time period and does not show circadian variation. On the basis of this and some other evidence, they suggested that the sensitivity of an enzyme's regulating system to inducing agents may be related to the inherent circadian rhythm of the enzyme.

The exact function, if any, of the pineal gland (epiphysis) is still in doubt. Because of its histology and the nature of its embryonic origin, it has been suspected for a long time that the structure has an endocrine function. This possibility, with special reference to neurohormonal control, seems to gain support from the demonstration (Quay and Halevy, 1962) that the pineal gland is rich in serotonin. Studies of the gland illustrate the complex interrelation that circadian rhythms may show in one small detail of mammalian physiology. In the rat the serotonin content of the gland shows a circadian rhythm (Quay, 1963; Snyder et al., 1964), which is somewhat modified by the estrus cycle (Quay, 1963). The rhythm persists in rats kept in the dark or in rats whose eyes have been removed, provided the animals are otherwise intact. The rhythm is abolished in intact rats by continuous light and also abolished by interruption of sympathetic innervation (Fiske, 1964; Snyder et al., 1964). The rhythm is changed in a matter of hours by change in photoperiods (Quay, 1963). The rhythm is not affected by removal of the pituitary, thyroid, adrenals, or ovaries (Snyder et al., 1965). The rat pineal gland also shows circadian rhythms for hydroxyindole O-methyltransferease (HIOMT) (Axelrod et al., 1965) and endogenous melatonin (Quay, 1964). However, these rhythms are opposite in phase to that of serotonin and also differ in that they do not persist in animals kept in the dark. The rhythms for HIOMT and melatonin are directly responsive to light. All three rhythms (HIOMT, melatonin, and serotonin) are interrupted by removal of the superior cervical ganglia (Fiske, 1964; Snyder et al., 1964; Wurtman et al., 1964). Since the nerve pathways are probably noradrenergic, McGeer and McGeer (1966) explored the possibility that there might be a circadian rhythm in the ability of the nerve endings of the pineal gland to form noradrenaline. They found such a rhythm in the activity of tyrosine hydroxylase, the rate-controlling enzyme in the synthesis of noradrenalin.

Some circadian rhythms involve reactions known to be of fundamental physiological importance. For example, Spoor and Jackson (1966) showed that the beating rate of rat atria decreased more in response to a standard concentration of acetylcholine if they were isolated at 1100 hours than if isolated at 2300 hours. The food intake of rats normally follows a circadian rhythm, the details and modification of which were studied by Siegel (1961).

The preceding examples involve rhythms with a single major peak and a single major trough during each 24-hour day. The rhythm is either a direct response to the periodicity of light or if endogenous, at least is synchronized by light. Lindsay and Kullman (1966) reported that the survival time of female mice given a standard dose of sodium pentabarbital varied during a 12-hour period in such a way that the graph showed several inflections. Although this result is unexplained and unconfirmed, it it not unique. A similar result was reported for the susceptibility of boll weevils to methyl parathion (Cole and Adkisson, 1964). The weevils showed greatest resistance at the beginning of the light period no matter whether that started at 0600 hours (14-hour photophase), 0700 hours (12-hour photophase), or 0900 hours (10-hour photophase). Regardless of the length of the photophase, peaks of resistance recurred at intervals of about 6 hours with intervening troughs of susceptibility. Why the 3-hour cycle corresponded with the sampling interval was unexplained. In any event, it is interesting that both examples of multiple peaks involve susceptibility to a foreign compound. Nothing is known of the enzymatic or other physiological basis of the reported phenomenon.

Typical circadian rhythms (one peak and one trough during a 24-hour day) are involved in the responses of several mammals to a number of foreign chemicals. Such cycles of susceptibility were observed at least as early as 1949 (Carlsson and Serin, 1950). As reviewed by Sollberger (1965), 24-hour rhythms in sensitivity of mammals to a number of drugs has been reported. Compounds involved include insulin, hormones, narcotics, sedatives, tranquilizers, bacterial toxins, and carcinogens. Other examples include lidocaine (Lutsch and Morris, 1967), methopyrapone (Ertel et al., 1964), nikethamide (Carlsson and Serin, 1950), and pentobarbital (Davis, 1962). Apparently, rhythmicity of response to a pesticide has not been demonstrated in a mammal, but this may be largely the result of limited observation.

Human circadian rhythms can persist in continuous darkness; social cues are sufficient to entrain them (Aschoff et al., 1971).

It is clear that circadian rhythms or the effects of light periodicity should be considered when there are unexplained differences in the results of different laboratories or in the results of the same laboratory at different times.

2.4.19 Other Factors Influencing Toxicity

Undoubtedly many other factors in addition to those discussed in the preceding sections may influence toxicity under certain circumstances. However, the other factors are not of major importance in mammalian toxicology.

2.4.19.1 Seasonal Differences. Seasonal differences are of tremendous importance in the physiology of coldblooded animals and in their responses to toxicants. Presumably, similar differences would hold for mammals that hibernate, but the question has received little attention.

2.4.19.2 Relative Humidity. Presumably relative humidity might influence the reaction of an animal to a toxin in any situation in which humidity was already critical for the animal's health, eg, maintenance of normal body temperature in a hot environment. Such an interaction would seem most likely in connection with compounds that increase heat production or influence temperature control. However, no instance of such an effect on toxicity seems to have been reported. What has been reported is an effect of relative humidity on the adsorption of insecticides and, therefore, on their availability for evaporation or absorption from surfaces. These matters are discussed in Sections 6.3.2.2 and 6.3.2.3.

It has been shown that parathion is absorbed more rapidly by the human skin at higher temperatures (Funckes et al., 1963; Wolfe et al., 1970). What part humidity (especially from sweat) may play in the process apparently is not known. It is conceivable that mammals may be able to absorb pesticides from their skin surfaces more readily if the surface is moist.

2.4.19.3 Aquatic Factors. Because it is sometimes suggested that fish or other aquatic organisms be used for bioassay of toxicants that might influence mammals, it is necessary to record that the welfare of aquatic organisms is influenced by several environmental factors that have little meaning for land animals.

pH. The influence of pH on toxicity often is explained easily in terms of the availability of toxicant. Toxic ions or alkaloids may be much more soluble or easily absorbable at one pH than at another.

Water Hardness. Henderson and Pickering (1957) found that water hardness had a significant effect on the toxicity of trichlorofon to fathead minnows but no significant effect on the toxicity of nine other organic phosphorus compounds they studied. Water hardness had little or no effect on the toxicity of chlorinated

Table 2-13

Summary of Information on the Importance of Different
Factors Influencing Toxicity

Expanded from Hayes (1967a) by permission of the Royal Society, London.

Factor	Total no. of compounds	Ratio of difference Range	Ratio of difference Mean	Increasing ratio indicates [a]
duration	22	0.5-20.0	---	2-year > 90-day
route	67	0.2-21 [b]	4.2 [b]	oral > dermal
species	20	0.2-11.8	1 [c]	other sp. > rat
	1	> 230		other sp. > rat
	1	> 1000		man > cat
individual [d]				
oral route	69	1.20-7.14	2.42	LD 50 > LD 1
dermal route	42	1.37-14.93	3.00	LD 50 > LD 1
sex				
oral route	65	0.21-4.62	0.94	male > female
dermal route	37	0.11-2.93	0.81	male > female
pregnancy	19	0.74-14.55	1.90	pregnancy > non-pregnancy
age	18	0.6-10.0	2.9	newborn > adult
	16	0.7-6.2	---	newborn > adult
	15	0.2-4.1	1.8	newborn > adult
	290	< 0.02-750	2.78 [e]	newborn > adult
temperature	1	10,000	---	cold > warm
nutrition	8	1.0-1.8	1.49	1/3 dietary protein > normal
	1	2,100	---	no protein > normal

a. > indicates greater toxicity of chemical or greater susceptibility of animal.

b. Compounds with very low or variable toxicity are not included.

c. Approximate value.

d. Same sex.

e. Geometric mean.

hydrocarbon insecticides to fish (Henderson *et al.*, 1959).

Chlorine Content. Ordinary tap water may contain enough free chlorine to kill some fish. This must be kept in mind in bioassays on fish.

2.4.20 Discussion of Factors Influencing Toxicity

The fact that a number of factors influence dosage-response relationships should not obscure the fact that these relationships are real and of paramount importance.

No special study seems to have been made of the interrelation of factors as regards ratios of difference. If the highest ratios observed for a series of factors were completely multiplicative in their effect the combined product would be very large. Although the possibility of such an occurrence cannot be excluded, none has been recognized. On the average, the ratios expressed as quotients differ little from 1.0, and since some are less than 1.0, they tend to cancel out.

Table 2-13 summarizes part of the information in the foregoing sections. It is clear from this summary and from additional information in Tables 2-8 and 2-9 that species differences may be more important under practical conditions than any factor except dosage in influencing toxicity of a particular compound. The largest ratio of difference found in connection with species was over 1,000 while the largest ratio associated with any other factor likely to be of practical importance was only 21. It is true that very large ratios have been observed in connection with age and temperature, respectively, but their rarity must be emphasized.

In summary, the maximal observed variation in effect associated with different factors is as follows: dosage, infinity (health vs death); compounds, 10^7; temperature, 10^4; age, 10^3; species, 10^3; other factors, 3×10^1 or less.

The numerical comparison regarding species ignores important phenomena that occur in man but are difficult or impossible to study in animals. One is forced to conclude that more emphasis should be placed on studies in man. This is particularly true when one considers that not only dosage and route but sometimes sex, age, temperature, duration of dosing, and other factors may be explored directly in volunteers or workers.

REFERENCES

Adolph, E. F. (1947). Tolerance to heat and dehydration in several species of mammals. Am. J. Physiol., 151:564–575.

Aldridge, W. N., and Barnes, J. M. (1961). Neurotoxic and biochemical properties of some triaryl phosphates. Biochem. Pharmacol., 6:177–188.

Aschoff, J., Fatranska, M., Giedke, H., Doerr, P., Stamm, D., and Wisser, H. (1971). Human circadian rhythms in continuous darkness; entrainment by social cues. Science, 171:213–215.

Axelrod, J., Wurtman, R. J., and Snyder, S. H. (1965). Control of hydroxyindole O-methyltransferase activity in the rat pineal gland by environmental lighting. J. Biol. Chem., 240:949–954.

Baetjer, A. M., and Smith, R. (1956). Effect of environmental temperature on reaction of mice to parathion, an anticholinesterase agent. Am. J. Physiol., 186:39–46.

Balazs, T., Murphy, J. B., and Grice, H. C. (1962). The influence of environmental changes on the cardiotoxicity of isoprenaline in rats. J. Pharm. Pharmacol., 14:750–755.

Barnes, J. M. (1968). Poisons that hit and run. New Sci., 38:619.

Barnes, J. M., and Denz, F. A. (1954). The reaction of sheep to diets containing octamethyl pyrophosphoramide (schradan) and O,O-diethyl-S-ethylmercaptoethanol thiophosphate ("Systox"). Br. J. Ind. Med., 11:11–19.

Barnes, J. M., and Heath, D. F. (1964). Some toxic effects of dieldrin in rats. Br. J. Ind. Med., 21:280–282.

Barnes, J. R., Smith, P. E., and Drummond, C. M. (1972). Urine osmolality and δ-aminolevulinic acid excretion. Arch. Environ. Health, 25:450–455.

Beck, S. D. (1963). Physiology and ecology of photoperiodism. Bull. Entomol. Soc. Am., 9(1):8–16.

Beliles, R. P. (1972). The influence of pregnancy on the acute toxicity of various compounds in mice. Toxicol. Appl. Pharmacol., 23:537–540.

Berti, T., and Cima, L. (1954). Concentrazione di Cloropromazine negli Organi ed Azione Farmacologica. Boll. Soc. Ital. Biol. Sper., 30:100–101.

Berti, T., and Cima, L. (1955). Einfluss der Temperatur auf die pharmakologische Wirkung des Chlorpromazins. Arzneim. Forsch., 5:73–74.

Bertrand, G. (1903). Les engrais complémentaires. Fifth Intern. Kongr. Angew Chem. (Berlin), 3:839–840.

Bertrand, M. D. (1962a). Physiologie végétale.—Sur une formule mathématique de la loi de l'optimum de concentration nutritive. C. R. Acad. Sci. [D] (Paris) 254:2810–2812.

Bertrand, M. D. (1962b). Expression mathématique logique de la loi de l'optimum de concentration nutritive. Son application à l'agriculture. C. R. Seances Acad. Agr. Fr., 422–428.

Bertrand, M. D. (1969). Anamorphose linéaire de la course dissymétrique de probabilité de Pearson-Volterra appli-

cations à l'agriculture. C. R. Seances Acad. Agr. Fr., 603–613.

Beyer, W. H. (ed.) (1966). Handbook of Tables for Probability and Statistics. Chemical Rubber Publishing Company, Cleveland.

Bliss, C. I. (1934a). The method of probits. Science, 79:38–39.

Bliss, C. I. (1934b). The method of probits—a correction. Science, 79:409–410.

Bliss, C. I. (1935a). The calculation of the dosage-mortality curve. Ann. Appl. Biol., 22:134–167.

Bliss, C. I. (1935b). The comparison of dosage-mortality data. Ann. Appl. Biol., 22:307–333.

Bliss, C. I. (1937). The calculation of the time-mortality curve. Ann. Appl. Biol., 24:815–852.

Bliss, C. I. (1938). Determination of the small dosage-mortality curve from small numbers. Q. J. Pharm. Pharmacol., 11:192–216.

Bliss, C. I. (1940). The relation between exposure time, concentration and toxicity in experiments on insecticides. Ann. Entomol. Soc. Am., 33:721–766.

Blum, H. F. (1941). Photodynamic Action and Diseases Caused by Light. Reinhold Publishing Corporation, New York.

Blum, H. F. (1945). The physiological effects of sunlight on man. Physiol. Rev., 25:483–530.

Bockel, P. (1957). Poisoning with an organophosphorus compound (basudin) of the diazinon group. Dtsch. Med. Wschr., pp. 1230–1231.

Bogdanovic, S. B. (1961). Effects of temperature on the action of drugs. Annu. Rev. Pharmacol., 1:65–78.

Boroff, D. A., and Fitzgerald, J. E. (1958). Fluorescence of the toxin Clostridium botulinum and its relation to toxicity. Nature, 181:751–752.

Boroff, D. A., and Fleck, U. (1966). Statistical analysis of a rapid in vivo method for the titration of the toxin of Clostridium botulinum. J. Bacteriol., 92:1580–1581.

Bough, R. G., Gurd, M. R., Hall, J. E., and Lessel, G. (1963). Effect of methaqualone hydrochloride in pregnant rabbits and rats. Nature, 200:656–657.

Boyd, C. E., and Boyd, E. M. (1962). The chronic toxicity of atropine administered intramuscularly to rabbits. Toxicol. Appl. Pharmacol., 4:457–467.

Boyd, E. M. (1959). The acute oral toxicity of caffeine. Toxicol. Appl. Pharmacol., 1:250–257.

Boyd, E. M. (1961). Toxicological studies. J. New Drugs, 1:104–109.

Boyd, E. M. (1968). Predictive drug toxicity. Assessment of drug safety before human use. Can. Med. Assoc. J., 98:278–293.

Boyd, E. M., Abel, M. M., and Knight, L. M. (1966). The chronic oral toxicity of sodium chloride at the range of the $LD_{50(0.1L)}$. Can. J. Physiol. Pharmacol., 44:157–172.

Boyd, E. M., and Carsky, E. (1969). The acute oral toxicity of the herbicide chlorpropham in albino rats. Arch. Environ. Health, 19:621–627.

Boyd, E. M., Carsky, E., and Krijnen, C. J. (1969). The effects of diets containing from 0 to 81 percent of casein on the acute oral toxicity of diazinon. Clin. Toxicol., 2:295–301.

Boyd, E. M., Chen, C. P., and Krijnen, C. J. (1969). Lindane and dietary protein. Pharmacol. Res. Commun., 1:403–412.

Boyd, E. M., and De Castro, E. S. (1968). Protein-deficient diet and DDT toxicity. Bull. WHO, 38:141–150.

Boyd, E. M., and Dobos, I. (1969). Acute toxicity of monuron in albino rats fed from weaning on different diets. J. Agric. Food Chem., 17:1213–1216.

Boyd, E. M., Dobos, I., and Krijnen, C. J. (1970). Endosulfan toxicity and dietary protein. Arch. Environ. Health, 21:15–19.

Boyd, E. M., Dolman, M., Knight, L. M., and Sheppard, E. P. (1965). The chronic oral toxicity of caffeine. Can. J. Physiol. Pharmacol., 43:995–1007.

Boyd, E. M., and Krijnen, C. J. (1969a). The influence of

protein intake on the acute oral toxicity of carbaryl. J. Clin. Pharmacol., 9:292–297.

Boyd, E. M., and Krijnen, C. J. (1969b). Dietary protein and DDT toxicity. Bull. Environ. Contam. Toxicol., 4:256–261.

Boyd, E. M., and Selby, M. J. (1962). The chronic oral toxicity of benzylpenicillin. Antibiot. Chemother., 12:249–262.

Boyd, E. M., and Shanas, M. N. (1963). The acute oral toxicity of sodium chloride. Arch. Int. Pharmacodyn. Ther., 144:86–97.

Boyd, E. M., and Taylor, F. I. (1971). Toxaphene toxicity in protein-deficient rats. Toxicol. Appl. Pharmacol., 18:158–167.

Brinkman, G. L., and Miller, R. F. (1961). Influence of cage type and dietary zinc oxide upon molybdenum toxicity. Science, 134:1531–1532.

Brodeur, J., and DuBois, K. P. (1963). Comparison of acute toxicity of anticholinesterase insecticides to weanling and adult male rats. Proc. Soc. Exp. Biol. Med., 114:509–511.

Brodie, B. B. (1967). Physiochemical and biochemical aspects of pharmacology. J.A.M.A., 202:600–609.

Brooks, C. M., Koizumi, K., and Malcolm, J. L. (1955). Effects of changes in temperature on reactions of spinal cord. J. Neurophysiol., 18:205–216.

Bryan, W. R., and Shimkin, M. B. (1943). Quantitative analysis of dose-response data obtained with three carcinogenic hydrocarbons in strain C3H male mice. J. Natl. Cancer Inst., 3:503–531.

Butler, W. H. (1965). Liver injury and aflatoxin. In: *Mycotoxins in Foodstuffs*, edited by G. N. Wogan, pp. 175–186. M.I.T. Press, Cambridge, Mass.

Carlsson, A., and Serin, F. (1950). Time of day as a factor influencing the toxicity of nikethamide. Acta Pharmacol. Toxicol. (Khb.), 6:181–186.

Carnaghan, R. B. (1967). Hepatic tumours and other chronic liver changes in rats following a single oral administration of aflatoxin. Br. J. Cancer, 21:811–814.

Casterline, J. L., Jr., and Williams, C. H. (1969). Effect of pesticide administration upon esterase activities in serum and tissues of rats fed variable casein diets. Toxicol. Appl. Pharmacol., 14:266–275.

Cavanagh, J. B., Davies, D. R., Holland, P., and Lancaster, M. (1961). Comparison of the functional effects of Dyflos, Tri-o-cresyl phosphate and tri-p-ethylphenyl phosphate in chickens. Br. J. Pharmacol., 17:21–27.

Cerf, J., Lebrun, A., and Dierichx, J. (1962). A new approach to helminthiasis control: The use of an organophosphorus compound. Am. J. Trop. Med. Hyg., 11:514–517.

Chance, M. R. A. (1947). Factors influencing the toxicity of sympathomimetic amines to solitary mice. J. Pharmacol. Exp. Ther., 89:289–296.

Chance, M. R. A., and Mackintosh, J. H. (1962). The effects of caging. Coll. Pap. Lab. Anim. Bur., 11:59–64.

Chen, K. K., Anderson, R. C., Steldt, F. A., and Mills, C. A. (1943). Environmental temperature and drug action in mice. J. Pharmacol. Exp. Ther., 79:127–133.

Christian, J. J., and Davis, D. E. (1964). Endocrines, behavior and population. Science, 146:1550–1560.

Civen, M., Ulrich, R., Trimmer, B. M., and Brown, C. B. (1967). Circadian rhythms of liver enzymes and their relationship to enzyme induction. Science, 157:1563–1564.

Clark, A. J. (1937). General pharmacology. Hnd. Exp. Pharmakol., 4:i–vi, 1–228.

Cole, C. L., and Adkisson, P. L. (1964). Daily rhythm in the susceptibility of an insect to a toxic agent. Science, 144:1148–1149.

Conney, A. H., Miller, E. C., and Miller, J. A. (1956). The metabolism of methylated aminoazo dyes. V. Evidence for induction of enzyme synthesis in the rat by 3-methylcholanthrene. Cancer Res., 16:450–459.

Cucinell, S. A., Odessky, L., Weiss, M., and Dayton, P. G. (1966). The effect of chloral hydrate on bishydroxycoumarin metabolism. J. A. M. A., 197:366–368.

Dadey, J. L., and Kammer, A. G. (1953). Chlordane intoxication. Report of a case. J. A. M. A., 153:723–725.

Dale, W. E., Gaines, T. B., and Hayes, W. J., Jr. (1962). Storage and excretion of DDT in starved rats. Toxicol. Appl. Pharmacol., 4:98–106.

Daniels, F., Jr. (1965). Diseases caused or aggravated by sunlight. Med. Clin. North Am., 49:565–580.

Danilevskii, A. S. (1965). *Photoperiodism and Seasonal Development of Insects*. Oliver & Boyd Ltd., Edinburgh.

d'Arcy, P. F. (1962). The conditioning of experimental animals. J. Pharm. Pharmacol., 14:411–428.

Dasgupta, B. R., Boroff, D. A., and Rothstein, E. (1966). Chromatographic fractionation of the crystalline toxin of *Clostridium botulinum* type A. Biochem. Biophys. Res. Commun., 22:750–756.

Datta, P. R., and Nelson, M. J. (1968). Enhanced metabolism of methylprylon, meprobamate, and chlordiazepoxide hydrochloride after chronic feeding of a low dietary level of DDT to male and female rats. Toxicol. Appl. Pharmacol., 13:346–352.

Davies, D. R., Holland, P., and Rumens, M. J. (1960). The relationship between the chemical structure and neurotoxicity of alkyl organophosphorus compounds. Br. J. Pharmacol. Chemotherap., 15:271–278.

Davies, D. R., Holland, P., and Rumens, M. J. (1966). The delayed neurotoxicity of phosphorodiamidic fluorides. Biochem. Pharmacol., 15:1783–1789.

Davies, G. M., and Lewis, I. (1956). Outbreak of food-poisoning from bread made of chemically contaminated flour. Br. Med. J., 2:393–398.

Davis, W. M. (1962). Day-night periodicity in pentobarbital response of mice and the influence of socio-psychological conditions. Experientia, 18:235–237.

Deichmann, W. B., and LeBlanc, T. J. (1943). Determination of the approximate lethal dose with about six animals. J. Ind. Hyg. Toxicol., 25:415–417.

DeMatteis, F. (1967). Disturbances of liver porphyrin metabolism caused by drugs. Pharmacol. Rev., 19:523–557.

Dickens, F., Jones, H. E. H., and Waynforth, H. B. (1966). Oral subcutaneous and intratracheal administration of carcinogenic lactones and related substances: The intratracheal administration of cigarette tar in the rat. Br. J. Cancer, 20:134–144.

Dinman, B. D. (1972). "Non-concept" of "no-threshold": Chemicals in the environment. Science, 175:495–497.

Drill, V. A., and Hiratzka, T. (1953). Toxicity of 2,4-dichlorophenoxyacetic acid and 2,4,5-trichlorophenoxyacetic acid: A report on their acute and chronic toxicity in dogs. Arch. Ind. Hyg. Occup. Med., 7:61–67.

Druckrey, H. (1943). Quantitative Grundlagen der Krebserzeugung. Klin. Wothenschr., 22:532–534.

Druckrey. H. (1959). Pharmacological approach to carcinogenesis. In: *Ciba Foundation Symposium on Carcinogenesis: Mechanisms of Action, London, 1958*, pp. 110–130. Little, Brown and Company, Boston.

Druckrey, H. (1967). Quantitative aspects in chemical carcinogenesis. In: *Potential Carcinogenic Hazards from Drugs: Evaluation of Risk*, edited by R. Truhaut, Vol. 7, pp. 60–78: U.I.C.C. Monograph Serv. Springer-Verlag, New York.

DuBois, K. P. (1972). Interactions of chemicals as a result of enzyme inhibition. In: *Multiple Factors in the Causation of Environmental Induced Disease*, edited by D. H. K. Lee and P. Kotin, pp. 95–107. Academic Press Inc., New York.

DuBois, K. P., and Geiling, E. M. (1959). *Textbook of Toxicology*. Oxford University Press, Oxford.

DuBois, K. P., Kinoshita, F. K., and Frawley, J. P. (1968). Quantitative measurement of inhibition of aliesterases, acylamidase, and cholinesterase by EPN and delnav. Toxicol. Appl. Pharmacol., 12:273–284.

Duggan, R. E. (1968). Residues in food and feed. Pesticide residue levels in foods in the United States from July 1, 1963 to June 30, 1967. Pestic. Monit. J., 2:2–46.

Durham, W. F. (1969). Body burden of pesticides in man. Ann. N. Y. Acad. Sci., 160:183–195.

Durham, W. F., Ortega, P., and Hayes, W. J., Jr. (1963). The effects of various dietary levels of DDT on liver function, cell morphology, and DDT storage in the rhesus monkey. Arch. Int. Pharmacodyn. Ther., 141:111–129.

Eagle, E., and Carlson, A. J. (1950). Toxicity, antipyretic and analgesic studies on 29 compounds including aspirin, phenacetin and 27 derivatives of carbazole and tetrahydrocarbazole. J. Pharmacol. Exp. Ther., 99:450–457.

Edson, E. F. (1964). No-effect levels of three organophosphates in the rat, pig, and man. Food Cosmet. Toxicol., 2:311–316.

Emmens, C. W. (1948). Principles of Biological Assay. Chapman & Hall Ltd., London.

Ertel, R. J., Halberg, F., and Ungar, F. (1964). Circadian system phase-dependent toxicity and other effects of methopyrapone (SU–4885) in the mouse. J. Pharmacol. Exp. Ther., 146:395–399.

Ferguson, H. C. (1966). Effect of red cedar chip bedding on hexobarbital and pentobarbital sleep time. J. Pharm. Sci., 55:1142–1143.

Finberg, L., Kiley, J., and Luttrell, C. N. (1963). Mass accidental salt poisoning in infancy. A study of a hospital disaster. J. A. M. A., 184:187–190.

Finney, D. J. (1952). Probit Analysis, Ed. 2. Cambridge University Press, Cambridge.

Fisher, R. A., and Yates, F. (1963). Statistical Tables for Biological, Agricultural, and Medical Research, Ed. 6. Hafner Publishing Company, New York.

Fiske, V. M. (1964). Serotonin rhythm in the pineal organ: control by the sympathetic nervous system. Science, 146:253–254.

Fitzhugh, O. G. (1966). Problems related to the use of pesticides. Can. Med. Assoc. J., 94:598–604.

Fitzhugh, O. G., and Nelson, A. A. (1947). The chronic oral toxicity of DDT (2,2-bis p-chlorophenyl 1,1,1-trichloroethane). J. Pharmacol. Exp. Ther., 89:18–30.

Food and Agriculture Organization and World Health Organization. (1965). Evaluation of the Toxicity of Pesticide Residues in Food. WHO/Food Add./27.65.

Food and Agriculture Organization and World Health Organization Expert Committee on Food Additives. (1958). Procedures for the Testing of Intentional Food Additives to Establish their Safety for Use. WHO Tech. Rep. Ser. No. 144.

Fouts, J. R., and Adamson, R. H. (1959). Drug metabolism in the newborn rabbit. Science, 129:897–898.

Frawley, J. P., Cook, J. W., Blake, J. R., and Fitzhugh, O. G. (1958). Effect of light on chemical and biological properties of parathion. J. Agric. Food Chem., 6:28–30.

Frawley, J. P., and Fuyat, H. N. (1957). Pesticide toxicity. Effect of low dietary levels of parathion and Systox on blood cholinesterase of dogs. J. Agric. Food Chem., 5:346–348.

Frawley, J. P., Weir, R., Tusing, T., DuBois, K. P., and Calandra, J. C. (1963). Toxicologic investigations on Delnav. Toxicol. Appl. Pharmacol., 5:605–624.

Friedman, B. (1959). The use of anticoagulants in the treatment of coronary and cerebral vascular disease. J. Tenn. Med. Assoc., 52:171–177.

Friedman, L. (1973). Problems of evaluating the health significance of the chemicals present in food. In: Proceedings of the Fifth International Congress on Pharmacology, edited by T. A. Loomis, Vol. 2, pp. 30–41. S. Karger, Basel.

Friend, M., and Trainer, D. O. (1970a). Polychlorinated biphenyl: interaction with duck hepatitis virus. Science, 170:1314–1316.

Friend, M., and Trainer, D. O. (1970b). Some effects of sublethal levels of insecticides on vertebrates. J. Wildl. Dis., 6:335–342.

Fuhrman, G. J., Weymouth, F. W., and Field, J. (1943). The effect of environmental temperature on the toxicity of 2,4-dinitrophenol in mice. J. Pharmacol. Exp. Ther., 79:176–178.

Funckes, A. J., Hayes, G. R., Jr., and Hartwell, W. V. (1963). Urinary excretion of paranitrophenol by volunteers following dermal exposure to parathion at different ambient temperatures. J. Agric. Food Chem., 11:455–457.

Gabliks, J., Bantug-Jurilla, M., and Friedman, L. (1967). Responses of cell structures to insecticides. IV. Relative toxicity of several organophosphates in mouse cell structures. Proc. Soc. Exp. Biol. Med., 125:1002–1005.

Gaddum, J. H. (1933). Reports on biological standards. III. Methods of biological assay depending on quantal response. Medical Research Council Special Report Series 183. H. M. S. O., London.

Gaddum, J. H. (1937). Discussion on pharmacological action. In: Clark, A. J. Discussion of the chemical and physical basis of pharmacological action, pp. 598–601. Proc. R. Soc. Lond. [Biol.], 121:580–609.

Gaddum, J. H. (1945). Lognormal distributions. Nature, 156:463–466.

Gaines, T. B. (1960). The acute toxicity of pesticides to rats. Toxic. Appl. Pharmacol., 2:88–99.

Gaines, T. B. (1962). Poisoning by organic phosphorus pesticides potentiated by phenothiazine derivatives. Science, 138:1260–1262.

Gaines, T. B. (1968). Personal communication.

Gaines, T. B. (1968). Unpublished results.

Gaines, T. B. (1969). Acute toxicity of pesticides. Toxicol. Appl. Pharmacol., 14:515–534.

Gaines, T. B., Hayes, W. J., Jr., and Linder, R. E. (1966). Liver metabolism of anticholinesterase compounds in live rats: Relation to toxicity. Nature, 209:88–89.

Gaines, T. B., Kimbrough, R., and Laws, E. R., Jr. (1967). Toxicology of Abate in laboratory animals. Arch. Environ. Health, 14:283–288.

Gajdos, A., and Gajdos-Török, M. (1961). Therapeutic action of adenosine-5-monophosphoric acid upon experimental porphyria of the white rat due to intoxication by hexachlorobenzene. Rev. Fr. Étud. Clin. Biol., 6(6):553–559.

Gajdos, A., and Gajdos-Török, M. (1971). Delta-aminolevulinic acid synthetase and adenosine triphosphate activity in acute saturnine intoxication in rabbits. Arch. Environ. Health, 23:270–274.

Galton, F. (1879). The geometric mean, in vital and social statistics. Proc. R. Soc. Lond. [Biol.], 29:365–367.

Garrett, R. M. (1947). Toxicity of DDT for man. Ala. State J. M. A., 17(2):74–76.

Gielen, J. E., and Nebert, D. W. (1971). Microsomal hydroxylase induction in liver cell culture by phenobarbital, polycyclic hydrocarbons, and p, p'-DDT. Science, 172:167–169.

Giese, A. C., and Crossman, E. B. (1946). Sensitization of cells to heat by visible light in presence of photodynamic dyes. J. Gen. Physiol., 29:193–202.

Gillett, J. W. (1968). No effect level of DDT in induction of microsomal epoxidation. J. Agric. Food Chem., 16:295–297.

Gillette, J. R. (1973). Factors that affect the covalent binding and toxicity of drugs. In: Proceedings of the Fifth International Congress on Pharmacology, edited by T. A. Loomis, Vol. 2, pp. 187–202. S. Karger, Basel.

Golberg, L. (1967). The amelioration of food—The Milroy Lectures. J. R. Coll. Physicians Lond. 1:385–426.

Golberg, L., Grasso, P., Feuer, G., and Gilbert, D. (1967). Activities of microsomal enzymes in relation to liver enlargement. Biochem. J., 103:12p.

Goldblatt, M. W. (1950). Organic phosphorus insecticides

and the antidotal action of atropine. Pharm. J., 164:229–233.

Goldenthal, E. I. (1971). A compilation of LD50 values in newborn and adult animals. Toxicol. Appl. Pharmacol., 18:185–207.

Graeve, K., and Herrnring, G. (1951). Über die Toxizitat des Gammahexachlorcyclohexan. Arch. Int. Pharmacodyn. Ther., 85(1–2):64–72.

Graffi, A. (1953). Unterschurchungen uber den Mechanismus der Cancerogenese und die Winkungweise cancerogener Reise. Abh. Dtsch. Akad. Wiss. Berlin, 53:1–27.

Granick, S. (1965). Hepatic porphyria and drug-induced or chemical porphyria. Ann. N. Y. Acad. Sci., 123:188–197.

Granick, S. (1966). The induction in vitro of the synthesis of δ-aminolevulinic acid synthetase in chemical porphyria: a response to certain drugs, sex hormones and foreign chemicals. J. Biol. Chem., 241:1359–1375.

Granick, S., and Levere, R. D. (1964). Heme synthesis in ethyroid cells. Prog. Hematol., 7:1–47.

Great Britain Ministry of Agriculture, Fisheries and Food (1966). Pesticides Safety Precautions Scheme Agreed Between Government Department and Industry. H. M. S. O., London.

Grob, D., Garlick, W. L., and Harvey, A. M. (1950). The toxic effects in man of the anticholinesterase insecticide parathion (p-nitrophenyl diethyl thionophosphate). Bull. Johns Hopkins Hosp., 87:106–129.

Grob, D., and Harvey, A. M. (1949). Observations on the effects of tetraethyl pyrophosphate (TEPP) in man, and on its use in the treatment of myasthenia gravis. Bull. Johns Hopkins Hosp., 84:532–567.

Gunn, J. A., and Gurd, M. R. (1940). Action of some amines related to adrenaline: Phenylallylamine, phenylbutenylamine, diphenylethylamine. J. Physiol. (Lond.), 98:424–441.

Guthrie, F. E., Monroe, R. J., and Abernathy, C. O. (1971). Response of the laboratory mouse to selection for resistance to insecticides. Toxicol. Appl. Pharmacol., 18:92–101.

Haber, F. (1924). Zur geschichte des gaskrieges. In: Fünf Vorträge aus den Jahren 1920–1923, pp. 76–92. Julius Springer, Berlin.

Haeger-Aronsen, B., Abdulla, M., and Fristedt, B. I. (1971). Effect of lead on δ-aminolevulinic acid dehydrase activity in red blood cells. Arch. Environ. Health, 23:440–445.

Hanson, H. B., and Hastings, A. B. (1933). The effect of smoking on the carbon monoxide content of blood. J. A. M. A. 100:1481.

Harbison, R. D., and Becker, B. A. (1970). Effect of phenobarbital and SKF 525A pretreatment on diphenylhydantoin teratogenicity in mice. J. Pharmacol. Exp. Ther., 175:283–288.

Hart, L. G., and Fouts, J. R. (1963). Effects of acute and chronic DDT administration on hepatic microsomal enzyme drug metabolism in the rat. Proc. Soc. Exp. Biol. Med., 114:388–392.

Hart, L. G., and Fouts, J. R. (1965). Further studies on the stimulation of hepatic microsomal drug metabolizing enzymes by DDT and its analogs. Naunyn Schmiedebergs Arch. Pharmacol., 249:486–500.

Hart, L. G., Shultice, R. W., and Fouts, J. R. (1963). Stimulatory effects of chlordane on hepatic microsomal drug metabolism in the rat. Toxicol. Appl. Pharmacol., 5:371–386.

Hatch, A., Balazs, T., Wiberg, G. S., and Grice, H. C. (1963). Long-term isolation stress in rats. Science, 142:507.

Hausmann, W. (1908). Über die sensibilisierende Wirkung tierischer Farbstoffe und ihre physiologische Bedeutung. Biochem. Zr., 14:274–278.

Hausmann, W. (1911). Die sensibilisierende Wirkung des Hamatoporphyrins. Biochem. Zr., 30:276–316.

Hausmann, W. (1914). Über die sensibilisierende Wirkung der Porphyrine. Biochem. Zr., 67:309–317.

Hayes, W. J., Jr. (1959). Pharmacology and toxicology of DDT. In: DDT, The Insecticide Dichlorodiphenyltrichloroethane and Its Significance, edited by P. Muller, Vol. 2, pp. 9–247. Birkhauser Verlag, Basel.

Hayes, W. J., Jr. (1963). Clinical Handbook on Economic Poisons. PHS Publ. No. 476, US Government Printing Office, Washington, DC.

Hayes, W. J., Jr. (1964). The toxicology of chemosterilants. Bull. WHO., 31:721–736.

Hayes, W. J., Jr. (1967a). Toxicity of pesticides to man: Risks from present levels. Proc. R. Soc. Lond. [Biol.], 167:101–127.

Hayes, W. J., Jr. (1967b). The 90-dose LD_{50} and a chronicity factor as measures of toxicity. Toxicol. Appl. Pharmacol., 11:327–335.

Hayes, W. J., Jr. (1968). Toxicological aspects of chemosterilants. In: Principles of Insect Chemosterilization, edited by G. C. LaBrecque and C. N. Smith, pp. 315–347. Appleton-Century-Crofts, New York.

Hayes, W. J., Jr. (1971). Editorial. Toxicol. Appl. Pharmacol., 20:iii.

Hayes, W. J., Jr., Dale, W. E., and Pirkle, C. I. (1971). Evidence of safety of long-term, high, oral doses of DDT for man. Arch. Environ. Health, 22:119–135.

Hayes, W. J., Jr., Durham, W. F., and Cueto, C., Jr. (1956). The effect of known repeated oral doses of chlorophenothane (DDT) in man. J. A. M. A., 162:890–897.

Hayes, W. J., Jr., and Gaines, T. B. (1959). Laboratory studies of five anticoagulant rodenticides. Public Health Rep., 74:105–113.

Hayes, W. J., Jr., Mattson, A. M., Short, J. G., and Witter, R. F. (1960). Safety of malathion dusting powder for louse control. Bull. WHO, 22:503–514.

Hazelton, L. W., and Holland, E. G. (1953). Toxicity of malathion. Summary of mammalian investigations. A. M. A. Arch. Ind. Hyg. Occup. Med., 8:399–405.

Heath, D. F., and Vandekar, M. (1964). Toxicity and metabolism of dieldrin in rats. Br. J. Ind. Med., 21:269–279.

Heinemann, B. (1971). Prophage induction in lysogenic bacteria as a method of detecting portneial mutagenic, carcinogenic, carcinostatic, and teratogenic agents. In:Chemical Mutagens, edited by A. Hollaender, Vol. 1, pp. 235–266. Plenum Press, New York.

Hemphill, F. E., Kaeberle, M. L., and Buck, W. B. (1971). Lead suppression of mouse resistance to Salmonella typhimurium. Science, 172:1031–1032.

Henderson, C., and Pickering, Q. H. (1957). Toxicity of organic phosphorus insecticides to fish. Trans. Am. Fish. Soc., 87:39–51.

Henderson, C., Pickering, Q. H., and Tarzwell, C. M. (1959). Relative toxicity of ten chlorinated hydrocarbon insecticides to four species of fish. Trans. Am. Fish. Soc., 88:23–32.

Hernberg, S., Nikkanen, J., Mellin, G., and Lilius, H. (1970). δ-Aminolevulinic acid dehydrase as a measure of lead exposure. Arch. Environ. Health, 21:140–145.

Herr, F., Borsi, J., and Pataky, G. (1953). Wirkung der Umwelttemperatur auf die Toxizität der Analgetika. Acta Physiol. Acad. Sci. Hung., 4:363–371.

Herr, F., Borsi, J., and Pataky, G. (1954). Wirkung der Umwelttemperatur auf die Toxicität der Analgetika. Arch Exp. Pathol. Pharmakol., 223:56–63.

Hill, E. V., and Carlisle, H. (1947). Toxicity of 2,4-dichlorophenoxacetic acid for experimental animals. J. Ind. Hyg., 29:85–95.

Hodgkinson, R. (1954). Blood dyscrasias associated with chloramphenicol. An investigation into the cases in the British Isles. Lancet, 1:285–287.

Hoffman, D. G., Worth, H. M., Emmerson, J. L., and Anderson, R. C. (1968). Stimulation of hepatic microsomal drug-metabolising enzymes by α-α-bis(p-chlorophenyl)-3-pyridinemethanol and a method for determining no-effect levels in rats. Toxicol. Appl. Pharmacol., 12:464–472.

Hoffman, D. G., Worth, H. M., Emmerson, J. L., and Anderson, R. C. (1970). Stimulation of hepatic drug-metabolizing enzymes by chlorophenothane (DDT): the relationship to liver enlargement and hepatotoxicity in the rat. Toxicol. Appl. Pharmacol., 16:171–178.

Hoffman, I., and Lendle, L. (1948). Zur Wirkungsweise newer insektizider Stoffe. Arch. Exp. Pathol. Pharmakol., 205:223–242.

Holmes, R. W., and Love, J. (1952). Suicide attempt with warfarin, a bishydroxycoumarin-like rodenticide. J. A. M. A., 148:935–937.

Holmstedt, B. (1959). Pharmacology of organophosphorus cholinesterase inhibitors. Pharmacol. Rev., 11:567–688.

Hoppe, J. O., Duprey, L. P., and Dennis, E. E. (1965). Acute toxicity in the young adult and the newborn mouse. Toxicol. Appl. Pharmacol., 7:486.

Hsieh, H. C. (1954). DDT intoxication in a family of Southern Taiwan. A. M. A. Arch. Ind. Hyg. Occup. Med., 10(4):344–346.

Hueppe, F. (1896). Naturwissenschaftliche Einfuhrung in die Bakteriologie. C. W. Kreidel's Verlag, Wiesbaden. (A translation by E. O. Jordan entitled The Principles of Bacteriology was published by the Open Court Publishing Co., Chicago, in 1899.)

Hutchinson, G. E. (1964). The influence of the environment. Proc. Natl. Acad. Sci. USA, 51:930.

Jackson, J. B., Drummond, R. O., Buck, W. B., and Hunt, L. M. (1960). Toxicity of organic phosphorus insecticides to horses. J. Econ. Entomol., 53:602–604.

Jaffé, E. R. (ed.) (1968). Porphyria and disorders of porphyrin metabolism. Semin. Hematol., 5:293–433.

Johnson, G. E., Sellers, E. A., and Schonbaum, E. (1963). Interrelationship of temperature on action of drugs. Fed. Proc., 22:745–749.

Jollow, D. J., Mitchell, J. R., Zampaglione, N., and Gillette, J. R. (1974). Bromobenzene-induced liver necrosis. Protective role of glutathion and evidence for 3,4-bromobenzene oxide as the hepatotoxic metabolite. Pharmacology, 11:151–169.

Käer, E., and Loewe, S. (1926). Über Kombinationswirkungen. II. Mitteilung: Wirkungen von Diäthylbarbitursäure-Pyramidon-Gemischen. Arch. Exp. Path. Pharmakol., 114:327–328.

Kaliser, L. A. (1968). An in vitro and in vivo study of the effect of DDT on the phagocytic activity of rat white blood cells. Toxicol. Appl. Pharmacol., 13:353–357.

Kalter, H. (1965). Species, stock, and strain differences in experimental teratogenesis. In: Supplement to Teratology Workshop Manual, edited by the Pharmaceutical Manufacturers Association, Berkeley, California.

Kanagaratnam, K., Boon, W. H., and Hoh, T. K. (1960). Parathion poisoning from contaminated barley. Lancet, 1:538–542.

Kappas, A., Bradlow, H. L., Gillette, P. N., Levere, R. D., and Gallagher, T. F. (1972). A defect of steroid hormone metabolism in acute intermittent porphyria. Fed. Proc., 31:1293–1297.

Karnofsky, D. A. (1965). Mechanisms of action of certain growth-inhibiting drugs. In: Teratology, Principles and Techniques, edited by J. G. Wilson and J. Warkany, pp. 145–184. University of Chicago Press, Chicago.

Kaufman, L., Swanson, A. L., and Marver, H. S. (1970). Chemically induced porphyria: Prevention by prior treatment with phenobarbital. Science, 170:320–322.

Kehoe, R. A. (1961). The metabolism of lead in man in health and disease. II. The metabolism of lead under abnormal conditions. J. R. Inst. Public Health Hyg., 24:129–143.

Keplinger, M. L., and Deichmann, W. B. (1967). Acute toxicity of combinations of pesticides. Toxicol. Appl. Pharmacol., 10:586–595.

Keplinger, M. L., Lanier, G. E., and Deichmann, W. B. (1959). Effects of environmental temperature on the acute toxicity of a number of compounds in rats. Toxicol. Appl. Pharmacol., 1:156–161.

Keppler, J. F., Maxfield, M. E., Moss, W. D., Tietjen, G., and Linch, A. L. (1970). Interlaboratory evaluation of the reliability of blood lead analyses. Am. Ind. Hyg. Assoc. J., 31:412–429.

Kinoshita, F. K., Frawley, J. P., and DuBois, K. P. (1966). Quantitative measurement of induction of hepatic microsomal enzymes by various dietary levels of DDT and toxaphene in rats. Toxicol. Appl. Pharmacol., 9:50513.

Koffler, H., and Markert, I. L. (1951). Effect of photodynamic action on the viscosity of desoxyribonucleic acid. Proc. Soc. Exp. Biol. Med., 76:90–92.

Koizumi, K. (1955). Tetanus and hyperresponsiveness of the mammalian spinal cord produced by strychnine, guanidine and cold. Am. J. Physiol., 183:35–43.

Krijnen, C. J., and Boyd, E. M. (1970). Susceptibility to captan pesticide of albino rats fed from weaning on diets containing various levels of protein. Food Cosmet. Toxicol. 8:35–42.

Krogh, A., and Hemmingsen, A. M. (1928). The assay of insulin on rabbits and mice. Det. Kgl. Danske Videnskebernes Selskab. Biol. VIII, 6.

Kueter, K. E., and Ott, J. N. (1964). Some observations on photo-biologic phenomena in animals. Lab. Anim. Care, 14:313.

Kun'ev, V. V. (1965). Influence of low DDT doses on the phagocytic state of the blood in albino rats. Vapr. Pitan., 24:74–78.

Labbe, R. F. (1967). Metabolic anomalies in porphyria. The result of impaired biological oxidation? Lancet, 1:1361–1364.

Lamanna, C., and Carr, C. J. (1967). The botulinal, tetanal, and enterostaphylococcal toxins: a review. Clin. Pharmacol. Ther., 8:286–332.

Lamanna, C., and Hart, E. R. (1968). Relationship of lethal toxic dose to body weight of the mouse. Toxicol. Appl. Pharmacol., 13:307–315.

Lange, P. F., and Terveer, J. (1954). Warfarin poisoning. Report of fourteen cases. US Armed Forces Med. J., 5:872–877.

Laug, E. P., Nelson, A. A., Fitzhugh, O. G., and Kunze, F. M. (1950). Liver cell alteration and DDT storage in the fat of the rat induced by dietary levels of 1 to 50 ppm in DDT. J. Pharmacol. Exp. Ther., 98:268–273.

Laug, E. P., Vos, E. A., Umberger, E. J., and Kunze, F. M. (1947). A method for the determination of cutaneous penetration of mercury. J. Pharmacol. Exp. Ther., 89:42–51.

Laws, E. R., Jr., Curley, A., and Biros, F. J. (1967). Men with intensive occupational exposure to DDT. A clinical and chemical study. Arch. Environ. Health, 15:766–775.

Lee, M., Harris, K., and Trowbridge, H. (1964). Effect of the level of dietary protein on the toxicity of dieldrin for the laboratory rat. J. Nutr., 84:136–144.

Lehman, A. J. (1965). Summaries of Pesticide Toxicity. Association of Food and Drug Officials of the United States, Topeka, Kansas.

Lensky, P., and Evans, H. L. (1952). Human poisoning by chlordane. Report of a case. J. A. M. A., 149:1394–1395.

Lichtenstein, L. M., and Osler, A. G. (1964). Studies on the mechanisms of hypersensitivity phenomena. IX. Histamine release from human leukocytes by ragweed pollen antigen. J. Exp. Med., 120:507–530.

Lindsay, H. A., and Kullman, V. S. (1966). Pentobarbital sodium: variation in toxicity. Science, 151:576–577.

Litchfield, J. T., Jr. (1949). A method for rapid graphic solution of time-percent effect curves. J. Pharmacol. Exp. Ther., 97:399–406.

Litchfield, J. T., Jr., and Wilcoxon, F. (1949). A simplified method of evaluating dose-effect experiments. J. Pharmacol. Exp. Ther., 96:99–113.

Loewe, S., and Muischnek, H. (1926). Über Kombinationswirkungen. I. Mitteilung: Hilfsmittel der Fragestellung. Arch. Exp. Pathol. Pharmakol., 114:313–326.

Lu, F. C., Jessup, D. C., and Levallee, A. (1965). Toxicity of pesticides in young rats versus adult rats. Food Cosmet.

Toxicol., 3:591–596.

Luckey, T. D. (1956). Mode of action of antibiotics: evidence from germfree birds, *Proceedings of First International Conference on Use of Antibiotics in Agriculture.* National Academy of Sciences, Washington, pp. 135–145.

Lutsch, E. F., and Morris, R. W. (1967). Circadian periodicity in susceptibility to lidocaine hydrochloride. Science, 156:100–102.

McAlister, D. (1879). The law of the geometric mean. Proc. R. Soc., 29:367–376.

McChesney, E. W., Golberg, L., and Harris, E. S. (1972). Reappraisal of the toxicology of ethylene glycol. IV. The metabolism of labelled glycollic and glyoxylic acids in the rhesus monkey. Food Cosmet. Toxicol., 10:655–670.

McDonald, F. F. (1948). The effect of environmental temperature on the toxicity of BAL. Br. J. Pharmacol., 3:116–117.

McGeer, E. G., and McGeer, P. L. (1966). Circadian rhythm in pineal tyrosine hydroxylase. Science, 153:73–74.

McIntosh, A. H. (1961). Graphical and other short statistical methods for "all-or-none" bioassay tests. J. Sci. Food Agric., 4:312–316.

McLean, A. E. M., and McLean, E. K. (1969). Diet and toxicity. Br. Med. Bull., 25:278–281.

Magee, P. N., and Barnes, J. M. (1962). Induction of kidney tumours in the rat with dimethylnitrosamine (N-nitrosodimethylamine). J. Pathol. Bacteriol., 84:19–31.

Mainland, D. (1963). *Elementary Medical Statistics.* W. B. Saunders Company, Philadelphia.

Mantel, N. (1963). The concept of threshold in carcinogenesis. Clin. Pharmacol. Ther., 4:104–109.

Mantel, N., and Bryan, W. R. (1961). "Safety" testing of carcinogenic agents. J. Natl. Cancer Inst., 27:455–470.

Marton, A. V., Sellers, E. A., and Kalow, W. (1962). Effect of cold on rats chronically exposed to malathion. Can. J. Biochem. Physiol., 40:1671–1676.

Mayer, P. S., Mosko, M. M., Schutz, P. J., Osterman, F. A., Steen, L. H., and Baker, L. A. (1953). Penicillin naphylaxis. J. A. M. A., 151:351–353.

Meneely, G. R. (1966). Toxic effects of dietary sodium chloride and the protective effect of potassium. In: *Toxicants Occurring Naturally in Foods,* NAS Publ. 1354. National Academy of Sciences, Washington, DC.

Meyer, B. J., and Karel, L. (1948). The effect of environmental temperature on alpha-naphthylthiourea (ANTU) toxicity to rats. J. Pharmacol. Exp. Ther., 93:420–422.

Meyer, U. A., and Marver, H. S. (1971). Chemically induced porphyria: Increased microsomal heme turnover after treatment with allylisopropylacetamide. Science, 171:64–66.

Milby, T. H., Ottoboni, F., and Mitchell, H. W. (1964). Parathion residue poisoning among orchard workers. J. A. M. A., 189:351–356.

Moeller, H. C., and Rider, J. A. (1962a). Plasma and red blood cell cholinesterase activity as indications of the threshold of incipient toxicity of ethyl-*p*-nitrophenyl thionobenzenephosphonate (EPN) and malathion in human beings. Toxicol. Appl. Pharmacol., 4:123–130.

Moeller, H. C., and Rider, J. A. (1962b). Threshold of incipient toxicity to Systox and methyl parathion. Fed. Proc., 21:451.

Moeschlin, S. (1965). *Poisoning—Diagnosis and Treatment.* Grune & Stratton, New York.

Monier-Williams, G. W. (1949). *Trace Elements in Food.* John Wiley & Sons, Inc., New York.

Moore, A. W., and Ward, J. C. (1935). The effect of altitude on the action of drugs. I. Strychnine. J. Am. Pharm. Assoc., 24:460–464.

Murphy, M. L. (1965). Factors influencing teratogenic response to drugs. In: *Teratology, Principles and Techniques,* edited by J. G. Wilson and J. Warkany, pp. 145–184. University of Chicago Press, Chicago.

Murphy, S. D., Anderson, R. L., and DuBois, K. P. (1959).

Potentiation of toxicity of malathion by triorthotolyl phosphate. Proc. Soc. Exp. Biol. Med., 100:483–487.

Murphy, S. D., and Cheever, K. L. (1968). Effect of feeding insecticides: Inhibition of carboxyesterase and cholinesterase activities in rats. Arch. Environ. Health, 17:749–758.

Murphy, S. D., and DuBois, K. P. (1957). Quantitative measurement of inhibition of the enzymatic detoxification of malathion by EPN (ethyl p-nitrophenyl thionobenzenephosphonate). Proc. Soc. Exp. Biol. Med., 96:813–818.

Murphy, S. D., and DuBois, K. P. (1958). The influence of various factors on the enzymatic conversion of organic thiophosphates to anticholinesterase agents. J. Pharmacol. Exp. Ther., 124:194–202.

National Academy of Sciences. (1960). *Problems in the Evaluation of Carcinogenic Hazard from Use of Food Additives.* NAS Publ. 749. Washington, DC.

National Academy of Sciences. (1969). Application of metabolic data to the evaluation of drugs. A report prepared by the Committee on Problems of Drug Safety of the Drug Research Board, National Academy of Sciences—National Research Council. Clin. Pharmacol. Ther., 10:607–634.

Neal, P. A., Sweeney, T. R., Spicer, S. S., and von Oettingen, W. F. (1946). The excretion of DDT (2,2-bis-(p-chlorophenyl-1,1,1-trichloroethane) in man, together with chemical observations. Public Health Rep., 61:403–409.

Ortega, P., Hayes, W. J., Jr., Durham, W. F., and Mattson, A. (1956). *DDT in the Diet of the Rat.* Public Health Monogr. No. 43, PHS Publ. No. 484.

Payton, J. (1953). Parathion and ultra-violet light. Nature, 171:355–356.

Pearson, E. W., and Hartley, E. O. (1958). *Biometrika Tables for Statisticians,* Ed. 2, Vol. 1. University Press, Cambridge.

Peterson, D. I., and Hardinge, M. G. (1967). The effect of various environmental factors on cocaine and ephedrine toxicity. J. Pharm. Pharmacol., 19:810–814.

Photinopoulos, N. J., Lorincz, A. L. (1965). The effects of copper salts on experimental porphyria. J. Invest. Dermatol., 45:510–515.

Pindyck, J., Kappas, A., and Levere, R. D. (1971). Recent advances in porphyrin metabolism. CRC Crit. Rev. Clin. Lab. Sci., 2:639–657.

Poland, A., Smith, D., Kuntzman, R., Jacobson, M., and Conney, A. H. (1970). Effect of intensive occupational exposure to DDT on phenylbutazone and cortisol metabolism in human subjects. Clin. Pharmacol. Ther., 11:724–732.

Polcik, B., Nowosielski, J. W., and Naegele, J. A. (1964). Daily sensitivity rhythm of the two-spotted spider mite, *Tetranychus urticae,* to DDVP. Science, 145:405–406.

Prendergast, J. A., Jones, R. A., Jenkins, L. J., Jr., and Siegel, J. (1967). Effects on experimental animals of long-term inhalation of trichloroethylene, carbon tetrachloride, 1,1,1-trichloroethane, dichlorodifluoromethane, and 1,1-dichloroethylene. Toxicol. Appl. Pharmacol., 10:270–289.

Price, P. J., Suk, W. A., and Freeman, A. E. (1972). Type C RNA tumor viruses as determinants of chemical carcinogenesis: Effects of sequence of treatment. Science, 177:1003–1004.

Princi, F. (1952). Human toxicity of certain chlorinated hydrocarbon insecticides. Third Int. Cong. of Phytopharmacy. Paris.

Pruzansky, J. J., Feinberg, S. W., and Kenniebrew, A. (1959). Passive anaphylaxis in the guinea pig and its inhibition by an extraneous antigen-antibody reaction. J. Immunol., 82:497–501.

Quay, W. B. (1963). Circadian rhythm in rat pineal serotonin and its modifications by estrous cycle and photoperiod. Ge.. Comp. Endocrinol., 1:473–479.

Quay, W. B. (1964). Circadian and estrous rhythms in pineal melatonin and 5-hydroxy indole-3-acetic acid. Proc. Soc. Exp. Biol. Med., 115:710–713.

Quay, W. B., and Halevy, A. (1962). Experimental modification of the rat pineal's content of serotonin and related indole amines. Physiol. Zool., 35:1–7.

Radeleff, R. D. (1964). *Veterinary Toxicology*. Lea & Febiger, Philadelphia.

Radeleff, R. D., Woodard, G. T., Nickerson, W. J., and Bushland, R. C. (1955). The acute toxicity of chlorinated hydrocarbon and organic phosphorus insecticides to livestock. US Dep. Agr. Tech. Bull. 1122.

Rapoport, M. I., Feigin, R. D., Bruton, J., and Beisel, W. R. (1966). Circadian rhythm for tryptophen pyrrolase and its circulating substrate. Science, 153:1642–1644.

Rask, E. N., and Howell, W. H. (1928). The photodynamic action of hematoporphyrin. Am. J. Physiol., 84:363–377.

Reeves, G. I. (1925). The arsenical poisoning of livestock. J. Econ. Entomol., 18:83.

Reid, W. D., and Krishna, G. (1973). Centrolobular hepatic necrosis related to covalent binding of metabolites of halogenated aromatic hydrocarbons. Exp. Mol. Path., 18:80–99.

Rider, J. A., Moeller, H. C., Swader, J., and Devereaux, R. G. (1959). A study of the anticholinesterase properties of EPN and malathion in human volunteers. Clin. Res., 7:81–82.

Robinson, J., Richardson, A., Bush, B., and Elgar, K. E. (1966). A photoisomerisation product of dieldrin. Bull. Environ. Contam. Toxicol., 1:127–132.

Roburn, J. (1963). Effect of sunlight and ultraviolet radiation on chlorinated pesticide residues. Chem. Ind. 38:1555–1556.

Rollo, I. M. (1955). The mode of action of sulphonamides, proguanil and pyrimethamine on *Plasmodium gallinaceum*. Br. J. Pharmacol., 10:208–214.

Roszkowski, A. P. (1965). The pharmacological properties of norbormide, a selective rat toxicant. J. Pharmacol. Exp. Ther., 149:288–299.

Roszkowski, A. P., Poos, G. I., and Mohrbacher, R. J. (1964). Selective rat toxicant. Science, 144:412–413.

Saffiotti, O., and Shubik, P. (1956). The effects of low concentration of carcinogen in epidermal carcinogenesis. A comparison with promoting agents. J. Natl. Cancer Inst., 16:961–969.

Schantz, E. J., and Sugiyama, H. (1974). The toxins of *Clostridium botulinum*. Essays in Toxicology, 5:99–119.

Schmid, R. (1966). The porphyrias. In: *The Metabolic Basis of Inherited Disease*, edited by J. B. Stanbury, J. B. Wyngaarden and D. S. Fredrickson, pp. 813–870. McGraw-Hill, New York.

Schmid, R., and Schwartz, S. (1952). Experimental porphyria. III. Hepatic type produced by sedormid. Proc. Soc. Exp. Biol. Med., 81:685–689.

Schoental, R., and Magee, P. N. (1957). Chronic liver changes in rats after a single dose of lasiocarpine, a pyrrolizidine (senecio) alkaloid. J. Pathol. Bacteriol., 74:305–319.

Scholz, J. (1965). Chronic toxicity testing. Nature, 207:870–871.

Schulz, H. (1888). Ueber Hefegifte. Pfluegers Arch. Ges. Physiol., 42:517–541, plus Plates III–VIII.

Schwabe, U., and Wendling, I. (1967). Beschleunigun des Arzneimittel-Abbaus durch kleine Dosen von DDT und anderen Chlorkohlen-Wasserstoff-Insecticiden. Arzneim. Forsch., 17:614–618.

Schwan, H. P., and Piersol, G. M. (1954). The absorption of electromagnetic energy in body tissues. A review and critical analysis. Part 1. Biophysical aspects. Am. J. Phys. Med., 33:371–404.

Schwan, H. P., and Piersol, G. M. (1955). The absorption of electromagnetic energy in body tissues. A review and critical analysis. Part II. Physiological and clinical aspects. Am. J. Phys. Med., 34:425–448.

Seabury, J. H. (1963). Toxicity of 2,4-dichlorophenoxyacetic acid for man and dog. Arch. Environ. Health. 7:202–209.

Shabad, L. M. (1971). Dose-response studies in experimentally induced lung tumors. Environ. Res., 4:305–315.

Shemano, I., and Nickerson, M. (1958). Effect of ambient temperature on thermal responses to drugs. Can. J. Biochem. Physiol., 36:1243–1249.

Shemano, I., and Nickerson, M. (1959). Mechanisms of thermal responses to pentylenetetrazol. J. Pharmacol. Exp. Ther., 126:143–147.

Siami, G. (1971). Personal communication.

Siegel, P. S. (1961). Food intake in the rat in relation to the dark-light cycle. J. Comp. Physiol. Psychol., 54:294–301.

Siegel, J., Rudolph, H. S., Getzkin, A. J., and Jones, R. A. (1965). Effects of experimental animals of long-term continuous inhalation of a triaryl phosphate hydraulic fluid. Toxicol. Appl. Pharmacol., 7:543–549.

Smith, M. I., Elvolne, E., and Frazier, W. H. (1930). The pharmacological action of certain phenol esters, with special reference to the etiology of so-called ginger paralysis. Public Health Rep., 45:2509–2524.

Smith, P. W., Mertens, H., Lewis, M. F., Funkhouser, G. E., Higgins, E. A., Crane, C. R., Sanders, D. C., Endecott, B. R., and Flux, M. (1972). Toxicology of dichlorovos at operational aircraft cabin altitudes. Aerosp. Med., 43:473–478.

Smyth, H. F., Jr. (1967). Sufficient challenge. Food Cosmet. Toxicol., 5:51–58.

Smyth, H. F., Jr., Carpenter, C. P., Weil, C. S., Pozzani, U. C., and Striegel, J. A. (1962). Range-finding toxicity data List VI. Am. Ind. Hyg. Assoc. J., 23:95–107.

Smyth, H. F., Jr., Weil, C. S., West, J. S., and Carpenter, C. P. (1969). An exploration of joint toxic action: Twenty-seven industrial chemicals intubated in rats in all possible pairs. Toxicol. Appl. Pharmacol., 14:340–347.

Snedecor, G. W. (1967). *Statistical Methods Applied to Experiments in Agriculture and Biology*, Ed. 6. The Iowa State University Press, Ames.

Snyder, S. H., Zweig, M., and Axelrod, J. (1964). Control of the circadian rhythm in serotonin content of the rat pineal gland. Life Sci., 3:1175–1179.

Snyder, S. H., Zweig, M., Axelrod, J., and Fischer, J. E. (1965). Control of the circadian rhythm in serotonin content of the rat pineal gland. Proc. Natl. Acad. Sci., 53:301–305.

Sollberger, A. (1965). *Biological Rhythm Research*. Elsevier Publishing Co., Amsterdam.

Sollmann, T. (1957). *A Manual of Pharmacology*, Ed. 8. W. B. Saunders Company, Philadelphia.

Southam, C. M., and Ehrlich, J. (1943). Effects of extract of western red-cedar heartwood on certain wood decaying fungi in culture. Phytopathol., 33:517–524.

Spoor, R. P., and Jackson, D. B. (1966). Circadian rhythms: variation in sensitivity of isolated rat atria to acetylcholine. Science, 154:782.

Steele, G. D., and Torrie, J. H. (1960). *Principles and Procedures of Statistics*. McGraw-Hill, New York.

Stein, A. A., Serrone, D. M., and Coulston, F. (1965). Safety evaluation of methoxychlor in human volunteers. Toxicol. Appl. Pharmacol., 7:499.

Stokinger, H. E. (1953). Size of dose; Its effect on distribution in the body. Nucleonics, 11:24–27.

Stokvis, B. J. (1895). Zur Pathogenese der Haematophorphyrie. Z. Klin. Med., 28:1–9.

Street, J. C., Mayer, F. L., and Wagstaff, D. J. (1969). Ecologic significance of pesticide interactions. Ind. Med. Surg., 38:409–419.

Su, M., Kinoshita, F. K., Frawley, J. P., and DuBois, K. P. (1971). Comparative inhibition of aliesterases and cholinesterase in rats fed eighteen organophosphorus insecticides. Toxicol. Appl. Pharmacol., 20:241–249.

Thiessen, D. D. (1963). Varying sensitivity of C57BL/Crgl mice to grouping. Science, 141:827–828.

Thomas, A. A. (1965). Low ambient pressure environments and toxicity. Arch. Environ. Health, 11:316–322.

Tio, T. H. (1956). Beschouwingen over de prophyria cutanea tarda. M. D. Thesis, University of Amsterdam.

Tio, T. H., Leijnse, B., Jarrett, A., and Rimington, C. (1957). Acquired porphyria from a liver tumor. Clin. Sci., 16:517–527.

Townsend, J. F., and Luckey, T. D. (1960). Hormoligosis in pharmacology, J. A. M. A., 173:44–48.

Tracy, R. L., Woodcock, J. G., and Chodroff, S. (1960). Toxicological aspects of 2,2-dichlorovinyl dimethyl phosphate (DDVP) in cows, horses, and white rats. J. Econ. Entomol., 53:593–601.

Treon, J. F., and Cleveland, F. P. (1955). Toxicity of certain chlorinated hydrocarbon insecticides for laboratory animals, with special reference to aldrin and dieldrin. J. Agric. Food Chem., 3:402–408.

Trevan, J. W. (1927). The error of determination of Toxicity. Proc. R. Soc. Lond. [Biol.] 101:483–514.

Velbinger, H. H. (1947). Zur Frage der "DDT"—Toxizitat fur Menschen. Dtsch. Gesundheitsw., 2(11):355–358.

Vesell, E. S. (1967). Induction of drug-metabolizing enzymes in liver microsomes of mice and rats by softwood bedding. Science, 157:1057–1058.

Vessey, S. (1967). Effects of chlorpromazine on aggression in laboratory populations of wild house mice. Ecology, 48:367–376.

Wade, A. E., Holl, J. E., Hilliard, C. C., Molton, E., and Greene, F. E. (1968). Alteration of drug metabolism in rats and mice by an environment of cedarwood. Pharmacology, 1:317–328.

Walters, M. N. I. (1957). Malathion intoxication. Med. J. Aust., 1:876–877.

Ward, J. C., Spencer, H. J., Crabtree, D. G., and Garlough, F. E. (1940). Red squill: VII. Influence of altitude upon toxicity to albino rats. J. Am. Pharm. Assoc., 29:350–353.

Warren, E. (1900). On the reaction of Daphnia magna (Straus) to certain changes in its environment. Q. J. Microsc. Sci., 43:199–224.

Wassermann, M., Wassermann, D., Gershon, Z., and Zellermayer, L. (1969). Effects of organochlorine insecticides on body defense systems. Ann. N. Y. Acad. Sci., 160:393–401.

Waud, D. T., Kottegoda, S. R., and Krayer, O. (1958). Threshold dose and time course of norepinephrine depletion of the mammalian heart by reserpine. J. Pharmacol. Exp. Ther., 124:340–346.

Way, J. L., Gibbon, S. L., and Sheehy, M. (1966). Effect of oxygen on cyanide intoxication. I. Prophylactic protection. J. Pharmacol. Exp. Ther., 153:381–385.

Webb, R. E., and Miranda, C. L. (1973). Effect of the quality of dietary protein on heptachlor toxicity. Food Cosmet. Toxicol., 11:63–67.

Weil, C. S. (1952). Tables for convenient calculation of median-effective dose (LD$_{50}$ or ED$_{50}$) and instructions in their use. Biometrics, 8:249–263.

Weil, C. S. (1970). Selection of the valid number of sampling units and a consideration of their combination in toxicological studies involving reproduction, teratogenesis or carcinogenesis. Food Cosmet. Toxicol., 8:177–182.

Weil, C. S., Carpenter, C. P., West, J. S., and Smyth, H. F., Jr. (1966). Reproducibility of single dose toxicity testing. Am. Ind. Hyg. Assoc. J., 27:483–487.

Weil, C. S., and Carpenter, C. P. (1969). Abnormal values in control groups during repeated-dose toxicologic studies. Toxicol. Appl. Pharmacol., 14:335–339.

Weil, C. S., and McCollister, D. D. (1963). Relationship between short-and long-term feeding studies in designing an effective toxicity test. J. Agric. Food Chem., 11:486–491.

Weil, C. S., and Scala, R. A. (1971). Study of intra- and interlaboratory variability in the results of rabbit eye and skin irritation tests. Toxicol. Appl. Pharmacol., 19:276–356.

Weil, C. S., Woodside, M. D., Bernard, J. R., and Carpenter, C. P. (1969). Relationship between single-peroral, one-week and ninety-day rat feeding studies. Toxicol. Appl. Pharmacol., 14:426–431.

Weil, C. S., and Wright, G. J. (1967). Intra- and interlaboratory comparative evaluation of single oral test. Toxicol. Appl. Pharmacol., 11:378–388.

Welch, B. L., and Welch, A. S. (1966). Graded effect of social stimulation upon d-amphetamine toxicity, aggressiveness and heart and adrenal weight. J. Pharmacol. Exp. Ther., 151:331–338.

Wiberg, G. S., and Grice, H. C. (1965). Effect of prolonged individual caging on toxicity parameters in rats. Food Cosmet. Toxicol., 3:597–603.

Wiepkema, P. R. (1966). Aurothioglucose sensitivity of CBA mice injected at two different times of day. Nature, 209:937.

Williams, M. W., Guyat, H. N., and Fitzhugh, O. G. (1959). The subacute toxicity of four organic phosphates to dogs. Toxicol. Appl. Pharmacol., 1:1–7.

Wilson, J. G. (1964). Teratogenic interaction of chemical agents in the rat. J. Pharmacol. Exp. Ther., 144:429–436.

Wogan, G. N., and Newberne, P. M. (1967). Dose-response characteristics of aflatoxin B, carcinogenesis in the rat. Cancer Res., 27:2370–2376.

Wolfe, H. R., Durham, W. F., and Armstrong, J. F. (1970). Urinary excretion of insecticide metabolites. Excretion of para-nitrophenol and DDA as indicators of exposure to parathion. Arch. Environ. Health, 21:711–716.

Wurtman, R. J., Axelrod, J., and Fischer, J. E. (1964). Melatonin synthesis in the pineal gland: effect of light mediated by the sympathetic nervous system. Science, 143:1328–1329.

Yeary, R. A., and Benish, R. A. (1965). A comparison of the acute toxicities of drugs in newborn and adult rats. Toxicol. Appl. Pharmacol., 7:504.

3

GENERAL PRINCIPLES: METABOLISM

The word *metabolism* may be used to designate the sum of chemical reactions that serve to maintain life. Parts of this integrated whole are spoken of as "protein metabolism," "fat metabolism," "enzyme-mediated metabolism," and the like. Some effects of pesticides and other foreign compounds on different aspects of initially normal metabolism are discussed in Chapter 4.

The word *metabolism* also may be used to designate the effect of an organism, through its enzymes, on the chemical structure of foreign compounds. These effects, also called *biotransformation,* are discussed in the present chapter.

3.1 Qualitative Aspects of Metabolism

3.1.1 Possibility of "External Metabolism"

The finding of a derivative of a compound in the tissues or excreta of an animal is not necessarily proof that the compound underwent biotransformation in that organism. Compounds, especially in thin films, may undergo chemical change when exposed to light or heat. Mitchell (1961) reported the effects of ultraviolet light on 141 pesticides. The enzymes of plants and microorganisms are responsible for a wide range of biotransformations (see Sections 6.1.2.2 and 6.3.2.2); therefore, an animal eating plants may ingest one or more derivatives as well as the compound applied to the plants or to the soil. At least one example is known of the interaction of two pesticides in soil to form a third compound (Bartha, 1969). Some toxicants may be metab-

olized by bacteria in the intestine—still external to the metabolism of the animal itself.

Although all these possibilities must be kept in mind, they are usually of secondary importance. Many derivatives known to be formed by light, plants, or microorganisms are formed by mammalian enzymes also. Thus, about 33% or more of the DDT-related material people consume is DDE (see Table 6-2), but man is capable of converting DDT to DDE (Hayes *et al.,* 1956), and DDE constitutes about 70% of the DDT-related material stored by people in the general population (see Table 7-10). Differences in the metabolism of a given compound by different animals and plants are often quantitative rather than qualitative.

3.1.2 Biotransformation

Biotransformation has been studied more thoroughly than any other aspect of the metabolism of foreign compounds. A number of books review the biotransformation of organic compounds generally (Williams, 1959) or specific aspects of it (Heath, 1961; Metcalf, 1955; O'Brien, 1960).

3.1.2.1 Known Reactions. Of the chemical reactions known to be involved in the biotransformation of one or more pesticides, only a portion have been traced to enzymes that have been at least partially purified and characterized. In many instances, all that is known is that one or more derivatives of a particular compound may be found in the tissues or excreta of animals dosed with the compound itself.

Chemical reactions reported to occur in the

metabolism of pesticides are illustrated in Table 3-1. The biotransformation of many, and probably most, pesticides involves a combination of chemical reactions. In some instances, some of the breakdown products become part of the general metabolic pool. For example, carbon tetrachloride is excreted partly as urea and partly as carbon dioxide. At least one compound, methylene chloride, apparently is metabolized in man partly to carbon monoxide (Stewart *et al.*, 1972a, 1972b).

Conjugation. Williams (1959) suggests that the metabolism of most foreign compounds occurs in two phases, the first involving oxidations, reductions, and hydrolyses, and the second involving synthesis or conjugation. This synthesis includes combination of the foreign compound or a derivative with a normal metabolite of the body to form a more water-soluble and, therefore, more readily excreted product. Conjugation may be simple, as in the case of phenol, but often it is a complicated process, and the final product is not derived by a single step from the natural metabolite it most resembles. The combination actually may arise from precursors of the natural metabolite. In spite of this possible complexity, it is useful to think of conjugation of foreign chemicals taking place with glucuronic acid to form glucuronides, cysteine (or N-acetylcysteyl residues) to form mercapturic acids, glycine to form hippuric and related acids, sulfate ions to form ethereal sulfates, thiosulfate ions to form thiocyanate, and glutamine to form conjugates of the same name. Conjugates involving glycine and glutamine may be formed by mammals with some foreign chemicals, but apparently have not been observed with pesticides. Conjugates of foreign chemicals that are rare in mammals, or known only in other classes or phyla, include glucosides, ribosides, ornithines, sulfides, and conjugates with serine, metal complexes, and methylated or acetylated compounds.

Conjugation is not only of general importance in toxicology, but it is of the greatest importance in the detoxication of some pesticides, notably cyanide. However, a number of pesticides or their metabolites are not known to form conjugates, and the nature of the complex is unknown for others. For example, Jensen *et al.* (1957) gave evidence that DDT-derived meterial in the bile of rats was in the form of an unidentified complex that was neither a glucuronide nor a sulfate.

3.1.2.2 Enzymatic Basis of Biotransformation.
Although some of the chemical changes pesticides undergo in the body have not been traced to enzymes, a great many of these changes in pesticides and other foreign chemicals have been traced to the microsomal enzymes. The most fascinating and perhaps single most distinctive property of these enzymes is their ability to be induced by certain foreign chemicals, and presumably by increased endogenous steroids. Because of this unusual property, any demonstration that the metabolism of a chemical can be induced or stimulated by another material is presumptive evidence that the metabolism is mediated by a microsomal enzyme. (An example of a different cause of increased rate of *in vivo* metabolism is given to Section 3.2.1.3.) Table 3-2 gives a list of reactions brought about by microsomal enzymes. Examples involving pesticides are given when possible. Undoubtedly (as indicated by the parallelism of Tables 3-1 and 3-2), many other biotransformations of pesticides are mediated by these enzymes, but the details have not been studied.

The stimulatory effect of foreign compounds on the liver microsomal enzymes was reported first in 1954 (Miller *et al.*, 1954; Brown *et al.*, 1954), and again independently in 1958 (Remmer, 1958). The phenomenon was explored throughly by the Millers and their group (Conney *et al.*, 1957). Because of the recentness of the discovery and the fascinating ramifications of the ensuing study, great emphasis has been placed during the last decade on this mechanism of drug interaction, and other mechanisms have been somewhat neglected. The amount of information now available on drug interaction mediated by microsomal enzymes is too extensive to cover here. Excellent reviews of the subject are those of Conney (1967), Gelboin and Conney (1968), and Gillette *et al.* (1972). A convenient tabulation of literature on drug enzyme induction and drug interactions for the period 1957 to 1970 was prepared by Sher (1971). Reviews of enzymes with emphasis on pesticides are those of Fouts (1963), Conney *et al.* (1967), Leibman (1968), Street *et al.* (1969), and DuBois (1969).

Suffice it to say that inducers have been shown to have profound effects on cell metabolism including: increased incorporation of ^{14}C-orotic acid into nuclear RNA, increased RNA/DNA ratio in the nucleus, increased messenger RNA in the nucleus, stimulation of RNA polymerase in the nucleus, increase of enzyme protein and activity in the microsomes, increased incorporation of amino acid into messenger RNA in the microsomes, and increased sensitivity to added messenger RNA in the microsomes. These effects are blocked by actinomycin-D, puromycin, and ethionine. Actinomycin-D is an inhibitor of DNA-dependent RNA synthesis. Puromycin blocks protein syn-

Table 3-1

Chemical Reactions in the Metabolism of Pesticides.
Pesticides for which abbreviated structural formulae
appear in the table are identified in Appendix I.

Reaction	Example

Oxidation

N-dealkylation

phosphamidon   → plants →   desethyl-phosphamidon   acetaldehyde

O-dealkylation

methyl parathion   →   desmethyl parathion   formaldehyde

epoxidation

aldrin   →   dieldrin

desulfuration

all double bond-S organic phosphorus compounds   →   oxygen analogs

hydroxylation of ring

carbaryl   →   4-hydroxyl-1-naphthyl N-methyl carbamate

hydroxylation of side chain

carbaryl   →   1-naphthyl N-hydroxylmethyl carbamate

N-oxidation

IPC   →   hydroxy IPC

sulfoxidation

$$R{-}S{-}R' \longrightarrow R{-}S{-}R' \longrightarrow R{-}S{-}R'$$

demeton   demeton sulfoxide   demeton sulfone

Table 3-1 (continued)

Reaction	Example

Reduction

reduction of nitro group

R—⟨ ⟩—NO$_2$ →(yeast) R—⟨ ⟩—N⟨^H_H⟩

parathion   aminoparathion

dechlorination

R—C(H)—R / Cl-C-Cl / Cl → R—C(H)—R / Cl-C-Cl / H

DDT   DDD

reduction of a double bond

R—C—R / H—C-Cl   + 2 H → R—C(H)—R / H—C-Cl / H

DDMU   DDMS

Hydration of a double bond

R—C—R / H—C—H   + HOH → R—C(H)—R / H—C—H / OH

DDNU   DDOH

Hydrolysis

hydrolysis of phosphate ester

R\R′(P=O)—O(S)—R′ → R\R′(P=O)—OH + HO(S) R′

most organic phosphorus esters   acid   alcohol

cleavage of amide

R—C(=O)—N⟨$^H_{CH_3}$⟩ → R—C(=O)—OH + H—N⟨$^H_{CH_3}$⟩

dimethoate   O,O-dimethyl-   methyl
(only part of a side chain shown)   S-carboxyl-   amine
                              methyl phos-
                              phorodithioate

cleavage of thioester

CH_3—CH_2—CH_2—S—C(=O)—N⟨$^{C_2H_5}_{C_4H_9}$⟩ → CH_3—CH_2—CH_2—SH

pebulate   propyl mercaptide

deamination

CH_3—O—P(=O)—N⟨$^H_{CH_3}$⟩ / O—⟨ ⟩Cl / CH_3—C(CH$_3$)—CH$_3$ →(hens) CH_3—O—P(=O)—OH / O—⟨ ⟩Cl / CH_3—C(CH$_3$)—CH$_3$

Ruelene ®   deaminomethyl Ruelene ®

Table 3-1 (continued)

Reaction	Example

Dehydrohalogenation

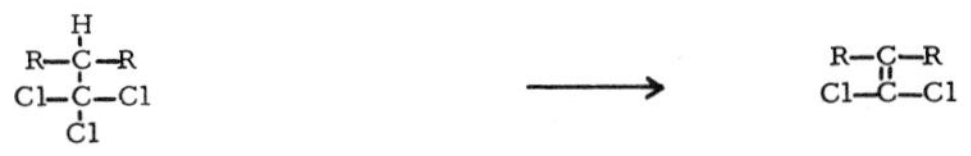

DDT   DDE

Isomerization

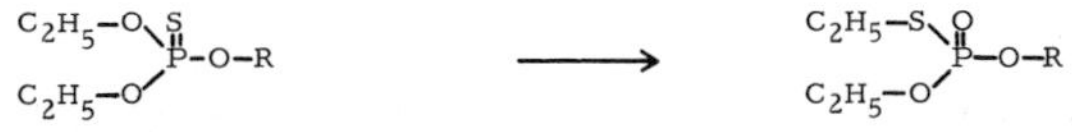

parathion   O, S-ethyl p-nitrophenyl
                                                      phosphate

Conjugation and Synthesis

  with glucuronic acid

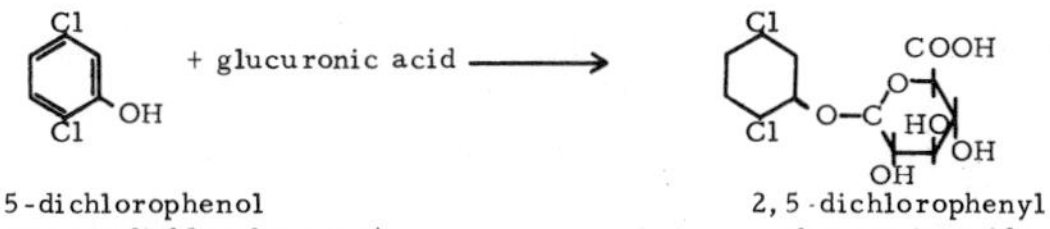

  2, 5-dichlorophenol   2, 5-dichlorophenyl
  (from paradichlorobenzene)   glucuronic acid

NOTE: Glucuronic acid also reacts with acid amines, and SH- groups,
      so the conjugated group may have the form:

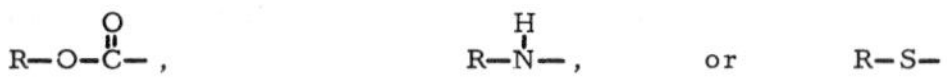

  with glutathion

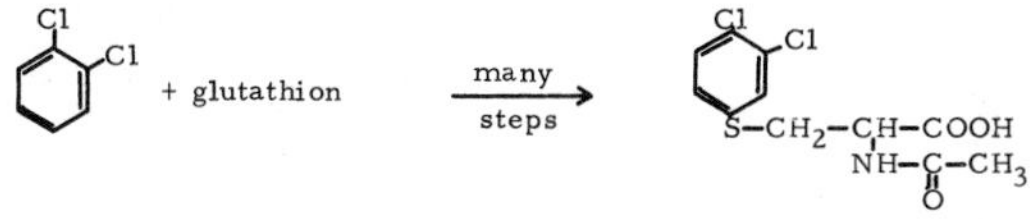

  o-dichlorobenzene   3, 4-dichlorophenyl
                                                        mercapturic acid

  with cystine

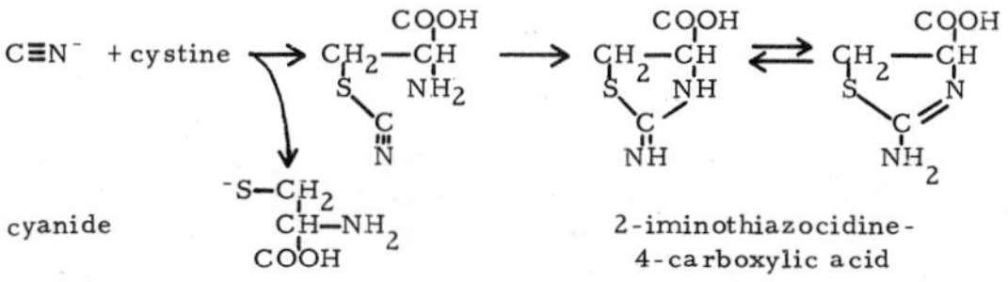

  cyanide   2-iminothiazocidine-
                                                      4-carboxylic acid

  with thiosulfate

CN^- $Na_2S_2O_3^=$ $\longrightarrow$ CNS^-

  cyanide   thiocyanate

  with sulfate

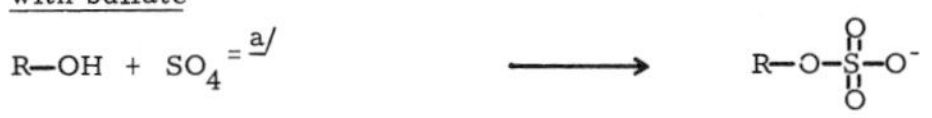

$R-OH + SO_4^=$ [a/] $\longrightarrow$

  4-hydroxybiphenyl   ethereal sulfate of
  (a metabolite of biphenyl)   4-hydroxybiphenyl

  with acetate

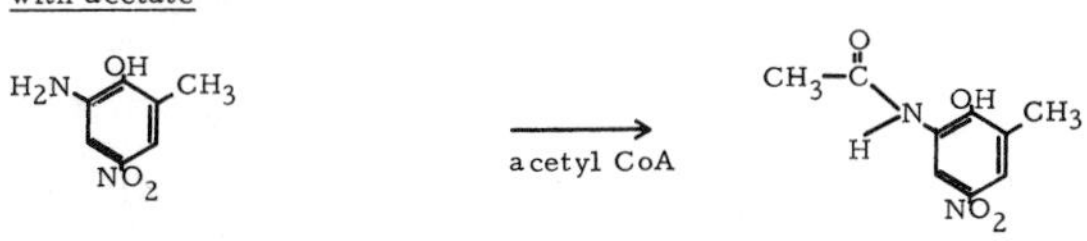

  2-amino-6-methyl-4-nitrophenol   2-acetamido-6-methyl
     (a metabolite of DNOC)   4-nitrophenol

a. Sulfate in the form of phosphoadenosine phosphosulfate (PAPS).

thesis at the microsomal level by preventing the transfer of soluble RNA-bound amino acid into polypeptide chains. Ethionine blocks pro-tein synthesis at several different levels by trapping adenosine triphosphate as S-adeno-sylethionine.

Table 3-2

Metabolic Pathways Catalyzed by Liver Microsomal Enzymes.
Pesticides are cited as examples wherever possible.

From Durham (1967) by permission of Springer Verlag.

Reactions	Examples	References
Oxidation		
N-dealkylation	N-methylaniline → aniline	LaDu et al., 1955
	aminopyrine → 4-aminoanti-pyrine	LaDu et al., 1955
	diphenamid → nordiphenamid → diphenylacetamide	McMahon, 1963
O-dealkylation (ether cleavage)	codeine → morphine	Axelrod, 1956
S-dealkylation	6-methylthiopurine → 6-mercaptopurine	Mazel et al., 1964
deamination	amphetamine → phenylacetone	Axelrod, 1955
epoxidation	aldrin → dieldrin	Wong and Terriere, 1965
exchange of O for S (desulfuration)	parathion → paraoxon	Davison, 1955
	azinphosmethyl → azinphos-methyl (oxygen analog)	DuBois et al., 1957
hydroxylation of ring	acetanilide → o- & p-hydroxyacetanilide	Mitoma et al., 1956
	zoxazolamine → 6-hydroxy-zoxazolamine	Conney et al., 1960
	1-naphthyl N-methyl carba-mate (carbaryl → 4- and 5-hydroxyl-1-naphthyl N-methyl carbamate	Dorough and Casida, 1964
hydroxylation of side chain	1-naphthyl N-methyl carba-mate (carbaryl) → 1-naphthyl N-hydroxy-methyl carbamate	Dorough and Casida, 1964
oxidation of N	trimethylamine → trimethylamine oxide	Baker and Chaykin, 1961
	schradan → schradan N-oxide[a]	DuBois et al., 1950
sulfoxidation	chlorpromazine → chlor-promazine sulfoxide	Gillette and Kamm, 1960
	demeton → demeton sulfoxide → demeton sulfone	March et al., 1955
Reduction		
nitro group	p-nitrobenzoic acid → p-aminobenzoic acid	Fouts and Brodie, 1957
azo compounds	azobenzene → aniline	Fouts et al., 1957
Hydrolysis		
de-esterification	procaine → 2-diethylamino-ethanol + p-aminobenzoic acid	Brodie, 1956
	acetanilide → aniline + acetic acid	Hollunger and Niklasson, 1962
Conjugation		
with glucuronic	o-aminophenol → o-amino-phenol glucuronide	Isselbacher and Axelrod, 1955

a. Other work (Heath et al., 1955) indicates that this product may be hydroxymethyl schradan.

Most of the biochemical effects listed above have been demonstrated with the common sedative phenobarbital and there is reason to think that all of them could be demonstrated in this way. Enzymes may also be induced by hormones and other normal constituents of the body (Conney, 1967) and by food (Wattenberg, 1971). Thus, the phenomenon of induction is a pervasive one, in no way restricted to toxic compounds.

Origin of Microsomal Enzymes. By definition, microsomal enzymes are those found in the microsomal fraction of a tissue following differential centrifugation. Fig. 3-1 shows a scheme for the isolation of microsomes and a number of other cell fractions. The principle of differential centrifugation underlies all such schemes, but the details of the suspending solutions and of the exact force and duration of centrifugation vary somewhat according to the tissue involved and the preferences of the investigator. A valuable book on the preparation of a wide variety of subcellular components is that edited by Birnie and Fox (1969).

The term *microsomal fraction* refers to a biochemical preparation and does not necessarily correspond to any particular cell structure. However, there is considerable evidence that the major component comes from the endoplasmic reticulum and its constituent ribosomes.

Quantitative and Qualitative Aspects of Biotransformation. Different inducers may activate different enzymes and, therefore, different metabolic pathways. Thus, Chadwick *et al.* (1971) showed that repeated doses of lindane and DDT increased oxidative hydrolysis, O-demethylase, dehydrochlorinase, and glucuronyl transferase activity, but to different degrees. Pretreatment of rats with lindane caused them to metabolize a single dose of radioactive lindane 2.5 times more than controls, and pretreatment with DDT caused a 3.5-fold increase in metabolism of radioactive lindane. Furthermore, the DDT pretreatment was followed by proportionally more neutral and weakly polar, but less free acid-type metabolites of the radioactive lindane. Thus, metabolism was qualitatively as well as quantitatively different following the two inducers. Subsequent study (Chadwick and Freal, 1972) confirmed these findings, including the increased excretion of metabolites following pretreatment with DDT. In addition, it was shown that rats pretreated with DDT plus lindane excreted more 2,4,5-trichlorophenol and 2,3,4,6- and 2,3,4,5- tetrachlorophenols by the second day of treatment than did rats receiving lindane alone. The results suggested that DDT treatment stimulates the metabolism of lindane through a selective effect on certain metabolic pathways involved in the oxidative degeneration of lindane, notably those leading to the formation of tetrachlorophenols, particularly 2,3,4,5-tetrachlorophenol.

Another example of qualitative difference in metabolism associated with induction by different compounds is given in Section 3.1.4.

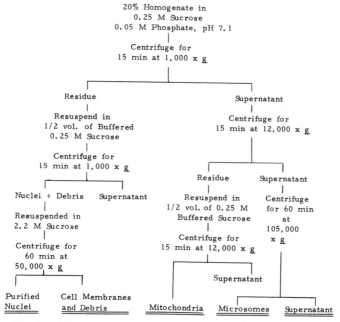

Fig. 3-1. Scheme for separation of subcellular fractions of tissue.

Factors Influencing Microsomal Enzyme Activity. It is important to recall that both the induction and the inhibition of enzymes exhibit clear dosage-response relationships. Some details are given in Section 2.3.8.

There is a strong suggestion that many factors in the metabolism of pesticides are mediated by microsomal enzymes; however, the relationship has been established in only a few instances. The mere fact that a particular pesticide is metabolized by a microsomal enzyme is not proof, for example, that observed variation in this metabolism between the sexes is mediated by these enzymes. Other influences may be involved. It has, therefore, appeared better to mention in this section a few examples in which it is established that the activity of microsomal enzymes may be influenced by age, sex, and species. A discussion of these same factors as they affect the toxicity and storage of pesticides may be found in Sections 2.4 and 3.2.3.3, respectively.

Microsomal enzymes are almost lacking in the fetus and the newborn of rats, but their activity increases rapidly during the early days or weeks of life (Fouts and Adamson, 1959). Sex differences in microsomal enzymes are much more pronounced in rats than in other species. In the absence of intentional stimulation, microsomal enzyme activity is higher in the adult male rat than in females or immature males. However, the stimulatory effect of foreign chemicals on these enzymes is usually greater in females and immature males than in the adult rat (Conney and Burns, 1962). It might be predicted on the basis of these findings that adult male rats would be more resistant than females or immature males to chemicals that are detoxified by microsomal enzymes, and less resistant to chemicals that are toxified by these enzymes. Whether there would be an age or sex difference in the toxicity of compounds not metabolized by microsomal enzymes of the liver would depend on the relative activity of other enzymes and mechanisms in animals of different age and sex.

Many species differences in the metabolism of lipid-soluble drugs can be explained in terms of species differences in activity of liver microsomal enzymes (Brodie and Maickel, 1962; Quinn *et al.*, 1958). Not only may differences in basic levels of enzyme activity be detected in different species, but this has also been accomplished in different strains of mice (Jay, 1955), rats (Quinn *et al.*, 1958) and rabbits (Cram *et al.*, 1965a).

Incidentally, when two inducers are involved, the resulting induction may be additive or slightly antagonistic. Thus, Geilen and Nebert (1971) found an additive effect when either phenobarbital or *p,p'*-DDT was present with a polycyclic hydrocarbon, but not when combinations of phenobarbital plus DDT, or one polycyclic hydrocarbon plus another were involved.

In Vitro Tests for Microsomal Enzymes. Microsomal fractions separated by centrifugation may, with or without further purification, be tested against one or more substrates chosen to demonstate one of the reactions listed in Table 3-2. Substrates commonly used in the study of pesticides are listed in Table 3-3.

The same tests may be carried out in human liver taken within 2 hours of death. This procedure is capable of demonstrating similarities and differences in the qualitative metabolism of man and that of laboratory animals. Although something can be learned of quantitative differences, it is not clear whether this information can be transferred with confidence to a comparison of metabolism in intact people and animals. *In vitro* study of enzymes from human and animal livers has been proposed as a method of selecting experimental animals whose metabolism of a compound under study is similar to that of man. Whether use of the procedure really leads to a more valid picture of the overall toxicity of a compound remains to be demonstrated.

In Vivo Tests for Microsomal Enzymes. In animals, the activity of microsomal enzymes may be tested by measuring a functional change caused by a drug known to be metabolized by one of these enzymes. For example, sleeping time may be measured following injection of hexobarbital. Any pretreatment leading to increased enzyme activity will hasten metabolism of the drug, and thus shorten the sleeping time following a standard dose of the barbiturate. Conversely, pretreatment that inhibits enzyme activity will retard metabolism of the drug and prolong sleeping time.

A somewhat different approach that sometimes may be used in man as well as animals is to measure the rate of disappearance of a drug from the blood following administration of a standard dose. The test drug must be metabolized by the enzyme under study and, of course, a method for measurement of the drug must be available. In man, it is preferable that the test drug in the dosage used produce no sedation or other sensory or clinical effect. In animals, one has a wider range of choice. Some of the test drugs and steroids that have been used in man are listed in Table 3-4. Although these *in vivo* tests have been used mainly for study of the classical inducers such as phenobarbital, there should be no difficulty in using the same technique to study pesticides, pro-

Table 3-3

Convenient In Vitro Tests for the Activity

of Certain Microsomal Enzymes

Reaction	Substrate	Reference
hydrolysis	EPN	Neal and DuBois, 1965
O-demethylation	p-nitroanisole	Netter and Seidel, 1964 as modified by Kinoshita et al., 1966
N-demethylation	aminopyrine	LaDu et al., 1955
hydrolysis	diethylsuccinate	DuBois, et al., 1968
hydrolysis	tributyrin	DuBois, et al., 1968
hydrolysis	acetanilide	DuBois, et al., 1968
decarboxylation	maloxon	Murphy and Dubois, 1957
reduction	p-nitrobenzoic acid	Hietbrink and DuBois, 1965
desulfuration	parathion	Neal, 1967

vided the same biochemical reaction is involved. Furthermore, by use of other test drugs, it might be possible to extend the technique to other biochemical reactions. To the list of test compounds already given to volunteers, one might add safely some, but not all, of the compounds that have been found to be acted on in patients (Sher, 1971).

Induction of Other Enzymes. Microsomal enzymes are not the only ones in the liver subject to induction. The synthetase of δ-aminolevulinic acid (ALA) is located in the mitochondria, and it increases 40 to 100 times in those structures on induction by certain compounds. The occurrence of small amounts of this enzyme in other parts of the cell cannot be ruled out. The *de novo* synthesis of ALA-synthetase is thought to resemble the induction of drug-metabolizing enzymes in four ways: (a) the response has so far been observed only in the liver; (b) a chemical may induce more than one activity; (c) the induction is not hormonal; (d) the induction does not occur rapidly in dividing liver cells. ALA-synthetase can be induced by a variety of chemicals including some that induce microsomal enzymes. However, it seems that chemicals that induce ALA-synthetase efficiently are poor inducers of microsomal enzymes and *vice versa* (Granick, 1965).

Interaction of the two kinds of induction is illustrated by the action of the pesticide *m*-dichlorobenzene in rats. Following daily doses at the rather high rate of 800 mg/kg, there is a biphasic stimulation of ALA-synthetase activity and of the excretion of urinary coproporphyrin, both of which peak by 3 days and then decline. The decrease in ALA-synthetase and in excretion of coproporphyrin at 5 days corresponds with the maximal stimulation of drug metabolism and with a decrease in the concentration of *m*-dichlorobenzene in the serum and liver at the time (Poland *et al.*, 1971).

In the supernatant fraction of homogenized rat liver, the activity of aldehyde dehydrogenase that is dependent on nicotinamide adenine dinucleotide (E.C. 1.2.1.2) is increased up to 10-fold after administration of phenobarbital for 3 days. The effect is genetically controlled and is inherited as an autosomal dominant characteristic. The mechanism is apparently unrelated to other drug-induced increases in enzyme activity such as those that occur in the hepatic microsomal systems for drug metabolism (Deitrich, 1971).

Biotransformation in Other Tissues. The liver is more important than other organs in the biotransformation of foreign chemicals. However, other organs and tissues may be active to some degree. For example, it was shown early that DDT is degraded by rat diaphragm, kidney, and brain *in vitro* (Judah,

Table 3-4

Test Compounds That Have Been Used to Demonstrate
Changes in Microsomal Enzymes or Related
Factors in Man In Vivo

Compound	Test	Reference
antipyrine	blood level[a/]	Kolmodin et al., 1969
"	halflife [b/]	Kampffmeyer, 1969
"	excretion	Chen et al., 1962
bishydroxycoumarin	blood level[a/]	Aggeler and O'Reilly, 1969
"	halflife[b/]	Dayton et al., 1961
cortisol	excretion of 6β-hydroxycortisol[c/]	Werk et al., 1964
"	"	Burstein and Klaiber, 1965
"	"	Kuntzman et al., 1966
"	"	Kuntzman et al., 1968
"	"	Poland et al., 1970
ethyl biscoumacetate	halflife[a/]	Garrettson et al., 1969
phenylbutazone	halflife[a/]	Poland et al., 1970
tolbutamide	halflife[a/]	Solomon and Schrogie, 1967
warfarin	prothrombin time	Udall, 1969

a. Reduced blood level or reduced area under curve.
b. Reduced plasma or serum halflife of administered drug.
c. From endogenous sources.

1949). Later study showed that these changes must be at a very slow rate *in vivo*. However, not all extrahepatic metabolism is inefficient. Organic phosphorus compounds may be rapidly degraded. For example, slices of rabbit skin hydrolyze paraoxon (at a concentration of 7.7×10^{-3} M) to the extent of 20% in 1 hour per gram of tissue. Since absorption of paraoxon and related compounds is slow, this metabolism may be an important defense mechanism (Fredriksson *et al.*, 1961). Furthermore, parathion is metabolized to paraoxon and diethylphosphorothioic acid by rabbit lung at about 20% of the rate in liver (Neal, 1972). Some carbaryl is hydrolyzed and the resulting naphthol is conjugated with glucuronic acid by the intestine (Pekas and Paulson, 1970).

Some enzymes outside the liver may be induced, but the matter has received little attention. Wattenburg (1971) demonstrated that the small intestines of rats fed a balanced purified diet or starved for 1 day possess virtually no benzpyrene hydroxylase activity, while the intestines of rats fed the same diet plus turnip greens, broccoli, cabbage, or brussel sprouts have marked activity of this enzyme. The same enzyme in human skin is induced by polycyclic hydrocarbons (Alvares *et al.*, 1973). Neal (1972) showed that mixed function oxidases of the lung active in the metabolism of parathion can be induced by phenobarbital.

Enzymatic Basis of Conjugation. Because conjugation is not known to be of importance in the metabolism of most pesticides, the enzymatic basis of conjugation is not discussed in this book. This matter has been reviewed in detail by Williams (1959). In many instances

the enzymatic relationships are very complicated.

3.1.2.3 Relation of Enzymes to Toxicity.

*Net Effect of the Liver in Biotransforma-
tion.* A useful measure of the net effect of the
liver in metabolizing a foreign compound may
be gained by infusing a solution of the material into a systemic vein and into a vien
entering the hepatic portal vein. After passing
through the heart, and provided it is not
removed earlier from the circulation, about 25
to 30% of material injected into a systemic
vein enters the liver either through the hepatic artery or through the hepatic portal vein
(see Section 3.2.3.1). On the contrary, 100% of
material injected into the hepatic portal system enters the liver. The distinction holds
only for the first complete circulatory cycle.
However, this one cycle can make the difference between life and death, as was shown for
nicotine and several other poisons at least as
early as 1877 (Lautenbach, 1877). A more
recent use (Gaines *et al.*, 1966) demonstrated
that the net effect of the liver is to detoxify
isolan and **dichlorvos** but to toxify parathion, as summarized in Table 3-5.

Adaptation and Injury. Although some
persons have tended to view even moderate
enlargement of the liver or of individual liver
cells as an injury, the evidence is very strong
that these changes are usually adaptive and
beneficial to the organism when they are the
result of an increase of smooth endoplasmic
reticulum and an associated increase in the
activity of liver microsomal enzymes (Barka

and Popper, 1967). However, simple logic indicates that any stimulus or effect may be harmful, if excessive. Hutterer *et al.* (1968) demonstrated how a distinction may be drawn between adaptation to dieldrin and decompensation resulting from excessive doses. Some of
the same authors, including Hans Popper,
have shown that the same distinction can be
drawn in connection with other sources of
potential liver injury.

It was found that a daily intraperitoneal
administration of dieldrin at the rate of 2 mg/
kg produced enlargement of the liver, hypertrophy of the smooth endoplasmic reticulum,
increase in microsomal protein and P-450
hemoprotein, and associated increase in the
activity of microsomal enzymes; furthermore,
normal activity of other enzymes not derived
from the microsomes was maintained. The
activity of microsomal enzymes per mole of
available P-450 hemoprotein remained unchanged. The highest level of activity of the
processing enzymes was reached after 14 days,
following which the new steady state was
maintained. Rats that had received dieldrin at
a rate of 2 mg/kg for 28 days were more
tolerant to dieldrin than normal rats, as shown
by the fact that they survived 25 consecutive
daily doses at the rate of 5 mg/kg, a dosage
that produced 70% mortality in previously
untreated rats. In spite of the ability of the
rats pretreated with a moderate dosage of
dieldrin to survive a large dosage, their livers
showed definite indications of decompensation
in response to the high dosage. Although the
smooth endoplasmic reticulum remained hy-

Table 3-5

Distinction Between the Effect of Systemic (Femoral) or Hepatic
Portal (Intestinal) Intravenous Injection on the Toxicity of Selected
Compounds when Each is Administered to Rats at a Fixed Rate for
1 Hour or Until Death

From Gaines et al. (1966) by permission of Nature.

Compound	Vein infused	Total dosage (mg/kg)	Time to death (min)	Mortality (died/ tested)
isolan	femoral	0.44 - 1.00	18 - 35	6/6
"	intestinal	1.35 - 1.95	1 at 60	1/6
dichlorvos	femoral	4.4 - 6.4	17 - 31	6/6
"	intestinal	12.5 - 17.0	lived	0/6
parathion	femoral	1.52 - 1.89	lived	0/6
"	intestinal	1.27 - 1.60	57 - 75	6/6

pertrophic and the microsomal protein and P-450 hemoprotein concentrations remained elevated, the enzyme activities per mole of available P-450 hemoprotein decreased, as did the activity of some enzymes not associated with the microsomes. Much of the excess smooth endoplasmic reticulum formed tightly packed clusters of tubular membranes with no glycogen and little hyaloplasm, and some of the mitochondrial membranes were injured. It was suggested that the phase of decompensation represented by hypertrophic but hypoactive smooth endoplasmic reticulum may serve as a sensitive criterion of toxic injury before light microscopic changes are recognizable (Hutterer *et al.*, 1968).

Other studies indicating not only the presence of adaptive change over a range of dosages but also the failure of adaptation and onset of injury at sufficiently high dosage levels have been reported for DDT (Hoffman *et al.*, 1970) and butylated hydroxytoluene (Gilbert and Golberg, 1967). The threshold of injury may be marked by an actual decrease in enzyme activity or merely by a failure to increase activity in response to increased dosage.

Some other compounds, notably phenobarbital, produce morphological changes in the liver entirely similar to those produced by some chlorinated hydrocarbon insecticides (Wright *et al.*, 1972). It seems possible that sufficiently high doses of phenobarbital, for example, may lead to a failure of adaptation and to levels of enzyme activity that do not correspond to dosage.

Pesticides in Relation to Microsomal Enzymes. Studies of pesticides in relation to microsomal enzymes are listed in Table 3-6, modified from a tabulation by Durham (1967). Most of the pesticides studied are stimulatory when given in sufficient dosage. None has been found exclusively inhibitory.

The results with enzymes serve to explain earlier findings regarding the effects of pesticides, especially chlorinated hydrocarbon insecticides, on the morphology of the liver. Considerable evidence has been given that the moderate enlargement of the liver and the characteristic changes in the liver cells of rats are adaptive rather than toxic (Walker *et al.*, 1969).

Many of the organic phosphorus compounds must be metabolized to an active form before they are significantly toxic. Both their toxication and detoxication are accomplished, at least in part, by liver microsomal enzymes. Their toxicity under any given set of conditions depends on the balance between their toxication and detoxication. It is, therefore,

probably not surprising that classical inducers of microsomal enzymes (eg, phenobarbital), and classical inhibitors (eg, SKF–525A), may not have opposite effects on the toxicity of organic phosphorous compounds, because the spectrum of enzymes induced or inhibited may not be the same.

Even the distinction between inducers and inhibitors is relative to the time at which observations are made. In the past, considerable emphasis has been put on the ability of piperonyl butoxide to inhibit microsomal enzymes. Later, evidence was presented that this insecticide synergist stimulates these enzymes. Earlier work was reviewed by Kamienski and Murphy (1971) who showed clearly that inhibition during the first 12 hours after administration of piperonyl butoxide or tropital was followed in a total of 24 to 48 hours by induction. There was some indication that the processes were completely separate, certain elements of inhibition persisting in the presence of stimulation.

3.1.3 Species, Strain, Individual, and Genetic Factors in Metabolism

It is a common observation that species, strains and individuals vary in their susceptibility to toxicants, including pesticides. These matters are discussed in Sections 2.4.7 and 2.4.8 with emphasis on measurement of toxicity. In many instances, the basis for the observed differences in susceptibility is unknown. In other instances, however, it has been possible to explain these differences by one of several causes, including differences in metabolism. Differences in metabolism, in turn, have been linked to genetic differences rather often in insects, but only occasionally in vertebrates.

3.1.3.1 Species Differences in Metabolism. Species vary in the way they metabolize drugs. Indeed it seems possible that, if they are examined in sufficient detail, no two species are identical both quantitatively and qualitatively in their metabolism of a single drug. A striking example is the ability of man and the rat to convert DDT to DDE and the inability of the rhesus monkey to produce more than a trace of the compound (Durham *et al.*, 1963).

3.1.3.2 Individual and Strain Differences in Metabolism. Strain and individual differences often are discussed conveniently in terms of "tolerance" and "resistance," both implying reduced susceptibility to a toxicant. The word *tolerance* is used when the observed decrease in susceptibility occurs in an individual organism as a result of its own previous or

Table 3-6

Summary of Studies of Stimulation of Liver Microsomal Enzyme Activity Involving a Pesticide as the Stimulating Agent or as the Test Compound[a]

Stimulating compound	Dosage regimen	Species	Test for enzyme effect			Reference
			Test compounds	Methods	Results	
Synergists						
piperonyl butoxide	50 mg/kg, ip	mouse	hexobarbital	sleeping time	increased	Fine and Molloy, 1964
sesoxane	"	"	"	" "	"	" " " "
piperonyl butoxide (PB)	200 mg/kg, ip	"	"	" "	increased at 12 hr or less after PB decreased at 24-72 hr after PB	Kamienski and Murphy, 1971
"	400 mg/kg, ip	"	parathion	toxicity in vivo	increased at 1 hr after PB decreased at 48 hr after PB	" " "
"	"	"	ethylguthion	"	increased at 1 hr after PB decreased at 48 hr after PB	" " "
"	"	"	methyl parathion	"	decreased	" " "
"	400 mg/kg, ip	mouse	azinphosmethyl	"	"	" "
"	"	"	dimethoate	"	decreased at 1 hr after PB increased at 48 hr after PB	" "
"	"	"	paraoxon	"	increased at 1 hr after PB decreased at 48 hr after PB	" "
"	"	"	ethygutoxon	"	increased at 1 hr after PB decreased at 48 hr after PB	" "
"	"	"	dimethoxon	"	no effect	" "
"	"	"	gutoxon	"	no effect at 1 hr after PB decreased at 48 hr after PB	" "
"	"	"	methyl paraoxon	"	no effect at 1 hr after PB decreased at 48 hr after PB	" "
"	5,000 ppm in diet for 15 days	rat	hexobarbital	sleeping time	decreased	Wagstaff and Short, 1971
safrole	10,000 ppm in diet for 15 days	"	" EPN	" detoxication	increased "	" " " "

Table 3-6 (continued)

Stimulating compound	Dosage regimen	Species	Test for Enzyme Effect			Reference
			Test compounds	Methods	Results	
Synergists						
safrole	5,000 ppm in diet for 15 days	"	hexobarbital	sleeping time	"	" "
Fumigants and Nematocides						
carbon tetra- chloride	inhalation, 239-1,276 ppm	"	"	"	"	Lal et al., 1970
Chlorinated Hydrocarbon Insecticides						
α, β, γ- BHC	γ--200 mg/kg β--200 mg/kg α--60 mg/kg	rat " "	" " scillicoside	in vitro metabolism sleeping time toxicity	increased[b] decreased decreased[c]	Koransky et al., 1964 "
phenobarbital	(not given)	dog, miniature swine	lindane	toxicity in vivo	decreased at first but still 3 times as lethal to dogs as to swine	Earl et al., 1970
lindane	15-16 mg/kg, ip or 0.5-800 ppm in diet	rat	hexobarbital	in vitro metabolism sleeping time	increased decreased	Kolmodin-Hedman et al., 1971 "
"	60 mg/kg single dose	"	antipyrine	in vitro metabolism	increased	"
DDT and related compounds						
DDT Trichloro- 237 γ-chlordan endrin	single oral dose. 25 mg/kg. for 1st 3 and 6.26 mg/kg for 4th	rat " " "	hexobarbital " " "	sleeping time " " "	no effect shortened " "	Hart and Fouts, 1963 " " "
DDT	500 ppm in diet for 0.5 to 4 mo.	"	" " aminopyrine aniline p-nitrobenzoic acid	in vitro metabolism " " "	" increased " no effect increased	Hart and Fouts, 1963 " " " "
"	25 to 100 mg/kg subcutaneously for 3 days	"	hexobarbital " aminopyrine aniline p-nitrobenzoic acid	sleeping time in vitro metabolism " " "	shortened increased " " "	Hart and Fouts, 1963 " " " "
"	5 and 50 ppm in diet for 10 weeks	"	dieldrin	storage of dieldrin in body	decreased	Street, 1964
"	5-50 ppm for 13 weeks " "	rat " "	EPN p-nitroanisole aminopyrine	detoxification O-demethylation N-demethylation	increased " "	Kinoshita et al., 1966 " "
toxaphene	5-50 ppm for 13 weeks "	"	EPN p-nitroanisole aminopyrine	detoxification O-demethylation N-demethylation	" " "	" " "
DDT	10 ppm x 5 (5 mg)	pigeon	estradiol	in vitro metabolism	"	Peakall, 1967
dieldrin	2 ppm x 5 (1 mg)	"	estrone	"	"	"

Table 3-6 (continued)

Stimulating compound	Dosage regimen	Species	Test for Enzyme Effects			References
			Test compounds	Methods	Results	

Chlorinated Hydrocarbon Insecticides

Stimulating compound	Dosage regimen	Species	Test compounds	Methods	Results	References
DDT	50 ppm	rat	dieldrin	excretion of metabolites	"	Street and Chadwick, 1967
"	0.04-0.10 mg/day for 4-20 wks	"	methyprylon meprobamate chlordiazepoxide hydrochloride	in vitro metabolism sleeping time	" decreased	Datta and Nelson, 1968
"	0.2-100 ppm in diet	rat	aldrin	epoxidation	increased	Gillett, 1968
DDT, lindane, chlordane	10-15 mg/kg, po	man	antipyrine	plasma half-life	decreased	Kolmodin et al., 1969
DPH (diphenyl-hydantoin)	250 ppm for 3-6 wks	rat	DDT	storage of DDT and DDE in vitro metabolism	" increased	Cranmer, 1970 "
DDT	4.50-90.00 mg/kg ip	mouse	pentobarbital	sleeping time	increased	Gabliks and Maltby-Askari, 1970
o,p'-DDD	4.50-90.00 mg/kg ip	mouse	"	"	"	"
DDT	90 mg/kg, ip	"	"	in vitro metabolism	decreased	"
o,p'-DDD	90 mg/kg, ip	"	"	"	"	"
DDT	90-180 mg/kg for 14 days	"	"	sleeping time	"	"
o,p'-DDD	90-135 mg/kg for 14 days	"	"	"	increased	"
"	180 mg/kg for 14 days	"	"	"	unchanged	"
DDT	0.5 and 2 mg/kg day for 14 days	rat	p-nitroanisole	O-demethylation	increased[d/]	Hoffman et al., 1970
"	5 gm in peanut oil, po	human	phenobarbital	CNS arousal	increased	Rappolt, 1970
"	25-50 ppm for 14 days	guinea pig	dieldrin	storage of DDT	decreased	Wagstaff and Street, 1970
"	5 mg/kg/day for 2-6 months	squirrel monkey	EPN p-nitroanisole	in vitro metabolism "	increased "	Cranmer et al., 1972 "
	0.5 mg/kg/day for 2-6 months	"	EPN p-nitroanisole	" "	no effect increased	" "
	0.05 mg/kg/day for 2-6 months	"	EPN p-nitroanisole	" "	no effect "	" "
o,p'-DDD	6-9 gm/day	man	cortizol (ex-ogenous or endo-genous)	excretion of metabolites	decreased	Bledsoe et al., 1964
"	300 mg/kg po for 5 days, then 50 mg/kg for 2 days	guinea pig	cortisol (endogenous)	excretion of metabolites	increased	Kupfer et al., 1964
"	subcutaneous (100 mg/kg/day & oral (300 mg/kg/day) for 2 day	rat	phenobarbital	sleeping time in vitro metabolism of phenobar-bital	shortened[c/] increased	Straw et al., 1965
methoxychlor	in diet	rat	dieldrin	storage of dieldrin in body fat	no effect	Street, 1964

Table 3-6 (continued)

Stimulating compound	Dosage regimen	Species	Test for Enzyme Effect			References
			Test compounds	Methods	Results	

Chlorinated Hydrocarbon Insecticides

Cyclodienes and related compounds

Stimulating compound	Dosage regimen	Species	Test compounds	Methods	Results	References
chlordane	10-100 mg/kg for 1 or 3 days, ip	rat	hexobarbital aminopyrine chlorpromazine	in vitro metabolism "	1 dose, no effect 3 doses, increased metabolism of all substrates[c]	Hart et al., 1963 "
"	50 mg/kg for 14 days;	dog	dicoumarol	toxicity in vivo	decreased	Welch and Harrison, 1966
DDT	50 mg/kg for 14 days	rat	phenylbutazone	"	"	"
chlordane	10 mg/kg/day, 7 ip	squirrel monkey	hexobarbital aminopyrine zoxazolamine	in vitro metabolism "	increased "	Cram et al., 1965b "
"	125-500 ppm in diet	rat	casein	in vitro metabolism	increased	Casterline and Williams, 1971
"	1-50 mg/kg	rat	estrone	in vitro metabolism	increased	Welch et al., 1971
lindane	15 mg/kg	"	estradiol-17ß	"	"	"
dieldrin	3 mg/kg	"	"	"	"	"
heptachlor	10 mg/kg	"	"	"	"	"
toxaphene	25 mg/kg	"	"	"	"	"
p,p'-DDD	25 mg/kg	"	"	"	"	"
p,p'-DDE	25 mg/kg	"	"	"	"	"
phenobarbital	50 mg/kg/day, ip	rat	dieldrin	storage of dieldrin in body fat	decreased	Cueto and Hayes, 1965
heptabarbital	40 and 225 mg/kg/day in diet for 10 days	rat	dieldrin	storage of dieldrin in body fat	decreased (47 to 80%)	Street et al., 1966
aminopyrine	75 and 350 mg/kg/day in diet for 10 days or 50 and 75 mg/kg/day ip for 10 days or 100 and 150 mg/kg/day ip for 5 days	"	"	"	decreased (63 to 81%; 22 to 42%; and 25 to 15%, respectively)	"
tolbutamide	60 and 290 mg/kg/day in diet for 10 days	"	"	"	decreased (13 to 57%)	"
phenylbutazone	50 mg/kg/day ip for 4 days	"	"	"	no effect	"
DDT	4 mg/kg/day in diet for 10 days	"	"	"	decreased (75%)	"
dieldrin	0.07 mg/kg/day for 6 years	rhesus monkey	chlorfenvinphos	in vitro metabolism	increased	Wright et al., 1972
"	2.0 mg/kg/day for 7 days	beagle	"	"	"	"
"	8.0 mg/kg/day for 28 days	rat	"	"	"	"
"	1.6 mg/kg/day for 350 days	mouse	"	"	"	"

Organic Phosphorus Insecticides

Stimulating compound	Dosage regimen	Species	Test compounds	Methods	Results	References
3-methylcholanthrene	20 mg/kg single dose	rat	azinphosmethyl	in vitro incubation with liver homogenate. Then cholinesterase inhibitory effect measured	increased[c]	Murphy and DuBois, 1958

Table 3-6 (continued)

Stimulating compound	Dosage regimen	Species	Test for Enzyme Effect			References
			Test compound	Methods	Results	
Organic Phosphorus Insecticides						
none	liver microsomal fraction incubated in vitro with pesticides listed	rat	coumaphos	change in cholinesterase inhibitory effect after incubation	increased[e/]	Dahm et al., 1962
		"	demeton (thiono)		no effect	" "
		"	diazinon		increased[e/]	" "
		"	dimethoate		no effect	" "
	"	"	azinphosmethyl		increased[e/]	" "
	"	"	malathion	"	"	" "
	"	"	menazon		no effect	" "
	"	"	methyl parathion	"	increased[e/]	" "
	"	"	phorate	"	no effect	" "
	"	"	ronnel	"	increased[e/]	" "
	"	"	carbophenothion	"	"	" "
parathion	1.0 to 25 mg/kg	mouse	hexobarbital	sleeping time	lengthened	Hart and Fouts, 1963
schradan	5 mg/kg	"	"	"	no effect	" "
EPN	12.5 mg/kg	"	"	"	lengthened	" "
malathion	25 mg/kg	"	"	"	"	" "
chlorcyclizine	25 mg/kg, b.i.d. for 4 days	mouse	parathion	toxicity in vivo; in vitro conversion to paraoxon	increased	Welch and Coon, 1964
"	25 mg/kg, b.i.d. for 4 days	mouse	paraoxon	toxicity in vivo	increased	" "
		"	tepp	"	"	" "
"	50 mg/kg, ip	mouse	paraoxon	paraoxonase content of liver and plasma	slight increase for liver, decrease for plasma	" "
phenobarbital	100 mg/kg, ip	"	"	"		" "
SKF-525A	50 mg/kg, ip	"	"	"	"	" "
chlorcyclizine	25-35 mg/kg, b.i.d., for 4 days	mouse	malathion	toxicity in vivo	decreased	" "
cyclizine	"	"	"	"	"	" "
phenobarbital	"	"	"	"	"	" "
SKF-525A	"	"	"	"	"	" "
chlorcyclizine	25-35 mg/kg, b.i.d., for 4 days	mouse	parathion	"	decreased	" "
cyclizine	"	"	"	"	"	" "
phenobarbital	"	"	"	"	"	" "
SKF-525A	"	"	"	"	"	" "
chlorcyclizine	25-35 mg/kg, b.i.d., for 4 days	mouse	EPN	"	decreased	" "
cyclizine	"	"	"	"	"	" "
phenobarbital	"	"	"	"	"	" "
SKF-525A	"	"	"	"	"	" "
phenobarbital	50 mg/kg/day for 5 days	rat and mouse	parathion	toxicity in vivo	decreased	DuBois, 1969
		"	methyl parathion	"	"	"
		"	demeton	"	"	"
		"	disulfoton	"	"	"
		"	azinphosmethyl	"	"	"
		"	dioxathion	"	"	"
		"	ethion	"	"	"
		"	carbophenothion	"	"	"
		"	mevinphos	"	"	"
		"	EPN	"	"	"
parathion	3.75-15.0 ppm in diet	rat	casein	in vitro metabolism	increased	Casterline and Williams, 1971
phenobarbital	50 mg/kg/day, ip	"	Hinosan®	anticholinesterase activity in vivo and in vitro	decreased	Chen et al., 1972
DDT	50 mg/kg/day, ip	"	"	"	"	"
3-methylcholanthrene	5 mg/kg/day, ip	"	"	"	"	"
testosterone	2 mg/kg/day, ip	"	"	"	"	"
Hinosan®	0, 5, 25 ppm in diet	"	malathion	"	increased	"

Table 3-6 (continued)

Stimulating compound	Dosage regimen	Species	Test compounds	Methods	Results	References
				Test for Enzyme Effect		
Carbamate Insecticides						
carbaryl	100-400 mg/kg po for 3-6 days	white leghorn cockerels	pentobarbital	sleeping time	decreased	Puyear and Paulson, 1972
"	10-50 mg/kg po for 3-6 days	"	"	"	no effect	"
Banol®	500-1,000 ppm in diet	rat	casein	in vitro metabolism	decreased	Casterline and Williams, 1971
Synthetic Organic Rodenticides						
heptabarbital	50 mg/kg po	man	dicoumarol	toxicity in vivo	"	Dayton et al., 1961
		dog	"	"	"	
		guinea pig	"	"	"	"
phenobarbital	2 mg/kg for 4 weeks	man	warfarin	action	"	Robinson and MacDonald, 1966
"	10 mg/kg/day for 8 days	dog	dicoumarol	toxicity in vivo	"	Welch et al., 1967
chloral hydrate	0.5 gm/day	man	"	"	"	Cucinell et al., 1967
phenyramidol	40 mg/kg	mouse	"	"	increased	Solomon and Schrogie, 1967
		rabbit	"	"	"	" "
		man	"	"	"	
acetylsalicylic acid	100 mg/kg, single dose	rat (Wistar)	"	prothrombin time	decreased	Coldwell and Zawidzka, 1968
heptabarbital	400 mg/day for 4 or 8 days	man	"	excretion of metabolites	increased	Aggeler and O'Reilly, 1969
Herbicides						
noruron	100-2,000 ppm po for 13 wks	rat	EPN p-nitroanisole aminopyrine	detoxification O-demethylation N-demethylation	increase 1-3 wks, then return to normal	Kinoshita and DuBois, 1967
diuron	100-2,000 ppm po for 13 wks	rat	EPN p-nitroanisole aminopyrine	detoxification O-demethylation N-demethylation	increase 1-3 wks, then return to normal <250 ppm no effect	"
Fungicides						
chloramphenicol	6.25-50 mg/kg ip	mouse	hexobarbital	sleeping time in vitro metabolism	increased decreased	Dixon and Fouts, 1962
"	100 mg/kg SC	rat	cyclophosphamide	toxicity in vivo	decreased	Dixon, 1968
phenobarbital (P)	30 mg t.i.d. for 3 days	man	griseofulvin (G)	elimination kinetics	no effect, but P decreased amount of G absorbed after oral administration	Riegelman et al., 1970
chloramphenicol	2 gm/day po for 4-10 days	man	tolbutamide diphenylhydantoin dicoumarol	in vitro metabolism " " "	decreased " "	Christensen and Skovsted, 1969
griseofulvin	1-2 gm/day	man	warfarin	action	decreased	Cullen and Catalano, 1967
Parnon®	15-100 ppm in diet for 4-28 days	rat	hepatic enzymes	in vitro metabolism	increased	Hoffman et al., 1968

a. Where possible, the table is arranged according to groups of pesticides, giving preference to the stimulating compound when it is a pesticide. However, where several pesticides have been reported in the same paper they are tabulated together sequentially and not separated out according to individual compounds.
b. All isomers had similar effects.
c. Stimulatory effect blocked by ethione.
d. Increase leveled off at 750 ppm.
e. Effect of enzymes blocked by SKF-525A and other inhibitors.

continuing exposure to the particular toxicant or to some other conditioning stimulus. The most common example of tolerance is that involving nicotine. The experienced smoker can inhale without concern a quantity of nicotine that would have caused him incapacitating illness as a young boy.

The word *resistance* refers to relative insusceptibility that is genetically determined. As discussed in greater length below, the genetic trait may preexist in a population so that it is obvious when the population is first exposed to the toxicant, or the trait may be brought to an observable level only through selection. Undoubtedly many instances of resistance are based on some difference of metabolism that distinguishes the resistant and nonresistant populations. Certainly some features of metabolism are known to be determined genetically (Section 3.1.3.3), and the origin of resistance through selection always strongly implies a genetic mechanism. However, in many instances, the metabolic basis of resistance is still unknown, and therefore resistance and genetic factors are discussed separately below.

Tolerance. Tolerance to a compound may be the result of an organism's increased ability to metabolize it. This is true, for example, in connection with the pesticides nicotine (Werle and Uschold, 1948) and dieldrin (Wright *et al.,* 1972). Some details on tolerance to dieldrin are discussed in connection with adaptation and injury in Section 3.1.2.3.

In a few instances, it has been shown clearly that the increased metabolism responsible for tolerance was mediated by increased activity of the microsomal enzymes of the liver. It seems likely that the same explanation will hold in connection with some other instances of tolerance. As recorded in Table 3-6, pesticides frequently act as inducers of microsomal enzymes. Since activity of these enzymes usually leads to detoxication, it seems likely that many of the compounds listed in Table 3-6 are capable of producing tolerance under suitable conditions.

Tolerance also may exist in situations in which it has been impossible to demonstrate any increased ability to metabolize the toxicant. In these instances, it is presumed that the receptor of the active form of the drug is somehow less reactive. Resistance to morphine is apparently an example of this form of tolerance, but the ultimate mechanism remains unknown.

Finally, there are instances of tolerance for which the mechanism is not only unknown but unexplored. For example, rodents may develop true tolerance (as distinguished from bait shyness) to ·a number of rodenticides, including arsenic oxide, zinc phosphide, strychnine, sodium fluoroacetate, antu, and norbormide (Lund, 1967). Certain populations of pine mice subjected to control with endrin have lost susceptibility to the compound, but sublethal exposure confers a degree of tolerance regardless of the past history of the population (Webb and Horsfall, 1967). The males were 11 times and the females 13 times less susceptible than corresponding members of relatively unexposed populations. Survivors of nonfatal doses were not as susceptible as previously untreated animals, but the possibility of inherited resistance was not investigated.

Resistance. When one thinks of resistance in the toxicological sense, one thinks immediately of insects and a variety of other lower forms that are pests. At least 104 species of public health importance are now resistant to one or more pesticides (Brown and Pal, 1971). A much larger number of agricultural pests are resistant to some degree. Resistance to a particular compound may not involve an entire species but only the population of a limited area; however, there is always a possibility that a less susceptible strain may extend its range. Although the picture is not as bleak as some would have us believe, the fact remains that resistance constitutes a tremendous public health and economic problem. Resistance is not confined to the newer synthetic, organic poisons. It has been recognized for years in connection with inorganic poisons, also. Although many species are or have become resistant to one or more pesticides, it does not follow that every species is genetically capable of developing resistance to every poison. On the contrary, there is no way to predict that resistance to a particular compound is impossible for any given species.

Some species are effectively resistant when they first encounter a particular compound (see Section 2.4.7). In a few instances, it has been recognized that resistance existed in one strain of a species before that strain was exposed, and in spite of the fact other strains were fully susceptible. More commonly, resistant strains are first recognized only after the parent population has been selected by killing off many of its susceptible members. In principle, there is no real difference between these three situations. In all of them, the organism has the power to develop a genotype that can cope successfully with the toxicant. It is of secondary importance whether the gene or genes necessary for resistance already exist in high frequency, whether they exist in low frequency, or even whether they are developed by mutation during the course of exposure. The ultimate result in each instance is a population that can withstand the toxicant more effectively.

Although most recognized examples of resistance involve populations of pests, there is no biological reason for supposing that the development of genetic resistance must be confined to one kind of organism. Of course, the possibility that a particular gene will actually occur at a particular time depends on the size of population, and the rate at which selection progresses depends not only on its intensity, but also on the duration of each generation. Therefore, it is not astonishing that resistance has often been observed among organisms such as bacteria or houseflies, characterized by vast numbers of individuals and a rapid rate of reproduction. However, resistance has been observed in species with relatively small populations and relatively slow multiplication.

Resistance of a vertebrate species to a pesticide apparently first was recognized in connection with Norway rats exposed to warfarin. This phenomenon was first reported from Scotland (Boyle, 1960). It has since been reported from Denmark (Lund, 1964, 1967), England and Wales (Drummond, 1966; Bentley, 1969), the Netherlands (Ophof and Langeveld, 1969), Germany (Telle, 1971), and the United States of America, specifically North Carolina and Idaho (Jackson and Kaukeinen, 1972; Brothers, 1972).

The extensive literature on the resistance of mammals to warfarin was reviewed by Lund (1967). Only a few points need be recorded here. So far, resistance is known to occur in four species, the Norway and roof rats, the house mouse, and man. In addition, in their original studies of coumarin compounds, Link and his students reported marked variation in susceptibility in rabbits as a Mendelian character (Campbell et al., 1941). The exact mechanism of inheritance of resistance to warfarin is not clear. In man, the facts are consistent with transmission by a single autosomal dominant gene (O'Reilly et al., 1964), but only one kindred has been studied. In rats, especially those of Denmark, and in mice, it seems that more than one gene is involved. The physiological basis of the resistance also is not clear and may be different in different instances. There is no evidence that resistant rats are more efficient in their use of vitamin K, but people resistant to warfarin were extremely sensitive to the antidotal action of the vitamin (O'Reilly et al., 1964). In every instance studied, including that in man, resistance extended to other coumarin anticoagulants and those based on indandione. Susceptibility to heparin is normal.

Another early report of resistance among vertebrates involved mosquito fish collected from insecticide-contaminated waters near cotton fields (Vinson et al., 1963). Further study revealed 2- to 1,500-fold levels of resistance to a variety of pesticides in mosquito fish and five other species of fish (Boyd and Ferguson, 1964a; 1964b; Ferguson and Boyd, 1964; Ferguson et al., 1964, 1965; Ferguson and Bingham, 1966a, 1966b). Resistance to chlorinated hydrocarbon pesticides was found in three species of frogs (Boyd et al., 1963). The degree of resistance may be so great in some instances that resistant species can withstand enough poison to kill their predators, as discussed in Section 11.2.3.1.

Ozburn and Morrison (1962) apparently were the first to produce resistance to a pesticide in a mammal under laboratory conditions. They divided a colony of white mice into two parts, one of which served as a control, while the other was selected by means of DDT administered to each mouse when it was 4 weeks old as a single intraperitoneal dose. By the ninth generation, resistance in the selected colony had increased by a factor of 1.7 as measured by the LD 50, while the susceptibility of the control colony remained identical to that originally measured in the parent colony. Although the factor of 1.7 is small, about half of the susceptible mice withstood a dose that was uniformly fatal to control mice. Further study (Ozburn and Morrison, 1965) revealed that the selected and control colonies differed in their rates of oxygen consumption. Undosed, DDT-resistant, young mice consumed more oxygen than controls. This difference rapidly disappeared with increasing age. When challenged by DDT, the resistant mice were more stable in their response; they showed less increase in oxygen consumption and returned to normal more quickly. This difference in response to DDT was most marked in older mice. The respiratory patterns of the two colonies were interpreted as indicating a physiological difference induced by selection but not by DDT per se. The resistant mice were fatter than the susceptible ones. Considerable evidence indicated that resistance depended on preferential deposit of DDT in the fat and consequently the avoidance of peak levels in sensitive tissues. The resistance was not specific for DDT but extended to lindane and dieldrin (Barker and Morrison, 1966).

Although resistance has been developed in mammals under laboratory conditions, success has not been uniform. Apparently some strains are not sufficiently heterozygous to respond to selection (Guthrie et al., 1971).

3.1.3.3 Genetic Factors. Considerable progress has been made in explaining the genetic basis of both inborn errors of metabolism and variation in the biotransformation of foreign chemicals. Study of these closely related matters has been recognized as a separate discipline in several names emphasizing one or another of its aspects. Interest was focused by a book by J. B. S. Haldane (1954) entitled, *The Biochemistry of Genetics.* Other books concerned with biochemical genetics (Harris, 1970) or chemical genetics (Strauss, 1960) have appeared. The term "pharmacogenetics" has been credited to both A. G. Motulsky and F. Vogel, in a book on the subject by Kalow (1962).

Section 2.4.7 describes a number of instances in which species or strains differ in their susceptibility to pesticides. In many instances, the resistance has been made observable through natural selection. In other instances, it has been possible to produce resistance in the laboratory through selection. The occurrence of species and strain differences, and especially the possibility of increasing resistance in populations through selection, whether in the laboratory or in nature, all argue for a genetic basis for the observed differences. In many instances it has been possible to define the genetic mechanisms responsible for observed differences in the metabolism of chemicals by organisms commonly studied by geneticists. It has even been possible to establish genetic mechanisms in connection with the metabolism of drugs by man or laboratory animals. A genetic mechanism has been defined only rarely in connection with metabolism of pesticides. This should be considered an indication for further study. Genetic mechanisms almost certainly are involved much more in different responses to pesticides than it has been possible to prove so far.

The mere existence of discontinuous or biphasic variation in the activity of enzymes that affect responses to chemicals is not a proof that the variation has a genetic mechanism. The variation could be associated with some factor in development. Specifically, it could be caused by tolerance developed in certain individuals through contact with the chemical (see Section 3.1.3.2). In spite of these reservations, the existence of discontinuous or biphasic variation is an indication of the possibility of genetic involvement. Some examples are given here in which such variation in enzyme activity within populations has been proved to be genetic in origin.

Enzymes that influence susceptibility to a chemical need not influence the metabolism of the chemical itself.

It has long been known that susceptibility to hemolytic anemia induced by eating fava beans is much more common among people of Mediterranean origin than among people from the northern part of Europe. Later it was found that a number of drugs, especially primaquine, produce acute hemolytic anemia in some persons when given at dosage rates easily tolerated by most others. The entire subject of drug-induced hemolytic anemia was reviewed by Beutler (1960). Briefly, it is now firmly established that this increased susceptibility to certain compounds is associated with a deficiency of the enzyme glucose-6-phosphate dehydrogenase (G–6–PD) in the red cells (Carson *et al.,* 1956). The exact mechanism by which a deficiency of G–6–PD leads to hemolysis in the presence of certain drugs in unknown; however, a number of *in vitro* tests are available for recognizing drug-sensitive cells. There is no evidence that G–6–PD influences the biotransformation of materials causing hemolytic anemia. Deficiency of the enzyme does make mature red cells more subject to hemolysis *in vivo,* but cells that are only 8 to 21 days old are not abnormally susceptible to primaquine, even though they are formed by susceptible persons. Thus, a patient who survives a hemolytic crisis may recover while continuing to take the drug. The abnormality in response to primaquine is quantitative rather than qualitative; high doses of primaquine cause hemolytic anemia in some persons in whom no abnormality of the enzyme can be demonstrated. In most instances, deficiency of G–6–PD is inherited as a sex-linked dominant of incomplete penetrance. However, there are some family histories that do not fit this pattern. It is not clear whether the variation depends on a modifying gene or whether two separate genetic patterns with currently indistinguishable phenotypes are involved.

The fungicide, ziram, caused hemolytic anemia with Heinz body formation in a man later shown to be deficient in erythrocyte G–6–PD. Ziram also caused one of the typical *in vitro* reactions (formation of Heinz bodies) in the blood of another person known to be deficient in this enzyme (Pinkhas *et al.,* 1963).

Another example involves atypical plasma cholinesterase, which is one of several causes of intolerance to succinylcholine. The atypical enzyme differs both quantitatively and qualitatively from the usual cholinesterase of the plasma (Kalow, 1956). The atypical enzyme is less efficient than the normal enzyme in the hydrolysis of succinylcholine, with the result that the effect of a given dose of this muscle relaxant is unusually intense and prolonged in persons with the atypical enzyme. The same clinical effect can result from a deficiency of normal plasma cholinesterase caused by liver damage or malnutrition. The occurrence of the atypical enzyme can be measured *in vitro* by measuring its sensitivity to inhibition by dibucaine.

Most family histories involving the atypical cholinesterase are consistent with an explanation based on a single autosomal dominant gene with incomplete penetrance. Persons with the defect fully developed are homozygous for the gene, but a milder defect in heterozygous persons can be demonstrated by special tests. The frequency of the homozygous condition in the population is one per 2,820 population with a range of 1:2,290 to 1:3,650. This construction of the inheritance is sufficiently accurate that there is good agreement between predicted frequencies and those observed in Canada and the United States of America, and in recent immigrants from Europe (Kalow and Gunn, 1959). However, there are a few family histories in which the apparent inheritance does not fit the simple hypothesis involving one normal and one abnormal allelomorphic gene. In these very unusual families, in which parentage has been confirmed by other genetic tests, it may be that a third allele or a modifying gene is involved. The difficulty in accepting the hypothesis of a third allele is that no homozygous condition has been observed (Kalow, 1962). The possibility that the third allele is lethal when homozygous would be logical, but apparently has not been explored.

The occurrence of atypical cholinesterase is of great practical importance in connection with therapeutic use of succinylcholine. It is only reasonable to ask whether the defect would influence susceptibility to organic phosphorus and carbamate insecticides; the possibility has been explored to some extent. Tabershaw and Cooper (1966) found no instance of atypical cholinesterase among 114 persons previously poisoned by organic phosphorus insecticides. This result shows that the abnormal enzyme is not an important condition for this kind of poisoning; it throws no light on what would happen if a person with atypical cholinesterase were exposed to as much organic phosphorus insecticide as the ordinary worker is. It is possible that nothing would happen, because *in vitro* tests show that the normal and atypical enzymes have the same response to tepp and DFP, even though their response to succinylcholine, decamethonium, and some other compounds is vastly different (Kalow and Davies, 1958). There is a greater chance that atypical cholinesterase would be important in connection with carbamate insecticides, because some carbamates are poorly hydrolyzed by it.

Human erythrocyte acetylcholinesterase also is subject to genetic variation, but in this instance there is no indication that the variation has any clinical importance. Pedigrees of the persons studied indicated that the three phenotypic forms of the stromal enzyme are expressions of two codominant alleles at a single locus (Coates and Simpson, 1972).

What little is known about the genetic basis of resistance to warfarin is stated in the foregoing section.

A defect known to be associated with increased susceptibility to chronic obstructive bronchopulmonary disease is deficiency of serum α_1-antitrypsin. The condition is inherited as a single, autosomal, recessive gene. There is essentially no overlapping in the concentration of the inhibitor in the blood of normal persons, those homozygous for the defect, and those heterozygous for it. The frequencies of the normal and abnormal genes are 0.976 and 0.024, respectively; the frequency of the homozygous phenotypes are these numbers squared, and the frequency of the heterozygous phenotype is twice the product of these numbers (Eriksson, 1965).

Incidentally, persons who have an inherited deficiency of serum α_1-antitrypsin have an inappropriately large amount of liver α_1-antitrypsin. Genetic variants of the molecule may be less able than normal molecules to leave their site of synthesis in the liver, even where no clinical disease of the liver is evident (Lieberman *et al.*, 1972).

Following a lecture a year earlier, Brieger (1963) concluded a review of the genetic basis of susceptibility and resistance to toxic agents with the broad suggestion that special procedures to detect genetic susceptibility become part of preemployment medical examinations in industries that present recognized hazards to defective genetic systems. In the same year, Mountain (1963) discussed three tests for G–6–PD deficiency and recommended one of them for use in occupational medicine.

Because a simple test for α_1-antitrypsin now is available, it has been suggested that the test be used to help distinguish whether cases of emphysema are job-related or not, and that the test be used as part of preemployment examinations in order to avoid hiring persons who are especially susceptible to emphysema for any job that involves even slight exposure to lung irritants that tend to cause the disease (Stokinger and Mountain, 1967; Stokinger *et al.*, 1968). So far, this test has not found use in connection with a pesticide, but the possibility of such use is not excluded.

3.1.4 Toxicity of Metabolites

In general, metabolites are less toxic than their parent compounds, if for no other reason than that they are usually more soluble and, therefore, more rapidly excreted. There are notable exceptions in which biotransformation results in an inherently more toxic product. The word "toxication" is used to describe this exceptional result of biotransformation and distinguish it from "detoxication," which may be used in the general sense of "metabolism" but usually connotes a lessening of toxicity. The metabolic production of a more toxic compound is sometimes called "lethal synthesis" to emphasize that biotransformation in this instance is the source of danger. The term *lethal synthesis* was introduced in a lecture given on June 7, 1951, by Peters (1952) in connection with fluoroacetic acid. This compound is not toxic to enzymes in itself, but it is converted by enzymes into a highly toxic material. Peters (1963) later reviewed and extended the concept of lethal synthesis.

Persons untrained in toxicology are sometimes confused by the phenomenon of toxication, supposing that discovery of an example requires a reevaluation of the parent compound. Actually, the inherent toxicity of a compound is not changed in the slightest by the discovery that it is metabolized to a particular, more toxic material. One may be certain that the phenomenon was present before its discovery. This is not to suggest that information on biotransformation is unimportant. Regardless of the toxicity of metabolites, information on biotransformation may throw light on the mode of action of the parent compound, and perhaps contribute to the development of antidotes.

Furthermore, the effects of metabolism may be complex, as illustrated by studies of bromobenzene. It has been known for some time that the liver necrosis associated with this compound is caused by one or more toxic metabolites. Stimulation of its biotransformation by phenobarbital potentiates the injury of toxic doses to the liver, and inhibition of its metabolism by SKF 525–A prevents this injury. However, although 3-methylcholanthrene causes a slight *in vitro* stimulation of the metabolism of bromobenzene and does not alter the overall rate *in vivo*, it does protect against the hepatotoxicity. Rats dosed with bromobenzene after induction with 3-methylcholanthrene excrete more bromophenyldihydrodiol, bromocatechol, and 2-bromophenol than do uninduced rats. Increase in the first two compounds suggests an increased capacity to detoxify the highly reactive epoxide. Increase in 2-bromophenol suggests that 3-methylcholanthrene diverts the metabolism of bromobenzene into a comparatively nontoxic pathway (Zampaglione *et al.*, 1973). Further details of the toxicity of bromobenzene are discussed in Section 2.2.7.4.

3.2 Quantitative Aspects of Metabolism

Investigators have given somewhat more attention to the identity of metabolites than to the quantitative aspects of the metabolism of foreign chemicals. When measurements are made, they often involve only one tissue or only one route of excretion. Even when a balance study is attempted, it is frequently impossible to account for the fate of all of the compound administered. The record is particularly poor for long-term studies, but it is these studies that are of greatest interest in connection with any compound absorbed repeatedly. The use of radioisotopes or chromatography may make it easier to complete a balance study successfully and may simultaneously make it possible to recognize metabolites. However, the use of these methods merely to demonstrate the existence of previously unrecognized metabolites is not a substitute for a complete balance study. The factor unaccounted for qualitatively or quantitatively may be the biologically significant one.

Knowledge of the metabolism of the most studied major pesticides is incomplete, and knowledge of the metabolism of many others is fragmentary by comparison. The broad biological significance, contribution to health, and economic importance of these compounds demand continuing study of their distribution and fate in the animal organism.

3.2.1 Factors Influencing the Transfer and Availability of Chemicals in the Body

At any given dosage, the availability of a compound for toxic action depends not only on dosage and the microsomal or other enzymes that serve to toxify or detoxify it, but also on the full availability of the compound or its active metabolites at specific reaction sites. Usually a toxic compound must penetrate one or more membranes to reach its site of action. Transfer across membranes often is conditioned by pH, for example in the stomach, the intestine, or the kidney tubules. Having once reached a reactive site, a compound may still be inactive because most of it is bound to toxicologically nonspecific protein, and only a tiny proportion is free to associate with the critical enzyme or other molecule. Protein binding, pH, and membrane permeability can be regulated to some degree. Thus, the mere fact that two compounds interact is not proof that their interaction depends on enzymes or any other single factor. The facts must be determined in each instance. A very thorough review of interactions that may influence the toxicity of warfarin and other anticoagulants is that of Koch-Weiser and Sellers (1971a and 1971b).

3.2.1.1 Properties of Membranes. Any material must penetrate one or more living membranes in order to enter the body and reach the circulating blood, or in order to pass from the blood into a cell, or from the cytoplasmic sap into a cytoplasmic organelle or the nucleus. Although living membranes are imperfectly understood and undoubtedly differ from one another in detail, they appear to have much in common. According to traditional models of membrane structure, both outer surfaces are composed of protein spread over the polar surface of a lipid bilayer (Eisenman, 1968). A more recent view holds that living membranes are protein lattices permeated by cylinders of lipid. Contact between protein subunits and between protein and lipid occurs in both polar and apolar regions of the membrane (Wallach and Gordon, 1968). These membranes are often about 100 Å in diameter. Such membranes are effective barriers to some compounds but not to others.

Some small, water-soluble, but nonionizable compounds such as urea readily traverse mammalian membranes, probably along with water, by way of the pores. This filtration process is particularly rapid between the capillaries and the extracellular fluid. At the arterial end of the capillary, water is forced out because the hydrostatic pressure in the lumen exceeds the osmotic pressure. At the venous end of the capillary, water is drawn back into the vessel because the osmotic pressure of the blood exceeds that of the extracellular fluid, and because the hydrostatic pressure is dissipated.

Even if there is no flow of water through a membrane, small molecules such as those of gases may diffuse through the pores, or those with some degree of fat solubility may pass through the substance of the membrane. These movements follow a concentration gradient. Finally, there are some molecules that require active transport in order to traverse membranes.

The question of membranes as sites of toxic action (in contrast to their importance in the transfer of toxicants) is discussed in Section 4.1.2.3.

3.2.1.2 Ionization. Another factor that limits the transfer of compounds across membranes is ionization.

The degree of ionization of an electrolyte in aqueous solution depends on the inherent nature of the compound and on the pH of the solution. For convenience, the dissociation constant usually is expressed in terms of its negative logarithm. Thus,

$$pK_a = \log \frac{1}{K_a} = -\log K_a$$

By convention, the dissociation of both acids and bases is usually expressed in terms of the acidic process. The pK_a of a compound may be derived from the Henderson-Hasselbach equation as follows:

$$pK_a \text{ for acids} = pH + \log \frac{\text{nonionized form}}{\text{ionized form}}$$

$$pK_a \text{ for bases} = pH + \log \frac{\text{ionized form}}{\text{nonionized form}}$$

From these equations it is evident that the pK_a for a given compound is that pH at which the compound in solution is exactly half dissociated (since the log of 0.5/0.5 is zero). The equations can also be used to calculate the ratio of nonionized to ionized compound if its pK_a and the pH of the solution are known. Strong acids have low pK_a values, while strong bases have high pK_a values. The higher the pK_a of an acid, the weaker the acid. The lower the pK_a of a base, the weaker the base.

The pH on both sides of most membranes in the body is essentially the same. Since only nonionized molecules are transferred through the major portion of these membranes, it follows that poorly ionized compounds or those incapable of being ionized usually will cross membranes more efficiently than those that are highly ionized at the pH of most body fluids. The nonionized and poorly ionized compounds tend to diffuse through membranes in the direction of the concentration gradient until equilibrium is reached. If these compounds are highly insoluble in lipids, their transfer across membranes will be efficient, and (except in special cases such as bone-seekers), the concentrations each compound reaches in different tissues at equilibrium will be of the same order of magnitude. If these compounds are highly soluble in lipids, they will cross membranes efficiently, but they will reach vastly higher concentrations in neutral fat than in the surrounding aqueous tissues.

Other anatomical locations in which vastly different concentrations may be expected on opposite sides of a membrane at equilibrium are the gastrointestinal tract and the kidney, respectively, as compared to the plasma. The pH of the lumen of the stomach is about 1.0, that of the intestinal lumen is about 5.3, while that of the lumen of the kidney tubules may be as high as 7.8 or as low as 5.2, all compared to 7.4, the pH of the plasma. These differences in pH may have an important influence on absorption of compounds from the gastrointestinal tract or their successful excretion by the kidney. Fig. 3-2, which is based on the Henderson-Hasselbach equation above, illustrates how great this difference can be in theory. The pK_a used for this exercise was that for 2,4–D, which is 2.6. Although the values given in the figure have not been corrected for protein binding, they help to explain important facts in the absorption and excretion of 2,4–D. The compound is rapidly absorbed from the stomach and somewhat less rapidly from the intestine. It is excreted much more efficiently in alkaline than in acid urine.

Unlike acids, but for fundamentally the same reason, alkalis and alkaloids are excreted more effectively in acid urine.

Because of protein binding and other complications, it may not be practical to calculate the exact benefit to be expected from appropriate adjustment of the pH of the urine, but it has been known for many years that the benefit may be considerable. For example, men given 500 mg each of quinine sulfate excreted twice as much in 48 hours when the urine was maintained acid with ammonium chloride than when it was kept alkaline with sodium bicarbonate (Haag *et al.*, 1943).

3.2.1.3 Protein Binding. Proteins are amphoteric; that is, they present both anionic and cationic reaction sites. Proteins are also capable of forming a variety of other combinations involving hydrogen bonding, Van der Waals' forces, electrostatic forces, and polarity. Many foreign compounds in the blood are bound to proteins, especially albumin. Compounds that are ionized at pH 7.4 or those that are lipid-soluble tend to be bound to a greater degree. Protein binding of a compound is measured by determining its concentration in blood and then finding how much can be removed by dialyzing the blood against buffered saline. Although the combination with blood protein formed by each compound is usually reversible, it often happens that only the unbound fraction is available directly for specific action. In view of the correspondence of the *in vitro* measurement with pharmacological action, it seems probable that the bound fraction is unavailable because it cannot cross membranes in the living organism.

The restriction of activity to the unbound fraction is illustrated by thyroxine. This thyroid hormone is normally bound to a globulin of the blood in a ratio of bound to unbound of about 999:1. Although there is an increase in the total concentration of thyroxine during pregnancy and a decrease during nephrosis, there is no change in basal metabolic rate, for the concentration of free thyroxine remains within the normal range in these conditions.

Most studies of protein binding have involved the blood because of the availability and convenience of samples. However, other proteins of the body also bind foreign compounds to a greater or lesser degree. Nonspe-

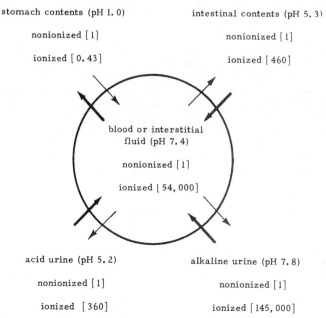

Fig. 3-2. Proportion of nonionized and ionized forms of 2,4–D (pK_a 2.6) at pH of body fluids.

cific binding to protein, in whatever tissue, reduces the concentration of compound available for reaction at a specific site. In some instances, the distribution of toxicant to the great mass of muscle and connective tissue may explain its rapid diminution in the brain and consequent termination of anesthesia or convulsions (see Section 3.2.3.1). Thus, the toxicological effect of protein binding is similar to that of storage in fat or bone. All of these processes reduce the amount of toxicant available for specific action, but they also form reservoirs from which a supply of toxicant may be drawn, with the result that its action is more prolonged than would be true otherwise.

The induction of enzymes is the most common but not the only way to increase the rate at which foreign compounds are metabolized *in vivo*. An example of another mechanism involves protein binding. Phenylbutazone binds to plasma albumin. Unlike the situation for many compounds, saturation is approached at therapeutic levels. At a plasma level of 100 ppm, only about 2% of the drug is free. At a plasma level of 250 ppm, about 12% is free, and biotransformation proceeds at 6 times the rate observed at the lower plasma level. The result is for the drug to remain at an unexpectedly uniform level, regardless of dosage (Burns *et al.*, 1953).

As already mentioned, proteins can bind foreign chemicals by several kinds of bonds. However, for any series of related chemicals, the bonding shows considerable specificity related to steric and spatial limitations of binding sites. Thus, nonspecific binding of foreign compounds to proteins has much in common with the reaction of these materials with their specific receptors. The principal difference is that the nonspecific reaction produces little or no recognizable pharmacological effect, while the specific toxic reaction produces a biochemical lesion in the intact animal, which interferes with function if the dose is sufficiently large. For example, various organic phosphorus compounds react with acetylcholinesterase to inhibit this enzyme. Phosphorylation of the enzyme constitutes the biochemical lesion. Some idea of the specificity of the reaction and the specificity of certain oximes and related compounds capable of reversing the inhibition by dephosphorylating the enzyme is given in Section 8.2.3.3.

Few pesticides have been studied to learn to what degree they are bound to plasma proteins. Part of the reason may be the difficulty of measuring the very small traces of some compounds that are unbound. In any event, Garrettson and Curley (1969) measured the protein binding of dieldrin by two methods.

Equilibrium dialysis at 25°C and a pH of 7.4 showed a ratio of 440:1 between serum and Sorensen's buffer. Because of the low protein content of the cerebrospinal fluid and the easy diffusion of many drugs into it, it is often in equilibrium with free drug in the plasma. Simultaneous sampling of serum and cerebrospinal fluid from a boy 48 days after he had ingested dieldrin gave a concentration ratio of 700:1. It was concluded that 99.8% or more of dieldrin in the blood is bound. Thus, the *in vitro* and *in vivo* methods agreed in showing a high degree of binding.

In the plasma, both aldrin and dieldrin are associated mainly with α- and β-lipoprotein fractions (Mick *et al.*, 1971).

Competition for binding sites is one mechanism for the interaction of compounds. For example, warfarin can be displaced from plasma protein by mefenamic acid, ethacrynic acid, diazoxide, and malidixic acid. At concentrations that may occur when these compounds are used as drugs, the increase in free warfarin can range from 66 to 400% with a corresponding increase in anticoagulant action (Sellers and Koch-Weiser, 1970). Because of the dosages involved, interactions are more likely to be important in patients treated with warfarin than in workers who use it as a pesticide, but the principle of interaction is the same.

Warfarin is a good example to discuss in connection with the transfer and availability of chemicals, because it illustrates how multiple factors may be involved. Whereas there is no evidence that barbiturates affect the distribution of warfarin in the body, the inherent activity of the blood coagulation process, or the response of the appropriate receptors to warfarin, they do induce warfarin-metabolizing enzymes that may reduce the plasma level of the compound associated with a particular dosage level (Levy *et al.*, 1970). Another example involves triclofos, a hypnotic that is metabolized to trichloroacetic acid. Daily administration of triclofos significantly prolonged prothrombin time in seven volunteers who previously and concurrently were treated with warfarin (Sellers *et al.*, 1972).

3.2.1.4 Passive and Specialized Transfer. When the observed transport of a compound across a membrane can be explained in terms of simple physics and present concepts of membrane structure, the transport is said to be passive because the membrane is inert. However, what is known of membranes fails to explain in simple physical terms the preferential uptake of potassium by cells or the observed transport of lipid-insoluble organic compounds. These and other situations are explained in terms of specialized transport in which the membrane has an active part in the transfer of material through it. The activity is thought to reside in portions of the membrane that act as carriers by forming a complex with the material at one surface of the membrane, after which the complex moves across the membrane and releases the material at the opposite surface.

Passive Transfer. Passive transfer may involve (a) simple diffusion, or (b) filtration. Diffusion explains the passage of lipid-soluble materials through the substance of membranes. Presumably the compound is dissolved in the lipid that constitutes the cores of the membrane. Once in solution, the compound diffuses at a rate determined by its lipid/water coefficient and the concentration gradient across the membrane. Simple diffusion may also involve the transfer of materials capable of passing through the pores of membranes. For these materials, the rate of diffusion is controlled by molecular size (small molecules and ions traveling faster than large ones), concentration gradient, and electrical charge (in the case of ions).

Filtration concerns the passage of molecules and ions capable of passing through the pores of membranes along with water that is propelled by hydrostatic or osmotic force. Filtration is most common at the arterial and venous ends of capillaries, as described in Section 3.2.1.1.

Specialized Transport. By definition, specialized transport involves participation of the membrane through some carrier mechanism. In active transport, the carrier complex may move across the membrane against a gradient of concentration or electrochemical potential. The system is characterized by the facts that (a) it can be saturated by solute; (b) it shows specificity for chemical structure; (c) if it carries two substances they will act as competitive inhibitors; (d) it is inhibited by anything that interferes with cellular metabolism; and, therefore, (e) it must require an input of energy.

Another recognized form of specialized transport is facilitated diffusion. This involves transport by a carrier mechanism but only in the direction of a concentration gradient. If this transfer does not require an input of energy it may be difficult to distinguish the carrier mechanism from an action of an inert membrane.

Pinocytosis is the process by which cells expend energy and engulf small droplets of the surrounding fluid. The possible bearing of this process on the gastrointestinal absorption of foreign compounds is discussed in Section 3.2.2.3.

3.2.2 Absorption

The three important, natural routes of absorption are oral, respiratory, and dermal. Some compounds are absorbed effectively by only one of these routes; others are absorbed by two routes, or by all routes. Viewed in another way, certain ecological situations favor one kind of exposure. Thus, the exposure of small children to solid and liquid poisons is most often oral, but sometimes dermal, and occasionally exclusively dermal. Many exposures involve more than one route, and then it is the character of the chemical involved that determines which of the routes will be of practical importance. The vast majority of industrial exposures are both respiratory and dermal. It is only the respiratory exposure that is significant in connection with silica, but the two kinds of exposure are about equally important in connection with aniline.

More people understand the importance of oral and respiratory absorption than understand dermal absorption. This is true not only of the laity, but also of some persons who should know better, as a result of medical training or industrial connection. The reason for this situation is that most of the older poisons are poorly absorbed from the skin and, therefore, this route of absorption generally could be ignored in the past. To be sure, there were some classical exceptions, such as the danger from excessive use of mercury ointment in the treatment of syphilis. However, in the main, there was much to justify the popular notion that chemicals were safe if the solids and liquids were not swallowed and the gases and vapors were not inhaled. The same view applied even to compounds such as strong acids and alkalis, in the sense that slight contact with the skin often gave a warning of danger before any real harm was done.

Such a complacent attitude about dermal exposure is no longer justified. Now there are industrial chemicals, pesticides, drugs, and even household chemicals that are effectively absorbed by the skin. Industrial standards (threshold limit values) for compounds are still stated in terms of air concentration. However, of the approximately 437 compounds for which threshold limits were recommended in 1972, at least 120 carried a notation indicating an important danger of skin absorption. Some of the others are absorbed by the skin but are not toxic enough to constitute a danger. This route of entry is especially important in connection with modern insecticides because many of them were selected as contact poisons, and the same chemical properties that make them able to penetrate the insect cuticle permit their absorption by mammals. A number of people have been made ill or even killed by exclusively dermal absorption of pesticides, including several organic phosphorus insecticides and at least one chlorinated hydrocarbon insecticide.

This emphasis on dermal absorption is not meant to detract from the importance of oral and respiratory absorption, whenever they are involved, but merely calls attention to a neglected subject. The skin you save may be your own.

3.2.2.1 Indirect Measurement of Absorption.

Inference of Absorption from Toxicity. The fact that a particular pesticide is toxic when administered by a certain route proves that it has been absorbed, but the mere fact of toxicity gives little information on the amount or rate of absorption.

Inference of Absorption by Consideration of Intravenous Toxicity. It would appear that some idea of the efficiency of absorption from the skin or from the gastrointestinal tract of vertebrates could be gained by comparing the dermal or oral toxicity with the intravenous toxicity. This method is based on the assumption that intravenous injection will make a compound freely available to the target organ, and thus exhibit the maximal or absolute toxicity of the dosage administered. Unfortunately, the method has serious limitations, as discussed in Section 3.2.2.6.

In addition to the possibility of sequestration of intravenously injected colloidal suspensions, determination of absorption by comparison often is complicated by difference of dosing schedule (see Section 2.4.3). A somewhat more valid comparison of the oral or dermal route with the intravenous route may be achieved through quantitative measurement of some effect associated with slow infusion into an appropriate vein. An example of the use of this technique for measuring dermal absorption in terms of cholinesterase inhibition is given in Section 3.2.2.5.

Obviously, any comparison involving intravenous injection must employ that portion of the venous system through which relevant absorption actually takes place. Failure to take this detail into account may lead to completely inaccurate results if the compound in question is actively metabolized in the liver (see Section 3.1.2.3).

Inference of Absorption from Disappearance. Absorption can also be inferred from disappearance or "remainder analysis." This method is commonly used in connection with all important natural routes of exposure, but there are subtle differences. Oral absorption is often equated to the dose minus unmetabolized compound excreted in the feces. Thus the proportion "lost" during passage through the gastrointestinal tract is assumed to be absorbed. When the fraction retained is large, the error of measurement is likely to be moderate or small. In a similar way, the amount of toxicant retained by the respiratory tract is often derived from its concentration in inhaled and exhaled air. Again, the error is likely to be small if the fraction retained is large. Dermal absorption also frequently is measured by rate of disappearance. However, since dermal absorption often is slow, the error of measurement may be relatively great.

3.2.2.2 Direct Measurement of Absorption.

Measurement in Blood or Lymph. Appropriate measurement of a compound in the blood or lymph draining an area offers the best and most direct information on its absorption from that area. So far, such studies of pesticides have been confined to the measurement of absorption from the intestinal tract via the lymphatic duct, the hepatic portal vein, or both. Examples of such measurements are studies by Rothe *et al.* (1957) and Laws (1966). Presumably, the method could be extended by suitable surgical techniques to measurement of absorption from the skin (Kjaersgaard, 1954; Ainsworth, 1960).

There is an inherent difference in sampling from the lymphatic duct and from an important vein such as the hepatic portal. During an experiment lasting several hours, the entire flow of the hepatic duct may be collected by cannula. The sample will contain all of the compound absorbed by that route during the sampling period. Of course, collection of the lymph alters the circulation of the blood, but not enough to have an important effect on the measurement under discussion. The only serious problem arises from the fact that the duct may have several channels in some species and part of the flow may be missed. On the other hand, one cannot collect all the blood from the hepatic portal vein without severe disturbance of the circulation and general physiology. Thus, one must be satisfied with a series of samples of such blood. Any calculation of the amount of compound absorbed during a measured interval must be based on the rate of flow of blood as well as the concentration of the compound in the samples.

Even compounds that seem chemically similar may be absorbed differently. For example, of the radioactive DDT administered orally to three rats with their thoracic ducts cannulated, 47 to 65% was recovered from the lymph (Rothe *et al.,* 1957). Absorption reached a peak about 1.5 to 2.5 hours after administration in two of the rats, but tended to maintain a plateau for several hours in the third rat. DDT was absorbed at rates as high as 381 μg/hr in rats weighing 325 to 375 g. Of the DDT-derived materials found in the lymph 50% was absorbed in the first 2.5 to 7 hours, and 95% in 18 hours. The total recovery of absorbed and unabsorbed DDT in this experiment varied from 89 to 118%. Although the possibility of some absorption of this compound from the intestine by the hepatic portal system was not ruled out, it appeared unlikely. The absorption of dieldrin is reported to be different from that of DDT, but the reason for the difference is not apparent from the physical characteristics of the two compounds. Of radioactive dieldrin administered orally, only 8% was recovered in the lymph (Heath and Vandekar, 1964). It seems likely that the mechanism of absorption is related closely to the mechanism of transport in the blood (see Section 3.2.3), but apparently the relation is unexplored.

Measurement from Storage in Solid Tissues. Obviously, any pesticide stored in the tissues must be considered to have been absorbed, provided exposure was by a natural route. This method of measuring absorption is relatively efficient in connection with a small number of doses, but becomes progressively less efficient as a steady state of storage is approached and maintained. The fat and muscle of pigs that had been fed DDT residues for 36 days were found to contain 49 to 57% of the total dose (Carter *et al.,* 1948). However, the dosage was measured by analysis of the residue in the food, and, if this analysis gave systematically low results, it would increase the apparent success of final recovery. The special case of the analysis of biopsy samples is discussed in Section 3.2.2.5.

Measurement from Excretion. Absorption may also be inferred from the measurement of true excretion. Because storage tends to reach a steady state at any given tolerated dosage, it should be possible (once the steady state has been reached) to account, on the average, for 100% of the daily intake in terms of elimination by mechanical passage of unabsorbed material plus true excretion by all routes. A comparison of fecal excretion following oral and intravenous dosage should permit recognition of excretory products resulting from absorbed material. A conclusion based on such a comparison cannot be absolute until two possibilities have been excluded. Following ingestion, there is a possibility that metabolites in the feces are the result of bacterial or enzyme action on unabsorbed compound, or conversely, that the original compound is absorbed but excreted unchanged, or only conjugated.

3.2.2.3 Gastrointestinal Absorption.
Factors responsible for gastrointestinal absorption are covered in Section 3.2.1 above. Lipid solubility appears to be the most important factor influencing the absorption of pesticides by this route. The stomach not only absorbs nonionized lipid-soluble materials, but also ionized lipid-soluble materials such as 2,4-D and 2,4,5-T. Such weak acids are largely nonionized in the presence of stomach acid (approximately pH 1). On the contrary, highly ionized weak bases such as paraquat and diquat presumably are little absorbed by the stomach.

Absorption by the intestine is similar to that by the stomach. The absorption of nonionized lipid-soluble material is favored. The greater the degree of ionization, the slower the absorption. Evidence from pharmacology indicates that in the rat the effective pH of the intestinal mucosal margin from which absorption occurs directly is about 5.3 rather than 6.6, which is the average pH of the intestinal contents.

Simple diffusion apparently accounts for most of the absorption of pesticides from the gastrointestinal tract. There is some evidence that 5-fluorouracil, which has been investigated as a chemosterilant, can be absorbed actively by the same process that ordinarily transports uracil and thymine.

Although the absorption of highly ionized materials such as paraquat and diquat is not efficient, it does occur. Absorption of these materials is favored by their lipid solubility, but this factor is inadequate to account for their absorption. It has been suggested that certain quaternary nitrogen drugs are absorbed by forming complexes with phospholipid peptides.

The intestinal mucosa of mammals engulfs droplets of fat that may be seen in the cytoplasm by means of the electron microscope. The droplets pass about halfway toward the base of the cell, after which no more are seen until they reappear in the intercellular spaces from which they presumably make their way into the lymphatic vessels. Imai and Coulston (1967) showed that electron-dense particles are associated with the fat droplets of the intestinal mucosa of rats following large oral doses of methoxychlor dissolved in oil. They suggest that the particles made visible by the electron microscope may represent a complex associated with methoxychlor. This mechanism of absorption in conjunction with fat would be consistent with the observation reported by a number of authors that several chlorinated hydrocarbon insecticides are absorbed more readily if administered in fat solutions.

3.2.2.4 Respiratory Absorption. Once non-particulate or soluble particulate material reaches the depths of the lungs, it is absorbed according to the principles described in Section 3.2.1. Absorption tends to be rapid compared with the rate by other portals because the alveolar membrane is thin and the blood supply abundant. However, it is not the absorptive membrane or the rate of blood flow that truly distinguishes the absorption of materials by the respiratory route; rather, it is the aerodynamics of the respiratory tract, which determines whether material will become available for absorption. In order to be inhaled at all by this route, a material must be in the form of a gas, vapor, or fine particulate.

Ways of measuring the quantity of pesticide that workers may inhale are discussed in Section 5.5.1, and the results of such measurements are described in Section 6.2.3.1.

For systemically acting toxicants, it makes little difference from what part of the respiratory system they may be absorbed. In general, the quantity of pesticide is proportional to the volume of the particle containing it, and absorption of inhaled active ingredient is prompt. Thus, for pesticides, greatest toxicological interest centers on the total retained dosage and not on the particular part of the respiratory tract in which deposition or absorption occurs. No pesticide is a primary lung irritant in the usual sense, although at least one (paraquat) has its most dramatic action on the lung regardless of the route of administration. Crystalline silica, of course, is avoided in all formulations of pesticides. The various clays and amorphous silicas used as carriers or as active ingredients are not known to have produced any pneumoconiosis; however, the possibility cannot be excluded completely. For this reason, and because of the great importance of inhaled particulates in toxicology generally, the fate of particles in the lungs requires brief notice here. The subject is covered at far greater length and from different points of view in books on pulmonary physiology and occupational health. Valuable symposia, reviews, and monographs include those by Blair (1964), Casarett (1972), Davies (1961, 1967), and Hatch and Gross (1964).

Physical Characteristics of Pesticides Especially at the Time of Application. A few of the fumigant pesticides are true gases; the others are liquids that readily vaporize at ordinary temperatures. A number of solid and liquid pesticides not ordinarily thought of as fumigants have a sufficiently high vapor pressure that their vapor in the thin layer of air in contact with their residues is of critical importance in their toxic action on pests, and their vapors are at least potentially important in mammalian toxicology.

Solid and liquid pesticides are applied commonly as dusts, sprays, mists, fogs, and aerosols. Unfortunately, as shown in Table 3-7, use of the terms is not uniform. In fact, not even the bases for measurement are uniform. Potts (1958) defined his terms according to the essentially complete range of particles issued from each applicator; thus, he called attention to the overlap of particle sizes designated by different words or phrases. The World Health Organization Expert Committee on Insecticides defined coarse sprays, fine sprays, mists, and aerosols in terms of their *volume median diameters,* that is, the particle diameter (measured in micrometers) such that half of the total volume of a particular dispersed material consists of smaller particles and half consists of larger particles. (Volume median diameter is essentially identical to mass median diameter.) A range of volume median diameters is not a complete range but is similar to a range of means. Such values do not suggest the great overall range of particles in pesticides at the moment of dispersal. It is important to remember that it requires many more small particles than large ones to constitute half of the volume of spray or other dispersed material. Thus, 80% of the particles from many commercial "aerosol bombs" are less than 30 μm in diameter, and the average is between 10 and 15 μm.

The nomenclature for particle sizes used by the World Health Organization is likely to be used in connection with vector control. With this exception, the meanings for "spray," "aerosol," and the like are indefinite unless defined.

The physical state of the active agent often is not limiting; solids may be applied as micronized particles and liquids may be sprayed directly. Solids may be dissolved and applied as sprays or aerosols. Even when a solid is applied as a dust, it may be that the dust is a carrier into which the active ingredient has been impregnated while in solution. Conversely, liquid pesticides may be impregnated on carriers and applied as dusts.

The size of droplets of purely liquid formulations depends entirely on the way in which they are applied. Of greatest importance is the form of the nozzle and the pressure of the liquid at the nozzle. The size of particles reaching the sprayman is also conditioned by his

Table 3-7

Size of Airborne Particles Applicators of Pesticides
May Encounter.   Two Classifications Based on
Different Parameters are Given

Parameter and formulation or application	Range (μm)	Mean (μm)	Reference or Authority
Diameter of particles			
dust	≲ 250		CIPAC[a]
fine dust	< 75		''
coarse dust	75 - 250		''
granule	1,000 - 2,000		''
granulette	250 - 1,000		''
spray	150 - 3,000	750	Potts, 1958
coarse mist	51 - 500	175	''
medium mist	60 - 350	75	''
fine mist	10 - 50	30	''
wet fog	10 - 50	35	''
dry fog	1 - 10	5	''
aerosol (coarse)	2 - 4	3	''
aerosol (fine)	1 and less	0.4	''
Volume median diameter of particles			
spray (coarse)	> 400		WHO, 1971
spray (fine)	100 - 400		''
mist	50 - 100		''
aerosol	< 50		''

a. Collaborative International Pesticide Analytical Council.

distance from the nozzle (length of wand) and by the character and nearness of the surface receiving spray. Spray droplets discharged at high speed against a nonabsorptive surface are shattered into smaller droplets. However, the smallness of particles in dusts and in sprays of water-wettable powders is limited by the original grind of the formulation. Application does not make the particles any finer, but may separate particles that otherwise would adhere to one another.

The wetness of particles as well as their size helps to determine whether they will stick to a surface, especially a dry one. Durham and Wolfe (1962) attached carbon-coated micro-scope slides to the hat brim of a sprayman applying water-wettable powder. Their paper contains a photomicrograph of one of the slides. The picture resembles that of snowballs that have fallen from different angles and with little velocity into fine dust. The photomicro-graph apparently shows that some droplets of water that reached the sprayman did not carry any particles, for the slide contained some empty craters on the carbon surface. The solid particles that did reach the slide were moist enough to pick up carbon, but not surrounded by enough water to make a crater very much larger than the solid particle itself. The parti-cles were usually single rather than aggregated. It was clear that the particles had only a small momentum when they reached the slide, for they made only feeble imprints on the soft film of carbon.

Some Characteristics of the Respiratory System. The respiratory system is so constructed that the volume, and especially the surface area, of the main parts increase progressively from the nose to the alveoli. As a consequence of this arrangement, the velocity of air flow is greatest in the nasopharyngeal region, somewhat less in the trachea and bronchi, even less in the bronchioles, and zero in the alveoli. By the same token, the change of direction of flow of air is very abrupt in the nasopharynx, less abrupt in the tracheobronchial tree, and very slight in the alveolar ducts.

The respiratory surface has been estimated as about 55 m^2.

The lining of much of the nasopharynx and all of the tracheobronchial tree is ciliated. This epithelium carries a continuous layer of mucus from the nose backward to the pharynx, or from the bronchioles up through the bronchi and the trachea to the pharynx. The mucus and whatever it may contain usually is swallowed but may be expectorated if sufficiently profuse.

Effect of Particle Size on Penetration. It is common experience that the inhalation of particles depends on their size. One does not inhale rain, but may inhale fog or smoke. Few particles larger than 30 μm are inhaled by a person at rest or at light work, because the velocity of air entering the nose is not great enough to divert their fall under the force of gravity. Some particles of this size are inhaled if work is sufficiently vigorous or if breathing is by the mouth.

Because of the high velocity of air back and forth in the nasal passages, many of the larger particles there are impacted on the mucous surface. Such impaction affects particles down to about 1 μm in diameter; it becomes progressively more efficient for larger particles and almost completely effective for those greater than 10 μm.

Because of the lower velocity of air in the tracheobronchial tree and because air remains there longer, particles there are more subject to gravity (settling) than to impaction. Here again, the deposition process is most efficient for larger particles, some of which may be as large as 10 μm. Smaller particles, especially those less than 0.1 μm, are little affected by gravity. Their mean settling time is very long. Those that deposit on the bronchial wall are most likely to do so by diffusion (Brownian motion).

Because only small particles reach the alveoli, diffusion is more important and settling less important there than in the bronchi as causes of deposition of particles.

Thus, inhaled particles larger than 5 to 10 μm are efficiently trapped in the upper respiratory tract. These particles impinge on the mucous layer continually carried upward from the respiratory tract into the pharynx by ciliary action. As the material is returned to the pharynx, it is swallowed. The efficiency of the upper respiratory tract in trapping particles decreases rapidly in the range between 5 and 1 μm, so that some particles 5 μm in diameter reach the alveoli and many particles 1 μm in diameter reach this level. Almost all particles 1 μm in diameter or greater that reach the alveolus are retained, and if they are eventually removed, it must be accomplished later by some special mechanism. Retention diminishes progressively for particles between 1 and 0.1 μm in diameter. In other words, these latter particles are so small that some of them never impinge even after reaching the alveolus, but are carried back into the ambient air by expiration. There is some evidence that retention increases again for particles less than 0.1 μm in size.

Although retention of particulate matter in the lungs depends on many factors—such as size, shape, hydroscopicity, and density of particles, the chemical form, and whether or not the material is inhaled by the nose or by the mouth—it may be assumed, in the absence of specific information, that about 25% of inhaled material is exhaled; about 50% is deposited in the upper respiratory passages and subsequently swallowed, and about 25% is deposited in the lower respiratory passages.

Retention of Smoke. At least some pesticides applied to tobacco in the field eventually pass into the smoke when the tobacco is used. The degree to which the smoke is inhaled has a marked influence on the degree of retention of insecticide. In a test with experimental cigarettes containing ^{14}C-DDD, one series was smoked by a machine, one series was smoked by noninhaling smokers, and a third series was smoked by inhaling smokers. All of the DDD in smoke from the machine was trapped and the radioactivity measured. The volunteers exhaled all smoke under slight vacuum into a tube connected with three solvent traps. Analysis showed that the mainstream smoke from the machine contained about 4.7% of the DDD in the cigarette. The noninhaling smokers exhaled essentially all the DDD brought into their mouths, whereas the inhaling smokers retained about 70% of the available DDD (that is, about 3% of that in the total cigarette)

(Bowery *et al.*, 1965).

Fate of Inhaled Material. Of the material reaching the lower respiratory passages, not all is absorbed. The initial rate of absorption of a gas or vapor depends on its chemical nature. The rate of absorption of very few pesticides has been measured. In the absence of measurement, it is only safe to assume that absorption is complete.

For compounds such as many anesthetic gases that undergo little chemical change in the body, the net rate of absorption will decrease as the concentration of material approaches a steady state in the tissues. In other words, the rate of diffusion from the blood into the lung will approach the rate of diffusion from the lung into the blood (Papper and Kitz, 1963).

It must be noted that the penetration and retention of a gas such as sulfur dioxide may be increased by simultaneous exposure to an otherwise inert aerosol such as those of sodium chloride or carbon (Amdur, 1957, 1961). This finding may be related to the fact that aerosols of sulfuric acid or sulfates are more irritant than the equivalent concentration of sulfur dioxide from which they may be formed in the atmosphere by oxidation (Amdur, 1971). Although sulfur dioxide is not an important pesticide, the principle illustrated may be important in connection with other vaporized pesticides that may adsorb on particles or in connection with aerosols that may vaporize partially.

Once particulate matter has been deposited in the lower respiratory tract, it must be retained or disposed of by some special mechanism. Since the rate of clearance of solid material from the lung is slow, most of what can be absorbed is eventually taken up. The problem of special clearance is concerned with relatively insoluble material. However, even highly insoluble material such as silica and asbestos may be toxic, and this may be associated with their limited solution in body fluids. Silicosis probably remains the most important single occupational disease. Recent evidence has pointed to asbestos as an inducer of cancer.

Brieger and LaBelle (1959) studied rats exposed to a dynamic atmosphere containing particles of a water-insoluble dye that had been carefully prepared for uniformity of particle size. The concentration of particles in the air was 20 mg/m³, a level only twice that now permitted for nuisance dusts in industry. Particles measuring 2 and 6 μm, respectively, were used in separate experiments; exposure was for 7 hours. Under these conditions, both sizes of particles reached a concentration of about 0.7 ppm in the lungs at the end of exposure. The concentrations in the gastrointestinal tract were about equal for the two sizes of particles, but higher than those in the lungs. The highest concentrations were reached on the skin, and the skin retained a higher concentration of the smaller particles. Loss of particles was most rapid from the skin. About 24 hours after exposure ended, the concentration of particles was greatest in the gastrointestinal tract. Clearance from the lungs, though measurable, was extremely slow. After a week or two, a relatively permanent phase began in which the highest concentration of particles was in the lungs; in fact, little material remained anywhere else. The initial rate of clearance was almost 6 times faster for 6-μm particles than for those measuring 2 μm.

Undissolved particles deposited in the lungs are partially cleared in two phases. The first phase lasts 24 to 48 hours and exhibits a halflife of 13 to 17 hours in the rat. The proportion of the total dose of toxic particles cleared during this first phase can be changed at will by increasing the total lung burden by the addition of inert particles, provided the clearance capacity of the lung is not overtaxed (LaBelle and Brieger, 1959). The increased clearance is accompanied by an increase in free-moving phagocytic cells in the lung, and these cells constitute the primary mechanism for removal of the particles (LaBelle and Brieger, 1960a, 1960b; LaBelle *et al.*, 1960). After ingesting the particles, these cells eventually are swept upward by ciliary movement to the pharynx and swallowed.

The first phase of clearance from the lung associated mainly with phagocytosis is, of course, accompanied by the even more rapid clearance from the nasopharynx and the tracheobronchial tree associated with ciliary action on particles caught in the overlying mucus. The second phase of lung clearance of relatively insoluble particles is very slow. Some authors (Casarett, 1972) divide the prolonged clearance into at least three subphases, emphasizing: (*a*) the declining importance over a period of 6 weeks or more of the movement of particle-laden macrophages to the ciliated epithelium and their transport to the pharynx; (*b*) the continuing process of lymphatic uptake over a period of months; and (*c*) the increasing relative importance of solubilization, which may persist for years. Regardless of any division of the clearance process into "phases," the continuity of the process and its rapid decline in rate after exposure has stopped must be emphasized.

Of the various factors leading to clearance of particles from the alveoli, phagocytosis is most important. Nearly all particles in the alveoli are found in macrophages only a short time after brief inhalation. The macrophages are thought to be derived from monocytes and from Type I pulmonary epithelial cells. Excessive concentrations of particles or particles that injure the macrophages that ingest them delay lung clearance.

3.2.2.5 Dermal Absorption. The importance of dermal absorption was pointed out in the introduction to Section 3.2.2. The relatively massive amounts of pesticides that men encounter by this route under actual working conditions are described in Section 6.2.3.1.

The following sections are concerned with methods for studying dermal absorption and with the major findings regarding absorption by this route. These matters were reviewed in detail by Malkinson and Rothman (1962) and by Tregear (1964, 1966). Techniques for measuring dermal exposure are discussed in Section 5.5.2. In the study of dermal absorption, the focus of attention is at least as much on the skin as on the compound involved. The interest is chiefly scientific and the welfare of the test animal is often irrelevant. In the measurement of dermal toxicity, attention is focused on the compound and its effects on the test animals. The interest is largely practical.

Dermal penetration of a compound may be demonstrated by the same indirect methods (Section 3.2.2.1) or direct methods (Section 3.2.2.2) already discussed in connection with the study of absorption by any route. However, practical considerations influence the relative value of different techniques. Dermal absorption is often slow and this increases the difficulty of its measurement. Dermal absorption also differs since it frequently happens that only a part of the skin becomes contaminated and, therefore, only that part participates in absorption. By contrast, oral dosing (unless very rapidly fatal) usually exposes the entire lumen of the gastrointestinal tract. Respiratory dosing usually exposes the entire respirator tract unless the exposure involves particulate matter too large to reach the depths of the lungs. Measurement of absorption in terms of surface area may be of basic interest in connection with any route of absorption, but it has special practical importance in connection with the skin.

The area of skin subjected to treatment may be limited by keeping the volume of all doses constant. For more refined studies, the treatment area may be limited by gluing metal or plastic rings to the skin, as described by Fri-

berg *et al.* (1961) and by Fredriksson (1963).

Indirect Methods for Studying Dermal Penetration. An indirect method for demonstrating absorption without the necessity for biopsy is the elicitation of local toxic, allergic, or pharmacological actions following dermal application. As far as pesticides are concerned, this method has been used in connection with some of the more toxic organic phosphorus compounds. It has been observed in the laboratory, or occasionally under field conditions, that areas of the skin exposed to paraoxon, parathion, or tepp responded by localized sweating and muscle fasciculation. The latter phenomenon is of particular interest when one considers that the blood supplies to the skin and the underlying muscle are largely independent. Localized response of the muscle is therefore an indication that some of the compound diffused directly through the skin and connective tissue into at least the superficial layer of muscle rather than all being taken up by the capillaries of the corium, and thus being carried off to the general circulation.

Absorption may be inferred from "remainder analysis" or disappearance; such analysis may be either chemical or radiological. In the first instance, the material must be contained in a closed vessel attached to the skin; the vessel may contain a gas or a solution of the compound under study. If serial analyses indicate a reduction of the concentration of the gas or solute, it may be concluded that the disappearance resulted from penetration into the skin; but the method does not necessarily distinguish between materials held in the superficial layer of skin and those that actually traverse the skin and pass into the general circulation. The applicability of remainder analysis is greatly extended by the use of radioactive materials. If this method of measurement is used, the material under study need not be in the form of a gas or solution, but may be in the form of a film applied directly to the skin. Measurement may be carried out at intervals of any length by means of windowless or thin end window counters.

Any form of remainder analysis suffers from the fault that all losses may be attributed to absorption. The importance of this limitation is great where absorption is small, so that the true rate of absorption approaches the experimental error inherent in whatever method of measurement is used. The method of remainder analysis is particularly valuable when emphasis is placed on the possibility of removal rather than on the possibility of absorption. This procedure, among others, was employed by Fredriksson (1961a) in connection with parathion. It was shown that some of the material remained on the skin in spite of thorough washing with soap and water for half a minute, followed by washing with alcohol. The alcohol removed material that the other washing failed to dislodge. Furthermore, the proportion of residue removed by the combination of procedures became progressively less as the time from application to washing was increased in separate tests.

O'Brien and Dannelley (1965) introduced a variation of technique that largely eliminated the usual criticism of the disappearance method. They used radioactive compounds applied at the rate of only 1 μg to 1 μl of solvent, and the full thickness of the skin was excised from a circular area large enough to permit recovery of approximately 100% of the dose immediately after application. The complication of binding or biotransformation within the skin was obviated by nitric digestion of the entire sample. It was found that, even in the same concentration in the same solvent, different compounds spread over the skin to different degrees; therefore, the exact area of skin to be removed had to be determined experimentally for each compound. Use of the method showed: (a) the following compounds were absorbed from intact rat skin in decreasing order, as follows: malathion > dieldrin > carbaryl > famphur > DDT; (b) the rate of absorption was not related to the olive oil/water partition coefficient; (c) the compounds varied in the proportion that could be recovered from the skin by washing with acetone; and (d) in general, the compounds were absorbed from different solvents in decreasing order as follows: acetone > benzene > corn oil. Since the actual area of skin covered by each dose was not predetermined or measured, it was impossible to measure the absorption rates in terms of skin area, and the effect ascribed to solvents was almost certainly a combined effect of variation in solvents and area. The very real value of this skin excision technique would be increased by ensuring that the treated area was (a) known, and (b) adequately covered by the test formulation at all times.

Another indirect method for studying dermal absorption involves dosage-response. An example is the determination of curves for depression of cholinesterase activity in the blood associated with (a) two or more uniform rates of intravenous infusion of an organic phosphorus compound, and (b) application of the same compound to a circumscribed area of skin. Largely by trial and error, intravenous dosage rates are selected that cause cholinesterase inhibition matching that caused by the dermal application. It is then concluded that the compound penetrated the skin and reached the blood at the same rate as the intravenous dosage that produced the same rate of enzyme inhibition. Fredriksson was one of the first to use the technique. His results for paraoxon in the cat are shown in Fig. 3-3. The numerical results are summarized in one line of Table 3-8. The graph (and other curves not shown) permitted calculation of the time necessary for paraoxon to penetrate the intact skin of the cat. As may be seen, it required between 10 and 15 minutes for the combined time necessary for the circulation of the blood and for the intravenously injected inhibitor to reach a concentration high enough to produce any measurable inactivation of enzyme activity. Following percutaneous absorption, the total latent period was 20 to 28 minutes. The difference between the latency period following percutaneous absorption and the one following intravenous absorption represents the time required for the compound to pass from the skin surface to the blood stream. When curves with approximately equal slope were chosen, the difference was found to be about 12 minutes (Fredriksson, 1962).

Direct Methods for Studying Dermal Penetration. General principles of the direct measurement are mentioned in Section 3.2.2.2; methods that have been applied to dermal absorption are discussed here. At intervals after a material has been applied to the skin, biopsies may be taken and distribution of the material or its metabolites within the skin may be studied by: (a) histochemical techniques; (b) fluorescent microscopy; or (c) autoradiography, depending on the nature of the applied material.

Something may be learned about the distribution of a compound by stripping off successive layers of the epidermis by means of the repeated application and removal of self-adhesive tape. If the compound is radioactive, it is easy to measure the activity of the succeeding samples by means of a densitometer. Such a study was made by Fredriksson (1961b) in connection with parathion. The results for the first six strips are shown in Fig. 3-4. There was a rapid decrease in the amount of radioactivity in the first four strips followed by a slower but steady decrease in the succeeding strips. Even in strip no. 25, the activity was greater than background. Autoradiographs of the same strips and of microscopic sections showed that the deep penetration was associated largely with the hair follicles and sebaceous glands, but not sweat glands. After skin had been exposed to parathion for 24 hours, there appeared to be increased spreading of material around the follicles and directly below the epidermis.

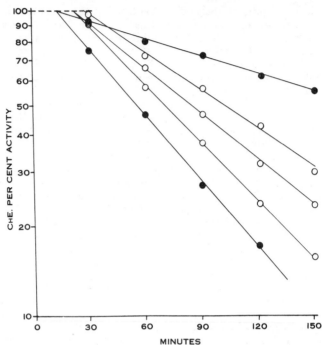

Fig. 3-3. Inhibition of plasma cholinesterase activity in five cats following cutaneous application (open circles) of 50 μl of paraoxon on 4.1 cm², and following intravenous infusion (filled circles) of paraoxon. The rates of infusion were 64 μg per hour (lower curve) and 32 μg per hour (upper curve). Time is in minutes after beginning of administration. From Fredriksson (1962) by permission of The Williams & Wilkins Co., Baltimore.

Under suitable conditions, the analysis of a compound or its metabolites in urine, feces, or exhaled air may serve as a direct measure of dermal absorption. Stewart and Dodd (1964) made such a study of people exposed to chlorinated hydrocarbon solvents. Application was topical, or the subject immersed his thumb or his entire hand for a predetermined period. Forced residual breath was collected at intervals and analyzed by gas chromatography. Marked differences were found in the rate of penetration of an equal area of skin by different compounds: methylene chloride was fastest, tetrachlorethylene was slowest, and 1,1,1-trichlorethane, carbon tetrachloride, and trichlorethylene were intermediate. The solvents also differed in the rate at which they disappeared from the breath, carbon tetrachloride and tetrachlorethylene being slowest. Absorption through a hand was about 20 times greater than absorption through a thumb. Although the authors were chiefly interested in comparing the five solvents, it should be possible to express their results numerically by taking the respiratory volume into account, and dividing the total weight of solvent recovered by the area of skin exposed and the duration of exposure. Assuming the subjects

were engaged in very light work throughout the period of measurement, and assuming that the area of a hand is 35 cm², it may be calculated from values read from the authors' second figure that the absorption of 1,1,1-trichloroethane during 30 minutes was about 62 μg/cm²/min. The true rate of absorption must have been greater because the subjects probably did some more active work during part of the 9-hour period of study, at least a small portion of the compound was metabolized and excreted in the urine, and respiratory excretion was not completed entirely during the period of observation.

Hayes et al. (1960), in testing the safety of malathion for the control of human lice, applied 1, 5, and 10% dust formulations daily to about 80% of the total skin surface of volunteers. Although the authors did not calculate the rate of absorption, they did recover malathion equivalent from the urine. For men receiving the 10% formulation, the average excretory rate was 1.99 mg/hr and the highest observed rate was 5.80 mg/hr. On the assumption that 80% of the body surface is 1,400 cm², these excretory rates correspond to average and maximal absorption rates of 0.027 and 0.069 μg/cm²/min, respectively. There is rea-

Table 3-8
Rate of Dermal Absorption of Selected Pesticides
and a Few Other Materials

Compound	Rate of absorption ($\mu g/cm^2/min$)	Technique [a]	Species	Reference
water	18	excretion	man	DeLong et al., 1954
water	27	disappearance I	man	Pinson, 1952
mercuric chloride	3.4	disappearance I	guinea pig	Skog and Wahlberg, 1964
1,1,1-trichloro-ethane	62[b]	direct	man	Stewart and Dodd, 1964
sarin	1-2	dosage-response	cat	Fredriksson, 1958
sarin	18	disappearance I	cat	Fredriksson, 1958
paraoxon	0.13-0.34 (0.23)[c]	dosage-response	cat	Fredriksson, 1962
	1.7	disappearance	cat	Fredriksson, 1964
	0.05-1.23 (0.32)	dosage-response	rabbit	Nabb et al., 1966
parathion	0.02-0.39 (0.06)	dosage-response	rabbit	Nabb et al., 1966
	1.4	disappearance I	cat	Fredriksson, 1961c
	0.005	disappearance E	cat	Fredriksson, 1961c
malathion	up to 0.30 (0.12)[b]	direct	man	Hayes et al., 1960

a. I - disappearance from intact animal; E - disappearance from excised skin.
b. Calculated by the reviewer.
c. Average values are shown in parentheses.

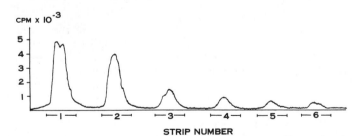

CPM x 10^{-3}

STRIP NUMBER

Fig. 3-4. Radioactivity as obtained from recorder in the first 6 tape strips from human skin, taken 1 hour following application of 6 μl of ^{32}P-labeled parathion. Scanning speed 3 in/min; slit opening 1/16 in; time constant 2 secs. From Fredriksson (1961b) by permission of Acta Dermato-Venerologica, Stockholm.

son to think that these estimates are low because, by the analytical method used, only 23% of a small oral dose of malathion was recovered, and failure of recovery seemed much more likely than failure of gastrointestinal absorption. Thus, in round numbers, the best estimate of average and maximal absorption of malathion is about 0.12 and 0.30 $\mu g/cm^2/min$, respectively. For what it may be worth, these estimates are of the same order of magnitude as those for parathion and paraoxon measured by dosage-response in animals (see Table 3-8).

Studies may be made of percutaneous absorption following more or less radical surgical procedures. Kjaersgaard (1954) took advantage of techniques developed earlier for physiological study in order to develop a technique for studying percutaneous absorption in perfused skin. He stated that material applied to the surface of such skin could be detected in the outgoing blood or other perfusion fluid. Further studies along the same lines have been made by Ainsworth (1960).

Treherne (1956) apparently introduced the use of excised skin for absorption studies. Although suitable for indirect measurements, excised skin is most used for direct measurements. Employment of isolated samples of skin taken by biopsy or autopsy makes it possible to extend studies of dermal absorption to man in connection with compounds too toxic to be studied by any other procedure. Movement of the sample within the skin can be studied microscopically following application of a compound to the unmounted skin. The usefulness of the technique may be extended by mounting the skin in a special chamber in such a way that the undersurface is exposed to fluid into which the chemical being investigated may diffuse, and from which it may be analyzed. The chamber may be arranged to permit a constant flow of fluid so that a sharp gradient is maintained between the fluid and the skin (see Fig. 1 in Tregear, 1966). Perhaps even more important than constant flow is the use of a fluid capable of accepting the compound under study. Substitution of serum or organic solvents for saline increased the measured rate of absorption of dieldrin by a factor of 10 (Tregear, 1966).

When investigators first learn about studies of isolated samples of skin, they generally condemn the technique on the basis that the skin is dead and, therefore, not representative of the situation in the intact organism. However, there are two extenuating circumstances: (a) the most important single factor limiting absorption is a nonliving membrane in the epidermis; and (b) the skin absorbs oxygen directly from the air, and it excretes carbon dioxide into the air. It probably would be best to regard a freshly isolated sample of skin as a special form of tissue culture rather than as a dead tissue. Although the possibility of differences between results obtained with isolated samples and the intact animal must be kept in mind, the fact remains that useful information can be obtained from isolated samples. Barnes (1968) considered the possibility that use of human skin for such testing could eliminate the problem of species difference without introducing other variables of perhaps even greater significance.

Units for Expressing Permeability. Permeability may be expressed in the following units: $\mu g/cm^2/min$, $m\mu M/cm^2/min$, and $\mu cm/min$.

Of these, the first is of most general use in toxicology because toxicity values are usually given simply in terms of weight. The first unit can be converted to the second (and *vice versa*) if the molecular weight of the compound under study is known, and of course the second unit cannot be used if this weight is not known. The use of moles (in this case millimicromoles) is valuable for comparing the absolute reactivity of compounds that combine stoichiometrically. Conversion of one of the first two units to the third or *vice versa* requires complete information on the particular experiment involved.

The last kind of unit is useful when it is desired to compare the absorption of different compounds applied to the skin in different concentrations. In instances in which the rate of penetration is proportional to the difference in concentration of the compound on the two sides of the membrane (that is, when it follows Fick's law), a permeability constant may be measured. If the compound is removed rapidly from the receiving side so that its concentration there is negligible compared to the applied concentration, the permeability constant, p, may be expressed as follows:

$$p = \frac{\text{steady penetration rate}}{\text{concentration}} = \frac{\mu g/cm^2/min}{g/cm^3}$$
$$= \mu cm/min = 0.1 \, \mu m/min$$

The dimensions of the permeability constant may be visualized as the depth of applied solution cleared of the penetrant per unit time (Tregear, 1966).

Although the permeability constant is invaluable for the purpose for which it is used, it has limited value in toxicology. In many practical situations, contamination of the skin is by an undiluted solid or liquid. Dosage and skin area are important variables but concentration is not involved. For undiluted compounds with a specific gravity essentially equal to 1.0 ($g/cm^3 = 1.0$), the "permeability constant" is equal to the steady rate of absorption within the limits of experimental error.

Discussion of Techniques. Comparison of values in Table 3-8 shows that the values for the intact animal determined by disappearance are generally greater than the corresponding values for the same compound and same species determined by dosage-response. In some instances, a part of the difference undoubtedly is caused by inactivation of the compound in the skin. This point was emphasized by Fredriksson (1964) in connection with paraoxon and sarin, which, according to independent studies, are inactivated by enzymes in the skin. However, this explanation cannot be applied to parathion, because all available evidence (Fredriksson *et al.*, 1961) indicates it is not inactivated or changed to paraoxon in the skin, and there is no *a priori* reason to suppose that the skin binds parathion more than paraoxon.

Although the disapperance technique tends to give higher values than the dosage-response method when both are used in the intact animal, the disappearance technique may give very low values when used with excised skin.

Obviously, many more compounds must be studied by different techniques before the relative value of these techniques can be assessed. An even greater amount of work, including measurement of the dermal exposure of workers in different situations, will have to be done before the rate of dermal absorption can be used with any precision in evaluating the hazard of dermal exposure. Barnes (1968) emphasized the importance of including in such studies compounds such as aniline that are known to penetrate the human skin very rapidly, and are known to present a definite hazard by that route.

The fact that an adequate comparison of different techniques is unlikely to be achieved soon should not obscure the value of using a single technique to compare the rate of absorption of different compounds. Thus, reference to Table 3-8 shows that the difference in rates of absorption undoubtedly is an important factor in determining the great hazard of sarin, a compound not much more toxic than paraoxon. This is especially clear when the difference in molecular weights is taken into account. Thus, the same author, by measuring disappearance in the cat in both instances, found that the rate of absorption of sarin is 129 mμM/cm^2/min (Fredriksson, 1958), while that of paraoxon is 6 mμM/cm^2/min (Fredriksson, 1964).

Pathways of Skin Absorption. Fig. 3-5 is a diagrammatic representation of the skin. Extensive study has shown that materials may penetrate directly through the epidermis or they may be absorbed after they have entered the skin appendages, namely, the sweat glands and the hair follicles and associated sebaceous glands. It appears that some compounds may be absorbed by one of these routes, some by another, some by both, and some by neither. However, transepidermal absorption is almost always accompanied by some degree of transappendageal absorption.

Factors that retard the two forms of skin absorption include (*a*) a superficial barrier within the epidermis, and (*b*) the physical difficulty of introducing some forms of material into the skin appendages. As described in more detail below, absorption may be promoted chiefly by injury of the superficial bar-

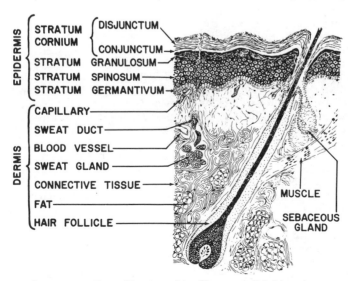

Fig. 3-5. Diagram of a cross section of human skin. The superficial barrier corresponds with the stratum corneum conjunctum.

rier or by anything that facilitates entry of the material under study into the skin appendages.

Although the concept of the superficial barrier is a functional one, there is ample evidence from different lines of investigation to indicate that it corresponds morphologically with the homogeneous membrane in the lower part of the corneum called the stratum conjunctum or stratum lucidum. The overlying portion of the stratum corneum (stratum disjunctum) is not a barrier. In fact, it is easily penetrated by a variety of materials, including molecular aggregates. Far from acting as a barrier, it may serve to absorb and hold materials that contact the skin so that they are not removable by washing but are available for gradual absorption. Szakall (1952) has shown that the superficial barrier has a fine fibrillar structure of great tensile strength and elasticity, permitting its separation from the remainder of the skin. The same author (Szakall, 1955) found that the barrier contained 42% water-soluble extractives and 58% insoluble keratinous material. Amino acids constituted 17.6% of the water-soluble compounds and were mainly responsible for the acetic pH of 4.62 to 5.17.

Wolf (1939) introduced a technique for removing the superficial layers of epidermis by means of repeated application of self-adhesive tape, especially ordinary cellophane tape. Twenty-four hours after this procedure, the stratum granulosum may be absent or only one cell layer of it may remain. Full reconstruction of the barrier in human subjects requires 48 to 72 hours or more (Malkinson, 1958).

After a substance has passed the superficial barrier from the outside, there is apparently no further hindrance to diffuse penetration of the epidermis. Once a compound reaches the dermis, it is available for absorption into the blood via the capillaries. Rapid removal by the blood is undoubtedly one reason why studies of many compounds have revealed little or none of the material in the dermis, even though it was entirely evident in the epidermis. In some instances, this very different distribution of material in the two layers has led to the hypothesis that a second barrier exists at the dermal-epidermal junction. Although the possibility of this second barrier cannot be denied, it must be pointed out that it has not been identified morphologically, nor has it been demonstrated functionally by means of removal or injury to alter its action.

The superficial barrier of the epidermis is apparently lacking over approximately the lower two-thirds of hair follicles, including the sebaceous glands. The barrier is also lacking in connection with the ducts and secretory portions of sweat glands. It seems clear that the hair follicles and associated sebaceous glands are more important for percutaneous absorption than are the sweat glands and their ducts. Passage of materials into the lumina of all of these structures has been demonstrated, and absorption from the hair follicles and sebaceous glands has been shown. According to Malkinson and Rothman (1962), actual absorption from sweat glands has not been seen so far. Undoubtedly, the resistance of skin appendages to the entrance of foreign material offers some protection against absorption. Application with pressure or the use of special ointment bases may be necessary to introduce materials effectively into the follicle.

Factors Affecting Percutaneous Absorption. The rate at which a particular compound is absorbed from a given area of skin is determined by the nature of the compound itself, the condition of the skin, and certain external factors, especially temperature.

A compound's solubility is the main factor determining whether it can be absorbed. Completely insoluble materials are not known to be absorbed from the skin. Water itself and a number of water-soluble materials are absorbed, but fat-soluble compounds are absorbed most readily. Treherne (1956) found that permeability of a small number of compounds through rabbit skin from aqueous solution was related to their ether/water partition coefficients; values near 1.0 appeared optimal for absorption. However, Tregear (1966) and others have pointed out exceptions.

O'Brien and Dannelley (1965) found no meaningful relation between penetration rates and olive oil/water partition coefficients. Their conclusion may be open to question because they failed to take skin area into account. However, they noted a more basic fact: the solvent selected for determining partition coefficients can be of importance. For example, paraoxon appears far less polar than malathion in chloroform but far more polar in hexane. It is just this kind of inconsistency that makes it possible to identify compounds through a system of *p*-values (Bowman and Beroza, 1965). The only conclusion appears to be that any correspondence between skin penetration of any foreign chemical and one of its partition coefficients would be fortuitous. If a meaningful relationship exists between skin penetration and partition coefficient, it must apply to the solvents involved, namely water and the lipids (especially neutral fat) of the animal body.

There seems to be a broad inverse relationship between molecular size and rate of dermal absorption. Helium is absorbed rapidly and proteins slowly. However, within the limited range of molecular size where most pesticides are found, there is no correlation between size and rate. Other factors are more important.

The rate of absorption is proportional to dosage within the range between zero and a dosage sufficient to really cover the skin. The application of liquid necessary to do this is about 1,000 $\mu g/cm^2$, or (for liquids of density 1.0) a depth of 10 μm. Blank *et al.* (1957) found no significant change in the rate of absorption when the dosage was increased 10-fold from a rate of 3,333 $\mu g/cm^2$. Dosages smaller than about 1,000 $\mu g/cm^2$ may be applied directly either by intent or as the result of some occupational exposures. More often, small but evenly distributed doses are the result of applying a solid or liquid in a solvent that evaporates promptly, leaving a thin film of the toxicant on the skin. For some compounds, a beautiful rectilinear relationship exists between absorption rate and dose per unit area over the range 0.1 to 100 $\mu g/cm^2$, and the same relationship presumably exists for other compounds (Tregear, 1966).

The concentration gradient also changes according to the concentrations of solutions applied to the skin in amounts sufficient to cover the area under test. If neither the solvent nor the solute affects the skin itself, there is again a rectilinear relationship between the rate of absorption and the concentration. This phenomenon is taken into account in calculating the penetration constant, p.

However, certain compounds injure the skin in such a way that they interfere with their own absorption. Thus, higher concentrations of phenol and mercuric chloride are absorbed less than weak concentrations. Silver ions are precipitated within the skin so that little or no silver is absorbed.

The skins of different species differ not only in the amount of hair, but also in the thickness of the different layers, the depth of the follicles, the presence of sweat glands, and many other features. Tregear (1964) reported a consistent difference in the permeability of the skins of different species to a fairly wide range of compounds. The skin of the rabbit was most permeable and that of man least, as follows: rabbit > rat > guinea pig > pig > man. The fact that permeability of the skin depends largely on a dead membrane, the stratum conjunctum, may explain this consistent difference. The consistency is in contrast to the randomicity of most species differences in toxicology. Even in connection with permeability of the skin, Tregear (1964) found no consist-

ency in the relative ease with which different compounds were absorbed; thus, of the compounds tested, the rat absorbed ethylene bromide most efficiently, but the pig absorbed it least efficiently.

The permeability of the skin decreases tremendously during the latter part of fetal life and then more slowly until weaning; further change after weaning is relatively slight (Hunt, cited by Tregear, 1966).

Different portions of the skin of the same species absorb compounds at different rates. In general, thin, delicate skin absorbs most readily, while the skin of the palms and soles absorbs at a lower rate. However, no part of the skin is completely impervious; the absorption of some compounds through the nails has been demonstrated. Studies in volunteers showed that absorption of parathion, malathion, and carbaryl by the palm was essentially the same as their absorption by the forearm. Areas rich in hair follicles absorbed various compounds at rates 3.5 to 13 times greater than those of the forearm. Compared to the forearm, the rate of absorption from the scrotum was 11.8 times greater for parathion and 42 times greater for hydrocortisone (Maibach *et al.*, 1971). Additional valuable details on the permeability of different skin areas are given in the same paper. It is, therefore, particularly unfortunate that a technical error (application of a correction factor for excretion following intravenous injection to data involving dermal absorption as well as excretion) invalidates use of the data to compare the rates of absorption of different compounds.

For any given compound and any kind of skin, absorption is proportional to skin area. Since most splashes are sufficient to wet whatever area they contact, it follows that it is of great practical importance how much of the skin is contaminated during an accident, or as the result of occupational contact. For the same reason, the area of application should be regulated in animal experiments (see Section 4.3.5.3).

By far the most important factor that may alter the rate of absorption per unit area is the presence and condition of the superficial barrier. As already mentioned, this barrier can be effectively removed by repeated application and removal of self-adhesive tape. Skin injured by the proper application of tape does not bleed and does not look especially irritated. Yet its permeability is completely different from that of normal skin. The barrier may be injured to some degree by a number of other agents, including prolonged immersion in water, washing with organic solvents, irradiation, thermal and chemical burns, and inflammation. The degree of change in permeability does not correspond with the degree of visible change. Mild abrasions or a mild burn may promote absorption, whereas severe abrasions or a severe burn may lead to the formation of a crust that is virtually impermeable.

One of the most dramatic demonstrations of the importance of the superficial barrier involves hydrocortisone-4 tagged by radioactive carbon. Only about 2% of the compound is absorbed from the normal human skin, but, after removal of the superficial barrier by the stripping technique, uptake of the hormone ranged from 70 to 90% within a period of 4 to 6 hours (Malkinson, 1958).

Vasoconstrictors, by reducing circulation, reduce the rate of dermal absorption. Increased circulation, whether caused by high ambient temperature, local inflammation, or some other cause, tends to increase the rate of absorption of chemicals from the skin. Hyperemia, of whatever cause, leads to a greater concentration gradient between the blood and the corium immediately surrounding the skin capillaries. By the same token, there is a greater concentration gradient between this part of the corium and the overlying epidermis.

If the hyperemia is caused by high ambient temperature or is accompanied by a fever, then the actual temperature of the skin is increased with a consequent increase in the rate of simple diffusion of gases and other compounds through the skin. For different compounds, the rate of absorption is increased by a factor of 1.4 to 3.0 for each increase of 10°C in the ambient temperature (Tregear, 1966).

A factor that may be introduced artificially for the purpose of therapy or investigation is electrophoresis. The skin will tolerate current densities of 0.5 to 1.0 milliampere per square centimeter (MA/cm^2) without showing any sign of injury. However, a potentially useful increase in the rate of absorption of many substances may be obtained with as little current density as 0.1 MA/cm^2. It is thought that, in the absence of skin damage, electrophoresis promotes absorption by the transfollicular route. The general principle was illustrated by an experiment performed by Leduc (1900), in which strychnine sulfate was applied to the skin of two rabbits electrically connected by a salt bridge. The animals whose skin was in contact with the anode moistened with the alkaloid salt died within a few minutes, while the rabbit in contact with the cathode moistened in exactly the same way showed no sign of injury. Not only do ions migrate in an electrical field but water migrates also. Water tends to move into the tissues from an anode

and out of the tissues into the skin of the cathode. Thus, gross shrinking of the skin may occur below the anode and swelling of the skin may occur at the cathode. This phenomenon called "electro-osmosis" tends to favor the absorption of metallic ions and alkaloid salts from the anode, because the water necessary for their solution moves with them. By the same token, electro-osmosis tends to oppose the passage of ions such as bromine and iodine into the skin from the cathode (Malkinson and Rothman, 1962).

Finally, dermal absorption may be increased by anything that increases the degree of contact between an absorbable material and the skin. The simplest illustration of this principle is the fact that very finely ground powders tend to be absorbed more readily than coarser powders rubbed on the skin in exactly the same way. Thus, it was found that very finely ground technical dieldrin was absorbed as readily as dieldrin applied to the skin in solution, even though coarsely ground dieldrin powder was not so well absorbed.

Although a vehicle may be able to promote absorption, no vehicle can carry an otherwise nonabsorbable material through the skin. The action of vehicles in promoting absorption involves transfollicular absorption almost entirely; the mechanism is mechanical. The incorporation of materials into certain ointment bases or their combination with wetting agents may facilitate their introduction into the follicle. The process of rubbing may expel air trapped in the follicles or the vehicle may absorb the air, thus permitting contact of the material with a larger surface and its penetration into the deeper portions of the follicle and the sebaceous glands. In any event, the importance of vehicles in promoting absorption through increased contact is not great.

A vehicle may also promote absorption through injury to the skin. Keratolytic compounds are especially active in this regard. Water promotes absorption by hydrating the stratum conjunctum. Some idea of the practical difference that different solvents can make in the rate of dermal absorption is given by Table 3-9, adapted from Brown (1968).

The presence and kind of skin covering used in dermal toxicity studies in animals constitutes an experimental variable that may influence skin temperature, skin moisture, the condition of the barrier, the amount of compound actually available for absorption (dosage), and perhaps other factors. The question of covering is considered in Section 4.3.5.3.

Classes of Compounds Known to be Absorbed. Materials known to be absorbed by the skin include: many gases; water; a number

Table 3-9

Comparison of the Single Dose Acute Percutaneous Toxicity
of Technical Bidrin and of Certain 10% w/v Solutions of it in
CFE Strain Rats 12 to 16 Weeks Old

From data of Brown (1968).

Solvent	LD 50 in mg/kg (limits at P = 0.95)			
	Males		Females	
none	136	(88-212)	111	(77-162)
water	140	(95-206)	208	(127-349)
isopropanol and water (equal parts)	286	(161-520)	148	(105-202)
isopropanol	190	(144-252)	82	(52-126)
dimethyl sulphoxide	150	(101-228)	78	(53-114)
cotton seed oil	51	(31-86)	50	(28-85)
xylene	50	(28-85)	58	(36-92)
methyl salicylate	43	(30-61)	38	(26-55)

of water-soluble, lipid-insoluble nonelectrolytes, including glucose, methanol, ethanol, urea, thiourea, and glycerol; a variety of electrolytes, including both cations and anions; and a wide range of lipid-soluble substances, including phenols, hormones, fat-soluble vitamins, organic bases, and many pesticides (Malkinson and Rothman, 1962). The absorption of fat itself, that is, various triglycerides, has not been demonstrated, but it may not have been studied by modern methods.

It is thought that material in the gaseous state is absorbed by simple diffusion through the epidermis and the follicles. The rate is determined by concentration gradient and temperature.

Gases and vapors known to be absorbed (or excreted) by the skin include oxygen, carbon dioxide, nitrogen, helium, radon, tritium, nitrobenzene, and dinitrotoluene.

Up to 1.9% of all the oxygen used by the body is absorbed from the skin, and about 2.7% of the carbon dioxide produced is excreted by this route. Under ordinary conditions, most of the oxygen absorbed by the skin is used in the metabolism of the epidermis. The absorption of carbon monoxide is said not to occur, but its absorption followed by oxidation within the epidermis has not been excluded.

The demonstration of the absorption of water was made by use of isotopes, both deuterium and tritium. The demonstration of absorption of cations such as sodium, calcium, nickel, cobalt, strontium, and thorium also was made with isotopes. The same is true of the anions sulfate and phosphate. Some metals, notably mercury, have been measured both chemically and radiologically following absorption by the skin.

Phenolic substances known to be absorbed include phenol, salicylic acid and a number of its salts and esters, and many phenolic derivatives, including several that are pesticides. The fat-soluble hormones, including estrogens, androgens, and various cortisones, are absorbed. The fat-soluble vitamins A, D, and K are absorbed from the skin, as are the lipid-insoluble vitamins, thiamine, riboflavin, calcium pantothenate, pyridoxine, and vitamin C. Organic bases known to be absorbed include a variety of alkaloids, antihistamines, and analgesics. Of these materials, strychnine and nicotine are pesticides. The salts of these materials are not readily absorbed by the skin, but as already noted, they may be made to enter the skin rapidly by electrophoresis.

Some materials may fit more than one of the classes just reviewed. For example, mercury and its salts not only produce mercury ions, but many of them are lipid-soluble.

The percutaneous absorption of a great many pesticides has been demonstrated by their systemic toxicity when applied to the skin. However, only a few of them have been studied quantitatively in such a way that their rate of absorption could be measured. Inspection of Table 3-8 shows there is a marked difference in the rates at which different pesticides and solvents penetrate the skin. Tregear (1966) tabulated the absorption of a much wider range of compounds but they showed only about 10 times more variation in reported rate.

3.2.2.6 Absorption by Other Routes.

Routes other than gastrointestinal, respiratory, or dermal may occasionally be important in the absorption of toxicants under practical conditions. A drop of tetraethyl pyrophosphate in the eye is generally fatal to rats and might easily be fatal to people. Although the pH of the eye, lacrimal duct, and nasal cavity is different from that of the gastrointestinal tract, there is little practical difference in absorption by this route and by the gastrointestinal tract. One difference involves the eye itself. The concentration of toxicant in the eye may be greater than that reached in the body as a whole, so that local effects may be produced in the eye in the absence of observable systemic effects. For example, Uphold *et al.* (1956) produced miosis in the eyes of volunteers with tetraethyl pyrophosphate without producing any systemic illness.

Absorption from the upper respiratory tract is also similar to absorption from the gastrointestinal tract. In fact, unless material that impinges in the upper respiratory tract is absorbed very rapidly, it will be carried to the pharynx and eventually swallowed.

Absorption can occur from the rectum and vagina. This is important in connection with a few drugs, but not of importance in connection with most toxicants.

Subcutaneous, intraperitoneal, and intravenous injections are frequently used in toxicological studies in the laboratory. Intramuscular and intra-arterial injections and injections into the ventricles of the brain are used much less frequently. All of these procedures assure that an entire, carefully measured dose can be administered without loss. It is this lack of loss that characterizes parenteral administration. Even if material is not absorbed, it is at least available for later recovery and analysis. However, the lack of loss is not the same as assurance of absorption. The absorption of material from subcutaneous deposits depends not only on the compound itself, but also on its vehicle and the rate of blood flow. Drugs may

be injected subcutaneously in oil to form a depot from which absorption continues at a relatively steady rate for days. The importance of blood flow is illustrated by the fact that it is entirely practical to delay the distribution of local anesthetic from a subcutaneous site by administering it with epinephrine. The epinephrine delays absorption by causing constriction of arterioles, capillaries, and possibly venules in the area in which the drug has been injected.

Sequestering of Injected Material. Water-soluble materials are distributed widely in the body following intravenous injection. However, many pesticides are not water-soluble, and if they are to be injected intravenously, they must be given in the form of homogenized emulsions or other colloidal suspensions. Although it is frequently assumed that such injections are evenly distributed, studies show this is not true. Many of the lipid droplets carrying dissolved toxicant are trapped in the first capillary bed they encounter. Thus, material injected into systemic veins tends to be trapped in the lungs. Some of the material that escapes this form of trapping is taken from the blood stream by the reticuloendothelial system, where it may be found in the liver and spleen.

After a single intravenous dose, as much DDT may be found stored in certain tissues as after a single oral or intraperitoneal dose at rates as much as 10 times greater (Judah, 1949), and yet the intravenous toxicity is only 3 to 5 times greater than the toxicity by the other two routes. The explanation lies in the sequestering of the material injected intravenously.

3.2.3 Dynamics of Distribution and Storage

Compounds that are water-soluble may be bound to plasma proteins (see Section 3.2.1.3). Other compounds, including many pesticides, require some form of binding if, as often happens, they reach concentrations in the blood higher than their solubility in water. It seems likely that the biochemical mechanism of transport of chemicals in the blood influences their distribution to other tissues, but this apparently is unexplored. What is clear is that compounds that seem similar in other ways may have very different mechanisms of transport. For example, telodrin and dieldrin appear in approximately equal concentrations in erythrocytes and plasma of rats and monkeys (Moss and Hathway, 1964), whereas less than 18% of p,p'-DDT and p,p'-DDE is carried in human erythrocytes (Morgan *et al.*, 1972).

It is of interest that, in nonlactescent plasma, chylomicrons carry less than 1% of all

DDT-related compounds. These compounds are associated with blood protein and are undetectable in plasma from which protein has been precipitated. Following ultracentrifugation, p,p'-DDT and p,p'-DDE are found mainly in the triglyceride-rich, low-density and very low-density lipoproteins. Following continuous electrophoresis, these compounds are found mainly in association with plasma albumin and α-globulins (Morgan et al., 1972).

3.2.3.1 Distribution after a Single Dose.

The blood serves to distribute most if not all poisons, regardless of the route of absorption. Even botulinal toxin, which has been thought to be transmitted by the nerves, may be isolated from the blood.

Distribution following Rapid Absorption. After a single, rapid, intravenous dose, distribution of a water-soluble compound within the blood may be considered almost instantaneous, and this is essentially true of the mobilized portion of an oil-soluble compound. There follows a period during which the compound is distributed to the tissues. The factors determining this distribution to each tissue include: (a) the rate (Q) blood flows to that tissue; (b) the mass (M) of the tissue; (c) the ratio (R) of equilibrium concentration of the compound in the particular tissue as compared to the blood (tissue/blood); and, of course, (d) the dosage (D). The rate of blood flow is most important in determining the initial distribution, and the inherent affinity of different tissues for the compound is most important in determining the final distribution.

Thus, tissues (eg, brain and liver) that have a relatively low affinity for a compound, but receive a high volume of blood flow in relation to their mass, may acquire a greater concentration of compound initially than tissues (eg, fat) that have an extremely high affinity for the compound, but a low rate of blood flow. Both the mass of the tissue and its inherent affinity for the compound are important in determining the quantity of the compound in the particular tissue at equilibrium, and the rate of blood flow is unimportant.

The rate of blood flow and the tissue mass are characteristic of animals of a given species, age, and sex. The rate of blood flow may be influenced by intoxication, but the following discussion is concerned with the usual situation in which tolerated doses of drugs do not significantly influence the relative blood flow to different tissues.

The ratio of equilibrium concentrations is characteristic of each compound and must be determined by measurement.

Early descriptions of the distribution of drugs were largely concerned with tissue affin-ity and with the distribution of each chemical at equilibrium; these descriptions tended to neglect the rate of blood flow. The importance of blood flow in determining distribution after a single rapid dose was emphasized in a now classical paper by Price et al. (1960) regarding thiopental. Their problem was to explain the brief duration of thiopental anesthesia following an intravenous dose. It was already known that the termination of anesthesia was associated with a fall in the concentration of the drug in the brain too rapid to be attributed to metabolism or excretion of the drug. The authors presented analytical evidence for discarding the then current theory that the loss of thiopental from the brain could be accounted for by its redistribution to fat. They showed instead that this loss was accounted for initially by redistribution to muscle and connective tissue. This conclusion was supported by actual chemical analysis of muscle, but considerably amplified by mathematical analysis of a model.

The model took into account the seven tissues, namely: central blood pool, central nervous system, myocardium, organs constituting the portal circulation, kidney, other aqueous tissues, and fat. The information on the weight of different organs listed in the first column of Table 3-10 is more detailed than that presented by Price et al., but is reasonably consistent with their values. A column showing blood flow expressed as milliliters per minute per kilogram of tissue is included in the table to emphasize the rapid flow of blood to the viscera, including the brain, and its slow flow to other aqueous tissues (muscle and connective tissue), and to fat. However, as shown in another column, the total amount of blood going to muscle and connective tissue is more than 5 times greater than that going to fat because of the difference in the mass of these tissues.

It is this difference in mass that accounts for the importance of muscle and connective tissue as a sink for thiopental soon after intravenous injection.

The mathematical solution for thiopental distribution given by Price et al. may be rewritten as follows:

$$D = M_A C_A + R_B M_B C_B + \ldots R_G M_G C_G \tag{1}$$

$$R_B M_B \frac{dC_B}{dt} = Q_B (C_A - C_B) \tag{2}$$

$$R_C M_C \frac{dC_C}{dt} = Q_C (C_A - C_C) \tag{3}$$

$$\text{similarly, for } D \text{ to } G, \tag{4-7}$$

Table 3-10

Characteristics of Human Body Compartments and Organs

Organ and compartment	Mass[a] (kg)	(kg)	Blood flow (ml/min)[b]	(ml/min/kg)
blood	5.40			
blood		5.40		
G.I. tract	2.00			
liver	1.70			
kidney	.30		1,000[b]	3333
spleen	.15			
pancreas	.07			
thyroid	.02			
lymphoid	.70			
thymus	.01			
brain	1.50		800[b]	522
spinal cord	.03			
bladder	.15			
salivary gland	.05			
eyes	.03			
prostate	.02			
adrenals	.02			
testes	.04			
heart	.30		250[b]	834
lung	1.00			
aqueous viscera[c]		8.09	3,750[b,d]	464
muscles	30.00			
bones	7.00			
red marrow	1.50			
teeth	.02			
skin	2.10			
connective tissues	4.10			
muscles and connective tissue		44.72	1,400[b]	31
fat	10.00		250[b]	25
yellow marrow	1.50			
lipid tissues		11.50		
total	69.71	69.71	5,400	77

a. From International Commission on Radiological Protection (1955).
b. From Price et al. (1960)
c. Organs contributing to the portal circulation weigh 2.24 kg; the portal circulation from these organs and to the liver is about 1,700 ml/min.
d. Excluding circulation to the lungs.
e. Cardiac output.

where C equals the concentration (w/w) of drug at any time in blood or lymph leaving any area (A to G), Q is the blood flow (ml/min), M is mass (kg), and R is the ratio (tissue/blood) of drug in these areas at equilibrium. Since the equations are simultaneous, they could be solved to yield estimates of the concentration of thiopental in various tissues at any time after its injection. Solution on a digital computer gave values in remarkable agreement with those measured chemically, and permitted a more detailed examination of the probable concentration of the drug in tissues from which it was difficult to obtain samples in living subjects.

A similar finding regarding the slow accumulation of a highly fat-soluble material in fat was reported by Dale et al. (1963) in connection with direct chemical analysis of DDT in rats (see Fig. 3-6).

Dieldrin poisoning in a boy was studied by Garrettson and Curley (1969) not only by chemical analysis but also by a model. Using the mathematical approach proposed by Price et al. (1960), they obtained calculated values in good agreement with those they measured chemically in fat and serum. They concluded on the basis of calculation, that the concentration in the brain and viscera reached a peak in minutes, while the concentration in muscle

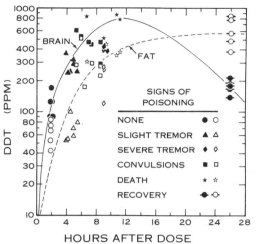

Fig. 3-6. Concentration of DDT in the lipids of brain (solid symbols) and fat (open symbols) of rats at different times after the administration of a single dose of the compound at a rate of 150 mg/kg. Different symbols indicate the clinical state of the animals when the samples were taken. After Dale *et al.* (1963), copyright 1963 by the American Association for the Advancement of Science.

reached its peak at 12 hours, and that between these times, the muscle compartment was the main reservoir for insecticide leaving the cerebral compartment. Correlated with this, it was concluded that the concentration of dieldrin in the brain was decreasing rapidly at 7.5 hours. Peak concentration in fat was not reached for 25 or 30 days.

However, no analysis of dieldrin in the sick boy's muscle was possible, and only one patient was available for study. Unlike the situation for the anesthetic thiopental, there could be no objective test of the hypothesis that dieldrin was first diverted from the brain to muscle and other poorly perfused aqueous tissues, and only later transferred to the fat. For this reason, a study was made in rats that were dosed by stomach tube to simulate rapid ingestion of a liquid formulation. The results did not confirm the hypothesis that muscle has any special significance in diverting dieldrin from the brain in this species. It was found that the highest concentration of dieldrin in muscle was reached at about 8 hours after administration, and at essentially the same time as the peaks for brain, liver, and kidney. Although the peak for fat came later (about 24 hours), the concentration in fat was higher than those in all other tissues 4 hours after administration, and it remained higher throughout the experiment. Thus, in the rat

and probably in man, body fat and not muscle is the important tissue for holding dieldrin that otherwise might be available to the nervous system (Hayes, 1974).

It seems unlikely that species difference would account for the kind of dissimilarity observed in the distribution of dieldrin and thiopental. Probably the major cause for the opposite results with the two compounds is the greater affinity of dieldrin for fat as compared to blood. For dieldrin, the ratio is certainly greater than 130:1 (Brown *et al.*, 1964; Hayes and Curley, 1968; Hunter and Robinson, 1967), and under certain circumstances may be very much higher (Garrettson and Curley, 1969). The ratio for thiopental is only 10:1 or 15:1 (Brodie *et al.*, 1952). A contributing cause of the difference is the slower absorption following oral administration, but that is the way dieldrin poisoning in children is acquired, not through intravenous injection. Although mathematical models can be of great value, the results ought to be confirmed by experiment.

Distribution following Slow Absorption. Slow delivery of a compound to the blood stream (either because it is given by slow injection, or because it is absorbed slowly by a natural route, or from a deposit in the body) will tend to suppress the high levels that otherwise would be reached in organs with a very rapid flow of blood. In spite of this tendency, absorption by any natural route may lead to dangerous blood levels of a sufficiently toxic compound in any susceptible tissue. Whatever toxicity is lost through more effective distribution to little affected tissues can be regained by increased dosage.

Distribution in Relation to Tissue. In the foregoing paragraphs, it has been taken as axiomatic that certain tissues have a greater affinity than others for certain compounds. In connection with many compounds, this difference is not great and has no demonstrable bearing on the pharmacological or toxicological properties of these materials. Although the difference for some compounds is tremendous, it may require considerable time for an equilibrium to be established between the concentrations in different tissues. For this reason, the matter is discussed in Section 3.2.3.3.

The distribution of compounds to the brain after a single dose is conditioned not so much by the affinity of the brain for them, or their rate of metabolism, as by the high rate of blood flow to the brain and by what is called the "blood-brain barrier." The term is used in a functional rather than a morphological sense. However, the brain does differ from other tissues in that the capillaries are completely surrounded in glial cells, and the sparse extracellular fluid (4 to 5%) is relatively free of protein. This means that compounds entering the brain not only must pass the thin capillary wall, but also the relatively thick specialized connective tissue cells. Furthermore, the lack of protein may interfere with the transport of some materials into the extracellular spaces of the brain. Nonionized, lipid-soluble materials usually penetrate easily. Materials that are not lipid-soluble, or are ionized, enter the brain or cerebrospinal fluid less easily, sometimes not in measurable amounts.

The distribution of drugs between the blood and cerebrospinal fluid is influenced by the rapid turnover of the cerebrospinal fluid, which is about 30% per hour. If a material does not enter the brain at a rapid rate, it will reach an equilibrium concentration less than that in the plasma. This is true because the cerebrospinal fluid appears to enter the blood in the arachnoid villi through pores that seem to behave as one-ways valves. Any drugs in the cerebrospinal fluid is thus carried into the blood along with the fluid.

The permeability of the blood-brain barrier may be influenced by chemicals so that the passage of other compounds into the brain is changed. Some electrolytes and some relatively lipid-soluble nonelectrolytes will open the barrier reversibly. Because of the reversibility, independence of specific drug action, direct dependence on increased osmolality or concentration, and inverse dependence on ability to penetrate cell membranes, it is considered that the action of these compounds consists in osmotically shrinking barrier cells and opening spaces between them to the passage of ions and large molecules. Lipid-soluble nonelectrolytes may damage the barrier irreversibly (Rapoport *et al.*, 1971).

3.2.3.2 Storage in Relation to Repeated Intake.

General Description of Storage. In the broadest sense, any foreign compound in the blood or other tissues may be said to be stored from the moment it enters the body until it leaves. This concept is necessary in any attempt to account for the entire exposure or dose in such a way that total exposure or dose equals unabsorbed compound, plus stored compound, plus excreted compound (all metabolites being expressed as equivalents of the original material). Thus, storage applies to all absorbed drugs and other foreign compounds.

Storage is usually expressed as a concentration, especially parts per million (ppm). Of course, parts per million is equivalent to milligrams per kilogram (mg/kg), but, as a convenience, the latter unit is generally reserved for expressing dosage, so there will never be any confusion about whether dosage or storage is referred to. Thus, dosage (mg/kg) leads to storage of a residue (ppm). In experiments, dosage is determined by volumetric or gravimetric measurement, but it may be inferred from the results of chemical analysis in connection with occupational exposure, accidents, and other "field" conditions. Residues are always measured by some form of chemical analysis.

Although storage *per se* is expressed as a concentration, the dynamics of storage involves time. No storage in a living organism is static, although it may reach a steady dynamic state, as discussed somewhat later. What must be established at this point is that compounds differ tremendously in the tenacity with which they are stored. At one end of a continuous spectrum are water-soluble drugs that are excreted easily, and consequently stored briefly after intake is stopped. At the other end of the spectrum are certain metals that are stored in bone; they are excreted very inefficiently and, therefore, are stored for long periods, even after intake is discontinued. The inherent differences in compounds are manifest not only in duration but also in degree of storage. At any particular continuous dosage level, the easily excreted ones reach relatively low concentrations in any tissue, while poorly excreted ones reach relatively high concentrations, especially in tissues for which they have a special affinity. Thus, it is impossible to discuss the dynamics of storage without reference to excretion.

The great majority of pesticides are excreted easily or they are metabolized efficiently to more water-soluble compounds that are excreted easily. Thus, most pesticides show no greater tendency to storage than do most drugs. However, some pesticides, notably lead, are stored with great tenacity. Although the chlorinated hydrocarbon insecticides are not stored to anything approaching the degree of lead, they are stored more tenaciously than most drugs, and this storage has been the subject of extensive measurement and some scientific study.

If a tolerated dosage is repeated at intervals for a sufficient period, the resulting storage may be observed to increase rapidly at first, and then more and more gradually until it reaches a steady state that continues until the dosage is changed. If dosage is stopped, storage decreases, and in some cases corresponds to an exponential function. If dosage is stopped before a steady state is reached, total body storage will decrease, but the storage in tissues with a high affinity for the compound, but that equilibrate only slowly with the circulating blood (whether because of a relatively slow circulation or some other reason), may remain unchanged or even increase for a time. The reason storage behaves in this way is the observed tendency for the rate of loss at a particular time to be directly related to the concentration stored at that instant.

Models Illustrating the Dynamics of Storage. Before exploring further the details of storage as observed in animals, it may be well to mention a monetary and a hydraulic analogy, which will help to make the overall situation clearer.

In Fig. 3-7 there are three curves (nos. 1, 2, and 3; open circles) showing the balances of three bank accounts in which the daily deposits were $1.00, $2.00, and $3.00, respectively, and the daily withdrawals were always half of the amount on deposit at the time. The oscillation caused by alternate deposit and withdrawal is shown for a portion of curve 3. The other curves show only the balance remaining at the end of each day's transaction. It may be seen that this balance reached a constant level after about the same length of time regardless of the size of the deposit. After depositing was stopped, the accounts decreased exponentially, as shown in the right-hand side of the figure.

A fourth curve (no. 1'; closed circles) in the same figure shows the successive balances in a bank account in which the daily deposit was $1.00 and the daily withdrawals were always one-fourth of the amount on deposit at the time. It may be seen that the balance reached a dynamic equilibrium more slowly where the proportion withdrawn daily was smaller, but the balance ($3.00) reached was higher than the balance ($1.00) in the other account (no. 1), in which the daily deposits were the same.

The curves in Fig. 3-7 are plotted on plain paper. If values of the kind involved are replotted on semilog paper, the general appearance of the portions representing increase and dynamic equilibrium are changed very little; however, the portion representing exponential decrease is converted from a curve to a straight line.

Fig. 3-8 shows the values of Fig. 3-7 replotted on semilog paper. It may be seen that the slope of those portions of curves nos. 1, 2, and 3 showing loss of storage are identical, while that for curve no. 1' is different. The rate of withdrawal for accounts nos. 1, 2, and 3 was the same, while that for account no. 1' was only half as great. At the same rate of withdrawal, it required longer to reach a particular level where the initial balance was greater. Thus, accounts nos. 1, 2, and 3 reached or fell below the $0.50 level on the 1st, 2nd, and 3rd days of uncompensated withdrawal. At a slower rate of withdrawal, it required longer to reach a particular level even though the initial balance was identical. Thus, account no. 3 fell from $3.00 to less than $0.50 on the 3rd day, but account no. 1' reached the same level on the 7th day of uncompensated withdrawal.

In these examples, deposit corresponds to dose, balance corresponds to storage, withdrawal corresponds to excretion, and each descending straight line (representing the decreasing balance remaining after depositing is stopped) has a slope corresponding to the rate of withdrawal or excretion.

The monetary examples serve to show what is meant by a dynamic equilibrium or steady state, and how it can be achieved. The monetary examples are defective because of the great oscillation that persists throughout the phases of increasing storage and of dynamic

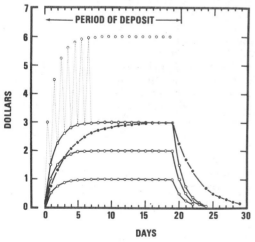

Fig. 3-7. Monetary illustration of (*a*) the equilibrium of storage during intake at a constant rate; and (*b*) the rate of loss of stored material following cessation of dosage. See text for explanation.

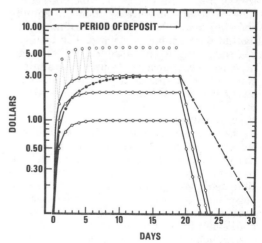

Fig. 3-8. Same values as those in Fig. 3-7 replotted on semilogarithmic paper. See text.

equilibrium (see curve 3 in Fig. 3-7). An illustration that is more realistic in some ways may be devised by allowing water from a faucet to flow into a vessel with an unobstructed hole of moderate size in the bottom. If the faucet is adjusted to a proper, constant rate of flow, the water level in the vessel will rise rapidly at first and gradually more slowly, until it becomes constant. At this stage, the rate at which water leaves by the hole is exactly equal to the rate at which water enters the system from the faucet. The equilibrium can be maintained indefinitely if the conditions do not change. If the faucet is closed, the water level in the vessel falls rapidly at first, and then more slowly until the vessel is empty. The oscillations seen in the monetary examples are absent in the hydraulic example, because "dosing" and "excretion" are simultaneous and continuous. The same arrangement of the faucet and vessel may be used to illustrate certain other features of storage. After a steady state is achieved, one may raise or lower the level by increasing or decreasing the rate of flow into the system; after a period of adjustment, a new equilibrium is achieved. Thus, each equilibrium corresponds to a rate of input or dosage. The rate of outflow is determined by the pressure, ie, the height of water above the opening. In a vessel with vertical sides, the amount of water stored is related directly to its height. By using vessels that are otherwise identical but have different sizes of openings, one may simulate different rates of excretion. If the vessel overflows, it corresponds to a situation in which high dosage exceeds the excretory powers and the tolerance of an organism and kills it.

Important Parameters of Storage. The important parameters of storage are illustrated in Fig. 3-9. These related parameters are: (*a*) time to achieve essentially complete equilibrium; (*b*) concentration at equilibrium; and (*c*) halflife after dosage is stopped. For tolerated dosages of any given compound, the excretion in a particular species tends to maintain a constant relationship to the concentration stored, but may be modified, as discussed below, by the action of microsomal enzymes or tissue damage.

The time necessary to reach a steady state of storage may be very great and, at least in theory, approaches infinity. However, the initial rise is relatively rapid, and much of the time required to achieve a steady state involves the last 5% of increase. Furthermore, in practice, one is not dealing with a perfect mathematical progression but with a biological system subject to many sources of real variation and also subject to some experimental

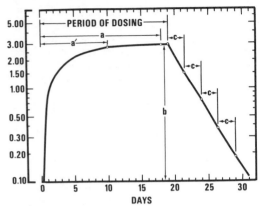

Fig. 3-9. Important parameters of storage: (a) time to achieve essentially complete equilibrium, (a') time to achieve 95% equilibrium, (b) concentration at equilibrium, and (c) halflife after dosage is stopped.

error of measurement. Under the circumstances, it is often reasonable to emphasize another parameter, (*a'*), the time required to reach 95% of the equilibrium value. Since the error of chemical measurement is often 5% or greater, and since biological variables are involved also, it may not be possible experimentally to distinguish between true equilibrium and its 95% approximation.

Insofar as excretion maintains a constant relation to storage, the term "halflife" is appropriate. If excretion is modified either by the level of storage or by progressive injury to the excretory mechanism, the term halflife is inaccurate to some degree. In any event, it is the efficiency of excretion that determines storage under any particular set of conditions. For example, as discussed under the heading of storage in relation to compound (Section 3.2.3.3), the storage of the isomers of BHC corresponds to their metabolism, not to their solubility. It is not so much that some compounds are stored avidly, as that they are excreted poorly, but the relative importance of slow metabolism and of unavailability for metabolism (binding) must be evaluated in each instance.

When excretion does not bear a constant relation to storage present at the time, the term "percent-per-day" is preferable to "halflife" in describing rate of storage loss or excretion. The distinction is especially important when the excretion factor changes rapidly, as it does in starvation. As an example of the rapid change that may occur, Heath and Vandekar (1964) found that about 5% of the dose of dieldrin was excreted in the bile daily following a single intravenous infusion of tagged material, but the rate increased to more than 10% after a few days in rats that were starved.

Relation of Storage to Dosage and Time. For each tolerated level of dosage of a compound, there is a characteristic equilibrium level of storage. The facts that (*a*) when first given, repeated doses at a constant rate lead to increasing storage; (*b*) constant dosage eventually leads to constant storage; but (*c*) different (increased) dosage rates produce different (increased) storage may lead to confusion. These relations of dosage and time to storage are shown in Fig. 3-10, representing the situation in which each increment of dosage produces an equivalent increment of storage. If excretion is more efficient at higher storage levels, then the slope of the curve relating equilibrium storage to dosage will be less. Conversely, if higher dosages are more poorly excreted because of the injury they produce, then the slope of the curve relating storage to dosage will be greater than that shown in part B of Fig. 3-10. In several species, storage of DDT is less efficient at higher dosage levels (Lehman, 1956; Hayes, 1959). In other words, the curve relating storage to dosage has a lower slope than the one shown in part B of Fig. 3-10. Lehman (1956) showed that, in varying degrees, the same is true of aldrin, dieldrin, endrin, and isodrin; on the contrary, lindane is stored with the same efficiency at all dosages studied, and methoxychlor, as already mentioned, shows a threshold and is stored only at higher dosage levels.

As we have seen, the relationship between excretion and tolerated levels of storage of a given compound tends to be constant in a particular species. The time necessary to reach a steady state depends on excretion and is essentially independent of dosage, provided the dosage remains constant. However, the rate at which a particular, nonequilibrium level of storage is reached does depend on dosage. This is illustrated by the fact that the slope of curves for bank balance from the 1st to the

2nd day in Fig. 3-7 increases in the order 1 < 2 < 3. Thus, the time necessary to reach a particular steady state can be regulated almost at will by manipulation of the dosage rate. By giving one or more large *loading doses,* it is possible to bring the storage up to the desired level in a short time; then that level may be continued as a steady state by repeated (usually daily) doses at a lower rate appropriate for the compound and species.

Mathematical Treatment of Storage. Mathematical treatments of the dynamics of storage have been offered from somewhat different points of view by a number of authors, including Webb (1963), Robinson (1969), Wagner *et al.* (1965), Wagner (1971), and Piotrowski (1971). Although there is general agreement about the form of equations, there is little agreement about the symbols to be used. In order to be consistent in this regard, it has been necessary in some instances to change the symbols used in an equation from those used when it was first introduced.

The applicability of the equations discussed below to drugs is admitted generally, but their applicability to pesticides is less well known. Therefore, Robinson (1969) rendered a great service when he reviewed the results of a series of original investigations on dieldrin and DDT and demonstrated step by step from the raw data that these compounds follow the same general rules as drugs follow. Specifically, he concluded: ". . . (1) the concentrations in a . . . tissue are related to the dietary intake; (2) the concentrations in different tissues are interrelated; (3) the concentrations in tissues are asymptotic functions of the time of exposure; (4) the rate of disappearance from a tissue is related to the concentration in that tissue. These conclusions are consistent with the mammillary-type compartmental model."

Mathematical Treatment of Storage during the Cumulative Stage. Available mathematical models of storage during the cumulative phase are based on the mathematically simplest situation in which the compound is introduced suddenly (as by rapid intravenous dose), and disappears by first order kinetics, that is at a rate proportional to the concentration. Under these conditions, the concentration at any time after administration is given by

$$C_{td} = C_0 \, e^{-kt} \qquad (8)$$

where:

C_{td} is the concentration at time td expressed as mg/kg (ie, ppm)

C_0 is the initial peak concentration

e is the base of natural logarithms

k is the first order rate constant for the disappearance process, and

td is time of dosing from C_0 to C_{td}.

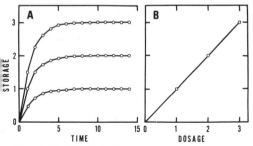

Fig. 3-10. (A) Relation of storage to time at three different, constant dosage levels and (B) relation of storage at equilibrium to dosage.

If a second dose is given before the first is eliminated, the maximal concentration reached will be the sum of what remains and what is added, as described in the monetary examples given earlier. Each additional dose will produce a progressively smaller increase, as was also described in the monetary model.

It may be shown that the concentration reached after the nth dose will be

$$C_n = C_0 [1 + e^{-k\tau} + e^{-2k\tau} + \ldots e^{-(n-1)k\tau}]$$

where: (9)

C_n is the concentration after n doses

τ is the interval between doses.

The geometrical series may be written in the form:

$$C_n = C_0 \frac{1 - e^{-nk\tau}}{1 - e^{-k\tau}}$$ (10)

The maximal constant level will be:

$$C_{max} = C_0 \frac{1}{1 - e^{-k\tau}}$$ (11)

According to this mathematical model, the time necessary to reach this maximal level would be infinite. However, the time necessary to reach a particular percentage may be calculated.

Mathematical Treatment of the Equilibrium State. It was shown many years ago that the concentration of a compound at storage equilibrium may be expressed by the equation:

$$\overline{C}_{max} = DF/VP$$ (12)

where:

$\overline{C}_{max}$ is the average concentration of the stored material after storage is maximal, expressed as ppm,

D is the daily dosage expressed as mg/kg,

F is the fraction absorbed,

V is the volume of distribution or fraction of the body in which storage occurs, and

P is the proportion of the storage lost per day expressed as a decimal fraction.

A more general form of the equation discussed by Wagner *et al.* (1965) is:

$$\overline{C}_{max} = DF/Vk\tau$$ (13)

where:

k is the first order rate constant for overall loss of the compound,

τ is the interval between doses, so that $k = P$ in the special case in which $\tau = 1$ day.

The other symbols have the same meaning as in equation (12). The expression $t_{1/2}$, signifies the biological halflife, ie, the time necessary to reduce the concentration of a compound in the body to half, in the absence of further intake. Since $k = 1/1.433 \, t_{1/2}$, equation (13) may be rewritten:

$$V\overline{C}_{max} = \frac{1.44 t_{1/2} DF}{\tau}$$ (14)

There are several known phenomena that partially invalidate use of these equations (Wagner *et al.*, 1965). The exceptions include: (a) The plasma level of the compound exceeds the protein binding capacity so that k increases and V decreases at high blood levels. (b) The volume of distribution (V) increases at high blood levels and k may increase or decrease. (c) An enzyme system metabolizing the drug becomes saturated, or a compound necessary for the conversion becomes exhausted at high blood levels so that the order of elimination may change from apparent first order to apparent zero order. (d) The compound's metabolism is inhibited by a compound not constantly present so that k decreases and V remains constant. (e) The compound's metabolism is stimulated by the compound itself or by another agent, so that k increases and V remains constant. (f) The fraction of the dose absorbed decreases as the dose is raised, so that F decreases as D increases.

Of these phenomena, it is unlikely that the first two will be important in connection with toxic compounds, simply because the toxicity of such compounds limits the blood levels at which an equilibrium may be achieved. The phenomena lettered c to f above are illustrated to some degree by various toxicants, for example: (c) An important factor in determining the toxicity of cyanide to a particular animal is the immediately available supply of sulfur compounds capable of forming thiosulfate. In other instances a critical enzyme may become saturated. (d) Inhibition of metabolism is usually a special case of enzyme exhaustion, and it often constitutes an example of potentiation. As discussed in Section 2.4.6.1, potentiation is not a common phenomenon, and when it does occur it usually involves toxic dosage levels rather than dosage levels at which a steady state of storage may be achieved. (e) Many pesticides especially the chlorinated hydrocarbon insecticides, stimulate their own metabolism and that of other compounds. (f) There is some evidence that the fraction of DDT absorbed decreases as the dose increases.

An additional phenomenon, (g), is sometimes listed as one of the conditions invalidating use of the equations under discussion. This phenomenon exists when a diffusion equilibrium is not maintained between the compound in blood and the compound in other compartments (Wagner *et al.*, 1965). However, under these conditions, an equilibrium does not exist and the premise on which the equations are based is not satisfied. The reason for failure to reach equilibrium may be merely a lack of sufficient time, or it may be that some com pounds, such as radium, injure the tissues in such a way that a true equilibrium is never achieved.

Even though the equations bear somewhat the same relation to the storage of toxicants as the gas laws bear to the behavior of ordinary gases, the equations are of considerable value for exploring the relation between dosage, metabolism, and storage. The equations, in one form or another, may be used to calculate any term when the others are fixed by measurement or hypothesis. If the observed C_{max} levels are not directly proportional to the dosage administered, then F, k, V, or some combination of them may not be constant. Knowledge of their relationships is useful in designing other studies to learn which factor or factors lack proportionality.

Insofar as the equations themselves are applicable, a number of useful relationships are defined. The slope of the plot of concentration against dosage will be $F/Vk\tau$. If a compound is not sequestered following intravenous administration, then $F = 1$ and the slope will be $1/Vk\tau$ from which the metabolic clearance rate, Vk, may be obtained. The ratio of the slopes obtained by the intravenous route and a nonintravenous route will yield the fraction, F, of the dose absorbed by the nonintravenous route.

The last two equations, especially (14), may be used to explore the consequences of giving different doses at different intervals. If the dosage interval is equal to the halflife, then the amount in the body at equilibrium will be 1.44 times greater than the amount absorbed following a single dose at the same rate. If the dosage interval is more than 1.44 times longer than the halflife, then the average amount in the body at equilibrium will be less than the total amount following a single dose—and the peaks and nadirs will be marked. To the extent that the dosage interval is shorter than the halflife, the storage at equilibrium will be greater than that following a single dose, and the peaks and nadirs will be small compared to the average height above the baseline.

The Concentration Index, a Measure of Cumulation of Storage. All compounds reach higher tissue levels when administered repeatedly at a sufficiently short interval than when administered only once at the same rate. However, the degree of increase varies greatly for different compounds. The *concentration index* (R_c) has been proposed by Wagner (1967) as a quantitative measure of the degree of buildup. The index, which is expressed as a quotient, is defined as a ratio between the average blood concentration at equilibrium and the average

blood concentration after a single dose, specifically:

$$R_c = \frac{\overline{C}_{max}}{\overline{C}} = \frac{\text{average blood concentration during one dosage interval (}\tau\text{ hours) at the equilibrium state}}{\text{average blood concentration during the first dosage interval, ie, 0 to }\tau\text{ hours after the first dose.}}$$

(15)

Since the concentration index is a ratio, it may be used to compare the tendency of different compounds to accumulate in the tissues regardless of the different ranges of dosage at which they are tolerated.

In the same paper, Wagner suggested several alternative ways of expressing the relationship between storage following a single dose and that following many doses. The variants include: (a) an index (R_1) based on a comparison of the average total amount of the compound present in the body during the first dosage interval and during a similar interval at equilibrium; and (b) the same index calculated from the biological halflife of the compound ($R_A = 1.44\ t_{1/2}/\tau$).

It is much easier to measure blood levels than to measure the total amount of a compound in the body at a given moment. Therefore, an index based on blood levels is more convenient and practical than one based on total storage. The calculation based on biological halflife involves certain conclusions that apparently are well established for drugs. The conclusions do not apply to some heavy metals and may not apply to certain other classes of compounds. It would seem best to base a standard measurement of the relation of storage at equilibrium to that following a single dose on direct measurement of the concentration of a compound in a tissue, for example, blood.

A particular tissue level of each toxicant has its characteristic effect no matter what schedule of dosage produced the concentration. Of course, the toxic effect persists insofar as an effective level of the compound or a toxic metabolite persists in the reactive tissue. However, some compounds with low concentration indices may have highly cumulative effects, as measured by the chronicity index (see Section 2.2.2). In other words, persistence of effect is found in connection with sufficient absorption of compounds that are stored effectively, but may not be limited to such compounds. We are forced to say "may," because the decisive measurements have been made in only a few instances. In the absence of quantitation, we are forced to depend on almost intuitive judgment of such apparent examples as the following: Warfarin is highly cumulative in its effect (chronicity index = 21) (Hayes, 1967), but it is rapidly metabolized in comparison with DDT, for example. The halflife for the disappearance of warfarin from human plasma varies from 15 to 58 hours and averages 42 hours (O'Reilley *et al.*, 1963). Hempa shows the greatest cumulation of effect of the few compounds measured in this way (chronicity factor > 200), but it seems unlikely that a compound of its structure would be stored to an important degree.

Patterns of Storage Loss after Dosing is Stopped. There are now two conventional ways to represent storage loss, one applicable to nearly all drugs, the other applicable to lead and other compounds that are stored predominantly in bone. In addition, it is now clear that the loss of some compounds, notably the chlorinated hydrocarbon insecticides and certain solvents, is not always represented properly by either convention. The storage of these insecticides and solvents has not been studied sufficiently, and there is no completely satisfactory mathematical way to represent their storage loss.

The disappearance from storage of a wide range of drugs and other water-soluble materials, such as creatinine, is represented satisfactorily by a straight line relating the logarithm of concentration to time (first order kinetics). This relationship indicates that these compounds are lost from storage with the same efficiency, no matter how long the loss may require. It must be noted, however, that the time required for their excretion is relatively short, usually being essentially complete in man in a few days or, at most, a few weeks. Evidence for these statements may be found in any good text on pharmacology and in a great number of papers on the quantitative aspects of drug metabolism.

The storage loss of lead and other bone-seekers is described infrequently in books on pharmacology and, therefore, is less generally known. If the loss of these compounds after dosing stops is plotted in the way conventionally used for drugs, the curve deviates upward from a straight line, indicating abnormal retention. It has been found convenient to describe the storage loss of these compounds in terms of a straight line relating the logarithm of concentration to the logarithm of time (Norris *et al.*, 1958). This relationship records quantitatively how the loss of these bone-seekers becomes progressively less efficient as time goes on. Of course, the time required for such loss is very long, often being measured in decades. Studies to explain the

behavior of lead storage apparently are not satisfactory. However, radium storage behaves in the same way, and the reason for the poor excretion of radium is understood better.

Retention of radium in rats, mice, and rabbits is directly proportional to dosage, and it has been suggested that the radium injures the mechanism necessary for its mobilization and excretion (Norris and Kisieleski, 1948). In fact, the injury to bone may be visualized histologically (Heller, 1948).

Storage Loss of Some Chlorinated Insecticides and Solvents. The storage loss of some chlorinated insecticides and solvents in some species has been found indistinguishable from that of drugs, at least following a brief period of equilibration. An example is the loss of dieldrin in the rat (Robinson *et al.*, 1969). However, a number of papers (Kunze *et al.*, 1949; Ambrose *et al.*, 1953; Durham, 1969; Gannon and Decker, 1960; Ware and Gilmore, 1959; Ludwig *et al.*, 1964; Daniel *et al.*, 1967; Stewart *et al.*, 1961; Morgan and Roan, 1972; Moubry *et al.*, 1968; McCully *et al.*, 1966) have presented data indicating that the storage loss or excretion of some chlorinated insecticides, solvents, and other compounds does not follow the general rule for drugs. In some instances, this fact was not mentioned in the paper and may be evident only after the values originally presented in tabular or some other form have been plotted on semilogarithmic paper. An example is shown in Fig. 3-11. Note that the

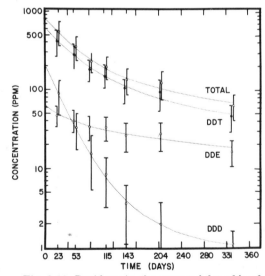

Fig. 3-11. Residues in the omental fat of beef steers at intervals after they had stopped eating forage bearing DDT at concentrations varying from 40 to 60 ppm dry weight for a period of 83 days. The points and their standard deviations are based on 20 animals. From data of McCully *et al.* (1966).

rate of loss from storage is fastest for DDD, intermediate for DDT, and slowest for DDE. Superficially, the storage loss of these compounds resembles that of the bone-seekers, but examination shows that their behavior is really opposite. The bone-seekers that have been studied in this regard interfere progressively with their own excretion. The insecticides and solvents under discussion stimulate their own metabolism. Thus, the most important variable in the storage of bone-seekers is time, while that for the insecticides and solvents is concentration. Of course, as the insecticides and solvents are gradually lost from storage, their concentration decreases and they stimulate the drug-metabolizing enzymes less. Thus, the change occurs in time, but as a result of concentration.

Proof that the behavior of bone-seekers and that of some chlorinated insecticides and solvents is opposite may be found in the effect of different dosage levels administered for the same length of time. As mentioned above, a lower proportion of radium is excreted per unit time if the dosage is large. For DDT, the proportion lost per unit time is greater when the dosage (within the tolerated range) is large.

Although the graphs in Fig. 3-11 are curved, the data show sufficient variation that one could not distinguish a short segment of any curve from a straight line. It is interesting to note that the characteristic storage behavior of carbon tetrachloride and tetrachloroethylene became evident only after gas chromatography made it possible to measure extremely low concentrations and thus follow storage loss for extended periods. Quite aside from sensitivity of analysis, there is a perfectly reasonable tendency to measure the loss of drugs from storage only for relatively brief periods, while they are at or near the therapeutic range. It is possible that, if the storage of drugs were measured for longer periods and to lower levels, some curvature of their storage loss curves would be detected. This is especially true of those that are known to stimulate microsomal enzymes of the liver.

Since the level of storage achieved at equilibrium in connection with any given rate of dosage is conditioned by the drug-metabolizing enzyme activity induced by that dosage, and since compounds differ in their ability to induce enzymes, it follows that there is a relationship between the form of the curve relating dosage to equilibrium storage (eg, part B of Fig. 3-10) and that relating time to storage after dosing is stopped (eg, Figs. 3-8 and 3-11). The simplest case is that in which equilibrium storage is directly related to dosage and the semilog plot of storage loss is a straight line. For compounds such as those under discussion, the slope of the curve relating storage to dosage is less, and the semilog plot of storage loss is curved—both reflecting that excretion is more efficient at higher storage levels.

The kind of prolonged curvature under discussion must be distinguished from the initial curvature often seen in the first few hours or days of storage loss or excretion following a single dose. The prolonged curvature is best seen when dosage is stopped only after storage equilibrium has been achieved. Unlike prolonged curvature based in a gradual slowing of metabolism, initial curvature may represent merely rapid clearing from blood followed by slower clearing from other compartments.

Mathematical Treatment of Storage Loss after Dosing is Stopped. When storage loss after the end of dosing follows first order kinetics, the concentration may be expressed as follows:

$$C_{tn} = \overline{C}_{max} (1 - e^{-kt}) \tag{16}$$

where C_{tn} is the concentration (ppm) at time t_n during which no dosing has occurred and the other symbols are the same as those used above.

3.2.3.3 Factors Other than Dosage and Time that Affect Storage.

As explained in the foregoing section, the primary factors determining storage of any given compound are: (a) dosage; and (b) time. Other factors influencing the dynamics of storage include (c) efficiency of absorption (really an aspect of dosage and already discussed in Section 3.2.2.5); (d) compound; (e) age; (f) sex; (g) species; (h) tissue; (i) the integrity of the detoxifying organs, especially the liver and kidneys; (j) nutrition, especially starvation; and (k) urinary pH discussed in Section 3.2.4.5. Although many of these factors are mediated by changes in liver microsomal enzymes (Section 3.1.2.3) or changes in protein binding (Section 3.2.1.3), the mechanism has not been established—or looked for—in many recognized examples of variation. Obviously, the underlying cause must be searched for objectively in each instance.

Storage in Relation to Compound. The dynamics of storage vary according to compound and may even be different for the isomers or metabolites of a single compound. The $\alpha, \beta, \gamma,$ and θ isomers of BHC are stored unaltered in the fat of rats and dogs (Davidow and Frawley, 1951). The γ-isomer is most toxic acutely, but at equivalent doses over 30 times more of the β-isomer is stored. The differences in the rates of storage of the isomers in the rat are remarkable and explain, at least in large measure, the lack of parallelism in the toxicity of the isomers following single and repeated doses. The difference in storage does not parallel the solubility of the isomers in rat fat (Sedlak, 1965), nor does it depend on difference of absorption, but it must be explained by different rates of biotransformation.

Theoretically at least, metabolites may not reach a steady state of storage at the same time as the parent compound. Thus, there is some evidence that DDE (Hayes et al., 1956) and DDD (Finley and Pillmore, 1963) reach equilibrium later than DDT.

Differences in storage also may depend on differences in excretion. Many solvents, including those used as anesthetics, are efficiently excreted by the respiratory tract as well as by the kidneys. This rapid excretion undoubtedly contributes to the relative speed with which they are removed from adipose tissue, for which their affinity is probably as great as that of chlorinated hydrocarbon insecticides.

However, the importance of the affinity of compounds for certain tissues must not be underestimated as a cause for prolonged storage. The storage of DDT in fat or the storage of lead in bone constitutes a form of binding, so that much of the compound in the body at any one time is not available for metabolism or excretion. Examination of Table 3-11 indicates that the blood levels of some compounds (DDT and dieldrin) noted for their storage in fat are similar to the blood levels of drugs when dosage is taken into account; it is only their marked affinity for tissue storage that distinguishes them. On the contrary, the storage of lead in both blood and bone is disproportionately high in relation to dosage.

DDT and dieldrin are stored in the fat at all accurately measurable or obtainable dietary levels. On the contrary, detectable storage of methoxychlor occurs only at dietary levels above a threshold (Kunze et al., 1950; Lehman, 1956). Detectable storage of heptachlor epoxide requires a dietary level of heptachlor in excess of 0.3 ppm in the male rat and 0.1 ppm in the female (Radomski and Davidow, 1953). However, it may be that the apparent difference in the storage of very small doses depends more on analytical technique than upon a qualitative pharmacological difference.

Gannon et al. (1959c) reported that, at comparable dosages, more dieldrin was stored in fat and excreted in milk of cows when aldrin was fed, than when dieldrin itself was fed at an equivalent rate. The explanation for this curious finding is not apparent.

Storage and the Interaction of Compounds. It is clear that the intake of one compound (at least at a relatively high level) can influence the storage of another. However, many details regarding factors that may influence the end result remain to be learned. For example, it is not clear whether the reported differences in the storage of DDT and cyclodiene insecticides in rats and dogs were caused by differences of species, dosage, compound, or some other factor. Briefly, Street (1964) found that storage of dieldrin in the adipose tissue of female rats was markedly depressed when DDT and dieldrin were fed simultaneously. The concentra-

Table 3-11

Comparison of the Storage of Selected Compounds

Compound	Dosage[a/] (mg/kg/day)	Route	Duration (days)	Storage Blood (ppm)	Storage Other (ppm)	Reference
aspirin	55	oral	14	150-200		Tainter and Ferris, 1969
phenobarbital	2-3	oral	12	18-33		Butler et al., 1954
p,p' - DDT	0.24	occupational[b/]	4,015	0.273	147.13[c/]	Laws et al., 1967
dieldrin	0.14	occupational[b/]	365	0.041	9.48[c/]	Hayes and Curley, 1968
lead	0[d/]	oral	life	0.23	0.80-3.59[e/]	Kehoe, 1961
	0.001[f/]	respiratory	616	0.45		"
	0[d/]	oral	life	0.30	0.80-3.59[e/]	"
	0.029[g/]	oral	644	0.65		"

a. Dosage in excess of unavoidable environmental exposure.
b. Mixed respiratory and dermal exposure.
c. Storage in fat.
d. Unavoidable dietary intake about 0.002 to 0.004 mg/kg/day.
e. Storage in femur for people in the general population, not for the particular persons whose blood values are shown immediately to the left.
f. Respiratory exposure 7.5 hrs per day, 5 days per week to 0.05µ particles of lead sesquioxide.
g. In form of solution of lead salt.

tion of dieldrin in the tissues of rats fed the compound at dietary levels of 1 ppm (about 0.053 mg/kg/day) was reduced 3-fold by the addition of DDT to the feed at a rate of 5 ppm (about 0.26 mg/kg/day) and 15-fold by the addition of DDT at a rate of 50 ppm (2.62 mg/kg/day). The corresponding reductions were 1.5-fold and 6-fold when the level of dieldrin intake was 10 ppm (0.525 mg/kg/day). There was no evidence that the different levels of dieldrin influenced the storage of DDT and DDE, which corresponded to the dosage of DDT. In a completely separate experiment, Deichmann et al. (1971) reported that the administration of capsules of aldrin to male and female beagles that had been receiving capsules of p,p'-DDT led to a rapid and progressive increase in the concentrations of DDT, DDE, and DDD in their blood and fat. The dosage of DDT was 12 mg/kg/day; that of aldrin, which is converted to dieldrin in the body, was 0.3 mg/kg/day. Over a period of 9 weeks after aldrin was started, the storage of total DDT-related compounds increased about two-fold in female dogs, and four- to five-fold in male dogs. Dosing with aldrin was begun 10 months after the storage of DDT had reached a plateau; control dogs that received only DDT maintained this plateau during all the remainder of the experiment.

Storage in Relation to Age. No age is immune from the storage of foreign compounds. It seems likely that all compounds absorbed by the mother are transferred to the fetus to some degree. However, there may be some discrimination, as has been demonstrated for strontium in comparison with calcium (Kulp and Schulert, 1962).

A number of pesticides are known to be stored in the fetus. For example, DDT is transferred to the fetus of the dog (Finnegan et al., 1949), rabbit (Pillmore et al., 1963), and man (Denes, 1962). Storage in the human fetus is discussed in Section 7.2.1.5, and age as a factor in storage in people is discussed in Section 7.2.4.1.

Storage in Relation to Sex. Possible differences in storage related to sex are well illustrated by findings with DDT and related compounds. At identical dosage levels of DDT in excess of about 0.05 mg/kg/day, the female rat stores more DDT and much more DDE than the male (Ortega et al., 1956; Durham et al., 1956). The female rat stores more DDD, more dicofol, more of each of the four common isomers of BHC, more chlordane, more aldrin, more endrin, more isodrin, and much more heptachlor epoxide. Female rats are said to store significantly more methoxychlor than males (Kunze et al., 1950).

The greater storage of chlorinated hydrocarbon insecticides in the female as compared with the male rat is characteristic of all tissues, and not of the fat only. This is documented by findings with DDT (Dale et al., 1962), and with aldrin, dieldrin, endrin, and isodrin (Kunze and Laug, 1953).

The difference in the storage of DDT and DDE between male and female rats fed DDT was reduced greatly, but not reversed by hormones of the opposite sex, gonadectomy, or a combination of these treatments (Durham et al., 1956). The effect was somewhat greater on DDE storage, so that the ratio of DDE to total DDT-derived material was actually reversed in hormone-treated animals though not in those gonadectomized but not injected with hormone.

The difference in DDT storage between the sexes is small or absent in the dog (Woodard et al., 1945), the hog (Harris et al., 1953), and the monkey (Durham et al., 1963).

Differences in DDT storage between men and women are so small that not all investigators have detected them. When a difference has been found, storage often was higher in the male. However, the possibility must be kept in mind that the difference in storage sometimes observed in men and women may not be due to sex *per se,* but to greater exposure of one sex or the other (see Section 7.2.4.1).

Storage in Relation to Species. So far as it is known, compounds stored by one species of mammal are stored to some degree by all species. Some difference related to species has been noted in the storage of DDT (Hayes, 1959), and especially dieldrin (Gannon et al., 1959b). It seems likely that many more species differences in storage exist than have been reported. Many studies of storage have been made without considering whether the animal had or had not reached a steady state of storage. For this reason, and because other factors in good experimental design frequently are neglected, no valid comparison between species can be made in connection with a great many published studies of storage.

Storage in Relation to Tissue. Storage in relation to tissue following a single dose was discussed in Section 3.2.3.1. Some of what was said there, especially about tissue affinity and the blood-brain barrier, applies to repeated doses also.

Differences in distribution following a single dose may be greatly exaggerated after repeated intake. Although the term "equilibrium" is often used in connection with the distribution of a compound measured several days or weeks after a single dose, this use of the word must be viewed with caution. It is certainly true that distribution approaches equilibrium after a single dose; but before there is time to reach true equilibrium, the concentration of material in one or more tissues may be so low that it cannot be measured. The only way to be certain that a steady state has been reached is to demonstrate it by repeated analyses.

The concentrations of a chlorinated hydrocarbon in blood and in adipose tissue both increase following the onset of daily dosing, and they both decrease after dosing is stopped. If dosing is stopped before equilibrium is achieved, a plot of the blood values against the fat values will constitute a loop, reflecting the fact that the concentration in blood relative to fat is higher while dosing continues and lower when dosing is discontinued, and the only source of the material in the blood is that stored in other tissues (Morgan and Roan, 1971). It seems likely that there is a relative decrease in blood values when dosing is stopped after equilibrium has been achieved, but this apparently has not been explored.

Under conditions of equilibrium in the storage of most chlorinated hydrocarbons, the concentration is between 150 and 350 times greater in adipose tissue than in blood. The high degree of fat solubility of these compounds and their relatively slow metabolism account fully for the great difference in concentration between fat and the aqueous tissues. Although the situation could not exist in the absence of the high degree of fat solubility, this solubility is not the determining factor, as was shown by a study of the isomers of benzene hexachloride. It was found that the highest degree of storage compatible with life was only a small fraction of the concentration that would be present if the fat were saturated. More important, it was shown that there was no parallelism between the storage of these isomers and their solubility in fat. It was concluded that the important factor in determining their relative storage at the same dosage rate was their ease of metabolism (Sedlak, 1965). In fact, considering chlorinated hydrocarbon insecticides as a class, no simple relationship appears to exist between their distribution in the tissues and either their liquid-liquid partition values or their R_f values as determined by thin-layer chromatography (Robinson and Roberts, 1968). A similar conclusion holds in connection with factors affecting percutaneous absorption (see Section 3.2.2.5).

Many pesticides tend to be stored more extensively in adipose tissue than in other tissues. There is some indication that the occurrence of DDT (Emmel and Krupe, 1946; Laug and Fitzhugh, 1946) and dieldrin (Gannon et al., 1959b) in other tissues is determined by their lipid content, and especially by their neutral fat content. The high DDT content of yellow bone marrow (Radeleff et al., 1952) is almost certainly explained by the high fat content of the tissue. The rather high levels of DDT reported for the adrenal (Lauger et al., 1945; Ludewig and Chanutin, 1946) and the ovary (Tauber and Hughes, 1950), may reflect a high fat content of these organs. DDD also shows high storage in the adrenal (Haag and Kampmeier, 1955). One report (Lackey, 1949) indicates that toxaphene or a derivative may be stored preferentially in the brain; the organic chloride content of acetone (but not ether) extracts of the brain was 20 times or more greater than that of controls. However, the distribution of DDT in the viscera before and after starvation suggests that fat content of the tissue may not be the only factor determining the relative concentration of DDT (Dale et al., 1962).

No difference was found in the concentration of DDT stored in the fat of different portions of the human body (Hayes et al., 1958). On the other hand, slightly more endrin was found in fat from the body cavities of lambs than in fat from the outer surface of the same animals (Long et al., 1961).

The storage of some of the heavy metals in bone is conditioned by their chemical similarity to the normal constituents of bone. Thus, strontium is similar to calcium in its chemical reactions, and it is stored tenaciously in bone (Kulp and Schulert, 1962). Undoubtedly, the rate of excretion is also important in determining to what extent materials will be stored in this tissue also.

The relatively low rate of blood flow to adipose tissue and bone is of importance in determining the distribution of compounds to these tissues following a single dose. However, it is doubtful that the rate of blood supply is of much importance in determining the level at which a steady state of storage is achieved in connection with repeated dosage.

Effect of Organ Function on Storage. Not every kind of injury to an organ interferes with its normal ability to detoxify or excrete foreign chemicals. However, when injury does interfere with one of these functions, it is axiomatic that it will lead to increased storage. A few examples are known. Laug and Kunze (1951) showed that rats fed methoxychlor stored 10 to 100 times as much of the material in their fat and liver, and suffered greater toxicity if given carbon tetrachloride concurrently, than did rats receiving no carbon tetrachloride. Undoubtedly, many other examples could be brought to light if suitable analytical studies were done in those situations in which it is known that injury to the liver or kidneys leads to greater toxicity of a compound. Thus, Truhaut *et al.* (1952) showed that rabbits whose kidneys had been injured by carbon tetrachloride were more susceptible than normal rabbits to poisoning by pentachlorophenol.

Effect of Nutrition, Especially Starvation. Although there is a recognized relationship between body fatness and susceptibility to one or a few large doses of chlorinated hydrocarbon insecticides (see Section 2.4.11.1), there is little or no quantitative information about the relationship between nutrition and the storage of these compounds. An interesting exception is the finding by Gannon *et al.* (1959a) that, at equivalent dosages, dieldrin was secreted in the milk at a generally lower rate by fat cows than by thin ones. This difference presumably reflects more complete storage in the fat cows, because there is no reason to suppose that excretion of the compound by fat ones was inherently less efficient. However, the animals may not have reached an equilibrium of storage and this may have influenced the result.

It is well known that some poisons such as lead, when stored in sufficient amounts, may be mobilized from storage with the result that clinical illness appears or recurs. This phenomenon was first demonstrated experimentally for DDT by Fitzhugh and Nelson (1947). They showed that rats that had been fed DDT at dietary concentrations of 600 ppm or more showed marked tremors when they were deprived of food completely. Rats deprived of all food after being fed DDT at a dietary level of 200 or 400 ppm showed increased irritability but no tremors. It was assumed that these clinical effects resulted from a mobilization of DDT concurrent with the mobilization of body fat.

The effect of starvation on the storage and excretion of DDT was studied quantitatively by Dale *et al.* (1962) before and immediately after a 10-day period of partial starvation, and again after 40 additional days of recovery. DDT and its metabolites were measured in the fat of rats fed traces of the insecticide, and in the fat, plasma, brain, liver, kidney, urine, and feces of rats fed the compound at the dietary rate of 200 ppm. Mobilization of the body fat during starvation resulted in an increased concentration of DDT-derived material in the remaining fat, and a corresponding increase in the concentration in the other tissues. An augmented excretion of metabolites occurred during starvation in spite of decreased intake of DDT. The increased excretion was inade-

quate to prevent the increase in concentration of DDT-derived material in the body, although it tended to do so. When sufficiently great, the augmented concentration of DDT in the brain associated with starvation produced signs of poisoning. Storage and excretion tended to return to prestarvation levels during recovery, but some lack of parallelism was observed between the concentration of DDT-derived materials in the brain, liver, and kidney, as compared with fat and plasma. Hukuhara (1962) later confirmed that starvation led to an increase in the concentration of DDT in the tissues of rats, but failed to study the effect of starvation on excretion.

Dale *et al.* (1962) concluded that their study did not support the view that DDT presents a hazard to people subject to starvation, whether as a result of dieting, deprivation, or disease. They pointed out that the concentration of DDT in men with the greatest occupational exposure—not to mention people in the general population—is less than what is necessary to produce the phenomenon in experimental animals. Furthermore, the metabolism of man is slower than that of the rat, so the phenomenon would be less likely to occur in man, even at the same concentration of DDT storage.

Heath and Vandekar (1964) reported that biliary excretion of radioactive dieldrin was doubled when rats were starved. Hunter and Robinson (1968) found no increase in the concentration of dieldrin in the whole blood of women who were dieting in order to lose weight, even though the rate of loss achieved was as great as 7.5 kg/week.

There seems little doubt that mobilization of fat will lead to mobilization of any compound stored in it. In a similar way, the mobilization of calcium from the bone will lead to the mobilization of strontium, which is stored much like calcium. Whether the mobilization of any particular material will lead to an increased concentration of it in the blood and tissues, will depend as much on the rate of its detoxication and excretion as on its rate of mobilization. Thus, the significance of mobilization following storage must be evaluated separately for each material and for each species.

Technical Considerations. Of course, analytical technique is the most important factor in obtaining an accurate estimate of the concentration of a substance in a particular sample. Whereas analytical methods are beyond the scope of this book, useful references are given in Section 1.7.2.

A rather unexpected complication in the sampling of adipose tissue must be mentioned, because this tissue is of such great importance in monitoring many pesticides. The concentration of dieldrin measured in samples of human subcutaneous fat was slightly but dependably greater in samples taken by needle biopsy than in those taken by open biopsy. The result was not conditioned by local anesthesia, there being no average difference when it was omitted (Hunter and Robinson, 1968). Since the needle involved use of negative pressure and the cutting or squeezing off of fat between a trocar and cannula, it seems likely that the procedure tended to select lipid and exclude connective tissue, to a small degree.

3.2.3.4 Storage in Relation to Toxicity. For any given compound, there is a direct relationship between its concentration (storage) in the target tissue and its toxicity. The same is often true for other tissues also, but striking exceptions can occur when the concentration in some nontarget tissues differs greatly following repeated doses, as compared with a single dose.

However, it must be reemphasized that, if one considers a range of compounds, there is no correlation between storage and toxicity. Some compounds (eg, cyanide) that show minimal storage are highly toxic. Other compounds (eg, DDT) that are stored tenaciously have a low or moderate toxicity, and are not outstanding for cumulative toxic effect when given repeatedly. Any compound, regardless of its storage characteristics, may produce toxicity if absorbed to a sufficient degree.

The relation of toxicity of a single compound to its concentration in the target tissue is illustrated by the following: the severity of signs of poisoning in rats after a single dose of DDT is directly proportional to the concentration of the compound in their brains. As shown in Table 3–12 (the first part of which is based on data used for Fig. 3-5), the concentrations in the brain associated with death after one large dose are about the same as those associated with death after many smaller doses (Dale et al., 1963; Hayes and Dale, 1964). A similar relationship was found for DDT in birds. See Table 3–13, in which the concentra-

Table 3-12

Storage of DDT in Rats (ppm in Lipid) -- Range, Mean, and Standard Error

Sex	No. Doses	Dosage (mg/kg/day)	Tissue	Pre-stress	Stress Died	Stress Lived	Recovery[a]
M	1	150	brain	<1	524 - 848 737 ± 73 N = 4	386 - 433 404[b] ± 15 N = 3	138 - 213 176 ± 12 N = 5
			fat	8	361	213	598
M	9	60 - 120	brain	<1	378 - 1301 600 ± 121 N = 7	194 - 981 589[b] ± 132 N = 5	197 - 382 268 ± 35 N = 5
			fat	8	6,660	2,484	5,359
M	90[c] 10[c] 40[c]	8.5 4.25 (starvation) 8.5	brain	74 - 106 92 ± 4 N = 8	205 - 985 595 N = 2	99 - 236 166[a] ± 18 N = 8	85 - 380 287 ± 44 N = 6
			fat	621	5,574	988	598
F	90[c] 10[c] 40[c]	10.5 5.25 (starvation) 10.5	brain	110 - 280 162 ± 25 N = 7	722 - 806 764 N = 2	124 - 523 230[a] ± 58 N = 7	148 - 224 169 ± 11 N = 6
			fat	892 - 2729 1447 ± 248 N = 8	9398 - 12143 10770 N = 2	1857 - 10204 4239[a] ± 1068 N = 8	1013 - 1982 1638 ± 150 N = 6

a. No sign of poisoning.
b. Moderate to severe tremor.
c. Sequence of dosing: 90 days at a dietary level of 200 ppm followed by 10 days on half rations c the same food, followed by 40 days of unrestricted intake of the same food.

Table 3-13

Effect of DDT in Relation to its Concentration in the Brain

Species	Concentration		No. of doses	Remarks	Reference
	Tolerated (ppm)	Fatal (ppm)			
rat	<0.07		0	usual colony level	Dale et al., 1962[a]
	15		1	no clinical sign	Dale et al., 1963[a]
	16-25		1	slight tremor	Dale et al., 1963[a]
	19-41		1	convulsions	Dale et al., 1963[a]
		35-52	1	died	Dale et al., 1963[a]
	13-25		9	survived	Hayes and Dale, 1964[a]
		26-88	9	died	Hayes and Dale, 1964[a]
	7-19		90	no clinical sign	Dale et al., 1962[a]
		13-63[b]	90	died	Dale et al., 1962[a]
robin		50-120		died	Bernard, 1963
sparrow		65-140		died	Bernard, 1963
"		18-38		died	Hill et al., 1971
cowbird[c]	6-21		11	survived	Stickel and Stickel, 1969
		27-77	2-11	died	Stickel and Stickel, 1969
bobwhite (reared)	10-15		5	survived	Hill et al., 1971
		19-32	5	died	Hill et al., 1971
bobwhite (wild)		17-29	5	died	Hill et al., 1971
cardinal		17-24	5	died	Hill et al., 1971
bluejay		12-20	5	died	Hill et al., 1971
bald eagle		58-86	15-62	died	Stickel et al., 1966

a. Values obtained from the original data are expressed in terms of the fresh weight of the brain in order to make them comparable with the values for birds.

b. Death due in part to starvation.

c. Female.

tions for rats are taken from the original data of the papers cited, and are based on wet weight to permit comparison with the values for birds. Although the concentrations of DDT in the brain associated with illness or death are slightly different in different species, the smallness of the species difference is striking.

Mortality of birds following dosing with DDD, DDE, and dieldrin also is correlated with the concentration of these compounds in the brain, but (compared to DDT) the lethal levels are high for DDD and DDE (Stickel *et al.*, 1970) and low for dieldrin (Stickel *et al.*, 1969).

Indirect evidence (Heath and Vandekar, 1964) indicates that the toxicity of dieldrin to rats is also related directly to the concentra-

tion of the compound present in the brain at the time. In dogs fed dieldrin, symptomatology correlates with blood levels, which undoubtedly reflect brain levels (Keane and Zavon, 1969).

Any result that fails to reveal a causal relation between toxicity and concentration of toxicant at the target immediately suggests that the primary target or the effective compound (perhaps a metabolite) has been misidentified, or that the analysis was faulty.

3.2.3.5 Storage in Relation to the Ecosystem. "Biological magnification," the progressive increase in storage of a compound in succeeding species of a food chain, might be considered the quintessence of storage. The nature of the process and its crucial importance for some forms of wildlife is discussed in Section 11.2.3.2.

3.2.4 Excretion

The elimination of unabsorbed pesticide, whether by vomiting or otherwise, is a protection from poisoning, and this elimination must be measured in any balance study. True excretion (elimination of previously absorbed material) may occur by way of expired air, urine, feces, milk, and dermal secretions. The passage of toxicant into eggs or the fetus has the effect of excretion for the parent. The presence of pesticides in eggs is discussed in Section 6.1.1.1, and the passage into the fetus is taken up in Section 7.2.1.5.

3.2.4.1 Respiratory Excretion. Respiratory excretion may be important in connection with certain fumigants. McCollister et al. (1950) found that, although monkeys eliminated 20% of absorbed radioactive carbon tetrachloride by exhalation during the first 18 hours following the end of exposure, ^{14}C continued to be measurable in samples of expired air for a period of 4 weeks. Material derived from carbon tetrachloride was found in the urine and feces, also. Recent developments in gas-liquid chromatography make it practical to measure fumigants and other solvents in the respired air of people for surprisingly long periods after occupational or accidental exposure (see Section 7.2.2.4).

3.2.4.2 Biliary and Fecal Excretion.
Fecal Excretion. For a wide range of compounds, urinary excretion has been studied more thoroughly than fecal excretion, yet fecal excretion is more important for many heavy metals and other compounds. True fecal excretion of DDT-derived material in guinea pigs and rats was established early (Wasicky and Unti, 1945; Judah, 1949), and later studies showed that in the rat, fecal excretion of DDT exceeds urinary excretion, irrespective of the route of administration. The same is true of Perthane® (Bleiberg and Larson, 1957), methoxychlor (Weikel, 1956), aldrin (Hunter et al., 1960; Ludwig et al., 1964), dieldrin (Hunter et al., 1960; Heath and Vandekar, 1964), and endrin (Hunter et al., 1960). In fact, 90% of excretion of dieldrin-derived material is via the feces (Heath and Vandekar, 1964). It may be that most residual chlorinated hydrocarbon insecticides are excreted chiefly in the feces. However, certain isomers of BHC are exceptions (Koransky et al., 1964).

The recovery of traces of DDT and DDE from human feces has been reported (Hayes et al., 1956) and denied (Hayes et al., 1971). Other metabolites have not been found in human feces, although most DDT metabolites excreted by rats occur in their feces in the form of DDA-like material.

Biliary Excretion and Enterohepatic Circulation. The fact of biliary excretion is proved for DDT (Jensen et al., 1957; Mattson et al., 1953), Perthane® (Bleiberg and Larson, 1957), methoxychlor (Weikel, 1956), aldrin (Mörsdorf et al., 1963), and dieldrin (Mörsdorf et al., 1963; Heath and Vandekar, 1964). The rate of biliary excretion may be considerable. Thus, Weikel (1956) recovered from rats as much as 40% of an intravenous dose of radioactive methoxychlor in 6 hours. The excretion reached a peak at about 30 minutes and then decreased rapidly for several hours; a slower excretion followed, and some activity still was present in the bile 48 hours after administration.

Burns et al. (1957) found that there is an increase in urinary excretion of radioactive material following ligation of the bile duct in rats fed radioactive DDT. Because the chief metabolite of DDT in the urine is DDA, the result is indirect evidence that some of the material ordinarily excreted in the bile is related to DDA. Unfortunately, the authors did not identify the DDT-derived material in the urine.

The existence of an enterohepatic circulation of the metabolites of these compounds appears certain. Bleiberg and Larson (1957) collected bile from two rats dosed intravenously with radioactive Perthane® and recovered in an 8-hour period 25 and 55%, respectively, of the ^{14}C. When the bile samples were combined and given orally to a third rat, about 70% of ^{14}C appeared in the feces and 13% in the urine over a 3-day period. This experiment also serves to illustrate the relatively rapid excretion of the metabolites as compared with the parent compound. Enterohepatic circulation of dieldrin itself was demonstrated by Heath and Vandekar (1964), who found that the proportion of dieldrin excreted unchanged could be increased from 3% of the total excretion to 10% by cannulation of the bile duct.

The bile appears to be the principal source of DDT metabolites in the feces. In a rat in which the bile duct was cannulated before the intravenous injection of radioactive DDT, 65% of the dose was recovered in the bile, 2% in the urine, and only 0.3% in the feces (Jensen et al., 1957), even though the possibility of some contamination of the feces by the urine could not be excluded.

The fact of biliary excretion of a metabolite suggests but does not prove that the liver is an important site for its production. In the case of aldrin and dieldrin, further evidence along this line is the high concentration of the parent compound, and especially its hydrophilic metabolite in the liver (Mörsdorf et al., 1963).

Rate of Bile Flow. Compounds excreted by the kidneys generally are considered to be more toxic in animals with impaired renal function. There has been far less study of the relationship between toxicity and impairment of bile flow, even though it is well known that some compounds or their metabolites are excreted in the bile. It is also well known that some compounds have little effect on the bile flow, while others increase it, and still others decrease it (Slater and Delaney, 1971). Studies published in 1967, and more recent ones, have demonstrated that the toxicity of some compounds that undergo biliary excretion is increased by ligation of the bile duct. When this relationship is found in one species, it frequently occurs in other species also, but striking exceptions are recognized. A number of compounds known to be excreted in the bile are more toxic to newborn than to adult rats. It has been suggested that a lesser facility for biliary excretion in the newborn may explain the difference in some instances. However, the same series of investigations revealed other instances in which biliary excretion was not an adequate explanation for observed age differences (Klaassen, 1973). (Other factors that may make newborns more susceptible than adults to some compounds include lesser biotransformation, lesser renal excretion, and greater permeability of the blood-brain barrier.)

Much remains to be learned about how interference with bile flow contributes to the toxicity of some compounds. This is especially true because many compounds excreted by this route are reabsorbed to a greater or lesser degree from the intestine, leading to an enterohepatic circulation. Clearly, such compounds have a more prolonged opportunity than others for microbial biotransformation in the gut. This biotransformation may be an important factor in determining their toxicity, and its interruption through cessation of bile flow may explain the latter's effect. Also, it seems impossible at this time to exclude the possibility that there may be even less direct ways in which interference with bile flow sometimes contributes to toxicity.

3.2.4.3 Urinary Excretion and Its Relation to Other Forms of Excretion. A higher proportion of some other chlorinated hydrocarbon insecticides is excreted in the urine of the rat than is true for DDT. Approximately 80% of radioactivity derived from both α- and γ-BHC was found in the urine and only about 20% in the feces (Koransky et al., 1964). Furthermore, a much higher percentage of DDT is excreted in the urine by man than by the rat. Volunteers who received technical DDT at the rate of 35 mg/man/day excreted on the average 16% (Hayes et al., 1971) to 19% (Hayes et al., 1956) of their total intake as DDA in the urine. Based on the dietary intake of 0.063 mg of all DDT-related material for a 16- to 19-year-old man (Duggan, 1968), an even higher proportion (43% as DDA and 45% as all DDT-related materials) could be recovered from the urine of people with ordinary exposure (Cranmer et al., 1969). This estimated recovery approaches 80 to 90%, if one recalls that the average person eats only about half as much as a 16- to 19-year old man. In any event, the proportion recovered in man is much higher than the 0.4 to 1.2% found in the urine of rats, and somewhat higher than the 17 to 23% of metabolized DDT found in the feces of these animals (Dale et al., 1962).

Trichloroethylene is expired from the lungs for 2 days after exposure, and traces may be present on the 3rd day. About 8% of the retained material is excreted as metabolites in the feces, but most is excreted in the urine (Bartoníček, 1962). Souček and Vlachová (1960) found that an average of 73% of the trichloroethylene retained by men and women after inhalation could be recovered in the urine as follows: monochloroacetic acid, 4%; trichloroacetic acid, 19%; and trichloroethanol, 50%.

The excretion of trichloroacetic acid in man is said to show a periodicity, reaching a maximum at 1300 hours each day. The other two metabolites show no such periodicity (Souček and Vlachová, 1960), and even the periodicity of trichloroacetic acid is denied by some (Gilchrist and Goldsmith, 1956). In man, excretion of the metabolites of trichloroethylene is fastest for monochloroacetic acid, intermediate for trichloroethanol, and slowest for trichloroacetic acid (Souček and Vlachová, 1960). Following the use of trichloroethylene as an anesthetic, trichloroacetic acid may be detected in the urine for 5 to 12 days (Gilchrist and Goldsmith, 1956). Following accidental ingestion of trichloroethylene, trichloroacetic acid was found in the serum and urine for 27 days (Abrahanssen, 1957).

As with some other fumigants, the excretion of metabolites of the dichlorobenzenes is regarded as "slow" because excretion is still incomplete after 6 days (Azouz et al., 1955), but the description is only relative. Following repeated high doses of DDT, urinary excretion may continue at a higher than normal rate in man for more than 3 years after the last dose (Hayes et al., 1971).

3.2.4.4 Excretion in Milk. The rate of excretion in the milk is proportional to dosage for DDT (Gannon et al., 1959c; Zweig et al., 1961), dieldrin (Gannon et al., 1959c, 1959a), aldrin, heptachlor, methoxychlor (Gannon et al., 1959c; Cluett et al., 1960), heptachlor epoxide (Bache et al., 1960; Huber and Bishop, 1962), and endrin (Kiigemagi et al., 1958). In fact, the slope of the lines relating concentration in milk to concentration in feed has been represented as identical for most of these compounds (Gannon et al., 1959c), although the data suggest that relatively less DDT is excreted in the milk at higher dosage levels.

The rate of excretion of bromide is also proportional to dosage, regardless of the source. Cows generally secrete bromides in their milk at the rate of 1 to 5 ppm, but may secrete somewhat more in areas such as tidewater Virginia, where there is a relatively high natural concentration of bromides in the soil (Young et al., 1959). Any addition of bromides to the diet, either in the form of inorganic bromide or bromide residues resulting from the fumigation of grain, produces increased concentrations of bromide in the blood and milk (Lynn et al., 1963). When sodium bromide was fed, 18% of the dose was recovered from the milk, but when residues from fumigation with methyl bromide were fed, 38% of the dose was secreted in the milk. Furthermore, there was a small but detectable difference in the relationship between the concentration of bromide in the blood and in the milk, depending on the original source of bromide (Lynn et al., 1963). The first difference could depend on incomplete analytical recovery of bromide from hay, but the second difference is more difficult to explain. Thus, although it is generally assumed that the bromide residues resulting from fumigation are inorganic (Lynn et al., 1963), there is some evidence that they are partly organic and metabolized differently from inorganic bromide. In any event, when dietary concentration of bromide is held constant, the concentration of bromide in the milk reaches a steady state in 20 to 30 days (Lynn et al., 1963).

It has been indicated by several authors (Smith, et al., 1948; Shepherd et al., 1949; Biddulph et al., 1950) that 10% or more of DDT derived from residues on forage is excreted subsequently in the milk. On some days certain cows secreted up to 32.5% of their daily DDT intake in their milk (Smith et al., 1948). However, these results must be viewed with caution, for they depend not only on analysis of DDT in milk, but also on analysis of DDT residues in hay. Any systematic failure to detect all of the residue in the hay would lead to an overestimate of the proportion of the dose recovered in the milk. It may be significant that Ely et al. (1952) were able to recover in the milk of cows only 1.8 to 7.0% of the DDT administered as an oil solution.

Huber and Bishop (1962) reported that cows fed heptachlor and heptachlor epoxide residues on hay secreted 20 to 29% in their milk in the form of heptachlor epoxide. Again, the accuracy of the percentage depends on the accuracy of the analysis of the residues in hay. Incidentally, the residues in the hay presumably resulted from translocation or some other indirect contamination, because heptachlor was applied to the soil very early in the season and not to the maturing crop. Methoxychlor appears in the milk of cows following large doses (Gannon et al., 1959c; Cluett et al., 1960), but according to Biddulph et al. (1952), the compound cannot be detected in the milk, blood, fat, kidney, liver, or muscle, under practical conditions of forage treatment with methoxychlor. Direct treatment of cows with methoxychlor leads to an increase of the compound in the milk, but an undetermined proportion of it may reach the milk by extraneous contamination rather than secretion (DeFoliart and Willett, 1961).

Incidentally, a comparison of ratios of concentrations of insecticides in fat to concentrations in milk is meaningless, unless it is made under standardized conditions—preferably a steady state of intake and storage.

Cows fed heptachlor reach a steady state of secretion of heptachlor epoxide in the milk in only 10 days (Huber and Bishop, 1962).

Cows fed on high doses of dieldrin continued to excrete the compound in their milk for more than 47 days after dosing was stopped (Ely et al., 1954). The concentration of heptachlor epoxide returned to pretreatment levels in 15 to 45 days, depending on the intensity of treatment (Huber and Bishop, 1962). Lindane requires less than 20 days to reach very low levels (Ware and Gilmore, 1959).

Secretion of several pesticides in human milk is described in Section 7.2.2.1.

3.2.4.5 Factors Changing the Rate of Excretion. Storage and excretion are so interrelated that any factor changing one is likely to influence the other. Thus, excretion may be influenced by dosage, time, rate of absorption, compound, age, sex, species, starvation, and, of course, the integrity of the excretory organs themselves. These factors were discussed in Section 3.2.3.3. Other factors that can affect excretion are drugs and pH (see Section 3.2.1.2).

Although some drugs influence excretion

through stimulation or inhibition of the microsomal enzymes (see Section 3.1.2.2), others change nonmicrosomal enzymes or affect the pH of urine. Interesting examples of changes of excretion associated with drugs involve trichlorethylene. The excretion of metabolites of this compound could be increased by approximately 22% by giving glucose and insulin (Souček and Vlachová, 1960). After trichlorethylene, the excretion of trichloroacetic acid drops almost to zero in animals given tetraethylthiuram disulfide ("Antabuse") (Forssman et al., 1955). In people treated with the same drug, urinary excretion of trichloroethanol was decreased 40 to 64%, trichloroacetic acid was decreased 72 to 87%, and there was a corresponding increase in the respiratory excretion of the unchanged trichloroethylene (Bartoníček and Teisinger, 1962). The use of Antabuse offers some promise in the treatment of poisoning by trichloroethylene because trichloroethanol is more toxic than the parent compound (Bartoníček and Teisinger, 1962).

3.2.5 Balance Studies

A balance study is an audit of quantitative metabolism. In finance, an audit may reveal hidden losses. In a similar way, an audit of quantitative metabolism may reveal that material is being lost by an unsuspected route. For example, a portion of the compound under study may be metabolized to carbon dioxide and exhaled. In another situation, convincing proof may be found that additional storage still is occurring in the tissues. Finally, it may be found that recognized daily excretion fully accounts for daily intake so that a steady state exists.

Presumably, all experiments are carried out with the greatest accuracy that the experimental methods permit. However, the results of inaccuracy, including the inevitable inaccuracy of chemical and radiometric analysis, may be especially evident in a balance study because the exact answer is known before the work is begun. By this we mean that the total dose, whether single or repeated, should be exactly equal to the sum of material remaining to be absorbed, accounted for in various tissues, and accounted for through excretion by one or more routes. Since there are inevitable errors under practical conditions, the best one can hope for is the close clustering of experimental results around the ideal, which is to account for 100% of the total dose. In spite of the tremendous difficulties involved, some balance studies are completed in which the apparent recovery ranges from 95 to 105% for different animals, or for replicates of the experiment.

There is often a great advantage in carrying out a balance study using radioactively tagged compound. This practice ensures that all metabolites involving the tagged portion of the molecule will be recognized, regardless of their chemical nature. Thus, by using isotopes, metabolites may be measured accurately in terms of the parent compound, even though their existence was previously unsuspected, or, as in the case of carbon dioxide, they are otherwise indistinguishable from compounds occurring naturally in the body.

Two kinds of balance studies may be recognized, depending on whether the study begins at the same time dosing begins, or whether the study is started after dosing has been in effect for an indefinite period. The first kind of study is inherently experimental. The investigator must have control of dosing. Such studies may be carried out in experimental animals and, depending on the nature of the material under study, in volunteers. The second kind of study may be made under experimental conditions in which the investigator controls dosing, or it may be made in situations in which it is impossible to control the dosage but is possible to measure it accurately. If analytical methods are sufficiently good, this kind of balance study can be carried out on persons with occupational exposure or those in the general population. Thus, it would be entirely feasible to undertake a balance study in connection with lead, because the element may be analyzed no matter what its chemical combination. By the same token, it is not feasible at this time to undertake a complete balance study of DDT in man, because there is considerable evidence that not all metabolites of DDT can be measured by chemical methods now available. At this time, a balance study with DDT requires the use of radioactively tagged material. This condition excludes the possibility of a balance study of DDT in workers, the general population, or even volunteers, because there is a real question whether the radioactivity which would have to be involved would be safe.

An excellent example of a balance study is that carried out by Ludwig et al. (1964) with aldrin. Aldrin-^{14}C was fed to male rats in doses of 4.3 μg/rat/day for 3 months. The steady state in which the daily dosage equaled the daily intake was reached after approximately 10 weeks of feeding. At the end of the feeding period, the rats had excreted approximately 90% of the total dose, the remainder being stored in their tissues. After feeding was discontinued, excretion decreased exponentially. Twelve weeks after the last dose, 99.5% of all the material administered had been excreted.

During the course of the study, it was found that the material excreted in feces and urine consisted of aldrin, dieldrin, and a mixture of hydrophilic metabolic products. The latter constituted 75% of the aldrin-related material in the feces and 95% of that in the urine.

3.3 Methods of Studying Metabolism

3.3.1 Tracers

Use of radioactive tracers has made a great contribution to the study of metabolism. Books have been devoted to their uses in the detection of pesticide residues (International Atomic Energy Agency, 1966, 1970).

At one time, radioactive substances could be measured with greater sensitivity than ordinary substances. This is no longer true of many compounds since the development of gas chromatography.

Even when chromatography is otherwise satisfactory, isotopes may offer the possibility of more rapid measurement.

The most important contribution of tracers is in the identification of metabolites. In order to detect a metabolite chemically, one must know what it is, or at least be able to show that its presence was introduced by exposure, generally intentional dosing under the conditions of a controlled experiment. If tracers are used, it may be assumed that all tagged materials are either the parent compound or metabolites in the broadest sense. This is true not only for metabolites that resemble the parent compound, but also for carbon dioxide and other compounds that may have resulted from entry of a fragment of the parent molecule into the general metabolic pool. In its simplest form, the technique may be used to overcome difficulties involving solvents; the total active material may be measured after the tissue in question has been destroyed by wet ashing, or some other harsh procedure likely to change the compound chemically. Conversely, tracers may be used to learn whether a compound and all its metabolites are extracted effectively by a particular solvent, or whether some remain behind in the extracted material.

3.3.2 New Chemical Techniques

Without doubt, the greatest single factor contributing to toxicology in the last decade is the development of chromatography. A detailed discussion of the techniques involved is beyond the scope of this book; fortunately, a number of books are available on the subject. A critical review of new problems and methods related to the analysis of pesticide residues is that of Lisk (1970).

Mass spectrography already has made the identification of unknown compounds, including metabolites, faster, easier, and more accurate. The combination of a mass spectrograph with a gas chromatograph to form a single system permits the identification of individual chromatographic peaks. The system even permits sampling of succeeding portions of the same peak to determine whether it represents a single substance, or a combination of substances that happen to be coming off the chromatographic column at otherwise indistinguishable times.

The resolution offered by gas-liquid chromatography using ordinary columns is remarkable. However, this resolution is feeble compared to that now achieved experimentally using capillary columns. There is good reason to think that the commercial introduction of equipment for capillary-tube, gas-liquid chromatography will constitute a new landmark in analytical chemistry. If use of this equipment is applied to the study of selected dosage levels so that the chemical basis of thresholds in dosage-response relationships can be defined (see Section 2.2.7.4), then we can be confident the findings will constitute a landmark in toxicology.

3.3.3 Metabolic Pool Technique

The metabolic pool technique consists of introducing radioactively tagged atoms into the normal metabolic pool and then observing what effect some experimental condition has on the identity and distribution of tagged compounds (Winteringham et al., 1953, 1955; Winteringham and Hellyer, 1954; Winteringham and Harrison, 1956). For example, phosphorus may be introduced as inorganic phosphate to experimental and control animals, which are then studied to detect any qualitative or quantitative differences in the way they utilize the material. The experimental condition may involve a toxicant, but it may also involve some other stress or some physiological condition. Thus, the metabolic pool technique constitutes a sort of biochemical microscope by which the tissues may be scanned for metabolic change. There is no guarantee that changes will be found, but that is true of the light and electron microscopes also.

Tracers, particularly radioactive tracers, have made feasible many studies of transfer rates and turnover rates of substances in living systems. Robertson (1957) reviewed the mathematical basis for the interpretation of such studies. Measurement of transfer rates and turnover rates is a basic problem in normal biochemistry. However, these rates may change under the influence of toxicants, and in this instance their measurement constitutes a special case of the metabolic pool technique.

REFERENCES

Abrahanssen, A. M. (1957). Alkaline pyridine reaction in serum in trichlorethylene poisoning. Scand. J. Clin. Lab. Invest., 9:406.

Aggeler, P. M., and O'Reilly, R. A. (1969). Effect of heptabarbital on the response to bishydroxycoumarin in man. J. Lab. Clin. Med., 74:229–238.

Ainsworth, M. (1960). Methods for measuring percutaneous absorption. J. Soc. Cosmet. Chem., 11:69–78.

Alvares, A. P., Kappas, A., Levin, W., and Conney, A. H. (1973). Inducibility of benzo[d]pyrene hydroxylase in human skin by polycyclic hydrocarbons. Clin. Pharmacol. Ther., 14:30–40.

Ambrose, A. M., Robbins, D. J., Christensen, H. E., and Rather, L. J. (1953). Toxicological and pharmacological studies on chlordane. A. M. A. Arch. Ind. Hyg. Occup. Med., 7:197–210.

Amdur, M. O. (1957). The influence of aerosols upon the respiratory responses of guinea pigs to sulfur dioxide. Am. Ind. Hyg. Assoc. J., 18:149–155.

Amdur, M. O. (1961). The effect of aerosols upon the response to irritant gases. In: Inhaled Particles and Vapours, edited by C. N. Davies. Pergamon Press, Inc., Oxford.

Amdur, M. O. (1971). Aerosols formed by oxidation of sulfur dioxide. Arch. Environ. Health, 23:459–468.

Axelrod, J. (1955). The enzymatic deamination of amphetamine (Benzedrine). J. Biol. Chem., 214:753–763.

Axelrod, J. (1956). Enzymatic cleavage of aromatic ethers. Biochem. J., 63:634–639.

Azouz, W. M., Parke, D. V., and Williams, R. T. (1955). Studies in detoxication. The metabolism of halogenobenzenes. Ortho and Paradichlorobenzenes. Biochem. J., 59:410–415.

Bache, C. A., Gyrisco, G. G., Feetig, S. N., Huddleston, E. W., Lisk, D. J., Fox, F. H., Trinberger, G. W., and Holland, R. F. (1960). Effects of feeding low levels of heptachloric epoxide to dairy cows on residues and off-flavors in milk. J. Agric. Food Chem., 8:408–409.

Baker, J., and Chaykin, S. (1961). The metabolism of trimethylamine-N-oxide. Fed. Proc., 20:47.

Barka, T., and Popper, H. (1967). Liver enlargement and drug toxicity. Medicine, 46:103–117.

Barker, P. S., and Morrison, F. O. (1966). The basis of DDT tolerance in the laboratory mouse. Can. J. Zool., 44:879–887.

Barnes, J. M. (1968). Percutaneous toxicity. In: Modern Trends in Toxicology, edited by E. Boyland and R. Goulding, pp. 18–38. Butterworths, London.

Bartha, R. (1969). Pesticide interaction creates hybrid residue. Science, 166:1299–1300.

Bartoníček, V. (1962). Metabolism and excretion of trichloroethylene after inhalation by human subjects. Br. J. Ind. Med., 19:134–141.

Bartoníček, V., and Teisinger, J. (1962). Effect of tetraethyl thiuram disulphide (disulfiram) on metabolism of trichloroethylene in man. Br. J. Ind. Med., 19:216–221.

Bentley, E. W. (1969). The warfarin resistance problem in England and Wales. Schriftenr. Ver. Wasser. Boden. Lufthyg., 32:19.

Bernard, R. F. (1963). Studies on the effects of DDT on birds. Mich. State Univ. Biol. Serv., 2:159–191.

Beutler, E. (1960). Drug-induced hemolytic anemia (primaquine sensitivity). In: The Metabolic Basis of Inherited Disease, edited by J. B. Stanbury, J. B. Nyngaarden, and D. S. Fredrikson, pp. 1031–1067. McGraw-Hill, New York.

Biddulph, C., Bateman, G. Q., Bryson, M. J., Harris, J. R., Greenwood, D. A., Binns, W., Miner, M. L., Harris, L. E., and Madsen, L. L. (1950). DDT in milk and tissues of dairy cows fed DDT-dusted alfalfa hay. Adv. Chem. Ser., 1:237–243.

Biddulph, C., Bateman, G. Q., Harris, J. R., Mangelson, F. L., Lieberman, F. V., Binns, W., and Greenwood, D. A. (1952). Effect of feeding methoxychlor-treated alfalfa hay to dairy cows. J. Dairy Sci., 35:445–448.

Birnie, G. C., and Fox, S. M. (eds.) (1969). Subcellular Components. Plenum Press, Inc., New York.

Blair, W. F., (ed.) (1964). Proceedings of the Hanford Symposium on Inhaled Radioactive Particles and Gases. Pergamon Press, Inc., London.

Blank, I. H., Griesemer, R. D., and Gould, E. (1957). The penetration of an anticholinesterase agent (Sarin) into skin. J. Invest. Dermatol., 29:299–309.

Bledsoe, T., Island, D. A., Ney, R. L., and Liddle, G. W. (1964). An effect of o,p'-DDD on extra-adrenal metabolism of cortisol in man. J. Clin. Endocrinol. Metab., 24:1303–1311.

Bleiberg, M. J., and Larson, P. S. (1957). Studies on derivatives of 2,2-bis(p-Chlorophenyl)-1,1-dichloroethane (DDD, TDE) with special reference to their effects on the adrenal cortex. J. Pharmacol. Exp. Ther., 121:421–431.

Bowery, T. G., Gatterdam, P. E., Guthrie, F. E., and Rabb, R. L. (1965). Fate of inhaled C^{14}-TDE in rabbits. J. Agric. Food. Chem., 13:356–359.

Bowman, M. C., and Beroza, M. (1965). Extraction p-values of pesticides and related compounds in six binary solvent systems. J. Assoc. Off. Anal. Chem., 48:943–952.

Boyd, C. E., and Ferguson, D. E. (1964a). Spectrum of cross-resistance to insecticides in the mosquito fish, Gambusia affinis. Mosquito News, 24:19–21.

Boyd, C. E., and Ferguson, D. E. (1964b). Susceptibility and resistance of mosquito fish to several insecticides. J. Econ. Entomol., 57:430–431.

Boyd, C. E., Vinson, S. B., and Ferguson, D. E. (1963). Possible DDT resistance in two species of frogs. Copeia, 1963:426–429.

Boyle, C. M. (1960). Case of apparent resistance of Rattus norvegicus Berkenhout to anticoagulant poisons. Nature, 188:517.

Brieger, H. (1963). Genetic bases of susceptibility and resistance to toxic agents. J. Occup. Med., 5:511–515.

Brieger, H., and LaBelle, C. W. (1959). The fate of inhaled particulates in the early post-exposure period. A. M. A. Arch. Ind. Health, 19:510–515.

Brodie, B. B. (1956). Pathways of drug metabolism. J. Pharm. Pharmacol., 8:1–17.

Brodie, B. B., Bernstein, E., and Mark, L. C. (1952). The role of body fat in limiting the duration of action of thiopental. J. Pharmacol. Exp. Ther., 105:421–426.

Brodie, B. B., and Maickel, R. P. (1962). Comparative biochemistry of drug metabolism. In: Metabolic Factors Controlling Duration of Drug Action. Proc. 1st Int. Pharmacol. Meeting (Stockholm, Aug. 22–25, 1961), 6:299–324.

Brothers, D. R. (1972). A case of anticoagulant rodenticide resistance in an Idaho Norway rat (Rattus norvegicus) population. Calif. Vector Views, 19:41–45.

Brown, A. W. A., and Pal, R. (1971). Insecticide Resistance in Arthropods, Ed. 2. World Health Organization, Geneva.

Brown, R. R., Miller, J. A., and Miller, E. C. (1954). The metabolism of methylated aminoazo dyes. IV. Dietary factors enhancing demethylation in vitro. J. Biol. Chem., 209:211–222.

Brown, V. K. (1968). Solubility and solvent effects as rate-determining factors in the acute percutaneous toxicities of pesticides. Soc. Chem. Ind. Monogr., 29:93–105.

Brown, V. K. H., Hunter, C. G., and Richardson, A. (1964). A blood test diagnostic of exposure to aldrin and dieldrin. Br. J. Ind. Med., 21:283–286.

Burns, E. C., Dahm, P. A., and Linquist, D. A. (1957). Secretion of DDT metabolites in the bile of rats. J. Pharmacol. Exp. Ther., 121:55–62.

Burns, J. J., Rose, R. K., Chenkin, T., Goldman, A., Schulert, A., and Brodie, B. B. (1953). The physiological disposition of phenylbutazone (butazolidin) in man and a method for its estimation in biological material. J. Pharmacol. Exp. Ther., 109:346–357.

Burstein, S., and Klaiber, E. L. (1965). Phenobarbital-induced increase in 6β-hydroxy-cortisol excretion. J. Clin. Endocrinol. Metab., 25:293–296.

Butler, T. C., Mahaffee, C., and Waddell, W. J. (1954). Phenobarbital: studies of elimination, accumulation, tolerance, and dosage schedules. J. Pharmacol. Exp. Ther., 111:425–435.

Campbell, H. A., Smith, W. K., Roberts. W. L., and Link, K. P. (1941). Studies on hemorrhagic sweet clover disease. II. Bioassay of hemorrhagic concentrates by following prothrombin level in plasma of rabbit blood. J. Biol. Chem., 138:1–20.

Carson, P. E., Flanagan, C. L., Ickes, C. E., and Alving, A. S. (1956). Enzymatic deficiency in primaquine-sensitive erythrocytes. Science, 124:484–485.

Carter, R. H., Hubanks, P. E., Mann, H. D., Zeller, J. H., and Hankins, O. G. (1948). The storage of DDT in the tissues of pigs fed beef containing this compound. J. Anim. Sci., 7:509–510.

Casarett, L. J. (1972). The vital sacs: Alveolar clearance mechanism in inhalation toxicology. Essays Toxicol., 3:1–36.

Casterline, J. L., Jr., and Williams, C. H. (1971). The effect of 28-day pesticide feeding on serum and tissue enzyme activities of rats fed diets of varying casein content. Toxicol. Appl. Pharmacol., 18:607–618.

Chadwick, R. W., Cranmer, M. F., and Peoples, A. J. (1971). Comparative stimulation of γHCH metabolism by pretreatment of rats with γHCH, DDT, and DDT + γHCH. Toxicol. Appl. Pharmacol., 18:685–695.

Chadwick, R. W., and Freal, J. J. (1972). Comparative acceleration of lindane metabolism to chlorophenols by pretreatment of rats with lindane or with DDT and lindane. Food Cosmet. Toxicol., 10:789–795.

Chen, T. S., Kinoshita, F. K., and DuBois, K. P. (1972). Acute toxicity and antiesterase action of O-ethyl-S,S-diphenyl phosphorodithioate (Hinosan®). Toxicol. Appl. Pharmacol., 23:519–527.

Chen, W., Vrindten, P. A., Dayton, P. G., and Burns, J. J. (1962). Accelerated aminopyrine metabolism in human subjects pretreated with phenylbutazone. Life Sci., 2:35–42.

Christensen, L. K., and Skovsted, L. (1969). Inhibition of drug metabolism by chloramphenicol. Lancet, 2:1397–1399.

Cluett, M. L., Lowen, W. K., Pease, H. L., and Woodhouse, C. A. (1960). Determination of methoxychlor and/or metabolites in milk following topical application to dairy cows. J. Agric. Food Chem., 8:277–281.

Coates, P. M., and Simpson, N. E. (1972). Genetic variation in human erythrocyte acetylcholinesterase. Science, 175:1466–1467.

Coldwell, B. B., and Zawidzka, L. (1968). Effect of acute administration of acetylsalicyclic acid on the prothrombin activity of bishydroxy-coumarin-treated rats. Blood, 32:945–949.

Conney, A. H. (1967). Pharmacological implications of microsomal enzyme induction. Pharmacol. Rev., 19:317–366.

Conney, A. H., and Burns, J. J. (1962). Factors influencing drug metabolism. Adv. Pharmacol., 1:31–58.

Conney, A. H., Miller, E. C., and Miller, J. A. (1957). Substrate-induced synthesis and other properties of benzpyrene hydroxylase in rat liver. J. Biol. Chem., 228:753–766.

Conney, A. H., Trousof, N., and Burns, J. J. (1960). The metabolic fate of zoxazolamine (Flexin) in man. J. Pharmacol. Exp. Ther., 128:333–339.

Conney, A. H., Welch, R. M., Kuntzman, R., and Burns, J. J. (1967). Effects of pesticides on drug and steroid metabolism. Clin. Pharmacol. Ther., 8:2–10.

Cram, R. L., Jachau, M. R., and Fouts, J. R. (1965a). Differences in hepatic drug metabolism in various rabbit strains before and after pretreatment with phenobarbital. Proc. Soc. Exp. Biol. Med., 118:872–875.

Cram, R. L., Jachau, M. R., and Fouts, J. R. (1956b). Stimulation by chlordane of hepatic drug metabolism in the squirrel monkey. J. Lab. Clin. Med., 66:906–911.

Cranmer, M. F. (1970). Effect of diphenylhydantoin on storage in the rat. Toxicol. Appl. Pharmacol., 17:315.

Cranmer, M. F., Carroll, J. J., and Copeland, M. F. (1969). Determination of DDT and metabolites, including DDA, in human urine by gas chromatography. Bull. Environ. Contam. Toxicol., 4:214–223.

Cranmer, M. F., Peoples, A., and Chadwick, R. (1972). Biochemical effects of repeated administration of p,p'-DDT on the squirrel monkey. Toxicol. Appl. Pharmacol., 21:98–101.

Cucinell, S. A., Odessky, L., Weiss, M., and Dayton, P. G. (1967). The effect of chloral hydrate on bishydroxycoumarin metabolism. J. A. M. A., 197:366–368.

Cueto, C., Jr., and Hayes, W. J., Jr. (1965). Effect of phenobarbital on the metabolism of dieldrin. Toxicol. Appl. Pharmacol., 7:481.

Cullen, S. I., and Catalano, P. M. (1967). Griseofulvin-warfarin antagonism. J. A. M. A., 199:150–151.

Dahm, P. A., Kopecky, B. E., and Walker, C. B. (1962). Activation of organophosphorus insecticides by rat liver microsomes. Toxicol. Appl. Pharmacol., 4:683–696.

Dale, W. E., Gaines, T. B., and Hayes, W. J., Jr. (1962). Storage and excretion of DDT in starved rats. Toxicol. Appl. Pharmacol., 4:89–106.

Dale, W. E., Gaines, T. B., Hayes, W. J., Jr., and Pearce, G. W. (1963). Poisoning by DDT: relation between clinical signs and concentration in rat brain. Science, 142:1474–1476.

Daniel, J. W., Gage, J. C., Jones, D. I., and Stevens, M. A. (1967). Excretion of butylated hydroxytoluene (BHT) and butylated hydroxyanisole (BHA) in man. Food Cosmet. Toxicol., 5:475–479.

Datta, P. R., and Nelson, M. J. (1968). Enhanced metabolism of methyprylon, meprobamate, and chlordiazepoxide hydrochloride after chronic feeding of a low dietary level of DDT to male and female rats. Toxicol. Appl. Pharmacol., 13:346–352.

Davidow, B., and Frawley, J. P. (1951). Tissue distribution, accumulation and elimination of the isomers of benzene hexachloride. Proc. Soc. Exp. Biol. Med., 76:780–783.

Davies, C. N. (ed.) (1961). Inhaled Particles and Vapours, Vol. 1. Pergamon Press, Inc., Oxford.

Davies, C. N. (ed.) (1967). Inhaled Particles and Vapours, Vol. 2. Pergamon Press, Inc., Oxford.

Davison, A. N. (1955). The conversion of schradan (OMPA) and parathion into inhibitors of cholinesterase by mammalian liver. Biochem. J., 61:203–209.

Dayton, P. G., Tarcan, Y., Chenkin, T., and Weiner, M. (1961). The influence of barbiturates on coumarin plasma levels and prothrombin response. J. Clin. Invest., 40:1797–1802.

DeFoliart, G. R., and Willett, D. N. (1961). Methoxychlor in milk of dairy cows dusted with wettable powder. J. Econ. Entomol., 54:781–783.

Deichmann, W. B., MacDonald, W. E., and Cubit, D. A. (1971). DDT tissue retention: sudden rise induced by the addition of aldrin to a fixed DDT intake. Science, 172:275–276.

Deitrich, R. A. (1971). Genetic aspects of increase in rat liver aldehyde dehydrogenase induced by phenobarbital. Science, 173:334–336.

DeLong, C. W., Thompson, R. C., and Kornberg, H. A. (1954). Percutaneous absorption of tritium oxide. Am. J.

Roentgenol. Radium Ther. Nucl. Med., 71:1038–1045.

Denes, A. (1962). Problems of food chemistry concerning residues of chlorinated hydrocarbons. Nahrung, 6:48–56.

Dixon, R. L. (1968). Effects of chloramphenicol on the metabolism and lethality of cyclophosphamide in rats. Proc. Soc. Exp. Biol. Med., 127:1151–1155.

Dixon, R. L., and Fouts, J. R. (1962). Inhibition of microsomal drug metabolic pathways by chloramphenicol. Biochem. Pharmacol., 11:715–720.

Dorough, H. W., and Casida, J. E. (1964). Nature of certain carbamate metabolites of the insecticide Sevin. J. Agric. Food Chem., 12:294–304.

Drummond, D. C. (1966). Rats' resistance to warfarin. New Sci., 30:771–772.

DuBois, K. P. (1969). Combined effects of pesticides. Can. Med. Assoc. J., 100:173–179.

DuBois, K. P., Doull, J., and Coon, J. M. (1950). Studies on the toxicity and pharmacological action of cotamethyl pyrophosphoramide (OMPA, Pestox III). J. Pharmacol. Exp. Ther., 99:376–393.

DuBois, K. P., Kinoshita, F. K., and Frawley, J. P. (1968). Quantitative measurement of inhibition of aliesterases, acylamidases, and cholinesterase by EPN and Delnav. Toxicol. Appl. Pharmacol., 12:273–284.

DuBois, K. P., Thursh, D. R., and Murphy, S. D. (1957). Studies on the toxicity and pharmacologic actions of the dimethoxy ester of benzotriazine dithiophosphoric acid (DBD, Guthion). J. Pharmacol. Exp. Ther., 119:208–218.

Duggan, R. E. (1968). Residues in food and feed. Pesticide residue levels in foods in the United States from July 1, 1963 to June 30, 1967. Pestic. Monit. J., 2:2–46.

Durham, W. F. (1967). The interaction of pesticides with other factors. Residue Rev., 18:21–103.

Durham, W. F. (1969). Body burden of pesticides in man. Ann. NY Acad. Sci., 160:183–195.

Durham, W. F., Cueto, C., Jr., and Hayes, W. J., Jr. (1956). Hormonal influences on DDT metabolism in the white rat. Am. J. Physiol., 187:373–377.

Durham, W. F., Ortega, P., and Hayes, W. J., Jr. (1963). The effect of various dietary levels of DDT on liver function, cell morphology, and DDT storage in the Rhesus monkey. Arch. Int. Pharmacodyn. Ther., 141:111–129.

Durham, W. F., and Wolfe, H. R. (1962). Measurement of the exposure of workers to pesticides. Bull. WHO, 26:75–91.

Earl, F. L., Van Loon, E. J., Melveger, B. E., Reinwall, J. E., Bierbower, G. W., Kass, R., and Miguez, W. (1970). Lindane toxicity: a comparative study in dogs and miniature swine with and without phenobarbital. Toxicol. Appl. Pharmacol., 17:287.

Eisenman, G. (1968). Ion permeation of cell membranes and its models. Fed. Proc., 27:1249–1251.

Ely, R. E., Moore, L. A., Carter, R. H., Hubanks, P. E., and Poos, F. W. (1954). Excretion of dieldrin in the milk of cows fed dieldrin-sprayed forage and technical dieldrin. J. Dairy Sci., 37:1461–1465.

Ely, R. E., Moore, L. A., Carter, R. H., Mann, H. D., and Poos, F. W. (1952). The effect of dosage level and method of administration of DDT on the concentration of DDT in milk. J. Dairy Sci., 35:266–271.

Emmel, L., and Krupe, M. (1946). Beitrage zur Kenntnis der Wirkungsweise des 4,4'-Dichlordiphenyl-trichlormethyl-methan beim Warmbluter. Z. Naturforsch., 1:691–695.

Eriksson, S. (1965). Studies in α_1-antitrypsin deficiency. Acta Med. Scand., 177 (Suppl):2–85.

Ferguson, D. E., and Bingham, C. R. (1966a). The effects of combinations of insecticides on susceptible and resistant mosquito fish. Bull. Environ. Contam. Toxicol., 1:97–103.

Ferguson, D. E., and Bingham, C. R. (1966b). Endrin resistance in yellow bullheads, Ictalurus natalis. Trans. Am. Fish Soc., 95:325–326.

Ferguson, D. E., and Boyd, C. E. (1964). Apparent resistance to methyl parathion in mosquito fish, Gambusia affinis. Copeia, 4:706.

Ferguson, D. E., Cotton, W. D., Gardner, D. T., and Culley, D. D. (1965). Tolerances to five chlorinated hydrocarbon insecticides in two species of fish from a transect of the Lower Mississippi River. J. Miss. Acad. Sci., 11:239–245.

Ferguson, D. E., Culley, D. D., Cotton, W. D., and Dodds, R. P. (1964). Resistance to chlorinated hydrocarbon insecticides in three species of fresh water fish. Bioscience, 14:43–44.

Fine, B. C., and Molloy, J. O. (1964). Effects of insecticide synergists on duration of sleep induced in mice by barbiturates. Nature, 204:789–790.

Finley, R. B., and Pillmore, R. E. (1963). Conversion of DDT to DDD in animal tissue. AIBS Bull., 13:41–42.

Finnegan, J. K., Haag, H. B., and Larson, P. S. (1949). Tissue distribution and elimination of DDD and DDT following oral administration to dogs and rats. Proc. Soc. Exp. Biol. Med., 72:357–360.

Fitzhugh, O. G., and Nelson, A. A. (1947). The chronic oral toxicity of DDT (2,2-bis-p-chlorophenyl-1,1,1-trichloroethane), J. Pharmacol., 89:18–30.

Fouts, J. R. (1963). Factors influencing the metabolism of drugs in liver microsomes. Ann. NY Acad. Sci., 104:875–880.

Fouts, J. R., and Adamson, R. H. (1959). Drug metabolism in the new born rabbit. Science, 129:897–898.

Fouts, J. R., and Brodie, B. B. (1957). The enzymatic reduction of chloramphenicol, p-nitrobenzoic acid and other aromatic nitro compounds in mammals. J. Pharmacol. Exp. Ther., 119:197–207.

Fouts, J. R., Kamm, J. J., and Brodie, B. B. (1957). Enzymatic reduction of prontosil and other azo dyes. J. Pharmacol. Exp. Ther., 120:291–300.

Forssman, S., Owe-Larsson, A., and Skog, E. (1955). Umsatz von Trichloräthylen im Organismus. Ein tierexperimentelle Untersuchung. Arch. Gewerbepathol. Gewerbehyg., 13:619–623.

Fredriksson, T. (1958). Studies on the percutaneous absorption of Sarin and two allied organophosphorus cholinesterase inhibitors. Acta Derm. Venereol. (Stockh.), 38:1–38.

Fredriksson, T. (1961a). Percutaneous absorption of parathion and paraoxon. IV. Decontamination of human skin from parathion. Arch. Environ. Health, 3:185–188.

Fredriksson, T. (1961b). Studies on the percutaneous absorption of parathion and paraoxon. II. Distribution of P32-labelled parathion within the skin. Acta Derm. Venereol. (Stockh.), 41:344–352.

Fredriksson, T. (1961c). Studies on the percutaneous absorption of parathion and paraoxon. III. Rate of absorption of parathion. Acta Derm. Venereol. (Stockh.), 41:353–362.

Fredriksson, T. (1962). Studies on the percutaneous absorption of parathion and paraoxon. V. Rate of absorption of paraoxon. J. Invest. Dermatol., 38:233–236.

Fredriksson, T. (1963). Influence of solvents and surface active agents on the barrier function of the skin towards sarin. Acta Derm. Venereol. (Stockh.), 43:91–101.

Fredriksson, T. (1964). Studies on the percutaneous absorption of parathion and paraoxon. VI. In vivo decomposition of paraoxon during the epidermal passage. J. Invest. Dermatol., 43:37–40.

Fredriksson, T., Farrior, W. L., Jr., and Witter, R. F. (1961). Studies on the percutaneous absorption of parathion and paraoxon. I. Hydrolysis and metabolism within the skin. Acta Derm. Venereol. (Stockh.), 41:335–343.

Friberg, L., Skog, E., and Wahlberg, J. E. (1961). Resorption of mercuric chloride and methyl mercury dicyandiamide in guinea pigs through normal skin and through skin pre-treated with acetone, alkylarylsulphonate and soap. Acta Derm. Venereol. (Stockh.), 41:40–52.

Gabliks, J., and Maltby-Askari, E. (1970). The effect of

chlorinated hydrocarbons on drug metabolism in mice. Ind. Med. Surg., 39:347–350.

Gaines, T. B., Hayes, W. J., Jr., and Linder, R. E. (1966). Liver metabolism of anticholinesterase compounds in live rats: relation to toxicity. Nature, 209:88–89.

Gannon, N., and Decker, G. C. (1960). The excretion of dieldrin, DDT, and heptachlor epoxide in milk of dairy cows fed on pastures treated with dieldrin, DDT, and heptachlor. J. Econ. Entomol., 53:411–415.

Gannon, N., Link, R. P., and Decker, G. C. (1959a). Pesticide residue in meat and milk: storage of dieldrin in tissues and its excretion in milk of dairy cows fed dieldrin in their diets. J. Agric. Food Chem., 7:824–826.

Gannon, N., Link, R. P., and Decker, G. C. (1959b). Pesticide residue in meat: storage of dieldrin in tissues of steers, hogs, lambs, and poultry fed dieldrin in their diets. J. Agric. Food Chem., 7:826–828.

Gannon, N., Link, R. P., and Decker, G. C. (1959c). Insecticide residues in the milk of dairy cows fed insecticides in their daily ration. J. Agric. Food Chem., 7:829–832.

Garrettson, L. K., and Curley, A. (1969). Dieldrin: studies in a poisoned child. Arch. Environ. Health, 19:814–822.

Garrettson, L. K., Perel, J. M., and Dayton, P. G. (1969). Methylphenidate interaction with both anticonvulsants and ethyl biscoumacetate. J. A. M. A., 207:2053–2056.

Gelboin, H. V., and Conney, A. H. (1968). Antagonism and potentiation of drug action. In: Modern Trends in Toxicology, edited by E. Boyland and R. Goulding, pp. 175–195. Butterworths, London.

Gielen, J. E., and Nebert, D. W. (1971). Microsomal hydroxylase induction in liver cell culture by phenobarbital, polycyclic hydrocarbons, and p,p'-DDT. Science, 172:167–169.

Gilbert, D., and Golberg, L. (1967). BHT oxidase. A liver-microsomal enzyme induced by the treatment of rats with butylated hydroxytoluene. Food Cosmet. Toxicol., 5:481–890.

Gilchrist, E., and Goldsmith, M. W. (1956). Some observations on the metabolism of trichlorethylene. Anaesthesia, 11:28–36.

Gillett, J. W. (1968). No effect level of DDT in induction of microsomal epoxidation. J. Agric. Food Chem., 16:295–297.

Gillette, J. R., Davis, D. C., and Sasame, H. A. (1972). Cytochrome P-450 and its role in drug metabolism. Annu. Rev. Pharmacol., 12:57–84.

Gillette, J. R., and Kamm, J. J. (1960). The enzymatic formation of sulfoxides. The oxidation of chlorpromazine and 4,4'-diaminodiphenyl sulfide by guinea pig liver microsomes. J. Pharmacol. Exp. Ther., 130:262–267.

Granick, S. (1965). Hepatic porphyria and drug-induced or chemical porphyria. Ann. NY Acad. Sci., 123:188–197.

Guthrie, F. E., Monroe, R. J., and Abernathy, C. O. (1971). Response of the laboratory mouse to selection for resistance to insecticides. Toxicol. Appl. Pharmacol., 18:92–101.

Haag, H. B., and Kampmeier, C. (1955). A review of toxicologic considerations pertinent to the safe use of 2,2-bis (p. chlorophenol)-1,1-dichloroethane (TDE, DDE, Rothane). Agric. Chem., 10:85, 123–126.

Haag, H. B., Larson, P. S., and Schwartz, J. J. (1943). The effect of urinary pH on the elimination of quinine in man. J. Pharmacol. Exp. Ther., 79:136–139.

Haldane, J. B. S. (1954). The Biochemistry of Genetics, Allen & Unwin Ltd., London.

Harris, H. (1970). The Principles of Human Biochemical Genetics. American Elsevier Publishing Co., Inc., New York.

Harris, L. E., Harris, J. R., Mangelson, F. L., Greenwood, D. A., Biddulph, C., Binns, W., and Miner, M. L. (1953). Effect of feeding DDT-treated hay to swine and of feeding the swine tissues to rats. J. Nutr., 51:491–505.

Hart, L. G., and Fouts, J. R. (1963). Effects of acute and

chronic DDT administration on hepatic microsomal drug metabolism in the rat. Proc. Soc. Exp. Biol. Med. 114:388–392.

Hart, L. G., Shultice, R. W., and Fouts, J. R. (1963) Stimulatory effects of chlordane on hepatic microsomal drug metabolism in the rat. Toxicol. Appl. Pharmacol., 5:371–386.

Hatch, T., and Gross, P. (1964). Pulmonary Deposition and Retention of Inhaled Aerosols. Academic Press, Inc., New York.

Hayes, W. J., Jr. (1959). Pharmacology and toxicology o DDT. In: DDT: The Insecticide Dichlorodiphenyl-Trich loroethane and Its Significance, edited by P. Müller, Vol 2, pp. 11–247. Birkäuser Verlag, Basel.

Hayes, W. J., Jr. (1967). The 90-dose LD50 and a chronic ity factor as measures of toxicity. Toxicol. Appl. Pharmacol., 11:327–335.

Hayes, W. J., Jr. (1974). Distribution of dieldrin following a single oral dose. Toxicol. Appl. Pharmacol., 28:485–492.

Hayes, W. J., Jr., and Curley, A. (1968). Storage and excretion of dieldrin and related compounds. Arch. Environ. Health, 16:155–162.

Hayes, W. J., Jr., and Dale, W. E. (1964). Concentration o DDT in brain and other tissues in relation to symptoma tology. Toxicol. Appl. Pharmacol., 6:349.

Hayes, W. J., Jr., Dale, E., and Pirkle, C. I. (1971) Evidence of safety of long-term, high, oral, doses of DD for man. Arch. Environ. Health, 22:119–135.

Hayes, W. J., Jr., Durham, W. F., and Cueto, C. J. (1956) The effect of known repeated oral doses of chlorophenothane (DDT) in man. J. A. M. A., 162:890–897.

Hayes, W. J., Jr., Mattson, A. M., Short, J. G., and Witter R. F. (1960). Skin absorption of malathion in man Safety of malathion dust: as powder for louse control Bull. WHO 22:503–514.

Hayes, W. J., Jr., Quinby, G. E., Walker, K. C., Elliott, J W., and Upholt, W. M. (1958). Storage of DDT and DD in people with different degrees of exposure to DDT. A M. A. Arch. Ind. Health, 18:398–406.

Heath, D. F. (1961). Organophosphorus Poisons. Anticholi nesterases and Related Compounds. Pergamon Press Inc., New York.

Heath, D. F., and Vandekar, M. (1964). Toxicity and metabolism of dieldrin in rats. Br. J. Ind. Med., 21:269–279.

Heath, D. F., Lane, D. W. J., and Park, P. O. (1955). The decomposition of some organophosphorus insecticide and related compounds in plants. Trans. R. Soc. 239B:191–214.

Heller, M. (1948). Bone. In: Histopathology of Irradiatio from External and Internal Sources, edited by W. Bloom pp. 70–161. McGraw Hill, New York.

Hietbrink, B. E., and DuBois, K. P. (1965). Influence of X radiation on development of enzymes responsible fo desulfuration of an organic phosphorothioate and reduc tion of p-nitrobenzoic acid in the liver of male rats Radiat. Res., 22:598–605.

Hill, E. F., Dale, W. E., and Miles, J. W. (1971). DD intoxication in birds: subchronic effects and brain res dues. Toxicol. Appl. Pharmacol., 20:502–514.

Hoffman, D. G., Worth, H. M., Emmerson, J. L., an Anderson, R. C. (1968). Stimulation of hepatic microso mal drug-metabolizing enzymes by α-α-bis (p-chloro phenyl)-3-pyridinemethanol and a method for determin ing no-effect levels in rats. Toxicol. Appl. Pharmacol 12:464–472.

Hoffman, D. G., Worth, H. M., Emmerson, J. L., an Anderson, R. C. (1970). Stimulation of hepatic drug metabolizing enzymes by chlorophenothane (DDT): th relationship to liver enlargement and hepatotoxicity i the rat. Toxicol. Appl. Pharmacol., 16:171–178.

Hollunger, G., and Niklasson, B. (1962). Solubilization an isolation of drug-hydrolysing enzymes from microsomes

In: *Metabolic Factors Controlling Duration of Drug Action*. Proc. 1st Int. Pharmacol. Meeting (Stockholm, Aug. 22–25, 1961), 6:149–158.

Huber, J. T., and Bishop, J. L. (1962). Secretion of heptachlor epoxide in milk of cows fed field-cured hay from soils treated with heptachlor. J. Dairy Sci., 45:79–81.

Hukuhara, T. (1962). Distribution of DDT between the brain and fatty tissue in experimental feeding in rats and behavior of fat-stored DDT in the starvation state. Naunyn Schmiedebergs Arch. Pharmacol. Exp. Pathol., 242:522–539.

Hunter, C. G., and Robinson, J. (1967). Pharmacodynamics of dieldrin (HEOD): I. Ingestion by human subjects for 18 months. Arch. Environ. Health, 15:614–626.

Hunter, C. G., and Robinson, J. (1968). Aldrin, dieldrin and man. Food Cosmet. Toxicol., 6:253–260.

Hunter, C. G., Rosen, A., Williams, R. T., Reynolds, J. G., and Worden, A. N. (1960). Studies of the fate of aldrin, dieldrin and endrin in the mammal. Mededel. Landbouwhogeschool Opzoekingsstat. Staat Gent., 25:1296–1307.

Hutterer, F., Schaffner, F., Klion, F. M., and Popper, H. (1968). Hypertrophic, hypoactive smooth endoplasmic reticulum: a sensitive indicator of hepatotoxicity exemplifed by dieldrin. Science, 161:1017–1019.

Imai, H., and Coulston, F. (1967). Ultrastructural study of the absorption of methoxychlor in rat jejunal mucosa. Toxicol. Appl. Pharmacol., 10:389.

International Atomic Energy Agency (1966). *Radioisotopes in the Detection of Pesticide Residues*. Vienna.

International Atomic Energy Agency. (1970). *Nuclear Techniques for Studying Pesticide Residue Problems*. Vienna.

International Commission on Radiological Protection (1955). Report of International Sub-committee II on Permissible Dose for Internal Radiation. Br. J. Radiol. (Suppl.) 6:23–59.

Isselbacher, K. J., and Axelrod, J. (1955). Enzymatic formation of corticosteroid glucuronides. J. Am. Chem. Soc., 77:1070–1071.

Jackson, W. B., and Kaukeinen, D. (1972). Resistance of wild Norway rats in North Carolina to warfarin rodenticide. Science, 176:1343–1344.

Jay, G. E., Jr. (1955). Variation in response of various mouse strains to hexobarbital (Evipal). Proc. Soc. Exp. Biol. Med., 90:378–380.

Jensen, J. A., Cueto, C., Dale, W. E., Roth, C. F., Pearce, G. W., and Mattson, A. M. (1957). Metabolism of insecticides. DDT metabolites in feces and bile of rats. J. Agric. Food Chem., 5:919–925.

Judah, J. D. (1949). Studies on the metabolism and mode of action of DDT. Br. J. Pharmacol., 4:120–131.

Kalow, W. (1956). Familial incidence of low pseudo-cholinesterase level. Lancet, 2:576–577.

Kalow, W. (1962). *Pharmacogenetics, Heredity and the Response to Drugs*. W. B. Saunders Company, Philadelphia.

Kalow, W., and Davies, R. O. (1958). The activity of various esterase inhibitors towards atypical human serum cholinesterase. Biochem. Pharmacol., 1:183–192.

Kalow, W., and Gunn, D. R. (1959). Some statistical data on atypical cholinesterase of human serum. Ann. Hum. Genet., 23:239–250.

Kamienski, F. X., and Murphy, S. D. (1971). Biphasic effects of methylenedioxyphenyl synergists on the action of hexobarbital and organophosphate insecticides in mice. Toxicol. Appl. Pharmacol., 18:883–894.

Kampffmeyer, H. G. (1969). Failure to detect increased elimination rate of phenacetin in man after treatment with phenobarbital. Klin. Woschenschr., 47:1237–1238.

Keane, W. T., and Zavon, M. R. (1969). Validity of a critical blood level for prevention of dieldrin intoxication. Arch. Environ. Health, 19:36–44.

Kehoe, R. A. (1961). The metabolism of lead in man in health and disease. Arch. Environ. Health, 2:418–422.

Kiigemagi, U., Sprowls, R. G., and Terriere, L. C. (1958). Endrin content of milk and body tissues of dairy cows receiving endrin daily in their diet. J. Agric. Food Chem., 6:518–521.

Kinoshita, F. K., and DuBois, K. P. (1967). Effects of substituted urea herbicides on activity of hepatic microsomal enzymes. Toxicol. Appl. Pharmacol., 10:410.

Kinoshita, F. K., Frawley, J. P., and DuBois, K. P. (1966). Quantitative measurement of induction of hepatic microsomal enzymes by various dietary levels of DDT and toxaphene in rats. Toxicol. Appl. Pharmacol., 9:505–513.

Kjaersgaard, A. R. (1954). Perfusion of isolated dog skin. J. Invest. Dermatol., 22:135–141.

Klaassen, C. D. (1973). Comparison of the toxicity of chemicals in newborn rats to bile duct-ligated and sham-operated rats and mice. Toxicol. Appl. Pharmacol., 24:37–44.

Koch-Weiser, J., and Sellers, E. M. (1971a). Drug interactions with coumarin anticoagulants. Part I. N. Engl. J. Med., 285:487–498.

Koch-Weiser, J., and Sellers, E. M. (1971b). Drug interactions with coumarin anticoagulants. Part II. N. Engl. J. Med., 285:547–558.

Kolmodin, B., Azarnoff, D. L., and Sjöqvist, F. (1969). Effect of environmental factors on drug metabolism: decreased plasma half-life of antipyrine in workers exposed to chlorinated hydrocarbon insecticides. Clin. Pharmacol. Ther., 10:638–642.

Kolmodin-Hedman, B., Alexanderson, B., and Sjöqvist, F. (1971). Effect of exposure to lindane on drug metabolism: decreased hexobarbital sleeping times and increased antipyrine disappearance rate in rats. Toxicol. Appl. Pharmacol., 20:299–307.

Koransky, W., Portig, J., Vohland, H. W., and Klempau, I. (1964). Aktivierung von mikrosomenenzymen durch hexachlor-cyclohexanisomere. Ihr einfluss auf die scillirosidvergiftung der ratte. Arch. Exp. Pathol. Pharmakol., 247:61–78.

Kulp, J. L., and Schulert, A. R. (1962). Strontium-90 in man. Science, 136:619–632.

Kuntzman, R., Jacobson, M., and Conney, A. H. (1966). Effect of phenylbutazone on cortisol metabolism in man. Pharmacologist, 8:195.

Kuntzman, R., Jacobson, M., Levin, W., and Conney, A. H. (1968). Stimulatory effect of N-phenylbarbital (phetharbital) on cortisol hydroxylation in man. Biochem. Pharmacol., 17:565–571.

Kunze, F. M., and Laug, E. P. (1953). Toxicants in tissues of rats on diets containing dieldrin, aldrin, endrin and isodrin. Fed. Proc., 12:339.

Kunze, F. M., Laug, E. P., and Prickett, C. S. (1950). Storage of methoxychlor in the fat of the rat. Fed. Proc., 9:293.

Kunze, F. M., Nelson, A. A., Fitzhugh, O. G., and Laug, E. P. (1949). Storage of DDT in the fat of the rat. Fed. Proc., 8:311.

Kupfer, T., Balazs, T., and Buyske, D. A. (1964). Stimulation of o,p'-DDD of cortisol metabolism in the guinea pig. Life Sci., 3:959–964.

LaBelle, C. W., and Brieger, H. (1959). Synergistic effects of aerosols. II. Effects on rate of clearance from the lung. A. M. A. Arch. Ind. Health, 20:100–105.

LaBelle, C. W., and Brieger, H. (1960a). The fate of inhaled particles in the early postexposure period. II. The role of pulmonary phagocytosis. Arch. Environ. Health, 1:423–427.

LaBelle, C. W., and Brieger, H. (1960b). Basic Physiologic Mechanisms in the Pulmonary Response to Inhaled Particulates. Proc. 13th Int. Congr. Occup. Health, pp. 730–735.

LaBelle, C. W., Brieger, H., Goddard, J. W., Rastatter, K. A., and Zinger, B. L. (1960). Retention and effect of radioactive particulates in the lung. Am. Ind. Hyg. Assoc. J., 21:195–200.

Lackey, R. W. (1949). Observations on the acute and chronic toxicity of toxaphene in the dog. J. Ind. Hyg. Toxicol., 31:117–120.

LaDu, B. N., Gaudette, L., Trousof, N., and Brodie, B. B. (1955). Enzymatic dealkylation of aminopyrine (Pyramidon) and other alkylamines. J. Biol. Chem., 214:741–752.

Lal, H., Puri, S. K., and Fuller, G. C. (1970). Impairment of hepatic drug metabolism by carbon tetrachloride inhalation. Toxicol. Appl. Pharmacol., 16:35–39.

Laug, E. P., and Fitzhugh, O. G. (1946). 2,2-Bis-(p-chlorophenyl) 1,1,1-trichloroethane (DDT) in the tissues of the rat following oral ingestion for periods of six months to two years. J. Pharmacol. Exp. Ther., 87:18–23.

Laug, E. P., and Kunze, F. M. (1951). Effect of carbon tetrachloride on toxicity and storage of methoxychlor in the rat. Fed. Proc., 10:318.

Lauger, P., Pulver, R., and Montigel, C. (1945). Uber die Wirkungsweise von 4,4'-Dichlordiphenyltrichlormethylmethan (DDT-Geigy) im Warmbluter Organismus. Helv. Physiol. Acta, 3:405–415.

Lautenbach, B. F. (1877). On a new function of the liver. Philadelphia Med. Times, 7:387–394.

Laws, E. R., Jr. (1966). Route of absorption of DDVP after oral administration to rats. Toxicol. Appl. Pharmacol., 8:193–196.

Laws, E. R., Jr., Curley, A., and Biros, F. J. (1967). Men with intensive occupational exposure to DDT. A clinical and chemical study. Arch. Environ. Health, 15:766–775.

Leduc, S. (1900). Introduction des substances médicamenteuses dans la profondeur des tissus par le courant électrique. Ann. Electrobiol., 3:545–560.

Lehman, A. J. (1956). The minute residue problem. Assoc. Food Drug Officials US Quart. Bull., 20:95–99.

Leibman, K. C. (1968). Actions of insecticides on drug activity. Int. Anesthesiol. Clin., 6:251–260.

Levy, G., O'Reilly, R. A., Aggeler, P. M., and Keech, G. M. (1970). Pharmacokinetic analysis of the effect of barbiturate on the anticoagulant action of warfarin in man. Clin. Pharmacol. Ther., 11:372–377

Lieberman, J., Mittman, C., and Gordon, H. W. (1972). Alpha₁ antitrypsin in the livers of patients with emphysema. Science, 175:63–65.

Lisk, D. J. (1970). The analysis of pesticide residues: new problems and methods. Science, 170:589–593.

Long, W. H., Newsom, L. D., and Mullins, A. M. (1961). Endrin residues in the fat of lambs grazed on endrin-treated pasture. J. Econ. Entomol., 54:605–606.

Ludewig, S., and Chanutin, A. (1946). Distribution of 2,2-(p-chlorophenyl)-1,1,1-trichlorethane (DDT) in tissues of rats after its ingestion. Proc. Soc. Exp. Biol. Med., 62:20–21.

Ludwig, G., Weis, J., and Korte, F. (1964). Excretion and distribution of aldrin-^{14}C and its metabolites after oral administration for a long period of time. Life Sci., 3:123–130.

Lund, M. (1964). Resistance to warfarin in the common rat. Nature, 203:778.

Lund, M. (1967). Resistance of rodents to rodenticides. World Rev. Pest Control, 6:131–138.

Lynn, G. E., Shrader, S. A., Hammer, O. H., and Lassiter, C. A. (1963). Grain fumigant residues: occurrence of bromides in the milk of cows fed sodium bromide and grain fumigated with methyl bromides. J. Agric. Food Chem., 11:87–91.

McCollister, D. D., Beamer, W. H., Atchison, G. J., and Spencer, H. G. (1950). Studies with low vapor concentrations of carbon tetrachloride labeled with carbon 14. I. Absorption, distribution, and elimination upon inhalation by monkeys. Fed. Proc., 9:300.

McCully, K. A., Villeneuve, D. C., McKinley, W. P., Phillips, W. E. J., and Hidiroglou, M. (1966). Metabolism and storage of DDT in cattle. J. Assoc. Off. Agric. Chem., 49:966–973.

McMahon, R. E. (1963). The demethylation in vitro of N-methyl barbiturates and related compounds by mammalian liver microsomes. Biochem. Pharmacol., 12:1225–1228.

Maibach, H. I., Feldmann, R. J., Milby, T. H., and Serat, W. F. (1971). Regional variation in percutaneous penetration in man. Arch. Environ. Health, 23:208–211.

Malkinson, F. D. (1958). Studies on the percutaneous absorption of C[14] labeled steroids by use of the gas-flow cell. J. Invest. Dermatol., 31:19–28.

Malkinson, F. D., and Rothman, S. (1962). Percutaneous absorption. In: Normale und Pathologische Physiologie der Haut I, edited by A. Marchionini and H. W. Spier, Vol. 1, Part 3, pp. 90–156. Springer Verlag, Berlin.

March, R. B., Metcalf, R. L., Fukuto, T. R., and Maxon, M. G. (1955). Metabolism of Systox in the white mouse and American cockroach. J. Econ. Entomol., 48:355–363.

Mattson, A. M., Spillane, J. T., Baker, C., and Pearce, G. W. (1953). Determination of DDT and related substances in human fat. Anal. Chem., 25:1065–1070.

Mazel, P., Henderson, J. F., and Axelrod, J. (1964). S-demethylation by microsomal enzymes. J. Pharmacol. Exp. Ther., 143:1–6.

Metcalf, R. L. (1955). Organic Insecticides—Their Chemistry and Mode of Action. Interscience Publishers, Inc., New York.

Mick, D. L., Long, K. R., Dretchen, J. S., and Bonderman, D. P. (1971). Aldrin and dieldrin in human blood components. Arch. Environ. Health, 23:177–180.

Miller, E. C., Miller, J. A., and Conney, A. H. (1954). On the mechanism of the methylcholanthrene inhibition of carcinogenesis by 3'-methyl-4-dimethylaminoazobenzene. Cancer Res., 51:32.

Mitchell, L. C. (1961). The effect of ultraviolet light (2537 Å) on 141 pesticide chemicals by paper chromatography. J. Assoc. Off. Agric. Chem., 44:643–704.

Mitoma, C., Posner, H. S., Reitz, H. C., and Udenfriend, S. (1956). Enzymatic hydroxylation of aromatic compounds. Arch. Biochem., 61:431–441.

Morgan, D. P., and Roan, C. C. (1971). Absorption, storage, and metabolic conversion of ingested DDT and metabolites in man. Arch. Environ. Health, 22:301–308.

Morgan, D. P., and Roan, C. C. (1972). Loss of DDT from storage in human body fat. Nature, 238:221–223.

Morgan, D. P., Roan, C. C., and Paschal, E. H. (1972). Transport of DDT, DDE, and dieldrin in human blood. Bull. Environ. Contam. Toxicol., 8:321–326.

Mörsdorf, K., Ludwig, G., Vogel, J., and Korte, F. (1963). Die Ausschiedung von Aldrin-C[14] und Dieldrin-C[14] sowie ihrer Metaboliten durch die Galls. Med. Expt., 8:90–94.

Moss, J. A., and Hathway, D. E. (1964). Transport of organic compounds in the mammal. Partition of dieldrin and telodrin between the cellular components and soluble proteins of the blood. Biochem. J., 91:384–393.

Moubry, R. J., Myrdal, G. R., and Sturges, A. (1968). Residues in food and feed. Rate of decline of chlorinated hydrocarbon pesticides in dairy milk. Pestic. Monit. J., 2:72–79.

Mountain, J. T. (1963). Detecting hypersusceptibility to toxic substances. Arch. Environ. Health, 6:357–365.

Murphy, S. D., and DuBois, K. P. (1957). Quantitative measurement of inhibition of the enzymatic detoxification of malathion by EPN (ethyl p-nitrophenyl thionobenzene phosphonate). Proc. Soc. Exp. Biol. Med., 96:813–818.

Murphy, S. D., and DuBois, K. P. (1958). The influence of various factors on the enzymatic conversion of organic thiophosphates to anticholinesterase agents. J. Pharmacol. Exp. Ther., 124:194–202.

Nabb, D. P., Stein, W. J., and Hayes, W. J., Jr. (1966). Rate of skin absorption of parathion and paraoxon. Arch. Environ. Health, 12:501–555.

Neal, R. A. (1967). Studies on the metabolism of diethyl 4-nitrophenyl phosphorothionate (parathion) *in vitro*. Biochem. J., 103:183–191.

Neal, R. A. (1972). A comparison of the *in vitro* metabolism of parathion in the lung and liver of the rabbit. Toxicol. Appl. Pharmacol., 23:123–130.

Neal, R. A., and DuBois, K. P. (1965). Studies on the mechanism of detoxification of cholinergic phosphorothioates. J. Pharmacol. Exp. Ther., 148:185–192.

Netter, K. J., and Seidel, G. (1964). An adaptively stimulated O-demethylating system in rat liver microsomes and its kinetic properties. J. Pharmacol. Exp. Ther., 146:61–65.

Norris, W. P., and Kisieleski, W. (1948). Comparative metabolism of radium, strontium, and calcium. Cold Spring Harbor Symp. Quant. Biol., 13:164–172.

Norris, W. P., Tyler, S. A., and Brues, A. M. (1958). Retention of radioactive bone-seekers. Science, 128:456–462.

O'Brien, R. D. (1960). *Toxic Phosphorus Esters. Chemistry, Metabolism and Biological Effects.* Academic Press, Inc., New York.

O'Brien, R. D., and Dannelley, C. E. (1965). Penetration of insecticides through rat skin. J. Agric. Food Chem., 13:245–247.

Ophof, A. J., and Langeveld, D. W. (1969). Warfarin-resistance in the Netherlands. Schriftenr. Ver. Wasser. Boden. Lufthyg., 32:39.

O'Reilly, R. A., Aggeler, P. M., Hoag, M. S., Leong, L. S., and Kropatkin, M. L. (1964). Hereditary transmission of exceptional resistance to coumarin anticoagulant drugs. N. Engl. J. Med., 271:809–815.

O'Reilly, R. A., Aggeler, P. M., and Leong, L. S. (1963). Studies on the coumarin anticoagulant drugs: the pharmacodynamics of warfarin in man. J. Clin. Invest., 4:1542–1551.

Ortega, P., Hayes, W. J., Jr., Durham, W. F., and Mattson, A. (1956). *DDT in the Diet of the Rat.* Public Health Monogr., 43:1–27.

Ozburn, G. W., and Morrison, F. O. (1962). Development of a DDT-tolerant strain of laboratory mice. Nature, 196:1006–1010.

Ozburn, G. W., and Morrison, F. O. (1965). The effect of DDT on respiratory metabolism of DDT-tolerant mice (*Mus musculus*). Can. J. Zool., 43:709–717.

Papper, E. M., and Kitz, R. J. (eds.) (1963). *Uptake and Distribution of Anesthetic Agents.* McGraw-Hill, New York.

Peakall, D. B. (1967). Pesticide-induced enzyme breakdown of steroids in birds. Nature, 216:505–506.

Pekas, J. C., and Paulson, G. D. (1970). Intestinal hydrolysis and conjugation of a pesticidal carbamate *in vitro*. Science, 170:77–78.

Peters, R. A. (1952). Lethal synthesis. Proc. R. Soc. [B], 139:143–170.

Peters, R. A. (1963). *Biochemical Lesions and Lethal Synthesis.* Macmillan, New York.

Pillmore, R. E., Keith, J. O., McEwen, L. C., Mohn, M. H., Wilson, R. A., and Ise, G. H. (1963). Cottontail rabbit: feeding test. US Fish Wildl. Serv. Circ., 167:47–50.

Pinkhas, J., Djaldetti, M., Joshua, H., Resnick, C., and DeVries, A. (1963). Sulfhemoglobinemia and acute hemolytic anemia with Heinz bodies following contact with a fungicide—zinc ethylene bisdithiocarbamate—in a subject with glucose-6-phosphate dehydrogenase deficiency and hypocatalasemia. Blood, 21: 484–494.

Pinson, E. A. (1952). Water exchanges and barriers as studied by the use of hydrogen isotopes. Physiol. Rev., 32:123–134.

Piotrowski, J. (1971). *The Application of Metabolic and Excretion Kinetics to Problems of Industrial Toxicology.* US Government Printing Office, Washington, DC.

Poland, A., Goldstein, J., Hickman, P., and Burse, V. W. (1971). A reciprocal relationship between the induction of δ-aminolevulinic acid synthetase and drug metabolism produced by *m*-dichlorobenzene. Biochem. Pharmacol., 20:1281–1290.

Poland, A., Smith, D., Kuntzman, R., Jacobson, M., and Conney, A. H. (1970). Effect of intensive occupational exposure to DDT on phenylbutazone and cortisol metabolism in human subjects. Clin. Pharmacol. Ther., 11:724–732.

Potts, S. F. (1958). *Concentrated Spray Equipment, Mixtures and Application Methods.* Dorland Books, Caldwell, NJ.

Price, H. L., Kovnat, P. J., Safer, J. N., Conner, E. H., and Price, M. L. (1960). The uptake of thiopental by body tissues and its relation to the duration of narcosis. Clin. Pharmacol. Ther., 1:16–22.

Puyear, R. L., and Paulson, G. D. (1972). Effect of carbaryl (1-naphthyl *n*-methylcarbamate) on pentobarbital-induced sleeping time and some liver microsomal enzymes in white leghorn cockerels. Toxicol. Appl. Pharmacol., 22:621–627.

Quinn, G. P., Axelrod, J., and Brodie, B. B. (1958). Species, strain and sex differences in metabolism of hexobarbitone, amidopyrine, aminopyrine, and aniline. Biochem. Pharmacol., 1:152–159.

Radeleff, R. D., Claborn, H. V., Wells, R. W., and Nickerson, W. J. (1952). Effects on beef cattle of prolonged treatment with a DDT spray. J. Vet. Med., 47:94–96.

Radomski, J. L., and Davidow, B. J. (1953). The metabolite of heptachlor, its elimination, storage and toxicity. J. Pharmacol. Exp. Ther., 107:266–272.

Rapoport, S. I., Hori, M., and Klatzo, I. (1971). Reversible osmotic opening of the blood-brain barrier. Science, 173:1026–1028.

Rappolt, R. T. (1970). Use of oral DDT in three human barbiturate intoxications: CNS arousal and/or hepatic enzyme induction by reciprocal detoxicants. Ind. Med. Surg., 39:319.

Remmer, H. (1958). Die Beschleunigung des Evipanabbaues unter der Wirkung von Barbituraten. Naturwissenchaften, 45:189.

Riegelman, S., Rowland, M., and Epstein, W. L. (1970). Griseofulvin-phenobarbital interaction in man. J. A. M. A., 213:426–431.

Robertson, J. S. (1957). Theory and use of tracers in determining transfer rates in biological systems. Physiol. Rev., 37:133–154.

Robinson, D. S., and MacDonald, M. G. (1966). The effect of phenobarbital administration on the control of coagulation achieved during warfarin therapy in man. J. Pharmacol. Exp. Ther., 153:250–253.

Robinson, J. (1969). The burden of chlorinated hydrocarbon pesticides in man. Can. Med. Assoc. J., 100:180–191.

Robinson, J., and Roberts, M. (1968). Accumulation, distribution and elimination of organochlorine insecticides by vertebrates. Soc. Chem. Ind. Monogr., 29:106–119.

Robinson, J., Roberts, M., Baldwin, M., and Walker, A. I. T. (1969). The pharmacokinetics of HEOD (dieldrin) in the rat. Food Cosmet. Toxicol., 7:317–332.

Rothe, C. F., Mattson, A. M., Nueslein, R. M., and Hayes, W. J., Jr. (1957). Metabolism of chlorophenothane (DDT): intestinal lymphatic absorption. A. M. A. Arch. Ind. Health, 16:82–86.

Sedlak, V. A. (1965). Solubility of benzene hexachloride isomers in rat fat. Toxicol. Appl. Pharmacol., 7:79–83.

Sellers, E. M., and Kock-Weser, J. (1970). Displacement of warfarin from human albumin by diazoxide and ethacrynic, mefenamic, and nalidixic acids. Clin. Pharmacol. Ther., 11:524–529.

Sellers, E. M., Lang, M., Koch-Weser, J., and Colman, R. W. (1972). Enhancement of warfarin-induced hypoprothrombinemia by triclofos. Clin. Pharmacol. Ther., 13:911–915.

Shepherd, J. B., Moore, L. A., Carter, R. H., and Poos, F. W. (1949). The effect of feeding alfalfa hay containing DDT residue on the DDT content of cow's milk. J. Dairy

Sci., 32:549–555.

Sher, S. P. (1971). Drug enzyme induction and drug interactions: literature tabulation. Toxicol. Appl. Pharmacol., 18:780–834.

Skog, E., and Wahlberg, J. E. (1964). A comparative investigation of the percutaneous absorption of metal compounds in the guinea pig by means of the radioactive isotopes: ^{51}Cr, ^{58}Co, ^{65}Zn, ^{110m}Ag, ^{115m}Cd, ^{203}Hg. J. Invest. Dermatol., 43:187–192.

Slater, T. F., and Delaney, V. B. (1971). The effects of various drugs and toxic agents on bile flow rate and composition in the rat. Toxicol. Appl. Pharmacol., 20:157–174.

Smith, R. F., Hoskins, W. M., and Fullmer, O. H. (1948). Secretion of DDT in milk of dairy cows fed low-residue alfalfa hay. J. Econ. Entomol., 41:759–763.

Solomon, H. M., and Schrogie, J. J. (1967). Effect of Phenyramidol and bishydroxy-coumarin on the metabolism of tolbutamide in human subjects. Metabolism, 16:1029–1033.

Souček, B., and Vlachová, D. (1960). Excretion of trichloroethylene metabolites in human urine. Br. J. Ind. Med., 17:60–64.

Stewart, R. D., and Dodd, H. C. (1964). Absorption of carbon tetrachloride, trichloroethylene, tetrachloroethylene, methylene chloride, and 1,1,1-trichloroethane through the human skin. Am. Ind. Hyg. Assoc. J., 25:439–446.

Stewart, R. D., Fisher, T. N., Hosko, M. J., Peterson, J. E., Baretta, E. D., and Dodd, H. C. (1972a). Experimental human exposure to methylene chloride. Arch. Environ. Health, 25:342–348.

Stewart, R. D., Fisher, T. N., Hosko, M. J., Peterson, J. E., Baretta, E. D., and Dodd, H. C. (1972b). Carboxyhemoglobin elevation after exposure to dichloromethane. Science, 176:295–296.

Stewart, R. D., Gay, H. H., Erley, D. S., Hake, C. L., and Schaffer, A. W. (1961). Human exposure to tetrachloroethylene vapor. Arch. Environ. Health, 2:516–522.

Stickel, L. F., Chura, N. J., Stewart, P. A., Menzie, C. M., Prouty, R. M., and Reichel, W. L. (1966). Bald eagle pesticide relations. In: Transactions of the Thirty-first North American Wildlife and Natural Resources Conference, edited by J. P. Trefethen, pp. 190–204. Wildlife Management Institute, Washington, DC.

Stickel, L. F., and Stickel, W. H. (1969). Distribution of DDT residues in tissues of birds in relation to mortality, body condition, and time. Ind. Med. Surg., 38:91–100.

Stickel, W. H., Stickel, L. F., and Coon, F. B. (1970). DDE and DDD residues correlated with mortality and experimental birds. In: Pesticides Symposia, edited by W. B. Deichmann, pp. 287–294. Halos and Associates, Inc., Miami.

Stickel, W. H., Stickel, L. F., and Spann, J. W. (1969). Tissue residues of dieldrin in relation to mortality in birds and mammals. In: Chemical Fallout: Current Research on Persistent Pesticides, edited by M. W. Miller and G. G. Berg, pp. 174–204. Charles C. Thomas, Springfield, Ill.

Stokinger, H. E., and Mountain, J. T. (1967). Progress in detecting the worker hypersusceptible to industrial chemicals. J. Occup. Med., 9:537–542.

Stokinger, H. E., Mountain, J. T., and Scheel, L. D. (1968). Pharmacogenetics in the detection of the hypersusceptible worker. Ann. NY Acad. Sci., 151:968–976.

Strauss, B. S. (1960). An Outline of Chemical Genetics. W. B. Saunders Company, Philadelphia.

Straw, J. A., Waters, I. W., and Fregly, M. J. (1965). Effect of o,p'-DDD on hepatic metabolism of pentobarbital in rats. Proc. Soc. Exp. Biol. Med., 118:391–394.

Street, J. C. (1964). DDT antagonism to dieldrin storage in adipose tissue of rats. Science, 146:1580–1581.

Street, J. C., and Chadwick, R. W. (1967). Stimulation of dieldrin metabolism by DDT. Toxicol. Appl. Pharmacol., 11:68–71.

Street, J. C., Mayer, F. L., and Wagstaff, D. J. (1969).

Ecological significance of pesticide interactions. Ind. Med. Surg., 38:409–414.

Street, J. C., Wang, M., and Blau, A. D. (1966). Drug effects on dieldrin storage in rat tissue. Bull. Environ. Contam. Toxicol., 1:6–15.

Szakall, A. (1952). Uber den Stand der Hautphysiologischen Forschung als Beitrag zu einem zielbewussten Arbeitsschutz. Arch. Dermatol. Syph. (Berlin), 194:376–391.

Szakall, A. (1955). Uber die Eigenschaften, Herkunft und physiologischen Funktionen der die H-Ionenkonzentration bestimmenden Wirkstoffe in der verhornten Epidermis. Arch. Klin. Exp. Dermatol., 201:331–360.

Tabershaw, I., and Cooper, W. C. (1966). Sequelae of organic phosphate poisoning. J. Occup. Med., 8:5–20.

Tainter, M. L., and Ferris, A. J. (1969). Aspirin in Modern Therapy. Bayer Company Division of Sterling Drug, Inc., New York.

Tauber, O. E., and Hughes, A. B. (1950). Effect of DDT ingestion on total cholesterol content of ovaries of white rat. Proc. Soc. Exp. Biol. Med., 75:420–422.

Telle, H. J. (1971). Resistance to warfarin of the brown rat (R. norvegicus) in Germany. WHO/VBC/71.331.

Tregear, R. T. (1964). The permeability of skin to molecules of widely-differing properties. In: Progress in the Biological Sciences in Relation to Dermatology, edited by A. Rook and R. H. Champion, Vol. 2, pp. 275–281. Cambridge University Press, London.

Tregear, R. T. (1966). Physical functions of skin. In: Molecular Movement, The Permeability of Skin, edited by R. T. Tregear, pp. 1–52. Academic Press, Inc., London.

Treherne, J. E. (1956). The permeability of skin to some non-electrolytes. J. Physiol., 133:171–180.

Truhaut, R., Vitte, G., and Boussemart, E. (1952). Recherches sur la toxicologie du pentachlorophénol. III. Etude des intoxications expérimentales aiguë et chronique chez le lapin. Influence de l'état rénal. Arch. Mal. Prof., 13:570–574.

Udall, J. A. (1969). Drug interference with warfarin therapy. Am. J. Cardiol., 23:143.

Upholt, W. M., Quinby, G. E., Batchelor, G. S., and Thompson, J. P. (1956). Visual effects accompanying TEPP-induced miosis. A. M. A. Arch. Ophthalmol., 56:128–134.

Vinson, S. B., Boyde, C. E., and Ferguson, D. E. (1963). DDT resistance in the mosquito fish (Gambusia affinis). Science, 139:217–218.

Wagner, J. G. (1967). Drug accumulation. J. Clin. Pharmacol., 7:84–88.

Wagner, J. G. (1971). Biopharmaceutics and Relevant Pharmacokinetics, Ed. 1. Drug Intelligence Pub., Hamilton, Ill.

Wagner, J. G., Northam, J. I., Alway, C. D., and Carpenter, O. S. (1965). Blood levels of drug at the equilibrium state after multiple dosing. Nature, 207:1301–1302.

Wagstaff, D. J., and Short, C. R. (1971). Induction of hepatic microsomal hydroxylating enzymes by technical piperonyl butoxide and some of its analogs. Toxicol. Appl. Pharmacol., 19:54–61.

Wagstaff, D. J., and Street, J. C. (1970). Dieldrin-DDT interactions in guinea pigs. Toxicol. Appl. Pharmacol., 17:276.

Walker, A. I. T., Stevenson, D. E., Robinson, J., Thorpe, E., and Roberts, M. (1969). The toxicology and pharmacodynamics of dieldrin (HEOD). Two-year oral exposures of rats and dogs. Toxicol. Appl. Pharmacol., 15:345–373.

Wallach, D. F. H., and Gordon (1968). Lipid protein interactions in cellular membranes. Fed. Proc., 27:1263–1268.

Ware, G. W., and Gilmore, L. O. (1959). Lindane in milk from sprayed cows. J. Econ. Entomol., 52:349–350.

Wasicky, R., and Unti, O. (1945). Dicloro-difenil-trichloroetano (DDT). Ulteriores pesquisas sobre as suas propriedades e aplicacoes. Arq. Hig. Sao Paulo, 10:49–64.

Wattenberg, L. W. (1971). Studies of polycyclic hydrocarbon hydroxylases of the intestine possibly related to cancer. Effect of diet on benzpyrene hydroxylase activity. Cancer, 28:99–102.

Webb, J. L. (1963). *Enzyme and Metabolic Inhibitors,* Vol. 1. Academic Press, Inc., New York.

Webb, R. E., and Horsfall, F., Jr. (1967). Endrin resistance in the Pine mouse. Science, 156:1762.

Weikel, J. H., Jr. (1956). The role of biliary excretion in the metabolism of methoxychlor [1,1,1-trichloro 2,2-bis (*p*-methoxychlor) ethane] in the rat. J. Pharmacol. Exp. Ther., 116:60–61.

Welch, R. M., and Coon, J. M. (1964). Studies on the effect of chlorcyclizine and other drugs on the toxicity of several organophosphate anticholinesterases. J. Pharmacol. Exp. Ther., 143:192–198.

Welch, R. M., and Harrison, Y. (1966). Reduced drug toxicity following insecticide treatment. Pharmacologist, 8:217.

Welch, R. M., Harrison, Y., and Burns, J. J. (1967). Hemorrhagic crises in the dog caused by dicumarol-phenobarbital interaction. Fed. Proc., 26:568.

Welch, R. M., Levin, W., Kuntzman, R., Jacobson, M., and Conney, A. H. (1971). Effect of halogenated hydrocarbon insecticides on the metabolism and uterotropic action of estrogens in rats and mice. Toxicol. Appl. Pharmacol., 19:234–246.

Werk, E. E., Jr., MacGee, J., and Sholiton, J. L. (1964). Effect of diphenylhydantoin on cortisol metabolism in man. J. Clin. Invest., 43:1824–1835.

Werle, E., and Uschold, E. (1948). Über fermentative Nicotinen giftung durch tierisches Gewebe. Biochem. Z., 318:531–537.

Williams, R. T. (ed.) (1959). Detoxication mechanisms. In: *The Metabolism and Detoxication of Drugs, Toxic Substances and Other Organic Compounds,* Ed. 2. John Wiley & Sons, Inc., New York.

Winteringham, F. P. W., Bridges, P. M., and Hellyer, G. C. (1955). Mode of insecticidal action studied with labeled systems. Phosphorylated compounds in the muscle of the adult housefly, *Musca domestica.* L. Biochem. J., 59:13–21.

Winteringham, F. P. W., and Harrison, A. (1956). Study of anticholinesterase action in insects by a labelled pool technique. Nature, 178:81–83.

Winteringham, F. P. W., and Hellyer, G. C. (1954). Effects of methylbromide, ethylenedibromide, and ethylenedichloride on phosphorus metabolism of *Musca domestica* L. Biochem. J., 58:xlv.

Winteringham, F. P. W., Loveday, P. M., and Hellyer, G. C. (1953). Phosphorus metabolism in the housefly *Musca domestica.* Biochem. J., 55:xxxiii–xxxiv.

Wolf, J. (1939). Die innere Struktur der Zellen des Stratum desquamativum der menschlichen Epidermis. Z. Mikrosk. Anat. Forsch., 46:170–202.

Wong, D. T., and Terriere, L. C. (1965). Epoxidation of aldrin, isodrin, and heptachlor by rat liver microsomes. Biochem. Pharmacol., 14:375–377.

Woodard, G., Ofner, R. R., and Montgomery, C. M. (1945). Accumulation of DDT in the body fat and its appearance in the milk of dogs. Science, 102:177–178.

World Health Organization (1971). *Application and Dispersal of Pesticides: Eighteenth Report of the WHO Expert Committee on Insecticides.* WHO Tech. Rep. Ser. No. 465.

Wright, A. S., Potter, D., Wooder, M. F., Donninger, C., and Greenland, R. D. (1972). Effects of dieldrin on mammaliam hepatocytes. Food Cosmet. Toxicol., 10:311–322.

Young, R. W., Miller, L. I., Hardison, W. A., and Engel, R. W. (1959). Bromide level of cows' milk as influenced by feeding peanut vines produced on soil fumigated with ethylene dibromide. Toxicol. Appl. Pharmacol., 1:384–390.

Zampaglione, N., Jollow, D. G., Mitchell, J. R., Stripp, B., Hamrick, M., and Gillette, J. R. (1973). Role of detoxifying enzymes in bromobenzene-induced liver necrosis. J. Pharmacol. Exp. Ther., 187:218–227.

Zweig, G., Smith, L. M., Peoples, S. A., and Cox, R. (1961). DDT residues in milk from dairy cows fed low levels of DDT in their daily rations. J. Agric. Food Chem., 9:481–484.

4

GENERAL PRINCIPLES: NATURE OF INJURIES AND TESTS FOR THEM

The expression, "mode of action," is used with different shades of meaning, depending partly on the nature of the action, but largely on the extent of our knowledge. Some compounds cause so many chemical changes and such diffuse injury that it is meaningless to select one specific action as most important. For these compounds the mode of action must be described in general terms.

When the action of a chemical is specific and our knowledge is relatively complete, "mode of action" refers to the inhibition of a critical enzyme or some other change at the molecular level. To emphasize its essentially chemical nature, such an injury is spoken of as a biochemical lesion (see Section 4.1.2). When the toxicity of a compound can be explained in this elegant way, the fact that it causes respiratory failure, hemolytic anemia, or some other disorder of form or function, is viewed as a manifestation of its basic action.

Some chemicals affect the function of a tissue or the structure of a particular kind of cell in a way so specific that—in the absence of any clue to its chemical basis—the observed change must be spoken of as the mode of action. However, each observation of this sort speaks for itself, and constitutes a challenge to discover the underlying physical or chemical mechanism that must exist.

Each exploration offers the hope not only of understanding the action of a particular chemical, but also of acquiring a better knowledge of the function of the normal body. Claude Bernard (1857) referred to toxic substances as kinds of physiological instruments more delicate than our mechanical ones, and destined to dissect, so to speak, one by one, the properties of the anatomical elements of the living organism. Based on this point of view, the second portion of this chapter offers a number of examples of highly specific, but in many instances unexplained, changes induced by chemicals (see Section 4.2).

4.1 Mode of Action

Just as important as how a compound produces injury is the question of the degree of reversibility of the injury. This question is considered mainly in Section 2.1.2.2 but is mentioned again here, because if we knew enough about the mode of action of each compound we presumably could predict its reversibility. Actually, such prediction is rarely possible and each compound ought to be tested directly.

In discussing mode of action, it must be pointed out that irreversibility of chemical action does not always lead to irreversibility of toxic action. For example, the drug echothiopate iodide causes essentially irreversible inhibition of cholinesterase, but it can be used therapeutically at appropriate dosage because the enzyme is replaced at a sufficiently rapid rate. Supposedly all compounds characterized by such a strong tendency to cause chronic toxicity that only one dose is sufficient, are also characterized by irreversible chemical reaction with some critical receptor. However, this generalization is unproved, because the mode of action of such compounds is poorly understood.

On the other hand, compounds that apparently cause only reversible chemical reactions can, if given in high dosage for a sufficient time, produce irreversible damage. Alcohol is an example.

4.1.1 Nonspecific Actions

4.1.1.1 Corrosive Action. Some compounds in suitable concentrations are corrosive poisons that denature proteins or cause other irreversible damage to any cell they contact. Examples include strong acids and alkalies, phenols, halogens, and the ions of heavy metals. The injuries they cause are meaningfully spoken of as chemical burns, for they are similar to thermal burns, and are resolved in much the same way by a surviving animal.

Although corrosive action is a drastic form of toxicity, many of the compounds that produce it are easily detoxified or excreted if presented in low concentration, and some, such as hydrochloric acid and iodine, are essential to normal function of the body.

Some other materials, notably the heavy metals, that are corrosive at higher concentrations are also highly toxic at low dosages. Lead, for example, affects many enzymes and tissues. Once a person has been poisoned by lead, it seems necessary only to make a new examination in order to find a previously undiscovered abnormality. Thus it was possible to demonstrate abnormality of thyroid function (Sandstead *et al.*, 1969b) and kidney function (Sandstead *et al.*, 1969a) among men who were clinically recovered from earlier lead poisoning.

4.1.1.2 Ferguson's Principle. Ferguson (1939) proposed the separation of toxic actions into two main classes—physical and chemical—and suggested that they be distinguished according to the ratio called the thermodynamic activity or chemical potential of each compound. He thus unified many earlier observations of lesser scope regarding the relationship between toxicity and some physical properties of certain toxic compounds. The application of the chemical potential to drug action has come to be known as Ferguson's principle.

Many organic vapors (eg, most hydrocarbon and chlorinated hydrocarbon solvents and alcohols) have activities in the range of 0.1 to 1.0 when the measurements are made under conditions in which the vapors are equally insecticidal or bacteriocidal, and in the range of about 0.01 to 0.1 under conditions in which they are equally narcotic; these compounds are considered to act physically. Some other compounds (eg, hydrogen cyanide and ammonia) have activities less than 0.001, even when measured at lethal concentrations; these compounds are considered to act chemically.

The thermodynamic activity of a compound can be estimated from any of the physical relationships listed in the second paragraph below. However, the relationship always involves a ratio. A conveniently determined ratio is that between the partial pressure just adequate to produce the observed effect and the saturation pressure under the same conditions of temperature and pressure—in other words, the relative humidity required to produce the characteristic toxic action. Another conveniently measurable ratio for estimating thermodynamic activity is that between the molar concentration of a solution just capable of producing a specific toxic effect and the molar concentration of a saturated solution under the same conditions.

It is characteristic of compounds acting physically that the action (*a*) reaches its maximum very rapidly after exposure begins, (*b*) remains at the same level of intensity while the organism is in contact with a constant, tolerated concentration, and (*c*) disappears rapidly when exposure is stopped. This behavior leads to the conclusion that an equilibrium must exist between the concentration of the substance in the external phase and its concentration at the site of action, no matter where that is. Since the thermodynamic activity or chemical potential must be the same in all phases involved in an equilibrium, it is possible to estimate it in the toxic solution or vapor to which an animal is exposed, with assurance that it is the same at the point of attack within the organism. By this procedure, the disturbing effect of phase distribution is eliminated from the comparison of toxicities of those compounds that exhibit the kind of equilibrium just described. Even though such compounds exert the same toxic action on a given kind of organism at widely different concentrations, the activities corresponding to these concentrations lie within a relatively narrow range. Thus, a series of normal primary alcohols kill the typhoid bacillus at concentrations ranging from 10.8 M (methyl) to 0.0034 M (octyl), but the corresponding activities range only from 0.33 (methyl) to 0.88 (octyl). This relatively small change in activity, increasing as the series is ascended, is generally observable in homologous series. However, if the rate of increase is maintained and the series is ascended far enough, the activity will reach 1.0, indicating saturation, and succeeding members of the series will show declining toxicity, simply because not enough of these compounds can be made available to the receptor to cause the characteristic action. This is the phenomenon of "cutoff" in the toxicity of a homologous series.

The thermodynamic activity or chemical potential of a compound may be estimated not only from vapor pressure and solubility, but also from adsorption, partition coefficient between water and oil, or the concentration reducing the surface tension of water. All of these properties vary in a parallel way for compounds in a homologous series. This means that the mere fact that a compound acts physically is not an argument that its action depends on fat solubility, or that it takes place at a lipid interface. The physical relationship offers no way to distinguish which of the related properties is critical in a particular instance. Thus, the exact mode of action must be sought by additional study. Although not mentioned by Ferguson, the physical phenomenon under discussion would seem not to exclude a biochemical action, but merely to indicate that the physical relationship is rate limiting. Certainly the phenomenon of physical action does not exclude the possibility that a single compound may have more than one action. In fact, the range of thermodynamic activity characteristic of a particular action of a homologous series of compounds can be shown to be even more narrow, if secondary actions can be distinguished and excluded (Brink and Posternak, 1948). The question of whether physical or chemical action will mask the other depends on the compound and the circumstances. The specificity of a compound that acts physically may be determined by its capacity to reach the site of action.

4.1.2 Specific Action

Most chemicals, whether toxicants or drugs, do not act physically, as judged by Ferguson's principle. Their effects appear at much lower concentrations relative to saturation than is true of nonspecific compounds, suggesting that they are much too potent to be merely solvents or foreign bodies. Some of these compounds react chemically with a known enzyme or a critical molecule such as hemoglobin, and their action on the body can be explained in terms of

this reaction with the specific receptor. In many other instances, no specific receptor is known, although it is supposed by analogy that one must exist.

Inherent in the concept of specific toxic action is the idea that this action is essentially chemical in nature, and that the initial injury is a chemical one. The term *biochemical lesion* was introduced by Peters and his colleagues (Gavrilescu and Peters, 1931) to convey this idea in connection with thiamine deficiency. In this deficiency, the biochemical lesion is quickly and completely reversible if corrected early, but it leads to permanent chemical and structural changes if permitted to persist. However, since its introduction, the term, biochemical lesion, has been applied to irreversible as well as reversible chemical injuries. Furthermore, the term is used to describe injuries caused by an excessive concentration of any chemical, as well as injuries caused by a deficiency of an essential nutrient. The book by Peters (1963), in which the concept of the biochemical lesion is elaborated fully, stands as a landmark in the history of toxicology.

4.1.2.1 Enzymes. The mere fact that a compound influences one or more enzymes does not necessarily explain its mode of action. To be meaningful, there must be appropriate qualitative and quantitative relationships between the enzymatic change and the change of body function which it is supposed to explain. In other words, the degree of enzyme change observed in affected animals must cause the observed degree and kind of functional change, and must do so even when the inhibition is produced by another mechanism. Furthermore, the compound must produce the specific enzymatic change *in vivo* when given in appropriate doses. The literature is full of reports of the *in vitro* inhibition of enzymes by high concentrations of compounds that produce *in vivo* effects at lower concentrations, but with no known relation to the enzyme in question.

Only a few biochemical lesions are clearly established. Of these, several involve the inhibition of enzymes including (a) SH-enzymes by arsenic, (b) acetylcholinesterase by organic phosphorus compounds and certain carbamates, and (c) cytochrome oxidase by cyanide ion. Almost in the same classification are the inhibition of oxidative phosphorylation by triethyltin and rotenone, and the uncoupling of this same phosphorylation by dinitrophenols and related compounds. The difficulty is that the relation of inhibition of oxidative phosphorylation to clinical effect remains unclear because of the wide variety of clinical effects involved. Although uncoupling of this phosphorylation is consistently associated with one clinical syndrome, the details of enzyme change leading to uncoupling remain obscure.

Knowledge of a biochemical lesion may suggest steps for its correction. Specific antidotes that repair the injury caused by arsenic and organic phosphorus compounds, respectively, were developed by application of information about their biochemical effects. A description of these and some other specific antidotes is given in Chapter 8.

Inhibition of SH-Enzymes by Arsenic. Arsenic inhibits pyruvate oxidase and the phosphatases. The blood level of pyruvate increases in poisoned animals or people. There is a reduction of tissue respiration leading to a wide range of functional and some morphological changes. Many other sulfhydryl-containing enzymes are involved also, and it is impossible to assign relative importance to them. However, studies on antidotes have made it clear that chemical reaction of trivalent arsenic with sulfhydryl groups, including those in susceptible enzymes, is the biochemical lesion (Peters, 1952). The fact that the same enzyme system is involved explains why there is considerable similarity between the polyneuropathy caused by arsenic and that associated with beriberi. Trivalent arsenic inhibits the pyruvate oxidase system through combination with —SH group of the enzyme itself, while thiamine deficiency deprives the system of an essential coenzyme.

Inhibition of Cytochrome Oxidase by Cyanide. The cyanide ion inhibits many enzymes, most but not all containing either iron or copper. The most sensitive of these enzymes is cytochrome oxidase, which is essential to tissue respiration. Cytochrome oxidase is 50% inhibited by a 10^{-8} M cyanide concentration. Inhibition of cytochrome oxidase prevents oxidation of reduced cytochrome C and, therefore, stops the use of oxygen by cells (Dixon and Webb, 1958).

Action of Anticholinesterases. The function of acetylcholinesterase is to hydrolyze acetylcholine. The initial, reversible complex formed between acetylcholinesterase and some organic phosphorus compounds, for example the drug echothiopate, is entirely analogous to that between the enzyme and its normal substrate. Most organic phosphorus pesticides lack a positive charge in the acidic group. These compounds react with the esteratic site on the acetylcholinesterase molecule but not with the anionic site. No matter whether the anionic site is involved or not, the splitting off of the esterifying group of the organic phosphorus compound is entirely analogous to the splitting off of choline from acetylcholine. However, the bond between the phosphorus atom and the esteratic site of the enzyme is firmer than the bond between the carbon atom of acetate and the same enzyme site. Spontaneous breaking of the phosphorus-enzyme bond requires hours to weeks, depending on the compound involved. Breaking of the carbon-enzyme bond from acetylcholine is complete in a few microseconds (Wilson, 1951). Thus, the phosphorylated enzyme is inhibited because its active site is occupied and, therefore, incapable of carrying out its normal function.

The anticholinesterase carbamates used as pesticides or as drugs carbamylate acetylcholinesterase and thus inactivate it. The chemical bond in this instance is intermediate in stability between that in the phosphorylated enzyme and the acetylated enzyme. Thus, poisoning by carbamates usually is briefer than that caused by organic phosphorus compounds.

The signs and symptoms caused by anticholinesterases are similar and are explained by the inhibition of acetylcholinesterase, which constitutes the biochemical lesion. Inhibition of the enzyme permits an abnormal accumulation of acetylcholine; a minimal excess causes (a) excessive activity of the parasympathetic system (miosis, sweating, profuse secretions in the upper respiratory tract, abdominal cramps and discomfort in chest from overactivity of smooth muscle, and nausea, vomiting, and diarrhea); (b) central nervous system effects (headache, giddiness, and nervousness); and (c) overreactivity of the voluntary muscles (fasciculations). A further accumulation of acetylcholine tends to increase the parasympathetic and central nervous system signs, but causes profound weakness of the muscles.

Knowledge of the phosphorylation of acetylcholinesterase permitted the development of oximes that greatly increase the rate at which the chemical bond to phosphorus is split and active enzyme is released (see Section 8.2.3.3).

4.1.2.2 Critical Molecules. Enzymes are protein catalysts to promote the interaction of two compounds that would occur anyway, but often at an infinitesimally slow rate in the absence of the enzyme. The reactions promoted by enzymes are both anabolic and catabolic. Other critical molecules promote the transfer of other molecules but, unlike enzymes, do not lead to the production of one or more new compounds. These critical molecules are similar to enzymes in regulating rate of change without themselves being consumed in the process.

Inactivation of Hemoglobin. The best example of a toxic action in which the receptor is a critical molecule is the combination of carbon monoxide with hemoglobin to form carboxyhemoglobin, which is incapable of transporting oxygen from the lungs to the tissues. The affinity of hemoglobin for carbon monoxide is between 210 and 300 times greater than its affinity for oxygen, the exact factor depending on pH of the blood and partial pressure of carbon dioxide (Lilienthal *et al.*, 1946; Joels and Pugh, 1958). As a result, when the concentration of carbon monoxide in air is only 0.1%, half of the hemoglobin in the blood will be in the form of carboxyhemoglobin and only half in the form of oxyhemoglobin. Furthermore, the presence of carboxyhemoglobin alters the dissociation of oxyhemoglobin so that the remaining oxyhemoglobin is somewhat less efficient in transporting oxygen. This explains why a person with 50% carboxyhemoglobin is at a greater disadvantage than an anemic person with only 50% the normal amount of hemoglobin. The result of carbon monoxide poisoning is hypoxia of the tissues, leading to acute cardiac dilatation and nerve damage.

4.1.2.3 Membranes. The crucial importance of membranes in determining the transfer and availability of chemicals in the body is discussed in Section 3.2.1.1. The following paragraphs concern membranes as possible sites of toxic action.

At least in theory, chemicals may act by altering the properties of a living membrane. Such action could be considered a special case of interaction with a critical molecule. However, no single kind of receptor molecule has been clearly identified in this situation. Furthermore, living membranes are certainly complex (see Section 3.2.1.1). The interference of a chemical with the permeability of a membrane might depend on physical change consistent with Ferguson's principle and involve alteration in the relationship of the molecules in the membrane, instead of a chemical reaction strictly limited to one kind of molecule.

One theory of the action of anesthetics, including some hydrocarbon and chlorinated hydrocarbon solvents used as pesticides, is that their depressant action is the result of a change in membrane permeability. The best understood toxic action on a living membrane is that involving the axon, but chemicals also can change conductance in a synthetic membrane. The potassium conductance which is induced by 10^{-6} M valinomycin in a lecithin-decane membrane is reversed by 3×10^{-6} M DDT. Such membranes not treated with valinomycin are not affected by DDT. This blockade of potassium conductance in a synthetic membrane parallels the effect of DDT on axonic conduction. Dieldrin and lindane, whose physiological actions are in some ways like those of DDT, do not affect valinomycin-induced conductance of lecithin-decane membranes (Hilton and O'Brien, 1970).

Derangement of the Sodium and Potassium Gates of the Nerve Axon. At least since the work of Domenjoz (1944), it has been known that DDT affects the nervous system. As a result of the classical work of Hodgkin and his colleagues (1949, 1958), it is known that each impulse along the axon is caused by: (*a*) a wave of permeability to sodium ions, which permits sodium to enter the axon rapidly and to produce a depolarization of the axon; and later, but separately, (*b*) a wave of permeability to potassium ions, which permits potassium to leave the axon rapidly and, thus, to restore the original polarization of the membrane. In 1960, Narahashi and Yamasaki (1960) found that the effect of DDT on the giant axons of the cockroach is limited to the recovery phase of the action potential, which is abnormally prolonged. They concluded that DDT influences the efflux of potassium ions from the axon, and added further evidence by showing that the effect of DDT could be accentuated by lowering the concentration of potassium ions in fluid surrounding the nerve. Later work by Narahashi and Haas (1967) showed that the action of DDT on giant axons of the lobster is more complex than formerly supposed. Investigations with the voltage clamp technique showed that DDT, at a concentration of 5×10^{-4} moles per liter of bathing medium, prolongs the flow of sodium ions as well as interfering with the flow of potassium ions; in other words, DDT delays shutting of the Na^+ gate and prevents full opening of the K^+ gate.

Matsumura and Patil (1969) showed that under certain conditions, DDT at concentrations as low as 10^{-8} M inhibits Na^+-, K^+-, and Mg^{2+}-adenosine triphosphatase derived from a nerve ending fraction of the rabbit brain. This enzyme is involved in ion transport in the nervous system. There is a good correlation between the degree of its inhibition by analogs of DDT and their toxicity to mosquito larvae. (Incidentally, inhibition of the different ATPase preparations studied by Koch (1969) showed no such correlation.)

Both the electrophysiological changes and the enzyme inhibition exhibit a negative temperature coefficient, an important feature of DDT poisoning in insects. It remains to be seen how the enzyme inhibition is related to the electrophysiological changes, particularly since Holan (1971) has shown that the toxic action of DDT analogs depends on a critical range of size of the cross section of the aliphatic side chain of the molecules, suggesting that this side chain has a critical physical relation to pores in the axonal membrane that serve as "gates." There is also some question whether the action of DDT is exactly the same in vertebrates as in arthropods. It is true that the symptomatologies in the two forms are as similar as the anatomical differences would seem to permit. Furthermore, the smallest toxic intravenous dosage in mammals is not greatly different from the smallest toxic dosage in arthropods (Hayes, 1959). However, it is reported that the effect of DDT on the vertebrate nerve is augmented rather than suppressed by potassium ions (Eyzaguirre and Lilienthal, 1949), and the temperature coefficient is not negative (Hoffman and Lendle, 1948; Deichmann et al., 1950).

4.2 Effects on Cells and Tissues

All of the pharmacological effects of drugs are examples of highly specific actions of chemicals—mainly foreign compounds—on the biochemistry of the body. It is sometimes said that all actions of drugs (except those that are nutrients) are toxic. For example, stimulation may be caused by suppression of a natural inhibitory mechanism. Be that as it may, drug actions, insofar as they are understood, serve to reveal underlying, normal functions. However, as mentioned in the introduction to this chapter, it was toxic substances in the ordinary sense that Claude Bernard thought of as "dissecting the properties of the anatomical elements of the living organism." Pesticides constitute a substantial proportion of all toxic substances found useful for this kind of study.

The following sections offer examples of toxic effects where the chemical mode of action often is unknown but the effects appear highly specific. The list is intended to illustrate the tremendous variety of astonishingly distinctive actions already recognized, and to suggest the challenge for finding the biochemical lesion corresponding to each one. The specificity of some of the effects (notably mutagenesis, carcinogenesis, and especially teratogenesis) may be more apparent than real, but a brief discussion of these phenomena and of their clinical implications is required anyway.

4.2.1 Cells

All toxic injuries to the body involve cells. Excluding such gross effects as physical and chemical burns, many toxic injuries are relatively specific for a particular kind of cell, and hence for the particular organ or tissue in which that kind of cell occurs. Some biochemically highly specific injuries, such as inhibition of respiration by the cyanide ion, affect all cells. Some other injuries, notably mutagenesis and carcinogenesis, potentially affect essentially any kind of cell and, therefore, any organ or tissue.

Although mutagenesis and carcinogenesis are certainly not understood, there is some evidence that both involve changes in DNA. One theory links the two by viewing carcinogenesis as a special form of mutagenesis. It has long been known that malignant neoplasms often have abnormal mitotic figures. Tyzzer (1916) may have been the first to propose that somatic mutation is involved in the origin of cancer. This concept was reinforced by Boveri (1929), who suggested that, regardless of how it arose, an abnormal chromosome complex would produce a tumor. The entire early history of the concept was reviewed by Strong (1949). The present status is that the molecular mechanism of action of no carcinogen (chemical, viral, or physical) is understood, and the molecular phenotype of no neoplasm is known. Carcinogens react with many cell constituents, but the critical target has not been identified and may be multiple. Many compounds that are carcinogenic in one system are mutagenic in another. However, there are many exceptions, and even where correspondence exists there is no proof that the same target is involved (Miller and Miller, 1971). In the relatively small proportion of instances in which both tests are carried out in the same species it cannot be argued that the difference is caused by a failure to activate an administered material or to inactivate that material or an active metabolite. In spite of the recognized lack of complete correspondence between carcinogens and mutagens, it is a fact that many of the active forms of both are electrophilic. On this basis, Miller and Miller (1971) suggested that mutagenic activity in a host-mediated test (which is relatively brief and cheap) be considered as one factor in selecting compounds for carcinogenic testing (which is necessarily prolonged and expensive).

4.2.1.1 Spindle Poisoning. The best known spindle poison is colchicine. Concentrations as low as 0.001 ppm are capable of inactivating spindles in tissue cultures (Bucher, 1945). However, some organisms such as Chlamydomonas are resistant, requiring concentrations as high as 2,000 ppm (Cornman, 1942).

The main use of colchicine is as a drug to treat gout. In an acute attack, the drug is usually given orally at the rate of 0.5 mg/hour. The total dose usually required to relieve an attack is 4 to 8 mg (about 0.057 to 0.114 mg/kg), and it is recommended that patients continue to take from 0.25 to 2.0 mg/day prophylactically. Toxicity can occur, but it is usually the result of overdosage and is generally neither so serious nor so frequent as to require discontinuation of the drug at an appropriate dosage (Woodbury, 1965).

The therapeutic and toxic levels, however, are close. Man may be highly sensitive, for one death was reported following a dose of 7 mg (Woodbury, 1965).

Neither the therapeutic effect on gout nor the toxic effects, with the possible exception of the blood dyscrasias, are related to the antimitotic action of colchicine. However, in addition to their other effects, toxic doses do stop mitosis at metaphase because these doses interfere with formation of the mitotic—or miotic—spindle. The first detailed autopsy in a fatal human case following discovery of the action of colchicine on cell division (Dustin, 1941), showed an abnormally high percentage of metaphase plates in the bone marrow, lymph glands, spleen, intestinal glands, liver, kidney, and both exocrine and endocrine tissues of the pancreas. The victim had survived 8 days following ingestion of 60 mg of colchicine with suicidal intent. Doses of the same order of magnitude (about 1 mg/kg) are used experimentally to disrupt spermatogenesis in mice.

Rotenone, an insecticide derived from derris, is also a spindle poison at concentrations ranging from 1×10^{-7} M to 1×10^{-5} M (Meisner and Sorensen, 1966).

The action of colchicine and rotenone on the spindle are special instances of the effects of chemicals on microtubules in living cells. This broader subject was reviewed in detail by Behnke (1970).

4.2.1.2 Mutagenesis.

The Nature of Mutation. By definition, mutation is a change of the genetic composition in a somatic or a germ cell. In this sense, the effect is specific. However, both the degree and the quality of the change are subject to variation. Two major kinds of genetic change are recognized. A *point mutation* involves a single gene and does not interfere otherwise with the integrity of the chromosome of which the gene is a part. From a genetic standpoint, knowledge that a gene exists depends on knowledge of at least two alternate forms, spoken of as alleles. Some genes are known to have more than two alternate forms. Many point mutations have been shown to be reversible. Back mutation was first reported by Timofeeff-Ressovsky (1929); it has since been found that the spontaneous rates for mutation and back mutation of a particular gene are generally different. Thus, in the absence of selection, a gene will occur chiefly in its most stable state. From a molecular standpoint, point mutations are conceived of as substitutions of base pairs, or the addition or deletion of as many as three base pairs.

A *chromosome aberration* is any change in the presence or morphology of a chromosome. One or more chromosomes may be lost as a result of abnormal cell division. Chromosomes that should separate at cell division may fail to do so, with the result that one daughter cell lacks a chromosome and the other has an extra one. Individual chromosomes are subject to deletion or addition of a portion, or to inversion or translocation of a segment without loss of material.

Both point mutations and chromosome aberrations are spontaneous. Their rates of occurrence differ from one species to another. In a given species, their rate of occurrence can be increased by shortwave radiation (Muller, 1927), increased temperature (Muller, 1928), or certain chemicals. The importance of the effect of chemicals was not fully realized at the time of the first report (Lobashow, 1937), and full realization awaited the work of Auerbach and Robson (1947a, 1947b). Infection has not been found to induce mutation unless one chooses to view carcinogenesis as a form of infection. Although radiation and chemicals may increase the rate of genetic change and even change the relative frequency of point mutations and chromosome aberrations, the kind of change produced is not altered. Furthermore, it is not always clear whether increased rate of genetic change is caused by direct action on genetic material, or is the indirect effect of injury to the normal repair mechanisms that are now beginning to be understood. An interesting review of the ways in which living cells repair their genetic material is that of Hanawalt (1972).

Mammals are not immune to chemical mutagenesis. Thirteen mutations involving coat color were reported by Strong (1945) among the untreated descendants of mice receiving methylcholanthrene. An extension of the same study revealed many additional mutations; the total mutation rate in the experimental animals was 1 in 557 compared with 1 in 26,250 in the colony (Strong, 1947). At about the same time, four mutants were produced by injecting mice with 1,2,5,6-dibenzanthracene (Carr, 1947).

Although one heritable recessive mutation in a mouse was reported (Auerbach and Falconer, 1949) in connection with studies of an alkylating agent, these compounds produce few point mutations. They do produce many dominant lethals or rearrangements in mice. This situation is opposite to that found in fruit flies; the difference has been interpreted as indicating the possible presence of a more efficient repair mechanism in mammals. It is easy to show that when male mammals are treated with certain alkylating agents they either produce no sperm, produce sperm incapable of generating a viable embryo, or produce young that are infertile to some degree. The rate is not one in several hundred but several in each litter. The kind of injury depends on the compound and the dosage, and is sometimes highly specific. A remarkable example of specificity is offered by busulfan and certain other members of a series of dimethanesulfonates of the form $CH_3-SO_2-O-(CH_2)_n-O-SO_2-CH_3$. At a suitable dosage, the n-1 analog acts on very late cells in spermatogenesis so that sterility occurs during the 1st week after dosage (Fox and Jackson, 1965). The n-2 analog acts on cells of intermediate age, producing sterility during the 2nd to 10th weeks following dosage. The n-4 analog (busulfan or Myleran®) acts on early cells only, producing sterility during the 7th and subsequent weeks after dosage (Jackson, 1964). It is thought that all these injuries are genetic, being caused by dominant lethal mutations, mainly chromosome aberrations.

An ingenious system for studying the *in vivo* incorporation of thymidine, uridine, and L-leucine into the DNA, RNA, and protein of different spermatogenic cells, and measurement of the incorporated material following separation of the different types of cells by the velocity sedimentation techniques, has been described by Lee and Dixon (1972). The system may be used to study animals pretreated with toxic compounds.

It recently has been shown that, under the conditions of study, semisterility of mice caused by tepa was associated with translocations (Epstein *et al.*, 1971). Lethality and sterility are self-limiting. Even semisterility is not heritable for more than a few generations, at most. Under these circumstances it is difficult to interpret the results of available tests. Of course, dosages capable of causing dominant lethals ought to be avoided. However, in practice this may not be restrictive; compounds studied so far that produce dominant lethals have other objectionable traits that limit their use.

Valuable general summaries of what is known about chemical mutagens are contained in books by Fishbein *et al.* (1970) and Hollaender (1971). A collection of essays on mutagenesis, mainly in lower forms, contains much of interest (Sobels, 1969).

Pesticides Studied as Mutagens. Pesticides and chemosterilants that have been studied as mutagens have been tabulated (Fishbein *et al.*, 1970; Epstein and Legator, 1971; Kalter, 1971). The tables include negative as well as positive findings in a wide range of tests.

Inheritance in Man. It has been known since ancient times that living organisms are subject to variation, and that some of this variation is inherited from one generation to another. The science of genetics has done much to explain how this transmission of differences occurs. Any observed condition may be determined by a single kind of gene, either in heterozygous or homozygous state, or it may be determined by multiple genes. Most of the genetically determined characteristics we value in domestic plants or animals depend on multiple gene effects. The same probably is true of man, but our knowledge is limited by the kinds of genetic observations that can be made. Some desirable features of domestic animals and plants depend on a single kind of gene.

There are excellent techniques for determining whether an observed human familial difference is or is not conditioned by one or a very few autosomal or sex-linked genes (Burdette, 1962; Hogben, 1946). Many genetically determined conditions are now known; they range from differences (such as those of eye color or blood group) that imply little or no advantage for survival, to differences that are fatal.

Many of the recognized human genetic differences, whether neutral or harmful in effect, have different frequencies in different racial groups or in people from different areas, such as the Mediterranean area. This distribution implies ancient origin. There is no reason to think that there has been any basic change in the picture. Of course, genes may be subject to selection; in limited populations they may be subject to the effects of inbreeding or outbreeding; in sufficiently small populations they are subject to genetic drift.

In spite of the large number of human conditions known to be genetic, the origin of none of them has been traced to radiation or to a chemical. The evidence from studies of lower organisms leaves no doubt that such origin is possible, but offers no hint about its probable frequency or importance.

Most human familial diseases and oddities, whose inheritance is understood, are based on point mutations. However, one important, potentially heritable condition involving multiple defects is known to involve an extra chromosome. Mongolism is evident in all who have the chromosomal defect. Since the affected persons rarely reproduce, the condition generally arises in each generation. However, its environmental cause, if any, is not known. The condition has been recognized for at least a century (Down, 1866), and it occurs in nonindustrial countries as well as in others.

It has been reported recently that a higher

proportion of lymphocytes cultured from nine persons with increased levels of mercury in their red blood cells may have shown chromosome breaks, than were present in similar lymphocyte-derived cells from four controls. The degree of difference failed to reach statistical significance, but a significant rank correlation was present. It was supposed that the mercury in the blood came from the eating of fish, rather than any contact with pesticides. Most of the persons studied were healthy, and the significance of the findings is unknown (Skerfving et al., 1970).

4.2.1.3 Carcinogenesis. The cause of neoplasia is unknown, but its incidence can be increased by radiation, viral infection, defective immune response, and at least some chemicals. The production of cancer by nearly pure compounds was reported in 1930, and the production by pure compounds was reported by the same team of investigators in 1932; the compounds were 1,2,5,6-dibenzanthracene (Heiger, 1930; Kennaway, 1930, Cook et al., 1932) and 6-isopropyl-1,2-benzanthracene (Cook, 1932).

There is no way at this time to exclude the possibility that every chemical is carcinogenic for some species under appropriate circumstances. Certainly, a number of pesticides have been reported to have this property, often when given in massive dosage. Table 4-1 lists compounds that have been studied specifically for tumorigenesis, as well as those found to cause tumors, regardless of the design of the study leading to the discovery. Thus, the table is biased in favor of positive results. In fact, some of the studies of carcinogenesis are themselves heavily biased by the selection of compounds for study that were suspect because of chemical resemblance to proved carcinogens, or for some other reason. All pesticides that may be used on food crops in such a way that they leave a finite residue at harvest have received 2-year studies in a rodent. This kind of study has served to reveal a tumorigenic tendency in a number of compounds, and they are included in Table 4-1. The value of conventional, long-term toxicity studies for identifying carcinogens has been recognized by those who specialize in the study of cancer (Shubik, 1970). Tests designed specifically for identifying carcinogens may differ from other long-term studies by using: (a) more experimental animals; (b) more highly susceptible strains; (c) higher dosages; (d) more prolonged administration, often beginning at weaning or before; and, sometimes, (e) artificial routes of administration. Such tests are of value in attempts to associate carcinogenesis scientifically with chemical structure, but they are extremely difficult to interpret in connection with any hazard to man.

As discussed in Section 2.3.4, the compounds known to induce cancer differ in the dosage required to do so, but the effect is always dosage-related. Chemical carcinogenesis may be influenced by any of the factors that influence toxicity generally (see Section 2.4). Of particular importance in evaluating the possible effect of multiple environmental exposures is the laboratory study of interaction between two or more compounds. A few materials are known to promote the action of certain carcinogens in specific tissues. This phenomenon of cocarcinogenesis is discussed in all general references on carcinogenesis. Apparently, this form of potentiation is as uncommon as potentiation generally. Certainly, studies of the interaction of carcinogens indicate slightly less than an additive effect (Deichmann et al., 1965). In a similar way, a study of certain pesticides (Aramite®, DDT, methoxychlor, thiourea, and aldrin) indicates slight antagonism (Deichmann et al., 1967).

Chemical Carcinogenesis in Man. It has been known since antiquity that people are subject to cancer and other malignant neoplasms. While always serious, this group of diseases has been of particular importance as a cause of morbidity and mortality since diseases known to be of infectious origin, and some of metabolic origin, were brought under improved control. Neoplastic disease now rates second in importance as a cause of death in the United States, approximately 16% of all mortality being due to this cause (see Table 7-1).

It is well established that ionizing radiation can increase the incidence of cancer in people. So far, it has not been proved that viruses induce cancer in man, although they do so in animals, and an epidemic of Hodgkin's disease spreading like an infection has been observed (Vianna et al., 1972). Furthermore, persons with certain congenital defects of their immune responses and those whose immune responses have been suppressed by drugs (eg, to permit organ transplants) have an increased susceptibility to cancer.

The fact that environmental exposure to a material can increase the incidence of a cancer was discovered in man. Potts (1775) reported that chimney sweeps were far more subject than other men to cancer of the scrotum. They were put to work as boys, and such was the intensity of their exposure that the cancer often appeared at puberty.

Materials found to cause cancer in man have proved carcinogenic in animals, but not in all species, or by any single or simple technique.

Table 4–1

Results of Studies of the Relation of Pesticides to Tumors

Compound	Species and sex	Dosage [a] (mg/kg/day)	Result	Reference
Inorganic and organometal pesticides				
cacodylic acid	mouse	15 – 46	not tumorigenic	Innes et al., 1969
phenyl mercuric acetate	mouse	3 – 24	not tumorigenic	Innes et al., 1969
fentin acetate	mouse	0.18 – 0.46	not tumorigenic	Innes et al., 1969
Pesticides derived from plants and other organisms				
rotenone	mouse	0.4 1.0	not tumorigenic	Innes et al., 1969
	rat	0.1 – 0.5	tumorigenic	Lehman, 1952
gibberellic acid	mouse	160-464	not tumorigenic	Innes et al., 1969
Synergists				
piperonyl butoxide	mouse	37-100	questionably tumorigenic	Innes et al., 1969
piperonyl butoxide in solvent	mouse	138-464	not tumorigenic	Innes et al., 1969
piperonyl butoxide with dichlorodifluoromethane	mouse	3,333 [b]	tumorigenic	Epstein et al., 1967
piperonyl sulfoxide	mouse	14-46	questionably tumorigenic	Innes et al., 1969
n-propylisome	mouse	744-2,000	not tumorigenic	Innes et al., 1969
sesame oil	mouse	10,000 [c]	tumorigenic	Morton and Mider, 1939
	mouse	12,000 [d]	tumorigenic	Dickens and Weil-Malherbe 1942
	mouse	20,000	not tumorigenic	Steiner, 1942
Fumigants and nematocides				
dichloroethyl ether	mouse	37-100	tumorigenic	Innes et al., 1969
calcium cyanamide	mouse	30-100	questionably tumorigenic	Innes et al., 1969
diphenatrile	mouse	69-215	not tumorigenic	Innes et al., 1969
Chlorinated hydrocarbon insecticides				
BHC	mouse, M	84	tumorigenic	Nagasaki et al., 1971 Nagasaki et al., 1972
	mouse, M	< 8.4	not tumorigenic	Nagasaki et al., 1971
β-BHC	mouse	26	tumorigenic	Thorpe and Walker, 1973
γ-BHC	mouse	52	tumorigenic	Thorpe and Walker, 1973
DDT and related compounds				
DDT, technical	rat	4.5-5.3	tumorigenic	Fitzhugh and Nelson, 1947
	rat, M	≥ 0.2-0.7	tumorigenic	Ortega et al., 1956
	rat, F	10.5	tumorigenic	Ortega et al., 1956
	rat, F	2-6	not tumorigenic	Ortega et al., 1956
	mouse	0.4-0.7	tumorigenic	Tarjan and Kemeny, 1969
	mouse	5.5	antitumorigenic	Laws, 1971
	mouse	15,000	not tumorigenic	Gargus et al., 1969
	mouse, M	2-250	tumorigenic	Tomatis et al., 1972
	mouse, F	10-250	tumorigenic	Tomatis et al., 1972
	mouse	0.25-33	tumorigenic	Tomatis, Turusov, Day, and Charles, 1972
	mouse	6.2-13.3	tumorigenic	Walker, Thorpe, and Stevenson, 1972
	mouse	12.4-13.3	tumorigenic	Thorpe and Walker, 1973
p, p'-DDT	mouse	0.4-0.7	tumorigenic	Innes et al., 1969
p, p'-DDD	mouse	37-100	questionably tumorigenic	Innes et al., 1969
o, p'-DDD	mouse	69-215	questionably tumorigenic	Innes et al., 1969
chlorobenzilate	mouse	75-215	tumorigenic	Innes et al., 1969
Perthane ®	mouse	101-215	questionably tumorigenic	Innes et al., 1969
Cyclodienes and related compounds				
aldrin	mouse	1.24-1.33	tumorigenic	Davis and Fitzhugh, 1962
dieldrin	mouse	1.24-1.33	tumorigenic	Davis and Fitzhugh, 1962
	mouse	0.01-2.6	tumorigenic	Walker, Thorpe, and Stevenson, 1972

Table 4–1 (continued)

Compounds	Species and sex	Dosage [a] (mg/kg/day)	Result	Reference
endosulfan	mouse	1.3	tumorigenic	Thorpe and Walker, 1973
endosulfan	mouse	0.37-1.0	not tumorigenic	Innes et al., 1969
isobenzan	mouse	0.08-0.22	not tumorigenic	Innes et al., 1969
mirex	mouse	3.2-10	tumorigenic	Innes et al., 1969
terpene polychlorinates	mouse	1.3-4.6	tumorigenic	Innes et al., 1969
Carbamates and related pesticides				
N-methyl carbamates				
carbaryl	mouse	1.7-4.6	questionably tumorigenic	Innes et al., 1969
isolan	mouse	0.007-0.022	not tumorigenic	Innes et al., 1969
Zectran ®	mouse	1.4-4.6	questionably tumorigenic	Innes et al., 1969
Other carbamates and thiocarbamates				
chloropropham (CIPC)	mouse	138-464	not tumorigenic	Innes et al., 1969
di-allate	mouse	69-215	tumorigenic	Innes et al., 1969
pebulate	mouse	40-100	not tumorigenic	Innes et al., 1969
propham (IPC)	mouse	70-215	not tumorigenic	Innes et al., 1969
Dithiocarbamates				
copper dimethyldithio-carbamate	mouse	21-46	not tumorigenic	Innes et al., 1969
ferbam	mouse	4-10	not tumorigenic	Innes et al., 1969
maneb	mouse	19-46	not tumorigenic	Innes et al., 1969
nabam	mouse	9-22	not tumorigenic	Innes et al., 1969
thiram	mouse	3.2-10	not tumorigenic	Innes et al., 1969
zineb	mouse	161-467	not tumorigenic	Innes et al., 1969
ziram	mouse	1.9-4.6	not tumorigenic	Innes et al., 1969
Phenolic and nitrophenolic pesticides				
dinocap	mouse	0.7-1.0	not tumorigenic	Innes et al., 1969
dihitrobutyphenol	mouse	0.9-2.2	not tumorigenic	Innes et al., 1969
pentachlorophenol	mouse	16-46	not tumorigenic	Innes et al., 1969
2,4,6-trichlorophenol	mouse	32-100	questionably tumorigenic	Innes et al., 1969
p-phenyphenol	mouse	173-464	not tumorigenic	Innes et al., 1969
o-phenyphenol	mouse	35-100	not tumorigenic	Innes et al., 1969
2,2-thiobis (4,6-dichlorophenol)	mouse	14-46	questionably tumorigenic	Innes et al., 1969
Miscellaneous pesticides				
Aramite ®	mouse	138-464	tumorigenic	Innes et al., 1969
Aramite ®	dog	18-32	tumorigenic	Sternberg et al., 1960
	rat	9.5-19.5	tumorigenic	Popper et al., 1960
	rat	78-250	tumorigenic	Oser and Oser, 1960
	rat	9.5-19.5	tumorigenic	Oser and Oser, 1962
	mouse	25-50	questionably tumorigenic	Oser and Oser, 1962
	dog	11-26	tumorigenic	Oser and Oser, 1962
	dog	34	questionably tumorigenic	Oser and Oser, 1962
chlorfenson	mouse	126-464	not tumorigenic	Innes et al., 1969
Genite ®	mouse	297-1,000	not tumorigenic	Innes et al., 1969
phenothiazine	mouse	185-464	not tumorigenic	Innes et al., 1969
tetradifon	mouse	32-100	not tumorigenic	Innes et al., 1969
Synthetic organic rodenticides				
antu	mouse	0.7-2.2	not tumorigenic	Innes et al., 1969
ethylene thiourea	mouse	80-215	tumorigenic	Innes et al., 1969
Herbicides and related compounds				
amitrole	mouse	274-1,000	tumorigenic	Innes et al., 1969
atrazine	mouse	10-22	not tumorigenic	Innes et al., 1969
chloroacetic acid	mouse	18-46	not tumorigenic	Innes et al., 1969
2-chloroethyl-trimethyl-ammonium chloride	mouse	8-22	questionably tumorigenic	Innes et al., 1969
2,4-D	mouse	14-100	not tumorigenic	Innes et al., 1969
	mouse	45-77 [e]	antitumorigenic	Walker et al., 1972

Table 4-1 (continued)

Compound	Species and sex	Dosage [a] (mg/kg/day)	Result	Reference
2, 4, 5-D	mouse	7.4-22	not tumorigenic	Innes et al., 1969
	mouse	62-85 [e]	antitumorigenic	Walker et al., 1972
dehydroacetic acid	mouse	30-100	not tumorigenic	Innes et al., 1969
dichlorprop	mouse	3.5-10	not tumorigenic	Innes et al., 1969
dicryl	mouse	9-22	not tumorigenic	Innes et al., 1969
diuron	mouse	174-464	not tumorigenic	Innes et al., 1969
2-hydroxyethylhydrazine	mouse	0.6-215	tumorigenic	Innes et al., 1969
indoleacetic acid	mouse	80-215	not tumorigenic	Innes et al., 1969
maleic hydrazide	mouse	374-1,000	not tumorigenic	Innes et al., 1969
	mouse, rat	500	not tumorigenic	Barnes et al., 1957
	rat	500	not tumorigenic	Barnes et al., 1957
monuron	mouse	64-215	questionably tumorigenic	Innes et al., 1969
1-naphthaleneacetamide	mouse	161-464	not tumorigenic	Innes et al., 1969
naptalam	mouse	64-215	not tumorigenic	Innes et al., 1969
norea	mouse	185-464	not tumorigenic	Innes et al., 1969
propazine	mouse	13-46	not tumorigenic	Innes et al., 1969
silvex	mouse	15-46	not tumorigenic	Innes et al., 1969
simazine	mouse	75-215	not tumorigenic	Innes et al., 1969
Fungicides and related compounds				
anthraquinone	mouse	150-464	not tumorigenic	Innes et al., 1969
azobenzene	mouse	7-22	questionably tumorigenic	Innes et al., 1969
captan	mouse	70-215	not tumorigenic	Innes et al., 1969
chloranil		80-215	questionably tumorigenic	Innes et al., 1969
copper 8-hydroxy quinoline	mouse	347-1,000	not tumorigenic	Innes et al., 1969
dichlone	mouse	3.7-10	not tumorigenic	Innes et al., 1969
dichloran	mouse	75-215	not tumorigenic	Innes et al., 1969
diphenyl	mouse	2.5-64	not tumorigenic	Innes et al., 1969
dodine	mouse	10-22	not tumorigenic	Innes et al., 1969
folpet	mouse	75-215	not tumorigenic	Innes et al., 1969
quintozene	mouse	150-464	tumorigenic	Innes et al., 1969
quinoline	mouse	347-1,000	not tumorigenic	Innes et al., 1969
8-quinolinol	mouse	pellet	tumorigenic	Boyland and Watson, 1956
	mouse	pellet	tumorigenic	Clayson et al., 1958
Chemosterilants				
metepa	rat, M	2.5	tumorigenic	Gaines and Kimbrough, 1966
	" "	0.625	not tumorigenic	Gaines and Kimbrough, 1966
tretamine	mouse	0.37 [e]	tumorigenic	Hendry et al., 1951
	rat	0.1	tumorigenic	Walpole et al., 1954
Repellants and attractants				
chloralose	mouse	3.5-10	not tumorigenic	Innes et al., 1969

a.   Oral except where noted otherwise.
b.   Subcutaneous.
c.   Accompanied by 10 mg/kg/day 3,4-benzypyrene.
d.   Accompanied by 12 mg/kg/day 3,4-benzypyrene.
e.   Intraperitoneal.

It is only relatively recently that it has been possible to produce bronchiogenic cancer in animals with cigarette smoke (Auerbach et al., 1970). The search for animal models and the screening of compounds for carcinogenicity, led to the discovery that many materials are capable of increasing the incidence of tumors in one species or another. Most of the testing has been done in small rodents. Tumors tend to appear in middle or old age, whether the animal has a long or a short life-span. Thus, rodents are more economical than large, long-lived species for cancer research because of low initial cost, low daily maintenance cost, and relatively short maintenance time.

Once a malignant neoplasm has developed, the extent of its differences from normal tissue seems to be limited only by the variety and refinement of the tests used for demonstrating the differences. From a biological standpoint, it is the invasiveness, or even metastasis, of the tumor that is striking. However, the differences extend to such obscure but fundamental properties as magnetic relaxation times. Thus, it has been reported that malignant tumors can be distinguished by nuclear magnetic resonance from both normal tissues and nonmalignant tumors (Damadian, 1971).

Much of the work on chemical carcinogenesis in animals has been done in the hope of gaining understanding of the neoplastic process, and in the implicit faith that this is a single process. It is supposed that this unique process can be characterized eventually in biochemical terms that will apply to all neoplasms in all tissues, in contrast to the necessity to explain the great array of infectious diseases by a corresponding, almost equally long list of diverse pathological organisms, each with its own biochemistry. It is not clear just how this unitary concept is to be related to the neoplasms induced by living organisms— or to the inhibition of chemical carcinogenesis by viral vaccines, as reported by Whitmire and Huebner (1972).

Be that as it may, the fact remains that, in almost all instances in which it is agreed that a chemical compound or mixture has induced cancer in any group of people, the relation was found epidemiologically first, and reproduced more or less faithfully in the laboratory only later. Furthermore, with the exception of a very small proportion of neoplasms of recognized occupational origin, there is little or no correlation of human cancer with industrialization, and therefore with industrial chemicals (Higginson, 1968).

Against this background, it is difficult to evaluate reports that large dosages of some pesticides have induced tumors and occasionally malignant neoplasms in experimental animals. This is especially true of DDT, which not only is reported to cause tumors of the liver in rodents, but also to discourage the transfer of an otherwise uniformly transplantable, lethal tumor in rats (see Table 4-1 for both effects). DDT failed to produce detectable tumors in men who absorbed DDT for 19 years or more at rates hundreds of times higher than those of the general population (Laws et al., 1967). Furthermore, the detection of tumors in these men did not depend exclusively on medical history and physical examination. When it was recognized that the presence of α-fetoprotein in the blood of adults provides evidence for the presence of carcinoma of the liver in man, 33 of the most heavily exposed workmen were examined for this protein; the results were negative for α-fetoprotein in all of them (Slomka, 1973).

For similar reasons, the reports (see Table 4-1) that aldrin and dieldrin are tumorigenic in mice have questionable relevance to man. Review of medical histories and of repeated physical and laboratory examinations, including tests of liver function, has failed to indicate any connection between these compounds and cancer in workers with prolonged occupational exposure (Jager, 1970). Twenty-one of these workers with the longest exposure were tested for α-fetoprotein, all with negative results. The highest concentration of dieldrin encountered

in the blood of these men was 0.190 ppm (Jansen, 1973).

As further evidence for the lack of correspondence between results in mice and people, one may consider the case of phenobarbital. Like dieldrin, it causes liver tumors in mice, and some of the tumors metastasize to the lungs (Walker et al., 1973; Thorpe and Walker, 1973). However, a study based on a complete tumor registry indicated no increase of tumors attributable to phenobarbital among men and women who received the heavy, essentially life-long dosage of this drug necessary for the control of epilepsy (Clemmesen et al., 1974).

4.2.2 Cardiovascular System

4.2.2.1 Blood and Lymph Vessels.

Induced Hypersensitivity to Cold. Extreme hypersensitivity to cold can be induced in a rat by a single subcutaneous injection of carrageenin at rates as low as about 500 mg/kg. In animals so treated, exposure at $-2°C$ for 2.5 hours induces necrotizing thrombohemorrhagic lesions in the nose, paws, and tail, accompanied by bilateral renal cortical necrosis resembling those of the generalized Sanarelli-Schwartzman phenomenon, and associated with high mortality. The lesions are associated with agglutination of erythrocytes and the formation of fibrin thrombi in the veins and capillaries of the nose, paws, and tail and in the glomerular capillaries of the kidney. Hemorrhages occur in the nose, paws, and tail, and perivascularly, in the renal medulla. If, instead of placing the animals in a refrigerated room, they are merely forced to walk on ice for 5 hours in a room of ordinary temperature, the lesions of the paws and tail become evident on the 2nd or 3rd day after injection, but lesions of the nose and kidneys do not occur and there is no mortality (Selye, 1965).

Hyperphagia and Obesity. Intraperitoneal injection of gold thioglucose causes lesions of the ventromedial region of the hypothalamus of mice, leading to hyperphagia and obesity. The size of the brain lesion is dosage-dependent. Convincing evidence has been presented that the action of gold thioglucose is on the rate of blood flow in the affected area and not directly on brain cells. There was no change in blood flow 4 hours after injection, but it was present 5 hours after injection. Following a single dose, the reduction of flow was still present 21 days later, the longest period studied (Arees et al., 1969).

4.2.3 Respiratory System

4.2.3.1 Lungs.

Fibrosis of the Lungs. In most rats, mice, and dogs, and some rabbits killed by a single dose of paraquat by any route, the important lesions are confined to the lungs. These show some consolidation, tend to be plum colored, and often sink in water. In most rats, the microscopic lesion involves proliferation of cells that at first appear as more or less typical fibroblasts arising from the adventitia of the vessels, and the fibrous tissue around the bronchi. This proliferation begins as early as the 3rd day after dosing and is accompanied by edema fluid in many alveoli, perivascular and peribronchial edema, and the presence of polymorphonuclear lymphocytes, mononuclear cells, macrophages, and occasionally, large numbers of eosinophils or a few giant cells. In animals that survive longer, the proliferating cells lose the appearance of fibroblasts, but proliferation continues and mitoses are very numerous. The mesenchymal cells extend into the alveolar walls, and hypertrophy of the epithelial cells of the alveoli contributes to thickening of the septa. In a smaller proportion of rats, epithelial hypertrophy and proliferation of either the alveolar cells, the terminal bronchial epithelium, or both, predominate over the fibrosis. Thus, in a series of animals, the histological pictures were very diverse (Clark et al., 1966; Kimbrough and Gaines, 1970).

The liver and kidney of poisoned rats occasionally show focal necrosis. The adrenals are congested; the thymus and spleen sometimes show lympholysis; the testis may show degenerative changes. None of these changes outside the lungs are adequate to explain death, which is due to gradual failure to aerate the blood.

4.2.4 Gastrointestinal System and Intermediary Metabolism

4.2.4.1 Liver. Partly because of their great importance for biotransformation and excretion, the liver and kidneys often show high concentrations of foreign chemicals or their metabolites. It is not astonishing, therefore, that these organs are more subject than others to chemical injury. It seems likely that each injury is specific, although in our present state of knowledge many of them appear similar. Necrosis followed by hyperplasia, and often by scarring, is common. However, some liver changes are characteristic. The alterations associated with the induction of microsomal enzymes were discussed in Sections 3.1.2.2 and 3.1.2.3. Interesting examples of specificity involve cuprizone and the endotoxin of *Escherichia coli*.

Mitochondria. Giant mitochondria as large as nuclei can be produced consistently in the livers of weanling mice by feeding them cuprizone (bis-cyclohexanone oxaldihydrazone). The compound also produces severe edema and enlargement of glial nuclei in the cerebellum and brain stem; it is not known which lesion is primary. The simplicity of the procedure and the consistency of the results make the feeding of cuprizone a new and useful experimental tool for the study of mitochondrial metabolism. The compound, a chelating agent used for quantitative determination of copper, is fed to the mice at a dietary level of 5,000 ppm (Suzuki, 1968).

Amyloid. One of the curious phenomena of human pathology is the deposition of amyloid, a homogeneous, eosinophilic, fibrillar glycoprotein in various tissues, especially the liver, spleen, and kidney. Its occurrence is generally secondary to chronic suppurative infections (including tuberculosis, osteomyelitis, and bronchiectasis), and sometimes secondary to certain tumors (multiple myeloma). Primary amyloidosis is a rare disease, not preceded by any other recognized illness, and characterized by deposits of amyloid in muscles, especially those of the heart and tongue, and on the endothelial surfaces of the heart and its valves. Amyloid can be induced experimentally by injection of living or killed bacteria, or by the repeated injection of proteins such as casein. However, only a very small dose (as little as 0.1 mg per mouse) of the endotoxin of *E. coli* is required to produce deposit of glycoprotein in mice. Twenty-five doses of 0.005 mg produced splenic amyloid in some white Swiss (G.P.) mice, and 15 doses of 0.5 mg produced it in all of them. Similar rates of administration were less effective in another strain. When the spleen was extensively involved, amyloid was found in the liver and kidneys, also. The glycoprotein may be detected as early as 1 week after dosing begins. Since endotoxin, a lipopolysaccharide, is rapidly localized in the reticuloendothelial system after parenteral injection, it may be that stimulation of the reticuloendothelial cells leads to amyloid production (Barth et al., 1968).

4.2.5 Urinary System

4.2.5.1 Kidneys. The fact that the kidney is subject to injury by a large number of materials has been remarked on already. An interesting example of specificity involves the collecting ducts.

Mitochondria of the Renal Collecting Ducts. Morfamquat dichloride, an herbicide, produces degeneration and necrosis of the proximal convoluted tubules of rats and dogs when administered in acutely toxic doses.

However, when rats are fed the compound at a dietary level of 150 ppm they develop an unusual lesion in the collecting ducts in the medullary-papillary zone, remote from the proximal convoluted tubules, which are of different embryological origin. Many of the cells of these ducts are abnormally large and have a strongly eosinophilic cytoplasm at least as early as 6 weeks after feeding begins (first examination). From the 13th week onward they are shed in small numbers into the lumen, but after 17 weeks of feeding they constitute about 80% of the cells of the affected region. Nuclei usually appear normal, but there are a few binucleate cells. Examination with the electron microscope reveals that the enlarged cells are packed with mitochondria, and there is a corresponding increase of certain enzymes of mitochondrial origin. Some of the mitochondria show constrictions, and some show vacuolation of the cristae and ballooning of the external membrane. There is some evidence that the cellular enlargement and associated increase of mitochondria affect only those cells of the collecting ducts that normally appear dark in electron micrographs. No functional disturbance has been identified with the condition, and the number of abnormal cells gradually declines, presumably as a result of shedding, after administration of morfamquat stops (Ferguson et al., 1969).

4.2.6 Muscles, Supportive Tissues, and Skin

4.2.6.1 Mesothelial Layers.

Acute Pericarditis. Acute pericarditis developed in three of four patients treated for at least 5 days with piscofuranine, a purine nucleoside analog, at rates of 10 mg/kg or higher (Costa et al., 1961). The same result occurred in three of nine other patients treated at a slightly lower rate for 6, 7, and 17 days, respectively (Yates and Olson, 1961). Apparently no animal model for this drug-induced pericarditis has been found.

4.2.7 Nervous System and Sense Organs

4.2.7.1 Central Nervous System.

Microcephaly. Development of the brain was defective in fetal rats whose mothers were injected with methylazoxymethanol at a total rate of 20 mg/kg in three divided doses, given on the 14th, 15th, and 16th days of gestation. All of the surviving young were microcephalic. They all had lower brain weights than control animals. The reduction in size was mostly in the neo- and paleocortex, without a proportionate reduction in brain stem structures and cerebellum. Microscopic inspection revealed no demyelination, gliosis, or inflammation. There

appeared to be some decrease in the number of neurons, particularly in the neocortex and hippocampus, as a result of a cytotoxic effect on neuroblasts in the fetus. The maze performance of the microcephalic rats was substantially and significantly inferior to that of normal ones, even though their learning patterns were similar, and they could not be distinguished by appearance (Haddad et al., 1968).

Hydrocephalus. Aqueductal stenosis and hydrocephalus were produced in 90% of male, weanling, albino Swiss mice that survived 8 weeks of dietary administration of a substituted hydrazine, cuprizone. Signs of illness included convulsions, and the skulls of surviving mice were dome-shaped. In some animals the hydrocephalus was so severe that only a thin mantle of cerebral cortex remained over the dilated lateral ventricles; the third ventricle was affected, also. Stenosis of the aqueduct of Sylvius was the result of pressure on the narrow tube by edematous mesencephalic tissue (Kesterson and Carlton, 1970). As noted in Section 4.2.4.1, the same compound affects mitochondria of the liver.

Mitochondrial Swelling and Axonal Dystrophy. The rodenticide, monosodium fluoroacetate (compound 1080), causes severe convulsions in some species when given by any route. It is generally agreed that its action is due to its conversion to the even more toxic fluorocitrate. Using the injection of only 3 to 50 μg of fluorocitrate into the subarachnoid space of the lumbar cord of the cat, Koenig (1969) showed that within as little as 15 minutes after injection and before the onset of focal convulsions, there is a localized accumulation of reactive lysosomes within the implantation cones and emergent axons. This is accompanied by swelling of the mitochondria in the cell body and its dendrites, but not at that time in the axon. These changes become more marked until and after the onset of convulsions. After convulsions begin, axonal balloons or dilatations develop, usually 3 to 4 hours after a small dose, or 1 to 2 hours after a large dose, and subsequently increase in size and number. The balloons are stuffed with mitochondria (many of which are swollen and degenerating), dense and multilaminated lysosome-like bodies, vesicles and other membranous structures, and neurofibrils. It is known that interference with the respiration-coupled generation of adenosine triphosphate leads to mitochondrial swelling. It is concluded that the mechanism underlying poisoning by fluoroacetate is the swelling of neuronal mitochondria secondary to disturbance of cell respiration, and that the swelling provides the propulsive force to expel cytoplasmic constituents from the cell body into the axon. Thus, the disorganization of the axon is considered secondary to the disgorgement of material from the cell body, and not a "primary axostasis," or obstruction of normal axoplasmic flow.

Mitochondrial swelling associated with axonal dystrophy is observed with several metabolic inhibitors with different modes of action, including cyanide, arsenious oxide, ouabain, and methionine sulfoximine (Koenig, 1969).

4.2.7.2 Peripheral Nervous System.
Both DDT and some anticholinesterases act on the central nervous system as well as on the peripheral system. However, it is their peripheral actions that are best understood. The specificity of these actions on axonal conduction and on acetylcholinesterase was discussed in Sections 4.1.2.3 and 4.1.2.1, respectively.

4.2.7.3 Eye.
Destruction of the Tapetum Lucidum. The intravenous injection of dithizone (diphenylthiocarbazone) at a rate of 100 mg/kg causes blindness in dogs within 24 hours. This dosage leads to destruction of the tapetum lucidum, followed by detachment of the retina. Other species are less susceptible (Weitzel et al., 1954). It is known that dithizone chelates zinc and other metals. The changes in the eye are accompanied, and presumably caused, by a rapid and permanent loss of zinc. It has been speculated that the observed action in dogs is related to the formation of a zinc dithizonate (Vallee, 1959).

Necrosis of the Retinal Ganglion Cells. Subcutaneous administration of monosodium L-glutamate at the rate of 4,000 to 8,000 mg/kg produces an acute degenerative lesion in the inner retina of neonatal mice. Chromatolysis and pyknosis of the nuclei of retinal ganglion cells may be demonstrated 1 hour after dosage (Lucas and Newhouse, 1957).

Cataract. Only a few compounds have produced cataracts under practical, or even under laboratory conditions. A valuable review of these compounds and of the chemical and physical properties that characterize them is that of Gehring (1971).

4.2.8 Endocrine Glands

4.2.8.1 Pancreas.
Diabetes Mellitus. In rabbits, the intravenous injection of dithizone at dosages of 30 to 200 mg/kg produces hyperglycemia in 1 to 2 hours, often followed by hypoglycemia in 8 to 12 hours, and finally, in those that survive, a state of permanent diabetes after 24 hours. Histochemically, the reaction of zinc gradually becomes negative during the acute phase of poisoning. These changes are accompanied by necrosis and disintegration of the beta cells of pancreatic islets. In permanent diabetes of this origin, the islets are reduced in size and number, and consist of alpha cells. Oral administration at a rate of 500 mg/kg causes only a transient hyperglycemia lasting 2 to 3 days (Kodota, 1950).

4.2.8.2 Thyroid.
Cretinism. Dwarfism and mental retardation similar to cretinism in people can be produced in rats by feeding the dams the antithyroid compounds, thiouracil and tricyanoaminopropene, either compound at a dietary level of 1,000 ppm (Davenport, 1970).

4.2.9 Reproductive System

4.2.9.1 Testis.
In some instances, injury to a particular tissue is secondary to injury in the associated blood vessels, but such injury is no less specific or puzzling, under these circumstances. An illustration is the injury to the testis and proximal end of the caput epididymis in rats given a single remote subcutaneous injection of cadmium chloride at a rate of 5.5 mg/kg. That the injury is vascular is shown by a blanching of the affected parts as early as 5 hours after injection, and their deep red-violet color about 48 hours after dosing. Injury restricted to the internal spermatic artery and associated pampiniform venous plexus serving the affected parts is inflammatory, as shown histologically. The injury may be prevented by zinc acetate injected subcutaneously at 100 times the molar rate of the cadmium chloride. Other blood vessels, including those to the main body of the epididymis and the vas deferens, and all vessels to the female reproductive tract, are uninjured by cadmium. Whatever it is in the susceptible blood vessels that makes them react differently from other vessels is under hormonal control. The testes of most mice preconditioned for 7 weeks or more by either of two estrogens were not injured by cadmium chloride (Gunn et al., 1961; 1963).

4.2.10 Embryo and Fetus

4.2.10.1 Teratogenesis.
The word *teratogenesis* is derived from the Greek words *teras*, a monster, and *genesis*, origin. Thus, teratogenesis is the production of freaks or monsters, that is, persons or animals born malformed. By general agreement the word *teratogenesis* refers to deformities resulting from abnormalities of embryonic development. Furthermore, the defects referred to in this way can be detected by inspection of babies or older persons during life, or by observations of their

organs at surgery or autopsy. The same kinds of deformities can be detected in rodent fetuses by direct inspection, or with the aid of a dissecting microscope. Teratogenic malformations are large enough to be visible because they begin during embryonic development, and subsequently are magnified by the growth of the organ involved or of the surrounding tissue. Ordinarily, the word teratogenesis does not include microscopic abnormalities. Many of these, such as sickle cell anemia, are hereditary and do not depend on abnormal embryonic development. The word teratogenesis does not include toxic injury to organs after they are fully formed, even though, if such injury occurs during the fetal period, the result is congenital. Examples of fetal toxicity include most of the malformations seen in congenital syphilis, or congenital injury from methyl mercury. At least some congenital malformations resulting from fetal toxicity may be distinguishable from teratogenic effects only by studies involving embryonic as well as fetal development, to determine when and how they arise. The term *fetal toxicity* designates not only visible injury to organs during the fetal period, but also the complete range of nondeforming injury, ranging from retardation of growth to increased mortality during any part of development. Another term, *inborn errors of metabolism*, is used to cover defects that can be detected biochemically soon after birth. Most inborn errors of metabolism are hereditary and have nothing to do with injury of the individual during its developmental period. An excellent review of teratology, offering far more detail than can be covered in this book, is that of Wilson (1972).

Classes of Teratogens. Injury to the adult organism may have many causes; in a similar way the developing embryo may be injured by: (a) infection; (b) radiation; (c) deprivation of an essential nutrient; (d) excess of a chemical (whether essential or not); and (e) its own genetic background. Although the word teratogenesis usually is restricted to nonheritable injuries, the distinction is somewhat artificial. This becomes apparent when one considers that genetic change may be caused by radiation and certain chemicals. Sterility and semisterility have been demonstrated in the offspring of mammals treated by certain alkylating agents. A few variations of eye color or hair color have been produced by other compounds (see Section 4.2.1.2), and perhaps deforming variations might be produced in the same way. Certainly heritable deformities are recognized, although the cause of the faulty inheritance is unknown.

Since ionizing radiation is an important cause of teratogenesis, it is not astonishing to learn that radiomimetic compounds, notably strongly alkylating compounds, are teratogenic. Since teratogenesis consists of interference with embryonic development, it might be correctly predicted that anything interfering with metabolism, growth, or tissue regulation (such as anoxia, vitamin deficiency, trace element deficiency, and some antibiotics) would be teratogenic. In addition to the classes of materials and other causes already named, there are many compounds that act as teratogens, but for reasons not so apparent. Thus, an excess of vitamin A, as well as a deficiency of it, is teratogenic. Even sodium chloride is teratogenic to rats if administered in sufficient dosage (Nishimura and Miyamoto, 1969). Some teratogens are plant alkaloids or belong to other groups that are often highly poisonous (Keeler, 1969). However, some compounds such as cortisones and salicylates that are extensively used as drugs are teratogenic in one or more experimental animals (Warkany, 1965). Karnofsky (1965) has proposed as a law, which cannot be disproved, that any drug administered at the proper dosage, and at the proper stage, to embryos of the proper species—and these include both vertebrates and invertebrates—will be effective in causing disturbances in embryonic development. Teratogenesis is merely a form of toxicity. Although certain classes of compounds mentioned above are often teratogenic, in the last analysis, each compound must be judged on its own merits in each species.

Relation of Teratogenesis to Toxicity in General. As discussed in Section 2.4.2, any compound is toxic if absorbed in excessive amount. This principle applies to experimental teratogenesis in its broadest sense (see Section 2.3.3). However, a mammalian mother must survive pregnancy, and a bird must survive egg laying and usually incubation, in order for her young to survive. The young, themselves, must survive if teratogenesis *per se* is to constitute a practical problem. Therefore, a compound that causes teratogenesis in a particular species under practical conditions must do so at a dosage that both the mother and the fetus can survive. Thus, suitably increasing dosage levels of a compound capable of causing teratogenesis will produce in groups of mothers: (a) no effect; (b) deformed young; (c) death of embryos; and (d) death of the mothers. What has just been said about this sequence of dosage relationships must be qualified in two ways: (a) the sequence can be changed by direct injection of the mammalian fetus or the bird's egg, or any other technique that artificially spares the mother; and (b) compounds vary greatly in the degree of overlap of their teratogenic and fatal dosage ranges. However, no matter how the dose is administered, and in spite of possible overlapping, there is a narrow *teratogenic zone* in which dosage is sufficient to interfere with specific developmental events without killing all embryos.

Murphy (1965) defined the *litter LD 50* as that dosage which is lethal to a majority of fetuses in 50% of treated mothers. She defined the *maternal LD 50* as that determined in pregnant animals. Defined in this way, it is clear that the litter LD 50 cannot exceed the maternal LD 50 for any given compound and experimental situation. Some idea of the range of variation may be gained by comparing certain antimetabolites. The ratio of litter LD 50 to maternal LD 50 is 1:530 for 6-diazo-5-oxo-L-norleucine, but only 1:6 for aminopterin, and 1:1 for 2-ethylamino-1,3,4-thiadiazole (Murphy, 1965).

The dosage relationships of teratogens and of compounds that exhibit only fetal toxicity tend to be opposite, especially during the latter two-thirds of gestation. During this period, the dosage of teratogens necessary to produce injury of any kind increases markedly as the period of great embryonal susceptibility is passed. During the same period, the dosage of some compounds, notably anticholinesterases, necessary to produce injury actually decreases, because the critical injury is not to cells, but to the integration of the whole organism.

Factors in Teratogenesis. The major factors in chemical teratogenesis include: (a) compound; (b) dosage; (c) species or strain of the mother; (d) genotype of the embryo; and (e) stage of development of the embryo. Temperature and humidity are important in birds. Other factors, including interaction of compounds, that influence toxicity in general may be of some importance here also.

Of all these factors, the one most characteristic of teratology is the stage of embryonic development. Although the zygote, cleavage stages, and early blastula or blastocyst may be killed *in situ* by certain chemicals that the mother survives, exposure of these stages usually produces no teratogenic response, regardless of the nature of the chemical. It has been postulated that this lack of teratogenic response of these very early stages is related to the demonstrated totipotency of the cells involved. It is supposed that if injury is limited enough to permit survival of the embryo, the remaining cells can regulate so that subsequent development is normal. In any event,

teratogenic susceptibility begins at about the time the germ layers are formed. Thus, susceptibility begins at about 8 days in the rat (7 days in connection with actinomycin D), 5 days in the mouse and hamster, 9 days in the rabbit, 10 days in the monkey, and 11 or 12 days in man (Wilson, 1965).

The different organs have periods of particular susceptibility to teratogenesis. This period begins in each organ when chemical differentiation begins, several hours or perhaps days before morphological differentiation is evident. For example, renal anomalies can be induced by irradiating rat embryos on the 9th day, but the first rudiment of the metanephros cannot be seen until the 12th day. The period of susceptibility gradually ends as organogenesis is completed. Injury after this time is not teratogenesis in a strict sense, because the embryonic processes can no longer be interrupted or diverted. Of course, as discussed above, the fetus may still be injured after the organs are formed, but such later injury of normally formed fetal structures is of the types that occur after birth or hatching. The formation of organs is complete in the rat at about the 17th day. With the exception of the external genitalia, organ formation is complete in human embryos at about the end of the 8th week.

The duration of the period of susceptibility is relative to dosage. The smallest dose capable of producing any teratogenesis does so at the time of maximal susceptibility, which for most compounds is 9 days in the rat. A larger dose within the teratogenic range not only will produce a higher incidence of injury at the time of greatest susceptibility, but also will tend to reveal a somewhat longer period of susceptibility. Some of these points are illustrated by Table 4-2, from data of Wilson (1965). Table 4-2 also shows that there may be a parallelism between the rates of malformation and embryonic death resulting from the same dose given on different days of embryonic development. For example, a large dose of actinomycin D produced little or no increase in mortality or deformity when given to rats on the 6th day or the 11th day of pregnancy, even though it produced substantial and about equal percentages of mortality and deformity of the survivors, when given at a high rate on the 7th, 8th, 9th, or 10th day, and when given at an intermediate dosage rate on the 8th, 9th, or 10th day.

The time of greatest susceptibility of an embryo to teratogenesis is simply the time when the greatest number of organs are highly susceptible. However, the susceptibilities of

Table 4–2

Effects of Actinomycin D in Developing Rats

From Wilson (1965) by permission of the University of Chicago Press.

Dos- age	Day of treatment	Proportion of total embryos		Proportion of survivors malformed
		Normal	Dead, resorbed	
(mg/kg)		(%)	(%)	(%)
0.1	9	92.0	7.1	1.0
0.2	7	86.9	11.5	1.9
0.2	8	80.8	4.2	16.0
0.2	9	48.7	32.5	28.1
0.2	10	83.8	12.3	4.4
0.2	11	92.3	7.7	0.0
0.3	6	87.2	10.3	2.8
0.3	7	77.4	13.0	11.2
0.3	8	10.8	84.8	26.6
0.3	9	0.0	99.2	100.0
0.3	10	14.7	57.9	65.2
0.3	11	87.1	12.1	0.9
none	--	95.5	3.6	0.9

the different organs reach their maxima at different times, and persist for different intervals. The time sequence of maximal susceptibility is in approximately the following order: eye, heart and aortic arches, brain, axial skeleton, palate, and urogenital organs. Furthermore, the development of each organ is complex, and different compounds may have different modes of action, even though they affect the same general structure. Therefore, by using different compounds, it may be possible to demonstrate more than one peak of susceptibility for the same organ.

Since compounds may differ in their mode of action, they often affect the development of different organs, even when administered on the same day of pregnancy. Thus, in spite of overlapping, the spectrum of injuries produced in a particular species tends to be characteristic of each compound (Wilson, 1965).

The susceptibility of each organ to terato-genic action varies according to the stage of development. This is true whether dosage is measured as the compound is administered to the mother or at the embryonic tissue level. However, it also is true that, in connection with maternal absorption by a normal route, most, if not all, of a compound that reaches the embryo does so by way of the placenta as soon as it becomes functional. The placenta has an active and selective role in chemical transfer mechanisms, and it is capable of biotransformation of some foreign chemicals. A useful review of placental drug transfer is that of Ginsburg (1971). Because development of the placenta corresponds with that of the embryo and fetus, any modifying action of the placenta in teratogenesis may be viewed as one aspect of the effect of the developmental stage.

The interactions of some compounds are understood easily, as in the teratogenic effects of a chelating agent and their prevention by zinc (Swenerton and Hurley, 1971). The reasons for other interactions are much less clear, as in the effects of cadmium, which also may be prevented by zinc.

4.2.10.2 Teratogenesis in Man. The thalidomide episode (Lenz et al., 1962) caused great public concern, and left no doubt of the necessity of testing the possible teratogenicity of compounds that may be encountered by pregnant women, especially compounds to be ingested in relatively large succinct doses. However, teratogenesis in man was well known before thalidomide was discovered, and a responsible and scientific assessment of the matter requires a review of teratogenesis and fetal toxicity as clinical problems. It is only in this way that aspects of the present problem that may have a toxic basis could find a solution.

In a prospective study of 5,964 human pregnancies, the incidence of congenital malformations was 7.0% among infants who survived the neonatal period, but less than half of these malformations were suspected or noted at birth. The incidence of deformities was higher if nonsurvivors were taken into account, being 7.5% among all products of conception weighing over 500g, 13.6% among antepartum deaths, 23.3% among intrapartum deaths, and 70.6% among deaths occurring between the ages of 1 and 12 months. Among children who survived the neonatal period, malformations were more common among males (8.4 vs 5.5%), among nonwhites (7.8 vs 6.3%), among infants weighing 2,500g or less (9.7 vs 6.7%), and among white infants of higher birth order (8.2 vs 5.3%). Maternal age had no detectable effect on congenital malformations (McIntosh et al., 1954). The real seriousness of the problem is indicated not so much by the fetal wastage, but by the fact that 5,964 pregnancies resulted in 374 babies still alive at 1 year of age, but deformed to some degree.

From this prospective study and many retrospective ones, it may be concluded that 2 to 3% of all infants born alive show one or more significant congenital malformations usually requiring medical attention soon after birth, and that by the end of 1 year this figure may be doubled by a careful search for lesser malformations not noticed at birth. These values do not include microscopic malformations or inborn errors of metabolism. Values for congenital deformities reported from different parts of the United States, from Japan, and from different European countries are similar. The most important factor determining a difference has been the method of collecting data; the more thorough the study, the more minor deformities are picked up, and the higher the total rate is found to be (Warkany and Kalter, 1961).

In their very scholarly review, Warkany and Kalter documented human malformations associated with: (a) defective inheritance transmitted from one generation to another according to Mendelian patterns; (b) chromosomal aberration in the affected child, but only rarely transmitted to a second generation; (c) infection with rubella, cytomegalic inclusion disease, syphilis, and toxoplasmosis; (d) drugs, including aminopterin, busulfan, and (at a lower frequency) tolbutamide and cortisone; (e) nutritional deficiency, especially iodine deficiency; (f) thyroid autoimmunization; (g) irradiation; and (h) possibly other causes. However, it was the authors' main point that in the great majority of cases, no cause for malformation, including those listed, is evident. They warn that any attempt to improve the situation must be based on knowledge of its causes. They further stress that no credence should be given to unitary, general, and simplified explanations of congenital malformations, whether they imply maternal disease, heredity, inborn errors of metabolism, or radiation.

Most human teratogenesis is endemic, and there is no evidence of an increase of incidence unexplained by more careful case finding, or by the relative decrease in many infectious diseases. There have been limited epidemics of teratogenesis caused by rubella, iodine deficiency, irradiation, and most recently, thalidomide. Of these epidemics, the last was best recorded but probably involved fewest cases.

Many microscopic malformations and inborn errors of metabolism are known to be inherited according to Mendelian patterns. It is not known that one of them in man is caused by exposure to radiation or chemiclas.

Few instances of fetal toxicity in man have been recorded. It has been observed following exposure of the mother to a methylmercury compound.

A recent book by Warkany (1971) is the most authoritative single source of information on teratogenesis in man.

4.3 Some Techniques for Measuring Different Kinds of Injury

There are several books providing useful information on a wide range of techniques in toxicology (European Society for the Study of Drug Toxicity, 1965; Boyland and Goulding, 1968; Paget, 1970). Some individual articles from them are referenced separately in connection with discussions in this and other chapters. There is reason to think that some, if not all, of these books will be revised or supplemented from time to time by the societies or editors responsible for them.

Most toxicological studies begin with an *acute toxicity test* to learn the kind and duration of illness associated with fatal and near fatal injury, and to learn the magnitude of the smallest dosages necessary to produce these effects. The acute toxicity test is basic to toxicological investigations. A number of valuable papers are available on the technique and objectives of the test (Hagan, 1959; Morrison *et al.*, 1968; Balazs, 1970; Boyd, 1972).

Thorough toxicological studies must consider the effects of repeated doses as well as the effects of a single dose, but the emphasis is the same: definition of illness and critical dosage. Tests involving repeated doses are commonly called *subacute toxicity tests* and *chronic toxicity tests,* depending on the number of doses involved. Again, valuable papers are available on the techniques and objectives of these tests (Fitzhugh and Schouboe, 1959; Fitzhugh, 1959; Benitz, 1970; Boyd, 1972).

In this book, acute, subacute, and chronic tests have not been considered separately. Instead, the tests usually have been broken down into their elements—compound, dosage, time, metabolism, and many others—and a discussion of these fundamentals constitutes Chapters 2 and 3. Unless there are legal requirements to be met in connection with some form of licensing, most can be gained by a creative application of the principles of toxicological testing, rather than by the routine application of some established protocol. The difficulty with any fixed protocol is that its application may leave unanswered questions regarding any particular compound and use situation.

From the very beginning of any study in toxicology, the investigator must be alert to learn how the compound affects the test organism. This same alertness ought to be maintained as long as study is continued. The fact that the action of a compound is reasonably well understood as the result of decades of study does not exclude the possibility that further details may be found, or that one of these details may be critical in understanding the mode of action, or in evaluating the safety of the toxicant. Conversely, recentness of discovery is no guarantee of importance.

It is impossible to overestimate the importance of what Boyd (1972) has called "cageside observation" in obvious reference to bedside observation of human patients. He listed 68 signs that can be distinguished in animals, and suggested that such a list be used to tabulate the time of appearance of each sign and its approximate intensity at suitable intervals. Ideally, the duration of each observation and the interval between them ought to be such that no change in the syndrome of toxicity is missed. Following each experiment, the incidences and also the intensities of tabulated signs should be analyzed statistically and reported in terms of differences from controls. Either tabular or graphic comparisons of the intensities of clinical findings may be made in relation to time and dosage. Accurate recording of signs prior to death gives a useful indication of its cause, which may be different for different dosage levels of the same compound. These signs, and those in survivors, offer leads for additional studies employing more specialized techniques.

At any given stage of investigation, the plan for future study ought to be determined by (*a*) what already has been learned about the compound, and (*b*) the conditions under which the compound may be used. For example, if the first animals tested suffer convulsions, attention clearly must be directed to the nervous system. A more detailed description of the effects and measurements of the concentrations of the compound and its possible metabolites in the brain will be needed. Voltage clamp studies should be considered early. If the compound is to be used as a drug administered in relatively large succinct doses, it is far more important to look for such side effects as teratogenesis than if the compound is to be contacted by male workers only, or is to be encountered by the general population in trace amounts only.

A creative approach to toxicological testing often will reveal problems involving routes of exposure or specific effects that require special techniques for effective study. Most of the remainder of this chapter is devoted to such techniques. It must be emphasized that the principles discussed in Chapters 2 and 3 apply to these special techniques, as well as to the more routine acute, subacute, and chronic tests.

Regardless of the particular kind of test, valuable information often can be obtained from a series of publications on laboratory animals for biomedical research issued by the National Academy of Sciences (1968, 1969a, 1969b, 1969c, 1969d, 1970a, 1970b, 1971a, 1971b).

Finally, much useful information on methodology, as well as specific guidance on regulatory requirements for testing, may be found in guides to safety evaluation. Perhaps the earliest of these guides was that of Woodard and Calvery (1943) of the US Food and Drug

Administration. This agency assumed leadership in this field and produced a series of guides (Calvery, 1944; Lehman et al., 1949, 1955, 1959). During the same period a number of other institutions, including the American Medical Association Council on Pharmacy and Chemistry (Van Winkle et al., 1944), the National Academy of Sciences (1956, 1960a, 1960b, 1964), health agencies of various western European countries (Tollenaar et al., 1952; Great Britain Ministry of Agriculture, Fisheries and Food, 1965, 1966), the Council of Europe (1962), and the Food and Agriculture Organization and the World Health Organization (FAO/WHO, 1958, 1961) produced guides on one or another aspect of safety testing. References to Russian guides of this same type are given by Medved and Kagan (1966) in their broad review of toxicology in the Soviet Union. In addition to guides issued by official agencies, several outstanding guides (Frazer, 1951; Boyd, 1968; Paget, 1970), or discussions of safety testing (Frazer, 1952), have been published by individual investigators or groups of them.

Some of the guides (Woodard and Calvery, 1943; Calvery, 1944; Lehman et al., 1949, 1955, 1959) were general in scope. Others were concerned with the toxicity of food additives (Frazer, 1951; Tollenaar et al., 1952; National Academy of Sciences, 1960a, 1960b; Great Britain, 1965; FAO/WHO, 1958), with some special aspect of this subject (World Health Organization, 1961), or with drugs (Van Winkle et al., 1944; Davey, 1965; Boyd, 1968), household substances (National Academy of Sciences, 1964), or pesticides (National Academy of Sciences, 1951, 1956; Council of Europe, 1962).

The critical reviews by Barnes and Denz (1954) and by Barnes (1960) made a very different kind of contribution to the problem. These classical papers should be consulted by anyone interested in the basic pharmacological principles that ought to be considered in safety testing.

4.3.1 Biochemical and Biophysical Investigations

Biochemical studies related to toxicology may be divided into (a) measurement of the action of the body on foreign chemicals, and (b) investigations of the action of foreign chemicals on the normal body metabolism. Techniques for using analytical chemistry to study the qualitative and quantitative changes in foreign chemicals were discussed in Section 3.3, and elsewhere in Chapter 3.

The action of foreign chemicals on normal metabolism is spoken of as their mode of action, a matter discussed in Section 4.1. Critical reviews of biochemical tests of body function are those of Frazer (1968) and Street (1970).

Biochemical and biophysical studies permit an understanding of different aspects of how chemicals exert their effects. A warning is necessary, however, lest every in vitro reaction be considered critical (see Section 4.1.2.1). The value of parallel studies in vivo and in vitro must be stressed. As Barnes (1969) remarked, "It is not always appreciated how much work is needed before it can be assumed that a change observed when an in vitro preparation is exposed to a toxic substance has any significance in respect to the effects of the same poison in the whole animal."

What is especially needed is thorough study of the effects of representative compounds on all aspects of metabolism at ranges of dosage below, as well as above, the smallest dosage observed to produce any toxic effect in the intact animal (see the discussion of the chemical basis of thresholds in Section 2.2.7.4).

4.3.2 Toxicological Studies on Isolated Cells

It is useful to divide studies on isolated cells into those that are mainly biochemical and those that are inherently toxicological. The use of red blood corpuscles to study membrane permeability is an example of a biochemical application. No special warning is needed in connection with such use. It is generally understood that, even if a compound affects the red cell membrane, further study is needed to learn what membrane, if any, in the intact animal is critical to the toxic action of the compound.

From a toxicological standpoint, compounds may be divided into those that affect cells in general, and those that interfere significantly with the integration of the body at a dosage well below what is required to injure isolated cells. This distinction does not depend on a basic difference in the modes of action, but rather on the biological significance of the reactive site involved in the biochemical lesion. For example, cytochrome oxidase and related enzymes inhibited by cyanide are essential to the respiration of all cells; therefore, cyanide affects isolated cells and intact organisms in a similar way. On the contrary, acetylcholinesterase has no known function in isolated cells, but is essential for integration of some higher organisms; many organic phosphorus and carbamate compounds that inhibit this enzyme kill mammals at concentrations that are harmless to isolated cells. Usually, only higher concentrations of organic phosphorus compounds injure isolated cells, and the mechanism may vary from compound to compound. By the same token, a metabolite that is less toxic than the original toxicant to intact animals may be more toxic to isolated cells. As a group, the dinitro compounds are more toxic to isolated cells than to intact animals. The chlorinated hydrocarbon compounds vary widely in their toxicity to cells, with no dependable relationship to their toxicity to intact animals. For the compounds that have been studied, toxicity to cells tends to increase with increasing solubility in water. Finally, different cell strains often vary in their susceptibility to the same compound. These relationships are illustrated by studies of a considerable variety of pesticides or their metabolites, as follows: organic phosphorus insecticides (diazinon, dimethoate, disulfoton, malathion, maloxon, parathion, paraoxon, paranitrophenol, and trichlorfon), carbamate insecticides (aldicarb, carbaryl, and 1-naphthol), nitro compounds (Bulan®, dinocap, dinitro-*o*-cyclohexylphenol, and Prolan®), and chlorinated hydrocarbon insecticides and acaricides (DDT, DDD, DDE, dicofol, methoxychlor, Perthane®, ovex, aldrin, dieldrin, chlordane, and heptachlor) (Gabliks and Friedman, 1965; Gabliks *et al.*, 1967; Wilson and Stinnett, 1969; Litterst *et al.*, 1969; Litterst and Lichenstein, 1971). Exposure of HeLa cells to aspirin or sodium chloride results in effects that are similar to those observed with some of the insecticides (Litterst *et al.*, 1969).

4.3.3 Tests of Mutagenesis

4.3.3.1 Background of Tests of Mutagenesis. Although genetics has its practical aspects in plant and animal breeding, the basic science has been developed largely through study of a wide variety of organisms that reproduce rapidly and easily in the laboratory and exhibit a large number of detectable, heritable characteristics. Some of these test organisms offer the additional advantage of having a small number of large chromosomes. Some Diptera even have giant chromosomes in some tissues, so that genes demonstrated genetically can be correlated with microscopically visible structures. Although each species has its own genetics, surprisingly few are really suitable for genetic study. For example, millions of houseflies are reared in laboratories each year in connection with studies of fly control, but very few genetic variations are known for this species. By contrast, the common fruit fly (*Drosophila melanogaster*), which also is reared easily, has thousands of genetic variations.

As each genetic phenomenon has been discovered, in one or another species, an effort has been made at once to confirm the finding in each species subjected to intense genetic study. The result has been the development of tests for genetic phenomena using bacteria, yeasts, bacterial viruses, a slime mold (*Neurospora crassa*), other fungi (eg, *Aspergillus*), small plants (eg, *Arabidopsis thaliana*), garden plants (onion, barley, wheat, beans, peas), fruit flies, parasitic wasps, and laboratory mammals, mainly mice. In addition, corn (maize) is important as an object of theoretical as well as practical study.

4.3.3.2 Outline of Tests. A number of books contain information on test systems for the detection and scoring of mutants (Fishbein *et al.*, 1970; Hollaender, 1971). A World Health Organization (1971) scientific group has reported on the evaluation and testing of drugs for mutagenicity. The emphasis on drugs seems wise, for compounds that are absorbed in large dosages, sometimes over extended periods, would seem to offer a hazard, if one exists.

Tests Based on Bacteria. Bacterial systems offer several advantages, including low cost, simplicity, and sensitivity. Mutant strains of *Salmonella typhimurium* are available that require particular nutrients for survival. If one of these mutants that requires histidine for survival is seeded in a Petri dish on a medium lacking histidine, and if about 1 mg of a test substance is placed in the center of the dish, only those bacteria will grow that have undergone back mutation. A circle of colonies will appear where the concentration of the mutagen is favorable. A count of the colonies indicates the number of mutations. The frequency of mutation need not be high to permit its detection, since about 5×10^8 bacteria are exposed on a single Petri plate. However, the sensitivity can be increased by using strains that are genetically deficient for the repair of excisions. Different strains are available in which the nutritional requirement depends on base pair substitution, insertion or deletion of one or two base pairs, or large deletions. Thus, compounds can be tested for each of several kinds of mutagenic action (Ames, 1971).

Tests Based on Neurospora crassa. Tests with slime mold employ two different genetically marked strains in what is called a two-compartment heterokaryon. The organism is exposed either *in vitro* or *in vivo* in the form of conidia; the conidia are then inoculated into a liquid medium where colonies grow to about 2 mm in diameter. Mutations at *ad-3A* or *ad-3B* locus result in the accumulation of a reddish purple pigment. The frequency of spontaneous *ad-3* mutations is only about 4×10^{-7}. Therefore, by counting white and colored colonies separately, it is possible to determine the rate of mutation directly. Thus, the mutagenic effects of different compounds and of different concentrations can be measured quantitatively. By subculturing and further genetic tests it is possible to characterize a variety of genetic injuries (de Serres and Malling, 1971).

Tests Based on Drosophila melanogaster. Tests of mutation commonly used in *Drosophila* include a two- or three-generation test for sex-linked recessives, a two-generation test for reciprocal translocations, a one-generation test for loss of sex chromosomes, and a one-generation test for detecting chromosome rearrangements. Each F_1 fly represents a treated gamete. Therefore, in the two-generation tests, it is necessary to culture each F_1 individual separately. The tests are objective and quantitative. However, they are time consuming (Abrahamson and Lewis, 1971). It is estimated in connection with the sex-linked recessive test that two or three highly skilled persons can screen between 5,000 and 10,000 chromosomes a month. With proper retesting 4 to 6 weeks are required to complete the translocation test. In the chromosome rearrangement test, a change is indicated by a recognizable phenotype, but the finding must be checked by the examination of chromosomes; one worker can analyze 4,000 to 8,000 chromosomes per week.

The tests mentioned and many others were described by Auerbach (1962) and by Muller and Oster (1963).

The Host-Mediated Test. Mammals may detoxify potential mutagens so that they do not reach critical tissues in an effective dosage. Conversely, compounds that are not mutagenic may undergo biotransformation to an active mutagen. These statements are made by analogy with other toxicants effective in other ways. What is actually observed is that some compounds mutagenic for lower forms are not all mutagenic for mammals, according to available tests. In any event, it has been proposed that mammalian metabolism may be taken into account, and advantage may be taken of the rapid screening of a large number of test cells by using a host-mediated assay. Cells that might be used in this way are *S. typhimurium, N. crassa,* and yeast (Legator and Malling, 1971), or mammalian cells from tissue culture (Miller and Miller, 1971). The microorganisms and the compound always are administered by different routes; usually the organisms are given intraperitoneally and the compound orally.

The host-mediated assay offers the advantages that it is relatively rapid, that it takes mammalian metabolism into account, and that it is capable of detecting point mutations (Legator and Malling, 1971). Of course, it must be pointed out that if lower forms are used in order to obtain point mutations, then it is these same lower forms that mutate, and a question of relevance may be raised. Even if human cells from tissue culture are used, the environment of these cells in the peritoneal cavity of an animal cannot be regarded as normal.

Cytogenic Study of Mammalian Cells. The chromosomes of mammalian cells may be examined for aberrations either after tissue (usually bone marrow) has been removed from intact treated animals, or after tissue cultures have been exposed to a compound or other experimental variable. Especially in the *in vivo* form of the test, the question of relevance is resolved in relation to compounds, but sometimes is ignored in relation to dosage.

An authoritative statement on chromosome methodologies in mutation testing has been issued by an Ad Hoc Committee (1972).

Genetic Studies of Mammalian Cells in Vitro. It has been possible to develop stable mutant tissue culture strains of Chinese hamster cells that require specific nutrients (proline, glycine, thymidine, hypoxanthine, inositol, or combinations of them) for growth. Such strains may be manipulated for genetic study in essentially the same way as genetically deficient microorganisms. The system is capable of detecting both point mutations and chromosome aberrations (Puck and Kao, 1967). Because of the versatility of this test, the attractiveness of nonmammalian, *in vitro* systems is reduced. On the other hand, the relative ease with which mutant strains may be developed and maintained is proof that the tissue cultures can be shielded from natural selection to a degree probably impossible for the intact animal, even under laboratory conditions.

The Specific Locus Test for Mutagenesis in Mammals. This test consists in mating wild-type animals to animals homozygous for a number of specific, visible recessives and observing the first generation offspring for mutations at any of these specific, marked loci. The mutation frequencies exhibited in the young of treated and untreated parents are then compared. The treated parent may be either male or female and either wild-type or homozygous recessive. Of course, the system is capable of detecting a variety of other mutations that may occur, as well as detecting the recessive point mutations missed by other systems. Examples of the specific locus test are those of

Russell (1971). Cytogenic examinations can be made of tissues from animals studied genetically. Use of the test for over 20 years has shown conclusively that the mutagenic effects of radiation in mice are very different from these effects in fruit flies. More recently, marked differences also have been found relative to chemical mutagens. The observed difference between the genetic behavior of mice and flies emphasizes the need to use mammalian models in estimating the effect of chemicals on human health.

Tests for Dominant Lethal Mutations in Mammals. Auerbach and Falconer (1949) reported temporary sterility in a mouse that survived treatment with nitrogen mustard, and they attributed the effect to translocation. Hendry *et al.* (1951) reported complete loss of spermatogenesis in a dog receiving 2,4,6-trisethyleneimino-1,3,5-triazine intravenously at the rate of 0.05 mg/kg/day up to a total of 0.45 mg without any evident clinical effect. They concluded that the ability of this and related compounds to inhibit tumors was correlated with their ability to injure chromosomes in dividing cells generally. Cattanach (1957) suggested that male sterility resulting from triethylenemelamine, which had been demonstrated earlier (Jackson and Bock, 1955), is due at least in part to dominant lethal mutation through chromosome breakage. In his own experiments, Cattanach confirmed that the compound causes male sterility, and showed that it also caused semisterility transmitted for a few generations in both the male and female line, and associated with translocations.

These early studies and many others reviewed by Jackson (1966) formed the basis for recent recommendations of tests for dominant lethal mutations in mammals. What is actually measured is the preimplantation loss of nonviable zygotes (inferred from an excess of corpora lutea compared to implantation sites), early fetal deaths (inferred from the number of unoccupied implantation sites), late fetal deaths (observed directly), and sterility and semisterility in the young of treated animals (inferred directly from the number and size of litters they are able to produce). Various shortcuts may be taken. For example, preimplantation losses may be inferred by comparing the average total number of implants in females mated to treated and control males. Compounds to be tested are administered to male mice or rats, because females are less susceptible in this test to most chemicals. The test may be extended by cytogenetic demonstration of translocations or other chromosome aberrations.

The range of techniques for studying antifertility compounds has been described by Jackson (1966). The search for dominant lethals may be made a part of the routine three-generation test of reproduction (see Section 4.3.5.6).

4.3.3.3 Toxicological Aspects of Tests of Mutagenesis.

It is sometimes argued that since mutations involve DNA, and since DNA of all organisms has the same double helical structure and the same four nucleotides, therefore, any organism may be used as an indicator system for mutagens. This argument suffers from the limitation of genetics itself, which is the study of detectable differences within breeding populations. The science makes no contribution to the unsolved question of why one organism is a slime mold and another is a man. The fact that they exhibit some common genetic and biochemical properties does not lessen their differences.

Toxicologists, familiar with the importance of species differences and the overriding importance of dosage, have some skepticism about any extrapolation of results, even from one mammalian species to another, and great skepticism about any procedure for which toxicological significance is claimed without taking dosage into account.

Some compounds react readily with DNA, and others have not been observed to react. Since chemical mutagenesis is thought to consist of the reaction of compounds with this one type of molecule, it is reasonable that some compounds are mutagens and others are not, as is commonly supposed. However, DNA is formed and repaired under the influence of enzymes. It is possible that toxicants may affect these enzymes. If this proved to be true, the reactions might involve a variety of sites on the enzymes and thus introduce doubt that any compound can be declared nonmutagenic except in a particular test system and under specific limitations of dosage.

It is difficult to evaluate the potential importance of chemical mutagenesis for man, since no instance of this kind of injury is known. The existence of genetically heritable disease in man is evidence for some instability of human genes and chromosomes, not for the importance of any extrinsic inducer. Direct experimentation with human beings to investigate this matter is unethical. Experiments with human cells in tissue culture or as part of a host-mediated test in animals suffer from the same limitations as do other *in vitro* toxicological tests (see Section 4.3.2).

Steps that might be taken toward the ultimate goal of evaluating tests of mutagenicity in relation to human health include: (a) emphasis on the dosage-response relationship; (b) systematic effort to determine the mutagenicity of commonly used and inescapable chemicals; and (c) increased effort to compare the mutagenic activity of a wide range of compounds in mammals and in lower forms. Of these items, the first requires no explanation. Since there is no evidence that human genetic disease has undergone any epidemiological change, it would be reasonable to explore those materials that people have used for generations, or those that cannot be avoided, either because they are essential to nutrition or are naturally occurring contaminants. The comparison of effects in mammals and in lower forms is of particular importance in connection with common or unavoidable materials, in order to evaluate the usefulness of tests based on lower forms. Furthermore, since caffeine produces dominant lethals in mice and induces chromatid breakage in human cells in vitro (Kuhlmann et al., 1968), it is urgent that the significance of these tests in mammals be evaluated. Perhaps the entire answer lies in the dosage-response relationship. In the lower experimental dosage ranges, the genetic injury is linearly dependent on dosage, and the concentrations used in the experiments have been 250 ppm or greater, that is more than 10 times the concentrations reported in human blood. If a safety factor of less than 100 is adequate for caffeine, perhaps it would be adequate for other mutagens also.

4.3.4 Tests of Carcinogenesis

There is general agreement regarding the procedures necessary to test the possible carcinogenicity of compounds. The procedures have been described by several official agencies (National Academy of Sciences, 1960a; Food and Drug Administration Advisory Committee on Protocols for Safety Evaluations, 1971; Food and Agriculture Organization and World Health Organization Expert Committee on Food Additives, 1961; World Health Organization, 1969), and by scientific authorities in the field (Boyland, 1957, 1968; Magee, 1970).

What is needed from a toxicological standpoint is more emphasis on dosage and an effort to gain some perspective on the relative carcinogenicity of common materials. To be sure, it is known that some of the classical laboratory carcinogens are effective when administered even once at a dosage of 1 mg/kg or less (see Table 2-4). However, many compounds are reported to be carcinogenic without any effort to learn the lowest effective dosage. Furthermore, there has been virtually no effort to test ordinary foods and other commonly encountered materials to see whether an excess will induce tumors. When comparing the lethality of compounds, careful studies on sodium chloride, caffeine, and other foods and beverages may be considered, as well as studies on war gases and bacterial toxins. Thus, the toxicity of a new compound can be viewed as one point on a broad spectrum. It cannot be argued—as some apparently suppose—that no common materials are carcinogenic. A diet high in oils routinely available in food stores induced chlorleukemia in rats (Kimbrough et al., 1964). This finding is not alarming, if for no other reason than that the proportion of fat in the experimental diet was so high that the food would never be consumed voluntarily. However, the finding does indicate the existence of a spectrum—one end of which is in great need of study.

There is also a need to evaluate the relation of lesions in animals to neoplastic disease in man. Such evaluation must involve not only consideration of species differences, but also evaluation of certain lesions per se. For example, in the past great emphasis has been placed on hyperplastic nodules in the liver of rodents. The position has been taken that it is impossible, or at least unwise, to distinguish them from carcinoma of the liver, even when metastasis has not been demonstrated and reversibility has not been tested. Some nodules seem to be related to the reversible increase in endoplasmic reticulum associated with induction of microsomal enzymes. Actually, nodules differ from carcinoma, even when both are produced by classical carcinogens. Cells from such nodules, unlike cells from the normal liver, can be grown in tissue culture. The same is true of cells from liver cancer, but the two kinds of abnormal cell behave differently (Slifkin et al., 1970).

4.3.5 Tests of Effects Specific to Certain Organs or Systems

4.3.5.1 Pharmacological Tests. Most pharmacological tests provide the same type of information acquired by direct observation, but in far greater detail than is possible without instrumentation. The emphasis is on definitions of drug action and side effects. However, the same tests are extremely valuable in defining clearly toxic effects. Use of pharmacological reagents, such as drugs known to block specific synapses or receptors, may help to define a biochemical lesion. Other tests that measure the effect of graded stimuli on sensation, secretion, muscle twitch, and the like ought not to be neglected when indicated by direct observation of the poisoned animal. Such tests seldom, if ever, reveal a biochemical lesion, but they provide a broad descriptive background of a compound's action that is essential in evaluating whether a particular action on an enzyme or transport mechanism ought to be regarded as a biochemical lesion or merely an incidental effect.

Although there were earlier guides for pharmacological study, the ones with greatest influence were those of Sollmann (1917) and Sollmann and Hanzlik (1928). Whereas much of the equipment described is outmoded and the list of phenomena discussed is incomplete, these classical guides are still worthy of review.

Newer reference works on pharmacological tests include those by DeJonge (1961), and Nodine and Siegler (1964). The latter is concerned with quantitative methods in pharmacology, and therefore has a bearing on the statistical aspects of many toxicological tests.

4.3.5.2 Tests of Respiratory Toxicity.

Tests of inhalation toxicity have been employed for many years and on a wide variety of compounds. The results in animals show a useful correspondence with the experience of people exposed to the same compounds. A review of these valuable tests is beyond the scope of this book, particularly since the techniques have been well described elsewhere. Useful reviews are those of Roe (1968) and Gage (1970).

Tests, whether on man or animals, must be accompanied by appropriate monitoring of the air they breathe. A valuable book on air sampling instruments for evaluating atmospheric contaminants is issued by the American Conference of Governmental Industrial Hygienists (1972). A fundamental paper on exposure chambers is that by Silver (1946). Ready sources of information on their design, construction, operation, and performance, are a monograph by Fraser et al. (1959), and a paper by Hinners et al. (1968). As discussed in Section 2.4.3, few studies of the effects of truly continuous exposure to a chemical have been carried out in such a way that these effects can be compared accurately with the effects of intermittent exposure to the same compound under otherwise identical circumstances. A contributing cause of this unfortunate situation is the complexity and expense of exposure chambers that permit truly continuous exposure. However, a few such chambers have been constructed. One group of them was designed primarily to permit investigation of low ambient pressures to be encountered by astronauts. Daily servicing of the continuous exposure chambers is done by one or more persons who enter each chamber through an airlock

system. Each chamber may be operated continuously for more than a year (Thomas, 1965; Back and Thomas, 1970).

For many purposes it may suffice to monitor air concentrations accurately and to express the results in terms of LC 50 values (see Section 2.2.4), or in terms of the product of concentration and time (see Section 2.2.3.2). However, it always is ideal to use methods that permit the results to be expressed in terms of the dosage (mg/kg) received by the test organism. Basically, this requires a way of measuring the retained dose. A classical procedure for doing this in dogs is that described by Tobias and Weston (1946), and Weston and Karel (1946). An adaptation suitable for use in small animals has been described by Leong and MacFarland (1965).

Tests of Respiratory Tract Irritants. Magné et al. (1925a; 1925b) reviewed the effects of irritants on the respiratory pattern in animals as reported by earlier authors (Kratschmer, 1870; Frank, 1876; Knoll, 1879; Brodie and Russel, 1900; Dixon and Brodie, 1903), and extended these findings by further experiments. By using tracheotomized animals, each compound can be tested separately on different parts of the airway. The results are summarized in Table 4-3. If intact animals are exposed to irritants, some compounds (eg, acrolein) elicit primarily an upper airway response, some (eg, phosgene) elicit primarily a lower airway response, and others (eg, chlorine) elicit a mixed response because they irritate the entire airway.

Using decrease of respiratory rate as an index, and body plethysmographs as a method for measuring it, Alarie (1966) developed an apparatus for testing compounds for their ability to irritate the upper respiratory tract of mice. The method is simple enough to permit its use in screening. It is reproducible, so that dosage-response curves and minimal effective dosage levels can be detected. It is sensitive enough to detect irritating effects at low concentrations that cause no pathological change. It can be used to detect the conditioned response of mice to a light or other stimulus they have come to associate with exposure to an irritant.

The plethysmographic method has not been evaluated fully as a method for screening irritants of the lower respiratory tract. It presumably is less sensitive than the measurement of airway resistance using the technique of Amdur and Mead (1955, 1958).

4.3.5.3 Tests of Dermal Toxicity, Irritation, and Sensitization.

The skin is an important route of entry for many systemic toxicants.

Table 4–3
Change in Various Parameters Following Exposure of
the Upper or the Lower Respiratory Tract to Irritants

Parameter	Upper airway	Lower airway
onset	rapid	slow
breathing rate	decreased[a]	increased
duration of expiration	increased	decreased
effect on larynx	spasm	unchanged
bronchial tone	increased	little change
pulmonary ventilation	decreased	increased
pulse rate	decreased	unchanged
blood pressure	increase	no change or slight decrease
pulmonary circulation	decreased	little change
recovery	rapid	slow

a.   There may be a transient increase in rate from time to time, sometimes accompanied by body movements.

Factors influencing dermal toxicity are discussed in Sections 3.2.2.5 and 6.2.3.1. Some of those factors, such as temperature (Section 2.4.15), are purposely eliminated in routine laboratory tests through standardization of conditions, although they may be important for human safety under some practical conditions. Some other factors influencing dermal toxicity are subject to considerable variation in what is intended to be routine testing procedure. Some of the following paragraphs with italicized headings discuss these important variations in technique.

To a far greater extent than applies in connection with other routes of entry, the skin is subject to local damage, sometimes accompanied by little or no systemic effect. The reason lies largely in the relatively unrestricted exposure of the skin and its relatively efficient barrier action. If the same amount of a given irritant were applied to the respiratory tract or the gastrointestinal tract, the resulting edema, respiratory embarrassment, or fluid loss might well cause such systemic effects that the reaction would be spoken of as "toxicity" rather than "irritation." Under the circumstances, it is necessary to pay special attention to strictly local effects on the skin.

The skin itself is subject to (a) primary irritation; (b) skin fatigue; (c) photosensitization; and (d) sensitization, all subject to dosage-response relationships. *Primary irritation* is similar to incipient inflammation. Evidence of it can be seen almost as soon as exposure begins. The injury ranges from only slight hyperemia to a combination of hyperemia, edema, and vesiculation, followed by suppuration and the formation of an eschar. *Skin fatigue* is similar to primary irritation except that it does not follow exposure promptly; it differs greatly from sensitization because it shows recovery rather than exacerbation if treatment is repeated after 10 to 14 days of rest. *Photosensitization* is an injury that becomes evident only after exposure to certain wavelengths of ultraviolet light (see Section 2.4.17.1). *Sensitization* is an allergic process; the injury appears—sometimes suddenly—

only after a number of exposures, and it may not be confined to the area of application.

Useful papers on irritation, sensitization, and related topics may be found in the proceedings of two symposia on cutaneous toxicity held jointly by the Society of Toxicology and the American Medical Association and published by the Society of Toxicology (1965, 1969).

Choice of Species. The most complete information on the dermal toxicity of a compound is obtained by testing it in as many species as possible. If limitation of time or budget dictate that only a single species is to be used, it may have to be chosen on the basis of statutory requirements for some official registration or approval. If this consideration is not limiting, these dermal tests should be made on a species used for studying toxicity by one or more other routes, so that a valid comparison can be made.

Some official test procedures require use of the rabbit, based on the claim that it is generally more susceptible than man (Draize, 1959). A number of examples of this relationship have been published, and it may be true on the average, not because the rabbit is regularly more susceptible to poisons, but because, as discussed in Section 3.2.2.5, its skin is generally more permeable to a wide range of compounds. In summary, Tregear (1964) concluded that the permeability of the skin of different species decreases in the order rabbit > rat > guinea pig > pig > man. Thus, the rat could be chosen for testing dermal toxicity on the basis of conservatism, as well as economy. It is the species most commonly used for testing oral toxicity, and it is entirely satisfactory for testing dermal toxicity also. Of course, the same strain, age, and sex should be used in tests intended to be comparable. The guinea pig is the common laboratory animal with skin permeability most nearly like that of man, and it is the animal of choice for studying skin sensitivity. However, it is relatively expensive and seldom used for oral testing.

Preparation of Animals. For reasons discussed in Section 3.2.2.5, great care should be exercised in preparing animals for dermal application of toxicants. Hair should be clipped from the application area 18 to 24 hours before dosing. An electric clipper is not only fast but easily controlled. Shaving or the use of a chemical depilatory should be avoided in order to prevent injury to the skin. The delay of 18 to 24 hours is important to permit healing of any unavoidable and often imperceptible injury that may result from clipping. As a further insurance against injury to the skin, the animals should be held in separate cages.

Before the application of toxicant, it may be desirable to wash the application area with a 1:1 mixture of acetone and 95% alcohol to remove dirt and excess oils. At least with parathion, removal of fat from the skin 24 hours before application had no effect on toxicity (Vandekar and Komanov, 1963).

The Question of Covering. Toxicologists are about equally divided in their preference as to whether dermal doses should be applied to the covered or the uncovered skin. In favor of covering the skin are the following: (a) Some compounds that otherwise would be partially lost by vaporization can be retained by a cover. (b) Since maceration of the skin promotes absorption, and since an impervious cover keeps the skin moist by preventing the evaporation of visible or imperceptible sweat, covering the skin ensures a test of the most hazardous conditions that might be encountered by people. (c) The use of a cover ensures that the test animal will not lick or otherwise ingest the toxicant. An animal that has interfered with the integrity of its covering is excluded from the test.

In favor of not covering the skin are the following: (a) People are most often and most severely contaminated by pesticides on their completely unclothed skin surfaces, and—with the all too common exception of the insides of rubber gloves and boots—contamination is rarely beneath a truly impermeable covering. (b) It is less work to use no covering; one operator can carry out the test without covering, but two operators are needed when a cover is used. Therefore, on the same budget, more tests can be run by the simpler technique. (c) Most compounds do not irritate or otherwise stimulate rats to licking or other activity leading to ingestion of the material from the shoulder area. (d) The same technique can be used for tests involving many daily doses. Thus, the results of single and repeated doses can be made truly comparable. By taping the animals firmly to wooden blocks, Gaines (1969a) showed that rats which could not scratch or lick any part of their bodies were equally as susceptible as rats kept in ordinary cages to parathion and dichlorovos applied to the skin of their backs. In the same series of tests, the restrained rats were oriented in a stream of air in such a way that they could not inhale any vapor that might be given off. Oral and respiratory exposure do not complicate the ordinary test of dermal toxicity, even when the toxicant is applied to the uncovered skin (Gaines, 1960; 1969a; Vandekar and Komanov, 1963).

A few compounds, for example arsenic trioxide, do cause animals to lick or scratch the area to which they were applied, and oral exposure does occur. However, this complication is clearly evident in these instances, and animals can be restrained in connection with the testing of such materials. One of the simplest ways to restrain a rat for this purpose is to place the animal in a cylinder of hardware cloth, about 4 cm in diameter (Gaines, 1960). However, because such wire often is rough and may injure the skin, a special cage devised by Bollman (1948) is preferable for restraint. Rats may be kept in such a cage for weeks without significant weight loss or other interference with their welfare. The cage consists of two end plates that hold a series of bars running parallel to the rat's body. A watering tube is presented through a hole in the front plate, and the rat's tail is passed out through a hole in the back plate. The rods constituting the floor of the cage are supported by a small crossbar in such a way that a food cup can be placed at the front of the cage and urine and feces may be collected without an objectionable contamination of the cage itself. The cage is especially adapted for holding a rat that has a draining cannula, such as one from the common bile duct (Bollman et al., 1949). However, the cage may be used also for holding a rat whose midsection is covered by an occlusive dressing. Fig. 4-1 shows a Bollman-type cage. Such cages are conveniently made from brass rods supported by clear plastic. The plastic may be drilled in such a way as to permit some selection in the placement of the rods and, therefore, the accommodation of larger or smaller rats. However, if rats of greatly different size are to be used, one must have cages of different lengths as well as different diameters.

If it is decided that covering of the skin will be standard in testing dermal toxicity, it is of the greatest importance that a truly impervious cover be used. Aluminum foil is best, except in those rare instances in which there is some reason to expect a reaction between aluminum and something in the formulation tested. Plastic coverings that may seem impervious to the casual observer may absorb a particular toxicant, and thus act as a partial protection to the animal by making a part of the dose unavailable for absorption by the skin. Such absorptive coverings have an effect exactly the opposite of that intended. Their use does not correspond to any situation people are likely to encounter.

Studies of parathion summarized in Table 4-4 offer an illustration of the variation in results that may be introduced by using different coverings in testing dermal toxicity. For this compound, no significant difference was found between the toxicity when no covering was

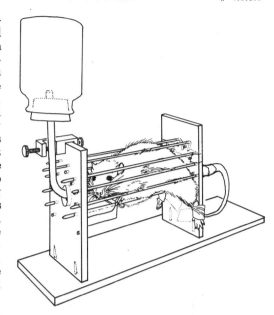

Fig. 4-1. Rat secured by adhesive tape in a Bollman-type cage.

used and that when the skin was covered by aluminum foil. Both studies were carried out near the thermoneutral range (21 to 24°C). The difference in results might have been greater if the ambient temperature had been higher and the maceration of the skin beneath the covering greater. Other coverings, including polyethylene, rubber, and adhesive plaster, absorbed parathion so that its effective toxicity was reduced by two-fold to 10-fold.

In contrast to parathion, compounds with sufficiently greater volatility do show a greater dermal toxicity if the skin is covered to prevent their loss. An example is offered by mercury in the form of calomel ointment, which was absorbed by rabbits during a 24-hour period about 3 times more effectively from covered skin than from uncovered skin. Volatility of the mercury was emphasized by the finding that almost 4% of the absorbed material entered by way of the respiratory tract. In rats, absorption of mercury from covered skin was about 1.6 times greater when the applied ointment was left in place than when the "excess" was removed by gentle wiping (Laug et al., 1947).

In tests in which the skin is covered, it is conventional to remove the covering after an interval (often 24 hours), and remove as much of the toxicant as possible by washing with detergent and water warmed to about body temperature. However, as discussed in Section 3.2.2.5, as the time after application increases, it becomes progressively more difficult to remove toxicant by washing. Although washing

Table 4–4
Dermal Toxicity of Parathion to Female Rats
Tested Under Different Conditions

Covering	Contact time (hrs)	LD 50 Male (mg/kg)	Female (mg/kg)	Reference
none	24+[a]	21	6.8	Gaines, 1960
"	24+[a]	30-39		Vandekar and Komanov, 1963
aluminum foil [b]	24		5.2	Noakes, 1964 [c]
aluminum foil [b]	4		8.8	Noakes, 1964 [c]
polyethylene sheet [b]	4		17.7	Noakes, 1964 [c]
" "	24+[a]	62.6		Vandekar and Komanov, 1963
rubber sheet [b]	4		41	Noakes, 1964 [c]
adhesive plaster	24		50	Noakes, 1964 [c]
" "	24+[a]	138.9		Vandekar and Komanov, 1963
adhesive plaster	4		70	Noakes, 1964 [c]

a. Single application without any attempt at removal.

b. Held in place by adhesive plaster.

c. D. N. Noakes, cited by V. K. Brown (1965).

delayed 24 hours may reduce further absorption, it certainly does not stop it.

Selection and Application of Formulation. The dermal toxicity of many compounds differs according to the formulation in which they are tested (Section 3.2.2.5). Therefore, formulations for testing should be selected knowingly. Ideally, each compound should be tested in every formulation in which it will be encountered by formulators, applicators, or others. Such testing will give a maximum of practical information.

However, if the dermal toxicity of a series of compounds is to be compared, it is unlikely that more than one formulation of each can be tested, and thought must be given to selection of a standard formulation. In choosing a solvent or suspending agent, attention may be given to: (*a*) similarity to formulations used by workers; (*b*) high solvent power for a wide range of compounds; (*c*) ability to promote absorption and thus reveal the maximal hazard; and (*d*) failure to injure the skin. The last two items are largely opposite in their implications. Which of the two will be chosen as a criterion depends on a value judgment. In other words, interest may be focused on testing toxicity under adverse conditions in order to be conservative in estimating safety, or interest may be focused on the more basic question of permeability of the normal skin.

Compounds that have been suggested as solvents or suspending agents in tests of dermal toxicity are xylene, dimethylphthalate, dimethylformamide, dimethylacetamid, dimethylsulfoxide, methyl salicylate, ethyl alcohol, isopropyl alcohol, *n*-octyl alcohol, propylene glycol, water and certain mixtures of them, especially aqueous solutions of alcohols.

Xylene was selected by a laboratory responsible for studying the safety of pesticides for vector control at a time when xylene was the principal solvent in formulations used for this purpose. The use was retained as a standard (Gaines, 1960; 1969a) on the basis that it is a good solvent and that it produces some skin injury and dilatation of blood vessels and thus promotes absorption. For some compounds, *n*-octanol is even more effective than xylene in promoting absorption (Brown, 1968).

Formulations should always be applied to the skin gently. (If the effect of mechanical injury is under study, the injury should be produced in a separate step before application.) Liquid formulations should be applied from a pipette or from a syringe with needle ending in a smooth metal bead. The pipette or syringe serves to measure the formulation and to distribute it as evenly as possible over a standard area. Dust formulations should be micronized before application, in order to ensure effective contact with the skin. Each dose is usually weighed but, if the volume is large enough, sufficient accuracy may be achieved by volumetric measurement (for example, with a selected kitchen measuring spoon filled exactly level). Depending on the size of the dose, it may be spread and brought into contact with the skin by means of a smooth glass rod or the tip of a gloved finger. Water-wettable powders may be made into a suspension in water and dispensed like any other liquid formulation.

No matter what formulation is chosen, it should be applied with due regard to known variables in dermal toxicity (see Section 3.2.2.5). This means (unless the variables themselves are under study) that all applications should be to the same part of the body and at the same rate in terms of volume per unit of body weight. If these things are done and the same solvent is used throughout, the proportion of body surface covered will be essentially constant. Exceptions to the rule are justified in the case of compounds of such low toxicity that a massive dose is required to produce an effect, or in the case of highly concentrated formulations such as emulsifiable concentrates, when dilution would destroy the purpose of the test.

Volume of Dose. A number of application rates have been employed. Gaines (1960, 1969a) used a rate of 0.0016 ml per gram of body weight. This rate was selected primarily on the basis that workers were subject to spills of which about 100 ml might remain on the skin. The assumption of less contamination was considered overoptimistic and the assumption of much greater retention was considered unrealistic. A rate of 100 ml/70 g is the same as 0.0014 ml/g. A slight modification of the

rate was made so that the formulations then in use for vector control could be expressed in even numbers in terms of milligrams of toxicant per kilogram of body weight. Thus, a 5% solution applied at the rate of 0.0016 ml/g results in a dosage of 80 mg/kg; four other solutions, each weaker by a factor of 2, also give dosages in even numbers, namely, 40, 20, 10, and 5 mg/kg (Hayes *et al.*, 1951).

Recent measurements showed that, when xylene solutions are applied to the skin of 200-g rats at the rate of 0.0016 ml/g, without any effort to spread the material, the area actually covered is about 24 cm^2, indicating a rate of 0.013 ml/cm^2 (Gaines, 1969b). Of course, liquids of different viscosities applied in the same way would cover different areas.

Tests of Primary Irritation. In many instances, adequate information on primary irritation may be obtained in the course of studies of dermal toxicity. Certainly, careful examination of the skin ought to be part of such studies. The question of covering the treated area was discussed above.

If separate tests of primary irritation are required for some form of licensing, it is important to follow the prescribed protocol in detail. The requirements of the US Food and Drug Administration involve a patch test applied to intact and abraded, closely clipped skin of albino rabbits. Either liquid (0.5 ml) or solid (0.5 g) is placed under a 1-inch patch which is then fastened by tape. The entire trunk of the rabbit is wrapped in a rubberized cloth and the animal is immobilized for 24 hours in a rack. At the end of the exposure period, the covering is removed and the reaction scored according to a fixed scheme. The results are scored again 72 hours after first application. The results for 24 and 72 hours and for intact and abraded skin are combined as a primary irritation index. Indices of 2 or less indicate only mild irritation; 2 to 5 indicate moderate irritation, and 6 or more indicate severe irritation (Draize, 1959).

In man, the same patch tests serve to measure primary irritation, skin fatigue, and sensitization. If the irritation is too severe, the test is terminated and sensitization is not explored, at least not with the strength of solution used at the beginning.

Tests of Photosensitization. Photosensitization and some factors that must be considered in its study were discussed in Section 2.4.17.

Tests of Skin Sensitization. No species of animal develops allergy to chemicals to the same degree as man does. Few species are suitable for testing sensitivity. The guinea pig is best for this purpose and is adequate for detecting compounds that are severe sensitizers. The Food and Drug Administration recommends white male guinea pigs weighing 300 to 500 g and maintained in a prescribed way. A 0.1% solution or suspension of the test material is injected intracutaneously using a 26-gauge needle along the clipped back or upper flanks. The first sensitizing dose is 0.05 ml, while the next nine are 0.1 ml. They are administered every other day or three times per week. Two weeks after the last sensitizing dose, a challenge dose of 0.05 ml of freshly prepared solution or suspension is given in an area just below the site where the sensitizing injections were given. The diameter, height, and color of the reaction is recorded 24 hours after each injection. The degree of increase in reaction following the challenge dose, as compared to the average of reactions following the sensitizing doses, is a measure of the degree of sensitization (Draize, 1959).

Davies (1970) has reviewed animal and *in vitro* tests suitable for detecting a wide range of allergic conditions.

Skin sensitization tests in man are done with volunteers. It is recommended that at least 100 men and 100 women of different ages be used in each test. Patches carrying 0.5 ml of fluid or 0.5 g of solid are applied for 24 hours to the arms or back. The reaction is read for erythema, edema, and vesiculation when each patch is removed. Following a day of rest, another patch is put on in another location, and the procedure is repeated until 10 sensitizing doses have been given. A challenge dose is given in exactly the same way but to a fresh area 10 to 14 days after the last challenge dose. As in the test with guinea pigs, the degree of sensitization is indicated by the increase in reaction after the challenge dose, as compared to the reactions after the sensitizing doses (Draize, 1959).

4.3.5.4 Tests of Irritation of the Eye. The rabbit is the most widely used animal for testing irritation of the eye. Equally good results may be obtained with other species, including cheaper ones. In any event, the test material is placed in one eye, while the other serves as a control.

The test prescribed by the Food and Drug Administration employs albino rabbits and a dose of 0.1 ml. Three animals receive this amount without further treatment; in three others the treated eye is rinsed with 20 ml of water at about body temperature 1 sec after treatment; and in three others washing with water is delayed a total of 4 sec. Readings are made at 24, 48, and 72 hours, and at 4 and 7 days, or as long as injury persists. A complex

scoring system is purposely weighted to emphasize injury to the cornea and iris because of their importance to vision (Draize, 1959). A brief atlas of eye injuries was published by Marzulli (1965).

The commonly used method has proved valuable but is undeniably subjective. A test of it in 25 laboratories revealed poor reproducibility. Inadequate training of some technicians in carrying out this particular test probably was the main factor contributing to excessive variability (Weil and Scala, 1971). However, it seems clear that a more objective test would be desirable.

Fortunately, a test based on measurement of the thickness of the cornea has been developed. The test requires use of a special depth-measuring attachment available as an accessory to a slit lamp. The accuracy of measurement is 0.01 mm. The results obtained agree well with those of the Draize test at its best. However, the new method is more easily standardized, and the results are more readily subjected to statistical analysis than are those of the Draize test (Burton, 1972). Use of the slit lamp is not confined to measurement of corneal thickness. A wide range of measurements may be made precisely and objectively with this instrument.

4.3.5.5 Tests of Behavior. A wide range of specialized behavioral tests are available, including learning and memory of a conditioned response, conditioned avoidance, passive avoidance, operant conditioning, and discriminative conditioning. These tests and their possible application to toxicology were reviewed by Brimblecombe (1968), who provided many references to other reviews and to papers on methods for carrying out specific procedures.

The biggest single difference between toxicological safety evaluation in Eastern Europe as compared to Western Europe and America concerns the emphasis placed on behavioral tests in general, and tests involving conditioned reflexes in particular. It is presumably for this reason that the hygienic standards for industrial chemicals often are more conservative in the Soviet Union than elsewhere. As discussed in Section 9.1.4.5, data are not available to permit an objective evaluation of the two approaches. It is not possible to compare the concentrations of the common industrial chemicals and waste products, such as carbon monoxide, actually realized under occupational conditions, much less to compare the health of workers protected by the different standards. Such comparisons would provide most valuable scientific information.

Under the circumstances, one is forced to

fall back on a comparison of the results of animal experiments. In doing so, it must be recognized that: (a) careful observation of the spontaneous activity of the experimental animals is a part of any good toxicological study; (b) some effects certainly involving behavior (such as lethargy, narcosis, change in drug-induced sleeping time ataxia, and convulsions, and a variety of electrophysiological phenomena) in animals and many of these same phenomena, as well as headache and other discomfort, in man have long been a recognized part of general toxicological evaluation; (c) an even wider range of behavioral tests, including some highly specialized ones, are a part of the pharmacological study of tranquilizers, stimulants, and other drugs intended to modify behavior; and (d) no limit should be placed on research regarding the effects of toxicants on any aspect of behavior. Discussion of the role of new behavioral tests in toxicology will be most meaningful if it compares them with tests that are already an established part of safety evaluation. The question is not whether behavioral effects exist, but whether they are significant if and when they occur at dosage levels below those causing one or more significant nonbehavioral toxicological effects. In considering the significance of altered behavior in animals, it is important—though perhaps difficult and seldom attempted—to learn whether the change depends on a real change in the nervous system or merely reflects the animal's awareness of a new stimulus or situation. Would a strange odor or a flashing light have a similar effect? It is likely that this kind of integrated information will be sought only by toxicologists familiar with the dosage-response relationship and the practical aspects of occupational medicine. However, in the absence of the comparisons of working conditions mentioned above, the only way to learn the practical value of the specialized behavioral tests is by a critical comparison of their results with the results of the complete range of presently accepted safety evaluation tests.

4.3.5.6 Tests of Reproduction. It is clear that a complex series of interrelated functions are involved in successful reproduction and that many of these functions are not involved to any important degree except in this connection. The most generally used method for evaluating the possible effect of compounds on reproduction is the three-generation test. Its use in toxicology was described by Lehman et al. (1949). An authoritative review of protocols for studying reproduction, including mutagen-

esis and teratogenesis, is that of the FDA Advisory Committee (1970).

The three-generation test is a direct outgrowth of nutritional studies. Jackson (1925) reviewed earlier studies on the effects of inanition and malnutrition on the survival and development of the fetus and of the young. It was found in due course that both deficiency and excess of some nutrients produce marked injury of the young. Thus, it was shown that a deficiency of vitamin A (Hale, 1933) or an excess of the same vitamin (Cohlan, 1953) are both teratogenic. Interest in injury from excess nutrients is closely related to interest in injury produced by an excess of other compounds.

In some of the nutritional studies it was found necessary to maintain animals on a deficient diet for more than one generation in order to deplete them of a trace element sufficiently to demonstrate an effect. In considering tests on the effects of foreign compounds on reproduction, it is reasoned that some compounds might lead to a specific deficiency while others may show greater cumulation of material or effect in succeeding generations. Even if there is no progression of depletion or increase of storage from one generation to another, any effect of continued exposure to a chemical that has its critical effect during development but its manifestation during adult life could be detected only by a multigeneration test. On these bases, the three-generation test is carried out according to the accompanying scheme (see page 216).

If properly adapted to follow up positive findings, the test permits gathering of information on effects of a compound on: (a) health of adults, including health of the mother during pregnancy; (b) fertility of the male; (c) fertility of the female; (d) gametogenesis; (e) genetic function (especially the dominant lethal effect); (f) implantation; (g) teratogenesis; (h) prenatal and perinatal toxicity; (i) parturition; (j) lactation; (k) growth, development, and sexual maturation of the young; and (l) gross and microscopic pathology. Some of these effects are conveniently expressed by indices.

The *fertility index* is the percentage of matings resulting in detectable pregnancy, regardless of the outcome of the pregnancy. Ideally, the fact of mating is established by daily vaginal examinations for copulatory plugs and sperm. Usually, each female is given a maximum of two males for two estrus cycles before being declared infertile. A *mating index* may be obtained by calculating the percentage of positive examinations for copulation (following one night of exposure) resulting in pregnancy.

The *gestation index* is the percentage of

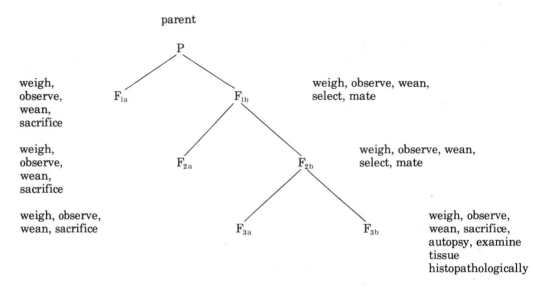

parent

weigh,
observe,
wean,
sacrifice

weigh,
observe,
wean,
sacrifice

weigh, observe,
wean, sacrifice

weigh, observe, wean,
select, mate

weigh, observe, wean,
select, mate

weigh, observe,
wean, sacrifice,
autopsy, examine
tissue
histopathologically

pregnancies that result in at least one living offspring. Any abnormality of the index should be explained by further observations, for example, prolongation of gestation beyond normal term, or some other abnormality of parturition.

The *survival index* is the percentage of young born alive that are able to survive 4 days. Lack of viability of the young can result from abnormality of the mother as well as abnormality of the young themselves. The distinction can be made by observation and by the early exchange of the litters of treated and untreated mothers. Items to consider include: (a) defects of the young; (b) inadequate production of milk; (c) excretion of a toxic substance in the milk; and (d) neglect by the mother, even though she is producing milk.

The term, *viability index,* is employed under two definitions, and therefore its meaning must be ascertained in connection with each report in which it is used. Most commonly, viability index means the same as survival index. Sometimes viability index is defined as the percentage of all young born that are able to survive 4 days.

The *lactation index* is the percentage of young alive at 4 days after birth that survive to weaning. In the case of the rat, survival is measured on the 21st day.

There is no doubt that some compounds interfere with reproduction and that this aspect of toxicity ought to be tested. It is also clear that one or a few doses of some compounds, including many that are teratogenic, interfere with reproduction while having little or no effect on the health of the mother (Murphy, 1965). It is far less clear (a) what proportion of compounds administered in small dosages over a long period injure reproduction without producing some detectable effect on the mother or even on nonpregnant animals given the same dosage, and (b) what proportion of compounds are really more toxic to reproduction in second and subsequent generations than in the first generation. Of 65 unnamed compounds that were studied from the standpoint of reproduction as well as ordinary toxicity, 15 affected reproduction. The lowest dosage that injured reproduction in these 15 instances also had some other toxic effect; however, in 5 of the 15, the reproductive injury was important (decreased fertility, viability, etc.), whereas the toxic effect was merely inhibition of cholinesterase (Food and Drug Administration Advisory Committee, 1970). Thus, studies of reproduction not only reveal kinds of injury that could not be found in other ways, but some of them reveal a lower toxic dosage than can be demonstrated in another way.

The question of the value of multigeneration tests of reproduction is more difficult to answer. It is not necessarily a valid argument that more information is gathered in a complete multigeneration test than is gathered in the first generation of the same test. After all, more information may be gained by repeating any test. The appearance of some injury in a second or subsequent generation may be a random occurrence, indicating that the dosage involved is a threshold one, or perhaps that the observed injury (if different from that produced by larger dosages) has a completely unrelated cause.

By the same token, injury may fail to appear

in subsequent generations after being observed in the first or second.

It is sometimes stated that compounds that are stored, notably the chlorinated hydrocarbon insecticides, are more injurious to reproduction in the second and third generation than in the first. However, experiments with these compounds are not immune to random effects. In fact, in a two-generation test, Ottoboni (1969) found slightly less response to DDT in the second generation than in the first. Thus, although the principle cannot be denied, its application to the chlorinated hydrocarbon insecticides is completely unproved.

Although the necessity to study three generations is not proved, there is objective evidence that three is enough. Keplinger et al. (1970) studied a number of chlorinated hydrocarbon insecticides and combinations of them for five or six generations, but found no reason for continuing beyond three.

4.3.5.7 Techniques for Study of Teratogenesis.
Teratology had its origin in experimental embryology, the main objectives of which have always been improved description and understanding of normal and abnormal embryonic development. Excellent techniques were worked out for producing, identifying, modifying, and enumerating developmental abnormalities, and their study became an end in itself. Some early studies, such as those on cretinism (De Quervain and Wegelin, 1936), had their inspiration in nutritional or other medical problems. However, it was not until the thalidomide disaster that the necessity of viewing teratogenesis from a toxicological standpoint became apparent in a startling way. This realization led to a series of workshops and corresponding books containing the lectures and demonstrations (Wilson and Warkany, 1965; Supplement to Teratology Workshop Manual, 1965). Reviews of teratological techniques are those of Robson and Sullivan (1968) and Delahunt (1970). These books and papers offer an excellent review of teratology and present the available techniques for its study in considerable detail. As pointed out most clearly by Karnofsky (1965), the tools for studying morphogenesis and embryonal toxicology are the same, but the objectives of the two kinds of study are different. In toxicology, particular attention must be paid to dosage-response relationships, and the possible importance of species differences must be kept in mind, for the objective is not only scientific understanding but also the prevention of injury in man.

Teratologists and toxicologists are alert to the practical aspects of teratology. However, it cannot be said that rigorous application of available techniques for animal study eliminates all possibility of introducing a compound capable of injuring the human fetus. The main problem is species difference. No one has thought of a test of teratogenesis in man that would be both safe and meaningful. Under the circumstances, toxicologists prefer multigeneration studies in animals as screening tests for teratogenesis and other disorders of reproduction. This is true even though the repeated administration of a compound may mask its teratogenic activity when given as a large single dose at a susceptible period. For example, Nishimura (1963) found that pretreatment of mice with mitomycin C before pregnancy reduces but does not eliminate the teratogenic effect of the compound given during pregnancy.

4.3.5.8 Tests of Oral Toxicity.
One or a Few Doses. Acute oral doses are often given by tube. Such tubes are commonly spoken of as "stomach tubes," even though they may not reach the stomach. It is important that the dose be given without injury and in such a way that it cannot be refused or regurgitated.

In the case of rats, these objectives can be achieved by skillful use of a 19-gauge needle about 100 mm long, with a spherical or ellipsoidal bead of silver solder about 2 mm in diameter at the end, to prevent perforation of the esophagus. The blunted needle is placed on a syringe of appropriate size, which is filled to the mark with the formulation to be administered, care being taken that the lumen of the needle, as well as that the syringe, is free of bubbles. The prepared syringe is laid aside. Use of the right hand to hold the rat by the tail permits the animal to be grasped firmly by the loose skin over the back and base of the neck in such a way that it can be held in an extended position and in the left hand only. Secured in this way with its head drawn slightly back, the rat is intubated. The syringe, held in the right hand, is introduced into the side of the rat's mouth, then moved to a midline position, and advanced its full length into the esophagus. Except in small rats, the metal tube does not reach the stomach, but the dose is delivered to the posterior part of the esophagus from which the rat cannot regurgitate.

Most other species are given liquid oral doses by means of rubber catheters introduced into the stomach. It is usually sufficient to place the dose in the rumen of ruminants or the crop of birds. It is often useful to prepare a rod of hard wood or plastic with a transverse hole through which the catheter may be passed easily. The rod is placed between the teeth in such a way that the jaws are held open and the catheter may be guided through the transverse hole into the esophagus. Two persons are usually required for intubating rabbits and larger animals.

A small volume of liquid or powder can be given to an animal by placing the dose in the center of a ball of food the animal will accept as a single mouthful. If the animal refuses even a portion of the food because it is distasteful or for any other reason, some other method of dosing must be used.

Carefully measured amounts of either liquid or powder may be placed in suitable capsules. An animal may swallow a capsule placed as far back in the pharynx as possible, or it may be necessary to push the capsule into the upper esophagus with a smooth rod or a special balling gun.

Volume of Dose. Regardless of how doses are given, all of them in a particular experiment should be of the same volume if possible. Unless the effect of volume is under study, concentration should be the only variable. Rats commonly are dosed orally at the rate of 0.005 ml per gram of body weight.

Many Doses. When many oral doses are to be given, one of the techniques used for single doses may be employed. However, it is more common to mix the compound into the animals' regular feed in such a concentration that they will consume it at the desired rate. This procedure has the advantages of (*a*) saving work, (*b*) avoiding injury from repeated intubation or balling, and (*c*) spreading the dose out over the day so that the period of absorption is similar to that resulting from occupational exposure or from residues in food.

The dietary concentrations of a toxicant may be held constant throughout an experiment, but the food intake ought to be measured so that the dosage can be calculated. An attempt may be made to keep the dosage constant by adjusting the dietary concentrations to compensate for differences in food intake resulting from maturation of the animals or any other cause. In this instance, food intake must be measured; dietary levels usually are adjusted each week and based on food consumption during the previous week. In either instance, the real dosage is calculated from the dietary level and food consumption measured while a particular dietary level is in use.

REFERENCES

Abrahmson, S., and Lewis, E. B. (1971). The detection of mutations in *Drosophila melanogaster.* In: *Chemical Mutagens: Principles and Methods for their Detection,* edited by A. Hollaender, Vol. 2, pp. 461–487. Plenum Press, New York.

Ad Hoc Committee of the Environmental Mutagen Society and the Institute for Medical Research (1972). Chromo-

some methodologies in mutation testing. Toxicol. Appl. Pharmacol., 22:269–275.

Alarie, Y. (1966). Irritating properties of airborne materials to the upper respiratory tract. Arch. Environ. Health, 13:433–449.

Amdur, M. O., and Mead, J. (1955). A method for studying the mechanical properties of the lungs in unanesthetized animals: application to the study of respiratory irritants. Proceedings of the Third National Air Pollution Symposium, Pasadena, California, pp. 150–159.

Amdur, M. O., and Mead, J. (1958). Mechanics of respiration in unanesthetized guinea pigs. Am. J. Physiol., 192:364–368.

American Conference of Governmental Industrial Hygienists, Air Sampling Instruments Committee (1972) *Air Sampling Instruments for Evaluation of Atmospheric Contaminants,* Ed. 4. ACGIH, Cincinnati.

Ames, B. N. (1971) The detection of chemical mutagens with enteric bacteria. In: *Chemical Mutagens: Principles and Methods for their Detection,* edited by A. Hollaender, Vol. 1, pp. 267–282. Plenum Press, New York.

Arees, E. A., Veltman, B. I., and Mayer, J. (1969). Hypothalamic blood flow following goldthioglucose-induced lesions. Exp. Neurol., 25:410–415.

Auerbach, C. (1962). *Mutation.* Oliver & Boyd, Inc., London.

Auerbach, C., and Falconer, D. S. (1949). A new mutant in the progeny of mice treated with nitrogen mustard. Nature, 163:678–679.

Auerbach, C., and Robson, J. M. (1947a). The production of mutations by chemical substances. Proc. R. Soc. Edinb. [Biol.] 62:271–283.

Auerbach, C., and Robson, J. M. (1947b). Tests of chemical substances for mutagenic action. Proc. R. Soc. Edinb. [Biol.] 62:284–291.

Auerbach, O., Hammond, E. C., Kirman, D., and Garfinkel, L. (1970). Effects of cigarette smoking on dogs. II. Pulmonary neoplasms. Arch. Environ. Health, 21:754–768.

Back, K. C., and Thomas, A. A. (1970). Aerospace problems in pharmacology and toxicology. Annu. Rev. Pharmacol., 10:395–412.

Balazs, T. (1970). Measurement of acute toxicity. In: *Methods in Toxicology,* edited by G. E. Paget, pp. 49–81. F. A. Davis Company, Philadelphia.

Barnes, J. M. (1960). Toxicity testing. In: *Modern Trends in Occupational Health,* edited by R. S. F. Shilling, pp. 20–32. Butterworths, London.

Barnes, J. M. (1969). Mechanisms of toxicity: introduction. Br. Med. Bull., 25:219–222.

Barnes, J. M., and Denz, F. A. (1954). Experimental methods used in determining chronic toxicity. Pharmacol. Rev., 6:191–242.

Barnes, J. M., Magee, P. N., Boyland, E., Haddow, A., Passey, R. D., Bullough, W. S., Cruickshank, C. N. D., Salaman, M. H., and Williams, R. T. (1957). Nontoxicity of maleic hydrazide for mammalian tissues. Nature, 180:62–64.

Barth, W. F., Gordon, J. K., and Willerson, J. T. (1968). Amyloidosis induced in mice by *Escherichia coli* endotoxin. Science, 162:694–695.

Behnke, O. (1970). Microtubules in disk-shaped blood cells. In: *International Review of Experimental Pathology,* edited by G. W. Richter and M. A. Epstein, Vol. 9, pp. 1–92. Academic Press, Inc., New York.

Benitz, K.-F. (1970). Measurements of chronic toxicity. In: *Methods in Toxicology,* edited by G. E. Paget, pp. 82–131. F. A. Davis Company, Philadelphia.

Bernard, C. (1857) *Leçons sur les Effets des Substances Toxiques et Medicamenteuses.* J. B. Baillière et Fils, Paris.

Bollman, J. L. (1948). A cage which limits the activity of rats. J. Lab. Clin. Med., 33:1348.

Bollman, J. L., Cain, J. C., and Grindlay, J. H. (1948). Techniques for the collection of lymph from the liver, small intestine, or thoracic duct of the rat. J. Lab. Clin. Med., 33:1349–1352.

Boveri, T. (1929). *The Origin of Malignant Tumors*. The Williams & Wilkins Company, Baltimore.

Boyd, E. M. (1968). Predictive drug toxicity. Assessment of drug safety before human use. Can. Med. Assoc. J., 98:278–293.

Boyd, E. M. (1972). *Predictive Toxicometrics*. Scientechnica, Bristol.

Boyland, E. (1957). The determination of carcinogenic activity. Acta Unio Int. Contra Cancrum, 13:271–279.

Boyland, E. (1968). Carcinogenicity. In: *Modern Trends in Toxicology*, edited by E. Boyland and R. Goulding, pp. 107–129. Butterworths, London.

Boyland, E., and Goulding, R. (eds.) (1968). *Modern Trends in Toxicology*. Butterworths, London.

Boyland, E., and Watson, G. (1956). 3-Hydroxyanthranilic acid, carcinogen produced by endogenous metabolism. Nature, 177:837–838.

Brimblecombe, R. W. (1968). Behavioural studies. In: *Modern Trends in Toxicology*, edited by E. Boyland and R. Goulding, pp. 149–174. Butterworths, London.

Brink, F., and Posternak, J. M. (1948). Thermodynamic analysis of the relative effectiveness of narcotics. J. Cell. Comp. Physiol., 32:211–233.

Brodie, G. T., and Russel, A. E. (1900). On reflex cardiac inhibition. J. Physiol., 26:92–106.

Brown, V. K. (1965). Some aspects of percutaneous toxicity testing. Overdruk Uit Mededel. Landbouwhogeschool Opzoekingsstat. Staat Gent., 30:1906–1912.

Brown, V. K. (1968). Solubility and solvent effects as rate-determining factors in the acute percutaneous toxicities of pesticides. Soc. Chem. Ind. Monogr. 29, pp. 93–105.

Bucher, O. (1945). Uber die Wirkung sehr kleinen Colchicindosen nach Untersuchungen an in vitro gezuchteten Bindgewebzellen. Schweiz. Med. Wochenschr., 75:715–718.

Burdette, W. J. (ed.) (1962). *Methodology in Human Genetics*. Holden-Day, Inc., San Francisco.

Burton, A. B. G. (1972). A method for the objective assessment of eye irritation. Food Cosmet. Toxicol., 10:209–217.

Calvery, H. O. (1944). Safeguarding foods and drugs in wartime. Am. Sci., 32:103–119.

Carr, J. G. (1947). Production of mutations in mice by 1:2:5:6 dibenzanthracene. Br. J. Cancer, 1:152–156.

Cattanach, B. M. (1957). Induction of translocation in mice by triethylenemelamine. Nature, 180:1364–1365.

Clark, D. G., McElligott, T. F., and Hurst, E. W. (1966). The toxicity of paraquat. Br. J. Ind. Med., 23:126–132.

Clayson, D. B., Jull, J. W., and Bonser, G. M. (1958). Testing of orthohydroxyamines and related compounds by bladder implantation and discussion of their structural requirements for carcinogenic activity. Br. J. Cancer, 12:222–230.

Clemmesen, J., Fugelsang-Fredericksen, V., and Plum, C. M. (1974). Are anticonvulsants oncogenic? Lancet, 1:705–707.

Cohlan, S. Q. (1953). Excessive intake of vitamin A as cause of congenital anomalies in rats. Science, 117:535–536.

Cook, J. W. (1932). The production of cancer by pure hydrocarbons. Part II. Proc. R. Soc. Lond. [Biol.], 111:485–496.

Cook, J. W., Hieger, I., Kennaway, E. L., and Mayneford, W. V. (1932). The production of cancer by pure hydrocarbons. Part I. Proc. R. Soc. Lond. [Biol.], 111:455–484.

Cornman, I. (1942). Susceptibility of *Colchicum* and *Chlamydomonas* to colchicine. Bot. Gaz., 104:50–61.

Costa, G., Holland, J. F., and Pickren, J. W. (1961). Acute pericarditis produced by piscofuranine, a nucleoside analogue. N. Engl. J. Med., 265:1143–1146.

Council of Europe (1962). *Agricultural Pesticides. Guidance to Manufacturers on Necessary Toxicity Data*. Strasbourg.

Damadian, R. (1971). Tumor detection by nuclear magnetic resonance. Science, 171:1151–1153.

Davenport, J. W. (1970). Cretinism in rats: enduring behavioral deficit induced by tricyanoaminopropene. Science, 167:1007–1009.

Davey, D. G. (1965). The study of the toxicity of a potential drug—basic principles. Eur. Soc. Stud. Drug Toxicity, 6 (Suppl.):1–13.

Davies, G. E. (1970). Detection of sensitizing potential. In: *Methods in Toxicology*, edited by G. E. Paget, pp. 197–214. F. A. Davis Company, Philadelphia.

Davis, K. J., and Fitzhugh, O. G. (1962). Tumorigenic potential of aldrin and dieldrin for mice. Toxicol. Appl. Pharmacol., 4:187–189.

Deichmann, W. B., Keplinger, M., Sala, F., and Glass, E. (1967). Synergism among oral carcinogens. IV. The simultaneous feeding of four tumorigens to rats. Toxicol. Appl. Pharmacol., 11:88–103.

Deichmann, W. B., Radomski, J., Glass, E., Anderson, W. A. D., Coplan, M., and Woods, F. (1965). Synergism among oral carcinogens. III. Simultaneous feeding of four bladder carcinogens to dogs. Ind. Med. Surg., 34:640–649.

Deichmann, W. B., Witherup, S., and Kitzmiller, K. V. (1950). *The Toxicity of DDT. I. Experimental Observations*. Kettering Laboratories, Cincinnati.

DeJonge, H. (ed.) (1961). *Quantitative Methods in Pharmacology*. Interscience Publishers, Inc., New York.

Delahunt, C. S. (1970). Detection of teratogenic actions. In: *Methods in Toxicology*, edited by G. E. Paget, pp. 132–157. F. A. Davis Company, Philadelphia.

De Quervain, F., and Wegelin, C. (1936). *Der Endemische Kretinismus*. Springer, Berlin.

de Serres, F. J., and Malling, H. V. (1971). Measurement of recessive lethal damage over the entire genome and at two specific loci in the ad-3 region of a two-component heterokaryon of *Neurospora crassa*. In: *Chemical Mutagens: Principles and Methods for Their Detection*, edited by A. Hollaender, Vol. 2, pp. 311–342. Plenum Press, New York.

Dickens, F., and Weil-Malherbe, H. (1942). Factors Affecting carcinogenesis. 1. The effect of lipid solvents on tumor production by 3,4-benzpyrene. Cancer Res., 2:560–566.

Dixon, M., and Webb, E. C. (1958). *Enzymes*. Academic Press, Inc., New York.

Dixon, W. E., and Brodie, G. T. (1903). Contributions to the physiology of the lungs. I. The bronchial muscles, their innervation and the action of drugs upon them. J. Physiol., 29:97–173.

Domenjoz, R. (1944). Experimentelle Erfahrungen mit einem neuen Insektizid (Neocid Geigy), ein Beitrag zur Theorie der Kontaktgiftwirkung Schweiz. Med. Wochenschr., 74:952–958.

Down, J. L. H. (1866). Observations on the ethnic classification of idiots. Lond. Hosp. Clin. Lect. Rep., 3:259–262.

Draize, J. H. (1959). Dermal toxicity. In: *Appraisal of the Safety of Chemicals in Foods, Drugs, and Cosmetics*, pp. 46–67. Association of Food and Drug Officials of the United States, Texas State Department of Health, Austin.

Dustin, P., Jr. (1941). Intoxication mortelle par la colchicine. Étude histologique et hématologique. Bull. Acad. R. Med. Belg., VIe Ser., 6:505–529.

Epstein, S. S., and Legator, M. S. (1971). *The Mutagenicity of Pesticides*. MIT Press, Cambridge, Mass.

Epstein, S. S., Bass, W., Arnold, E., Bishop, Y., Joshi, S., and Adler, I. D. (1971). Sterility and semisterility in male progeny of male mice treated with the chemical mutagen TEPA. Toxicol. Appl. Pharmacol., 19:134–146.

Epstein, S. S., Joshi, S., Andrea, J., Clapp, P., Falk, H., and Mantel, N. (1967). Synergistic toxicity and carcinogenicity of 'freons' and piperonyl butoxide. Nature, 214:526–528.

European Society for the Study of Drug Toxicity (1965).

Advances in Toxicological Methodology. Proceedings of the meeting held in Bad Homburg, January 1965. Excerpta Medica Foundation, International Congress Series No. 90, New York.

Eyzaguirre, C., and Lilienthal, J. L., Jr. (1949). Veratrinic effects of pentamethylenetetrazol (Metrazol) and 2,2-bis (*p*-chlorophenyl)-1,1,1-trichloroethane (DDT) on mammalian neuromuscular function. Proc. Soc. Exp. Biol. Med., 70:272–275.

Ferguson, D. M., Etherton, J. E., and Hayes, M. J. (1969). Mitochondrial increase after long-term feeding of morfamquat. Nature, 224:83–84.

Ferguson, J. (1939). The use of chemical potentials as indices of toxicity. Proc. R. Soc. Lond. [Biol.], 127:387–404.

Fishbein, L., Flamm, W. G., and Falk, H. L. (1970). *Chemical Mutagens*. Academic Press, Inc., New York.

Fitzhugh, O. G. (1959). Chronic oral toxicity. In: *Appraisal of the Safety of Chemicals in Foods, Drugs, and Cosmetics*, pp. 36–45. Association of Food and Drug Officials of the United States, Texas State Department of Health, Austin.

Fitzhugh, O. G., and Nelson, A. A. (1947). The chronic oral toxicity of DDT 2,2-bis(*p*-chlorophenyl-1,1,1-trichloroethane). J. Pharmacol. Exp. Ther., 89:18–30.

Fitzhugh, O. G., and Schouboe, P. J. (1959). Subacute toxicity. In: *Appraisal of the Safety of Chemicals in Foods, Drugs, and Cosmetics*, pp. 26–35. Association of Food and Drug Officials of the United States, Texas State Department of Health, Austin.

Food and Agricultural Organization and World Health Organization Expert Committee on Food Additives (1958). Procedures for the testing of intentional food additives to establish their safety for use. WHO Tech. Rep. Ser. No. 144.

Food and Agricultural Organization and World Health Organization Expert Committee on Food Additives (1961). Evaluation of the carcinogenic hazards of food additives. WHO Tech. Rep. Ser. No. 220.

Food and Drug Administration Advisory Committee on Protocols for Safety Evaluations (1970). Panel on Reproduction report on reproduction studies in the safety evaluation of food additives and pesticide residues. Toxicol. Appl. Pharmacol., 16:264–296.

Food and Drug Administration Advisory Committee on Protocols for Safety Evaluation (1971). Panel on Carcinogenesis report on cancer testing in the safety evaluation of food additives and pesticides. Toxicol. Appl. Pharmacol., 20:419–438.

Fox, B. W., and Jackson, H. (1965). *In vivo* effects of methylene dimethanesulphonate on proliferating cell systems. Br. J. Pharmacol. Chemother., 24:24–28.

Frank, F. (1876). Recherches experimentales sur les effets cardiaques, vasculaires et respiratoires des excitations douloureuses, Presenté par Cl. Bernard. C. R. Acad. Sci., 83:1109–1111.

Fraser, D. A., Bales, R. E., Lippmann, M., and Stokinger, H. E. (1959). Exposure chambers for research in animal inhalation. Public Health Monogr. No. 57.

Frazer, A. C. (1951). Synthetic chemicals and the food industry. J. Sci. Food Agric., 2:1–7.

Frazer, A. C. (1952). Problems arising from the use of chemicals in food. Pharmacological aspects: Chem. Ind., May 24, pp. 456–458.

Frazer, A. C. (1968). Function tests. In: *Modern Trends in Toxicology*, edited by E. Boyland and R. Goulding, pp. 130–148. Butterworths, London.

Gabliks, J., Bantug-Jurilla, M., and Friedman, L. (1967). Responses of cell cultures to insecticides. IV. Relative toxicity of several organophosphates in mouse cell cultures. Proc. Soc. Exp. Biol. Med., 125:1002–1005.

Gabliks, J., and Friedman, L. (1965). Responses of cell cultures to insecticides. I. Acute toxicity to human cells. Proc. Soc. Exp. Biol. Med., 120:163–168.

Gage, J. C. (1970). Experimental inhalation toxicity. In: *Methods in Toxicology,* edited by G. E. Paget, pp. 258–278. F. A. Davis Company, Philadelphia.

Gaines, T. B. (1960). The acute toxicity of pesticides to rats. Toxicol. Appl. Pharmacol., 2:88–99.

Gaines, T. B. (1969a). Acute toxicity of pesticides. Toxicol. Appl. Pharmacol., 14:515–534.

Gaines, T. B. (1969b). Personal communication.

Gaines, T. B., and Kimbrough, R. D. (1966). Toxicity of metepa to rats. With notes on two other chemosterilants. Bull. WHO, 34:317–320.

Gargus, J. L., Paynter, O. E., and Reese, W. H., Jr. (1969). Utilization of newborn mice in the bioassay of chemical carcinogens. Toxicol. Appl. Pharmacol., 15:552–559.

Gavrilescu, N., and Peters, R. A. (1931). Biochemical lesions in vitamin B deficiency. Biochem. J., 25:1397–1409.

Gehring, P. J. (1971). The cataractogenic activity of chemical agents. CRC Crit. Rev. Toxicol., 1:93–118.

Ginsburg, J. (1971). Placental drug transfer. Annu. Rev. Pharmacol., 11:387–407.

Great Britain Ministry of Agriculture, Fisheries and Food (1965). *Memorandum on Procedure for Submissions on Food Additives and on Methods of Toxicity Testing*. H.M.S.O., London.

Great Britain Ministry of Agriculture, Fisheries and Food (1966). *Pesticides Safety Precautions Scheme Agreed Between Government Departments and Industry*. H.M.S.O., London.

Gunn, S. A., Gould, T. C., and Anderson, W. A. (1961). Zinc protection against cadmium injury to rat testes. Arch. Pathol. 71:274–281.

Gunn, S. A., Gould, T. C., and Anderson, W. A. (1963). The selective injurious response of testicular and epididymal blood vessels to cadmium and its prevention by zinc. Am. J. Pathol., 42:685–702.

Haddad, R. K., Rabe, A., Laqueur, G. L., Spatz, M., and Valsamis, M. P. (1968). Intellectual deficit associated with transplacentally induced microcephaly in the rat. Science, 163:88–90.

Hagan, E. C. (1959). Acute toxicity. In: *Appraisal of the Safety of Chemicals in Foods, Drugs, and Cosmetics*. pp. 17–25. Association of Food and Drug Officials of the United States, Texas State Department of Health, Austin.

Hale, F. (1933). Pigs born without eyeballs. J. Hered., 24:105–106.

Hanawalt, P. C. (1972). Repair of genetic material in living cells. Endeavour, 113:83–87.

Hayes, W. J., Jr. (1959). Pharmacology and toxicology of DDT. In: *DDT, The Insecticide Dichlorodiphenyltrichloroethane and Its Significance*, edited by Paul Muller, Vol. 2, pp. 9–247. Birkhauser Verlag, Basel.

Hayes, W. J., Jr., Ferguson, F. F., and Cass, J. S. (1951). The toxicology of dieldrin and its bearing on field use of the compound. J. Trop. Med. Hyg., 31:519–522.

Heiger, I. (1930). The spectra of cancer-producing tars and oils and of related substances. Biochem. J., 24:505–511.

Hendry, J. A., Homer, R. F., Rose, F. L., and Walpole, A. L. (1951). Cytotoxic agents. III. Derivatives of ethyleneimine. Br. J. Pharmacol., 6:357–410.

Higginson, J. (1968). Pattern of cancer in industrialized and non-industrialized communities. Food Cosmet. Toxicol., 6:585–586.

Hilton, B. D., and O'Brien, R. D. (1970). Antagonism by DDT of the effect of valinomycin on a synthetic membrane. Science; 168:841–843.

Hinners, R. G., Burkhart, J. K., and Punte, C. L. (1968). Animal inhalation exposure chambers. Arch. Environ. Health, 16:194–206.

Hodgkin, A. L. (1958). Ionic movements and electrical activity in giant nerve fibres. Proc. R. Soc. Lond. ≼Biol.√, 148:1037.

Hodgkin, A. L., Huxley, A. F., and Katz, B. (1949). Ionic

currents underlying activity in the giant axon of the squid. Arch. Sci. Physiol., 3:129–150.

Hoffman, I., and Lendle, L. (1948). Zur Wirkungsweise neuer insektizider Stoffe. Arch. Exp. Pathol. Pharmakol., 205:223–242.

Hogben, L. (1946). *An Introduction to Mathematical Genetics.* W. W. Norton & Company, Inc., New York.

Holan, G (1971). Rational design of insecticides. Presented at the International Conference on Alternative Insecticides for Vector Control, Atlanta, Georgia, Feb. 15–19.

Hollaender, A. (ed.) (1971). *Chemical Mutagens. Principles and Methods for Their Detection,* Vols. 1 and 2. Plenum Press, New York.

Innes, J. R. M., Ulland, B. M., Valerio, M. G., Petrucelli, L., Fishbein, L., Hart, E. R., Pallotta, A. J., Bates, R. R., Falk, H. L., Gart, J. J., Klein, G. M., Mitchell, I., and Peters, J. (1969). Bioassay of pesticides and industrial chemicals for tumorigenicity in mice: a preliminary note. J. Natl. Cancer Inst., 42:1101–1114.

Jackson, C. M. (1925). *Effects of Inanition and Malnutrition upon Growth and Structure.* Blakiston, Philadelphia.

Jackson, H. (1964). The effects of alkylating agents on fertility. Br. Med. Bull., 20:107–114.

Jackson, H. (1966). *Antifertility Compounds in the Male and Female.* Charles C Thomas, Springfield, Ill.

Jackson, H., and Bock, M. (1955). The effect of triethyleneamine in the fertility of rats. Nature, 175:1037–1038.

Jager, K. W. (1970). *Aldrin, Dieldrin, Endrin and Telodrin.* Elsevier Publishing Co., Amsterdam.

Jansen, J. D. (1973). Personal communication.

Joels, N., and Pugh, L. G. C. E. (1958). The carbon monoxide dissociation curve of human blood. J. Physiol. (Lond.), 142:63–77.

Kalter, H. (1971). Correlation between teratogenic and mutagenic effects of chemicals in mammals. In: *Chemical Mutagens: Principles and Methods of Their Detection,* edited by A. Hollaender, Vol. 1, pp. 57–82. Plenum Press, New York.

Karnofsky, D. A. (1965). Mechanisms of action of certain growth-inhibiting drugs. In: *Teratology—Principles and Techniques,* edited by J. G. Wilson and J. Warkany, pp. 185–213. University of Chicago Press, Chicago.

Keeler, R. F. (1969). Toxic and teratogenic alkaloids of western range plants. J. Agric. Food Chem., 17:473–482.

Kennaway, E. L. (1930). Further experiments on cancer-producing substances. Biochem. J., 24:497–504.

Keplinger, M. L., Deichmann, W. B., and Sala, F. (1970). Effects of combinations of pesticides on reproduction in mice. In: *Pesticides Symposia,* edited by W. B. Deichmann, pp. 125–138. Halos and Associates, Inc., Miami.

Kesterson, J. W., and Carlton, W. M. (1970). Aqueductal stenosis as the cause of hydrocephalus in mice fed the substituted hydrazine, cuprizone. Exp. Mol. Pathol., 13:281–294.

Kimbrough, R. D., and Gaines, T. B. (1970). Toxicity of paraquat to rats and its effect on rat lungs. Toxicol. Appl. Pharmacol., 17:679–690.

Kimbrough, R. D., Gaines, T. B., and Sherman, J. D. (1964). Nutritional factors, long-term DDT intake, and chloroleukemia in rats. J. Natl. Cancer Inst., 33:215–225.

Knoll (1879). Über die Wirkung von Chloroform und Aether auf Athmung und Blutkreislauf. Acad. Sci. Vienne, Soc. Medic., 223–252.

Koch, R. B. (1969). Chlorinated hydrocarbon insecticides: Inhibition of rabbit brain ATPase activities. J. Neurochem., 16:269–271.

Kodota, I. (1950). Studies on experimental diabetes mellitus, as produced by organic reagents. J. Lab. Clin. Med., 35:568–591.

Koenig, H. (1969). Acute axonal dystrophy caused by fluorocitrate: The role of mitochondrial swelling. Science, 164:310–312.

Kratschmer, F. (1870). Über Reflexe von der Nasen-

schleimhaut auf Athmung und Kreislauf. Sitzber Akad. Wiss., 62:147–170.

Kuhlmann, W., Fromme, H., Heege, E. M., and Ostertag, W. (1968). The mutagenic action of caffeine in higher organisms. Cancer Res., 28:2375–2389.

Laug, E. P., Vos, E. A., Umberger, E. J., and Kunze, F. M. (1947). A method for the determination of cutaneous penetration of mercury. J. Pharmacol. Exp. Ther., 89:42–51.

Laws, E. R., Jr. (1971). Evidence of antitumorigenic effects of DDT. Arch. Environ. Health, 23:181–184.

Laws, E. R., Jr., Curley, A., and Biros, F. J. (1967). Men with extensive occupational exposure to DDT. Arch Environ. Health, 15:766–775.

Lee, I. P., and Dixon, R. L. (1972). Antineoplastic drug effects on spermatogenesis studied by velocity sedimentation cell separation. Toxicol. Appl. Pharmacol., 23:20–41.

Legator, M. S., and Malling, H. V. (1971). The host-mediated assay, a practical procedure for evaluating potential mutagenic agents in mammals. In: *Chemical Mutagens: Principles and Methods for Their Detection,* edited by M. Hollaender, Vol. 2, pp. 569–589. Plenum Press, New York.

Lehman, A. J. (1952). Chemicals in foods: a report to the Association of Food and Drug Officials on current developments. Part II. Pesticides. Section III. Subacute and chronic toxicity. Assoc. Food Drug Off. Q. Bull., 16:47–53.

Lehman, A. J., Laug, E. P., Woodard, G., Draize, J. H., Fitzhugh, O. G., and Nelson, A. A. (1949). Procedures for the appraisal of the toxicity of chemicals in foods. Food Drug Cosmet. Law Q., 4:412–434.

Lehman, A. J., Patterson, W. I., Davidow, B., Hagan, E. C., Woodard, G., Laug, E. P., Frawley, J. P., Fitzhugh, O. G., Bourke, A. R., Draize, J. H., Nelson, A. A., and Vos, B. J. (1955). Procedures for the appraisal of the toxicity of chemicals in foods, drugs and cosmetics. Food Drug Cosmet. Law J., 10:679–748.

Lehman, A. J., Vorhes, F. A., Jr., Ramsey, L. L., Hagan, E. C., Fitzhugh, O. G., Schouboe, P. J., Draize, J. H., Goldenthal, E. I., D'Aguanno, W. D., Laug, E. P., Umberger, E. J., Gass, G. H., Zwickey, R. E., Davis, K. J., Braun, H. A., Nelson, A. A., and Vos, B. J. (1959). *Appraisal of the Safety of Chemicals in Foods, Drugs, and Cosmetics.* Association of Food Drug Officials of the United States, Texas State Department of Health, Austin.

Lenz, W., Pfeiffer, R. A., Kosenow, W., and Hayman, D. J. (1962). Thalidomide and congenital abnormalities. Lancet, 1:45.

Leong, K. J., and MacFarland, H. H. (1965). Pulmonary dynamics and retention of toxic gases. Arch. Environ. Health, 11:555–563.

Lilienthal, J. L., Jr., Riley, R. L., Proemmeland, D. D., and Frane, R. E. (1946). The relationships between carbon monoxide, oxygen and hemoglobin in the blood of man at altitude. Am. J. Physiol., 145:351–364.

Litterst, C. L., and Lichtenstein E. P. (1971). Effects and interactions of environmental chemicals on human cells in tissue culture. Arch. Environ. Health, 22:454–459.

Litterst, C. L., Lichtenstein, E. P., and Kajiwara, K. (1969). Effects of insecticides on growth of HeLa cells. J. Agric. Food Chem., 17:1199–1203.

Lobashow, M. E. (1937). Über die Natur der Einwirkung der chemischen Agentien auf den Mutationsprozess bei *Drosophila melanogaster.* Genetica, 19:200–241.

Lucas, D. R., and Newhouse, J. P. (1957). The toxic effect of sodium L-glutamate on the inner layers of the retina. Arch. Ophthalmol., 58:193–201.

McIntosh, R., Merritt, K. K., Richards, M. R., Samuels, M. H., and Bellows, M. T. (1954). The incidence of congenital malformations: a study of 5,964 pregnancies. Pediatrics, 14:505–522.

Magee, P. N. (1970). Tests for carcinogenic potential. In:

Methods in Toxicology, edited by G. E. Paget, pp. 158–196. F. A. Davis Company, Philadelphia.

Magné, H., Mayer, A., and Plantefol, L. (1925a). Recherches sur les actions réflexes produites par l'irritation des voies respiratoires. Ann. Physiol., 1:394–427.

Magné, H., Mayer, A., and Plantefol, L. (1925b). La mort par l'inhibition et l'irritation des prèmieres voies respiratoires. Ann. Physiol., 1:428–443.

Marzulli, F. N. (1965). New data on eye and skin tests. Toxicol. Appl. Pharmacol., 7:79–85.

Matsumura, F., and Patil, K. C. (1969). Adenosine triphosphatase sensitive to DDT in synapses of rat brain. Science, 166:121–122.

Medved, L. I., and Kagan, J. S. (1966). Toxicology. Annu. Rev. Pharmacol., 6:293–308.

Meisner, H. M., and Sorensen, L. (1966). Metaphase arrest of Chinese hamster cells with rotenone. Exp. Cell Res., 42:291–295.

Miller, E. C., and Miller, J. A. (1971). The mutagenicity of chemical carcinogens: correlations, problems, and interpretations. In: *Chemical Mutagens: Principles and Methods for Their Detection,* edited by A. Hollaender, Vol. 1, pp. 83–119. Plenum Press, New York.

Morrison, J. K., Quinton, R. M., and Reinert, H. (1968). The purpose and value of LD 50 determinations. In: *Modern Trends in Toxicology,* edited by E. Boyland and R. Goulding, pp. 1–17. Butterworths, London.

Morton, J. P., and Mider, G. B. (1939). Effect of petroleum ether extract of mouse carcasses as solvent in production of sarcoma. Proc. Soc. Exp. Biol. Med., 41:357–360.

Muller, H. J. (1927). Artificial transmutation of the gene. Science, 66:84–87.

Muller, H. J. (1928). The measurement of gene mutation rate in *Drosophila,* its high variability, and its dependence upon temperature. Genetics, 13:279–357.

Muller, H. J., and Oster, I. I. (1963). Some mutational techniques in *Drosophila.* In: *Methodology in Basic Genetics,* edited by W. J. Burdette, pp. 249–278. Holden-Day, Inc., San Francisco.

Murphy, M. L. (1965). Factors influencing teratogenic response to drugs. In: *Teratology—Principles and Techniques,* edited by J. G. Wilson and J. Warkany, pp. 145–184. University of Chicago Press, Chicago.

Nagasaki, H., Tomii, S., Mega, T., Marugami, M., and Ito, N. (1971). Development of hepatomas in mice treated with benzene hexachloride. Gann, 62:431.

Nagasaki, H., Tomii, S., Mega, T., Marugami, M., and Ito, N. (1972). Hepatocarcinogenic effect of α-, β-, γ, and δ-isomers of benzene hexachloride in mice. Gann, 63:393.

Narahashi, T., and Haas, H. G. (1967). DDT: interaction with nerve membrane conductance changes. Science, 157:1438–1440.

Narahashi, T., and Yamasaki, T. (1960). Mechanism of increase in negative after-potential by dicophanum (DDT) in the giant axon of the cockroach. J. Physiol. (Lond.), 152:122–140.

National Academy of Sciences, Food Protection Committee (1956). *Safe Use of Pesticides in Food Protection.* NAS Publ. 470, Washington, DC.

National Academy of Sciences (1960a). *Problems in the Evaluation of Carcinogenic Hazard from Use of Food Additives.* NAS Publ. 749, Washington, DC.

National Academy of Sciences, Food Protection Committee (1960b). *Principles and Procedures for Evaluating the Safety of Food Additives.* NAS Publ. 750, Washington, DC.

National Academy of Sciences (1964). *Principles and Procedures for Evaluating the Toxicity of Household Substances.* NAS Publ. 1138, Washington, DC.

National Academy of Sciences (1968). *Nonhuman Primates.* NAS Publ. 1677, Washington, DC.

National Academy of Sciences (1969a). *Coturnix.* NAS Publ. 1703, Washington, DC.

National Academy of Sciences (1969b). *Genetics in Labora-*

tory Animal Medicine. NAS Publ. 1724, Washington, DC.

National Academy of Sciences (1969c). *Animal Models for Biomedical Research II.* NAS Publ. 1736, Washington, DC.

National Academy of Sciences (1969d). *Rodents.* SBN 0-309-01758-0, Washington, DC.

National Academy of Sciences (1970a). *Gnotobiotes.* SBN 0-309-01858-7, Washington, DC.

National Academy of Sciences (1970b). *Animal Models for Biomedical Research III.* SBN 309-0185404, Washington, DC.

National Academy of Sciences (1971a). *Defining the Laboratory Animal.* SBN 0-309-01862-5, Washington, DC.

National Academy of Sciences (1971b). *Animals for Research.* Ed. 8, SBN 0-309-01864-1, Washington, DC.

Nishimura, H. (1963). Interstrain differences in susceptibility to the teratogenic effects of mitomycin C in mice. Paper presented at 3rd Annual meeting of the Teratology Society, St. Adele, Quebec.

Nishimura, H., and Miyamota, S. (1969). Teratogenic effects of sodium chloride in mice. Acta Anat. Nippon, 74:121–124.

Nodine, J. H., and Siegler, P. E. (1964). *Animal and Clinical Pharmacologic Techniques in Drug Evaluation.* Year Book Medical Publishers, Inc., Chicago.

Ortega, P., Hayes, W. J., Jr., Durham, W. F., and Mattson, A. (1956). DDT in the diet of the rat. Public Health Monogr. 43, Public Health Service Publ. 484.

Oser, B. L., and Oser, M. (1960). 2-(p-tert-Butylphenoxy) isopropyl 2-chloroethyl sulfite (aramitè). I. Acute, subacute, and chronic oral toxicity. Toxicol. Appl. Pharmacol., 2:441–457.

Oser, B. L., and Oser, M. (1962). 2-(p-tert-Butylphenoxy) isopropyl 2-chloroethyl sulfite (aramite). II. Carcinogenicity. Toxicol. Appl. Pharmacol., 4:70–88.

Ottoboni, A. (1969). Effect of DDT on reproduction in the rat. Toxicol. Appl. Pharmacol., 14:74–81.

Paget, G. E. (1970). *Methods in Toxicology.* F. A. Davis Company, Philadelphia.

Peters, R. A. (1952). British anti-lewisite. J. R. Inst. Public Health, 15:89–103.

Peters, R. A. (1963). *Biochemical Lesion and Lethal Synthesis.* Pergamon Press, Inc., Oxford.

Popper, H., Sternberg, S. S., Oser, B. L., and Oser, M. (1960). The carcinogenic effect of aramite in rats. A study of hepatic nodules. Cancer, 13:1035–1046.

Potts, P. (1775). *Chirurgical Observations Relative to the Cataract, the Polypus of the Nose, the Cancer of the Scrotum,* etc. T. F. Carnegy, London.

Puck, T. T., and Kao, F. T. (1967). Genetics of somatic mammalian cells. V. Treatment with 5-bromodeoxyuridine and visible light for isolation of nutritionally deficient mutants. Proc. Natl. Acad. Sci. U. S. A., 58:1227–1234.

Robson, J. M., and Sullivan, F. M. (1968). Teratology. In: *Modern Trends in Toxicology,* edited by E. Boyland and R. Goulding, pp. 86–106. Butterworths, London.

Roe, F. J. C. (1968). Inhalation tests. In: *Modern Trends in Toxicology,* edited by E. Boyland and R. Goulding, pp. 39–74. Butterworths, London.

Russell, W. L. (1971). Definition of functional units in a small chromosomal segment of the mouse and its use in interpreting the nature of radiation-induced mutations. Mutat. Res., 11:107–123.

Sandstead, H. H., Michelakis, A. M., and Temple, T. E. (1969a). Chronic lead intoxication, its effect on the reninaldosterone response to sodium deprivation. Arch. Environ. Health, 20:356–363.

Sandstead, H. H., Stant, E. G., Brill, A. B., Arias, L. I., and Terry, R. T. (1969b). Lead intoxication and the thyroid. Arch. Intern. Med., 123:632–635.

Selye, H. (1965). Induced hypersensitivity to cold. Science, 149:201–202.

Shubik, P. (1970.) Symposium on the evaluation of the

safety of food additives and chemical residues. III. The role of the chronic study in the laboratory animal for evaluation of safety. Toxicol. Appl. Pharmacol., 16:507–512.

Silver, S. D. (1946). Laboratory methods. Constant flow gassing chambers. Principles influencing design and operation. J. Lab. Clin. Med., 31:1153–1161.

Skerfving, S., Hansson, K., and Lindsten, J. (1970). Chromosome breakage in humans exposed to methyl mercury through fish consumption. Arch. Environ. Health, 21:133–139.

Slifkin, M., Merkow, L. P., Pardo, M., Epstein, S. M., Leighton, J., and Farber, E. (1970). Growth in vitro of cells from hyperplastic nodules of liver induced by 2-fluorenylacetamide or aflatoxin B₁. Science, 167:285–287.

Slomka, M. B. (1973). Personal communication.

Sobels, F. H. (ed.) (1969). Studies in mutagenesis. J. Mutat. Res., 8:111–125.

Society of Toxicology (1965). Cutaneous toxicity. Toxicol. Appl. Pharmacol. 7 (Suppl. 2):1–106.

Society of Toxicology (1969). Evaluation of safety of cosmetics. Toxicol. Appl. Pharmacol. (Suppl. 3):1–139.

Sollmann, T. H. (1917). A Laboratory Guide in Pharmacology. W. B. Saunders Company, Philadelphia.

Sollman, T. H., and Hanslik, P. J. (1928). An Introduction to Experimental Pharmacology. W. B. Saunders Company, Philadelphia.

Steiner, P. E. (1942). The induction of tumors with extracts from human livers and human cancers. Cancer Res., 2:425–435.

Sternberg, S. S., Popper, H., Oser, B. L., and Oser, M. (1960). Gallbladder and bile duct adenocarcinomas in dogs after long-term feeding of aramite. Cancer, 13:780–789.

Street, A. E. (1970). Biochemical tests in toxicology. In: Methods in Toxicology, edited by G. E. Paget, pp. 313–337. F. A. Davis Company, Philadelphia.

Strong, L. C. (1945). Genetic analysis of the induction of tumors by methylcholanthrene. XI. Germinal mutations and other sudden biological changes following the subcutaneous injection of methylcholanthrene. Proc. Natl. Acad. Sci. U.S.A., 31:290–293.

Strong, L. C. (1947). The induction of germinal mutations by chemical means. Am. Naturalist, 81:50–59.

Strong, L. C. (1949). The induction of mutations by a carcinogen. Br. J. Cancer, 3:97–108.

Supplement to Teratology Workshop Manual. (1965). Edited by the Pharmaceutical Manufacturers Association, Berkeley, California.

Suzuki, K. (1968). Giant hepatic mitochondria: production in mice fed with cuprizone. Science, 163:81–82.

Swenerton, H., and Hurley, L. S. (1971). Teratogenic effects of a chelating agent and their prevention by zinc. Science, 173:62–64.

Tarján, R., and Kemény, T. (1969). Multigeneration studies on DDT in mice. Food Cosmet. Toxicol., 7:215–222.

Thomas, A. A. (1965). Low ambient pressure environments and toxicity. Arch. Environ. Health, 11:316–322.

Thorpe, E., and Walker, A. I. T. (1973). The toxicology of dieldrin (HEOD). II. Comparative long-term oral toxicity studies in mice with dieldrin, DDT, phenobarbitone, β-BHC, and γ-BHC. Food Cosmet. Toxicol., 11:433–442.

Timofeeff-Ressovsky, N. W. (1929). Rückgenovariationen und die Genovariabilität in verschiedenen Richtungen. I. Somatische Genovariationen der Gene W, wᵉ, und w Drosophila melanogaster unter dem Einfluss der Röntgenbestrahlung. Arch. Entwicklungsmech. Org. (Wilhelm Roux), 115:620–634.

Tobias, J. M., and Weston, R. E. (1946). An apparatus for measuring the retained dose of inhaled substances. J. Lab. Clin. Med., 31:806–814.

Tollenaar, F. D., Mossel, D. A. A., and Van Genderen, H. (1952). Non-nutrient chemicals in foods. Chem. Ind., Sept. 20, pp. 923–924.

Tomatis, L., Turusov, V., Day, N., and Charles, R. T. (1972). The effect of long-term exposure to DDT on CF–1 mice. Int. J. Cancer, 10:489–506.

Tregear, R. T. (1964). The permeability of skin to molecules of widely-differing properties. In: Progress in the Biological Sciences in Relation to Dermatology, edited by A. Rook and R. H. Champion, Vol. 2, pp. 275–281. Cambridge University Press, London.

Tyzzer, E. E. (1916). Tumor immunity. J. Cancer Res., 1:125–155.

Vallee, B. L. (1959). Biochemistry, physiology, and pathology of zinc. Physiol. Rev., 39:443–490.

Vandekar, M., and Komanov, I. (1963). Study of dermal toxicity of organophosphorus compounds. I. Parathion toxicity in relation to the skin surface and the technique of application. Arh. Hig. Rada Toksikol., 14:7–12.

Van Winkle, W., Jr., Herwick, R. P., Calvery, H. O., and Smith, A. (1944). Laboratory and clinical appraisal of new drugs. J. A. M. A., 126:958–961.

Vianna, N. J., Greenwald, P., Brady, J., Polan, A. K., Dwork, A., Mauro, J., and Davies, J. N. P. (1972). Hodgkin's disease: cases with features of a community outbreak. Ann. Intern. Med., 77:169–180.

Walker, A. I. T., Thorpe, E., and Stevenson, D. E. (1973). The toxicology of dieldrin (HEOD). I. Long-term oral toxicity studies in mice. Food Cosmet. Toxicol., 11:415–432.

Walker, E. M., Gadsden, R. H., Atkins, L. M., and Gale, G. R. (1972). Some effects of 2,4-D and 2,4,5-T on Ehrlich ascites tumor cells in vivo and in vitro. Ind. Med., 41:22–27.

Walpole, A. L., Roberts, D. C., Rose, F. L., Hendry, J. A., and Homer, R. F. (1954). Cytotoxic agents. IV. The carcinogenic actions of some monofunctional ethyleneimine derivatives. Br. J. Pharmacol., 9:306–323.

Warkany, J. (1965). Development of experimental mammalian teratology. In: Teratology—Principles and Techniques, edited by J. G. Wilson and J. Warkany, pp. 1–20. University of Chicago Press, Chicago.

Warkany, J. (1971). Congenital Malformations. Notes and Comments. Year Book Medical Publishers, Inc., Chicago.

Warkany, J., and Kalter, H. (1961). Congenital malformations. N. Engl. J. Med., 265:993–1001; 1046–1052.

Weil, C. S., and Scala, R. A. (1971). Study of intra- and inter-laboratory variability in the results of rabbit eye and skin irritation tests. Toxicol. Appl. Pharmacol., 19:276–360.

Weitzel, G., Strecker, F. J., Roester, U., Buddecke, E., and Fretzdorff, A. M. (1954). Zink im Tapetum lucidum. Z. Physiol. Chem., 296:19–30.

Weston, R. E., and Karel, L. (1946). An application of the dosimetric method for biologically assaying inhaled substances. The determination of the retained median lethal dose, percentage retention, and respiratory response in dogs exposed to different concentrations of phosgene. J. Pharmacol. Exp. Ther., 88:195–207.

Whitmire, C. E., and Huebner, R. J. (1972). Inhibition of chemical carcinogenesis by viral vaccines. Science, 177:60–61.

Wilson, B. W., and Stinnett, H. O. (1969). Growth and respiration of monolayer cell structures of chick embryo heart and skeletal muscle: action of malathion and malaoxon. Proc. Soc. Exp. Biol. Med., 130:30–34.

Wilson, I. B. (1951). Acetylcholinesterase. XI. Reversibility of tetraethylpyrophosphate inhibition. J. Biol. Chem., 190:111–117.

Wilson, J. G. (1965). Embryological considerations in teratology. In: Teratology—Principles and Techniques, edited by J. G. Wilson and J. Warkany, pp. 251–277. University of Chicago Press, Chicago.

Wilson, J. G. (1972). Environmental effects on development—teratology. In: Pathophysiology of Gestation, edited by N. S. Assali, Vol. 2, pp. 269–320. Academic Press, Inc., New York.

Wilson, J. G., and Warkany, J. (eds.) (1965). Teratology—

Principles and Techniques. University of Chicago Press, Chicago.

Woodard, G., and Calvery, H. O. (1943). Acute and chronic toxicity—public health aspects. Ind. Med., 12:55–59.

Woodbury, D. M. (1965). Analgesics and antipyretics. Salicylates and congeners; phenacetin and congeners; antipyrine and congeners; colchicine. In: *The Pharmacological Basis of Therapeutics,* edited by L. S. Goodman and A. Gilman, pp. 321–344. Macmillan, New York.

World Health Organization (1969). Principles for the testing and evaluation of drugs for carcinogenicity. Report of a WHO Scientific group. WHO Tech. Rep. Ser. No. 426.

World Health Organization (1971). Evaluation and testing of drugs for mutagenicity: principles and problems. WHO Tech. Rep. Ser. No. 482.

Yates, R. C., and Olson, K. B. (1961). Drug induced pericarditis: report of three cases due to 6-amino-9-D-piscofuranosylphurine. N. Engl. J. Med., 265:274–277.

5

STUDIES IN MAN

It seems likely that more has been written about drugs and other chemicals than about any other aspect of clinical research, except actual disease. This is borne out by extensive recent collections of papers on human research (Ladimer and Newman, 1963; National Academy of Sciences, 1967; American Academy of Arts and Sciences, 1969).

The reason for making some studies in man rather than limiting them to animals is that species are not identical. Under practical conditions (see Sections 2.4.7 and 2.4.20) the factor of species is likely to involve a greater quantitative difference than any other factor in toxicity, except dosage. Furthermore, species differences may be qualitative as well as quantitative. Phenomena of mental state or of allergic sensitivity can be studied in animals only with great difficulty.

Because man is unique, there is a question whether it is right to introduce a biologically active chemical into commercial use without first submitting it to careful observation in a limited number of people exposed to it, under conditions controlled as carefully as possible. The only alternative is to introduce the chemical directly from the laboratory to the public under conditions that necessarily minimize control and discourage observation.

Information about different aspects of the effect of a chemical on man can be obtained in four situations: (a) cases of poisoning; (b) use experience, especially that involving occupational exposure; (c) use of the compound as a drug; and (d) administration of the compound to volunteers. The value of information derived from cases, therapeutic use, and occupational medicine is generally recognized, and no special discussion of the techniques required for gathering it is needed here.

In this chapter, special emphasis is placed on studies of volunteers, simply because this kind of study is less used and less well understood. This emphasis should not detract from the fact that the scientific requirement is for study in man, not necessarily for studies in volunteers. If the requisite information can be obtained from people with occupational exposure, so much the better.

Each of the four kinds or sources of information on toxicology in man has its own advantages and limitations. In general, cases of poisoning constitute our only source of information on symptomatology in man. The fact that poisoning occurred is evidence that the dose was large, but its measurement is often unsatisfactory. Very detailed information on a limited but known dosage range is available for pesticides that have been used as drugs, but the number of these compounds is limited. Use experience (whether at the relatively high dosage rates of workers or the lower dosage rates of other groups) has the advantage of involving relatively large and diverse groups of people for extended periods. It has the disadvantage that the dosage is difficult to determine. Studies of volunteers offer the great advantage that their dosage can be determined accurately. Unfortunately, such studies are usually limited to small groups and a short duration. The fact that volunteers cannot be given dosages high enough to cause harm is a strict limitation, but not one that seriously interferes with the value of this source of information.

This chapter is concerned with technique. It also lists or refers to pesticides that have been studied in man, whether in connection with cases of poisoning, use as drugs, exposure of workers, or investigations in volunteers.

5.1 Cases

Everyone recognizes the need to study cases of poisoning. They are our only source of information on the exact form of illness that adequate doses of most pesticides produce in people. They are also the only source of information on the dosage of most pesticides required to produce illness.

Since there is no way to predict when poisoning will occur, its study must be opportunistic. However, the general quality of reporting has improved because facilities for measuring pesticides and their metabolites have improved. Further progress could be made if more attention were given to the collection of appropriate samples. A specimen of the formulation supposed to have caused illness should be sent to the laboratory in a completely separate container from other specimens. Grossly contaminated clothing should be shipped separately also, lest vapor of the chemical contaminate other specimens. Specimens of vomitus, stomach washings, urine, feces, blood, and organs are always appropriate. Where possible, serial samples should be obtained. In addition, samples should be selected from those materials that, on an epidemiological basis, seem to have been the cause of trouble. For example, if the clothing was contaminated, collect samples of it and analyze soiled and unsoiled portions. If food appears to have been responsible, collect what remains of some that led to illness, and also collect samples of the ingredients of that particular food. Always sample selectively and in reference to cases of illness.

A list of pesticides that have caused illness in man is given in Chapter 7 (Table 7-2). The table does not distinguish cases that arose from accidental, occupational, or therapeutic overexposure. Section 7.1.1 is a summary of the relative importance of different compounds as causes of poisoning.

5.2 Medical Use

Although only a small proportion of pesticides has been used as drugs, it may be astonishing that at least 21 have been administered by the oral or respiratory route; a dozen are still in use in this way; and at least as many are applied dermally for control of external parasites.

Table 5-1 lists pesticides that have been or are now used as drugs. After some of the older materials such as arsenic and phosphorus had been used widely, it was realized that their toxicity far outweighed any therapeutic value they might have, and they were gradually withdrawn from medical use.

More recently, it has become customary, and later required, to study chemicals thoroughly before they are released for sale as drugs. Pesticides that have been studied in volunteers in connection with their use as drugs (and in other connections also) are listed in Table 5-3. A few of them, such as warfarin, eventually came into widespread use. Most of them were found to offer no real advantage over other available drugs, and they were never licensed for regular use. Thus, a somewhat different kind of information is available on the old and new pesticides used as drugs.

5.3 Use Experience

As suggested in the introduction to this chapter, the term "use experience" can be thought of as including total experience in the use of a compound. It would include any clinical findings and the results of measuring residues in peoples' environments (see Chapter 6), and in their tissues and excreta (see Chapter 7). It would even include such useful but negative information as the observation that a compound has been produced at a measured rate for many years, but is not known to be stored in tissues or to be the cause of any illness in man.

However, at this point we shall discuss only the portion of use experience that involves relatively high dosages and leads to some quantitative information—for practical purposes this limits the subject to studies in workers.

The major disadvantage in using workers for tests is the difficulty in regulating or even measuring the dosage. However, this is not a handicap in many biochemical studies, especially where the results can be related to measurement of the compound or its metabolite(s) in blood or excreta (see Sections 3.2 and 8.1.4.1). Furthermore, if the compound or its metabolite(s) can be measured, the results of the study can be used directly in interpreting the safety of other persons exposed under different circumstances that lead to the same—or different—blood levels or excretory levels.

If the dosage is unknown, it may not be possible to determine what proportion of the

Table 5-1

Pesticides That Have Been or Are Administered by
the Oral or Respiratory Route [a] as Drugs for Man or Animals [b]

Compound	Purpose
Pesticides formerly used as drugs	
Inorganic and organometal compounds	
arsenic trioxide [c]	tonic
antimony potassium tartrate	emetic
copper sulfate	emetic
mercurous chloride	cathartic
thallium acetate	depilatory
white phosphorus	rickets
Compounds derived from plants and other organisms	
strychnine	tonic
Solvents, fumigants, and nematocides	
chloroform	anaesthetic
Phenolic and nitrophenolic compounds	
2, 4-dinitrophenol [c]	weight reduction
Pesticides now used as drugs	
Inorganic and organometal compounds	
ferrous sulfate	mineral supplement
Chlorinated hydrocarbon insecticides	
DDD	corticoid reduction
DDT	stimulation of drug metabolism
Compounds derived from plants and other organisms	
chloramphenicol	antibiotic
griseofulvin	antifungal agent
streptomycin	antibiotic
Synthetic organic rodenticides	
warfarin	anticoagulant
Solvents, fumigants and nematocides	
tetrachlorethylene	anthelmintic
Organic phosphorus insecticides	
coumaphos	anthelmintic
dichlorvos	anthelmintic
ronnel	anthelmintic
Ruelene®	anthelmintic
trichlorfon	anthelmintic

a. Pesticides applied dermally to man to control bacteria, insects, or
    other parasites on the surface include: coal tar, boric acid, pyrethrum,
    DDT, lindane, hexachlorophene, dichlorvos, malathion, carbaryl, and
    the complete range of insect repellants.

b. A few other pesticides that were investigated as possible drugs but did
    not achieve continuing use for that purpose are listed in Table 5-3.

c. Some other compounds of the same class have been used as drugs.

compound or metabolite(s) is actually detected. Even so, it may be possible to show that the results are exposure-related by comparing them with results of environmental measurements (see Section 5.5).

Often, the ideal scheme is to use volunteers to relate carefully measured dosages to the dynamics of storage and excretion, and then to carry out other studies, especially very prolonged ones, in workers. Certainly, the exposures of workers often last much longer than any it would be practicable to arrange for volunteers.

Table 5-2 lists epidemiological, clinical, or chemical studies that have been made on workers exposed to pesticides. It includes studies of mixers, spraymen, and the inhabitants of houses they sprayed in connection with testing the effectiveness and/or safety of compounds for the control of vector-borne diseases (mainly malaria). Each paper dealing with this subject is distinguished by underlining its reference. The table does not include studies of environmental exposure, a matter discussed in Section 6.2.3.

5.4 Volunteers

5.4.1 Introduction

Table 5-3 lists pesticides that have been studied in volunteers.

The most important advance that has been made in our times regarding planned tests in man is the recognition that they constitute established medical practice, at least for evaluating the effectiveness of drugs. Testing, as such, is not new. It has been carried on in one degree or another since organized medicine came into existence. Occasional systematic tests were carried on at least as early as 1835, when Dr. Louis (1835) investigated the effect of bleeding on the survival of patients with pneumonia. He found that the longer bleeding was delayed after the onset of illness, the higher the proportion of patients who survived. He concluded quite rightly that if bleeding had not been carried out at all, the results would have been even better. Most people in the medical profession are familiar with the fact that tests on the efficacy of drugs are routine. It is also generally known within the profession that such studies are being done with improved design and increasing skill. If the frequency of these tests is not sufficient evidence that they constitute established medical practice, then certainly this status was achieved in October, 1962, when the "Drug Amendments Act of 1962," which amends the Federal Food, Drug, and Cosmetic Act (21 USC 321 *et seq.*), was passed in the United States of America, requiring that the effectiveness of all new drugs must be tested in man before the drug can be licensed for sale.

Strangely enough, the law requiring that the effectiveness of drugs be tested in man does not require specifically that their safety be tested in this way. It does demand that safety be tested in animals, and that any untoward effects in man be reported promptly. If injury of sufficient importance is demonstrated, license for sale of the drug will be withheld or withdrawn, depending on whether or not the drug has actually reached the market. The fact that testing of effectiveness in man is required directly but testing of safety in man is required only indirectly could be a matter of semantics, but the difference probably reflects a certain general ambivalence in present thinking about tests in man. This ambivalence may be explained on the one hand by an ever present awareness that such tests are needed, and on the other hand by a combination of fear they will be misused and ignorance of the manner in which these tests are carried out under proper scientific supervision. The ambivalence can be relieved by increasing attention to the ethical necessity of testing chemicals purposefully, scientifically, and safely in man, rather than leaving the matter to accident.

5.4.1.1 Kinds of Studies. A number of authors have recognized tacitly (Medical Research Council, 1964) or expressly (Académie Nationale de Médecine, 1952; Hayes, 1965) that there are different kinds of studies in volunteers. Although different terms may be used, all authors seem agreed that the basic distinction is between: (*a*) studies of diagnostic procedures or therapy; and (*b*) studies of physiology in the broadest sense.

Diagnostic or Therapeutic Studies. Subjects for the first kind of study are usually sick at the time of the study. They or their representatives freely consent to a calculated risk in undertaking the study, but they do so in the hope that the diagnostic procedure or treatment will be of benefit to their own health. They usually receive no other reward. Such studies are generally carried out according to a sophisticated design, frequently by the double blind technique. An early example of a controlled study of this kind was that by which James Lind (1753) compared the value of oranges and lemons, vinegar, sea water, cider, and a variety of other preparations as cures for scurvy among 12 patients he selected for the experiment on the 20th of May, 1747. However, it is generally recognized that if the disease being diagnosed or treated is sufficiently rare, such studies must be carried out

Table 5-2

Studies of Pesticides in Workers [a]

Kind of pesticide and compound	Reference
Fumigants and nematocides	
p-dichlorobenzene	Pagnotto and Walkley, 1965
ethylene dichloride	Brzozowski et al., 1954
trichloroethylene	Frant and Westendorp, 1950
Chlorinated hydrocarbon insecticides	
BHC or lindane	Boguskevskii and Burkatskaya, 1951; Brzozowski et al., 1954; Burkatskaya et al., 1959; Milby et al., 1968; Schüttman, 1968; Milby and Samuels, 1971
chlordane	Alvarez and Hyman, 1953; Fishbein et al., 1964
DDT	Gordon, 1946; Quinby et al., 1965; Ortelee, 1958; Krasnyuk, 1958, 1964a, 1964b; Aleksieva et al., 1959; Burkatskaya et al., 1961; Laws et al., 1967b; Jovčič and Ivanuš, 1968; Paramonchik, 1968; Paramonchik and Platonova, 1968; Model, 1968; Schuttman, 1968; Edmundson et al., 1969a, 1969b, 1970; Poland et al., 1970
dieldrin and related compounds	Carrillo, 1954; Hayes, 1957, 1959; Fletcher et al., 1959; Hoogendam et al., 1962, 1965; Hayes and Curley, 1968
Organic phosphorus insecticides	
azinphosmethyl	Simpson, 1965
bromophos	Vandekar and Svetličić, 1966
demeton	Kagan et al., 1958
dichlorvos	Witter, 1960; Gratz et al., 1963; Funckes et al., 1963b; Stein et al., 1966; Zavon and Kindel, 1966
fenitrothion	Vandekar, 1965; Vandekar and Svetličić, 1966
fenthion	Taylor, 1963
malathion	Elliot and Barnes, 1963; Grech, 1965; Milby and Epstein, 1964; Najera et al., 1967
methyl demeton	Asribekova, 1963
naled	Edmundson and Davies, 1967
parathion	Brown and Bush, 1950; Ingram, 1951; Kay et al., 1952; Lieben et al., 1953; Quinby and Lemmon, 1958; Simpson and Beck, 1965
tepp	Sutton et al., 1960
thiometon	Rosival and Rajnoha, 1961
Carbamates and related pesticides	
carbaryl	Best and Murray, 1962; Vandekar, 1965
mobam	Pant et al., 1969
o-isopropylphenyl-N-methylcarbamate	Vandekar, 1965; Vandekar and Svetlicic, 1966; Vandekar et al., 1968
3-isopropylphenyl-N-methylcarbamate	Vandekar, 1965
propoxur	Wright et al., 1969
Phenolic and nitrophenolic pesticides	
pentachlorophenol	Casarett et al., 1969
nitro compounds	Batchelor et al., 1956; Wolfe et al., 1961
Herbicides	
2,4-D and 2,4,5-T	Poland et al., 1971
Fungicides	
dichloran	Edmundson et al., 1967

Table 5-2 (continued)

Kind of pesticide and compound	Reference
Combinations of compounds	Stein and Hayes, 1964; Barnes and Davies, 1951; Princi and Spurbeck, 1951; Fowler, 1953; Sumerford et al., 1953; Culver et al., 1956; Bruaux, 1957; Hayes et al., 1957; Paulus et al., 1957; Quinby et al., 1958; Vengerskaya et al., 1959; Wassermann et al., 1960; Klhufkova and Pospisil, 1961; Lyubetskii and Vengerskaya, 1961; Ruprich, 1961; Davignon et al., 1965; Hartwell and Hayes, 1965; Bezuglyi and Kaskevich, 1969

a. References underlined are for papers dealing with mixers, spraymen, or the occupants of houses treated with insecticides for the control of vector-borne diseases.

with a less formal plan, although with no less skill. For example, a promising new treatment for an unusual form of poisoning must be used when the opportunity arises, or it will not be used at all.

In the case of patients who are unable to give consent because of their age or medical condition, consent should be obtained from the parents or next of kin, just as is true in connection with any diagnostic procedure or therapy for such patients. It is agreed (Freund, 1965) that parents or guardians may consent for a child (or other legal incompetent) in connection with acts for the welfare or benefit of the child (or other legal incompetent).

Physiological Studies. Subjects for the second kind of study may be sick or well, but in either event the state of their health is not in itself critical to the study, and the subjects have no reason to suppose they will be healthier because of the test. They are often paid, or given some other benefit, in exchange for their service and the calculated risk to which they freely consent. (Minors and mental incompetents should not be accepted as volunteers, or should be accepted only with caution and with the consent of their guardians. Married women should be accepted as volunteers only with the consent of their husbands in states where this consent is required by law.)

Here again, the formality of the plan of study has to depend on the situation. For example, preselected groups of men—including one or more control groups—have been studied in regard to critical ambient concentrations of oxygen and carbon dioxide (Consolazio et al., 1947), and the safety of the insecticide mala-

thion (Golz, 1959; Hayes et al., 1960). On the other hand, Beaumont (1833) had no possibility of using controls or of checking his observations in a number of preselected subjects, for there was only one Alexis St. Martin.

Although the separation of tests in man into the two kinds just described is generally valid, it implies a certain defect of logic already hinted at above. To be sure, tests of safety or pharmacological action are not in themselves therapeutic or diagnostic, even if they involve a drug. However, patients selected as controls in therapeutic studies receive no benefit to their own health. The contradiction lies in the fact that certain authors contend that the only permissible tests are those that potentially benefit the health of every individual who participates in them. Strict application of this concept would rob therapeutic tests of much of their clinical value and scientific worth. It is true that the rewards to the participant in the two kinds of studies described above are often different, requiring different administrative approaches. However, the time has come to emphasize the basic similarity of the aim and contribution of both kinds of studies—ultimate improvement of human health. The basic similarity in risk of the two kinds of studies should be emphasized also. There is no way to exclude potential danger from any study. The simplest procedure, such as venipuncture, occasionally causes serious injury, even when proper precautions are observed. However, this is no more true of studies involving pharmacology or safety than of those involving diagnosis or therapy. The probable risk must be judged for each test individually.

STUDIES IN MAN

Table 5-3

Studies of Pesticides in Volunteers

Kind of pesticide and compound	Parameter or condition[a]	Reference
Inorganic and organometal pesticides		
thallium	distribution and excretion	Barclay et al., 1953
Pesticides derived from plants and other organisms, including their synthetic analogs		
barthrin	primary irritation, sensitization and allergic response	Ambrose, 1963
derris	dermatitis	Ambrose and Haag, 1936
pyrethrum	dermatitis	Feinberg, 1934; Lord and Johnson, 1947; Martin and Hester, 1941
	scabies	Sweitzer and Tedder, 1935
	intestinal helminthiasis	Chevalier, 1930
Synergists		
piperonyl butoxide	metabolism of antipyrine	Conney et al., 1972
Solvents, propellants, fumigants, and nematocides		
carbon tetrachloride	concentration in blood, urine, and expired air	Stewart et al., 1961a
isobornyl thiocyanoacetate	excretion, primary irritation sensitization effects, and symptomatology	Keplinger, 1963
methylene chloride	concentration in blood and expired air	Stewart et al., 1972
tetrachloroethylene	concentration in blood and expired air	Stewart et al., 1961b; Stewart et al., 1970
	symptomatology	Rowe et al., 1952
1,1,1-trichloroethane	concentration in blood and expired air	Stewart et al., 1961c
trichloroethylene	excretion in urine	Barret and Johnston, 1939; Souček and Vlachová, 1960; Bartoniček, 1962; Bartoniček and Teisinger, 1962; Bartoniček, 1963;
	concentration in blood	Bartoniček, 1962; Stewart et al., 1962
	concentration in saliva and sweat	Bartoniček, 1962
	concentration in expired air	Stewart et al., 1962
Chlorinated hydrocarbon insecticides		
aldrin	symptomatology	Baker et al., 1959
DDD	skin irritation, sensitization	Haag et al., 1948
	Cushing's syndrome	Sheehan et al., 1953; Southren et al., 1961; Wallace et al., 1961; Weisenfeld and Goldner, 1962; Bar-Hay et al., 1964; Danowski et al., 1964; DeFossey et al., 1968

Table 5-3 (continued)

Kind of pesticide and compound	Parameter or condition[a]	Reference
Chlorinated hydrocarbon insecticides (cont'd.)		
	metabolism of steroids	Bradlow et al., 1963; Bledsoe et al., 1964
	adrenal tumors	Molnar et al., 1961; Nichols et al., 1961; Verdon et al., 1962; Hutter and Kahoe, 1966; Hartwig et al., 1968
	metastatic carcinoma, especially of prostate and breast	Zimmerman et al., 1956; Weisenfeld and Goldner, 1962
	diabetes	Törnblom, 1959
	storage and excretion	Morgan and Roan, 1971; Roan et al., 1971
DDT	symptomatology	Domenjoz, 1944; Neal et al., 1944; Cameron and Burgess, 1945; Case, 1945; Dangerfield, 1946; Velbinger, 1947a, 1947b; Stammers and Whitfield, 1947
	general systemic effect	Neal et al., 1944, 1946; Cameron and Burgess, 1945; Case, 1945; Velbinger, 1947a, 1947b; Stammers and Whitfield, 1947
	sensitization	Draize et al., 1944; Wasicky and Unti, 1944; Cameron and Burgess, 1945; Wigglesworth, 1945; Chin and T'ant, 1946; Haag et al., 1948; Kailin and Hastings, 1966
	storage and excretion	Neal et al., 1946; Hayes et al., 1956, 1971; Thompson et al., 1969; Apple et al., 1970; Morgan and Roan, 1971; Roan et al., 1971
	pediculosis	Domenjoz, 1944; MacCormack, 1945; Kaiser, 1946; Zein-El-Dine, 1946
	scabies	Zein-El-Dine, 1946
dieldrin	skin irritation, sensitization	Suskind, 1959
	absorption, storage and excretion	Abery et al., 1959; Robinson and Hunter, 1966; Hunter and Robinson, 1967, 1968; Hunter et al., 1969; Robinson and Roberts, 1969
lindane and BHC	symptomatology	Batterman, cited by Halpern et al., 1950
	skin irritation, sensitization	Halpern et al., 1950
	pediculosis	Cannon and McRae, 1948; Gardner, 1958; Munster et al., 1962
	scabies	Cannon and McRae, 1948; Wooldridge, 1948; Halpern et al., 1950; Panja and Choudhury, 1969
methoxychlor	symptomatology and pathology	Stein et al., 1965; Stein, 1968
Perthane ®	17-hydroxycorticosteroids and clinical effect in tumor patients	Taliaferro and Leone, 1957; Weisenfeld and Goldner, 1962
toxaphene	symptomatology and general systemic effect	Keplinger, 1963

Table 5-3 (continued)

Kind of pesticide and compound	Parameter or condition[a/]	Reference
Chlorinated hydrocarbon insecticides cont'd.)		
mixture of lindane and DDT	symptomatology	Baker et al., 1959
Organic phosphorus insecticides		
demeton	cholinesterase	Upholt et al., 1954; Rider and Moeller, 1960, 1964; Moeller and Rider, 1959, 1962b, 1963; Rider et al., 1969
DFP	cholinesterase	Leopold and Comroe, 1946; Comroe et al., 1946b; Grob et al., 1947a; Rowntree et al., 1950; Munkner et al., 1961; Spiers and Juul, 1964
	intestinal mobility	Grob et al., 1947b
	labelling of blood cells	Bratteby and Wadman, 1968; Cooney et al., 1968
	mental effects in normal people and psychotic patients	Rowntree et al., 1950
	central nervous system effects	Grob et al., 1947c
	EEG	Grob et al., 1947c; Rowntree et al., 1950
	neuromuscular function	Harvey et al., 1946, 1947
	general systemic effect	Grob et al., 1947a; Spiers and Juul, 1964
	visual functions	Leopold and Comroe, 1946; Scholz and Wallen, 1946
	myasthenia gravis	Harvey et al., 1946, 1947; Comroe et al., 1946a, 1947b; Grob et al., 1947a; Gaddum and Wilson, 1947; Buchthal and Engbaek, 1948
	glaucoma	Comroe et al., 1946b; Marr, 1947; Leopold and McDonald, 1948; Grant, 1950; Stone, 1950
	abdominal distention	Grob et al., 1947b
diazinon	creeping eruption	Hayes, 1963, p. 30
dichlorvos	cholinesterase	Durham et al., 1959; Witter et al., 1961; Rasmussen et al., 1963; Smith et al., 1972
	visual and respiratory functions, reaction time	Rasmussen et al., 1963; Smith et al., 1972
	function of sweat glands	McLaughlin and Sonnenschein, 1960; Smith et al., 1972
difenphos	excretion, cholinesterase	Laws et al., 1967a
dimefox	cholinesterase	Edson, 1956; Edson, 1964
dimethoate	excretion, cholinesterase	Sanderson and Edson, 1964; Edson et al., 1967
dioxathion	cholinesterase	Frawley et al., 1963
EPN	cholinesterase	Rider et al., 1959; Moeller and Rider, 1959, 1962a; Rider and Moeller, 1960
HETP	myasthenia gravis	Westerberg and Luros, 1948
malathion	cholinesterase	Golz, 1959; Gutentag, 1959; Moeller and Rider, 1959, 1962a; Rider et al., 1959; Hayes et al., 1960; Mattson and Sedlak, 1960; Rider and Moeller, 1960

Table 5-3 (continued)

Kind of pesticide and compound	Parameter or condition[a/]	Reference
Organic phosphorus insecticides (cont'd.)		
malathion (cont'd.)	excretion	Hayes et al., 1960; Mattson and Sedlak,1960
	pediculosis	Cole et al., 1958; Barnes et al., 1962; Shawarby et al., 1963
	sensitization	Kligman, 1966; Milby and Epstein, 1964
maloxon	function of sweat glands	McLaughlin and Sonnenschein, 1960
methyl demeton	cholinesterase	Klimmer and Pfaff,1955
methyl parathion	cholinesterase	Moeller and Rider,1959, 1961, 1962b, 1963; Rider and Moeller, 1960, 1964; Rider et al., 1969
naled	dermatitis	Kohn, 1962
paraoxon	function of sweat glands	McLaughlin and Sonnenschein, 1960
parathion	cholinesterase	Edson, 1957; Rider et al., 1958; Rider and Moeller, 1960; Moeller and Rider, 1961; Funckes et al., 1963a; Hartwell et al., 1964; G. R. Hayes et al., 1964; Edson, 1964; Rider et al., 1969
	general systemic effect	Goldblatt, 1950
	absorption	Fredriksson, 1961a, 1961b
	excretion	Funckes et al., 1963a; Hartwell et al., 1964; G. R. Hayes et al., 1964
	cholinesterase	Edson, 1955; Edson, 1964
	myasthenia gravis	Rider et al., 1951; Gregory et al., 1952; Schulman et al., 1953; Osserman and Kaplan, 1954; Rider and Moeller, 1960; Hayes, 1963, p. 39; Rider et al., 1969
tepp	cholinesterase	Grob and Harvey, 1949; Upholt et al., 1956
	symptomatology	Grob and Harvey, 1949
	visual effects	Grant, 1948; Marr and Grob, 1950; Upholt et al., 1956
	myasthenia gravis	Burgen et al., 1948; Grob and Harvey, 1949; Stone and Rider, 1949; Rider and Moeller, 1960
	glaucoma	Grant, 1948, 1950; Marr and Grob, 1950
trichlorfon	cholinesterase	Lebrun and Cerf, 1960; Hanna et al., 1966
	symptomatology	Cerf et al., 1962
	helminthiasis	Beheyt et al., 1961; Cerf et al., 1962; Talaat, 1964
	bilharziasis	Hanna et al., 1966
Carbamate insecticides		
carbaryl	general systemic effect	Hayes, 1963
	excretion in urine	Knaak et al., 1968
propoxur	excretion	Dawson et al., 1964
Phenolic and nitrophenolic pesticides		
DNOC	concentration in blood and excretion in urine	Harvey et al., 1951

Table 5-3 (continued)

Kind of pesticide and compound	Parameter or condition [a]	Reference
Synthetic organic rodenticides		
warfarin	thromboembolic disease	Shapiro, 1953; Pollock, 1955; Friedman, 1959; Wolff et al., 1953; Clatanoff et al., 1954; Baer et al., 1958; Fremont et al., 1963
	absorption and excretion	O'Reilly et al., 1963
Herbicides		
2,4-D	coccidioidomycosis	Seabury, 1963

a. Therapeutic studies in volunteers are underlined.

5.4.2 Legal Considerations

5.4.2.1 Codes of Practice.

Most past discussions of tests in man have been concerned mainly with codes of practice. Although stated in different ways, these discussions add little to the Ten Points laid down by the Nuremberg Military Tribunal (1947) as follows:

(1) Voluntary consent of the subject is absolutely essential. Consent must be based on knowledge and understanding of the elements of the study and awareness of possible consequences. The duty of ascertaining the quality of consent rests on the individual scientist and cannot be delegated. [The original document, which was prepared by Leo Alexander in 1947 and which served as a basis for much of the Nuremberg Code, contained provisions for valid consent of mentally sick persons to be obtained from the next of kin or legal guardian and also from the patient, whenever possible. These special provisions were omitted from the Code, probably because this kind of consent did not apply in the specific cases under trial (Alexander, 1966).]

(2) The test should seek some benefit to society unobtainable by any other method.

(3) The investigation should be designed and based on prior animal study, and the natural history of the disease or problem, and other data, so that anticipated results may justify the action taken.

(4) It should be so conducted as to avoid unnecessary physical and mental suffering.

(5) No test should be undertaken where there is reason to believe that death or lasting disability will occur, except perhaps where the investigator may serve as his own subject.

(6) The degree of risk should never exceed that which the importance of the problem warrants.

(7) There should be preparation and adequate facilities to protect the subject against even remote possibility of injury, disability, or death.

(8) Only scientifically qualified persons, exercising a high degree of skill and care, should conduct investigations on human beings.

(9) The subject should be permitted to end the test whenever he reaches a mental or physical state in which its continuation seems to him impossible.

(10) The investigator must be prepared to end the test if he has reason to believe that its continuation is likely to result in injury, lasting disability, or death.

Put more succinctly by the American Medical Association (1946), tests in man must meet three requirements: (1) There must be voluntary consent of the person on whom the investigation is to be performed. (2) The danger of each study must be previously investigated by animal experimentation. (3) The investigation must be performed under proper medical protection and management.

In the last analysis, the conduct of tests in man depends on the good sense, integrity, and freedom of the participaing scientists, rather than on an elaborate code of ethics. In fact, the only instances in which tests in man were grossly abused involved Nazi physicians who were under military orders to carry out experiments that by their nature excluded any possibility of voluntary participation and, therefore, required coercion of the subjects. It is true that some irregularities of a far lesser magnitude have been alleged (Beecher, 1966), even though the scientists involved were free agents. There is no intimation that the patients or other subjects were coerced or knowingly injured in these instances, but consent either was not obtained or, if obtained, was not recorded in publication.

Any promulgation of a code or any discussion of principles for tests in man is evidence for acceptance of such tests under certain conditions. It is therefore significant that in several countries, codes or discussions of principles, which are basically similar and consistent, have been prepared by important persons or institutions including: Pope Pius XII (1952), the Medical Research Council (1964), the Public Health Council of the Netherlands (1957), the National Academy of Sciences (1965), the American Medical Association (1946), the US Public Health Service (Stewart, 1966a), and the World Medical Association (1964).

Approval of tests in man is most clearly implicit in those codes of practice that set forth administrative regulations for conduct of such tests in a particular institution, or in laws that require such tests. Examples are discussed in the next sections.

5.4.2.2 Regulation of Clinical Research and Investigations.

The US Public Health Service has emphasized the importance of group review in connection with nonstandard, potentially hazardous procedures, and any involving normal subjects (Sessoms, 1958). This pattern was extended by a resolution of the National Advisory Health Council on December 3, 1965 and formalized by a policy decision issued by the Surgeon General on February 8, 1966 (Stewart, 1966a) from which the following is quoted:

"No new, renewal, or continuation research or research training grant in support of clinical research and investigation involving human beings shall be awarded by the Public Health Service unless the grantee has indicated in the application the manner in which the grantee institution will provide prior review of the judgment of the principal investigator or program director by a committee of his institutional associates. This review should assure an independent determination: (1) of the rights and welfare of the individual or individuals involved, (2) of the appropriateness of the methods used to secure informed consent, and (3) of the risks and potential medical benefits of the investigation. A description of the committee of the associates who will provide the review shall be included in the application."

It was pointed out that such a "committee of institutional associates" would need to be: (a) acquainted with the investigator under review; (b) free to assess his judgment without placing in jeopardy their own goals; (c) sufficiently mature and competent to make the necessary assessment; and (d) composed in part of members drawn from different disciplines or inter-

ests that do not overlap those of the investigator under review. The policy was implemented by a number of administrative issuances (US Public Health Service, Division of Research Grants, PPO No. 129, February 8, April 7, July 1, 1966) that established the coverage, form, and timing of the assurance each institution must furnish before it may receive additional grants or extensions of existing grants. It is required that the grantee make and keep written records of group reviews and decisions, and obtain and keep documentary evidence of informed consent. The policy was also extended to intramural and contract research carried out by the Public Health Service (Stewart, 1966b).

That portion of the Public Health Act concerned with research and investigations generally (42 USC 241) requires the Surgeon General to conduct and encourage research and authorizes him, among other things to: "Make grants-in-aid . . ." and "For purposes of study, admit, and treat at institutions, hospitals, and stations of the Service, persons not otherwise eligible for such treatment." (Certain groups [eg, commissioned officers of the Public Health Service, some merchant seamen, and others] are eligible for medical care as distinct from "study.")

It is worth noting that the requirement for review committees represents an extension and formalization of consultation, which was recommended long ago by Percival (1803) as a preparation for testing "new remedies and new methods of chirurgical art."

5.4.2.3 A Law Permitting Tests in Man.

A law that permits tests in man is the "Armed Forces Act" of August 10, 1956 (10 USC 4503), representing the revision, codification, and enactment of pre-existing laws relating to the military services. Army Regulations No. 70-25 (Use of Volunteers as Subjects of Research, Washington, DC, 26 March 1962) cites the "Armed Forces Act" as its basis. Army Regulations No. 70-25 refers only to tests on man that pertain to military research and specifically exclude ". . . investigations involving the basic disease process or new treatment procedures conducted by the Army Medical Service for the benefit of patients." With the exception of any specific reference to prior studies in animals, the regulations restate the Ten Points laid down by the Nuremberg Military Tribunal (see Section 5.4.2.1). In addition, the regulations impose a number of other limitations, as follows: Prisoners of war will not be used under any circumstances. A physician approved by the Surgeon General of the Army will be responsible for the care of volunteers. (The physician may or may not be project leader, but he will have authority to terminate the study at any time.) Appropriate consultants will be available at all times. No studies will be done prior to approval of each protocol by the Surgeon General of the Army and the Chief of Research and Development; for certain classes of studies, approval by the Secretary of the Army is required.

5.4.2.4 Legal and Other Requirements for Tests in Man. It is clear that all countries that are successful in developing new drugs find some way to test them in man.

United States of America. Apparently the only law clearly requiring tests in man as a condition for the licensing of new drugs is the "Drug Amendments Act of 1962" mentioned in Section 5.4.1. The law provides, among other things, that a license will be refused for any new drug if "there is a lack of substantial evidence that the drug will have the effect it purports or is represented to have under the conditions of use prescribed, recommended, or suggested in the proposed labeling thereof." According to the law, "the term 'substantial evidence' means evidence consisting of adequate and well controlled investigations, including clinical investigations, by experts qualified by scientific training and experience to evaluate the effectiveness of the drug involved, on the basis of which it could fairly and responsibly be concluded by such experts that the drug will have the effect it purports or is represented to have under the conditions of use prescribed, recommended, or suggested in the labeling or proposed labeling thereof."

The same law also provides that a license will be refused for any new drug if the reports that are required to be submitted to the Secretary "do not include adequate tests by all methods reasonably applicable to show whether or not such drug is safe for use under the conditions prescribed, recommended, or suggested in the proposed labeling thereof."

Having provided that no new drug will be licensed without prior tests in man for efficacy, the act conditions all such tests "upon the manufacturer, or the sponsor of the investigation, requiring that experts using such drugs for investigational purposes certify to such manufacturer or sponsor that they will inform any human beings to whom such drugs, or any controls used in connection therewith, are being administered, or their representatives, that such drugs are being used for investigational purposes and will obtain the consent of such human beings or their representatives, except where they deem it not feasible or, in their professional judgment, contrary to the best interests of such human beings."

It is interesting that the law requires the consent of persons who serve as controls, as well as those who take or receive candidate drugs. The fact that provision is made for professional judgment in the matter of consent is noteworthy. As pointed out by Cady (1965), the discussion of this matter of consent by the legislators who passed the law (Congressional Record, 1962) will probably be considered if the question of professional judgment in connection with consent should ever be involved in an action in federal court.

France. The French law on new drugs (de Gaulle *et al.,* 1959), as explained in its preamble, was made necessary by the "Stalinon" catastrophe. This circumstance probably explains the emphasis accorded to safety in Article L. 601 of the law. The law does not specifically require tests in man, but clinical trials are required by a regulation (Article R. 5119) issued under the law. Article R. 5119 outlines a wide range of reports that must be submitted in the form of two dossiers in connection with each application for a registration or "visa." Among these reports, the one on clinical trials must specify any necessary contraindications and define the conditions of use. This regulation implies that those making clinical trials will be alert to untoward reactions during the course of the work. However, the separate paragraphs of Article R. 5119 dealing with toxicology and proof of safety do not mention tests in man. In fact, the requirement (Article R. 5.20-4) that the clinical experts will be furnished reports of all trials of toxicity before beginning clinical trials suggests that the toxicity tests are limited to animals.

An important feature of the French law is the requirement, set forth in Article L. 605, that compliance of a candidate drug with the requirements of Article L. 601 must be verified by experts chosen by the manufacturer from a list established by the minister of public health and population. Article R. 5122 sets the term of office of the experts and establishes the composition of a commission to nominate them.

For further details of the workings of the French law see Guillot (1964). It is interesting that the French law and regulations apparently do not require, or even mention, consent by patients taking part in clinical trials.

United Kingdom. Apparently no law in the United Kingdom requires or specifically regulates tests in man. However, somewhat the same thing is accomplished by the Committee on Safety of Drugs (1965) through a "Memorandum to manufacturers and other persons developing or proposing to market a drug in the United Kingdom." In one sense, this brief Memorandum is broader than the American or

French laws, for its refers to "pharmacological studies on healthy human volunteers" as a part of the preclinical investigation of a new drug. The Memorandum goes on to state that the results of clinical trials should include: "(a) human pharmacological findings; (b) therapeutic activity; (c) any hazards, contra-indications, side effects and necessary precautions."

Although the Committee on Safety of Drugs is not a part of the Ministry of Health, it is financed by the Ministry. The Committee would seem to be in an excellent position to sponsor legislation that would give protection from tort claims to the medical scientist who carefully and properly conducts medical research on human beings in accordance with prescribed standards. Under such legislation, the acts of the scientists, within specifically prescribed limits, would be those of the government, and "sovereign immunity" would be waived in cases where unforeseen or unpredictable harm resulted to a subject.

Sweden. Rydin (1965) and Lönngren (1965) have discussed toxicity testing of drugs in Sweden and its relation to laws concerning drugs in Sweden. New drugs must be registered before use. The National Pharmaceutical Laboratory is in charge of the main part of the control work. The Council on Drug Acceptance is the consulting organ, and the National Board of Health determines whether or not a drug can be accepted for registration. Clinical trials include pharmacological and toxicological as well as therapeutic considerations. Emphasis is placed on individual handling of each application for registration.

Discussion. American regulations place more restrictions on the investigator of new drugs than apparently are imposed by medical ethics and custom in some other countries, where greater emphasis is given to the discretion of the physician and less to the consent of the patient. Oddly enough, a relative disregard for the consent of patients subjected to new drugs may be linked with customs forbidding all tests in man that do not contribute, at least potentially, to the health of the subject. As already pointed out, strict insistence on direct medical benefit to the patient rules out not only studies devoted primarily to pharmacology, or the safety of chemicals including drugs, but also rules out the use of placebos in tests of efficacy. Thus, truly scientific testing of drug efficacy would be prevented by a requirement that all tests contribute, at least potentially, to the health of every subject.

5.4.2.5 Court Action.

Malpractice. Until recently there has never been a court case involving tests in man, as discussed in this paper. Of course, negligence (malpractice) may be a basis for suit at any time. Since the generally accepted landmark case of Slater v. Baker in 1767, English and American courts generally have held that human experimentation is at the peril of those who conduct the tests. In the case of Slater v. Baker, tried in English courts (King's Bench) under the jury system, it was established (presumably on the assumption that the physician deviated from the then current method of treating a fractured tibia) that the physician lacked proper skill and failed to disclose his intention or to obtain the patient's consent in using a previously untested procedure. The case established a precedent that has been followed in English and American law and, in various degrees, in other parts of the world.

In any case in which negligence is alleged, the true issue of investigation does not arise. Should a claim arise in the course of a planned test in man, the best defense is proof that the subject assumed the risk knowingly and voluntarily (Monthly Summary from the Office of General Counsel, US Department of Health, Education, and Welfare, December, 1959). Certainly, the mere fact of investigation is no longer considered evidence of negligence. As Cady (1965) has pointed out, the question is not whether a study is made, but how well it is made.

In France, a physician found guilty of malpractice may be subject to fines or a prison sentence under Articles 319, 320, and R. 4, 4th paragraph of the penal code, or to damages under Article 1382 of the civil code.

A Case Involving Scientific Tests in Man. The only case brought to trial involving scientific tests in man was the matter of Hyman v. Jewish Hospital (15 NY 2d 317), in which Hyman, a member of the board of directors of the Jewish Chronic Disease Hospital, sought the right to examine the records of 22 patients who had taken part in a test. The petition was granted by the trial court, reversed by the lower State appeals court, but finally upheld by the Court of Appeals of New York, the highest court in that state. The final decision ruled that the director was entitled to examine the medical records in connection with the study because of the possibility of liability of the hospital, although no opinion whatever was expressed on whether such liability would indeed exist.

The court contest attracted interest in the case from the New York State Department of Education, and the professional conduct of the two physicians primarily concerned with the study was reviewed by the Regents of the University of the State of New York, acting under their responsibility for licensing the medical profession. The findings of fact in the case were published by Freund (1965) and discussed at length by Langer (1966); Langer has also reproduced the body of the Regents' decision. Briefly, the study involved subcutaneous injection of living cancer cells into 19 very debilitated patients suffering from non-malignant chronic disease, and into three equally debilitated controls who had cancer. The patients were told that a cell suspension would be injected as a test for immunity or response. The patients were also told that within a few days a lump would form at the site of injection, but that it would gradually disappear after a few weeks. This is exactly what happened. The record indicates that all the patients approached agreed to the injection and, further, that none suffered any ill effects other than the transient discomfort of the injection and the nodule it produced. The study showed that the sick and debilitated patients with nonmalignant disease rejected cancer transplants as promptly (6 to 8 weeks) as healthy volunteers who had been tested earlier. The test also confirmed that cancer patients are deficient in their ability to reject cancer transplants, the rejection requiring 6 weeks to several months. The court noted that these findings open up the possibility of stimulating defense against cancer, either before it strikes or perhaps even later when it has taken hold.

In spite of these considerations, the Regents found the two physicians guilty of "unprofessional conduct" and of "fraud and deceit in the practice of medicine," because the patients had not been told that living cancer cells were to be injected and, therefore, the patients could not give informed consent. The physicians' medical licenses were suspended for a year, but the sentence was stayed, and the men continued to practice while on probation for 1 year. The Regents held that: (a) it is the volunteer, and not the physician, who has the right to decide what factors are or are not relevant to consent—hence all details must be revealed; and (b) when acting as an investigator, the physician has no claim in the doctor-patient relationship that in a therapeutic situation would give him the generally acknowledged right to withhold information if he judged it in the best interest of the patient. The desirability of obtaining consent in writing was emphasized.

Perhaps the most important aspect of the entire proceedings was that the legality and propriety of the study itself were never challenged; only the failure to obtain informed consent was condemned. This is a strong indication of the public support that medical research enjoys. Further evidence may be found in the informed and constructive comments on the case appearing in some parts of the lay press (Carley, 1966), as well as in some scientific journals (Freund, 1965; Langer, 1966; Halpern, 1966).

5.4.2.6 Consent. Although consent has been mentioned in preceding sections and must be referred to in later ones also, several aspects of the matter need to be emphasized at this point.

Informed consent for a particular project ought to be based on knowledge of need for the rsearch, as well as on knowledge of real and potential hazards. A person's consent will be more complete if it is based on his conviction that he is contributing to the welfare of others, as well as contributing in one or more ways to his own benefit.

Since the vast majority of investigators have the welfare of their subjects uppermost in their minds, it seems likely that the greatest contribution of the concept of consent is not in protecting subjects—although this is a real contribution—but rather in providing a device for justifying studies that do not offer direct benefit to the participant. If informed consent is the yardstick by which adequate protection of the subject is measured, there is no logical difficulty in undertaking studies of the safety of drugs and a wide range of other chemicals. All of these tests are excluded if one insists, as in France, that every study must be of potential value to every participant. Thus, the concept of consent offers an intellectual basis for a truly scientific study of drugs and other chemicals, whereas insistence on personal benefits fails to offer the same intellectual basis and, if adhered to, rules out the use of placebos and double blind study.

It is argued by some that only persons trained in medicine or closely related disciplines are capable of really understanding an investigation. Although this statement contains an element of truth, it is basically misleading. Any adult of normal intelligence can be instructed so that he understands the most drastic potential hazards of an investigation, even though he does not comprehend the details or have any clear idea of the probability of injury. Few laymen would admit they failed to understand a release from liability for "any injury, fatal or otherwise, that may result." Most laymen recognize that a release from liability for "any results that may occur" carries the same implications (see Section 5.4.3.5). A great many studies have been completed by volunteers who signed such releases as a condition of participation. Thus, an intelligent layman is capable of informed consent, as well as many other complex decisions of which those who question democracy seem eager to divest him.

These considerations cover most situations involving studies of pesticides and other industrial chemicals in volunteers, inasmuch as nearly all of these studies involve adults capable of both understanding and legal consent. A minor exception may involve the use of new drugs in the treatment of persons who have been poisoned, but who because of age, unconsciousness, or some other condition are incapable of giving legal consent. However, because of the clear need of the patient for medical assistance, this small number of cases falls naturally within the ordinary patient-physician relationship and has offered no practical problem of consent.

It rarely happens that there is any need to carry out nontherapeutic tests of chemicals in children, or in persons who are mentally disturbed or incompetent. However, there is a very real need to use such subjects in connection with studies of nutrition, pediatric disease, psychiatric disease, and some other important conditions. The question of consent in these instances is beyond the scope of this book, but information on the subject may be found in reviews (Ladimer and Newman, 1963; National Academy of Sciences, 1965, 1967; Stumpf, 1966, 1967; American Academy of Arts and Sciences, 1969).

5.4.3 Design of Studies

5.4.3.1 Selection of Parameters. Tests in man should be carried out only after whatever tests may be possible in animals have revealed one or more parameters suitable for study in man. Even the most superficial study in animals often will reveal which organ system is involved predominantly in toxic action. One may then determine by further study which of the functional tests appropriate for exploring this organ system in man is best able to measure the alteration produced in animals. Thus, an *index test* may be found. Emphasis should be placed on the appropriateness and thoroughness of the studies, not on the use of large numbers of animals. Every effort must be made to avoid producing in man any clinical illness or any irreversible subclinical change. Therefore, in preliminary animal studies, emphasis must be placed on finding tests to detect the earliest, mildest, reversible change that indicates action of the chemical under study. A valuable discussion of tests of the various organ systems of man is given in a book entitled *Animal and Clinical Pharmacologic Techniques in Drug Evaluation*, edited by Nodine and Siegler (1964). A few illustrations may be helpful at this point.

With few exceptions, research has failed to turn up a test for any effect of organic phosphorus or carbamate insecticides that is more sensitive than a test for depression of blood cholinesterase activity. This is true even if the comparison is made with alterations of conditioned reflexes (Letavet, 1961), or other behavioral change (Carpenter et al., 1961). Therefore, any study of an organic phosphorus or carbamate insecticide in man ought to include the measurement of plasma and red cell cholinesterase as an index test.

The recognized exceptions to the generalization about the sensitivity of cholinsterase include the inhibition of aliesterases by low dosages of some organic phosphorus pesticides and the neurotoxicity of one organic phosphorus compound that is not a pesticide. The implication of these two kinds of exceptions is entirely different.

Some organic phosphorus compounds (eg, EPN, TOCP, dioxathion, carbophenothion, fenthion, coumaphos, ronnel, tributyl phosphorotrithioite, and schradan) inhibit aliesterases (diethylsuccinase and tributyrinase) at substantially lower daily dosage levels than they require to inhibit cholinesterases to the same degree. Other organic phosphorus compounds (eg, parathion) inhibit aliesterases and cholinesterases at about the same dosage levels (Su et al., 1971). Compounds that inhibit aliesterases much more efficiently than they inhibit cholinesterases are likely to potentiate the toxicity of malathion and other compounds whose toxicity is highly dependent on their rate of detoxication. Compounds that inhibit aliesterases and cholinesterases to about the same degree are likely to be additive in their toxicity. Any study of an organic phosphorus compound or carbamate in man offers an opportunity to learn its ability to inhibit aliesterases, but this measurement is less important than measurement of cholinesterases.

All potential insecticides that produce neurotoxicity (delayed, irreversible paralysis) also produce cholinesterase inhibition. Measurement of cholinesterase activity used as an index test in any investigation in man concerned with an organic phosphorus or carbamate compound may give warning before a neurotoxic dosage is reached. However, at least one organic phosphorus compound (tri-*p*-ethylphenyl phosphate) that is not insecticidal and does not inhibit cholinesterase is neurotoxic in chickens (Cavanagh et al., 1961). Clearly, the possibility that an organic phosphorus compound is neurotoxic should be thoroughly studied in chickens, and compounds that are positive should not be tested in man.

Some functions may be measured mechanically rather than biochemically. Complex reaction time was found by Durham *et al.* (1965) to be affected in persons sufficiently exposed to organic phosphorus insecticides. It seems reasonable that the same would be true of airway resistance. Depth perception was affected by traces of tetraethylpyrophosphate in one eye, but not in both eyes (Upholt *et al.*, 1956). In general, even those functions that are relatively simple to measure mechanically in man are difficult or impossible to measure in animals, and yet, like the ones just mentioned, they may be critical to the safety of workers or others.

An effort should be made to measure the effect, if any, of a compound on the critical functions of those who may use it, whether or not there is a pharmacological reason to think it will affect those functions. For example, drugs or other chemicals to which pilots may be exposed should be tested for their effect on vision and reaction time.

Any test of pharmacological action is of potential value in judging the safety of a chemical not intended for use as a drug. No action is expected under ordinary conditions of use, and if one occurs, its significance must be evaluated. On the contrary, pharmacological action must be present if a compound is a drug. Thus, a drug is judged unsafe only if it leads to discomfort or dysfunction incommensurate with the benefits its produces.

Whenever either drugs or other chemicals are tested in man, an effort should be made to measure the compound or its metabolite(s) in blood and excreta. Such measurements permit use of information gained during the test in the solution of diagnostic and other practical problems. For example, if a person is suspected of being poisoned by a particular compound, it is of great interest to know whether the concentration of it in his blood is merely equal to or is significantly greater than that previously found in healthy volunteers or workers. By much the same token, it is valuable to learn as much as possible about the metabolism of compounds in man. Information on this matter may help to explain observed similarities or differences in the pharmacological or toxicological action of the compound in man and animals (Brodie, 1964). In particular, such information may help in selection of the best species of experimental animal for further exploration of the compound. It often happens, not only in connection with metabolism, but also in connection with other parameters, that studies in man will raise a question that can be explored best in animals before it is returned to man a second time for further evaluation.

No matter what special parameters are selected for study, every test in man must include a medical history and general physical and laboratory examinations. These studies must be made before the chemical under investigation is administered, and they must be repeated at suitable intervals. This general surveillance should detect unexpected reactions, including sensitization that may be peculiar to man. The surveillance should also detect illness that is etiologically unrelated to the chemical under study. Such basically unrelated illness may influence the reaction of the body to the compound under study or, if not detected early, it may serve to confuse the study.

5.4.3.2 Selection of Dosage. The highest dosage selected for a test in volunteers should be one that is believed to be (*a*) harmless on the basis of animal studies and all other available information, and (*b*) capable of influencing some measurable parameter. For compounds of low toxicity, measurement of excretion of the compound or its metabolites may be the only parameter influenced. For compounds of moderate or high toxicity, it may be desirable to use a graduated series of dosages beginning with a very low one, and gradually approaching the highest dosage that produced no significant injury in animals.

Regardless of the toxicity, it is usually desirable to have more than one dosage, either in a single test or in succeeding tests, in order to determine whether responses are dosage related. Even if dosage-response is not under investigation, it is necessary that a control group be included in every study. Its use may serve to detect laboratory error and other factors that might influence the results, without having any relation to the agent under study.

5.4.3.3 Choice of Volunteers. Selection of volunteers is determined by (*a*) the number of people required, and (*b*) the duration of the study. People from any group including the general population may be recruited for short periods of testing, especially if the tests involve little inconvenience. In studies in which each individual need be tested only once, and then only briefly, one could eventually study large numbers of people enrolled from the general population. However, for studies requiring a substantial number of volunteers for an extended period, the only practical method is to recruit volunteers through employment or through appeal to some special interest of the candidates. Thus, depending on the nature of their interests, volunteers for most studies of safety may involve the following groups: (*a*) patients; (*b*) paid employees from the general population, groups of workers, or other groups; (c) laboratory staff; (d) medical or other students; (e) military personnel, including conscientious objectors; (f) persons with some occupational interest in the problem under study; and (g) prisoners.

If patients wish to volunteer for a test having no relation to relief of their own condition, they may do so, provided they are capable of giving consent. In fact, there are a few studies that in man can be carried out only in patients. An example would be measurement after death of the distribution of a chemical in all tissues of the body. Another example would be any study involving debility or a specific metabolic disorder as a necessary condition.

In any study of patients as volunteers, the investigator should not be the personal physician for any volunteer, and a personal physician as well as the investigator should be able to discontinue the participation of one or more volunteers, as required. Of course, each patient should be able to stop his own participation at will.

Fully paid employees have been utilized in small numbers, and usually for special purposes. Although perhaps not typical, Alexis St. Martin, who was studied by Beaumont (1833), is the most famous employee hired in order that he might be studied. This method of obtaining volunteers deserves more consideration. It offers a particularly good opportunity to choose the desired distribution of persons of different age and sex.

A number of studies have been carried out using laboratory staff. This method has the advantage that the volunteers are conveniently available for repeated brief examinations, which under other circumstances would require far more of their time and of the investigator's time. Another advantage is that such volunteers, because of their technical background, are in an unusually good position to understand the nature of the test and its potential risks. This means that the investigator need not exaggerate the danger of the study in order to be sure he has not underestimated it. The chief disadvantage of using staff as volunteers is that it is difficult to avoid subtle coercion. Many staffs are not large enough to provide a numerically adequate group for study even if everyone participates. The result is social pressure to be one of the group. The pressure may increase as the study progresses and the volunteers develop an *esprit de corps*. By the same token, a volunteer cannot leave such a study without attracting special attention. There is a certain danger that because of their social and economic rela-

tions to the investigator, these volunteers may be more likely than some others to behave as they think they should. Obviously, this danger is greater in connection with subjective tests, and should be essentially nonexistent in connection with chemical or physical measurements. All the disadvantages of studies using laboratory staff are accentuated in studies in which the investigator is also a subject.

The comments in the preceding paragraph apply with equal force to medical or other students used as volunteers. This is especially true if the students come from the same school or department as the investigator. The disadvantages would be lessened if the volunteers were drawn from a large student body so that, although the participants become known to one another, they are not generally recognized as a group by the student body.

The use of military personnel or civilian personnel of military installations in medical studies is limited to the armed forces and to the problems peculiar to their mission.

People may volunteer for tests because of an occupational interest in the problem under study. In this respect, they are like military volunteers, because they know they may contribute directly to their own future welfare if they can help in the solution of a problem peculiar to their work. For example, crop duster pilots volunteered during the winter season, when they were not flying, for a study to learn how tetraethylpyrophosphate affects vision, and especially why, when pilots had gotten it in their eyes, it had interfered with their ability to judge distance and thus to control their planes (Upholt *et al.*, 1956).

Prisoners offer many advantages as candidates for medical study. The population of a single prison is often large enough to permit an adequate number of volunteers of the desired range of age. In many instances, both men and women will be available through the same prison administration, though seldom at the same installation. If the institution is large enough, sufficient volunteers may be obtained without exerting any social pressure on them, and a volunteer can stop participating without drawing special attention from his fellow prisoners. With proper scheduling, the studies may be carried out with efficient use of the investigator's time, and without interfering with the prisoners' regular duties. The disadvantages of using prisoners include their erratic motivation and their often considerable variation in ability to understand the nature and risks of a study. A major disadvantage is that all doses or other treatments must be given under observation. By contrast, staff members not only may take their own doses, but may do so during travel or other inconvenient circumstances.

Those without personal familiarity with tests in man sometimes express doubts that volunteers act without some form of coercion. The doubt is probably most often expressed about prisoners, but may be referred to medical students or any other group from which volunteers may be drawn. The most convincing argument against this sort of doubt is active experience with a properly conducted study.

5.4.3.4 Studies of Workers.

In the preceding section on volunteers, workers might be included under several headings, especially "paid employees," although the pay in question is that received for medical study and not that for whatever duty makes the person a "worker." The distinction between participation of an employee in a study as a volunteer or as a worker lies in the nature of the exposure. Regardless of his employment status, a person is a volunteer if he agrees to receive an exposure administered for the purpose of making a study. On the contrary, a worker is not a volunteer in the usual sense if he agrees to undergo medical study in relation to an exposure or some other factor that is a necessary condition of his regular employment.

One might ask how participation of a worker in the kinds of tests under discussion differs from that ordinarily involved in good industrial medicine. The difference is one of emphasis; there is no clear dividing line. Tests in man emphasize our ignorance of how chemicals or other environmental factors act in man; hence, these tests seek new information. They seek safety by trying to identify and define unexpected dangers. Industrial medicine emphasizes our wealth of knowledge of how chemicals or other environmental factors act in man. Like any good medical practice, industrial medicine attempts to prevent—and if necessary, cure—injury by taking all known dangers and signs of danger into account.

Some opposition to tests in man seems to be based on a desire of industry to limit the extent of tests, of whatever nature, that are required for official acceptance of a product. This opposition might be reduced if it were understood fully that many of the tests that need to be done regarding pharmacology and safety can be carried out in workers as a part of good occupational medicine.

It is a curious fact that, in studies of workers, no question is raised about consent for exposure, although consent for diagnostic procedures should be obtained by the investigator.

It is assumed that consent for exposure exists if a person is employed in the manufacture or formulation of a chemical, provided the management takes conventional measures to limit exposure and no illness occurs as a result of the exposure. This is true even in those instances in which the amount of chemical absorbed is equal to or greater than that adequate for studies in volunteers.

5.4.3.5 Protocol and Conduct of the Study.

Function and Content of the Protocol. The plans for every study in man should be put in writing. Before this is done, it may be well to reach an informal agreement with the administration of any institution where the study is to be made. Such preliminary discussion may save a great deal of inconvenience by bringing to light requirements of the institution that, although of no scientific importance, may be of crucial practical significance. In general, the writing of a protocol forces the investigator to face not only the scientific but also the technical and administrative logistics of the study. Once the document is prepared, it may be used as a basis for approval of the project by (a) management or custodial authorities for administrative feasibility, or (b) academic or comparable authorities for scientific merit and safety.

The protocol should cover at least the following topics: (a) summary of the problem that justifies the study, (b) specific purpose of the study; (c) experimental design; (d) safety of the study; (e) rewards to volunteers; and (f) proposed contract or other form to document consent.

The "problem" referred to in item (a) may be very broad. It is often ill defined, but never unimportant. An example would be the need to control the vector of urban yellow fever, dengue, and hemorrhagic fever. The fact that the vector, *Aedes aegypti,* is not yet fully controlled only adds to its importance as a medical problem.

By contrast with the problem, the purpose of any study in man should be clearly defined and is frequently very limited. Thus, study of a candidate insecticide such as difenphos to help to control *A. aegypti* might be limited to investigation of its metabolism and storage in normal people.

The section of the protocol dealing with experimental design should state the number of people to be studied, their distribution into experimental groups, the rate and duration of dosage, and the observations to be made. The groups should be large enough to permit statistically valid conclusions, even if some of the participants drop out before the study is complete. The protocol should state clearly what measurements are to be completed before dosage or some other experimental situation is instituted, and how long this preliminary period will be. The protocol should also state what observations are to be made after dosage is discontinued. The duration of study need not be predetermined, but the schedule may be defined in terms of some pharmacological constant. For example, the study may be continued after dosage is stopped until the excretion of a metabolite of the chemical under study reaches the level found in the controls.

The section on experimental design should give particular attention to things that concern the volunteers directly. Thus, the protocol should state the kind and approximate number of samples that will be taken from each person. It is just as important to enumerate procedures that may involve inconvenience or interference with institutional routine as it is to define those that may involve pain, discomfort, or even risk. The author and his colleagues almost lost a project because the way in which the urine samples were collected interfered with the employment of a few of the volunteers in a weaving mill, which was a part of the occupational training and therapy program of the prison. Fortunately, it was possible to change the schedule for collecting samples without decreasing their number or scientific value, and the study was saved. Not all difficulties can be foreseen, but they can be reduced by careful planning.

The section on safety is one of the most important parts of the protocol. If possible, this section should be brief and inescapably clear. The major points may be supported by published reports of animal experiments or by other appropriate documents presented as appendices. In any event, this section must define: (a) the nature of any hazard; (b) the probability of danger; (c) the means availble to detect or, if possible, predict injury; and (d) the possibility of specific treatment if injury should occur. The section on safety must include a statement that individual volunteers or the entire group will be withdrawn from active participation if circumstances require it. Of course, a volunteer whose active participation is stopped will continue under observation, and he will receive therapy if needed.

The protocol should specify the rewards (eg, money and a certificate) the investigator is prepared to give the volunteers. It may also list other compensations that would be appropriate although they are not under the control of the investigator. For example, if the work is done at an institution which is able to offer some other form of reward, then that, too, should be mentioned. Some prison systems routinely give a reduction in sentence for good behavior, including but not restricted to participation in medical research.

The last section of the protocol should refer to the agreement or contract to be used in connection with the study. The American Medical Association (1973) has supplied a model release form (Form P-30) for use with an experimental procedure or treatment, and another (Form P-31) for use with an investigational drug. The latter form is reproduced by permission of the American Medical Association.

The author and his colleagues have used a more elaborate contract in connection with studies in institutions. The contract includes the following features: (a) date; (b) name of organization (or persons) making the study; (c) name of institution where study is made; (d) name of applicant; (e) description of the study; (f) kind and approximate number of services applicant will be expected to contribute, and the approximate duration of service; (g) statement by the applicant that the procedure, value, and danger of the study have been explained to him, and that he is fully aware that there can be no guarantee that he will not become ill (in a study in which illness really is anticipated, its nature should be defined in the contract); (h) statement by the applicant that he knowingly and voluntarily accepts the risks, and agrees to cooperate in the work; (i) amount of money and other rewards the applicant will receive in exchange for his services, provided his participation is satisfactory; (j) applicant's statement on behalf of himself, his representatives, and heirs that he releases the investigators and the organization they represent from all liability, including claims, and suits at law or in equity for any injury, fatal or otherwise, that may result from his participation in the investigation; (k) signature of the applicant; (l) signature of witnesses; (m) signature of responsible investigator who accepts the applicant as a volunteer; (n) signature of officer who approves the contract for the institution where the work is done.

The contract always omits any statement that the applicant agrees to remain in the project. In some instances, the signatures mentioned above were followed by a statement signed by an officer of the institution: "I attest that the purposes, procedures, and inherent risks of this study were fully explained to the applicant by the officer in charge of the investigation. I am convinced of the applicant's complete understanding of the study and of his willingness to participate in it. I am confident that no duress of any kind was present in the

AUTHORIZATION FOR TREATMENT WITH

DRUG UNDER CLINICAL INVESTIGATION

A.M.
Date_____ Time_____P.M.

I authorize Dr._____, the attending

physician, to treat_____with
             (name of patient)

the drug presently identified as _____

for the following condition: _____

_____
    (Describe symptoms of disease to be treated)

It has been explained to me that the safety and usefulness of

the drug in the treatment of patients for the above condition are now

being investigated and that the manufacturer or distributor has

supplied the drug for the purpose of providing further evidence of

its safety and usefulness.

I voluntarily consent to treatment with the drug and release the

attending physician from liability for any results that may occur.

Signed_____
          (Patient or person authorized
          to consent for patient)

Witness_____

proceedings leading to the signing of this con-tract."

Initiation of a Study. The method of obtaining volunteers must vary with circumstances. If the study involves members of a laboratory staff, they will be generally familiar with the need for the study and the character of the risk, if any, as the preliminary work progresses in experimental animals. If the work is to be done with a group of people who have no preliminary introduction to it, it is best that a completely impersonal notice be issued, and that the candidates consist only of those persons who show enough interest to seek further information. Such a notice should state briefly the purpose and nature of the study and invite anyone interested to attend a meeting at a specified time and place, at which a further explanation will be offered. If the work is done in a prison the custodial staff should screen those who propose to attend the introductory meeting in order to exclude those who are unsuitable by reason of a short sentence, a reputation for making trouble, or some special duty that would conflict with participation in the study.

At the meeting, the principal investigator and others, if necessary, should explain the study in detail. Emphasis should be placed on: (*a*) the value of the work; (*b*) what each volunteer will be asked to do; and (*c*) the hazards, no matter how remote, that the volunteer may encounter. Of course, the rewards, the agreement, and other administrative arrangements should be explained. When questions from the candidates have been answered, the candidates are asked whether they wish to volunteer. A list is made of those who do, and they are instructed when and where to report for preliminary medical examination.

The preliminary examination consists of a complete medical history and appropriate physical and laboratory examinations of each applicant. The examination also involves special tests, including the index test, dictated by the nature of the study. One or more parts of the preliminary examination may serve to exclude some applicants from the study, and all parts are used as a baseline for judging future findings in the others. Those candidates who are found completely satisfactory are asked to sign the agreement or contract, and they are not considered volunteers until they have done so.

Although candidates for a study should be told its complete design, it should be understood that no volunteer is to be told the dosage group to which he belongs. A useful device is to give placebos to all dosage groups for about a week at the beginning of a study. Appropriate samples are taken during this period when each volunteer serves as his own control. It sometimes happens that more complaints are received during the period when placebos are given to everyone than during all the remainder of the study. This is entirely understandable, because the volunteers have been told about risks which the investigator felt morally obliged to mention, although he considered that the chance they would materialize was really nonexistent. Furthermore, it is fair to say that volunteers think that their appetite or general health has improved about as often as they think they have suffered some injury. In any event, it is absolutely necessary to have one or more control groups throughout the study. Such a group permits a random distribution of complaints that have no real connection with the experimental conditions. It also permits immediate recognition of the cause if some unexpected finding is the result of laboratory error. Some measurements tend to vary even when made in the best laboratories. An example is the potentiometric measurement of blood cholinesterase. If it is found that the blood cholinesterase of all groups, including the control, drops sharply for a day or two and then returns to normal, the result may be safely ignored as being unrelated to the variable under study.

Double Blind Studies. The double blind technique requires that neither the subjects nor the investigators responsible for recording their reactions be aware of which volunteers receive different chemicals or different dosage levels (including placebo) of the same chemical. It follows that a third party will be responsible for assigning dosages but have no direct contact with the volunteers during the course of the study. The third party is usually a member of the team of investigators; he may take major responsibility for design of the study and interpretation of the results, but not for collection of the data.

The great value of the double blind technique in many situations should not lead to a routine demand for it in all studies. Need for the technique diminishes as the degree of difference to be measured increases. Furthermore, the need is inversely proportional to the objectivity and repeatability of the measurements required. Finally, the double blind technique is contraindicated in connection with early studies of really new materials. Under these circumstances, the investigator should have every opportunity to discontinue or otherwise modify the study in response to the first hint of injury.

Contrary to the opinion of some authors, use of the single or the double blind technique has no necessary bearing on the matter of consent. Candidates for studies by the author and his colleagues were always told what dosage levels were planned, including the fact that some volunteers would receive a preparation containing none of the chemical under study. The only information withheld was who got which dosage. The candidates were told not to volunteer unless they were willing to receive the highest dosage.

Closing Ceremony. It is almost always wise to have a closing ceremony to recognize the contribution of the volunteers. The main purpose is to say "thank you" and to emphasize the contribution of the volunteers toward solution of a scientific problem. Each volunteer completing some studies carried out by the Public Health Service was presented with an engraved certificate, signed by the Surgeon General and other important persons.

5.4.3.6 Protection of the Volunteer. Protection of the volunteer, to summarize what has already been said in other contexts, includes: (a) guarantee that no study is made without valid consent—that is, continuing consent freely given by a person legally capable of giving it. The recognized ability of the volunteer to withdraw from the study at any time, even without reason, is a part of this concept; (b) qualification of the investigator; (c) freedom of the investigator to stop the participation of volunteers if he thinks their continuation in the project might injure them; and (d) care in the event of injury.

Department of Health, Education, and Welfare

Public Health Service

presented to

FULL NAME

in grateful appreciation of services as a volunteer in a

research study of broad significance to the advancement

of medical science and the ultimate

benefit of mankind

Seal

_____   _____

Signatures   Signatures

Tests in man should not be done in situations that do not permit medical care of a volunteer if he becomes ill. For some large medical institutions, this presents no problem. For example, provisions for care of whatever duration necessary is made in the Army Regulations cited above. For smaller institutions, insurance may be the best method to prepare for the unlikely eventuality of injury. Zavon (1964) reported that, in a study of the irritant effect of air pollution on the eyes, insurance for $3 million was purchased for $278.90.

5.4.3.7 Protection of the Investigator.
Protection of the investigator should be built into the design of every test in man. Of course, the most important protection of the investigator consists of demonstrable evidence that he has done everything possible to protect the volunteer.

Proof of Consent. As we have seen, the matter of consent was the only thing brought into question in the case of Hyman v. Jewish Hospital (15 NY 2d 317). Proof of consent involves not only evidence of the fact, but also evidence that the volunteer was legally capable of giving consent. The fact of consent is best established by a written document as discussed under Section 5.4.3.5 above. While written consent will not protect the investigator against liability for his negligence, it will constitute a defense against claims for injuries resulting from foreseeable and assumed risks (Monthly Summary from the Office of General Counsel, US Department of Health, Education, and Welfare, December, 1959).

Proof of Qualifications. Any investigator or team of investigators who undertakes tests in man should be fully qualified not only from a general medical standpoint, but also from the special standpoint of the problem under study. Evidence of qualification may include consultantships, membership in learned societies, and papers published in the field. Proof of qualification for a particular study is strengthened by a signed permit from the investigator's institution and/or another agency involved. Such approval would, of course, be conditioned on other relevant factors as well as the qualifications of the investigator.

Proof of Value of the Research. In many instances the value of research on man is evident to a layman and requires no justification. Even in such instances, the reason should be outlined clearly in the protocol. Again, official approval offers additional evidence that the work is considered valuable. Because the word "experimentation" carries the legal implication of malpractice, it is only common sense to avoid its use in connection with proper medical investigation.

Insurance. Insurance is not only a protection for the volunteer but also for the investigator (Beecher, 1969). Ballard (1964) has discussed the possibility of legal and financial support from the manufacturer of a compound in the event that an authorized investigator of the compound is sued.

Tort Claims Act. For many years there has been a need for tort claims acts to protect government-employed physicians and other medical personnel acting within the scope of their employment, including the conduct of medical investigations (Hayes, 1965, 1968). Such a law for "Defense of Certain Malpractice and Negligence Suits" now has been approved in the United States of America. It is a portion of the "Emergency Health Personnel Act of 1970" and constitutes Section 223 of Public Law 91-623 approved December 31, 1970 (42 USC 233). The Act provides protection from suit ". . . for damage for personal injury, including death, resulting from the performance of medical, surgical, dental, or related functions, including the conduct of clinical studies or investigation, by any commissioned officer or employee of the Public Health Service while acting within the scope of his office or employment. . . ." The law does not provide protection of medical personnel in connection with the private practice of medicine, voluntary treatment of patients who lack a legal right to such treatment by the Public Health Service, or duties while on assignment to states, foreign countries, or nonprofit institutions. However, paragraph 223(f) authorizes the Secretary to ". . . hold harmless or provide liability insurance for any officer or employee of the Public Health Service for damage for personal injury, including death, negligently caused by such officer or employee while acting within the scope of his office or employment and as a result of the performance of medical, surgical, dental or related functions, including the conduct of clinical studies or investigations, if such employee is assigned to a foreign country or detailed to a State or political subdivision thereof or to a non-profit institution. . . ."

This law sets a pattern that may be extended to the protection of government-employed physicians generally. Although the law and foreseeable extensions of it apply directly only to government employees, it may be expected to influence legal action at all levels. The specific inclusion of the "conduct of clinical studies and investigations" in the Act is a substantial evidence of confidence in medical research in general.

5.4.4 Motivation of Volunteers

Different people participate in research for different reasons or different combinations of reasons, including: (a) tangible rewards; (b) a desire for new experience; (c) occupational or other specialized interest in a specific project; (d) interest in science generally; and (e) a desire to contribute to society.

Tangible rewards may include money and (in the case of prisoners) reduction of prison term. Reduction of sentence may be guaranteed or potential, that is, it may be prorated according to the duration of each volunteer's participation in the study, or it may consist of the hope that participation will influence parole or the dropping of detainers by another court. Although tangible rewards may be critical for participation in some instances, the importance of this factor is easily overestimated. The author and his colleagues have carried out a number of studies successfully even though we could afford only token payments. We have recruited prisoner volunteers without difficulty when no reduction in sentence could be offered.

A general interest in science is probably the most important overall reason leading people to become volunteers in medical studies. Many people want to help in solving any problem they understand. If the problem involves their occupation, there is every reason they will understand its importance, and they may even have some technical insight into it.

Of course, prisoners share with people in general an interest in science, a need for money, and a desire for new experience. In fact, the desire for new and varied experience may be especially strong in people who are confined. However, the main feature that distinguishes prisoners from others in this connection is an unrecognized urge to do something useful. Either on a conscious or subconscious level, many prisoners wish to compensate for records indicating little positive contribution to society and, consequently, little positive recognition from society. Few prisoners will admit this urge to contribute except in time of war, when any worthwhile act can be attributed to patriotism. A partial exception was revealed by one prisoner who told the author that participation in a project had led to his reinstatement in his family. His father was pleased that he had finally done something commendable. Even though prisoners generally deny it, I believe that an urge to serve society is the most important single motivation for their participating in projects.

Continuation in a project requires an element of steadfastness which is not necessary for initial recruitment. This steadfastness seems to be characteristic of the individual; it has little or no relation to the nature of the study, or to whether discomfort is or is not involved. Dropping out must be permitted, but in the author's experience it usually occurs very early in a project, frequently before anything has happened. Once a project has settled down to a routine, it is most unusual for a volunteer to drop out. In studies such as those on antimalarial drugs, in which production of the disease was a necessary part of the work, the men accepted their illness with true heroism.

5.4.5 Conclusion

The limited ability of animal tests to predict human reactions to chemicals is recognized generally. Tests in man represent a logical step to full-scale use of a chemical. The fact that even hypersensitivity is basically dosage related emphasizes the importance of a continuing surveillance of workers or other persons whose exposure is intensive and prolonged in order to detect idiosyncrasy as well as overt toxicity at the earliest possible moment.

Many countries accept the necessity for orderly testing of the effectiveness of new drugs in man. Such testing of drugs for effectiveness implies, but does not require, that the safety of therapeutic doses will be observed critically, and that some pharmacological studies of the drug will be made in man. Furthermore, testing for effectiveness does not necessarily mean that possible adverse reactions will be looked for systematically after a drug is released for prescription use. Thus, studies of the safety of drugs in man often are not required by law or custom in exactly the same way that tests of effectiveness are required. There is even less recognition of the need to test in man the safety of other chemicals to which people will be exposed. In fact, little thought seems to have been given to the question of whether it is ethical to release a new chemical for general use before it has been tested under controlled conditions in a limited population. However, there is some evidence—including circumstances surrounding the case of Hyman v. Jewish Hospital—suggesting that not only investigators but many other educated people consider that, as long as the subjects of research are uninjured, it is ethically more important to gather knowledge leading to human welfare than to observe legalistic limitations of informed consent.

If it is decided that general release of a new chemical under conditions that defy orderly study is unwise—or, in fact, if studies of therapeutic effect are to be done scientifically using proper controls—then one must abandon the notion that tests in man can be justified only if they are of possible direct benefit to each person participating in the test. Countries apparently vary widely in the tenacity with which they support this notion. Certainly, tests of great value to society have been carried out without injury, but also without any medical benefit to the volunteers involved. However, only in special situations, especially in the military, are such studies clearly permitted by law.

Great progress was made by the recent passage of a law to protect any commissioned officer or employee of the Public Health Service against suit for damage resulting from action within the scope of his office or employment, including those actions involving clinical studies or investigations. Further progress could be made by passage of additional tort claims acts to protect all government employees with medical duties, including duties of medical research. This would serve not only to protect the employees but to establish the legitimacy of their proper activities. Such laws might serve as devices to define standards of conduct for investigations. However, the present law makes no such attempt, and this may be just as well. In the last analysis, as we have said, the proper conduct of tests in man depends on the good sense, integrity, and freedom of the participating scientists, rather than on an elaborate code of ethics.

5.5 Measurement of Exposure under Practical Conditions

Because of the crucial importance of dosage in all toxicological matters, it is imperative that dosage be known wherever possible. This measurement is relatively easy in connection with medication with drugs, but difficult in connection with occupational or accidental exposure to industrial chemicals, including pesticides. It can be argued that the only really important dosage is one at the tissue level, and that it is just as easy to measure this level following one kind of exposure as another. However, it is also important to know the dosage of a compound encountered by the entire body, and to know the relative importance of different routes by which it may be absorbed.

This section describes methods for the direct measurement of exposure and certain special applications of indirect measurement aimed at evaluating the separate contributions from different routes of exposure.

Practical methods of indirect measurement of exposure resulting from occupation or accident include direct measurement of storage (Section 3.2.3.2) or urinary excretion (Section 3.2.4). Another method, measurement of respiratory excretion by breath analysis, although relatively new, has been brought to a high degree of perfection for many solvents and fumigants. It deserves far wider use than it has received. Because of its importance in diagnosis, it is discussed in Section 8.1.4.1. However, respiratory excretion can be used in studies of volunteers or as a part of good occupational medicine (Stewart, 1974).

5.5.1 Measurement of Respiratory Exposure

Respiratory exposure cannot be separated completely from oral exposure because some inhaled material is likely to be retained on the mucous membranes of the upper respiratory tract. This material may be absorbed directly from these membranes or swallowed so that it becomes available for absorption from the gastrointestinal tract. The depths which inhaled material will reach in the respiratory tract are determined largely by its particle size. This and related matters are discussed in Section 3.2.2.4.

5.5.1.1 Estimation of Respiratory Exposure from Air Concentration.

It is common practice to estimate the respiratory exposure of workers in factories and mines by measuring the concentration of toxicant in samples of ambient air, and by assuming that the samples are representative of the air inhaled. This assumption is generally valid when the concentration of toxicant in the air is relatively constant and when the toxicant itself is either a gas, vapor, or extremely fine particulate. The assumption that ambient air is representative of inhaled air may be misleading when the concentration of toxicant in it varies greatly from time to time, or when at least a portion of the toxicant is present in the form of relatively large particles. If the toxicant enters the air in the form of clouds that quickly drift away, it may be extremely difficult to obtain a representative sample. If the cloud lasts only a very short time, the worker may be able to hold his breath or turn his head so that he inhales little of the material. If a cloud of whatever duration is made up mostly of relatively large particles, then only a small portion of the toxicant present can reach the lung even if the large particles are inhaled. In spite of these necessary limitations, measurement of air concentration is an important way of estimating respiratory exposure.

Air sampling equipment is discussed in Section 4.3.5.2. No matter what device is used in collecting air samples for analysis, an effort should be made to obtain samples with the same spectrum of particle size as is picked up by the nostrils in breathing. One approach is to imitate the aerodynamics of human respiration. For example, it may be possible to have the position and size of the collecting orifice similar to that of the nose, and to make the rate of air flow similar to that in human respiration. In all sampling, the collecting orifice should be as near the breathing zone of workers as is practically possible. If very large particle sizes are involved, it is important that the orifice be inverted so that large particles will not fall in simply mechanically. After all, some spray droplets approach the size of fine rain droplets, which are too heavy to be diverted from their free fall and caught up in the respiratory stream.

Regardless of what collecting equipment is chosen, it is wise to use all glass fittings.

Traces of material obtained from rubber or plastic produce false positive results for many pesticides when measured by gas-liquid chromatography.

In selecting a liquid to use in impingers or fritted glass absorbers, it is necessary to consider a vapor pressure as well as solubilizing action. Ether and acetone generally are not satisfactory, even for collecting compounds highly soluble in them, because these solvents evaporate too rapidly. The material to be sampled may codistill with the solvent. On the other hand, use of a too viscous solvent will impede the flow of air through the sampling device. Miles (1965) has shown the value of ethylene glycol as a medium for collecting parathion. Although this particular solvent might not be ideal for other materials, the principle of seeking maximal dissolving power and minimal evaporation is always valid.

Another approach is to use some kind of a filter instead of a solvent. It might appear that filters would act mechanically and trap only particles larger than the pores of the filter, thus failing to capture smaller particles, gases, and vapors. Actually, the situation is far more complex. Extremely fine solid particles are more difficult to trap than larger particles on the one hand, or vapors on the other. In some situations, a high proportion of small particles will be carried directly through an impinger filled with a solvent in which the material composing the particles is soluble. On the contrary, vapors and gases may be adsorbed on filters or dissolved in solvent. Surface area is the most important single factor in determining whether adsorption will occur. Thus, filters made of glass wool usually adsorb less gas or vapor than columns packed with alumina. Of course, the specific properties of the adsorbent are also important; therefore, the efficiency of a filter or column packing should be tested before it is selected for a particular purpose.

After the concentration of the toxicant in the air has been measured, the respiratory exposure of workers or others can be calculated by using an assumed tidal volume and respiratory rate. The average values for lung ventilation in adults are given in Table 5-4. An even more accurate calculation can be made if lung ventilation is actually measured under the conditions of work being studied.

Collection of Particulates by Impaction on Screens. It may be desirable to learn something, either qualitatively or quantitatively, about the dustiness of an environment in situations in which ordinary air sampling equipment is not suitable, either because of a lack of power to run sampling equipment, or because the air flow associated with such equipment

Table 5-4

Average Lung Ventilation in Young Athletes
From data of Taylor (1941).

Sex	Condition	Rate (liters/min)	
male	rest	7.4	(5.8 - 10.3)
	light work (500 kg-m/min)	28.6	(27.3 - 30.9)
	heavy work (800 kg-m/min)	42.9	(39.3 - 45.2)
female	rest	4.5	(4.0 - 5.1)
	light work (300 kg-m/min)	16.3	(15.9 - 16.8)
	heavy work (600 kg-m/min)	24.5	(17.3 - 31.8)

would introduce an important, undesirable bias. Collecting screens have been used to meet problems of this sort. Apparently, the first use of screens in this way and certainly the most thorough study of their properties was that of Blifford et al. (1956). Their initial studies were with metal screens, which they compared with "an efficient filter apparatus" and with standard, gummed paper fallout sheets. They concluded that the screens were about 1% efficient in the absence of rain, and also that ordinary cheesecloth screens lost less material during rain. Their screens were mounted on rotating vanes to direct them toward the wind. However, no such mounting is required if screens are used to sample particulate material outdoors where the wind is always from the same direction, or indoors where dust is carried by imperceptible, random air currents. The lack of quantitation is a disadvantage, but it may be outweighed by other features of the system. The use of screens is a valid way to compare the dustiness of indoor situations, or to compare the composition of dust in different situations.

Fabric used for screens should offer little restriction to the passage of air and (following suitable cleaning) the fabric itself should not produce peaks on analysis. Nylon chiffon has been found suitable. The amount of dust retained may be increased by pretreating the clean fabric with 10% ethylene glycol in acetone (Tessari and Spencer, 1971).

5.5.1.2 Estimation of Respiratory Exposure from Trapping Toxicant in Inhaled Air.
A different approach for estimating respiratory exposure avoids some of the complications just discussed, by relating the sampling directly to the worker or other subject. The method, which apparently was introduced by Batchelor and Walker (1954), involves determination of the amount of toxicant trapped by the filter system of a respirator worn by the worker during an accurately timed period of exposure. The nature of the apparatus is shown in Fig. 5-1. If a properly fitted face piece is used, all inhaled air must pass through the filter system; thus, the volume of inhaled air does not have to be measured or estimated. The equipment is so designed that the air enters it through holes similar to the nostrils in placement and size. This may be achieved by firmly taping a modified funnel to the retaining ring of the respirator. The stem of the funnel is shortened and plugged, and two holes 12 mm in diameter and 6 mm apart are drilled midway between the base and the apex of the funnel. In use, the holes of the funnel are directed downward. The special funnel prevents the direct impingement of large particles on the filter and, by controlling the velocity of the air, also regulates the particle size of the material having access to the filter.

The same authors reported studies showing that, under some circumstances, omission of a special funnel from the apparatus could lead to a value about 30% higher than the true value because so much material impinged directly on the filter pad. They also showed that measurment made with the special funnel in place gave results in satisfactory agreement with estimates made in the same situation by measuring the concentration of the toxicant in the ambient air.

The fully developed equipment described by Durham and Wolfe (1962) has a filter consisting of 32 layers of surgical gauze stapled to an α-cellulose respirator pad. It was found that such a multilayer filter was efficient for trapping both sprays and dust.

Tests indicate the filter pads could be relied upon to be about 90% efficient in removing parathion from air under the conditions ordinarily encountered in the field.

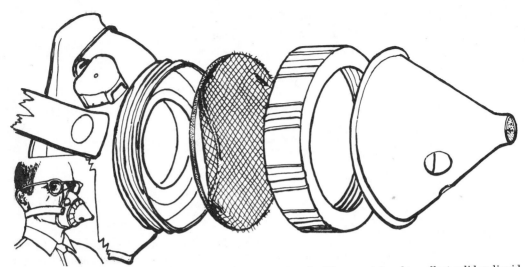

Fig. 5–1. Expanded view of a single-unit respirator equipped with a special pad to collect solid or liquid spray aerosols from inhaled air. On the front of the respirator is taped a plastic funnel with its stem plugged and with two openings 12 mm in diameter to admit at the same velocity that the air enters the nostrils. The complete assembly as worn is shown at the lower left of the illustration. After Durham & Wolfe (1962) by courtesy of the World Health Organization.

Before filter pads are used, they should be pre-extracted with a suitable solvent to remove any material that might later interfere with chemical analysis. To recover the toxicant after exposure, the entire filter pad is extracted in a Soxhlet apparatus. The amount of toxicant removed from the pad, plus that rinsed from the inside of the funnel, is considered the amount to which the worker would have been exposed by the respiratory route during the selected exposure period. The amount of toxicant received per hour, per working day, or per operational cycle can then be calculated.

5.5.2 Measurement of Dermal Exposure

The classical problems of industrial toxicology involve respiratory absorption of heavy metals, toxic gases, and silica. All these materials are absorbed so much more efficiently by the respiratory tract than by the skin that dermal exposure to them may be ignored under practical conditions. Some of them such as silica have no systemic dermal toxicity regardless of the intensity of exposure. These classical problems of industrial toxicology remain of tremendous importance, even today. However, there is a growing list of industrial chemicals that may be absorbed from the skin efficiently enough that exposure to them by this route is dangerous under practical conditions of occupational exposure. Many of the pesticides fall into this class, and it is mainly in connection with pesticides that methods for

measuring dermal exposure have been developed.

In general, dermal absorption is far less efficient than respiratory absorption. Compounds vary greatly in the ease with which they are absorbed by the skin. In spite of these facts, dermal absorption is of crucial importance in some situations. It may happen that there is practically no opportunity for respiratory exposure in a situation that permits dangerous dermal exposure. More often, the ratio of respiratory to dermal exposure is such that the dosage resulting from absorption of all inhaled material is less than the dosage from absorption of even a small percentage of the material contaminating the skin.

Certain properties of aerosol particles that are important in understanding the measurement of dermal exposure are discussed in Section 3.2.2.4.

5.5.2.1 Estimation of Dermal Exposure from Air Concentration.

Edson (1956) proposed a table for conversion of air concentration values to surface contamination rates at various wind velocities. The table was based on the assumption that the surface would retain all spray particles approaching it at right angles. The table was used by Edson to show that, for various aerodynamic reasons, the surface contamination he measured was, in the absence of splashing, much less than would be predicted on the basis of the assumptions used. Even if more realistic assumptions were made, the prediction of dermal exposure from air concentration would be difficult, because the many different surfaces and movements involved would create an extremely complicated aerodynamic situation.

Because of the complexities involved, it seems impractical to use measurements of air concentration in estimating dermal exposure.

5.5.2.2 Estimation of Dermal Exposure from Absorbent Samplers.

Dermal exposure may be estimated directly be measuring the amount of toxicant trapped by absorbent pads or absorbent clothing worn by the operator in the course of his work. These samplers can be attached to the hands, face, and other parts of the body that are normally unclothed. The samplers can also be attached to protective clothing to measure the exposure that the clothing obviates, or the samplers may be placed above and below ordinary clothing in order to estimate the degree of protection such clothing offers. No matter for what purpose they are used, the absorbent samplers are exposed for a carefully measured interval, usually one or more complete cycles of work. For example, measurements may be made from the time a sprayman begins to fill his spray tank with pesticide until he has completely used up that tankful of material.

Detailed instructions for using absorbent pads have been stated by Durham and Wolfe (1962). Briefly, it has been found practical to use pads made of α-cellulose for measuring sprays and pads backed by filter paper and made from 32 thicknesses of surgical gauze for measuring dust. Whatever material is chosen must be pre-extracted, using the same solvent to be used later during extraction of samples for analysis. It has not been found possible to remove inks and oils completely from samplers, so pads and gauze marked or treated with these materials should not be used.

The exact size of pads is not important, but they should be uniform in size—small enough to put conveniently on the parts of the body to be studied, and large enough to provide a margin by which they may be attached without interfering with a central portion later used for analysis. Square pads of α-cellulose (10.2 cm on each edge) have been found convenient. Gauze pads are backed by a single sheet of white filter paper and bound with pressure-sensitive tape on all four edges in order to prevent raveling. When bound in this way, the gauze pad is slightly larger than the α-cellulose pad but not enough larger to interfere with use. Laboratory tests have shown that gauze pads retain approximately 90% of dust applied to them, even though they are held in an inverted position and shaken in a

mechanical shaker after application of the dust (Durham and Wolfe, 1962). Of course, in practice, all pads are handled with care to avoid loss of toxicant on the one hand, or unintentional contamination on the other. It has been found practical to place exposed pads between the folds of a piece of quantitative white filter paper, which is then placed in a waxed paper sandwich bag for transport to the laboratory.

In the laboratory, each exposure pad is removed from the fold of filter paper inside the waxed paper bag. The margins of each pad are cut away with a paper trimmer leaving a central area 5 cm on each edge. The 25-cm^2 portion of the pad is then extracted in a Soxhlet apparatus. The total amount of toxicant finally measured in the extract is a measure of the exposure of the 25-cm^2 area under the condition of the test.

A shortcoming of the pad technique is the necessity of assuming that the area covered by the pad is representative of the entire body part being studied. This difficulty may be overcome by using knit white cotton garments that cover the entire body part during exposure. Gloves have been used for the hands, short sleeved undershirts for the upper part of the body, socks for the feet, and the tops of socks for both ankles and wrists. The short sleeved undershirts are of particular use for measuring the amount of toxicant that penetrates outer clothing, whether this be ordinary work clothing or special protective clothing. In a similar way, socks can be used to measure the amount of toxicant that penetrates the shoes, and cotton gloves may be used to estimate the amount of exposure resulting from misuse of rubber gloves. Gloves may be more permeable than supposed, or they may become contaminated on the inside through improper use.

Occasionally, a garment may have to be cut off the subject in order to avoid its contamination by some part of the body over which it would normally be slipped in the process of removal. This is nearly always the case with the short sleeved undershirt. However, the upper portion of a sock that has been used to measure exposure of the lower arm and wrist may be removed by slipping it over a plastic bag used to cover the hand. Uncut or resewn garments can be laundered and reused after they have been extracted to remove the toxicant under study.

5.5.2.3 Estimation of Dermal Exposure from Washing.

It must be recognized that the ability of the skin to collect and hold a particular formulation of a toxicant may not be identical to that of an absorbent sampler chosen to study exposure. Some of the water-wettable powder that impinges on the skin may later dry completely and fall away. The degree of loss may vary depending on how wet the skin is with sweat. Thus, the efficiency of the skin as a collecting surface may not be constant. One approach to this problem is to use the skin itself as the collecting surface and to remove the toxicant from it by means of some kind of washing following a predetermined period of exposure. Although perfect in theory, this method, too, has some practical difficulties. For example, there is the difficulty of determining that the skin is completely clean before exposure starts, and the difficulty of knowing that all of the toxicant that impinged upon the skin during exposure is removed in the washing process. The skin is not inactive. In addition to possible loss through evaporation, the toxicant may be absorbed by the skin. Fredriksson (1961b) showed that, whereas 80 to 92% of radioactive parathion applied to the skin of volunteers could be removed by ordinary washing 30 minutes after application, only 50 to 70% could be removed if the washing was delayed 300 minutes after the application.

In spite of recognized limitations, the method of washing has an important place in measuring the dermal exposure of occupationally exposed persons. There is a certain tendency for the two kinds of error mentioned above to cancel one another out. During relatively brief cycles of exposure dermal absorption, though real, is minimal. In other words, because absorption is slow, the material that cannot be removed from the skin in preparation for measuring exposure may be almost the same as the material that cannot be removed after the exposure is complete. Thus, the quantity washed from the skin following exposure is a reasonable measure of the dosage received during the interval under study.

Any part of the body can be washed with swabs even if the area chosen for study is small, large, or irregular. Durham and Wolfe (1962) recommended that each swab be made by placing two, 8-ply, approximately 10 by 10-cm pre-extracted, surgical gauze sponges together and folding them twice to form an approximately 5 by 5-cm square which is stapled near the folded edge. The swabs to be used for a single area of skin are placed in a jar and saturated with 95% ethyl alcohol. The lid of the jar is lined with aluminum foil to prevent any possible extraction of the original liner. In the field, the sealed jar is opened and each swab is grasped at the stapled edge with ring forceps. The excess alcohol is squeezed off against the inside of the jar, and the area of skin to be studied is cleaned by rubbing the cloth back and forth over the surface with light pressure. After all the swabs have been used and placed back in the jar, it is sealed and returned to the laboratory for analysis. Durham and Wolfe (1962) found that one swab was insufficient, but four swabs were adequate to remove about 90% of parathion from an area of skin the size of the back of a man's hand.

It is difficult to clean between the fingers and around the fingernails with swabs. Durham and Wolfe (1962) described the use of plastic bags that they had introduced somewhat earlier for washing the hand and wrist or foot and ankle. In use, the hand is thrust into one of the bags containing about 200 ml of 95% ethyl alcohol, or some other harmless solvent. While the open end of the bag is held tightly around the arm or wrist to prevent leakage, the thumb and fingers are rubbed briskly against one another and against the palm of the hand. Then the hand and bag are shaken vigorously about 50 times. The bags are carried to the place of sampling and back again to the laboratory in 0.5-liter wide-mouthed canning jars. Both before and after use, the top of the bag is twisted to form a tight seal that is held with a clamp. Two bag rinses were found to remove an average of 96% of parathion from one hand when sampling was carried out soon after exposure, and two rinses were adopted as standard for this purpose. However, four rinses were found necessary to remove 90% of the recoverable toxicant one or more days after exposure. Durham and Wolfe (1962) found no significant difference in the efficiency of α-cellulose pads and swabbing for removing insecticides from the dorsal surface of the forearm. However, bag rinses were approximately twice as effective as swabs in removing insecticides from the hands.

5.5.2.4 Conventions for Measuring Dermal Exposure. Careful workers applying highly dangerous pesticides in a temperate climate will use protective clothing in such a way that their dermal exposure is slight. By contrast, some workers in tropical countries may wear little clothing regardless of the nature of the material they are applying. Their dermal exposure may be very great. Because of the wide variation in the kind and amount of clothing worn by workers, it is necessary to establish some standard for comparison so that measurements made under different circumstances

Table 5-5

Surface Area of the Body and of Portions Frequently
Contaminated by Pesticides

	Area (m^2)	Proportion (%)
whole body	1.85[a]	100
face	0.065[b]	3.5
hands	0.082[b]	4.4
forearms	0.121[b]	6.5
back of neck	0.011[b]	0.6
front of neck and "V" of chest	0.015[b]	0.8

a.   Surface area of a man 180 cm high weighing 70 kg according to
Sendroy and Cecchini (1954).

b.   Values from Durham and Wolfe (1962); the calculated proportions
are similar to those of Berkow (1931).

may be evaluated. Thus, it has become conventional to calculate dermal exposure values on the assumption that the exposed person wore long pants, a short sleeved, open neck shirt, shoes and socks, but no gloves or hat, and that his clothing gave complete protection of the areas covered. This convention corresponds to approximately the smallest amount of protection used by workers in the developed countries. According to convention, the surfaces of the face, the back of the neck, the "V" of the chest, the forearms, and the hands are considered to be unclothed. The areas of these and other parts of the body are shown in Table 5-5. By use of published measurement of dermal exposure under standard conditions and the values for the surface area of different parts of the body shown in Table 5-5, one may get a rough idea of the added protection to be obtained from wearing protective clothing or the added danger that would follow the use of less than standard clothing.

5.5.3 Measurement of Oral Exposure

It is common to warn workers against smoking or eating during work, lest they ingest pesticides transferred from their hands or clothing. Another more certain source of oral exposure involves blowing out clogged spray nozzles or the like. Although it is only common sense to avoid oral exposure, few studies have been made to learn how much real danger is involved.

The analysis of vomitus or of stomach washings gives a minimal measure of the amount of toxicant swallowed. Lavage may be done experimentally as well as therapeutically. However, the ordinary worker cannot be expected to cooperate by permitting gastric lavage merely for study.

Durham and Wolfe (1962) proposed that methylene blue be combined with a formulation, and that urinary excretion of the dye be used as a measure of oral ingestion, inasmuch as dermal absorption of the dye is minimal. Apparently, the method has not been tested.

Another method suggested for measurement of oral exposure involves analysis of food or objects that commonly are placed in the mouth after these things have been handled by formulators or spraymen while at work. Thus, Wolfe et al. (1963) asked workers to remove cigarettes from the package and handle them in the usual way in preparation for smoking. In some instances the worker also smoked the cigarette halfway. The unsmoked or partially smoked cigarettes were then protected from further contamination and taken to the laboratory for analysis. It was assumed that the amount of pesticide in the cigarettes might have been ingested or inhaled, depending on whether the contamination was on a portion that would have touched the lips (unsmoked cigarettes) or was on a portion that ordinarily would have been smoked (all cigarettes).

In a similar way, spraymen were provided with sandwiches and other box lunch-type foods, which they carried into the field. After a predetermined period, each worker unwrapped his food and ate half of it. The other half, with which the worker's hands had come in contact, was returned to the laboratory for analysis (Armstrong *et al.*, 1973). Results of some of these studies are outlined in Section 6.2.3.2.

5.5.4 Problems of Measuring Separate Contributions from Different Routes of Exposure

In comparing the importance of different routes of exposure, one can, of course, use the results of independent measurements of exposure by each route during the same operation. However, direct measures of exposure fail to take absorptive ability into account. It is possible that heavy contamination which is little absorbed by one route is less dangerous than light contamination which is efficiently absorbed by another route. Durham and Wolfe (1963) called attention to two special methods that may be of use when a question arises regarding the relative amount of toxicant absorbed by two routes. Both methods depend on measuring absorption in terms of urinary excretion of the toxicant or one or more of its metabolites. As described, both methods produce minimal measures of absorption by the dermal route.

5.5.4.1 Smyth Technique. The first of these special methods apparently was first published by Durham and Wolfe (1963), but they attributed it to Dr. Henry Smyth, Jr. and spoke of it as the Smyth technique. The method consists in measuring the excretion of a toxicant or one of its metabolites and comparing the result with respiratory exposure estimated on the basis of respiratory volume and the measured concentration of toxicant in the air. If the amount found in the urine after a day, or some other definite unit of exposure, is fully accounted for by the amount of toxicant that would have been inhaled during the corresponding period of work, it simply is concluded that respiratory exposure accounts for all absorption that can be measured within the accuracy of the method. The same conclusion is reached if the amount of toxicant or metabolite excreted is less than the amount that would have been inhaled during the test interval. However, if the amount excreted is greater than can be accounted for by respiratory exposure, it is concluded that another route of exposure, usually the dermal, accounts for the difference. The method is not well adapted for measuring small differences of exposure, but it is a valuable technique for measuring larger differences. The method involves an assumption that oral exposure is trivial, but this assumption us-

ually is valid. The method is limited by the efficiency of measuring excretion, which is why it gives only a minimal measure of dermal exposure. The method is biased in favor of respiratory exposure because it assumes that all of the toxicant in the air would be inhaled regardless of particle size, and that all the inhaled material would reach the depths of the lungs and be retained. Actually, many particles in pesticidal aerosols and dusts are too large to be inhaled. Particles that are inhaled may impinge on the upper respiratory tract and eventually be swallowed. Gases, vapors, and extremely fine aerosols may be only partially retained. The special merit of the Smyth technique is that it permits the collection of useful quantitative data from measurements that may already be available, or at least are easy to make. It can be carried out without any interference with the worker's activity except that involved in the periodic collection of samples of urine.

Results obtained by the Smyth technique are discussed in Section 6.2.3.1.

5.5.4.2 Differential Protection Technique. The second method of measuring the separate contribution of different routes of exposure referred to by Durham and Wolfe (1963) has been used by Dutkiewicz (1961) in his studies of aniline, but it still is not well known. As a minimal measure of dermal absorption and as used by Dutkiewicz, the method can be considered a refinement of the Smyth technique, in which respiratory exposure and absorption are kept at zero by use of a supplied air respirator. Under these conditions, all of the excreted toxicant—including any that remains undetected—must have been absorbed from the skin.

An extension of the latter method involves the use of a rubber suit, gloves, boots, and a complete plastic cover for the head with all potential openings sealed with tape so as to permit no air to enter, except through two small vents below the nose. In this form the method offers an accurate measure of respiratory absorption, provided the chosen measure of excretion is a good index of absorption. Unfortunately, this method of measuring respiratory absorption can be used only in certain circumstances. A person will be injured seriously if he stays long in the sun or in a hot place while sealed in rubber and plastic.

Although the two forms of complete protection may be used separately, they can be employed to greatest advantage in experiments designed to exploit both, namely, what may be called the "complete differential protection technique". Groups of workers carrying out essentially identical operations may be divided into three groups who receive complete respiratory, complete dermal, and no special protection, respectively. The latter group serves as a control and is given only such protection as ordinary clothing or whatever protective devices are considered standard for the operation under study. When exposed in this way for a work cycle or other predetermined period, the average absorption experienced by the controls should equal approximately the average absorption of one of the experimental groups plus that of the other. In case absorption by one route is relatively very large, it may not be possible to distinguish the absorption in that group from absorption in the control.

Results obtained by the differential protection technique are discussed in Sections 6.2.3.1 and 7.2.4.1.

REFERENCES

Abery, P., Goodwin, E., Goulden, R., and Reynolds, J. G. (1959). *Dieldrin—Absorption through Skin after Dermal Exposure to Dieldrin Wettable Powder.* Woodstock Agricultural Centre, Sittingbourne, Kent.

Académie Nationale de Médecine (1952). Conclusions de l'académie à propos de l'experimentation sur l'homme. Bull. Acad. Natl. Med. (Paris), 136:562–563.

Aleksieva, T., Vasilev, G., and Spasorski, M. (1959). Study of the toxic effects of DDT. Hig. Epidemiol. Microbiol., 5:8–15.

Alexander, L. (1966). Limitations in experimental research on human beings. Lex et Scientia, 3:8–24.

Alvarez, W. C., and Hyman, S. (1953). Absence of toxic manifestations in workers exposed to chlordane. Arch. Ind. Hyg. Occup. Med., 8:480–483.

Ambrose, A. M. (1963). Toxicologic studies on pyrethrin-type esters of chrysanthemumic acid. I. Chrysanthemumic acid, 6-chloropiperonyl ester (barthrin). Toxicol. Appl. Pharmacol., 5:414–416.

Ambrose, A. M., and Haag, H. B. (1936). Toxicological study of derris. Ind. Eng. Chem., 28:815–821.

American Academy of Arts and Sciences (1969). Ethical aspects of experimentation with human subjects, Daedalus, 98:v–xiv, 219–603.

American Medical Association (1946). Supplementary report of the Judicial Council. J. A. M. A., 132:1090.

American Medical Association, Office of the General Counsel (1973). *Medicolegal Forms with Legal Analysis.* American Medical Association, Chicago, Illinois.

Apple, G., Morgan, D. P., and Roan, C. C. (1970). Determinants of serum DDT and DDE concentrations. Bull. Environ. Contamin. Toxicol., 5:16–23.

Armstrong, J. F., Wolfe, H. R., Comer, S. W., and Staiff, D. C. (1973). Oral exposure of workers to parathion through contamination of food items. Bull. Environ. Contam. Toxicol., 10:321–327.

Asribekova, T. A. (1963). Occupational hygiene in the aircraft spraying of methylmerkaptophose. Gig. Sanit., 28:28–34.

Baer, S., Yarrow, M. W., Kranitz, C., and Markson, V. (1958). Clinical experiences with warfarin (coumarin) sodium as an anticoagulant. J. A. M. A., 167:704–708.

Baker, A. H., Whitney, G. F. H., and Worden, A. N. (1959). The toxic hazard associated with continuous-flow heat-volatilized insecticidal and acaricidal aerosols. Lab. Pract., 8:3–10.

Ballard, R. W. (1964). Patient consent in experimental

drug therapy. Presented at the International Academy of Law and Sciences, Las Vegas, Nevada, June 19.

Barclay, R. K., Peacock, W. C., and Karnofsky, D. A. (1953). Distribution and excretion of radioactive thallium in the chick embryo, rat, and man. J. Pharmacol. Exp. Ther., 107:178–187.

Bar-Hay, J., Benderly, A., and Rumney, G. (1964). Treating of a case of nontumorous Cushings syndrome with o,p′-DDD. Pediatrics, 33:239–244.

Barnes, J. M., and Davies, D. R. (1951). Blood cholinesterase levels in workers exposed to organo-phosphorus insecticides. Br. Med. J., 2:816–819.

Barnes, W. W., Eldridge, B. F., Greenberg, J. H., and Vinona, S. (1962). A field evaluation of malathion dust for the control of body lice. J. Econ. Entomol., 55:391–394.

Barrett, H., and Johnston, J. (1939). The fate of trichloroethylene in the organism. J. Biol. Chem., 127:765–770.

Bartoniček, V. (1962). Metabolism and excretion of trichloroethylene after inhalation by human subjects. Br. J. Ind. Med., 19:134–141.

Bartoniček, V. (1963). The effect of some substances on the elimination of trichloroethylene metabolites. Arch. Int. Pharmacodyn. Ther., 144:69–85.

Bartoniček, V., and Teisinger, J. (1962). Effect of tetraethyl thiuram disulphide (disulfiram) on metabolism of trichloroethylene in man. Br. J. Ind. Med., 19:216–221.

Batchelor, G. S., and Walker, K. C. (1954). Health hazards involved in use of parathion in fruit orchards of North Central Washington. A. M. A. Arch. Ind. Hyg. Occup. Med., 10:522–529.

Batchelor, G. S., Walker, K. C., and Elliott, J. W. (1956). Dinitroorthocresol exposure from apple-thinning sprays. Arch. Ind. Health, 13:593–596.

Beaumont, W. (1833). *Experiments and Observations on the Gastric Juice and the Physiology of Digestion.* F. P. Allen, Printer, Plattsburg, New York. (Reprinted: Dover Publications, Inc., New York, 1959.)

Beecher, H. K. (1966). Ethics and clinical research. N. Engl. J. Med., 274:1354–1360.

Beecher, H. K. (1969). Human studies. Science, 164:1256–1258.

Beheyt, P., Leburn, A., Cerf, J., Dierickx, J., and Degroote, V. (1961). Étude de la toxicité pour l'homme d'un insecticide organophosphore. Bull. WHO, 24:465–473.

Berkow, S. G. (1931). Value of surface area proportions in the prognosis of cutaneous burns and scalds. Am. J. Surg., 11:315–317.

Best, E. M., Jr., and Murray, B. L. (1962). Observations on workers exposed to Sevin insecticide: a preliminary report. J. Occup. Med., 4:507–517.

Bezuglyi, V. P., and Kaskevich, L. M. (1969). Some indices of the functional state of the liver in flying personnel engaged in aerial chemical operations. Gig. Tr. Prof. Zabol., 13:52–53.

Bledsoe, T., Island, D. P., Ney, R. L., and Liddle, G. W. (1964). An effect of o,p′-DDD on the extra-adrenal metabolism of cortisol in man. J. Clin. Endocr., 24:1303–1311.

Blifford, I. H., Jr., Lockhart, L. B., Jr., Baus, R. A. (1956). Collection of atomic bomb debris from the atmosphere by impaction on screens. Science, 123:1120–1121.

Bogushevskii, S. M., and Burkatskaya, E. N. (1951). Labor hygiene in agriculture in work with benzene hexachloride. Gig. Sanit., 4:30–34.

Bradlow, H. L., Fukushima, D. K., Zumoff, B., Hellman, L., and Gallagher, T. F. (1963). A peripheral action of o,p′-DDD on steroid biotransformation. J. Clin. Endocrinol. Metab., 23:918–922.

Bratteby, L. E., and Wadman, B. (1968). Labelling of red blood cells in vitro with small amounts of DFP. Scand. J. Clin. Lab. Invest., 21:197–201.

Brodie, B. B. (1964). Of mice, microsomes and man. Pharmacologist, 6:12–26.

Brown, H. V., and Bush, A. F. (1950). Parathion inhibition

of cholinesterase. Arch. Ind. Hyg. Occup. Med., 1:633–636.

Bruaux, P. (1957). Toxicité de deux insecticides organophosphores (Diazinon et Malathion) chez les travailleurs utilisant ces insecticides. Ann. Soc. Belg. Med. Trop., 37:789-800.

Brzozowski, J., Czajke, J., Dutkiewicz, T., Kesy, I., and Wojcik, J. (1954). Higiena pracy i stan zdrowis zatrudnionych przy zwalczaniu stonki aiemniaczanej hekasachlorocyklokeksanem, dwuchloroetanem. Med. Pracy, 5:89–98.

Buchthal, F., and Engbaek, L. (1948). On the neuromuscular transmission in normal and myasthenic subjects. Acta Psychiat. Neurol., 23:3–11.

Burgen, A. S. V., Keele, C. A., and McAlpine, D. (1948). Tetraethylpyrophosphate in myasthenia gravis. Lancet, 1:519–521.

Burkatskaya, E. N., Ivanova, E. V., and Krasniuk, E. P. (1959). Gigiena truda i sostojanie zdorovja rabotajuscih pri proizvadostve desinekciomyh preparatov soderzascih geksahloran. Gig. Sanit., 24(5):17–22.

Burkatskaya, E. N., Voitenko, V. A., and Krasnyuk, E. P. (1961). Working conditions and health status of workers at DDT production plants. Gig. Sanit., 26:24–29.

Cady, E. L., Jr. (1965). Medicolegal facets of clinical experimentation. Gen. Pract., 31:187–197.

Cameron, G. R., and Burgess, F. (1945). Toxicity of 2, 2-bis (p-chlorophenyl) 1,1,1-trichlorethane (DDT). Br. Med. J., 1:865–871.

Cannon, A. B., and McRae, M. E. (1948). Treatment of scabies. Report of one hundred patients treated with hexachlorocyclohexane in a vanishing cream base. J. A. M. A., 138:557–560.

Carley, W. M. (1966). Patient consent to research: rules set. Wall Street J., January 21.

Carpenter, C. P., Weil, C. S., Palm, P. E., Woodside, M. W., Nair, J. H., III, and Smyth, H. F., Jr. (1961). Mammalian toxicity of 1-naphthyl-N-methylcarbamate (Sevin insecticide). J. Agric. Food Chem., 9:30–39.

Carrillo, S. J. (1954). El empleo del dieldrin en Venezuela. Bol. Of. Sanit. Panam., 37:76–81.

Casarett, L. J., Bevenue, A., Yauger, W. L., Jr., and Whalen, S. A. (1969). Observations on pentachlorophenol in human blood and urine. Am. Ind. Hyg. Assoc. J., 30:360–366.

Case, R. A. M. (1945). Toxic effects of 2, 2-bis (p-chlorophenyl) 1,1,1-trichlorethane (D.D.T.) in man. Br. Med. J., 2:842–850.

Cavanagh, J. B., Davies, D. R., Holland, P., and Lancaster, M. (1961). Comparison of the functional effects of dyflos, tri-o-cresyl phosphate and tri-p-ethylphenyl phosphate in chickens. Br. J. Pharmacol., 17:21–27.

Cerf, J., Lebrun, A., and Dierichx, J. (1962). A new approach to helminthiasis control: the use of an organophosphorus compound. Am. J. Trop. Med. Hyg., 11:514–517.

Chevalièr, J. (1930). Le préthre (chrysanthème insecticide). Activité pharmacodynamique et thérapeutique. Bull. Sci. Pharmacol., 37:154–165.

Chin, Y., and T'ant, C. (1946). The effect of DDT on cutaneous sensations in man. Science, 103:654.

Clatanoff, D. V., Triggs, P. O., and Meyer, O. O. (1954). Clinical experience with coumarin anticoagulants warfarin and warfarin sodium. Arch. Intern. Med., 94:213–220.

Cole, M. M., Clark, P. H., and Weidhass, D. E. (1958). Sleeve tests with malathion powders against DDT-resistant body lice. J. Econ. Entomol., 51:741–742.

Committee on Safety of Drugs (1965). Memorandum to manufacturers and other persons developing or proposing to market a drug in the United Kingdom. Mimeographed report.

Comroe, J. H., Jr., Todd, J., and Koelle, G. B. (1946b). Pharmacology of di-isopropyl fluorophosphate (DFP) in man. J. Pharmacol. Exp. Ther., 87:281–290.

Comroe, J. H., Jr., Todd, J., Gammon, G. D., Leopold, I. H., Koelle, G. B., Bodansky, O., and Gilman, A. (1946a). The effect of di-isopropyl-fluorophosphate (DFP) upon patients with myasthenia gravis. Am. J. Med. Sci., 212:641–651.

Congressional Record 108 (1962). 17395–17401, 17403–17405 (August 23); 22038, 22042–22043 (October 3). (Selected portions reprinted in: Hearings before the Subcommittee on Reorganization and International Organization. Interagency Coordination in Drug Research and Regulation. Part 5, Exhibit 276, pp. 2432–2444, June 19, 1963.)

Conney, A. H., Chang, R., Levin, W. M., Garbut, A., Munro-Faure, A. D., Peck, A. W., and Bye, A. (1972). Effects of piperonyl butoxide on drug metabolism in rodents and man. Arch. Environ. Health, 24:97–106.

Consolazio, W. V., Fisher, M. B., Pace, N. Pecora, L. J., Pitts, G. C., and Behnke, A. R. (1947). Effects on man of high concentrations of carbon dioxide in relation to various oxygen pressures during exposures as long as 72 hours. Am. J. Physiol., 151:479–503.

Cooney, D. P., Smith, B. P., and Fawley, D. E. (1968). Use of [32]DFP as a platelet label. Blood, 31:791–805.

Culver, D., Caplan, P., and Batchelor, G. S. (1956). Studies of human exposure during aerosol application of malathion and Chlorthion. Arch. Ind. Health, 13:37–50.

Dangerfield, W. G. (1946). Toxicity of D.D.T. to man. Br. Med. J., 1:27.

Danowski, T. S., Sarver, M. E., Moses, C., and Bonessi, J. V. (1964). o,p'-DDD therapy in Cushing's syndrome and in obesity with Cushingoid changes. Am. J. Med., 37:235–250.

Davignon, L. F., St.-Pierre, J., Charest, G., and Tourangeau, F. J. (1965). A study of the chronic effects of insecticides in man. Can. Med. Assoc. J., 92:597–602.

Dawson, J. A., Thain, E. M., and Ward, J. B. (1964). The excretion by humans of the phenol derived in vivo from 2-isopropoxyphenol N-methylcarbamate. Bull. WHO, 30:127–134.

de Fossey, B. M., Luton, J.-P., and Bricaire, H. (1968). Notre expérience de l'op' DDD dans le traitement des hypercorticismes. Ann. Endocrinol., 29:93–102.

de Gaulle, C., Derbré, M., Michelet, E., Pinay, A., Jeanneney, J. M., Bacon, P., and Chenot, B. (1959). Ordonnance No. 59-250 du 4 février 1959 relative à la réforme du régime diverses modifications du code de la santé publique. J. Off. Republique Française, pp. 1756–1759. 8 February.

Domenjoz, R. (1944). Experimentelle Erfahrungen mit einem neuen Isektizid (Neocid-Geigy), ein Beitrag zur Theorie der Kontaktgiftwirkung. Schweiz. Med. Wochenschr., 74:952–958.

Draize, J. H., Nelson, A. A., AND Calvery, H. O. (1944). The percutaneous absorption of DDT (2, 2-bis (p-chlorophenyl) l, l, l-trichloroethane) in laboratory animals. J. Pharmacol. Exp. Ther. 82:159–166.

Durham, W. F., Hayes, W. J., Jr., and Mattson, A. M. (1959). Toxicological studies of O,O-dimethyl-2, 2-dichlorovinyl phosphate (DDVP) in tobacco warehouses. Arch. Indu. Health, 20:202–210.

Durham, W. F., and Wolfe, H. R. (1962). Measurement of the exposure of workers to pesticides. Bull. WHO, 26:75–91.

Durham, W. F., and Wolfe, H. R. (1963). An additional note regarding measurement of the exposure of workers to pesticides. Bull. WHO, 29:279–281.

Durham, W. F., Wolfe, H. R., and Quinby, G. E. (1965). Organophosphorus insecticides and mental alertness. Arch. Environ. Health, 10:55–66.

Dutkiewicz, T. (1961). Absorption of aniline vapors in men. In: Proceedings of the 13th International Congress on Occupational Health, July 25–29, pp. 681–686. Book Craftsmen Accociates, Inc., New York.

Edmundson, W. F., and Davies, J. E. (1967). Occupational dermatitis from naled. Arch. Environ. Health, 15:89–91.

Edmundson, W. F., Davies, J. E., and Cranmer, M. (1970).
DDT and DDE in blood and DDA in urine of men
exposed to 3 percent DDT aerosol. Public Health Rep.,
85:457–463.

Edmundson, W. F., Davies, J. E., Cranmer, M., and Nachman, G. A. (1969a). Levels of DDT and DDE in blood
and DDA in urine of pesticide formulators following a
single intensive exposure. Ind. Med. Surg., 38:145–150.

Edmundson, W. F., Davies, J. E., Nachman, G. A., and
Roeth, R. L. (1969b). p,p'-DDT and p,p'-DDE in blood
samples of occupationally exposed workers. Public
Health Rep., 84:53–58.

Edmundson, W. F., Freal, J. J., and Davies, J. E. (1967).
Identification and measurement of dichloran in the
blood and urine of man. Environ. Res., 1:240–246.

Edson, E. F. (1955). The Effect of Prolonged Ingestion of
Low Dosages of Schradan in Humans. Mimeographed
report from the Medical Department, Fisons Pest Control Ltd.

Edson, E. F. (1956). The Effects of Prolonged Administration of Small Daily Doses of Dimefox in the Rat, Pig and
Man. Mimeographed report from the Medical Department, Fisons Pest Control Ltd.

Edson, E. F. (1957). The Effects of Prolonged Administration of Small Daily Doses of Parathion in the Rat, Pig
and Man. Mimeographed report from the Medical Department, Fisons Pest Control Ltd.

Edson, E. F. (1964). No-effect levels of three organophosphates in the rat, pig and man. Food Cosmet. Toxicol.,
2:311–316.

Edson, E. F., Jones, K. H., and Watson, W. A. (1967).
Safety of dimethoate insecticide. Br. Med. J., 4:554–555.

Elliot, R., and Barnes, J. M. (1963). Organophosphorus
insecticides for the control of mosquitos in Nigeria. Bull.
WHO, 28:35–54.

Feinberg, S. M. (1934). Pyrethrum sensitization. Its importance and relation to pollen allergy. J. A. M. A.,
102:1557–1558.

Fishbein, W. I., White, J. V., and Isaacs, H. J. (1964).
Survey of workers exposed to chlordane. Ind. Med. Surg.,
33: 726–727.

Fletcher, T. E., Press, J. M., and Wilson, D. B. (1959).
Exposure of spray-men to dieldrin in residual spraying.
Bull. WHO, 20:15–25.

Fowler, R. E. L. (1953). Insecticide toxicology. Manifestations of cottonfield insecticides in the Mississippi Delta.
J. Agric. Food Chem., 1:469–473.

Frant, R., and Westendorp, J. (1950). Medical control on
exposure of industrial workers to trichloroethylene.
Arch. Ind. Hyg. Occup. Med., 1:308–318.

Frawley, J. P., Weir, R., Tusing, T., DuBois, K. P., and
Calandra, J. C. (1963). Toxicologic investigations on
Delnav. Toxicol. Appl. Pharmacol., 5:605–624.

Frear, D. E. H. (ed.) (1969). Pesticide Index, Ed. 4. College
Science Publishers, State College, Pa.

Fredriksson, T. (1961a). Studies on the percutaneous absorption of parathion and paraoxon. III. Rate of absorption of parathion. Acta Derm. Venereol., (Stockh.)
41:353–362.

Fredriksson, T. (1961b). Percutaneous absorption of parathion and paraoxon. IV. Decontamination of human skin
from parathion. Arch. Environ. Health, 3:185–188.

Fremont, R. E., Wiedman, M., and Lubell, D. (1963). A
comparison of bishydroxycoumarin and warfarin sodium
in terms of coagulation factor changes and bleeding
complications. Am. J. Med. Sci., 246:265–276.

Freund, P. A. (1965). Ethical problems in human experimentation. N. Engl. J. Med., 273:687–692.

Friedman, B. (1959). The use of anticoagulants in the
treatment of coronary and cerebral vascular disease. J.
Tenn. Med. Assoc., 52:171–177.

Funckes, A. J., Hayes, G. R., Jr., and Hartwell, W. V.
(1963a). Insecticide activity in man. Urinary excretion
of paranitrophenol by volunteers following dermal exposure to parathion at different ambient temperatures. J.

Agric. Food Chem., 11:455–457.

Funckes, A. J., Miller, S., and Hayes, W. J., Jr. (1963b).
Initial field studies in Upper Volta with dichlorvos
residual fumigant as a malaria eradication technique.
Bull. WHO, 29:243–246.

Gaddum, J. H., and Wilson, A. (1947). Treatment of
myasthenia gravis with di-isopropylfluorophosphonate.
Nature, 159:680–681.

Gardner, J. (1958). Pediculosis capitis in preschool and
school children: control with a shampoo containing
gamma benzene hexachloride. J. Pediatr., 52:448–450.

Goldblatt, M. W. (1950). Organic phosphorus insecticides
and the antidotal action of atropine. Pharm. J., 164:229–
233.

Golz, H. H. (1959). Controlled human exposures to malathion aerosols. Arch. Ind. Health, 19:516–523.

Gordon, I. (1946). The occupational hazard of DDT spraying. Br. J. Ind. Med., 3:245–249.

Grant, W. M. (1948). Miotic and antiglaucomatous activity
of tetraethyl pyrophosphate in human eyes. Arch.
Ophthalmol., 39:579–586.

Grant, W. M. (1950). Additional experiences with tetraethyl pyrophosphate in treatment of glaucoma. Arch.
Ophthalmol. 44:362–364.

Gratz, N. G., Bracha, P., and Carmichael, A. (1963). A
village-scale trial with dichlorvos as a residual fumigant
insecticide in Southern Nigeria. Bull. WHO, 29:251–270.

Grech, J. L. (1965). Alterations in serum enzymes after
repeated exposure to malathion. Br. J. Ind. Med., 22:67–
71.

Gregory, L., Jr., Futch, E. D., and Stone, C. T. (1952).
Octamethyl pyrophosphoramide in the therapy of myasthenia gravis. Am. J. Med., 13:423–427.

Grob, D., and Harvey, A. M. (1949). Observations on the
effects of tetraethyl pyrophosphate (TEPP) in man, and
on its use in the treatment of myasthenia gravis. Bull.
Johns Hopkins Hosp., 84:532–567.

Grob, D., Lilienthal, J. L., Jr., and Harvey, A. M. (1947b).
The administration of di-isopropyl fluorophosphate
(DFP) to man. II. Effect on intestinal motility and use in
the treatment of abdominal distention. Bull. Johns Hopkins Hosp., 81:245–256.

Grob, D., Harvey, A. M., Langworthy, O. R., and Lilienthal, J. L., Jr. (1947c). The administration of di-isopropyl fluorophosphate (DFP) to man. III. Effect on the
central nervous system with special reference to the
electrical activity of the brain. Bull. Johns Hopkins
Hosp., 81:257–266.

Grob, D., Lilienthal, J. L., Jr., Harvey, A. M., and Jones, B.
F. (1947a). The administration of di-isopropyl fluorophosphate (DFP) to man. I. Effect on plasma and erythrocyte cholinesterase; general systemic effects; use in
study of hepatic function and erythropoiesis; and some
properties of plasma cholinesterase. Bull. Johns Hopkins
Hosp., 81:217–244.

Guillot, M. (1964). Exigences actuelles de la legislation
française. Farmacia, 12(3):175–180.

Gutentag, P. J. (1959). Cutaneous application of 1.1%
malathion powder to volunteers. US Army Chem. Warfare Lab. Tech. Rept. CWLR 2290.

Haag, H. B., Finnegan, J. K., Larson, P. S., Dreyfuss, M.
L., Main, R. J., and Riese, W. (1948). Comparative
chronic toxicity for warm-blooded animals of 2, 2-bis-(p-
chlorophenyl)-1, 1, 1-trichloroethane (DDT) and 2, 2-bis-
(p-chlorophenyl)-1, 1-dichloroethane (DDD). Ind. Med.,
17:477–484.

Halpern, L. K., Wooldridge, W. E., and Weiss, R. S. (1950).
Appraisal of the toxicity of the gamma isomer of hexachlorocyclohexane in clinical usage. Arch. Dermatol.,
62:648–650.

Halpern, P. B. (1966). Ce qu'un médecin doit risquer.
Moniteur Pharmacol., 716:469–472.

Hanna, S. Basmy, K., Selim, O., Shoeb, S. M., and Awny,
A. Y. (1966). Effects of administration of an organophosphorus compound as an antibilharzial agent, with

special reference to plasma cholinesterase. Br. Med. J., 1:1390–1392.

Hartwell, W. V., and Hayes, G. R., Jr. (1965). Respiratory exposure to organic phosphorus insecticides. Arch. Environ. Health, 11:564–568.

Hartwell, W. V., Hayes, G. R., Jr., and Funckes, A. J. (1964). Respiratory exposure of volunteers to parathion. Arch. Environ. Health, 8:820–825.

Hartwig, W., Massalski, W., Kasperlik-Zatuska, A., Migdalska, B., Szamatowicz, M., and Jakowicki, J. (1968). Hormonally active carcinoma of the adrenal cortex treated with o,p'-DDD. Pol. Endocrinol., 19:57–69.

Harvey, A. M., Jones, B. F., Talbot, S., and Grob, D. (1946). The effect of diisopropyl fluorophosphate (DFP) on neuromuscular transmission in normal individuals and in patients with myasthenia gravis. Fed. Proc., 5: 182.

Harvey, A. M., Lilienthal, J. L., Jr., Grob, D., Jones, B. F., and Talbot, S. A. (1947). The administration of diisopropyl fluorophosphate to man. IV. The effects of neuromuscular fuction in normal subjects and in myasthenia gravis. Bull. Johns Hopkins Hosp., 81:267–292.

Harvey, D. G., Bidstrup, P. L., and Bonnell, J. A. L. (1951). Poisoning by dinitro-ortho-cresol: Some observations on the effects of dinitro-ortho-cresol administered by mouth to human volunteers. Br. Med. J., 2:13–16.

Hayes, G. R., Jr., Funckes, A. J., and Hartwell, W. V. (1964). Dermal exposure of human volunteers to parathion. Arch. Environ. Health, 8:829–833.

Hayes, W. J., Jr. (1957). Dieldrin poisoning in man. Public Health Rep., 72:1087–1091.

Hayes, W. J., Jr. (1959). The toxicity of dieldrin to man. Bull. WHO, 20:891–912.

Hayes, W. J., Jr. (1963). Clinical Handbook on Economic Poisons. PHS Publ. No. 476, US Government Printing Office, Washington, DC.

Hayes, W. J., Jr. (1965). Experiences with the exposure of human subjects to agricultural chemicals and a discussion of the legal position of investigations using people. In: Research in Pesticides, edited by C. O. Chichester, pp. 329–355. Academic Press, Inc., New York.

Hayes, W. J., Jr. (1968). Tests in man. In: Modern Trends in Toxicology, edited by E. Boyland and R. Goulding, pp. 198–230. Butterworths, London.

Hayes, W. J., Jr., and Curley, A. (1968). Storage and excretion of dieldrin and related compounds. Effect of occupational exposure. Arch. Environ. Health, 16:155–162.

Hayes, W. J., Jr., Dale, W. E., and Pirkle, C. I. (1971). Evidence of safety of long-term, high, oral doses of DDT for man. Arch. Environ. Health, 22:119–135.

Hayes, W. J. Jr., Dixon, E. M., Batchelor, G. S., and Upholt, W. M. (1957). Exposure to organic phosphorus sprays and occurrence of selected symptoms. Public Health Rep., 72:787–794.

Hayes, W. J., Jr., Durham, W. F., and Cueto, C., Jr. (1956). The effect of known repeated oral doses of chlorophenothane (DDT) in man. J. A. M. A., 162:890–897.

Hayes, W. J., Jr., Mattson, A. M., Short, J. G., and Witter, R. F. (1960). Safety of malathion dusting powder for louse control. Bull. WHO, 22:503–514.

Hoogendam, I., Versteeg, J. P. J., and deVlieger, M. (1962). Electroencephalograms in insecticide toxicity. Arch. Environ. Health, 4:86–94.

Hoogendam, I., Versteeg, J. P. J., and deVlieger, M. (1965). Nine years' toxicity control in insecticide plants. Arch. Environ. Health, 10:441–448.

Hunter, C. G., and Robinson, J. (1967). Pharmacodynamics of dieldrin (HEOD). I. Ingestion by human subjects for 18 months. Arch. Environ. Health, 15:614–626.

Hunter, C. G., and Robinson, J. (1968). Aldrin, dieldrin and man. Food Cosmet. Toxicol., 6:253–260.

Hunter, C. G., Robinson, J., and Roberts, M. (1969). Pharmacodynamics of dieldrin (HEOD): ingestion by human subjects for 18 to 24 months, and postexposure for eight

months. Arch Environ. Health, 18:12–21.

Hutter, A. M., and Kayhoe, D. E. (1966). Adrenal cortical carcinoma. Am. J. Med., 41:572–580.

Ingram, F. R. (1951). Health hazards associated with use of airplanes for dusting crops with parathion. Am. Ind. Hyg. Assoc. Q., 12:165–170.

Jovčič, B., and Ivanus, J. (1968). Variations in the electroencephalogram in workers exposed to insecticides. Zentralbl. Arbeitsmed., 18: 270–272.

Kagan, Y. S., Kundiev, Y. I., and Trotsenko, M. A. (1958). Gigiena truda pri primenenii sistemnykh fosfororganicheskikh insektitsidov. Soobschenie vtoroe. Gig. Sanit., 23(6):25–31.

Kailin, E. W., and Hastings, A. (1966). Electromyographic evidence of DDT-induced myasthenia. Med. Ann. DC, 35:237–244.

Kaiser, A. D. (1946). Treatment of Pediculus capitis in school children with DDT powder. Am. J. Public Health, 36:1133–1134.

Kay, K., Monkman, L., Windish, J. P., Doherty, T., Pare, J., and Racicot, C. (1952). Parathion exposure and cholinesterase response of Quebec apple growers. Arch. Ind. Hyg. Occup. Med., 6:252–262.

Keplinger, M. L. (1963). Use of humans to evaluate safety of chemicals. Arch. Environ. Health, 6:342–349.

Klhufkova, E., and Pospisil, R. (1961). Poznatky sledovani hladiny cholinesterazy v krvi u pracovniku s organofosfaty. Prak. Lek., 13: 406–407.

Kligman, A. M. (1966). The identification of contact allergies by human assay. III. The maximization test: a procedure for screening and rating contact sensitizers. J. Invest. Dermatol., 47:393–409.

Klimmer, O. R., and Pfaff, W. (1955). Untersuchungen uber die Toxicat des neuen Kontaktinsekticides O,O-Dimethylthiophosphorsaure-O-(B-s-athyl)-ester ('metasystox') Arzneim. Forsch., 5:584–587.

Knaak, J. B., Tallant, M. J., Kozbelt, S. J., and Sullivan,. L. J. (1968). The metabolism of carbaryl in man, monkey, pig, and sheep. J. Agric. Food Chem., 16:465–470.

Kohn, F. E. (1962). Research report on Dibrom. Report to the Ortho Division, California Chemical Company.

Krasnyuk, E. P. (1958). Vliyanic DDT na organizm rabochikh, zanyatykh ego proizvodstvom. Vrach. Delo, 5:519–522.

Krasnyuk, E. P. (1964a). Some indications of the functional condition of the glands of internal secretion in persons working with organochlorine compounds. Vrach. Delo, 1:115–119.

Krasnyuk, E. P. (1964b). Electrorcardiographic changes in persons working with organic chlorine insecticides. Sov. Med., 28:134–137.

Ladimer, I., and Newman, R. W. (1963). Clinical Investigation in Medicine: Legal, Ethical and Moral Aspects. An Anthology and Bibliography. Law-Medicine Research Institute, Boston University.

Langer, E. (1966). Human experimentation: New York verdict affirms patient's rights. Science, 151:663–666.

Laws, E. R., Jr., Ramos Morales, F., Hayes, W. J., Jr., and Romney Josph, C. (1967a). Toxicology of Abate in volunteers. Arch. Environ. Health, 14:289–291.

Laws, E. R., Jr., Curley, A., and Biros, F. J. (1967b). Men with intensive occupational exposure to DDT. A clinical and chemical study. Arch. Environ. Health, 15:766–776.

Lebrun, A., and Cerf, C. (1960). Note preliminaire sur la toxicité pour l'homme d'un insecticide organophosphore (Dipterex). Bull. WHO, 22:579–582.

Leopold, I. H., and Comroe, J. H., Jr. (1946). Effect of diisopropyl fluorophosphate (DFP) on the normal eye. Arch. Ophthalmol., 36:17–32.

Leopold, I. H., and McDonald, P. R. (1948). Di-isopropyl fluorophosphate (DFP) in treatment of glaucoma. Arch Ophthalmol., 40:176–188.

Letavet, A. A. (1961). Scientific Principles for the Establishment of the Maximum Allowable Concentration of

Toxic Substances in the U.S.S.R. Proc. 13th Int. Congr. Occup. Health, pp. 983–987.

Lieben, J., Waldman, R. K., and Krause, L. (1953). Urinary excretion of paranitrophenol following exposure to parathion. Arch. Ind. Hyg. Occup. Med., 7:93–98.

Lind, J. (1753). *A Treatise of the Scurvey.* Edinburgh. (Edited by Stewart, C. P. and Guthrie, D., and reprinted at the University Press, Edinburgh, 1953.)

Lönngren, R. (1965). Toxicological aspects and the law concerning drugs in Sweden. IN: *Experimental Studies and Clinical Experience—The Assessment of Risk.* Proceedings of the European Society for the Study of Drug Toxicity, Vol. VI, pp. 245–247. Excerpta Medica Foundation, Amsterdam.

Lord, K. A., and Johnson, C. G. (1947). The production of dermatitis by pyrethrum and attempts to produce a nonirritant extract. Br. J. Dermatol., 59:368–375.

Louis, P. C. A. (1835). *Recherches sur les Effets de la Saignee.* J. B. Baillière et Fils, Paris.

Lyubetskii, K. Z., and Vengerskaya, K. Y. (1961). Sravitel'naya otsenka uslovii truda pri obrabotke khlopchatnika merkaptofosom, metilsistoksomi preparation M-81. Gig. Sanit., 26:36–39.

MacCormack, J. D. (1945). Infestation and D.D.T. Ir. J. Med. Sci., 6:627–634.

McLaughlin, J. T., and Sonnenschein, R. P. (1960). Action of paraoxon (diethyl 4-nitrophenyl phosphate) on human sweat glands and the sympathetic axone reflex. Acta Pharmacol., 17:7–17.

Marr, W. G. (1947). The clinical use of di-isopropyl fluorophosphate (D.F.P.) in chronic glaucoma. Am. J. Ophthalmol., 30:1423–1426.

Marr, W. G., and Grob, D. (1950). Some occular effects of a new anticholinesterase agent. Tetraethyl pyrophosphate (TEPP) and its use in the treatment of chronic glaucoma. Am. J. Ophthalmol., 33:904–908.

Martin, J. T., and Hester, K. H. C. (1941). Dermatitis caused by insecticidal pyrethrum flowers (Chrysanthemum cineraufolium). Br. J. Dermatol., 53:127–142.

Mattson, A. M., and Sedlak, V. A. (1960). Measurement of insecticide exposure. Ether-extractable urinary phosphates in man and rats derived from malathion and similar compounds. J. Agric. Food Chem., 8:107–110.

Medical Research Council (1964). Responsibility in investigations on human subjects. Br. Med. J., 2:178–180. (Originally published in the Annual Report of the Medical Research Council for 1962–63, H.M.S.O. 1964.)

Milby, T. H., and Epstein, W. L. (1964). Allergic contact sensitivity to malathion. Arch. Environ. Health, 9:434–437.

Milby, T. H., and Samuels, A. J. (1971). Human exposure to lindane. Comparison of an exposed and unexposed population. J. Occup. Med., 13:256–258.

Milby, T. H., Samuels, A. J., and Ottoboni, F. (1968). Human exposure to lindane. J. Occup. Med., 10:584–587.

Miles, J. W. (1965). Collection and determination of trace quantities of pesticides in air. Presented at the 149th meeting of the American Chemical Society, Detroit, Michigan, April 5–8.

Model, A. (1968). Peculiarities of neurological symptoms in chronic DDT poisoning. Sov. Med., 31:110–114.

Moeller, H. C., and Rider, J. A. (1959). The effects of various organic phosphate insecticides on RBC and plasma cholinesterase in humans. Fed. Proc., 18:424.

Moeller, H. C., and Rider, J. A. (1961). Studies on the anticholinesterase effect of parathion and methyl parathion in humans. Fed. Proc., 20:434.

Moeller, H. C., and Rider, J. A. (1962a). Plasma and red blood cell cholinesterase activity as indications of the threshold of incipient toxicity of ethyl-p-nitrophenyl thionobenzenephosphonate (EPN) and malathion in human beings. Toxicol. Appl. Pharmacol., 4:123–130.

Moeller, H. C., and Rider, J. A. (1962b). Threshold of incipient toxicity to Systox and methyl parathion. Fed.

Proc., 21:451.

Moeller, H. C., and Rider, J. A. (1963). Further studies on the toxicity of Systox and methyl parathion. Fed. Proc., 22:189.

Molnar, G. D., Nun, S. L., and Tauxe, W. N. (1961). The effect of o,p′-DDD therapy on plasma cholesterol in adrenal carcinoma. Proc. Staff Meet. Mayo Clin., 36:618–620.

Morgan, D. P., and Roan, C. C. (1971). Absorption, storage, and metabolic conversion of ingested DDT and DDT metabolites in man. Arch. Environ. Health, 22:301–308.

Munkner, T., Matzke, J., and Videback, A. (1961). Cholinesterase activity of human plasma after intermuscular diisopropyl fluorophosphate (DFP). Acta Pharmacol., 18:170–174.

Munster, A. J., Bollman, H., and Saunders, J. C. (1962). Hexachlorocyclohexane in the treatment of pediculosis. Arch. Pediatr., 79:94–95.

Najera, J. A., Shirdawi, G. R., Gibson, F. D., and Stafford, J. S. (1967). A large-scale field trial of malathion as an insecticide for antimalarial work in Southern Uganda. Bull. WHO, 36:913–935.

National Academy of Sciences (1965). *Some Considerations in the Use of Human Subjects in Safety Evaluation of Pesticides and Food Chemicals.* NAS-NRC, Publ. 1270, Washington, DC.

National Academy of Sciences (1967). *Use of Human Subjects in Safety Evaluation of Food Chemicals.* NAS-NRC, Publ. 1491, Washington, DC.

Neal, P. A., Sweeney, T. R., Spicer, S. S., and von Oettingen, W. F. (1946). The excretion of DDT (2,2-bis-(p-chlorophenyl)-1,1,1-trichloroethane) in man, together with clinical observations. Public Health Rep., 61:403–409.

Neal, P. A., von Oettingen, W. F., Smith, W. W., Malmo, R. B., Dunn, R. C., Moran, H. E., Sweeney, T. T., Armstrong, D. W., and White, W. C. (1944). Toxicity and potential dangers of aerosols,, mists and dusting powders containing DDT. Public Health Rep. (Suppl.) 177.

Nichols, J., Prestley, W. F., and Nichols, F. (1961). Effects of m,p′-DDD in a case of adrenal cortical carcinoma. Curr. Ther. Res., 3:266–271.

Nodine, J. H., and Siegler, P. E. (eds.) (1964). *Animal and Clinical Pharmacologic Techniques in Drug Evaluation.* Year Book Medical Publishers, Inc., Chicago.

Nuremberg Military Tribunal (1947). United States versus Karl Brandt et al. ("The Medical Case"). In: *Trials of War Criminals,* Vol. 2, pp. 181–184. US Government Printing Office, Washington, DC.

O'Reilly, R. A., Aggeler, P. M., and Leong, L. S. (1963). Studies on the coumarin anticoagulant drugs: the pharmacodynamics of warfarin in man. J. Clin. Invest., 42:1542–1551.

Ortelee, M. F. (1958). Study of men with prolonged intensive occupational exposure to DDT. Arch. Ind. Health, 18:433–440.

Osserman, K., and Kaplan, L. I. (1954). Studies in myasthenia gravis: Present status of therapy with octamethyl pyrophosphoramide. (OMPA). Ann. Intern. Med., 41:108–111.

Pagnotto, L. D., and Walkley, J. E. (1965). Urinary dichlorophenol as an index of para-dichlorobenzene exposure. Am. Ind. Hyg. Assoc. J., 26:137–142.

Panja, R. K., and Choudhury, S. (1969). A clinical trial with gamma benzene hexachloride in scabies. Indian J. Dermatol., 14:136–137.

Pant, C. P., Rosen, P., Joshi, G. P., Pearson, J. A., Ramasamy, M., Renaud, P., and Vandekar, M. (1969). A village-scale trial of OMS-708 (Mobam) for the control of *Anopheles gambiae* and *Anopheles funestus* in Northern Nigeria. Bull. WHO, 41:316–319.

Paramonchik, V. M. (1968). Liver function in workers engaged in the production of certain organochlorous chemical poisons. Sov. Med., 31:62–65.

Paramonchik, V. M., and Platonova, V. I. (1968). Functional condition of the liver and stomach in persons exposed to effects of organochlorous chemical poisons. Gig. Tr. Zabol., 12:27–31.

Paulus, H. J., Lippmann, M., and Cohen, A. E. (1957). Evaluation of potential health hazards in fumigation of shelled corn with a mixture of carbon disulfide and carbon tetrachloride. Am. Ind. Hyg. Assoc. Q., 18:345–350.

Percival, T. (1803). *Medical Ethics*. London. (Republished by Leake, C. D., and part of his book *Percival's Medical Ethics*, The Williams & Wilkins Company, Baltimore, 1927.)

Pius XII (1952). The moral limits of medical research and treatment. Acta Apostolicae Sedis, 44:779.

Poland, A., Smith, D., Kuntzman, R., Jacobson, M., and Conney, A. H. (1970). Effect of intensive occupational exposure to DDT on phenylbutazone and cortisol metabolism in human subjects. Clin. Pharmacol. Ther., 11:724–732.

Poland, A. P., Smith, D., Metter, G., and Possick, P. (1971). A health survey of workers in a 2,4-D and 2,4,5-T plant. Arch. Environ. Health, 22:316–327.

Pollock, B. E. (1955). Clinical experience with warfarin (coumarin) sodium, a new anticoagulant. J. A. M. A., 159:1094–1097.

Princi, F., and Spurbeck, G. H. (1951). A study of workers exposed to the insecticides chlordane, aldrin, dieldrin. Arch. Ind. Hyg. Occup. Med., 3:64–72.

Public Health Council of the Netherlands (1957). Report on human experimentation. World Med. J., 4:299–300.

Quinby, G. E., Hayes, W. J., Jr., Armstrong, J. F., and Durham, W. F. (1965). DDT storage in the U. S. population. J. A. M. A., 191:175–179.

Quinby, G. E., and Lemmon, A. B. (1958). Parathion residues as a cause of poisoning in crop workers. J. A. M. A., 166:740–746.

Quinby, G. E., Walker, K. C., and Durham, W. F. (1958). Public health hazards involved in the use of organic phosphorus insecticides in cotton culture in the Delta area of Mississippi. J. Econ. Entomol., 51:831–838.

Rasmussen, W. A., Jensen, J. A., Stein, W. J., and Hayes, W. J., Jr. (1963). Toxicological studies of DDVP for disinsection of aircraft. Aerosp. Med., 34:594–600.

Rider, J. A., and Moeller, H. C. (1960). Effects of various organic phosphate anticholinesterase agents on serum and red blood cell cholinesterase and their relation to the treatment of myasthenia gravis. In: *Thymectomy for Myasthenia Gravis*, edited by H. R. Viets and R. S. Schwab, pp. 556–580. Charles C Thomas, Springfield, Ill.

Rider, J. A., and Moeller, H. C. (1964). Studies on the anticholinesterase effects of Systox and methyl parathion in humans. Fed. Proc., 23:176.

Rider, J. A., Moeller, H. C., Pulletti, E. J., and Swader, J. I. (1969). Toxicity of parathion, systox, octamethyl pyrophosphoramide, and methyl parathion in man. Toxicol. Appl. Pharmacol., 14:603–611.

Rider, J. A., Moeller, H. S. Swader, J., and Devereaux, R. G. (1959). A study of the anticholinesterase properties of EPN and malathion in human volunteers. Clin. Res., 7:81–83.

Rider, J. A., Moeller, H. C., Swader, J., and Weilerstein, R. W. (1958). The effect of parathion on human red blood cell and plasma cholinesterase. Section II. Arch. Ind. Health, 18:442–445.

Rider, J. A., Schulman, S., Richter, R. B., Moeller, H. C., and DuBois, K. P. (1951). Treatment of myasthenia gravis with octamethyl pyrophosphoramide. J. A. M. A., 145:967–972.

Roan, C., Morgan, D., and Paschal, E. H. (1971). Urinary excretion of DDA following ingestion of DDT and DDT metabolites in man. Arch. Environ. Health, 22:309–315.

Robinson, J., and Hunter, C. G. (1966). Organochlorine insecticides: Concentrations in human blood and adipose tissue. Arch. Environ. Health, 13:558–563.

Robinson, J., and Roberts, M. (1969). Estimation of the exposure of the general population to dieldrin (HEOD). Food Cosmet. Toxicol., 7:501–514.

Rosival, L., and Rajnoha, F. (1961). Ochrana zdravia pri vyrobe intrationu. Cs. Hyg., 6:287–289.

Rowe, V. K., McCollister, D. D., Spencer, H. C., Adams, E. M., and Irish, D. D. (1952). Vapor toxicity of tetrachloroethylene for laboratory animals and human subjects. Arch. Ind. Hyg. Occup. Med., 6:566–579.

Rowntree, D. W., Nevin, S., and Wilson, A. (1950). The effects of diisopropylfluorophosphonate in schizophrenia and manic depressive psychosis. J. Neurol. Neurosurg. Psychiatry., 13:47–62.

Ruprich, J. (1961). Zkusenosti ze zdravotnitkeno zabezpecni provadeni postriku a zalivky organickymi fosforovymi insekticidy. Prak. Lek., 13:408–409.

Rydin, H. (1965). Experience with the preliminary Swedish recommendations for toxicity tests. In: *Experimental Studies and Clinical Experience—The Assessment of Risk*. Proceedings of the European Society for the Study of Drug Toxicity, Vol. VI, pp. 242–244. Excerpta Medica Foundation, Amsterdam.

Sanderson, D. M., and Edson, E. F. (1964). Toxicological properties of the organo-phosphorus insecticide dimethoate. Br. J. Ind. Med., 21:52-64.

Scholz, R. O., and Wallen, L. J. (1946). Effects of diisopropyl fluorophosphate on normal human eyes. J. Pharmacol. Exp. Ther., 88:238–245.

Schulman, S., Rider, J. A., and Richter, R. B. (1953). Use of octamethyl pyrophosphoramide in the treatment of myasthenia gravis. J. A. M. A., 152:1707–1711.

Schüttman, W. (1968). Chronic liver diseases after occupational exposure to dichlorodiphenyltrichloroethane (DDT) and hexachlor cyclohexane (BHC). Int. Gewerbepath. Gewerbehyg., 24:193–210.

Seabury, J. H. (1963). Toxicity of 2,4-dichlorophenoxyacetic acid for man and dog. Arch. Environ. Health, 7:202–209.

Sendroy, J., Jr., and Cecchini, L. P. (1954). Determination of human body surface area from height and weight. J. Appl. Physiol., 7:1–12.

Sessoms, S. M. (1958). What hospitals should know about investigational drugs; guiding principles in medical research involving humans. Hospitals, 32:44, 58, 60, 62, 64.

Shapiro, S. (1953). Warfarin sodium derivative: (coumarin sodium). Angiology, 4:380–390.

Shawarby, A. A., El-Refai, A.-R., El-Hawary, M. F. S., and Ed-Essawi, M. (1963). Field and laboratory studies on the use of malathion for control of body-lice in Egypt. Bull. WHO, 28:111–120.

Sheehan, H. L., Summers, V. K., and Nichols, J. (1953). D.D.D. therapy in Cushing's syndrome. Lancet, 1:312–314.

Simpson, G. R. (1965). Exposure to Guthion during formulation. Arch. Environ. Health, 10:53–54.

Simpson, G. R., and Beck, A. (1965). Exposure to parathion. Arch. Environ. Health, 11:784–786.

Smith, P. W., Mertens, H., Lewis, M. F., Funkhouser, G. E.. Higgins, E. A., Crane, C. R., Sanders, D. C., Endecott, B. R., and Flux, M. (1972). Toxicology of dichlorvos at operational aircraft cabin altitudes. Aerosp. Med., 43:473–478.

Soucek, B., and Vlachová, D. (1960). Excretion of trichloroethylene metabolites in human urine. Br. J. Ind. Med., 17:60–64.

Southren, A. L., Weisenfeld, S., Laufer, A., and Goldner, M. G. (1961). Effect of o,p′-DDD in a patient with Cushing's syndrome. J. Clin. Endocrinol., 21:201–208.

Spiers, F., and Juul, P. (1964). Cholinesterase activity in plasma and erythrocytes. Acta Ophthalmol., 42:696–712.

Stammers, F. M. G., and Whitfield, F. G. S. (1947). The

toxicity of DDT to man and animals. Bull. Entomol. Res., 38:1–73.

Stein, A. A. (1968). Comparative methoxychlor toxicity in dogs, swine, rats, monkeys and man. Ind. Med. Surg., 37:540–541.

Stein, A. A., Serrone, D. M., and Coulston, F. (1965). Safety evaluation of methoxychlor in human volunteers. Toxicol. Appl. Pharmacol., 7:499.

Stein, W. J., and Hayes, W. J., Jr. (1964). Health survey of pest control operators. Ind. Med. Surg., 33:549–555.

Stein, W. J., Miller, S., and Fetzer, L. E., Jr. (1966). Studies with dichlorvos residual fumigant as a malaria eradication technique in Haiti. III. Toxicological studies. Am. J. Trop. Med. Hyg., 15:672–675.

Stewart, R. D. (1974). The use of breath analysis in clinical toxicology. Essays Toxicol. 5:121–147.

Stewart, R. D., Baretta, E. D., Dodd, H. C., and Torkelson, T. R. (1970). Experimental human exposure to tetrachloroethylene. Arch. Environ. Health, 20:224–229.

Stewart, R. D., Fisher, T. N., Hosko, M. J., Peterson, J. E., Baretta, E. D., and Dodd, H. C. (1972). Experimental human exposure to methylene chloride. Arch. Environ. Health, 25:342–348.

Stewart, R. D., Gay, H. H., Erley, D. S., Hake, C. L., and Peterson, J. E. (1961a). Human exposure to carbon tetrachloride vapor. J. Occup. Med., 3:586–590.

Stewart, R. D., Gay, H. H., Erley, D. S., Hake, C. L., and Schaffer, A. W. (1961b). Human exposure to tetrachloroethylene vapor. Arch. Environ. Health, 2:516–522.

Stewart, R. D., Gay, H. H., Erley, D. S., Hake, C. L., and Schaffer, A. W. (1961c). Human exposure to 1,1,1-trichloroethane vapor: relationship of expired air and blood concentrations to exposure and toxicity. Am. Ind. Hyg. Assoc. J., 22:252–262.

Stewart, R. D., Gay, H. H., Erley, D. S., Hake, C. L., and Peterson, J. E. (1962). Observations on the concentrations of trichloroethylene in blood and expired air following exposure of humans. Am. Ind. Hyg. Assoc. J., 23:167–170.

Stewart, W. H. (1966a). Clinical research and investigation involving human beings. Memorandum from the Surgeon General, Public Health Service to the Heads of Institutions Conducting Research with Public Health Service Grants, February 8.

Stewart, W. H. (1966b). Clinical investigations using human beings as subjects. Memorandum from the Surgeon General, Public Health Service to the Bureau Chiefs, March 30.

Stone, C. T., and Rider, J. A. (1949). Treatment of myasthenia gravis. J. A. M. A., 141: 107–111.

Stone, W. C. (1950). Use of di-isopropyl fluorophosphate (DFP) in treatment of glaucoma. Arch. Ophthalmol., 43:36–42.

Stumpf, S. E. (1966). Some moral dimensions of medicine. Ann. Intern. Med., 64:460–470.

Stumpf, S. E. (1967). Momentum and morality in medicine. Ann. Intern. Med., 67:10–14.

Su, M., Kinoshita, F. K., Frawley, J. P., and DuBois, K. P. (1971). Comparative inhibition of aliesterases and cholinesterase in rats fed eighteen organophosphorus insecticides. Toxicol. Appl. Pharmacol., 20:241–249.

Sumerford, W. T., Hayes, W. J., Jr., Johnston, J. M., Walker, K., and Spillane, J. (1953). Cholinesterase response and symptomatology from exposure to organic phosphorus insecticides. Arch. Ind. Hyg. Occup. Med., 7:383–398.

Suskind, R. R. (1959). *The Cutaneous Appraisal of Several Fabrics Treated with Dieldrin.* The Kettering Laboratory, Cincinnati, Ohio.

Sutton, W. L., Terharr, C. J., Miller, F. A., Scherberger, M. S., Riley, E. C., Roudabush, R. L., and Fassett, D. W. (1960). Studies on the industrial hygiene and toxicology of triphenyl phosphate. Arch. Environ. Health, 1:33–46.

Sweitzer, S. E., and Tedder, J. W. (1935). Pyrethrum in treatment of scabies. Minn. Med., 18:793, 795.

Talaat, S. M. (1964). *The Treatment of Schistosomiasis and Other Intestinal Parasites with Dipterex.* United Arab Republic, Cairo.

Taliaferro, I., and Leone, L. (1957). Inhibitory effect of Perthane (2,2-bis-(para-ethylphenyl)-1,1-dichloroethane) on adrenocortical function in human subjects. N. Engl. J. Med., 257:855–860.

Taylor, A. (1963). Observations on human exposure to the organophosphorus insecticide fenthion in Nigeria. Bull. WHO, 29:213–218.

Taylor, C. (1941). Studies in exercise physiology. Am. J. Physiol., 135:27–42.

Tessari, J. D., and Spencer, D. L. (1971). Air sampling for pesticides in the human environment. J. Assoc. Off. Anal. Chem., 54:1376–1382.

Thompson, R. P. H., Stathers, G. M., Pilcher, C. W. T., McLean, A. E. M., Robinson, J., and Williams, R. (1969). Treatment of unconjugated jaundice with dicophane. Lancet, 2:4–6.

Törnblom, N. (1959). Administration of DDD (2,2-bis(parachlorophenyl)-1,1-dichloroethane) to diabetics with hyaline vascular changes and hyperpolysaccharidemia. Acta Med. Scand., 164:23–37.

Upholt, W. M., Quinby, G. E., and Batchelor, G. S. (1954). Eating Systox-treated fruit under controlled conditions. Proc. 50th Annu. Meet. Wash. St. Horticul. Assoc., 50:217–220.

Upholt, W. M., Quinby, G. E., Batchelor, G. S., and Thompson, J. P. (1956). Visual effects accompanying TEPP-induced miosis. Arch. Ophthalmol., 56:128–134.

Vandekar, M. (1965). Observations on the toxicity of carbaryl, Folithion and 3-isopropylphenyl N-methylcarbamate in village scale trail in Southern Nigeria. Bull. WHO, 33:107–115.

Vandekar, M., Hedayat, S., Plestina, R., and Ahmady, G. (1968). A study of the safety of O-isopropoxyphenylmethylcarbamate in an operational field-trial in Iran. Bull. WHO, 38:609–623.

Vandekar, M., and Svetlićić, B. (1966). Observations on the toxicity of three anticholinesterase insecticides in a village-scale trial and comparison of methods used for determining cholinesterase activity. Arh. Hig. Rada Toksikol., 17:135–150.

Velbinger, H. H. (1947a). Zur Frage der "DDT"—Toxizitat fur Menschen. Dtsch. Gesundheitsw., 2:355–358.

Velbinger, H. H. (1947b). Beitrag zur Toxikologie des DDT-Wirkstoffes Dichlor-diphenyl-trichlormethyl methane. Pharmazie, 2:268–274.

Vengerskaya, Kh. Y., Liubetskii, Kh. Z., and Tareva, G. A. (1959). Uslovija truda pri ispytanii novyh fosfor-organischeskih insekticidov. Gig. Sanit., 24(5):12–17.

Verdon, T. A., Bruton, J., Herman, R. H., and Beisel, W. R. (1962). Clinical and chemical response of functioning adrenal cortical carcinoma to ortho, para'-DDD. Metabolism, 11:226–234.

Wallace, E. Z., Silverstein, J. N., Villadolick, L. S., and Weisenfeld, S. (1961). Cushing's syndrome due to adrenocortical hyperplasia. N. Engl. J. Med., 265:1088–1093.

Wasicky, R., and Unti, O. (1944). Dichloro-difenil-tricholoroetano (DDT) no combate às larvas de Culicideos. Arg. Hig., Sao Paulo, 9(21):87–102.

Wassermann, M., Iliescu, S., Mandric, G., and Horvath, P. (1960). Toxic hazards during DDT- and BHC-spraying of forests against Lymantria Monacha. Arch. Ind. Health, 21:503–508.

Weisenfeld, S., and Goldner, M. G. (1962). Treatment of advanced malignancy and Cushing's syndrome with DDD. Cancer Chemother. Rep., 16:335–339.

Westerberg, M. R., and Luros, J. T. (1948). The clinical use of hexaethyl tetraphosphate in myasthenia gravis. Univ. Hosp. Bull., Ann Arbor, 14:15–17.

Wigglesworth, V. B. (1945). DDT and the balance of nature. Atlantic Monthly, Dec., p. 107.

Witter, R. F. (1960). Effects of DDVP aerosols on blood cholinesterase of fogging machine operators. Arch. Ind. Health, 21:7–9.

Witter, R. F., Gaines, T. B., Short, J. G., Sedlak, V. A., and Maddock, D. R. (1961). Studies on the safety of DDVP for the disinfection of commercial aircraft. Bull. WHO, 24:635–642.

Wolfe, H. R., Durham, W. F., and Armstrong, J. F. (1963). Health hazards of the pesticides endrin and dieldrin. Hazards in some agricultural uses in the pacific Northwest. Arch. Environ. Health, 6:458–464.

Wolfe, H. R., Durham, W. F., and Batchelor, G. S. (1961). Health hazards of some dinitro compounds. Effects associated with agricultural usage in Washington State. Arch. Environ. Health, 3:468–475.

Wolff, J. M., Barker, N. W., Gifford, R. W., Jr., and Mann, F. D. (1953). Experience with a new intravenous coumarin anticoagulant (warfarin, sodium derivative). Proc. Staff Meet. Mayo Clin., 28:489–497.

Woolridge, W. E. (1948). The gamma isomer of hexachlorocyclohexane in the treatment of scabies. J. Invest. Dermatol., 10:363–366.

World Medical Association (1964). Human experimentation. Br. Med. J., 2:177.

Wright, J. W., Fritz, R. F., Hocking, K. S., Babione, R., Gratz, N. G., Pal, R., Stiles, A. R., and Vandekar, M. (1969). Orthoisopropoxyphenyl methylcarbamate (OMS-33) as a residual spray for control of anopheline mosquitos. Bull. WHO, 40:67–90.

Zavon, M. R. (1964). Personal communication.

Zavon, M. R., and Kindel, E. A., Jr. (1966). Potential hazard in using dichlorvos insecticide resin. Adv. Chem. Ser., 60:177–186.

Zein-El-Dine, K. (1946). The insecticide DDT. J. R. Egypt. Med. Assoc., 29:38–54.

Zimmerman, B., Block, H. S., Williams, W. L., Hitchcock, C. R., and Hoelscher, B. (1956). The effects of DDD (1,1-dichloro-2,2-bis-(p-chlorophenyl)ethane) on the human adrenal. Cancer, 9:940–948.

6

RECOGNIZED AND POSSIBLE EXPOSURE TO PESTICIDES

This chapter is concerned with the magnitude of human contact with pesticides, ranging from exposures that are questionably detectable by the most sensitive modern methods—and, in fact, may not exist at all—to the heavy exposures of workers who make, formulate, or apply tons of concentrated material. The major exposure of most people involves residues on food. This exposure is large enough to be easily measurable but smaller than the exposure of workers, often by a factor of several hundred. These great differences in magnitude must be kept in mind in evaluating the significance of any particular residue.

This chapter also is concerned with the physical, chemical, and biological factors that determine how great residues will be and how long they will last. The human factors limiting exposure through choice of compound and formulation, good sanitation, engineering, medical and environmental surveillance, law, and other means are discussed in Chapter 9.

6.1 Residues in Food

Before a pesticide can be registered in the United States of America for any use that might lead to the contamination of food, an adequate method for its analysis in food must be presented to the Environmental Protection Agency. Thus, it is illegal to sell a pesticide for use on crops unless the residues can be identified and measured. In recent scientific surveys carried out by the Food and Drug Administration, a search has been made for all important compounds, using methods capable of measuring concentrations far less than those of any biological significance. The results of this important surveillance are discussed in Section 6.1.5.1. The intervening sections are concerned with residues in different classes of foods and with factors that influence these residues.

Different kinds of food require different pesticides in their production, and may vary in their retention of compounds that do reach them. Furthermore, different kinds of food are eaten in different amounts by the general adult population of a particular country, and the proportion may vary widely for infants or other special groups in the same country, or for the general adult populations of different countries. Under the circumstances, both investigators and administrators have found it necessary to classify foods in connection with residues of pesticides. The categories used by the US Food and Drug Administration are employed in the following paragraphs. These categories are based largely on raw agricultural products, making it possible to relate information about residues to variations of agricultural practice on the one hand and diet on the other.

In addition to residues, whether legal or illegal, that may occur in food sold on the open market, there are those residues resulting from a wide variety of experimental conditions. For example, before any pesticide is registered for use on a particular crop, extensive tests must be done to learn what residues will occur following different dosage schedules and at different intervals after application. This chapter is concerned almost entirely with residues that may lead to human exposure. However, the residues produced under experimental conditions are important in other connections. Information on them may be found in agricultural and entomological publications. Results of this kind related to DDT have been reviewed (Hayes, 1959).

6.1.1 Residues in Animal Products

6.1.1.1 Observed Residues. Although many compounds are stored in tissue or secreted in the milk if administered to cows in sufficient dosage, it is unusual for residues arising from pesticides, other than the chlorinated hydrocarbon insecticides, to be detectable in more than trace amounts in marketed food of animal origin. The regular occurrence of the chlorinated hydrocarbon insecticides is remarkable, because their application to forage or to dairy cows, or to animals prior to slaughter, was abandoned long ago. The residues that do occur are thought to result mainly from the contamination of forage by the drift of pesticides intended for other crops.

Dairy Products. This category consists of milk, buttermilk, processed milks, butter, and cheese.

The pesticides that have actually been found in dairy products under practical conditions are almost entirely chlorinated hydrocarbon insecticides. The concentrations of these materials in different products from the same herd correspond to the butterfat content of the material. However, this would not be true of all classes of compounds that might occur in milk if available to cows at sufficient dosage.

Monitoring of milk was carried out on several occasions by the US Food and Drug Administration (FDA) (Clifford, 1957; Clifford et al., 1959). Although traces of DDT were found, the proportion of samples that were positive and the concentration of DDT in these samples gradually decreased over a period of years. Before DDT was regulated more strictly during the 1950's, the amount of it in the total diet and the proportion of it in dairy products

were both greater (Walker et al., 1954; Durham et al., 1965).

Recent studies (Duggan and Weatherwax, 1967) indicate that of DDT and its analogs in the total diet, about 9 to 12% comes from dairy products. Other chlorinated hydrocarbon insecticides are found in dairy products in smaller amounts, but in about the same proportion.

In the past, very small quantities of herbicides occasionally were found in dairy products. Other classes of compounds have not been found in market samples.

In the most recent survey, DDE levels exceeded 0.1 ppm in only 15% of domestic milk samples, and other chlorinated hydrocarbon insecticides exceeded 0.1 ppm in 5% or less of these samples. BHC was found in greater concentration in imported dairy products, exceeding 0.1 ppm in 26% of such samples (Duggan et al., 1971).

It is entirely too early to determine how rapidly the recent curtailment in the use of DDT will be reflected in further reductions in residues in food.

At least in the majority of instances, residues in excess of actionable levels are caused by something not under the control of the dairy farmer. Such sources include drift onto pastures or forage crops of pesticides applied to other crops of neighboring farmers. In at least one instance, DDT that drifted probably was intended for municipal mosquito control. Another source of residues is feed or forage, especially ensilage, purchased from an outside source. Dieldrin residues have been found in hay raised on soil treated earlier with aldrin or dieldrin for control of soil or other insects attacking another crop. In a very few instances, residues in milk probably were the result of the mislabeling of a formulation (Moubry et al., 1968).

After absorption of a chlorinated hydrocarbon insecticide following ingestion or dermal application, the concentration of the compound or its metabolite declines rapidly at first and then more slowly (Moubry et al., 1968). For milk, a graph of the logarithm of concentration against time is not straight, but similar to that for storage loss from tissue (see Section 3,2,-3,2). The time necessary to reach a nonactionable level varies, of course, with the initial dosage, but tends to be less in the following order: dieldrin > DDT and related compounds > BHC > lindane > endrin > methoxychlor. After DDT is applied dermally, its concentration in milk is approximately equal to that of DDD, but after ingestion, the concentration of DDD in milk is much greater than that of DDT. This relationship, which undoubtedly reflects the metabolism of microorganisms in silage and rumen contents, is useful in predicting the source of residues in milk.

Meat, Fish, Poultry, and Eggs. The first study of total diet (Walker *et al.*, 1954) showed that most of the DDT found was in meats or in foods cooked with animal fat. This remains true of DDT and its analogs. To some degree it is true of other chlorinated hydrocarbon insecticides, although a slightly greater proportion of these materials may be found on fruits. From 35 to 40% of DDT and its analogs in the total diet are found in meat, fish, and poultry (Duggan and Weatherwax, 1967).

Except for the chlorinated hydrocarbon insecticides, and occasionally arsenic, other pesticides either do not occur in meats or are found at concentrations determining an intake of less than 0.001 mg/man/day.

In the most recent survey, 12 chlorinated hydrocarbon insecticides and traces of herbicide MCPA were found in the fat of red meat. The highest average residue was that of DDT, 0.39 ppm on a fat basis. The other compounds exceeded 0.1 ppm in 3% or less of samples of domestic meat. The residue levels of DDT compounds, dieldrin, and MCPA were higher in imported than in domestic meats (Duggan *et al.*, 1971).

In the same survey, eight chlorinated hydrocarbon insecticides in addition to the DDT compounds were found in poultry. Other classes of compounds were not found even in trace amounts. The incidences of DDT, dieldrin, and heptachlor plus its epoxide exceeded those found in any other class of foods. However, residues of DDT exceeded 0.1 ppm in only 23% of samples, and residues of the other compounds exceeded 0.1 ppm in 1% or less of samples. The findings for eggs were essentially similar, except that the incidence of samples in which the concentration of DDT or related compounds exceeded 0.1 ppm was 5% or less. Twelve chlorinated hydrocarbon insecticides but not other pesticides have been found in fish and/or shellfish. In shellfish no compound exceeded 0.1 ppm in more than 3% of samples. The same was true of most compounds in fish, but the incidence of samples containing more than 0.1 ppm was 5% for dieldrin, 17% for DDD, 24% for DDT, and 28% for DDE. The average DDE residue was 0.5 ppm. However, it was pointed out that many of the fish samples were taken from known problem areas (Duggan *et al.*, 1971).

Data for fish collected at 50 nationwide freshwater monitoring stations by the Bureau of Sport Fisheries and Wildlife are not presented in the same way as those for fish sold for food. However, it is clear that many samples of freshwater fish contain higher concentrations of chlorinated hydrocarbon insecticides (mainly DDT and dieldrin) than do commercial fish, most of which are of marine origin. Whereas many samples of freshwater fish contain no detectable polychlorinated biphenyls (PCB's), a substantial number of these samples contain PCB's at concentrations as high or higher than those of insecticides in the same samples (Henderson *et al.*, 1971).

6.1.1.2 Factors Influencing Residues in Animal Products. The factors influencing residues in animal products used by man as food are the same as the factors that determine the absorption, distribution, and storage of pesticides in laboratory animals or even in man himself (see Section 3.2.3.3).

6.1.2 Residues in Vegetable Products

6.1.2.1 Observed Residues. To a large extent, pesticide residues on plants are the result of direct application or, especially in the case of root vegetables, the result of absorption from the soil. Chemical change of the applied material may occur through the action of heat, moisture, radiation, or the enzymes of plants or microorganisms. As in animals, much of the chemical change that occurs leads to water-soluble compounds that are not recovered and measured as residues. A few compounds such as aldrin and heptachlor are metabolized to other insoluble, toxic compounds.

Grain and Cereals. This class consists not only of whole and ground grain and prepared cereals, but also macaroni, bread, cakes, crackers, and fresh and processed corn (maize). Not more than 5% of DDT and its analogs and less than 10% of all chlorinated hydrocarbon insecticides in the total diet are found in grain and grain products.

Small amounts of a wide range of other pesticides may be found in grain. The only materials likely to be present in more than trace amounts are malathion and bromides, both of which are used extensively for the disinfestation of grain. The average daily intake of malathion by an adolescent boy from this source may be as high as 0.008 mg, and the intake of bromides may be as high as 4.2 mg. The method used in surveys does not distinguish bromine derived from methyl bromide and related compounds from bromine of inorganic origin (Duggan and Weatherwax, 1967).

In the most recent survey, trace or greater concentrations of 13 chlorinated hydrocarbon insecticides, three organic phosphorus insecticides, one carbamate, and one herbicide, were found in grains or cereals for human use; bromides were not reported. The incidence of chlorinated hydrocarbon insecticides in this class of food has been decreasing for several years, but malathion residues are increasing in incidence and concentration. With the exception of malathion, residues of individual compounds exceed 0.1 ppm in 5% or less of samples. Malathion residues exceed 0.1 ppm in 11% of samples (Duggan *et al.*, 1971).

The use of chlorinated hydrocarbon insecticides to prevent the destruction of staple foods by insects may produce very high residues. In the past, DDT was found in market wheat in India in concentrations as high as 16 ppm (Sharangapani and Pingale, 1954).

Potatoes. Irish and sweet potatoes constitute a separate class from root vegetables, not because they are tubers, but because they constitute such an important part of the diet. Actually, potatoes are not an important source of residues, but a day's ration may contain up to 0.005 mg of the fungicide, trichloronitrobenze, and the herbicide, chlorpropham, which are rarely found in other foods. Potatoes may also contain bromides, but not to the extent found in grain.

Potatoes, like other roots and tubers, may absorb various chlorinated hydrocarbon insecticides from the soil. This proved to be a practical problem soon after the introduction of BHC, because mere traces of that compound taint the flavor of potatoes and some other foods. Absorption from the soil was also a problem in connection with aldrin in the Columbia Basin area of Washington. The compound had been applied in bands, a practice which favored uptake by potatoes planted along the bands. Residues in excess of 0.1 ppm were common, and some shipments of potatoes were seized by the Food and Drug Administration. This use of aldrin was discontinued promptly. Now less than 0.001 mg of various chlorinated hydrocarbon insecticides are found in the potatoes eaten daily by a 16- to 19-year-old boy (Duggan and Weatherwax, 1967).

The use of insecticides to prevent insect damage during storage may lead to very high residues. Some years ago DDT was found in potatoes in India in concentrations as high as 169 ppm (Sharangapani and Pingale, 1954).

Root Vegetables. The residue picture in root vegetables is similar to that in potatoes except that no trace of fungicide or herbicide is found. Various chlorinated hydrocarbon insecticides may reach amounts as great as 0.001 mg in a day's ration (Duggan and Weatherwax, 1967).

In the most recent survey of root vegetables including potatoes, 12 chlorinated hydrocarbon insecticides and three organic phosphorus insecticides were found in trace or greater concentrations. These residues exceeded 0.1 ppm in 5% or less of samples except for DDT, where the proportion was 8%. The highest average residue (0.04 ppm) was for DDT. The average concentration of the residues in this class of food prepared for the table is only about one-tenth as great as in the fresh produce; it is 0.002 ppm for DDT (Duggan *et al.*, 1971). The difference is due to the fact that the residues generally are concentrated in the peel, which often is discarded during preparation of the food.

Leafy Vegetables. This class includes not only leafy vegetables in the usual sense, but broccoli, cauliflower, asparagus, and mushrooms. Since leafy vegetables have a large surface-to-volume ratio, it might be predicted that they would be likely to carry residues of pesticides applied directly to them. In fact, small amounts of various chlorinated hydrocarbon insecticides, organic phosphorus insecticides, and carbamates have been found. A few herbicides have also been reported, but their presence in healthy plants is difficult to explain. In any event, the largest residue found in a recent study was 0.002 mg of DDT in a day's ration (Duggan and Weatherwax, 1967).

In the most recent survey, residues of 13 chlorinated hydrocarbon insecticides, three organic phosphorus insecticides, one herbicide, and one fungicide were found in leaf and stem vegetables in trace or greater concentrations. The levels of most chlorinated hydrocarbon insecticides in this class of foods has declined during the past several years; residues of toxaphene have shown some increase, while those of DDT and BHC have shown no change. Residues exceed 0.1 ppm in 7% or less of samples, except that 14% of residues of DDT exceed this level (Duggan *et al.*, 1971).

Legume Vegetables. Some legumes, such as green beans and snow peas, are eaten pod and all. In other instances the pod is not eaten. Residues of bromides and chlorinated hydrocarbon insecticides have been reported in amounts as high as 0.002 mg in a day's ration (Duggan and Weatherwax, 1967). It appears that in the United States of America, legumes contain less residue than any other class of food. In some countries, at least in the past, the direct addition of DDT and BHC to staple foods to prevent their destruction by insects during storage has led to very high residues in dried beans and pulses.

The most recent survey in the USA revealed

10 chlorinated hydrocarbon and two organic phosphorus insecticides in beans and peas. The concentrations in ready-to-eat legumes is substantially lower than in the fresh produce. Except for DDT, residues exceed 0.1 ppm in only 6% of fresh produce; 10% of DDT residues exceed this level.

Garden Fruits. Garden fruits include peppers, tomatoes, cucumbers, eggplants, and squash. These foods contribute more than other plant products (nearly 10%) of the DDT and its analogs in the total diet. Average amounts of DDT, as high as 0.006 mg, have been reported from this source in 1 day's food. Traces of organic phosphorus compounds and carbamates may be present also (Duggan and Weatherwax, 1967). However, only two organic phosphorus compounds and no carbamates were found in the last survey, even though 12 chlorinated hydrocarbon insecticides were encountered. Except for DDT, residues exceed 0.1 ppm in 6% or less of samples; the proportion of DDT samples exceeding this level was 22% (Duggan *et al.*, 1971).

Fruits. Fruits now contribute only a small proportion of the DDT in the total diet, but they contribute about 10% of total chlorinated organic pesticides. Organic phosphorus compounds, carbamates, bromides, and arsenic may be found. In 1 year, carbaryl on fruit averaged 0.008 mg per daily ration (Duggan and Weatherwax, 1967).

The most recent survey revealed essentially similar findings for large and small fruits. Both contained residues of 13 chlorinated hydrocarbon insecticides, three or four organic phosphorus insecticides and (in the case of large fruits) one carbamate. For each of these compounds, the residue exceeded 0.1 ppm in 10% or less of the samples (Duggan *et al.*, 1971).

Plant Oils and Fats. With the exception of oil from treated olives, plant oils with or without hydrogenation contain little chlorinated hydrocarbon insecticides. Average amounts of DDT leading to rates as high as 0.002 mg/man/day have been reported. Small amounts (0.001 to 0.003 mg) of some organic phosphorus insecticides and herbicides have been reported. Bromides have been found in amounts as high as 1.19 mg in the oils and fats consumed in 1 day (Duggan and Weatherwax, 1967).

The most recent survey showed that eight chlorinated hydrocarbon insecticides occurred in one or more common kinds of refined food oil. The highest average concentration was 0.120 ppm for toxaphene in cottonseed oil. The next highest was 0.073 ppm for DDT in peanut oil. The highest average concentration in oleomargarine was 0.034 for DDE. Most residues are substantially lower in refined seed oil than in the crude oil. The proportion of residues exceeding 0.1 ppm of any pesticide was 10% or less, except that 27% of samples of peanut oil had higher levels of DDT (Duggan *et al.*, 1971).

Sugars and Adjuncts. This class includes sugar, jams and jellies, syrups, candy, and some condiments. The largest amount of any chlorinated pesticide found in a day's ration of this class was 0.001 mg of DDT. Some other pesticides have been found in the following maximal amounts in this class consumed in a single day: herbicides, 0.004 mg; carbaryl, 0.005 mg; arsenic, 0.001 mg; and bromides 0.41 mg (Duggan and Weatherwax, 1967).

Beverages. Beverages (excluding milk, already covered under dairy products) are not an important source of pesticide residues.

6.1.2.2 Factors Influencing Residues on Plants and Plant Products. Some pesticides are applied directly to the leaves of plants. Some are absorbed by the foliage and translocated to all parts of the plant or, if applied to the soil, they may be absorbed by the roots and translocated to tubers or to the entire plant. Residues may also result from the condensation of vapor evaporated from the soil. The amount of residue remaining at harvest is conditioned by one or more of the following factors: (*a*) dosage and numbers of applications; (*b*) time from application to harvest; (*c*) nature of compound; (*d*) character of the formulation; (*e*) character of the plant; (*f*) migration from soil; (*g*) weather; (*h*) volatilization; and (*i*) method of harvest. An understanding of these variables seldom will permit accurate prediction of residues at harvest, but often will give some idea of their probable order of magnitude. Finally, (*j*) possible intentional or unintentional postharvest application; and (*k*) method of storage must be considered as factors in determining pesticide residues on plant products at the time they are eaten by man or domestic animals.

Factors influencing residues on plants at harvest were reviewed by Hayes (1959) in connection with DDT. Interaction of the factors was illustrated by a six-page, fully referenced table. Actually many of the principles apply to a wide range of compounds; the important points may be summarized as follows:

Dosage and Number of Applications. If the number and timing of applications is the same, then higher dosages produce higher residues. If the total dosage is constant and first applications are at the same time, then several small doses (the last one necessarily close to harvest) will produce a higher residue at harvest than a single large dose. If the dosage per application is constant, then each application represents an increase in total dosage, and tends to produce a higher residue at any given time after the last application. However, the proportion of the total dosage that can be recovered is greatest for a single dose. These relationships are illustrated in Table 6-1.

Certain compounds and certain application rates of other compounds are inappropriate for treating crops. If the dosage is sufficiently high, the residue remaining after about a month after the last application may reflect more the ability of the plant to hold the compound firmly, rather than the details of application. Thus, the plant may reach a kind of saturation. This, too, is illustrated in Table 6-1.

Time from Application to Harvest. Reduction of residue begins after each application of pesticide. This reduction involves two factors: (*a*) actual loss of pesticide, and (*b*) growth of the plant. Loss is due to mechanical removal by wind and rain; vaporization; chemical change in the thin film of pesticide under the influence of oxygen, water vapor, and sunlight; and biochemical change under the influence of plant enzymes. Growth of the plant reduces the rate of contamination in a relative sense by increasing the weight and surface area of the plant. Growth of the plant may also reduce the residue in an absolute sense, insofar as residues are on old leaves or other structures that wither and drop off.

In general, residues on plants decrease expo-nentially, at least during the first few weeks. Many examples may be found in data reported by Frear *et al.* (1963), although the same publication offers some unexplained exceptions in which the recorded rate of loss became more rapid in succeeding weeks. Regardless of the exact form of the curve during the first few weeks, the rate of loss generally becomes slower after that time. The form of the curve is explained at least in part by the relative importance of different factors influencing reduction. Early losses are largely mechanical and due to wind and rain, whereas later losses result more from chemical change and growth of the plant.

For any given compound and plan of application, the rate of loss from last application to harvest is dependable. Most regulation of pesticides in Europe has been in terms of dosage and required interval from last application to harvest (concepts that farmers can understand), rather than in terms of published tolerance levels.

Nature of Compound. Compounds vary greatly in their tendency to form and maintain residues. The more volatile ones evaporate to a measurable degree in the process of application. Thus, when applied under identical conditions, volatile pesticides form relatively small residues that (other things being equal) disappear relatively fast. Compounds also vary in stability; the metallic poisons are completely stable in toxicity, while some organic phosphorus insecticides undergo extensive hydrolysis

Table 6-1

Recovery of DDT from Alfalfa Hay after Treatment at
10-Day Intervals of Wet Foliage with 3%
DDT Dust at the Rate of 3,363 mg/m^2

The calculated residue of 543 ppm per application is based on the rate of application and the final yield of 750 kg of dry alfalfa per acre. The table is based on data of Eden and Arant (1948) and is reproduced by permission of the Entomological Society of America.

Number of appli-cations	Calculated total application (ppm)	DDT recovered after stated period following last application of dust									
		0 days		10 days		20 days		30 days		40 days	
		(ppm)	(%)	(ppm)	(%)	(ppm)	(%)	(ppm)	(%)	(ppm)	(%)
3	1629	162	9.9	70	4.3	40	2.5	36	2.2	32	2.0
2	1086	147	13.5	70	6.4	65	6.0	60	5.5	50	4.6
1	543	132	24.3	60	11.0	50	9.2	41	7.5	32	5.9
Average		147	15.9	67	7.3	52	5.9	46	5.1	38	4.1

in a few hours and form harmless compounds.

Compounds also differ in their ability to be absorbed and translocated by plants. Some compounds such as aldicarb, demeton, dimethoate, disulfoton, phosphamidon, and trichlorofon are so active in this regard that they are intentionally used as systemic insecticides. Some (eg, demeton) are commonly applied to the leaves from which they are absorbed and transferred to other parts of the plant. Others (eg, aldicarb) are commonly applied to the soil from which they are absorbed and distributed to the whole plant. Aldicarb may be absorbed by mint in sufficient concentration that the plants not only become toxic to pests, but also highly dangerous to people who eat small amounts of them.

Some other compounds are not absorbed by plants to an extent useful for pest control, but they are absorbed enough to offer a potential problem, if not to health, at least in connection with the regulation of residues. Thus, some chlorinated hydrocarbon insecticides (notably, aldrin, heptachlor, and BHC, but not DDT) are absorbed by the roots of many plants. Apparently they are not translocated to the upper portions of plants but they may form unwanted residues in potatoes, peanuts, carrots, and other plants of which the edible portion grows underground.

Interaction of Compounds. Nothing is known yet about the practical importance of the interaction of compounds as a factor influencing residues. However, experiments suggest that an accidental combination of residues (eg, through drift) might produce completely unexpected and perhaps undesirable effects. On the other hand, as the experimenters have indicated, the purposeful combination of compounds might be of value for controlling the persistence of residues on crops.

When applied at low concentrations to plant foliage, rotenone catalyzes the photoisomerization of dieldrin and other cyclodiene insecticide residues. A measurable increase in photochemical activity occurs when the concentration of rotenone is only 0.3 ppm, based on the fresh weight of leaves bearing the residues. Activity is increased by a further factor of about 12 times when the residue is increased from 0.3 to 30 ppm. Photodieldrin is somewhat more toxic than dieldrin and also more persistent on leaves. However, photodecomposition was the predominant effect when residues of rotenone were combined with those of methylcarbamate and phosphothionate insecticides. Rotenone is highly active but short-lived as a photosensitizer. It is speculated that less active compounds, if stable and persistent, might be considerably more effective under practical conditions (Ivie and Casida, 1970).

Character of Formulation. When applied at the same rate, dusts usually give lower initial residues than liquid formulations. However, dusts give higher than expected residues if they are applied when the plants are moist, as from dew. Granules are designed to pass through vegetation without leaving a residue. However, some individual granules are caught by whorls of grass and other pockets. Thus, granules produce little residue on plant surfaces, but they may produce significant residues from the standpoint of an animal that eats the whole plant. Although surface residues resulting from the application of granules are initially small and remain small relative to those applied in other ways, a redistribution of the pesticide may produce a small, absolute increase in surface residue for a few days after application. An example involving the use of diazinon granules on tomatoes was reported by Frear *et al.* (1963).

When the initial residues are the same, residues applied as dusts are lost most rapidly, while those resulting from oil solutions are lost least rapidly.

The initial uptake of DDT by cotton leaves is increased by amine stearates in the formulation, but after a time an equilibrium is reached that depends on the deposit density regardless of formulation (Phillips and Gilham, 1971).

Character of Plant. The texture of a plant surface influences the residue it will hold. Waxy surfaces are difficult to wet. Hairy leaves, such as those as those of soybeans, retain a relatively high proportion of the spray or dust that reaches them. Some compounds, such as the chlorinated hydrocarbon insecticides, are stored in plant oils just as they are in animal fats. In general, storage does not occur in seed oils that are separated from the plant surface by tissue. However, oils in olives and in the peels of citrus fruits readily absorb DDT and related insecticides.

Other things being equal, plants with extensive surface will receive more insecticide than those with less surface. If only a part of the plant is used for food, then the surface-volume relationships of that part are important. Residues on fruits are frequently much smaller than residues on leaves from the same plant. Leafy vegetables eaten by people and forage eaten by animals have a large surface-to-volume ratio and, therefore, tend to receive large deposits relative to what is applied. Sometimes people and animals eat different portions of the same plant. Thus, pea vines are commonly used for silage after the peas have been removed. Although corn (maize) is frequently raised entirely for animals, it sometimes happens that the leaves and stems are used for forage or silage after the ears have been removed for human consumption. Since peas and the ears of corn are covered, they rarely constitute a problem from the standpoint of residues. However, the same is not true of the leaves and stems of the same plants. Consequently, certain pesticides cannot be used for these crops if they are to serve as animal food.

Not only do various root crops differ in their propensity for absorbing pesticides from the soil, but this difference may extend to strains of the same vegetable. Thus, Lichtenstein et al. (1965a) found that some crops did not absorb detectable amounts of aldrin or heptachlor from treated soil. Carrots absorbed more than any other crop tested. Absorption by five varieties of carrots differed by factors as high as 2.5, even when the carrots were grown in the same soil, and distribution of insecticide between peel and pulp also differed among the varieties of carrots.

Migration from Soil. The presence of pesticides in soil may lead to residues of them in plants grown in the soil. The degree to which this will occur depends not only on (*a*) species and strain of plant (just referred to), but also on (*b*) compound, (*c*) concentration, and (*d*) type of soil.

Persistence of a pesticide in the soil is a necessary condition of its absorption from the soil by a plant. However, compounds that are about equally persistent may differ in rate of absorption. Thus, heptachlor is absorbed more readily than aldrin (Lichtenstein et al., 1965b).

For some, and perhaps most, compounds mixed evenly in soil, the rate of transport in the soil is unlikely to limit their uptake by plants roots (Graham-Bryce, 1968). This does not contradict the finding of Lichtenstein et al. (1965a) that some relationship exists between residues in soil and residues in plants grown in the soil. This dosage-response relationship extended to soil layers. The vertical distribution of residues within carrot tissue corresponded to the vertical distribution of the compound in the soil.

On the other hand, residues in carrots and potatoes definitely increased in the 2d and 3rd year of application of aldrin and heptachlor, respectively, even though the soil residues apparently reached maximum in the 1st year. When insecticide application was stopped after the 5th year, residues in plants decreased at a rate similar to the rate of decrease in the soil in which they were grown (Lichtenstein et al., 1970).

The correspondence of residues in layers of soil and in some root crops indicates that the pesticide passes directly from the soil to these plant tissues. Not all residues that pass from soil to plants are transferred in that way. Lichtenstein et al. (1965b) found that cucumber plants absorb aldrin or heptachlor from soil treated with one of these compounds. However, the concentration was only very slightly greater in cucumbers that lay on the ground while they developed than in others that were supported on racks, and the concentration was the same in the top and bottom halves of the fruit. In this instance, it was concluded that the compound was absorbed by the roots and translocated through the stems to the cucumbers.

The volatilization of compounds from the soil surface and their subsequent condensation on plants are discussed below.

The efficiency with which certain crops absorb some compounds is remarkable. The concentration of heptachlor plus heptachlor epoxide in one variety of carrot at harvest was 61% of the concentration of the compound in the surrounding soil. So much was removed from the soil into which it had been mixed evenly that less insecticide was found along the carrot rows than in areas where no carrots had grown (Lichtenstein et al., 1965a). Although the proportion of different insecticides taken up by different crops varies widely, measurement of the relationship may be of some value for predicting the residue a particular crop will bear following a given regimen of soil treatment (Lichtenstein, 1966). For example, residue concentrations in or on alfalfa grown on aldrin-treated soils were $0.88 \pm 0.23\%$ of their concentrations in the soils at harvest, and $3.01 \pm 0.85\%$ for alfalfa grown in heptachlor-treated soils. Once these percentages are known, they may be used together with information on the rate of decay of residues in soil to predict residues in the same kind of crop following different schedules of application.

Pesticides are absorbed into crops most readily from sandy soils and least readily from muck soils, which have a high content of organic matter (Lichtenstein, 1959). The same is true of absorption by insects; the same concentration of insecticide is more effective in sandy soil than in muck soil. In fact, pesticides are bound so firmly to muck soils that they persist longer in such soils (Lichtenstein and Schulz, 1959b). It was even possible to change the adsorptive properties of silt loam by the addition of carbon at the rate of 2,000 ppm. Uptake of aldrin-dieldrin residues from the treated soil by carrots and potatoes was reduced more than 50%, and the uptake of heptachlor, heptachlor epoxide, and γ-chlordane was reduced more than 60%. One application of carbon was effective for the duration of study, ie, 4 years (Lichtenstein *et al.,* 1971a). Nutrients, including micronutrients, influence the penetration of pesticides into plants and translocation of the compounds after they have been absorbed (Talekar and Lichtenstein, 1971).

Weather. Rain soon after the application of a pesticide dislodges a significant proportion of the compound, but rain late in the season has little effect on the more firmly attached residues persisting at that time.

Volatilization. Volatilization plays a double role in influencing pesticides on plants. Residues on plants tend to be lost by volatilization, but the same compounds volatilized from the soil may condense on plants and thus increase their residues. Compounds vary greatly in this regard. For example, residues of DDT on soybeans arise mostly from vapor from contaminated soil, but residues of dieldrin, endrin, and heptachlor result primarily from root uptake and translocation to all parts of the plants (Nash and Beall, 1970).

Factors influencing volatilization are discussed in Section 6.2.2.3, and the rate of mobilization is discussed in Section 6.2.2.1, where it is pointed out that vaporization begins at the instant sprays or dusts are applied to crops. It must be mentioned here that one of these factors, temperature, may be higher and is subject to more variation in connection with plants than often is realized. According to Mauney (1973), a wilted cotton leaf may reach 4°C above air temperature of the leaf canopy. Air temperature of the canopy is generally about 1°C below weather station records, which in the southwestern part of the United States of America may reach 48°C. Thus, maximal leaf tissue temperatures may reach 51°C in a wilted leaf. A turgid leaf is generally 2 to 3°C below air temperature. Thus, maximal turgid leaf temperature would be about 45°C. Minimal leaf temperature at night is usually very close to canopy air temperature. During the cotton growing season, minimal night temperatures range from 5°C in the early season to 30°C in mid-July and August. Most crop plants adjust to the local temperature in approximately the way cotton does.

Method of Harvest. The ordinary handling of crops associated with harvesting may remove appreciable quantities of pesticides.

Postharvest Application. It is often necessary to fumigate or otherwise treat staple foods sometimes after harvest to prevent their destruction by insects. Eventually, it may prove necessary to treat certain staples with fungicides in much the same way, in order to minimize the less obvious but more dangerous effects of fungal toxins.

At the moment, most postharvest insecticidal treatments involve fumigants, many of which have been in use for many years. These compounds have no residual action on insects. Grain may be fumigated several times before it reaches the consumer. When DDT first became available, its use as a residual, postharvest insecticide was considered. According to a review (Hayes, 1959), concentrations of 30 to 50 ppm were required to protect grain. Flour from such grain contained residues in the order of 15 ppm, whereas bran and other byproducts contained residues of more than 100 ppm. The use of DDT in this way was reported or at least discussed in several European countries, but this use of DDT was never extensive and was soon discontinued in Europe. There is evidence that the practice was more general and retained longer in some developing countries.

To prevent invasion by insects, DDT also was considered for treating the surface of bags containing grain, the outside of piles of grain, or the inside of bins or elevators in which grain was later stored. However, the degree of contamination under these circumstances was greater than expected. After 3 or more months of storage, grain from the center of treated elevators was found to contain DDT at average concentrations of 1.5 to 2.4 ppm. In a similar way, it was found that DDT migrated from cloth bags into the food they contained. The transfer was fastest when the food was finely ground or had a high fat content. Experiments showed that these transfers could be accounted for, at least in part, by the diffusion of DDT vapor.

Storage of packages of food on shelving covered with insecticide-impregnated paint or varnish has not been an important source of contamination. However, such storage could lead to heavy contamination, as· shown by Dyte and Tyler (1960) in studies of endrin and dieldrin.

The continuing need for an insecticide with some residual action to control insects in staple food has led to the use of malathion and pyrethrum. Not only are these compounds less persistent than DDT under ordinary grain storage conditions, but they are rapidly hydrolyzed by cooking.

The use of many grain fumigants was introduced when the study of residues was less extensive than it is now. Since the materials were highly volatile and were dissipated readily by adequate ventilation, it was supposed that no residue remained. However, further study showed that some fumigants react with the proteins of grain or other foods and the resulting metabolites are persistent. For example, trichloroethylene can react with cysteine to form dichlorvinylcysteine (McKinney et al., 1959), and dichloroethane can react with trimethylamine to form choline chloride (Munro and Morrison, 1967).

Method of Storage. Most forms of storage compatible with food preservation have little effect on pesticides persistent enough to last until harvest. Ensilage constitutes a striking exception to the rule; this kind of storage leads to a significant reduction in the residues of certain compounds that are otherwise highly persistent. The phenomenon was reported as early as 1946 in connection with DDT (Wilson et al., 1946a, 1946b). A number of studies have confirmed the original finding. Very much later (Kallman and Andrews, 1963), it was shown that DDT is converted efficiently to DDD by yeast.

The preparation of sauerkraut is similar to the preparation of silage. Apparently no studies have been made of pesticide residues in cabbage and in kraut made from it.

6.1.3 Residues in Water

6.1.3.1 Residues in Potential Drinking Water. Water is really a part of our food. A substantial proportion of the measurements of pesticides in water have involved streams or ponds to which pesticides were added intentionally; most others concerned water suspected of being contaminated, for example, by runoff from fields where crops had been treated by economic poisons. Such analyses would tend to indicate a higher concentration of pesticides than would be expected in the average drinking water. Although pesticides have been found in raw drinking water (Breidenbach and Lichtenberg, 1963; Nicholson et al., 1964; Rosen and Middleton, 1959; Weaver et al., 1965), and in finished drinking water (Nicholson et al., 1964), and even in rainwater (Wheatley and Hardman, 1965; Abbott et al., 1965; Tarrant and Tatton, 1968), the concentrations were usually extremely small. The highest concentration of any chlorinated hydrocarbon insecticide in the rainwater of an urban area during any month was 0.0004 ppm for DDT (Abbott et al., 1965).

Apparently, the highest concentration (0.02 ppm) in potable water was that reported quite early for DDT in certain rivers and lakes (Middleton and Lichtenberg, 1960). The highest concentration reported for any insecticide in a comprehensive survey during the mid-1960's was 0.00012 ppm for dieldrin (Weaver et al., 1965), and many of the samples contained no detectable pesticide. Six insecticides or metabolites (aldrin, dieldrin, endrin, DDT, DDE, and DDD) were found in measurable amounts in some samples, and heptachlor and BHC were presumably present in a few samples. The average concentration for the six compounds combined was 0.000023 ppm for the entire survey (Weaver et al., 1965). Based on this concentration, and the usual assumption that each person drinks 2 liters of water each day, it may be calculated that the intake of chlorinated hydrocarbon insecticides from water would be 0.000046 mg per person. Even an estimate based on the highest concentration of any pesticide in water reported in recent years, ie, 0.001 ppm for BHC (Nicholson et al., 1964), would be only 0.002 mg per day per person.

According to a recent survey of pesticides in surface waters, the number of occurrences of measurable residues reached a peak in 1966 and then dropped sharply in 1967 and in 1968, in spite of improved analytical methods. The highest values for either of those years was 0.00084 ppm for DDD and 0.00041 for dieldrin. The concentrations found were 1/10 to 1/500 of the permissible levels for drinking water supplies (Lichtenberg et al., 1970).

In the case of heavy metals and some other inorganic pesticides, the finding of a toxic element may not indicate that its source is a pesticide or even an industrial chemical. For example, mercury in fish from waters with no known industrial or agricultural contamination may exceed the actionable level of 0.5 ppm for mercury, probably as a result of natural deposits of mercury (Sumner et al., 1972).

6.1.3.2 Residues in Other Water and Sediments.

Residues in Nonpotable Water. Residues may be high at least temporarily in some nonpotable water. In fact, a pesticide may be added to water purposely to control insects, especially vectors of disease, breeding in it. In recent years, such additions have involved mainly organic phosphorus compounds. Some compounds that have proved too toxic for application to the interior walls of houses for malaria control may be entirely safe for application to polluted water to prevent breeding of mosquitoes that transmit other diseases. The problem has been to find materials that persist long enough to be effective. One such compound is fenthion.

Residues in Sediments. Residues in sediments are unlikely to contribute directly to residues in potable water, which nearly always is filtered. Sediments may contribute indirectly, for in situations quiet enough to permit the deposit of sediment, an equilibrium will be approached between residues in the sediment and those in the overlying water. Furthermore, sediments may be ingested by bottom feeding organisms and they may contribute to the transport of pesticides, including eventually transport into the sea.

In a 3-year study of the chlorinated hydrocarbon insecticide content of sediments and water from the lower Mississippi River and its tributaries, residues were detected from both agricultural and industrial sources. No evidence was found of a general buildup of these compounds from farm use, although DDT and related compounds were found in some tributaries where no known formulating plants were located. They must have arisen from municipal or agricultural uses. Higher concentrations and a far wider range of compounds, including aldrin, dieldrin, endrin, keto-endrin, isodrin, chlordane, heptachlor, lindane, DDT and related compounds, and several precursors or metabolites, were found downstream from manufacturing or formulating plants. The major conclusion was that the large amounts of chlorinated hydrocarbon insecticides previously applied to crops in the Mississippi River Delta have not created widespread contamination of streambed materials (Barthel *et al.,* 1969).

In a similar way, there has been no consistent upward or downward trend in pesticide levels in estuaries. Distinct seasonal, geographic, and regional differences in levels are apparent. Although each sample is screened for 10 or more pesticides, DDT (including its metabolites) is the only one commonly found. Other pesticides in decreasing order of frequency in estuaries are: dieldrin > endrin > toxaphene > mirex. The residues are not large enough to constitute a human health problem (Butler, 1969). Whereas various minor, or local, disasters to estuarian life have been reported, no major ecological disruption has been detected.

In fact, as a result of changing patterns of use of pesticides, residues may be decreasing. For example, repeated study showed that the introduction of pesticides into a Louisiana estuary associated with the Mississippi River decreased strikingly from the early 1960's to the late 1960's (Rowe *et al.,* 1971).

6.1.4 *Removal of Residues from Food and Water*

6.1.4.1 **Removal of Residues from Food.** According to Frisbie (1936), spray residues resulting from the use of lead arsenate were a problem as early as 1915. In 1919 the Boston Health Department embargoed a ship-

ment of western pears, some of which contained arsenic on a single fruit "equivalent to half a medical dose." Efforts were made for years thereafter to develop effective methods to remove the lead and arsenic. Washing and brushing removed some of the material, but not all. Certain stronger measures, such as acid washes, were more effective but tended to injure the fruit.

DDT proved valuable, not only for control of the codling moth in apples, but also for many other agricultural pests against which the inorganic insecticides were useless. As reviewed elsewhere (Hayes, 1959), a number of studies were made to find ways of removing DDT from food or to learn the effects of ordinary processing on its residues. Briefly, it was found that under agricultural conditions, a portion of the residue on apples is so feebly attached that care must be exercised in gathering apples to prevent its loss. Ordinary fruit handling procedures remove this loosely adherent part, but leave a portion that cannot be completely removed by methods that leave the fruit intact.

Contamination of the product consumed by people is often greatly reduced or undetectable, even though it was intimately mixed with a contaminated part of the crop during processing. Thus, it is possible to separate DDT-free juice from grapes bearing residues, and it is possible to make uncontaminated jam from contaminated grape pomace. From a practical standpoint, these separations are not different from the reduction of residues on fruit by peeling or, on lettuce and cabbage, by removing outside leaves. In a similar way, residues in meat can be reduced by cutting away fat either during preparation or when the meat is served; some reduction is also accomplished by forms of cooking that remove part of the fat. The milling of contaminated grain produces flour with low residues, but bran and related products with high residues. Thus, the selection of food that is preferred by people and incidentally is low in residues leads to the production of byproducts that would be suitable for animal food were it not for their high residues. One of the best examples involves apple pomace, which was formerly an important food supplement for dairy cattle but cannot be used if DDT, for example, is applied to apples.

Residues not only may be separated and discarded but, at least in some instances, they may be driven off or destroyed. For example, baking leads to some loss of DDT from the crust of bread, presumably as the result of vaporization. Ordinary commercial canning produces some loss of DDT residues in apples, peaches, and tomatoes; the reaction is presumably catalyzed by metal, for it did not occur in Pyrex tubes. Although the losses of chlorinated hydrocarbon insecticide residues through cooking are of academic interest, they are of little practical importance. On the contrary, residues of organic phosphorus insecticides—which generally are small or absent to begin with—are efficiently hydrolyzed to harmless materials through cooking.

The reduction of residues as a result of storage, especially ensilage, is discussed in Section 6.1.2.2.

6.1.4.2 Removal of Residues from Water. Residues of pesticides that commonly occur in water are low (Section 6.1.3), and constitute only a small proportion of the traces of pesticides absorbed by ordinary people (Section 6.4.1). Thus, there usually is no need to remove pesticides from water to be used for drinking, although, as it happens, routine water purification does reduce residues of many compounds. If an accident or other unforeseen circumstance should lead to residue levels much higher than those yet observed, removal of the residues might be indicated. Studies of methods for removal are justified only as a preparation for emergency or as a source of basic information.

It was shown as early as 1945 that DDT is gradually lost from clear water by adsorption on surfaces, and from turbid water by the sedimentation of particulate matter on which it adsorbs also (Carollo, 1945). The same study showed that conventional water treatment involving coagulation, sedimentation, and filtration would remove 80 to 98% of DDT from a water supply containing from 0.1 to 10.0 ppm. Removal to < 0.001 ppm was possible if activated charcoal was added to the water for 15 minutes after coagulation and sedimentation, but before filtration. The last trace of DDT could also be removed from water by storage for 4 or 5 days or by filtration through anion and cation zeolites.

This result for DDT has been amply confirmed, but not all pesticides are dealt with so easily. It seems there is a close relationship between the way in which compounds migrate in soil and the ease with which they may be removed from water. Those like DDT that are tightly bound to soil are easily removed from water; those like lindane that migrate in the soil, through leaching or some other mechanism, are removed from water with some difficulty. An exception would be any compound that migrates in soil but is destroyed chemically by chlorination or some other chemical treatment used in water purification.

The effects of water purification on residues of DDT, lindane, dieldrin, endrin, 2,4,5-T, and parathion were studied by Robeck et al. (1965). The compounds were added at rates of 0.001 to 0.025 ppm, levels much higher than any found in natural water in recent times. It was found that routine coagulation and filtration removed 98% of DDT, 80% of parathion, 65% of a 2,4,5-T ester, 55% of dieldrin, but only 35% of endrin, and less than 10% of lindane. Chlorination had little effect on chlorinated pesticides but did remove 75% of parathion. Other oxidizing agents had essentially similar results except that large, probably impractical concentrations of ozone produced substantial reduction of chlorinated pesticides. Although the authors assumed that the entire conversion of parathion by chlorination was to paraoxon, they failed to identify any product, and a mixture of derivatives would be expected. Most of the investigation was concerned with the action of charcoal. More than 99% of all the compounds studied were removed by passing pesticide-containing river water through granular activated carbon at a rate of 0.5 gallons per minute per cubic foot. The effectiveness of charcoal slurries depended on the concentration of charcoal. The effectiveness of charcoal was always greater in distilled water than in river water because other materials in river water competed with pesticides for adsorption. At the concentrations studied, one pesticide usually did not interfere with adsorption of another. Even 5 ppm removed over 99% of parathion from river water, but was somewhat less efficient for the other compounds. Powdered charcoal at a rate of 20 ppm was almost as efficient as the bed of granular charcoal. Furthermore, the efficiency of the process could be improved by using two separate small applications of charcoal rather than a single large application.

Further evidence for the effectiveness of charcoal for clearing water is its use in analytical chemistry for quantitative sampling of organic compounds in raw or filtered surface waters (Braus et al., 1951). When used in this way, the water to be tested is taken directly from the pipe, through a large column packed with charcoal, and finally through a meter. After an appropriate volume of water has been processed, the column is opened and the charcoal is extracted with organic solvents after being dried.

6.1.5 Residues in Total Diet

6.1.5.1 Regular Diet.
Historical and General Considerations. A review (Hayes, 1959) shows that the occur

rence of DDT residues on crops to which the insecticide was applied was recognized and measured at least as early as 1945 (Harman, 1946). Apparently, the earliest effort to learn how much DDT the average man obtains from his daily food was that of Walker and his colleagues (1954), which is summarized, together with some later surveys, in Table 6-2. In 1953 and 1954, these investigators analyzed the individual items constituting typical restaurant meals. DDT was found in every meal but not in every kind of food. The greater proportion was in meat and other food of animal origin. The average amount in the three meals a person would eat each day was 0.184 mg.

Later, the famous "Market Basket" studies were carried out by the US Food and Drug Administration (FDA) (Corneliussen, 1969; Cummings, 1965; Duggan, 1967, 1968a, 1968b; Duggan and Corneliussen, 1972; Duggan and McFarland, 1967; Duggan and Lipscomb, 1969; Duggan et al., 1966, 1967; Duggan et al., 1971; Mills, 1963; and Williams, 1964). A wide range of foods constituting a balanced diet and sufficient to feed a 16- to 19-year-old boy for a week was purchased from ordinary grocery stores in cities in different parts of the country. This particular plan was selected because it is known that on the average 16- to 19-year-old boys eat more than other individu-

als in the population. The results again showed traces of DDT in some, but not in all, total diet samples. Although the authors originally failed to calculate the rate of intake of DDT, which would be determined by the Market Basket samples, these rates have been calculated from data they supplied (Durham et al., 1965) and are shown on Table 6-2. The daily intakes of different pesticides indicated by recent, more comprehensive Market Basket samples are recorded in Table 6-3.

In repeating the earlier work of Walker et al. (1954), Durham et al. (1965) found that a person who ate regularly in the restaurants sampled would receive DDT at an average rate of 0.038 mg/man/day. This represented less than one-fourth of the average rate of intake measured 11 years earlier in the same laboratory. Furthermore, the results for DDT in the Market Basket samples during the mid-1960's are in good agreement with those found in the second study of complete restaurant meals. Thus, it appears that there was a marked reduction in DDT residues in food after 1955, but there has been no further change of similar magnitude in recent years.

Duggan (1968b) expressed the opinion that there had been no significant change in the incidence or levels of pesticides in food since 1964. However, more recent results shown in Table 6-3 indicate that there may have been a

Table 6-2

Early Estimates of the Daily Content of DDT and DDE in Complete Meals in the United States of America

From Hayes (1966) by permission of the National Academy of Sciences.

Year	Location	Source	Number	Total daily content (mg)			DDE as DDT (% of total)	Reference
				DDT	DDE as DDT	Total as DDT		
1953-1954	Wenatchee, Wash.	restaurant	18	0.178	0.102	0.280	37	Walker et al., 1954
	Tacoma, Wash.	prison	7	0.116	0.063	0.179	35	" " "
1954-1955	Tallahassee, Fla.	prison	12	0.202	0.056	0.258	21	Hayes et al., 1956
1956-1957	Walla Walla, Wash.	college dining room for meat abstainers	11	0.041	0.027	0.068	39	Hayes et al., 1958
1959-1960	Anchorage, Alaska	hospital	3	0.184	0.029	0.213	14	Durham et al., 1961
1961-1962	Washington, D. C. Baltimore, Md. Atlanta, Ga. Minneapolis, Minn. San Francisco, Calif.	Market Basket survey	36[a]	0.026[b]	0.017[b]	0.043[b]	40[b]	Mills, 1963
1962-1964	Wenatchee, Wash.	restaurant	12	0.038	0.049	0.087	56	Durham et al., 1965
	Wenatchee, Wash.	household	17	0.314	0.193	0.507	40	" " "
1962-1964	Atlanta, Ga. Baltimore, Md. Minneapolis, Minn. St. Louis, Mo. San Francisco, Calif.	Market Basket survey	23[a]	0.023[b]	0.013[b]	0.036[b]	36[b]	Williams, 1964

a. This figure refers to the number of diet samples, each consisting of the total normal 14-day food intake for males 16 to 19 years old, which were tested. In some instances, additional diet samples were taken and aliquots were analyzed for pesticide content of various classes of foodstuffs, but no composite value was given.

b. The author did not calculate the daily DDT or DDE intake. However, using the author's mean dietary concentrations of DDT and DDE and the mean daily food intake of 3.78 kg from the Market Basket survey, the reviewer has calculated the values shown.

Table 6-3

Comparison of Residues of Pesticides in the Total Diet with Available Standards

All values except those in the last column are expressed as mg/man/day.

Pesticides (by group)	Daily intake of pesticides in the United States of America[a]						Acceptable daily intake[b]	Largest oral dosage tested in man without clinical effect	
	1965	1966	1967	1968	1969	1970		Rate	Days fed
Inorganic and organometal pesticides									
arsenic	.069	.005	.03	.14	.075	.057			
bromides	27.0	14.9	20.3	27.9	16.8	16.3	70		
Chlorinated hydrocarbons									
lindane	.004	.004	.005	.003	.00	.001	.88		
BHC	.002	.004	.002	.003	.001	.001			
DDT	.031	.041	.026	.019	.016	.015	0.35[c]	35[d]	630
DDE	.018	.028	.017	.015	.011	.010			
DDD	.013	.018	.013	.011	.005	.004			
dicofol (Kelthane®)	.003	.002	.012	.010	.007	.004	1.75[e]		
Perthane®	<.001	.001		.001	.004				
methoxychlor		<.001	.001	.001	<.001	.001	7.0[e]	140[f]	56
aldrin	.001	.002	.001	<.001	<.001	<.001	.007[g]		
dieldrin	.005	.007	.004	.004	.005	.005	.007[g]	0.221[h]	730
endrin	<.001	.001	<.001	.001	<.001	<.001			
heptachlor	<.001		<.001	<.001	<.001	<.001			
heptachlor epoxide	.002	.003	.001	.002	.002	.001	.035[i]		
endosulfan		<.001	<.001	<.001	.001	.001	.525[e]		
toxaphene		.002		.002	.004	.001			
Organic phosphorus compounds									
diazinon		.001	<.001	<.001	<.001	.001	.14[e]		
ethion		<.001	<.002	.001	.003	.004			
malathion		.009	.010	.003	.012	.013	1.40[e]	24[l]	56
parathion		<.001	.001	<.001	<.001	.001	.35	7.2[k]	42
Other compounds									
2,4-D	.005	.002	.001	.001	<.001	<.001		500[l]	21
pentachlorophenol	<.001	.006	.001	.001	.002				
carbaryl	.150	.026	.007		.003		.7[e]		
dithiocarbamates	.026		.005	.003		<.001	1.75[e]		

a. From Duggan and Weatherwax, 1967; Duggan, 1968b; Duggan and Lipscomb, 1969; Duggan, personal communication, 1969; and Duggan and Corneliussen, 1972.
b. FAO/WHO (1970) values expressed in terms of a 70 kg man.
c. For DDT, DDE, DDD, or a combination.
d. Hayes et al., 1971.
e. Temporary value.
f. Stein et al., 1965.
g. For dieldrin, aldrin, or a combination.
h. Hunter et al., 1969.
i. Includes heptachlor plus its epoxide.
j. Moeller and Rider, 1962.
k. Edson, 1964.
l. Mitchell et al., 1946. A patient was given 12 intravenous 800 mg doses of 2,4-D without clinical effect (Seabury, 1963).

small increase in residues of dicofol, Perthane®, ethion and small but real decreases in residues of DDT, DDE, DDD, carbaryl, dithiocarbamates, and 2,4-D.

Compounds Now Found in Residues. Residues of 83 different pesticide chemicals were found in 111,296 samples of domestic food examined during the period of July 1, 1963, to June 30, 1969, in connection with the Market Basket Survey. Many of these compounds were found infrequently. Only 22 organic pesticides were found in as much as 1% of composite samples of food

during any 2 years. These compounds are listed in Table 6-4, along with the percentage of composite samples that contained detectable levels of each material. Only 30 pesticides were found in as much as 1% of the samples of any food class for even a single year. These 30 compounds include, in addition to the 22 listed in Table 6-4, two chlorinated hydrocarbon insecticides (chlorbenside and chlordane), three organic phosphorus insecticides (carbophenothion, methyl parathion, and tetradifon), two herbicides (DCPA and MCPA), and one fungicide (DCNB) (Duggan et al., 1971).

Table 6-4

Average Proportion of Composite Samples
Positive for 22 Pesticides Arranged in
Approximate Order of Decreasing Frequency.

From data of Duggan and Corneliussen (1972).

Compound	1965 [a] (%)	1966 [b] (%)	1967 [c] (%)	1968 [c] (%)	1969 [c] (%)	1970 (%)
DDT	37.5	37.3	38.6	44.2	48.9	55.6
DDE	31.5	33.0	31.1	37.5	39.4	50.6
TDE (DDD)	19.4	25.7	28.9	31.1	28.1	32.8
dieldrin	18.5	21.3	15.3	15.6	25.3	31.3
lindane	15.8	12.3	10.6	15.3	13.3	13.3
heptachlor epoxide	13.4	12.0	8.9	13.1	12.2	11.1
BHC	6.5	6.0	8.9	9.7	10.6	13.6
malathion	--	5.3	3.6	1.9	5.8	11.1
carbaryl	7.4	2.7	1.1	--	0.8	--
aldrin	5.6	3.7	3.3	3.9	1.4	0.8
2,4-D	4.2	3.0	1.7	0.6	0.3	0.3
diazinon	--	3.0	0.3	0.3	3.9	5.8
dicofol (Kelthane®)	0.5	3.7	5.6	4.7	3.6	4.4
PCP	1.4	3.3	2.2	1.9	2.8	--
endrin	2.8	2.0	1.7	1.1	3.3	1.4
methoxychlor	--	1.6	0.8	1.1	0.3	1.9
heptachlor	1.9	--	0.3	0.3	1.7	0.3
toxaphene	--	1.0	--	1.1	3.6	1.1
Perthane®	0.5	1.3	--	0.6	1.1	--
parathion	--	1.0	1.4	0.6	3.3	5.0
endosulfan	--	1.6	0.3	0.8	4.2	5.3
ethion	--	0.3	1.1	1.7	1.7	4.4

a.　216 composites examined.

b.　312 composites examined.

c.　360 composites examined.

Table 6-3 shows the amount of various pesticides consumed by the average 16- to 19-year-old boy in the United States of America during different years. DDT and its analogs account for about half of the total daily intake of chlorinated organic compounds. DDT, DDE, and DDD are followed by dieldrin, lindane, and heptachlor epoxide, in that order. These six compounds now account for approximately half of the total dietary intake of organic pesticides, with the possible exception of bromides. Other chlorinated organic pesticides are too low to be meaningful as individual residues; their daily combined intake is less than 0.020 mg. The quantity of organic phosphorus compounds in the total diet is low; much of it consists of malathion used for the protection of grain. Only small residues of herbicides are present in the diet. Residues of carbaryl showed a marked decrease from 1964 to 1969. A high percentage of all food composites contain some bromide, but the analytical method that has been used does not distinguish between naturally occurring bromide residues and those resulting from treatment with organic bromine fumigants. However, the fact that the highest bromine residues are in grain may be significant. Methyl bromide and, to a lesser extent, other organic bromides are used to fumigate a great variety of foods, but their most important use is for grain. Residues of arsenic are low in recent years (Duggan and Weatherwax, 1967; Duggan, 1968b; Duggan et al., 1971).

Table 6-3 also shows the acceptable daily intake levels established by WHO-FAO. The amount of pesticide in the diet of 16- to 19-year-old boys—about twice the intake of the average person—is well below these stand-ards, except for dieldrin and aldrin combined. The daily intake for these compounds has been about equal to the FAO-WHO acceptable daily intake for the last 5 years (Duggan, 1968b; Duggan and Lipscomb, 1969; Duggan et al., 1971). However, the standards are con-servative, and those for aldrin and dieldrin are particularly so.

Geographical Distribution of Residues in the United States of America. Almost every sep-arate kind of food is produced in more than one geographical area of the United States of America. In many instances, the crop reaches maturity at different times in different areas, so that the supply is essentially constant but the source varies with the season. The distri-bution system that brings food to market is rapid and the market is sensitive to supply and demand. Under these conditions, the great majority of the population consume food that is not produced locally and often is shipped great distances. This statement ap-plies even to a high proportion of the farm population, because many farms are confined to one or a few crops and lack kitchen gar-dens. Therefore, it is not astonishing that residues found in food in one part of the country are generally similar to those found in food from all other parts. However, small differences do exist even for food sold through general commerce. Duggan and Weatherwax (1967) found that residues in all diet samples collected in the Minneapolis area were quite low during 1966 and 1967. The same was true the following year (Duggan and Lipscomb, 1969). Examination of available data shows that food sold in the northern regions contains somewhat less DDT-related material than food sold in southern regions. Correlation of

the residue values shown in Table 6-5 with the latitudes of the cities that are headquar-ters for the regions where the samples were collected yields coefficients of -0.63 and -0.59 for the two sampling periods. The use of latitude for this purpose is justified by the generality that pesticides are used to a greater extent in the South, especially since cotton is an exclusively southern crop. The correlation might be improved if it could be based on regional use of pesticides, instead of latitude; however, no data are available to permit this comparison.

It may be speculated that the small ob-served regional differences are explained at least in part by the following facts: (a) About half of the observed residues are found in products of animal origin, even though these products constitute only about one-fourth of the total diet (Duggan and Lipscomb, 1969). (b) Cattle are raised now in all regions of the country. (c) Much animal food is produced on the same farm where the animal is raised, and feed, especially hay, that is shipped is often not shipped as far as vegetable food intended for people. (d) Unlike the situation for many field crops, there is no striking relationship between region of the country and time of "harvest" for meat. (e) Meat is shipped less widely than many other foods.

Quite aside from the exact mechanism by which regional differences in pesticide resi-dues are maintained, it is necessary to recog-nize their reality on the one hand and their small magnitude on the other. The situation is similar to that observed in connection with selenium. General uniformity in the concentra-tions of this essential trace metal in human blood is more striking than the small regional differences that are observed. These small reg-

Table 6-5

Average Daily Intake of DDT and Related Compounds by
Region and Year as Reported by Duggan and Lipscomb (1969)

Headquarters of region	North latitude	Intake (mg/man/day)	
		1966–1967	1967–1968
Los Angeles	34.1°	0.092	0.059
Kansas City	39.1°	0.045	0.086
Baltimore	39.3°	0.032	0.026
Boston	42.4°	0.071	0.035
Minneapolis	45.0°	0.031	0.017

ional differences in people reflect established regional differences in the concentrations of selenium in crops so closely that exceptions to the rule raise the possibility of unknown environmental sources (Allaway *et al.*, 1968).

In contrast to the small differences in residues of pesticides in food grown and sold commercially, large variations may be found in home grown foods, and there are a few people in nearly every part of the country whose diet consists of such food to a significant degree. This is of no importance when the agricultural practices are standard. If the conditions under which the food is produced are unusual, the residues at harvest may be high, as discussed in a part of Section 6.1.5.2.

The concentrations of pesticides in foods imported into the United States of America are essentially the same as those found in food produced in the country and shipped in interstate commerce (Duggan, 1968b; Duggan *et al.*, 1971).

Canada. Although the daily intake for Canada has not been calculated, both the frequency and the concentration of pesticides in whole meals there apparently are even lower than in the USA (Swackhamer, 1965).

England. The results of a study of whole meals collected in southeast England during the period March, 1965, through March, 1966, were remarkably similar to those of studies in the United States of America during the same period. The intakes determined by residues found in the total diet in England were: DDT, 0.030; DDE, 0.025; total DDT-related material, 0.072; and dieldrin, 0.021 mg/man/day. DDE constituted 39% of the total DDT-related material, a proportion similar to that in the United States of America. It was found that cooking had little effect on the insecticidal content of the diet (McGill and Robinson, 1968). A similar survey during March through October, 1967, revealed a significant decrease in the daily intake of dieldrin from an arithmetic average of 0.021 to 0.014 mg/man/day (or from a geometric average of 0.019 to 0.013 mg/man/day) (McGill *et al.*, 1969).

Japan. In total diet samples, pesticide residues were essentially the same in overall amount as those in the USA. The proportion of compounds differed; there was more BHC than DDT. The average concentration of all pesticides consumed was 0.03 ppm, but the resulting daily intake was not stated (Nishimoto *et al.*, 1966).

6.1.5.2 Special Diet.

Prepared Foods for Babies. During the period July 1, 1963, through June 30, 1967, the US Food and Drug Administration examined 684 samples of prepared baby foods chosen at random from commercial stores. Approximately one-fourth of the samples contained detectable residues. Chlorinated pesticides accounted for 275 (93%) of the 297 residues found. About 97% of the values were below 0.51 ppm, and 86.5% were below 0.11 ppm. On the average, the incidence and the levels of residues found were lower than those from raw agricultural products, other processed foods, and samples examined in the Market Basket study (Lipscomb, 1968). Although it was clearly shown that the amounts of various pesticides an infant might receive in its total diet are small, the report unfortunately does not permit estimation of numerical values.

The study was continued, and by 1969, 2,078 samples had been examined. During the entire period, only 25.5% contained detectable residues. The average residue for DDE and for DDD was 0.01 ppm, each. The average residues for DDT, dieldrin, aldrin, lindane, and heptachlor epoxide were less than 0.005 ppm; those for other compounds were undetectable (Duggan *et al.*, 1971).

Health Foods. So called "health foods" are sold in special stores and are represented as more "natural," nutritious, and safe than food available elsewhere. It is generally implied and sometimes stated that they are free of pesticides. Durham *et al.* (1965) found no significant difference in the DDT and DDE contents of such foods and corresponding items purchased from ordinary grocery stores. They did record that the price of different "health foods" was about twice that of similar items in other stores. Apparently no study has been made to determine whether the residues present on "health foods" are the result of drift, or whether these products are drawn from the same wholesale market as other foods.

Home Grown Foods. Pesticide residues on home grown foods may differ from those on commercially grown crops under at least three circumstances: (*a*) no pesticides are used; (*b*) pesticides are used but not according to label directions; and (*c*) pesticides are used for a totally different purpose so that contamination of the home grown food is incidental. Obviously, the first situation involves no toxicological problem.

One hears a great deal about the overenthusiastic and ill advised use of pesticides by home gardeners. There are a small number of examples (Section 7.1.2.4) in which spraying of a vegetable with a compound not recommended for that use led to poisoning. In the single instance in which the residue was measured, it was 3,315 ppm compared to a legal level of zero. However, the few known examples could be considered accidents. There has been no systematic study to learn whether there is really a residue problem associated with the use of pesticides in home gardens. There is, of course, a real problem in the care and storage of all hazardous materials—whether drugs, household chemicals, or pesticides—to prevent their ingestion by children (see Section 7.1.4.7).

By contrast, high residues have been found in food raised in or near orchards, or in association with cotton. Thus, Durham et al. (1965) found an average DDT residue of about 21 ppm in samples of eggs from hens kept by orchardists. Commercially grown eggs available in the same area contained an average of only 0.11 ppm. The importance of a difference of this kind would depend on whether the food involved formed an important part of the diet for a significant period. However, such high residues in a beef or hog raised by a family and later frozen for their continuing use would contribute substantially to their pesticide intake.

Food of Alaskan Natives. No DDT or DDE was found in native Alaskan foods with the exception of two white owls, both of which contained low levels of DDE. Eskimos who eat such food store considerably less DDT and DDE in their body fat than do people of the general population of the mainland USA. The limited storage found in Eskimos is explained readily by the fact that a part of their diet consists of items "imported" from the contiguous states and produced according to ordinary agricultural practices (Durham et al., 1961).

6.2 Residues in Air

6.2.1 Observed Residues in Community Air

The highest concentration of DDT reported in the air of Pittsburgh, Pa was 0.00000236 mg/m³. This city is far from any important agricultural area, and it had no community mosquito control program. The samples consisted of dust separated according to particle size. DDT was detected somewhat more frequently in samples of respirable than nonrespirable particles. Some samples contained no detectable insecticide in particles of either size range (Antommaria et al., 1965).

In six small communities in an agricultural area, DDT was found in concentrations ranging from 0.000001 to 0.000022 mg/m³. Aldrin, chlordane, and toxaphene were found at slightly lower concentrations in many samples, and traces of thiophosphates were found in some samples. On the assumption that breathing is at an average rate of 1 m³/hour, the highest observed concentration of DDT would lead to respiratory exposure at the rate of 0.0005 mg/man/day (Tabor, 1965, 1966). This rate may be compared with the maximal rate of 0.00006 mg/man/day in Pittsburgh, calculated on the same basis.

Tabor (1965, 1966) found that the concentrations of insecticide in the air of communities with antimosquito fogging programs may be essentially the same as those found in the drift from agricultural applications. The maximal concentrations he reported in these situations, 0.0080 and 0.0085 mg/m³, respectively, were really rather low as compared with those shown in Table 6-7 (p. 289), probably because the sampling period was long and tended to average out the peak values.

The most complete survey of atmospheric levels of pesticides was one carried out in four urban areas (Baltimore, Md; Fresno, Calif; Riverside, Calif; and Salt Lake City, Utah), and five rural areas located up to 32 km from Buffalo, NY; Dothan, Ala; Iowa City, Iowa; Orlando, Fla; and Stoneville, Miss. Samples were taken for 12 or 24 hours each, so that any peak concentrations were averaged out and a value characteristic of the particular locality for that day was obtained. The sampler was operated at a rate of 29 liters per minute, giving a sample of about 40 m³ in 24 hours. Of 19 pesticides for which analysis was made in 880 composite samples, only p,p′-DDT and o,p′-DDT were found at all localities (but not necessarily in all samples). DDD, heptachlor epoxide, chlordane, and 2,4–D esters were found in no sample. p,p′-DDE, o,p′-DDE, aldrin, dieldrin, endrin, heptachlor, four isomers of BHC, 2,4-D salt, malathion, parathion, and methyl parathion were found in a variable number of samples, sometimes as few as one. In addition to the 19 compounds originally sought, toxaphene and DEF also were encountered. The organic phosphorus insecticides and defoliant were found only in southeastern, rural areas. Concentrations of pesticides were generally lower in urban areas, but the rural area near Iowa City averaged at least as low as those of any urban area studied. Strangely, isomers of BHC were found more frequently and in greater variety in urban areas. In rural areas, highest concentrations of pesticides were found when spraying was reported in the area, and the lower concentrations often found on rainy days were due to lack of spraying rather than to rain, *per se*. Especially in rural areas, the distribution of the compounds in the initial filter of the air sampling device suggested that much of the pesticide was adsorbed on particulate matter. The residues found in air varied from the lower limit of detection of 0.1×10^{-6} mg/m^3 to a maximum of 0.002520 mg/m^3 for toxaphene, encountered near Orlando among at least 99 samples, of which 9 were positive for the compound. No effort was made to estimate average intake. However, even if all the pesticide in inhaled air were retained in the body, the intake from the highest level of DDT in a rural area near Orlando would be 0.037 mg/man/day, which is of the same order of magnitude as dietary exposure to this compound (Stanley *et al.*, 1971).

6.2.2 Drift and Related Matters

6.2.2.1 Local Drift. Simple observation of the application of pesticides to crops or forests often demonstrates the reality of drift. The same thing is true on a smaller scale in connection with some other uses of these compounds. However, the fact that a cloud is seen to hover over the target area and then gradually drift away with the wind offers little hint regarding the fate of what is lost. Furthermore, in addition to the visible particulate material, one must consider vapor that may evaporate from airborne spray or dust, or from deposits on plants, soil, or other surfaces for an indefinite period after application.

Whereas the ways in which pesticides may enter the air are known and the factors influencing this entrance are outlined reasonably well, the rate at which different compounds actually are mobilized into air under practical conditions is unknown.

Rate of Loss of Applied Material. It was found very early that only a small portion of DDT applied to crops actually reached the plants for which it was intended. It was recognized that part of the material is lost by drift and part sifts down between the leaves and falls to the ground. Even under special test conditions, recovery of 24% of the applied material immediately after application of DDT dust to wet alfalfa was unusually high (Eden and Arant, 1948). More typical of general agricultural conditions was the recovery of 7.5% from plants just after application of DDT dust (Wilson *et al.*, 1946b). A similar situation was found in the early studies of DDT applied for mosquito control.

Measurements of the proportion of applied material that remain on field crops usually

have ignored what fell to the ground and, therefore, offer no help in estimating the proportion lost to the air. However, the fact that the proportion reaching the target plant is inversely proportional to the volatility of the compound applied (Decker *et al.*, 1950) strongly suggests that a considerable proportion is vaporized at the time of application.

Additional information about net loss has been obtained from attempts to measure the proportion of applied material that can be recovered from typical target areas. Such measurements have been made to determine the efficiency of different kinds of application, or because of an interest in the possible effects of environmental contamination on wildlife. In studies of aircraft applying a thermal aerosol of DDT, recovery at the center of the swath was only 12.5% of the nominal rate of 11.2 mg/m^2 and, of course, even less at increasing distances from the center (Hess and Keener, 1947). In another study, an average of only 8% could be recovered following application of a thermal aerosol, whereas an average of 46% was recovered following application of a spray under otherwsie similar conditions (Scudder and Tarzwell, 1950). In another situation, the seasonal average recovery of DDT applied as a thermal aerosol ranged from 10 to 12%, while seasonal recoveries following spray ranged from 56 to 76% (Tarzwell, 1950). The following lower recoveries of spray have been reported: 30% (Hoffman and Merkel, 1948), 39% (Hoffman and Surber, 1948), and 27% (Surber and Friddle, 1949).

Following a single application of DDT to a forest, about 26% reached the forest floor immediately, and an additional 6% came down during a period of 36 months on falling leaves and other litter (Tarrant *et al.*, 1972).

Local Fallout. Since pesticides are almost always finely dispersed at the time of application, there is an excellent opportunity for volatilization as long as the particles remain in the air. Part of the vapor might be expected to travel great distances. On the other hand, most of the particles themselves, carrying some fraction of their original load of pesticide, may be expected to fall out in the general area of application. An indication that this is exactly what happens may be gained from a study of chlorinated insecticide residues in soil and wildlife as a function of distance from application. The samples were taken in an essentially desert area with little or no agriculture, but downwind from an area of intense agriculture. A nearly straight line inverse relationship was found between the logarithm of distance from point of application and the logarithm of the concentration of DDT-related material in the soil. The soil level at 10 meters was about 1 ppm; at 100,000 meters the residue approached 0.001 ppm. The concentrations found in the tissues of wildlife were directly proportional to the soil levels of their habitat (Laubscher et al., 1971). These observations are consistent with the finding that uncultivated fields interspersed among cultivated ones have only slightly less pesticide residues in their soils than do the cultivated ones (see Section 6.3.1.1).

A different kind of measure of the general dispersion of some pesticides within 100 km or less of their point of manufacture or use is their occurrence in rainwater in large urban areas (see Section 6.1.3).

Fate of Residues in Air. As just stated, much of the pesticidal material that finds its way into the air is returned to earth in the same general area, largely downwind from the source. This is especially true of particulate material. The transport of such material for more than 100 km must be slight except in connection with unusual storms (see Section 6.2.2.2).

Hartley (1969) pointed out that much of any pesticide vapor escaping to 50 meters or more above the ground will ascend even higher by eddy diffusion and eventually reach the photochemically active ionosphere. The rapid destruction of pesticides by ultraviolet light under laboratory conditions has been demonstrated. An example is the breakdown of DDT (Mosier et al., 1969; Plimmer et al., 1970; Miller and Narang, 1970). Hartley considered that the destructive reactions in the upper atmosphere are of great importance in the detoxification not only of synthetic compounds, but of ordinary biological waste products.

6.2.2.2 Worldwide Drift. The visible scattering of pesticides beyond the target area, their measurable volatility, and the persistence of certain ones open the logical possibility that some of them can stay suspended as dust or vapor long enough to become mixed (not necessarily evenly) into the air over the entire surface of the earth. Proof that worldwide distribution actually occurs must depend on direct measurement. The demonstration of pesticides in species confined to the open ocean or to the polar areas (see Section 11.1.2) is not evidence for worldwide distribution of pesticides by air, unless the possibility can be excluded in each instance that the animals acquired the compounds via ocean currents, their food chains, or both.

Evidence that pesticides can be blown about 1,600 km was apparently provided by the finding of arsenic, DDT, DDE, chlordane, heptachlor epoxide, dieldrin, 2,4,5-T, and ronnel in dust collected in Ohio and thought to have originated in Texas. The concentrations reported on the basis of dry weight of dust were 26 ppm for arsenic, 0.6 ppm for DDT, and lesser amounts of the other compounds (Cohen and Pinkerton, 1966). The sample was identified by its association with a dust storm of such intensity and novelty that its progress across the country was described in newspapers. The sample was collected on a galvanized roof that had recently been cleaned by rain; after the dust had settled, it was flushed with tap water into a stainless steel tank and recovered by filtration. The dust obtained in this way weighed 175 g, equivalent (in view of the area of the collecting surface) to 4.8 tons per square mile, or about 16.8 kg/ha.

That precipitation and perhaps impingement may be important factors in removing residues from air is suggested by a study in California. The more than 485-km long Sierra Nevada Mountains lie east of the Central Valley of California; the distance of the crest from the eastern edge of the valley varies from about 32 to 130 km. The prevailing winds blow from the Pacific Ocean across the valley and against the western face of the mountains, which are of sufficient height that much of the moisture in the air is removed as precipitation on the western face. The crest of the Sierra Nevada marks the western boundary of a great desert. Using residues of DDE in frogs as a measure of environmental contamination, it was found that in the Central Sierra, the average concentrations were 3.46 ppm at low altitudes, and 3.19 ppm at altitudes above 1,640 m on the western face, but only 0.97 ppm just across the crest (Cory et al., 1970).

Pesticides have been measured in rainwater. In most instances, the collections were made in agricultural or urban areas where the residues found might be of local origin (see Section 6.1.3.1). In reporting on samples collected mainly in London, Abbott et al. (1965) remarked that the residues were extremely low, near the limit of sensitivity of the delicate electron-capture detection system, and that two samples taken from remote areas of Scotland during periods of heavy rainfall showed "practically no residue." However, in more recent studies (Tarrant and Tatton, 1968), a more equal distribution of residues was found. In addition to cities and farming areas, extensive collections were made in two remote, sparsely populated areas where some sheep farming was essentially the only agricultural activity. The places were Eskdalemuir in Scotland and Lerwick in the Shetland Islands.

Especially in the latter place, it is difficult to see how any but the most minute residues in rainwater could be of local origin. A possible exception would be residues of dieldrin used for a time on sheep. However, the residues actually found in both remote places were not significantly lower than those found in agricultural and urban areas sampled in the same study. In fact, in one or more of the places where residues might be expected from local sources, the concentrations of α-BHC, dieldrin, p,p'-DDT, p,p'-DDE, and p,p'-DDD actually were lower than in either of the remote places. This was not true of γ-BHC; the lowest average value for that isomer was found in Scotland, but the highest average value was found in the Shetland Islands. The evidence, then, not only suggests a worldwide distribution of certain chlorinated hydrocarbon insecticides in the air, but suggests that the mixture is rather evenly distributed and not dependably high in agricultural and urban areas of the United Kingdom, where local use exists but is of moderate intensity.

Worldwide distribution is indicated, perhaps even more persuasively, by a report of 0.00004 ppm of DDT in water melted from Antarctic snow (Perterle, 1969).

Identification and measurement of pesticides in dust collected on the island of Barbados in the West Indies, and thought to come from Europe and Africa, a distance of over 4,850 km, has been reported (Risebrough et al., 1968). The dust was collected on nylon nets treated with a 50% aqueous solution of glycerine. The identity of p,p'-DDT, $p.p'$-DDE, o,p'-DDT, DDD, and dieldrin were indicated by use of two chromatographic columns, by thin layer chromatography, and (in the case of p,p'-DDT, o,p'-DDT, and p,p'-DDD) by dehydrochlorination followed by gas chromatography, with detection of the expected derivatives. The compound encountered most frequently and in greatest concentration was p,p'-DDT. The concentration of pesticide in the trapped dust ranged from 0.001 to 0.164 ppm and averaged 0.041 ppm, but there was not much dust. The volume of air filtered by the nets could not have been measured accurately, but the average concentration of all pesticides in it was estimated to be 0.000,000,000,078 mg/m^3.

Unfortunately, analysis at very low levels is subject to numerous errors. There is a question whether any thin layer plate can be considered absolutely blank. Gas chromatographic columns must be conditioned by the compounds they are to measure; unfortunately, various extractives may upset the equilibrium and release trace amounts of pes-

ticide from the column, which are detected as such to give a false positive—a process called "ghosting." Under the circmstances, the existence of even persistent pesticides in the general atmosphere may be questioned. A similar precaution applied to traces of "insecticides" in other materials that may be dispersed as dust in the air. On one chromatographic column or another, apparent traces of several chlorinated hydrocarbon insecticides, especially aldrin and heptachlor epoxide, were found in many samples of soil collected and sealed in 1910, many years before the compounds were invented (Frazier et al., 1970).

6.2.2.3 Factors Influencing Residues in Community Air. Factors influencing residues in air are best understood and the resulting concentrations are most predictable when the source of contamination is single, close, and clearly defined, and when air currents are simple or essentially absent. Thus, it usually is possible to understand and control airborne vapors and particulates in factories and mines. A great deal is known also about the distribution of waste from smoke stacks, and even about general community air pollution in which the source of contamination is within the community. These matters are not covered in this book, but information on them may be found in texts on air pollution, including a three-volume work edited by Stern (1968).

Factors influencing local drift of pesticides are essentially identical to those influencing the distribution of wastes from stacks. Factors influencing drift over great distances from many, poorly defined sources are themselves poorly understood. To be sure, a great deal of information is available on the worldwide fallout from nuclear explosions. However, what has been learned about radioactive fallout is not necessarily valid for pesticides. Because the products of a nuclear explosion can be identified and measured with accuracy even at very low concentrations, it has been possible to recognize and measure fallout from a single explosion pinpointed in time and space. By contrast, the concentrations of pesticides said to result from worldwide drift present tremendous analytical difficulties, and the applications from which the residues are thought to result are certainly widely scattered in time and space. In connection with pesticides, there is nothing comparable to the detailed studies of the chronological and spatial distribution of the fallout following a nuclear explosion at a single point of time and space. Under the circumstances, only very general principles can be stated regarding the drift of pesticides over long distances. It is apparent from simple logic that such distribution will be influenced by: (a) dosage, (b) compound, and (c) winds.

Dosage. Considering even the minimal dilution factors involved, it is evident that a compound must be applied in tremendous amounts if the application is to be the true cause of finding a recognizable part of the material in the air of a distant place. It seems possible that if dilution factors are taken into account, certain reports of residues in remote places require (a) the application of more pesticide than has ever been produced, or (b) some yet undefined channeling from source to final location. Under these circumstances, unrecognized contamination of samples or of some other error of analysis must be considered, unless some reasonable mechanism for delivery can be found.

Compound. Two properties of compounds that may influence their distribution to distant places are: (a) stability, and (b) volatility. In order to reach a distant point by way of the air, a compound must resist oxidation and hydrolysis in the presence of oxygen, water vapor, and sunlight long enough to make the trip. Compounds that are reasonably stable during storage may be unstable when dispersed as a vapor or as fine particles. This requirement for stability is completely satisfied in connection with metallic poisons, because there is so little difference in the toxicities of different compounds of the same metal. However, the oxidative and hydrolytic products of many organic pesticides are of insignificant toxicity.

Presumably any pesticide could be blown by the wind as dust derived from the original formulation, or consisting of soil particles to which the compound was adsorbed. However, compounds differ greatly in vapor pressure, and this difference may be critical in determining whether a particular compound will enter the air in significant amount. Table 6-6 offers some idea of the range of vapor pressure of pesticides. Moreover, different compounds are influenced differently by the same factor. Lichtenstein (1966) concluded that a significant proportion of chlorinated hydrocarbon insecticides are vaporized into the air after they are displaced from soil by water. By contrast, when organic phosphorus compounds are displaced in the same way, their hydrolysis is more prominent than their evaporation.

Wind. Wind may carry off vapor and fine particles of pesticide during application, or even after the material has become attached to plant surfaces or the soil. Vaporization from a surface is increased if the gradient is kept high through constant removal of the vapor.

If a pesticide remained in the air for a significant period, its ultimate distribution would depend on where the release occurred and the height reached by the material. In spite of considerable turbulence, the winds of the temperate zones blow mainly from west to east, while those near the equator blow from east to west.

Volatilization. Pesticides evaporate from sprays and dusts at the time of their application and at any time that dust impregnated with these compounds is mobilized by the wind. Volatilization is an important factor in removing some residues from plants (Section 6.1.2.2), and from soil (Section 6.3.2.1). Since pesticides are applied extensively to plants and soils, it follows that considerable amounts of some of these compounds enter the air from these sources, at least temporarily. Once evaporation has occurred, the compound may condense on a nearby object, but it also may drift. Because of the importance of drift, this seems a good place to discuss factors that influence vaporization.

The evaporation of pesticides has been reviewed in detail by Hartley (1969). Briefly, the rate at which simple evaporation takes place depends on: (a) the vapor pressure of each compound (see Table 6-6); (b) the diffusion coefficient of each compound; (c) the surface temperature; and (d) the rate of air exchange across the surface. In addition, (e) the presence of moisture in soil and other adsorptive materials partially releases them for evaporation. Finally, (f) water can affect volatilization of soluble materials from porous surfaces in a second way called wick evaporation, provided the water evaporates. The rate of evaporation of water under field conditions can lead to mass flow in capillaries of soil. Although the concentration of most pesticides in soil water is low, it is sufficient that capillary flow of the solution leads to more rapid passage of the dissolved compound through the soil than is possible by diffusion alone. Thus, capillary flow can bring pesticides to the surface, available for evaporation at a higher rate than would occur otherwise. These compounds increase to concentrations at which their rates of evaporation balance their rates of arrival. (The possibility that a pesticide will reach sufficient concentration at the soil surface to reduce the rate of water loss or to form crystals is remote, although these effects can be the result of wick action involving other compounds.)

It is important to note that, in wick evaporation, it is only the delivery of compound to the surface that depends on water; the actual evaporation of compound is independent of the

Table 6-6

Vapor Pressure of Selected Pesticides

Compound	Vapor pressure (mm Hg)	Temperature (C°)	Reference
DDT	1.9×10^{-7}	20	Dickinson, 1956
dieldrin	2.7×10^{-6}	20	Spencer and Cliath, 1969
lindane	9.4×10^{-6}	20	Balsom, 1947
parathion	3.78×10^{-5}	20	Bright, 1950
dichlorvos	2.0×10^{-2}	25	Miles and Sedlak, 1960
nicotine	4.25×10^{-2}	25	Norton et al., 1940
p-dichlorobenzene	1.0×10^{0}	25	Shepard, 1951
carbon tetrachloride	1.14×10^{2}	25	Shepard, 1951
methylbromide	1.42×10^{3}	20	Merck Index

evaporation of water. Evaporation of water influences the evaporation of solute only when the rate is sufficiently great to provide bulk flow of vapor, and thus overcome the effect of the stagnant air layer that otherwise would cover the surface and impede release of compound to the open air. This is the process involved in steam distillation. It is practical for the extraction and distillation of some pesticides under laboratory conditions. However, during evaporation from moist soil, there is no distillation in this sense.

Pesticides evaporate from the surface of water in which they are dissolved or suspended. This came to special attention in connection with certain unexplained results of bioassays with mosquito larvae (Bowman et al., 1959). According to Acree et al. (1963), the observed loss of DDT can be explained on the basis of codistillation and by the further assumption that DDT has a great affinity for the air-water interface, or, to state it another way, by the heterogeneous distribution of the compound in quiet water. The authors emphasized that the DDT and water were lost together and clearly implied that the loss of DDT depended on the loss of water. The same authors (Bowman et al., 1964) studied the loss of other chlorinated hydrocarbon insecticides from water and concluded that this loss is inversely proportional to their polarity.

No one has challenged the observed facts, namely, the loss of chlorinated hydrocarbon insecticides from water and the simultaneous loss of water—which, on a simple etymological basis, is codistillation. However, the implication that evaporation of pesticide depends on the evaporation of water (that is, on codistillation in the chemical sense) has been questioned. It seems likely that classical physico-chemical theory of evaporation is adequate to account for the observed loss (Hartley, 1969; Spencer and Cliath, 1969). While admitting the correctness of the criticism as related to the evaporation of water, it is only fair to point out that the criticism does not exclude small deviations from theoretical expectation, nor contribute any evidence on the question of whether chlorinated hydrocarbon insecticides and similar compounds do or do not concentrate at the air interface of quiet, dilute suspensions. Such concentration has been reported in nature. Duce et al. (1972) used a polyethylene screen to collect selectively the surface microlayer of water from Narragansett Bay, south of Providence, R.I. They found concentrations of lead, iron, nickel, copper, fatty acids, hydrocarbons, and chlorinated hydrocarbons enriched 1.5 to 50 times in the top 20 to 100 μm relative to the water 20 cm below the surface. The trace metal enrichment involved the particulate and organic fractions but not the inorganic fraction. If the enrichment involves a film only a few molecules thick, then the enrichment in the film itself may be greater than 10^4.

It has been reported (Bowman *et al.*, 1964) that the rate of loss of a wide range of chlorinated hydrocarbon insecticides from water is inversely proportional to their polarity and, therefore, directly proportional to their tendency to concentrate at the air-water interface. It seems reasonable to assume that, if such concentration occurs, it would influence the rate of evaporation. Lichtenstein and Schulz (1970) found no clearcut relationship between water solubility and volatilization from aqueous media. They did find that the rate of volatilization from water is much greater than that from soil, and the addition of soil, algae, or detergents retards the volatilization of some compounds from water. The evaporation of pesticides from water probably is complex and certainly requires further experimental study.

A detail that has been studied is the retarding effect of monolayers on evaporation. The reduction in the steady state of evaporation of water by hexadecanol monolayers depends only on the air velocity above the surface, and is independent of the absolute rate of evaporation up to air velocities of 40 cm/sec. This indicates that the monolayer does not affect the vaporization step but increases the size of the diffusion boundary layer (MacRitchie, 1969).

Although it is possible to demonstrate the volatilization of pesticides under field conditions (see Section 6.3.2.2), it is extremely difficult to measure the rate. Furthermore, the process is subject to so many variables that the rate defies exact calculation. On the other hand, the order of magnitude can be calculated, and this is adequate to account for the mobilization of vast quantities of pesticides on a worldwide basis. Based on considerations too complex to review here, Hartley (1969) estimated that the rate of loss of DDT from glass plates is 1.2 lbs/acre/year (134.5 mg/m²/year or 1.345 kg/ha/year).

6.2.3 Exposure of Workers

Discussion of the exposure of workers in a section on residues in air is not meant to imply that absorption of pesticides is restricted to the respiratory route. The route of absorption must be evaluated separately for each compound and, to some degree, for each occupational situation. However, ambient air is the source not only of inhaled material, but also a portion of the material that finds its way onto the worker's skin or onto the food he may eat. Therefore, it is reasonable to discuss the exposure of workers in connection with residues in air.

As explained in Sections 5.5 and 3.2.2.2, the dermal, respiratory, and oral exposure of people to pesticides may be measured directly, or total occupational exposure may be inferred indirectly from the concentration of these materials in the air, or from the measurement of the compounds or their metabolites in body tissues or excreta. The following paragraphs are concerned with the results of direct measurement. Information on levels found in tissue and excreta is presented in Section 7.2.

6.2.3.1 Respiratory and Dermal Exposures of Workers.

Observed Values. Respiratory and dermal exposures of workers have been reviewed by Wolfe *et al.* (1967), and Table 6-7 is modified from one they prepared. Where possible, the same measurements are presented in terms of air concentration and hourly exposure. Clearly, the air concentrations of pesticides ordinarily encountered by workers are of a totally different order of magnitude from those occurring in community air, as described in Section 6.2.1. Much higher values than any shown in the table have been reported, although rarely, and the reason for their occurrence is not understood. Thus, Wassermann *et al.* (1960) reported air concentrations between 2.6 and 12.5 mg/m³ for γ-BHC, and between 4.6 and 25.5 mg/m³ for DDT during application of these insecticides to forests.

Another important point illustrated by Table 6-7 is that dermal exposure is generally greater than respiratory exposure, and sometimes very much greater. Wolfe *et al.* (1967) found that respiratory exposure ranged from 0.02 to 5.8%, or a mean of only 0.75% of the total dermal plus respiratory exposures to a number of pesticides. As reviewed in the same paper, other investigators also have found that occupational exposure to pesticides is mainly dermal. It is no wonder that measurements described in Section 5.5.4.2 often reveal that the amount of pesticide actually absorbed from the skin is much greater than that absorbed from the respiratory tract. This is true, even though only a small percentage of

Table 6-7

Summary of Published Studies on Potential Exposure of Workers to
Pesticides Using Direct Methods

Compound	Activity	Exposure [a]				Reference
		Respiratory		Dermal	Total	
		(mg/m^3)	(mg/hr)	(mg/hr)	(% toxic dose/hr)	
Chlorinated Hydrocarbon Insecticides						
BHC	spraying forests		(3.06)	(70.3)	(0.29)	Wassermann et al., 1960
BHC	hand spraying for mosquitoes		(4.29)	(10.2)	(0.15)	Wassermann et al., unpublished data
DDT and related compounds						
DDT	indoor house spraying			543	(>0.31)	Hayes, 1959
DDT	indoor house spraying	7.1	3.4[b]	1,755	(1.02)	Wolfe et al., 1959
DDT	outdoor house spraying			84	(>0.05)	Hayes, 1959
DDT	outdoor house spraying		0.11	243	(0.14)	Wolfe et al., 1959
DDT	spraying forests		(4.92)	(212)	(0.15)	Wassermann et al., 1960
dicofol	air blast spraying fruit orchards		0.05[b]	30.5	0.04	Wolfe et al., 1972
dilan	air blast spraying fruit orchards		0.26[b]	75.1	0.02	Wolfe et al., 1972
Perthane®	air blast spraying fruit orchards		0.14[b]	59.4	<0.01	Wolfe et al., 1972
Cyclodienes and related compounds						
dieldrin	hand-spraying of dwellings for disease vector control			(18.6)	(>0.33)	Fletcher et al., 1959
dieldrin	spraying pear orchards		0.25 (0.03)[b,f]	14.2	0.24	Wolfe et al., 1963
dieldrin	operating power air blast machine spraying fruit orchards		0.03[a]	15.5	0.25	Wolfe et al., 1967
dieldrin	power hand gun spraying fruit orchards from portable machine		0.03[b]	15.1	0.25	Wolfe et al., 1967
endosulfan	air blast spraying fruit orchards		0.02[b]	24.7	0.27	Wolfe et al., 1972
endrin	spraying orchard cover crops for mouse control		0.01[b]	2.6	0.21	Wolfe et al., 1963
endrin	high pressure power hand gun spraying orchard cover crops for mouse control		0.01[b]	3	0.25	Wolfe et al., 1967
endrin	operating power air blast or boom sprayers treating orchard cover crops for mouse control		0.01[b]	2.5	0.21	Wolfe et al., 1967
endrin	dusting potatoes		0.41[b]	18.7	1.5	Wolfe et al., 1963
endrin	spraying row crops		ND[b,c]	0.15	(0.01)	Jegier, 1964b
endrin	piloting airplane during air application of spray	0.05	0.08[b]	1.18	0.29 (0.16)[d]	Jegier, 1964b

Table 6-7 (continued)

Compound	Activity	Exposure [a]				Reference
		Respiratory		Dermal	Total	
		(mg/m^3)	(mg/hr)	(mg/hr)	(% toxic dose/hr)	

Organic Phosphorus Insecticides

Dimethoxy compounds

Compound	Activity	(mg/m^3)	(mg/hr)	(mg/hr)	(% toxic dose/hr)	Reference
azinphosmethyl	checking cotton for insect damage		0.02[b]	5.4	(0.04)	Quinby et al., 1958
azinphosmethyl	air blast spraying fruit orchards during night		0.47	541	6.5 (3.5)[d]	Wassermann et al., 1963
azinphosmethyl	air blast spraying fruit orchards during day	1.1	0.54	755	8.4 (4.9)	Wassermann et al., 1963
azinphosmethyl	air blast spraying fruit orchards	0.6	0.26[b]	12.5	(0.1)	Jegier, 1964a
azinphosmethyl	air blast spraying fruit orchards		0.1	9.9	0.15	Simpson, 1965
azinphosmethyl	air blast spraying fruit orchards		0.04[b]	27.2	0.18	Wolfe et al., 1967
azinphosmethyl	filling spray tank (dust)	2.8	1.27[b]	52.9	0.72 (0.46)[e]	Jegier, 1964a
azinphosmethyl	working in formulating plant (dust)	(4.2)	0.56[b]	10.1	(0.1)	Jegier, 1964a
chlorthion	operating aerosol machine for mosquitoes		(0.3)[b]	(3)	(0.003)	Culver et al., 1956
malathion	operating aerosol machine		(0.3)[b]	(6.6)	(0.003)	Culver et al., 1956
malathion	air blast spraying fruit orchards	0.6	0.08[b]	2.5	0.002 (0.001)[d]	Jegier, 1964b
malathion	air blast spraying fruit orchards		0.11[b]	30	0.01	Wolfe et al., 1967
malathion	persons outdoors during air application of spray to populated area	0.067	(0.055)	(0.89)	(<0.001)	Caplan et al., 1956
malathion	persons indoors during air application of spray to populated area	0.014	(0.012)	(0.25)	(<0.001)	Caplan et al., 1956
methyl parathion	checking cotton for insect damage		<0.01[b]	0.7	(0.02)	Quinby et al., 1958

Diethoxy compounds

Compound	Activity	(mg/m^3)	(mg/hr)	(mg/hr)	(% toxic dose/hr)	Reference
carbophenothion	air blast spraying fruit orchards		0.11[b]	41.3	1.12	Wolfe et al., 1972
diazinon	air blast spraying fruit orchards		0.06[b]	23.4	0.04	Wolfe et al., 1972
ethion	air blast spraying fruit orchards		0.04[b]	44.2	0.26	Wolfe et al., 1972
parathion	air blast spraying fruit orchards	0.09	0.06[b]	77.7	(5.4)	Batchelor and Walker, 1954
parathion	air blast spraying fruit orchards	0.15	0.03[b]	2.4	0.43 (0.18)[d]	Jegier, 1964b
parathion	air blast spraying fruit orchards		0.02[b]	19	1.33	Wolfe et al., 1966
parathion	concentrate air blast spraying fruit orchards		0.06[b]	28	1.95	Wolfe et al., 1966
parathion	high pressure power hand gun spraying fruit orchards	0.03	0.19[b]	55.8	(3.9)	Batchelor and Walker, 1954
parathion	hand knapsack mist spraying tomato bushes		0.29[b]	9.1	(0.82)	Simpson and Beck, 1965

Table 6-7 (continued)

Compound	Activity	Exposure[a] Respiratory (mg/m^3)	Exposure[a] Respiratory (mg/hr)	Exposure[a] Dermal (mg/hr)	Exposure[a] Total (% toxic dose/hr)	Reference
Carbamates and Related Pesticides						
carbaryl	air blast spraying fruit orchards	0.6	0.29[b]	25.3	0.03	Jegier, 1964b
carbaryl	air blast spraying fruit orchards		0.48	24.9	0.02	Simpson, 1965
Phenolic and Nitrophenolic Pesticides						
binapacryl	air blast spraying fruit orchards		0.07[b]	29.6	0.05	Wolfe et al., 1972
dinobuton	air blast spraying fruit orchards		0.02[b]	31.0	0.03	Wolfe et al., 1972
dinoseb	herbicide spraying corn and pea fields with boom ground sprayers		0.12[b]	88.7	(0.57)	Wolfe et al., 1961
DNOC	spray-thinning apples		0.4[b]	63.2	(0.25)	Batchelor et al., 1956
DNOC	spray-thinning apples		2.75	57.5	0.20	Wassermann et al., 1963
DNOC	spray-thinning apples		0.03[b]	24.4	(0.1)	Wolfe et al., 1961
DNOC	chemical thinning apple blossoms by power hand gun spraying		0.13[b]	55.1	0.13	Wolfe et al., 1967
DNOC	chemical thinning apple blossoms by power air blast spray machine		<0.05[b]	22.5	0.05	Wolfe et al., 1967
Miscellaneous Pesticides						
tetradifon	air blast spraying fruit orchards		0.07[a]	36.4	<0.01	Wolfe et al., 1972
Fungicides and Related Compounds						
chinomethionate	air blast spraying fruit orchards		0.02[a]	23.7	0.02	Wolfe et al., 1972

a. All values shown in parentheses were not included in the original paper but were calculated.

b. Measurement by respirator pad technique.

c. Not detectable.

d. Calculations based on the original authors' published dermal and respiratory exposure data indicated that the correct total exposure as a percentage of the toxic dose per hour should be the values shown in parentheses rather than the figures originally published.

e. These original values were calculated on the basis of maximum exposure. The recalculated values shown in parentheses are based on mean exposure.

f. Study of the original data on which the published respiratory value (0.25 mg/hr) was based indicated that this figure was derived in error and should have been 0.03 mg/hr.

the material impinging on the skin may be absorbed. The observed rates of absorption as they relate to routes of exposure are discussed in Section 7.2.4.1.

Factors Influencing Respiratory and Dermal Exposure. Exposure of workers to a particular compound may be influenced by: (a) type of formulation; (b) concentration of formulation;

(c) method of application; (d) duration of application; (e) type of work; (f) wind; and (g) attitude of worker.

Although it is not always possible to determine the relative importance of different factors, it is important to remember that individual measurements may indicate great differences in the exposure of men doing the same work with a given pesticide. Thus, Wolfe et al. (1967) reported up to about 200-fold variation in dermal exposure associated with applying parathion to fruit trees with an air blast, dilute spray machine, and up to almost a 300-fold variation for respiratory exposure associated with the same compound applied for the same purpose as a concentrate. However, in spite of the wide variations that sometimes occur, dependable trends may be recognized.

Respiratory and dermal exposures of workers to aerosols and dusts have been studied less than their exposure to sprays. Based on numerous pesticides and work situations they studied, Wolfe et al. (1967) prepared a table to compare exposure to these different particulates, and it is reproduced with slight simplification as Table 6-8. Respiratory exposure was found highest for aerosols, intermediate for dusts, and low for dilute spray formulations. These results were consistent with those reported earlier and reviewed by these authors. Thus, the smaller the particles, the higher the proportion of the total dispersed material that can be expected to be inhaled.

The kind of particulate to which the applicator is exposed is determined in part by the formulation and in part by the method of application. The fineness of a dust depends almost entirely on its formulation (especially its original grind). Whether a liquid formulation will form a spray or aerosol depends largely on how it is applied, except that the particle size of water-wettable powders cannot be made any smaller than the original grind.

Presumably, the exposure of men doing the same kind of work is directly proportional to the concentration of formulation applied. However, there is no objective evidence on the matter because, under comparable circumstances, formulations of similar concentrations generally are used. The effects of such small variations as may occur are easily obscured by other factors.

The size and number of particles encountered by an applicator depend not only on the state of the formulation as it leaves the nozzle, but also on whether the spray stream strikes a wall or other sufficiently solid object. Contamination of men who spray houses for control of vector-borne disease is largely the result of particles that have bounced back from the wall against which they were directed. If the formulation is completely liquid, the drops will be further subdivided by the impact. Thus, the average size of particles reaching the house sprayman is often smaller than the average size dispersed by the sprayer. How much smaller depends on the velocity of the impact, and this, in turn, depends on the pressure at the nozzle. Thus, the exposure of spraymen may be reduced somewhat by the use of pressure regulators, and by the use of long spray wands that permit them to work at a greater distance from the treated surface.

The method of application may influence

Table 6-8

Relative Respiratory Exposure (expressed as the percentage of total dermal and respiratory exposure) for Workers Applying Different Types of Pesticide Formulations.

Adapted from Wolfe et al. (1967) by permission of the authors and the American Medical Association.

Type of formulation	Respiratory Exposure	
	Range (%)	Mean (%)
dilute spray	0.02 - 0.05	0.23
aerosol	0.3 - 5.8	2.87
dust	0.05 - 3.2	0.94

not only the particle size of the dispersed pesticide but also the total rate of exposure to it. The height of application is especially important, whether it involves a distinction between air and ground application, or between ground application directed upward and that directed downward from a relatively low initial level. Thus, Wolfe *et al.* (1967) found that an air blast sprayer that directed formulation upward into fruit trees led to 12 times greater exposure of the operator than resulted from a boom-type sprayer that directed a comparable formulation downward into row crops. In a similar way, spraying that includes the ceiling or underside of the roof of houses leads to greater exposure of the operator than spraying confined to the walls (Wolfe *et al.*, 1959).

As pointed out by Wolfe and his colleagues, the application of pesticides to agricultural crops is usually seasonal and often is broken up into separate periods of application, each lasting a few days or even less. If spraying is interrupted by wind or some other adverse condition, the spray period is extended but the number of hours per day is reduced. Brief intermittent exposure favors the detoxification and excretion of absorbed toxicant. However, this factor must be balanced against the great variation in degree of exposure that often characterizes agricultural application. Thus, the factory worker may have more continuous but much less variable exposure susceptible to control by built-in ventilation. The degree of exposure actually associated with any given work situation must be determined by measurement, although the experienced toxicologist often can make a useful estimate on the basis of observation related to earlier measurements in similar situations.

Different members of a spray team may receive different average exposures determined by their type of work. For example, in airplane application of 1% tepp dust to a fruit orchard, the loader received about 3 times as much exposure as the pilot and 4.5 times as much as the flagman. Activities that do not involve direct contact with a formulation before or during application usually produce relatively low exposures. In general, the exposure of checkers, irrigators, cultivators, and pickers who work in treated crops is less than that of the worker who applied the pesticide initially. The apparent exception, in which isolated groups of cropworkers exposed to aged residues of parathion have become ill (see Section 7.1.2.4), is not understood, and may reflect unrecognized factors.

Wind makes a great difference in the exposure of workers out of doors. Paradoxically,

the absence of wind indoors leads to greater exposure in indoor than in outdoor house spraying. Wolfe *et al.* (1967) considered wind the most important environmental condition in determining exposure. Pesticides should not be applied if wind is detectable without instrumentation. At higher wind speeds, drift is increased so that less spray is deposited on the treated crop and more is carried to areas where it may be harmful. In theory, it would be safer for the operator to apply pesticides at higher wind speeds if he could always keep his back to the wind. In practice, higher wind speeds lead to greater exposure because the worker has only limited choice of the direction in which he sprays and, furthermore, the direction of the wind may change in a moment while the direction of spraying remains unchanged.

Men spraying indoors receive about 7 times more dermal exposure and 65 times more respiratory exposure than those applying the same formulation to the outside of houses. The difference is due in part to the greater height of spraying indoors, and in part to the fact that there is no drift indoors, whereas even an imperceptible breeze outdoors will dissipate some of the spray that otherwise would contact the applicator.

Although it was difficult to document, Wolfe *et al.* (1967) noted that workers differed in their attitude toward safety, so that some consistently received greater exposure than others in similar situations. These investigators observed differences in the care with which concentrated and dilute formulations were mixed or dispensed, differences in the use of protective equipment, and differences in personal hygiene. Furthermore, careless operators sometimes sprayed on windy days or in other adverse situations, while careful spraymen waited for better conditions.

Relation of Exposure to the Toxic Dose. It is obvious that the danger of exposure to a pesticide by a particular route depends on the toxicity of the compound by that route, as well as on the dosage received. It would be desirable to take both factors into account in a single unit, and Durham and Wolfe (1962) attempted to do so by expressing exposure in terms of "percentage of toxic dose received per hour." The exposure was that outlined in this section measured by techniques described in Section 5.5. The toxic doses for man were extrapolated from LD 50 values measured in rats. In the large number of studies carried out by Wolfe and his colleagues (1967), only three compounds (endrin, parathion, and tepp) were used in such a way that the average percentage of the toxic dose potentially absorbed per hour exceeded 1%. They noted that, of the compounds they had studied, only these three and demeton were known to have caused poisoning under the conditions of work they had investigated. Some of percentages for these three compounds were very high. Thus, one man averages 44% of the toxic dose per hour in loading airplanes with 1% tepp dust.

Wolfe *et al*. (1967) considered that the morbidity of occupationally exposed persons is no greater than it really is because : (*a*) Some of the more dangerous jobs they studied occupied only a few hours per day or per week, thus allowing detoxication between periods of exposure. (*b*) The measurements of exposure were expressed in terms of "standard conditions," and therefore represented potential exposure. Actually, the workers usually gave much more attention to protective clothing and devices when handling highly toxic compounds. (*c*) The proportion of material absorbed under field conditions may be less than that absorbed by laboratory animals. Laboratory conditions often are selected to favor absorption, whereas workers not only may limit exposure, but also may limit absorption by bathing and change of clothing.

In summary, occupational poisoning has occurred in situations similar to those in which the fraction of the toxic dose was found to be high. Conversely, occupational poisoning associated with certain compounds and situations has not been reported, and the hazard of exposure to them (expressed as percentage of toxic dose per hour) is so low that it is doubtful occupational poisoning will occur. It must be concluded that the expression of exposure in terms of fraction of toxic dose may constitute a useful, objective measure of hazard, but, because of the number of variables involved, this measure cannot be expected to be exact.

6.2.3.2 Oral Exposure of Workers. Strictly oral exposure has not been found to be an important source of absorption of pesticides by workers regardless of the compound or work situation involved. This does not mean that exposure and absorption may not be by the gastrointestinal tract. Depending on particle size, a high proportion of inhaled particulate material impinges in the upper respiratory tract and eventually is swallowed (See Section 3.2.2.4).

Of course, if workers were to be sufficiently careless in keeping food near the work area, contaminated food might contribute a major part of their exposure and even lead to poisoning. This seemed to be what had happened in

a case reported by Quinby and his colleagues (Quinby *et al*., 1963) in which serious poisoning of a worker was traced to eating a candy bar he had carried partially opened in his shirt pocket while spraying parathion. However, Quinby (personal communication) later found that suicidal intent may have been involved.

Measurements have been made of the exposure that might result from a degree of carelessness that, while undesirable, undoubtedly occurs. The methods used are discussed in Section 5.5.3.

In a study of workers spraying endrin, Wolfe *et al*. (1963) found a maximum of only 0.002 mg per cigarette, even when the man's hands had been damp with formulation when he removed the cigarette from its package.

Armstrong *et al*. (1973) found an average of 0.02 mg or more of parathion on those portions of sandwiches which workmen held in their hands while eating the other halves. The men had worked for 1 to 5 hours thinning apples sprayed 24 to 48 hours earlier with the compound. In eating an entire lunch of sandwiches, cookies, and pickles, the men would have ingested an average of 0.16 mg of the pesticide. Similar values were obtained with candy bars carried partially open in the pocket during spraying. However, one candy bar handled after contact with parathion concentrate contained 2.07 mg of the poison, or almost as much as volunteers can tolerate daily without cholinesterase inhibition. Although the degree of contamination involved in this kind of oral exposure usually is not great, it is in addition to less avoidable, occupational exposure by other routes, and ought to be prevented.

6.3 Residues in Soil

Residues of pesticides in soil are rarely important as a source of direct exposure of people, although there is at least one case in which a child was poisoned by eating soil that had been contaminated by a concentrate of parathion. However, ordinary residues in soil constitute a reservoir from which crops, air, and water may acquire residues. Some of these materials may be absorbed by the roots of plants and possibly be translocated to other parts. Some residues on soil evaporate into the air, from which they may condense on plants, or dust to which they adhere may be blown by the wind. All residues in soil may be subject to runoff in the presence of heavy rain, and some are subject to leaching. Thus, it is important to know what residues of pesticides occur in the soil following agricultural and other uses and what changes each material undergoes in soil.

6.3.1 Observed Residues in Soil

Although studies of the fate of pesticides in the soil have been under way for many years, most of them were concerned with identification and evaluation of the factors involved. Until 1964, there was little reported study of the extent and duration of residues under different practical conditions of use.

6.3.1.1 Residues Following Application to Crops.

Cotton Culture. Cotton is a crop subject to severe damage by insects; it usually requires heavy applications of pesticides if it is to be raised profitably. In 1964, extensive monitoring of soil, sediment, and water was carried out on selected farms in the Mississippi Delta area of Mississippi and Arkansas, USA (US Department of Agriculture, 1966). The three major crops were cotton, soybeans, and rice. As a part of the survey, records of pesticide applications to each field during the preceeding 10 years were tabulated. The soil of both cultivated and uncultivated fields was sampled systematically. Each soil sample consisted of 25 cores taken to a depth of 7.5 cm. An effort was made to measure all of the pesticides that had been used at one time or another. Most of the analytical work was under the direction of William Barthel. Herbicides, carbamate insecticides, and sulfur were rarely detectable. Only traces of organic phosphorus compounds were found. However, chlorinated hydrocarbon insecticides were found in many samples and arsenic was found in essentially all.

The main, positive results for the soil of six farms are summarized in Table 6-9. Although there had been considerable variation in the extent to which different pesticides had been used on different farms, the major results were repeated from one to the other.

Although there had been little use of arsenic during the last 10 years, arsenic was found in all samples of soil considered in the table. Average concentrations in cultivated soils were 2.85 to 12.90 ppm on different farms. Average concentrations (1.20 to 5.90 ppm) were lower in uncultivated soils, but even here every sample contained some arsenic.

On most of the farms, DDT was used during 1964 and had been applied at a cumulative rate of more than 11.2 kg/ha over a period of years. It was found in 67% or more of samples of cultivated land, and in 15.5 to 92.3% of samples of uncultivated land. The average

concentrations were 0.75 to 2.03 ppm in cultivated land, and 0.10 to 0.91 ppm in uncultivated land. Most DDT is found near the soil surface, chiefly in the top 2.54 cm. The samples under discussion were taken to a depth of 7.5 cm and thus contained essentially all the DDT present. It is, therefore, of particular interest to note that an application rate of 1.12 kg/ha will produce a concentration of 1.0 ppm if evenly distributed to a depth of 7.62 cm in soil with a specific gravity of 1.47. Of course, the density of soil varies with its type and degree of hydration. Under standard conditions the specific gravities of soils range from 0.4 to 2.0. A density of 2 million pounds per 6-inch acre (specific gravity = 1.47) is often used as standard. In any given area the mean value may be somewhat different. Decker *et al.* (1965) reported that the specific gravities of soils used for growing corn in Illinois ranged from 1.23 to 1.39, with a mean of 1.35.

Thus, under the conditions of sampling used in the Mississippi Delta study, the application of DDT at rates greater than 11.2 kg/ha would result in residues greater than 10 ppm if all the DDT entered and remained in the soil. The concentration found was far less than would be predicted on this basis. For this and other compounds, numerous examples of the lack of progressive accumulation of residues in soil were found.

Of the various chlorinated hydrocarbon insecticides, endrin showed the least cumulation. Even on farms where it was used at a cumulative rate of more than 11.2 kg/ha, the compound could be detected in less than 40% of samples of treated, cultivated land, and the residues that did occur were low. In most instances, no endrin was found in uncultivated land.

As the result of recent, heavy applications, methyl parathion was found in occasional samples from all the farms. However, the number of positive samples was so small that no percentage was expressed. In general, the concentrations measured in samples from uncultivated fields (presumably as a result of drift) were lower than the corresponding values for cultivated fields. The presence of one exception for methyl parathion and a somewhat similar one for dieldrin point to the erratic nature of drift.

National Soil Monitoring. Monitoring of pesticides in the cropland soil of 43 states, and in noncropland soil of 11 states during 1968 and 1969 has been reported (Wiersma *et al.*, 1972b). In addition to arsenic and the chlorinated hydrocarbon insecticides, a search was made for organic phosphorus compounds, and

Table 6-9

Pesticide Residues in the Soils of Farms in Mississippi Sampled in 1964

From a U. S. Department of Agriculture (1966) Report.

Compound	Area	Treated Cultivated				Untreated Uncultivated		
		Cumulative application (kg/ha)	Samples positive (%)	Mean total (ppm)	Mean positive (ppm)	Samples positive (%)	Mean total (ppm)	Mean positive (ppm)
arsenic	CHA	- - a/	100	2.93	2.93	100	1.20	1.20
	CHB	- -	100	2.85	2.85	100	2.68	2.68
	GRA	- -	100	4.31	4.31	100	3.64	3.64
	GRB	- -	100	8.37	8.37	100	2.83	2.83
	SCA	0.65	100	10.28	10.28	100	4.76	4.76
	SCB	0.50	100	12.90	12.90	100	5.90	5.90
DDT	CHA	36.50	84.7	1.46	1.72	35.7	.36	.10
	CHB	12.37	67.1	0.5	.75	15.5	.09	.60
	GRA	- -	82.7	1.23	1.49	16.7	.07	.41
	GRB	25.60	100	2.17	2.17	58.3	.28	.48
	SCA	22.08	97.6	1.70	1.74	36.4	.11	.30
	SCB	7.17	97.2	1.97	2.03	92.3	.84	.91
dieldrin	CHA	.90	6.9	0.01	0.09	8.6	0.01	0.14
	CHB	- -	5.7	<.01	.08	2.4	< .01	.08
	GRA	- -	25.0	.02	.10	0.0	ND b/	ND
	GRB	2.04	7.3	<.01	.11	0.0	ND	ND
	SCA	- -	33.6	.04	.10	0.0	ND	ND
	SCB	- -	2.8	<.01	.08	7.7	< 0.01	0.08
endrin	CHA	.69	0	ND	ND	0.0	ND	ND
	CHB	.66	0	ND	ND	0.0	ND	ND
	GRA	3.05	16.0	.05	0.29	0.0	ND	ND
	GRB	6.72	5.2	.01	0.15	0.0	ND	ND
	SCA	14.35	26.5	.09	0.33	0.0	ND	ND
	SCB	11.81	39.4	.34	0.86	7.7	0.02	0.28
BHC	CHA	8.18	19.4	0.02	0.12	2.8	0.01	0.23
	CHB	.35	1.4	<.01	.08	0.0	ND	ND
	GRA	- -	9.6	.01	.12	0.0	ND	ND
	GRB	- -	7.3	.01	.08	0.0	ND	ND
	SCA	- -	12.1	.01	.08	0.0	ND	ND
methyl parathion	CHA	16.82	- -	- -	0.29	- -	- -	0.12
	CHB	13.24	- -	- -	0.17	- -	- -	0.10
	GRA	- -	- -	- -	0.04	- -	- -	0.08
	GRB	5.00	- -	- -	0.35	- -	- -	0.19
	SCA	25.30	- -	- -	0.29	- -	- -	0.16
	SCB	17.10	- -	- -	0.18	- -	- -	ND

a. In general, records of the application of pesticides covered the period 1955 to 1964. Thus, there were fewer records of pesticides such as BHC and especially arsenic, use of which was largely replaced ten years or more before the study began.

b. ND = not detectable

for atrazine, 2,4-D, and several other herbicides. Twenty-five pesticides and certain isomers and metabolites of some of them were found in one or more samples. Application records indicated the use of 130 pesticides on cropland and three pesticides on noncropland. Many of these compounds were not present in detectable quantities in any sample. The most commonly used but undetected compounds were mirex, captan, and methylmercury dicyandiamide. The proportion of sites positive for different compounds that were detected varied from 0.1% each for DCPA, DEF, methoxychlor, and PCNB to 26.1% for DDT-related

compounds, 27.8% for dieldrin, and 99.3% for arsenic. Although analysis was made for many compounds not listed in Table 6-9, substantial residues of other pesticides were not found. Some regional differences were evident. For example, aldrin was found more frequently and in higher concentration in the maize region, more DDT-related material was found in the vegetable and fruit regions, and more toxaphene was found in association with cotton.

Comparison of Different Crops. Trautman et al. (1968) studied a wide range of soils collected in 1967 from Wisconsin and eight states west of it. Only chlorinated hydrocarbon insecticides were measured. For these compounds, most of the results were of the same order of magnitude as the values in Table 6-9. A striking exception involved some samples from muck soils in Wisconsin used for raising vegetables; these soils contained residues as high as 23.70 ppm for DDT, or 42 ppm for DDT plus related compounds. Of the 41 soils sampled from nine states, 22 contained no detectable insecticide. It appeared that all major contamination was associated with soils growing specialty, high value crops. Endrin and methoxychlor were not found in any sample, pointing to the rapid breakdown of these materials.

The trend to use high levels of pesticides on high value crops apparently was confirmed by a study of root crops in the eastern states in 1965. However, the selection of fields on the basis of a history of heavy recent use of chlorinated hydrocarbon insecticides undoubtedly resulted in higher values than would have been found in a random selection. In soils used for raising peanuts, potatoes, and carrots, DDT was found in 48 of 49 fields, in concentrations ranging from 0.10 to 12.8 ppm, and averaging 2.8 ppm. Dieldrin was present in 28 of the fields in concentrations ranging from 0.05 to 0.26 ppm. Endrin, heptachlor epoxide, and endosulfan were found in a smaller proportion of the soils at average concentrations of 0.46 ppm or less (Seal et al., 1967).

In samples of crop loams taken in five states at the end of a growing season, Lichtenstein (1957) found 0.0 to 4.6 ppm of DDT, or only 0.612 times the average annual application. By contrast, the same study revealed residues of 1.5 to 106 ppm of DDT in orchard soils in four states. The average recovery in 14 orchards was 2.37 times the average annual application, and 0.266 times the total amount applied over a period of 10 years. The cumulative rates of application to the crop soils had ranged from 3.4 to 47.8 kg/ha, while those for orchard soils ranged from 67.3 to 630 kg/ha. The higher rate of application and the lower rate of cultivation undoubtedly influenced the higher retention rate in orchard soils.

A 2-year moratorium on the use of DDT in Arizona quickly reduced the residues on green alfalfa and in beef to about half of their former levels. However, the moratorium had virtually no effect on residues of DDT-related material in the soil of alfalfa fields or desert, indicating a very long persistence of the compound (Ware et al., 1971).

Pesticide Residues in City Soil. Only a few papers have reported measurement of pesticides in city soil. Analysis indicates higher concentrations in the soils of lawns and gardens that in the soils of waste areas. In this sense grass and flowers are crops. In almost all instances, the concentrations of arsenic exceed those of DDT-related compounds combined (Wiersma et al., 1972a).

6.3.1.2 Residues Following Direct Application to Soil.
Most residues of pesticides in the soil are unintentional. They are there because part of the spray applied to crops or forests failed to impinge on the plants, or because leaves and other portions of the treated plants eventually became incorporated into the soil. However, some residues are intentionally applied to soil for the control of such pests as grubs, termites, or weeds.

The heaviest applications of insecticides to the soil are made under buildings to protect them from termite damage. The building protects the treated soil from rain and mechanical diturbance, and (in the case of concrete slab construction) prevents evaporation of the pesticide. A test was made to see how rapidly DDT is lost from soil and how far it moves when not protected by an overlying building. The equivalent of 2,300 ppm of technical DDT was applied; after 20 years, 35 to 50% could be recovered from the treated soil. However, only 2 ppm was detected 30 cm directly below the treated surface, and none was detected in samples taken 10 cm or more below the surface and as much as 50 cm away from the treated soil. Thus, there appeared to be a maximum of 50 cm of lateral movement of DDT below the soil surface in 20 years. In the top 10 cm of soil, less than 0.5 ppm of DDT and about the same concentration of DDE were found 76 to 91 cm from the treated area. Most of the insecticide was in the top inch, indicating distribution by rain splash and other erosion of soil particles. The most distant movement of DDT detected was about 300 cm, undoubtedly caused by erosion (Smith, 1968). DDT always shows some binding to soil from which it is at least partially displaced by water. When the moisture content was 2.5% or less, the DDT lost its effectiveness against termites. Not only did the DDT fail to move in the soil to an important degree, but in the course of 20 years it became more firmly bound to soil constituents and ineffective against termites, even when the soil was moist. So tenacious was this final binding that the same concentration of DDT found, after thorough extraction with an organic solvent, would have protected against termites for 4 years or more if added freshly to the soil (Smith, 1973).

Over 60% of dieldrin applied as granules to soil for control of the Japanese beetle was recovered immediately after treatment, and there was no detectable decrease after 7 months of weathering (Fahey *et al.*, 1968).

The schedule of application may have a marked effect on the concentration of pesticide remaining in the soil after a specified interval. Thus, Murphy *et al.* (1962) found that the residue following two successive 0.28 kg/ha treatments of soil with heptachlor for control of the fire ant was equivalent, after 10 months, to that following a single 1.12 kg/ha treatment. The total concentration found in either case was about 0.25 ppm, mostly in the form of the epoxide.

In a study of aldrin and heptachlor applied to soil in the usual way and therefore concentrated in the surface layer, Lichtenstein *et al.* (1965a) found the same time-dosage relationships as those observed in plants (Section 6.1.2.2). Higher dosages produced higher residues. A single large dose produced a high residue, but in 5 years it was reduced to a level lower than that reached after each of five successive doses at one-fifth the rate of the large dose.

6.3.2 Physical and Chemical Changes of Pesticides in the Soil

6.3.2.1 Nature of Changes.

Qualitative Changes. Pesticides in the soil are far from static. They may undergo physical change including evaporation, diffusion, and leaching. They may undergo chemical change under the influence of heat, light, oxygen, and moisture. Finally, they may undergo biochemical change under the influence of enzymes of soil microorganisms and higher plants. The range of biotransformation in this situation is similar in general to that carried out in mammals (see Section 3.1.2), but the exact routes of metabolism for a particular compound are often different in soil and in the animal body (Lichtenstein and Corbett, 1969). The net result is the same. Organic compounds are rendered simpler, more water-soluble, and ultimately less toxic.

Quantitative Changes. The behavior of pesticides in soil is analogous to their behavior in animals. The mathematical treatment of their residence (storage) in soil and their elimination from it also is the same as that for animals (see Section 3.2.3.2). The mathematical prediction of cumulative levels of pesticides in soil was discussed by Hamaker (1966) who emphasized the steady state achieved following repeated applications.

As discussed in the following section, excessive levels of pesticides in the soil inhibit the enzymes responsible for their breakdown, and in this and perhaps other ways account for the slow rate of disappearance of many pesticides when concentrates are spilled on the soil. However, when organic pesticides are applied at ordinary agricultural rates, the concentration in the soil tends to reach an equilibrium whereby the total amount lost each year is equal to the amount applied. The various changes undergone by pesticides in the soil, especially their volatilization and biotransformation, explain the observations set forth in the preceding sections.

6.3.2.2 Factors Influencing Residues in Soil.
A number of factors have been observed to influence the changes mentioned in the preceding section. Some of the factors may affect more than one change. Thus, temperature influences many physical and all chemical and biochemical changes. The relative importance of different factors may differ for different compounds and even for the same compound under different circumstances.

Factors known to influence residues in soil may be divided into three general categories, namely *those involving pest control practices:* (a) time-dosage relationships, (b) compound, and (c) formulation and mode of application; *those involving field conditions:* (d) moisture, (e) temperature, (f) air movement, (g) cover crops, and (h) cultivation; and finally *those factors involving removal or chemical change of the applied compound:* (i) leaching, (j) volatilization, (k) microbiological activity, and (l) absorption and transport. These factors, some of which are interrelated, are discussed briefly in the following paragraphs. Those interested in further detail should consult the review by Lichtenstein (1966) and the references cited in it.

Time-Dosage Relationships. A distinction must be made between (a) agricultural soils to the surface of which relatively small amounts of pesticide are applied annually or more frequently, and (b) soils to which a large dose of pesticide is applied deeply either once or at long, irregular intervals.

In the case of agricultural soils, monitoring has produced many examples of a dynamic equilibrium whereby the level of a particular pesticide remains stable in spite of continuing application of the compound. In at least one study (Decker *et al.*, 1965), first-order kinetics (see Section 6.2.3.2) were used to calculate the long-term residues from repeated treatment of soil with aldrin in 35 locations in Illinois. The existing residues could be accounted for by the assumption that 80 to 90% of the relatively volatile aldrin was lost fairly rapidly after each application, that 30 to 70% of the remaining aldrin was converted to less volatile dieldrin, and that the halflife for dieldrin in Illinois soil is similar to that found by Lichtenstein and Schultz (1965) in Wisconsin soil. There is, then, some reason to believe that chlorinated hydrocarbon insecticides not only reach a dynamic equilibrium in soil but that they do so according to first-order kinetics.

Hamaker (1966) considered that investigators should be alert for examples of Michaelis-Menton kinetics according to which the rate of loss is first-order at lower concentrations but zero-order at higher concentrations because (at the high level) the enzyme necessary for biotransformation is completely complexed and the rate of conversion cannot be increased further. It may be that something of this kind is involved when very high concentrations of pesticides are added to soil. In fact, Decker and his colleagues found an indication of this effect, for they observed that epoxidation proceeded most rapidly when application rates were low and became progressively slower as the dosage rate increased. Lichtenstein and Schultz (1959b) observed the same relationship in connection with the diappearance of DDT, lindane, and aldrin from field plots treated at the rate of 112 to 224 kg/ha, as compared to 11.2 to 22.4 kg/ha.

Although it is clear that high levels of various pesticides interfere with their own loss from soil, the level at which this interference commences is not known. It does not involve concentrations likely to be found intentionally except in connection with termite control. In a study of insecticides applied to turf soils, no increase in persistence was observed in connection with application rates of chlordane up to 28 kg/ha, lindane up to 5.6 kg/ha, heptachlor up to 22.4 kg/ha, or aldrin up to 84 kg/ha. Increased persistence of lindane applied at the rate of 11.2 kg/ha was indicated but not proved (Lichtenstein and Polivka, 1959).

Nash and Woolson (1967) investigated a number of chlorinated hydrocarbon insecticides that were thoroughly mixed with soil to a depth of 23 to 38 cm in different experiments, but always in such a way that leaching, volatilization, photodecomposition, mechanical removal, and probably biological decomposition were minimal. They presented their data graphically. For aldrin, dieldrin, BHC, chlordane, heptachlor (including epoxide), toxaphene, dilan, and DDT, the observed values fell reasonably well along straight lines, at least from the 1st or 2nd year through the 15th to 17th year, when the percentage remaining was plotted against the log of time. The results for isodrin and endrin apparently did not fit this scheme, but their values gave reasonably straight lines after the first 6 months or so, when the percentage remaining was plotted against time. In many instances, the rate of loss was apparently more rapid during the 1st year or during the 1st and 2nd years than it was later. This was especially true of lower dosage rates. Neither of the graphic relationships described corresponds with the pattern of loss of drugs or bone-seekers in mammals (see Section 3.2.3.2).

Replotting of the original data for dieldrin kindly supplied by Dr. Nash showed that values for that compound defined a fairly straight line when the log of remaining residue was plotted against the log of time, as for a bone-seeker. The plot on semilog paper was a curve that fell more rapidly at first and more slowly afterward. This behavior on semilog paper seemed similar to that of several chlorinated hydrocarbons in mammals, but the resemblance was apparently superficial. After all, a curve of somewhat the same form is obtained when the unexcreted residues of a bone-seeker are plotted as the log of storage against time.

It is too early to reach a conclusion about the kinetics of the loss of pesticides from soil, especially after very heavy applications. A declining rate of loss of a particular dose with time is consistent either with an improvement of elimination at higher concentrations (for example through stimulation of soil microorganisms), or with a decline in rate that is inherently time dependent. The more rapid initial decline associated with lower (as well as higher) rates of application and the tendency of the values to form a straight line when the log of remaining storage is plotted against the log of time both suggest that the decline in rate is inherently time dependent. Theoretically, this could be associated with injury to soil microorganisms or with increasingly firm adsorption of the compounds to soil constituents over a period of years. There is no clear evidence for progressive injury to soil organisms, although there is some evidence indicating that very high initial levels of some pesticides have a prompt and continuing inhibitory effect. There is clear evidence for a gradual increase in bonding of some pesticides to some soils (see Section 6.3.1.2), but the nature of the new bond is unknown.

Numerous examples of adaptation of microorganisms for the metabolism of foreign chemicals are known. The number of bacteria in soil frequently rises when pesticides are added, just as happens when nutrients are added. However, this does not exclude the possibility that organisms—even adapted ones—will be injured by excessive concentrations. It must be kept in mind that the kinetics of loss of a particular pesticide may be entirely different for different rates of application. For a soil, there is nothing that corresponds exactly to illness and death of an animal. However, one or more species of microorganisms in the soil may decline and die. The fate of residues in soil after very high rates of application may be similar to the fate of residues in a corpse. Unfortunately, much of what is known about the fate of residues in soil involves concentrations and other conditions that (although they may be representative of subterranean termite control and gross spillage and disposal of pesticides) are not typical of most practical situations.

Compound. There is tremendous variation in the stability of different pesticides in the soil. The metals are extremely persistent. The chlorinated hydrocarbon insecticides are moderately persistent. The organic phosphorus and carbamate pesticides are less persistent, although even these compounds may remain in the soil for months. Furthermore, there are marked differences between members of the same chemical group. For example, under similar conditions, residues of malathion in soil were reduced to about 3% of their original concentration in 8 days, whereas those of parathion were reduced to only about 50% in 20 days and required 90 days for reduction to 3% (Lichtenstein and Schultz, 1964).

In the soil, each pesticide is subject to both chemical and biochemical change depending on its own chemical properties. All metabolites of the metallic poisons are of essentially equal toxicity. In general, the metabolism of organic pesticides reduces their toxicity. However, there are exceptions not only in connection with mammalian metabolism (Section 3.1.4), but also soil metabolism. In general, compounds that undergo lethal synthesis in mammals are the ones likely to become more toxic as the result of changes they undergo in the soil. Whether such changes within the soil actually lead to an increase in toxicity depends on the balance between production of the more toxic compound on one hand, and the production of less toxic materials combined with loss through evaporation or leaching on the other hand.

To show the complexity that may be involved, Lichtenstein (1966) recalled a study in which residues of phorate extracted from standard samples of soil produced a mortality in fruit flies of 100% immediately after application of the insecticide, and mortalities of 89, 65, and 27% at intervals of 1, 2, and 5 months after application. This was true even though only the initial sample contained any phorate. The initial sample collected about an hour after application already contained more phorate sulfoxide than phorate. The amount of phorate sulfoxide gradually decreased, but some of it was slowly converted to the sulfone, which constituted a relatively high percentage of later samples. The sulfoxide and sulfone are not as toxic to fruit flies as the parent phorate, but they are sufficiently toxic to account for the mortalities reported. Furthermore, the metabolites are slightly more toxic to mammals than the parent compound.

The marked difference in the effective volatility of different compounds was illustrated by laboratory and field studies showing that vapors toxic to two species of flies were given off by soils treated with aldrin, heptachlor, phorate, lindane, heptachlor epoxide, and dieldrin (in order of decreasing effectiveness), but not from soils treated with DDT, carbaryl, malathion or parathion (Harris and Lichtenstein, 1961).

Formulation and Mode of Application. The loss of a pesticide from soil may be delayed by formulations that are not themselves lost by evaporation or otherwise and that bind the compound. Thus, Barthel *et al.* (1960) showed that heptachlor was lost from soil less rapidly when it was formulated with Aroclor or rosin than when it was formulated in heavy aromatic naphtha.

Some pesticides are subject to diffusion or leaching in the soil; thus, they gradually move beyond the portion of soil to which they are applied. However, many compounds remain in the portion of soil to which they are distributed mechanically. This distribution may involve the original application or the mixing of soil during cultivation, or it may involve lateral movement at the surface caused through erosion by water or wind. For example, the chlorinated hydrocarbon insecticides show very little spontaneous migration in the soil. When applied to forests or rangeland, they remain confined to the upper inch of soil. In cultivated cropland, they remain confined to the plowed layer. In soil treated for termite control, they extend to whatever depth they are injected. The manner of application influences not only the distribution, but also the rate of loss from the soil, for the material near the surface is more subject to evaporation, photochemical change, and biochemical destruction.

In a 3-year field test, the persistence of aldrin and heptachlor in soil was 10 times greater when the compounds were mixed into the top 12.7 cm of soil at the time of application, rather than being applied to the surface without mixing (Lichtenstein et al., 1962).

Soil Type. Pesticides last longer in soils of higher organic content. Three and a half years after field treatment, 1.43 times more DDT, 4.25 times more aldrin, and 8.45 times more lindane were recovered from muck soil than from a silt loam treated in the same way (Lichtenstein and Schulz, 1959b). The degree of difference tends to be greater for more volatile compounds. Essentially similar results have been obtained in other studies (Lichtenstein et al., 1960).

The force of adsorption that binds a compound to soil particles tends to prevent absorption of the compound by pests or by the roots of crops. Thus, at any given concentration, insecticides are less effective in muck soil (organic content about 50%) than in sandy soil (Lichtenstein and Schulz, 1959a). In fact, there is an orderly progression in the LD 50 for insects as the percentage of organic matter in the soil is increased (Edwards et al., 1957). In a similar way, roots, including the root crops, absorb least pesticide from muck soil and most from sandy soil (Lichtenstein, 1959).

Moisture. Moisture can influence the loss of pesticides in at least three ways: (a) by displacing them from adsorption on soil surfaces so they can vaporize more easily; (b) by permitting nonenzymatic hydrolysis; and (c) by permitting activity and growth of soil microorganisms responsible for a wide range of biochemical changes. The relative importance of each effect depends on the volatility and chemical stability of each compound and on various soil factors.

High moisture content of soil promotes the loss of volatile pesticides. Little or no volatilization occurs from dry soils when the air passing over them is dry. However, when the air passing over dry soil is humid, some evaporation occurs. Maximal volatilization is found when humid air is passed over wet soil (Harris and Lichtenstein, 1961; Lichtenstein, 1966) (see Section 6.2.2.3).

Temperature. Temperature influences loss of pesticides through volatilization and through chemical and biochemical changes. No loss of aldrin or heptachlor was observed from soils kept frozen for 6 months. However, loss occurred at 6°C and was progressively more rapid in samples held at 26°C and at 46°C. For example, the proportion of the applied dose of aldrin remaining after 56 days at the four temperatures was 100, 63, 38, and 10%, respectively (Lichtenstein and Schultz, 1959b).

Actual measurement of evaporated material has established the importance of increasing temperature in increasing the volatility of pesticides from soils (Harris and Lichtenstein, 1961).

The temperature of soils at the surface may be higher than one might think. The temperature of soils may reach 59 to 62°C (Bartholic et al., 1972; Wiegand et al., 1968). The surface of desert soil may be over 70°C, but such soil is less likely than crop soils to be treated with pesticides.

Air Movement. The rate of pesticide volatilization from soil is dependent on the rate at which air passes over it. Under laboratory conditions, the proportions of aldrin that evaporated from soil samples during a fixed interval under standardized conditions were <0.5, 4.4, and 6.3%, when the rates of airflow were 0.0, 0.5, and 1.5 liters per minute, respectively.

Cover Crops. Cover crops tend to retard the loss of pesticides from soil, presumably by reducing surface temperature and air movement, and thus reducing volatilization. In a 3-year field test, alfalfa reduced loss of aldrin and heptachlor by two- to three-fold (Lichtenstein et al., 1962). The difference was accentuated when the experiment was extended 7 or more years (Lichtenstein et al., 1971b).

Cultivation. Cultivation of the soil promotes evaporation of pesticides. Daily discing of a loam soil for 3 months after the application of insecticides at the rate of 4.5 kg/ha resulted in a reduction after 4 months of 71% in a residue of aldrin plus resulting dieldrin, and 44% in a residue of DDT as compared to losses of 53 and 26%, respectively, from fields that were not disced repeatedly, but were mixed initially to the same depth (Lichtenstein and Schulz, 1961). Even a single discing in the course of a 15-year period following single applications of DDT and aldrin produced a significant reduction of the residue recoverable from the soil 10 years later (Lichtenstein et al., 1971c).

The fact that cover crops and cultivation have so much effect on soil residues is evidence for the importance of volatilization (see Section 6.2.2.3), as a factor in removing pesticides from soil and dispersing them in the air.

Leaching. Whether water that passes through soil containing a pesticide residue will remove any of the compound depends on its solubility and concentration (Lichtenstein *et al.*, 1966). Leaching is most noticeable in sandy soil and least noticeable in muck soils (Lichtenstein, 1958). The mobility of compounds in each kind of soil can be learned rapidly by measuring their R values following chromatography with water on thin layers of that soil. The results correlate well with measurements under field conditions (Helling and Turner, 1968).

Not all downward movement of pesticides in soil can be attributed to leaching. Volatile compounds such as lindane and parathion disperse in soils even in the absence of water. This movement is not only downward but upward and sideways also (Lichtenstein, 1958).

Volatilization from Soil. Factors that determine volatilization are discussed in Section 6.2.2.3.

It is common knowledge that biotransformation products of pesticides produced by microorganisms can be extracted from soils and identified and measured in the usual way. It is not so well known that, whereas volatilization is frequently deduced from the observed disappearance of pesticides from soils, the evaporated materials have been collected from the air and measured chemically and by bioassay. Such studies have established the fact of volatilization under field conditions, and have made it possible (at least under laboratory conditions) to account for essentially 100% of a pesticide in terms of the sum of material remaining in the soil and the material progressively lost by evaporation. The quantitative importance of volatilization may be great. For example, in 7 days under laboratory conditions at a temperature of only 22°C, 16% of the original residue of aldrin was recovered from air passed over loam, and 38% was recovered from air passed over sand (Harris and Lichtenstein, 1961).

Even after mixing with soil to a depth of 15.24 cm, some chlorinated hydrocarbon insecticides could be recovered from the air above test plots for long periods. The concentrations of all the compounds studied were relatively high the day after application. The concentrations of endrin fell rapidly at first, and then more gradually throughout the 77-day period of observation. The concentrations of DDT and DDD fell precipitously by the second day, and only very slowly and irregularly thereafter, being easily measurable over 6 months later. No study was made to determine when these concentrations became undetectable, but concentrations 30 cm above the surface were consistently lower than those at 10 cm, indicating concentration gradients (Willis *et al.*, 1971).

Once DDT and DDD had been applied to the soil of test plots, they could be detected in slightly higher concentrations above non-flooded than above flooded plots (Willis *et al.*, 1971).

Microbiological Activity. Many pesticides are metabolized by microorganisms. In some instances, a pesticide may be used as a source of energy by bacteria or yeasts. Selection may lead to the formulation of a strain more efficient than the original population in metabolizing a given compound or group of compounds, but, as discussed below, use of such strains offers practical difficulty.

Anything that limits the activity of soil microorganisms will delay the loss of pesticides from the soil. Thus, drying, autoclaving, chilling (Lichtenstein and Schultz, 1959b, 1960, 1964; Guenzi and Beard, 1967), or the application of various bactericides reduces the loss of residues. Laboratory studies show that relatively high levels of many insecticides inhibit the growth of soil fungi. The degree of inhibition may or may not be sufficient to interfere with the breakdown of pesticides. The concentration of aldrin, lindane, parathion, phorate, and carbaryl that failed to cause significant inhibition of two species of fungus varied from 1 to 20 ppm (Cowley and Lichtenstein, 1970).

The rate at which degradation of pesticides can occur in some soils is astonishing. For example, using radioactive DDT and incubation at 30°C under anaerobic conditions (20% CO_2 and 80% N_2) the proportion of added p,p'-DDT recovered in the form of metabolites was 8.5% after 2 weeks and 37.6% after 4 weeks, with no degradation detected in an autoclaved control. DDD was by far the most abundant metabolite found (35% of original material at 4 weeks), but the following additional compounds (listed in decreasing order of abundance) were found also: p,p'-dichlorobenzophenone, dicofol, p'-chlorobenzoic acid, DDA, DDE, and p,p'-dichlorodiphenylmethane. An increasing proportion of the original material was not measured at each successive sampling; total measured recovery was only 57% at 4 weeks. At least part of the loss resulted from further metabolism of DDT, for some radioactivity was found in the water layer after the other products had been partitioned into hexane. The water-soluble materials were not isolated and identified. Volatilization presumably was not involved in the loss; no radioactivity was found in a hexane trap or in NaOH trap for CO_2, through which the mixture of carbon dioxide and nitrogen passed over the soil had been bubbled during incubation (Guenzi and Beard, 1967).

Different microorganisms may promote different reactions of the same compounds. Thus, yeast is primarily responsible for the reduction of parathion to aminoparathion; bacteria apparently have no effect on this reduction, although they are active in other reactions leading to complete decomposition of the compound (Lichtenstein and Schulz, 1964).

Because the toxicity of metabolites may be different from that of the parent compound, biotransformation of a pesticide may lead to a lack of correspondence between the results of chemical analyses and bioassays of treated soil. Thus, it was found that lindane in soil became progressively less toxic than the results of wet chemical analysis indicated, because the chemical method detected the nontoxic metabolites formed by soil organisms. Conversely, aldrin-treated soil became temporarily more toxic because of the greater toxicity of the dieldrin formed from it (Lichtenstein and Schulz, 1959, 1960).

The reason that soils in nature are not even more effective in breaking down pesticides was explained largely or perhaps completely by Anderson and Lichtenstein (1972). To do this they used a strain of *Mucor alternans* that had been isolated from DDT-contaminated soil and that, in pure culture, was able to degrade DDT to water-soluble metabolites (Anderson *et al.*, 1970). When the spores of this fungus were added to DDT-contaminated soil, its insecticide-degrading capacity was no longer evident. Of various insecticides and related compounds added separately to cultures of *M. alternans*, only lindane, parathion, and Dyfonate caused a reduction of DDT degradation by the fungus without severely reducing its vegetative growth. However, eight other fungi, including some capable of degrading DDT, partially or completely inhibited degradation by *M. alternans*. Although the cell-free media from the stale cultures of some fungi, including *M. alternans*, degrade DDT, the addition of these filtrates from some fungi inhibited degradation by pure cultures of *M. alternans* (Anderson and Lichtenstein, 1972).

The ultimate explanation may lie in the availability of nutritional factors to organisms inherently capable of degrading a particular compound. For example, in pure culture, *M. alternans* is not capable of using DDT as its only source of carbon, but is efficient in degrading it in the presence of glucose and ammonium nitrate. When other sugars (except ribose) are substituted for glucose, or

other sources of nitrogen are substituted for ammonium nitrate, the production of metabolites is reduced. The kind of metabolites produced is the same in the presence of different sugars but varies in connection with some sources of nitrogen (Anderson and Lichtenstein, 1971).

Since there is no practical possibility of maintaining a pure culture of one microorganism in natural soils, and since many kinds of microorganisms interfere with the degradation of pesticides, the problem of achieving and maintaining a favorable ecological balance obviously is extremely complex.

Absorption and Translocation. These factors are discussed in Section 6.1.2.2.

6.3.2.3 Distribution of Residues in the Mud Walls of Houses.

An astonishingly high proportion of homes in the world are made of mud. The distribution and fate of insecticides in dried mud used for this purpose are not different from those that would be in effect if the same compound were applied in the same way to the same soil held under the same conditions—but for a different purpose. However, the practical requirements and conditions relevant to insecticidal residues on walls are so different from those associated with residues in agricultural soils, or in soils treated for termite control, that some special discussion is required.

The soils available for building purposes vary greatly in their adsorptive properties, but many of them, especially red lateritic soils, adsorb DDT, BHC, dieldrin, and a wide range of other chlorinated hydrocarbon, organic phosphorus, and carbamate insecticides so rapidly that soon only a nonlethal concentration remains at the surface available to insects. Thus, adsorption of 10 to 20-μm crystals of BHC by an Uganda clay required only 24 hours at 25°C, and DDT disappeared in a few days. Almost the entire dosage could be recovered from the clay, chiefly the top 2.5 mm. The adsorption was more rapid when the relative humidity of the ambient air was low, and slower when the humidity was high (Hadaway and Barlow, 1951; 1963a, 1963b; Barlow and Hadaway, 1955; 1958; Miles and Pearce, 1957). Early analyses of successive layers of clay showed that the depth to which dieldrin penetrated was greatest when the humidity was high (Barlow and Hadaway, 1956), but later measurements (Miles and Pearce, 1957; Miles, 1969) showed a more consistent result; greater penetration and less DDT remained at the surface when the humidity was low. The inconsistency cannot be explained on the basis of available data; the difference may have been related to the difference in compound, differences in the kinds of soil, or both. It may be that some compounds are so strongly adsorbed by certain soils that they are free to diffuse only when the humidity is high.

Compounds of low volatility such as DDT become unavailable to insects when their crystals are no longer microscopically visible on the clay surface, but more volatile compounds such as BHC retain a fumigant action after the crystals are no longer seen (Hadaway and Barlow, 1951).

Under absolutely dry conditions, DDT is catalytically decomposed to DDE in soil with a high iron content (Hadaway and Barlow, 1951). Although this indicates that the insecticide is present in the clay as a highly reactive surface layer, it is generally considered (Barlow and Hadaway, 1955) that adsorption rather than decomposition is more important in the inactivation of insecticides on mud walls. It was observed first in the field (Pal and Sharma, 1952), and later in the laboratory (Hadaway and Barlow, 1963a; Barlow and Hadaway, 1956), that the leathality of an insecticide-treated, dried mud surface to insects could be restored or increased by increasing the relative humidity of the surrounding air, and the change was almost complete in 24 hours. The increase in biological activity occurs at about the same rate as the increase in water content of the dry clay exposed to air of high humidity (Barlow and Hadaway, 1958). The logarithms of the LT 50 of a number of insecticides decreased linearly with increasing humidity (Gerolt, 1961; Hadaway and Barlow, 1963a). It is not certain whether the concentration of insecticide is increased, or whether the compound already at the surface is merely more available to the insect. Some evidence indicates that the concentration at the surface is actually decreased (Barlow and Hadaway, 1956), basically unchanged (Gerolt, 1961), or slightly increased (Miles and Pearce, 1957). It may be that the observed differences were caused by the obviously different conditions of the experiments. The two latter experiments were based on radiological techniques, ensuring that only the surface layer was measured. In the study by Miles and Pearce, the insecticide was applied to the surface as is true in house spraying and, therefore, it was unequally distributed in the clay. In the study by Gerolt, the distribution of insecticide in the clay was initially homogeneous. Gerolt concluded that the pesticide moved only in association with water vapor, so that the concentration at the surface returned to its original level when the water content of the clay reached equilibrium with that of the air, regardless of whether the air was moist or dry. In any event, it is clear that insects actually pick up more insecticide from a particular residue when the humidity is high (Gerolt, 1963).

Although the method apparently never has become popular, the availability of insecticides on sorptive mud surfaces may be increased by formulating them as water-wettable powders ground from a resin or similar material with which the poison has been melted to form a homogeneous mass. The resin holds the insecticide against the adsorptive force of the clay. Even with such resin formulations, release to insects is promoted by high humidity (Gerolt, 1957, 1963).

6.4 Importance of Residues in Different Media

6.4.1 Importance to Man

Campbell and his colleagues (1965) estimated that over 90% of the DDT stored by the general population is obtained from food. This is consistent with the measured intake from food and water at about the time Campbell had in mind, that is, 0.04 mg/man/day from food, and less than 0.000046 mg/man/day from water. It is also consistent with the fact that, at most, only traces of DDT have been measured in air except the air of work places. Actual exposure of ordinary people must be somewhat less than estimates for cities (0.00006 mg/man/day), or for small agricultural communities (0.00050 mg/man/day), based on the highest concentrations measured in the air of these places. A number of other investigators (Durham et al., 1965; Morgan and Roan, 1970) have concluded independently that food is the major source of intake of pesticides for the general population.

Dietary intake of pesticides found as residues in ordinary food constitutes a base to which other kinds of exposure may be added, but if there is exposure in excess of the average, that, too, may be dietary. The fact that ordinary commercial food tends to have slightly less DDT in some states than in others is discussed in Section 6.1.5.1. In some instances, locally produced foods contain high residues, either as a result of direct application of a pesticide to the crop, or because the "crop" is contaminated secondarily. An example of secondary contamination was reported in connection with eggs laid by chickens raised for home use in an orchard area where

DDT was used extensively (see Section 6.1.5.2).

Of course, not all additional exposure is dietary. The major exposure of applicators and formulators is not oral (see Sections 6.2.3.1 and 6.2.3.2). Clearly, a variety of possibilities exist for different groups of people. Considerable evidence indicates that populations are not homogeneous in relation to pesticide intake. Deichmann and his colleagues (Deichmann and Radomski, 1968; Radomski *et al.*, 1968) in a study of the general population reported that persons of unstated race who stored DDT, and especially DDE, in relatively high concentrations were found, on retrospective investigation, to have used household insecticides much more consistently that was true of persons whose storage of DDT and DDE was low. The same relationship was not detectable for dieldrin and heptachlor epoxide, compounds not normally found in formulations intended for home usage. Working in the same community, Davies and Edmundson (Davies *et al.*, 1969; Edmundson *et al.*, 1970) found that high storage of DDT and especially DDE was characteristic of Negroes, and that these people, in turn, were heavy users of household insecticides. They are heavy users of household insecticides in other USA communities also (Keil *et al.*, 1969).

Edmundson *et al.* (1970) considered that environmental contamination, especially in the house, contributes substantially to the magnitude of storage levels, even when the occupants fail to recall using pesticides. The authors reported a study in which a cat was placed in a home where the occupants all had relatively low blood levels of DDE, and another cat from the same litter was put in a home where the children all had high DDE levels. Both cats were fed the same commercial cat food. Of course, both cats licked their fur and thus ingested whatever dust they picked up. After 4 months of exposure, the blood levels of the first cat remained low and constant, while those of the second cat showed a 10-fold increase of DDT and a 3-fold increase of DDE.

In another study, the correlations between residues of DDT in serum of people in the general population and either residues in their food or residues in dust collected in their homes were reported to be of the same order of magnitude but both slightly less than required to give statistical significance (Warnick, 1972). The meaning of these findings is difficult to determine, particularly since details were not published.

Even when the importance of household insecticides as a source of increased storage has been demonstrated, one cannot conclude without further evidence that the significant, added exposure is by one particular route. Use of aerosols would permit respiratory exposure, but improper use of aerosols might contaminate food and greatly increase oral exposure. Residues of some compounds can be absorbed dermally from sprayed surfaces. In the last analysis, the importance of different residues and different exposures must be determined separately in each instance.

A different kind of evidence for absorption by the respiratory route and, by the same token, the possibility of a different approach to the question of the importance of respiratory exposure was offered by the observations of Casarett *et al.* (1968). They reported a greater concentration of DDT-related compounds in the lungs and pulmonary lymph nodes than would be predicted on the basis of their lipid content, and in some individuals they found a higher proportion of unmetabolized DDT in these than in other tissues. They considered both observations as indirect evidence of respiratory intake.

A discussion of criteria of the safety of pesticides under different conditions of exposure constitutes Section 7.5.

6.4.2 Importance to Other Organisms

6.4.2.1 Domestic Animals. Domestic animals are not unlike man in the ways in which they obtain pesticides. In general, feed constitutes their most important source of intake. Residues in the feed (whether in the form of pasture or harvested crops) may come from direct, intentional application or from drift, just as is true of man's food. Animals to which pesticides are applied for control of external parasites absorb these materials dermally to a degree depending on the individual compound and its dosage. In addition, some species, especially cats and cattle, lick themselves and thus ingest pesticides sprayed or dusted on them. In fact, Claborn *et al.* (1950) showed years ago that nearly all DDT sprayed on cattle and absorbed by them is ingested; experimentally absorption could be prevented almost entirely by preventing licking. Of course, not all compounds are so poorly absorbed by the skin. The respiratory tract has not been found an important route of exposure of domestic animals under ordinary circumstances. Acute poisoning by the respiratory route is rare but has been reported (see Section 10.1.2.2).

6.4.2.2 Wildlife. Because of the great differences among organisms spoken of as wildlife, and because of the great variety in habits even among those of the same class, few useful generalizations can be made about the importance of residues of pesticides in different media as sources of injury to wildlife. It is true that problems have been somewhat more frequent and severe in aquatic environments. In some instances, this is associated with the ability of some organisms to concentrate compounds directly from water, either by adsorption or by filtering from the water particulate matter on which compounds already are adsorbed. It is also true that biological magnification is a more important factor in connection with the food of many forms of wildlife than it is in connection with the food of man or domestic animals. This is mainly because the food chains of some wildlife are long and not subject to control (see Section 11.2.3), while those of man and domestic animals are short and supervised.

6.5 Degradation of Poisons in Nature

In this book, the breakdown of pesticides is considered in connection with the situations in which it occurs, that is, mainly in the mammal (much of Chapter 3), in the air (Section 6.2.2), and in the soil (Section 6.3.2). This arrangement permits a relevant discussion of other processes associated with elimination of these compounds in each situation, for example, excretion by the mammal and volatilization from the soil. The tests for biodegradability, the use of which should prevent future introduction of compounds that exhibit significant biological magnification, are mentioned in connection with wildlife (Section 11.2.3.2).

It remains to state that the degradation of natural, pesticidal, and other organic compounds in nature is an important matter in its own right, and it has been the subject of an excellent conference (National Academy of Sciences, 1972). There are striking similarities in the chemical mechanisms through which compounds synthesized by organisms or by man are broken down by mammals, insects, plants, microbes, or even by photooxidation. The similarities certainly are more important than the differences, but interesting differences do exist. For example, plants synthesize compounds better than they degrade them. Tyrosine and tryptophan are thought to be the only benzenoid compounds completely oxidized by mammals, which possess a far more restricted range of catabolic enzymes, especially ring-fission dioxygenases, than do

microorganisms. Collectively, microorganisms are more efficient than other organisms in degrading synthetic compounds of whatever origin. There is no way at this time to evaluate the relative importance of photooxidation and microorganisms in the degradation of even a single pesticide under the practical conditions of its use. However, it does seem clear that susceptibility of a compound to attack by microbes is not sufficient to prevent its accumulation in food chains. Metabolism by at least some organisms in each chain is required.

REFERENCES

Abbott, D. C., Harrison, R. B., Tatton, J. O'G., and Thomson, J. (1965). Organochlorine pesticides in the atmospheric environment. Nature, 208:1317–1318.

Acree, F., Jr., Beroza, M., Bowman, M. C. (1963). Codistillation of DDT with water. J. Agric. Food Chem., 11:278–280.

Allaway, W. H., Kubota, J., Losee, F., and Roth, M. (1968). Selenium, molybdenum, and vanadium in human blood. Arch. Environ. Health, 16:342–348.

Anderson, J. P. E., and Lichtenstein, E. P. (1971). Effect of nutritional factors on DDT-degradation by *Mucor alternans*. Can. J. Microbiol., 17:1291–1298.

Anderson, J. P. E., and Lichtenstein, E. P. (1972). Effects of various soil fungi and insecticides on the capacity of *Mucor alternans* to degrade DDT. Can. J. Microbiol., 18:553–560.

Anderson, J. P. E., Lichtenstein, E. P., and Whittingham, W. F. (1970). Effect of *Mucor alternans* on the persistence of DDT and dieldrin in culture and in soil. J. Econ. Entomol., 63:1595–1599.

Antommaria, P., Corn, M., and DeMaio, L. (1965). Airborne particulates in Pittsburgh: Association with p,p'-DDT. Science, 150:1476–1477.

Armstrong, J. F., Wolfe, H. R., Comer, S. W., and Staiff, D. C. (1973). Oral exposure of workers to parathion through contamination of food items. Bull. Environ. Contam. Toxicol., 10:321–327.

Balson, E. W. (1947). Studies in vapour pressure measurement, part III.—An effusion manometer sensitive to 5×10^{-6} millimetres of mercury: vapour pressure of D.D.T. and other slightly volatile substances. Trans. Faraday Soc., 43:54–60.

Barlow, F., and Hadaway, A. B. (1955). Studies on aqueous suspensions of insecticides. Part V. The sorption of insecticides by soils. Bull. Entomol. Res., 46:547–559.

Barlow, F., and Hadaway, A. B. (1956). Effect of changes in humidity on the toxicity and distribution of insecticides sorbed by some dried soils. Nature, 178:1299–1300.

Barlow, F., and Hadaway, A. B. (1958). Studies on aqueous suspensions of insecticides. Part VII. The influence of relative humidity upon the sorption of insecticides by soils. Bull. Entomol. Res., 49:333–354.

Barthel, W. F., Hawthorne, J. C., Ford, J. H., Bolton, G. C., McDowell, L. L., Grissinger, E. H., and Parsons, D. A. (1969). Pesticides in water. Pesticide Residues in sediments of the lower Mississippi River and its tributaries. Pestic. Monit. J., 3:8–66.

Barthel, W. F., Murphy, R. T., Mitchell, W. G., and Corley, C. (1960). The fate of heptachlor in the soil following granular application to the surface. J. Agric. Food Chem., 8:445–447.

Bartholic, J. F., Namken, L. N., and Wiegand, C. L. (1972). Aerial thermal scanner to determine temperatures of soils and of crop canopies differing in water stress.

Agron. J., 64:603–608.

Batchelor, G. S., and Walker, K. C. (1954). Hazards involved in use of parathion in fruit orchards of North Central Washington. Arch. Ind. Hyg., 10:522–529.

Batchelor, G. S., Walker, K. C., and Elliott, J. W. (1956). Dinitroorthocresol exposure from apple-thinning sprays. Arch. Ind. Health, 13:593–596.

Bowman, M. C., Acree, F., Jr., Lofgren, C. S., and Beroza, M. (1964). Chlorinated insecticides: Fate in aqueous suspensions containing mosquito larvae. Science, 146:1480–1481.

Bowman, M. C., Acree, F., Jr., Schmidt, C. H., Beroza, M. (1959). Fate of DDT in larvacide suspensions. J. Econ. Entomol., 52:1038–1042.

Braus, H., Middleton, E. M., and Walton, G. (1951). Organic chemical compounds in raw and filtered surface waters. J. Anal. Chem., 23:1160–1164.

Breidenbach, A. W., and Lichtenberg, J. J. (1963). DDT and dieldrin in rivers—a report of the National Water Quality Network. Science, 141:899–901.

Bright, N. F. H., Cuthill, J. C., and Woodbury, N. H. (1950). The vapour pressure of parathion and related compounds. J. Sci. Food Agric. 1:344–348.

Butler, P. A. (1969). Monitoring pesticide pollution. Bio. Sci., 19:889–891.

Campbell, J. E., Richardson, L. A., and Schafer, M. L. (1965). Insecticide residues in the human diet. Arch. Environ. Health, 10:831–836.

Caplan, P. E., Culver, D., and Thielen, W. C. (1956). Human exposures in populated areas during airplane application of malathion. Arch. Ind. Health, 14:326–332.

Carollo, J. A. (1945). The removal of DDT from water supplies. J. Am. Water Works. Assoc., 37:1310–1317.

Casarett, L. J., Fryer, G. C., Yauger, W. L., Klemmer, H. W. (1968). Organochlorine pesticide residues in human tissues—Hawaii. Arch: Environ. Health, 17:306–311.

Claborn, H. V., Beckman, M. F., Wells, R. W., Radeleff, R. D., and Nickerson, W. J. (1950). Excretion of DDT and TDE in milk from cows treated with these insecticides. J. Econ. Entomol., 43:850–852.

Clifford, P. A. (1957). Pesticide residues in fluid market milk. Public Health Rep., 72:729–734.

Clifford, P. A., Bassen, J. L., and Mills, P. A. (1959). Chlorinated organic pesticide residues in fluid milk. Public Health Rep., 74:1109–1114.

Cohen, J. M., and Pinkerton, C. (1966). Widespread translocation of pesticides by air transport and rainout. Adv. Chem. Ser., 60:163–176.

Corneliussen, P. E. (1969). Residues in food and feed. (IV) Pesticide residues in total diet samples. Pestic. Monit. J., 2:140–152.

Cory, L., Fjeld, P, and Serat, W. (1970). Distribution patterns of DDT residues in the Sierra Nevada Mountains. Pestic. Monit. J., 3:204–211.

Cowley, G. T., and Lichtenstein, E. P. (1970). Growth inhibition of soil fungi by insecticides and annulment of inhibition by yeast extract or nitrogenous nutrients. J. Gen. Microbiol., 62:27–34.

Culver, D., Caplan, P., and Batchelor, G. W. (1956). Studies of human exposure during aerosol application of malathion and chlorthion. Arch. Ind. Health, 13:37–50.

Cummings, J. G. (1965). Total diet study. Pesticide residues in total diet samples. J. Assoc. Off. Anal. Chem., 48:1177–1180.

Davies, J. E., Edmundson, W. F., Maceo, A., Barquet, A., and Cassady, J. (1969). An epidemiologic application of the study of DDE levels in whole blood. Am. J. Public Health, 59:435–441.

Decker, G. C., Bruce, W. N., and Bigger, J. H. (1965). The accumulation and dissipation of residues resulting from the use of aldrin in soils. J. Econ. Entomol., 58:266–271.

Decker, G. C., Weinman, C. J., and Bann, J. M. (1950). A preliminary report on the rate of insecticide residue loss from treated plants. J. Econ. Entomol., 43:919–927.

Deichmann, W. B., and Radomski, J. L. (1968). Retention of pesticides in human adipose tissue—preliminary report. Ind. Med. Surg., 37:218–219.

Dickinson, W. (1956). The ionization constants of phenol and of some substituted phenols. Trans. Faraday Soc., 52:31–35.

Duce, R. A., Quinn, J. G., Olney, C. E., Piotrowicz, S. R., Ray, B. J., and Wade, T. L. (1972). Enrichment of heavy metals and organic compounds in the surface microlayer of Narragansett Bay, Rhode Island. Science, 176:161–163.

Duggan, R. E. (1967). Residues in food and feed: Chlorinated pesticide residues in fluid milk and other dairy products in the United States. Pestic. Monit. J., 1(3):2–8.

Duggan, R. E. (1968a). Residues in food and feed: Pesticide residues in vegetable oil seeds, oils, and by-products. Pestic. Monit. J., 1(4):2–7.

Duggan, R. E. (1968b). Residues in food and feed. Pesticide residue levels in food in the United States from July 1, 1963 to June 30, 1967. Pestic. Monit. J., 2:2–46.

Duggan, R. E., Barry, H. C., and Johnson, L. Y. (1966). Pesticide residues in total-diet samples. Science, 151:101–104.

Duggan, R. E., Barry, H. C., and Johnson, L. Y. (1967). Residues in food and feed: Pesticide residues in total diet samples. Pestic. Monit. J., 1(2):2–14.

Duggan, R. E., and Cornelliussen, P. E. (1972). Dietary intake of pesticide chemicals in the United States (III), June 1968–April 1970. Pestic. Monit. J., 5:331–341.

Duggan, R. E., and Lipscomb, G. Q. (1969). Dietary Intake of Pesticide Chemicals in the United States (II), June 1966–April 1968. Pestic. Monit. J., 2:153–162.

Duggan, R. E., Lipscomb, G. Q., Cox, E. L., Heatwole, R. E., and Kling, R. C. (1971). Residues in food and feed. Pesticide residue levels in foods in the United States from July 1, 1963 to June 30, 1969. Pestic. Monit. J., 5:73–212.

Duggan, R. E., and McFarland, F. J. (1967). Residues in food and feed. Assessments include raw food and feed commodities, market basket items prepared for consumption, meat samples taken at slaughter. Pestic. Monit. J., 1(1):1–5.

Duggan, R. E., and Weatherwax, J. R. (1967). Dietary intake of pesticide chemicals: Calculated daily consumption of pesticides with foods is discussed and compared with currently accepted values. Science, 157:1006–1010.

Durham, W. F., Armstrong, J. F., Quinby, G. E. (1965). DDT and DDE content of complete prepared meals. Arch. Environ. Health, 11:641–647.

Durham, W. F., Armstrong, J. F., Upholt, W. M., and Heller, C. (1961). Insecticide content of diet and body fat of Alaskan natives. Science, 134:1880–1881.

Durham, W. F., and Wolfe, H. R. (1962). Measurement of the exposure of workers to pesticides. Bull. WHO, 26:75–91.

Dyte, C. E., and Tyler, P. R. (1960). The contamination of flour by insecticidal lacquers containing endrin and dieldrin. J. Sci. Food Agric., 11:745–750.

Eden, W. G., and Arant, F. S. (1948). DDT residues on alfalfa. J. Econ. Entomol., 41:383–387.

Edmundson, W. F., Davies, J. E., Maceo, A., and Morgade, C. (1970). Drug and environmental effects on DDT residues in human blood. South. Med. J., 63:1440–1441.

Edson, E. F. (1964). No-effect levels of three organophosphates in the rat, pig, and man. Food Cosmet. Toxicol., 2:311–316.

Edwards, C. A., Beck, S. D., and Lichtenstein, E. P. (1957). Bioassay of aldrin and lindane in soil. J. Econ. Entomol., 50:622–626.

Fahey, J. E., Butcher, J. W., and Turner, M. E. (1968). Pesticides in soil. Pestic. Monit. J., 1(4):30–33.

FAO/WHO (1970). Pesticide Residues in Food. WHO Tech Rept. Ser. No. 458.

Fletcher, T. E., Press, J. M., and Wilson, D. B. (1959). Exposure of spraymen to dieldrin in residual spraying. Bull. WHO, 20:15–25.

Frazier, B. E., Chesters, G., and Lee, G. B. (1970). "Apparent" organochlorine insecticide contents of soils samples in 1910. Pestic. Monit. J., 4:67–70.

Frear, D. E. H., Connell, W. A., Fertig, S. N., and Pepper, B. B. (1963). *Pesticide Residue Investigations on Raw Agricultural Commodities*. Pennsylvania State University, University Park, Pa.

Frisbie, W. S. (1936). Federal control of spray residues on fruits and vegetables. Am. J. Public Health, 26:369–373.

Gerolt, P. (1957). Improved persistence of dieldrin deposits on sorptive mud surface. Nature, 180:394–395.

Gerolt, P. (1961). Investigation into the problem of insecticide sorption by soils. Bull. WHO, 24:577–592.

Gerolt, P. (1963). Entomology: influence of relative humidity on the uptake of insecticides from residual films. Nature, 197:721.

Graham-Bryce, I. J. (1968). Movement of systemic insecticides through soil to plant roots. Soc. Chem. Ind. Monogr., 29:251–267.

Guenzi, W. D., and Beard, W. E. (1967). Anaerobic biodegradation of DDT to DDD in soil. Science, 156:1116–1117.

Hadaway, A. B., and Barlow, F. (1951). Sorption of solid insecticides by dried mud. Nature, 167:854.

Hadaway, A. B., and Barlow, F. (1963a). The influence of environmental conditions on the contact toxicity of some insecticide deposits to adult mosquitos, *Anopheles Stephensi List*. Bull. Entomol. Res., 54:329–344.

Hadaway, A. B., and Barlow, F. (1963b). The residual action of two organophosphorus compounds and a carbamate on dried muds. Bull. WHO, 28:69–76.

Hamaker, J. W. (1966). Mathematical prediction of cumulative levels of pesticides in soil. In: *Organic Pesticides in the Environment*, pp. 122–131. American Chemical Society, Washington, DC.

Harman, S. W. (1946). DDT for codling moth control in Western New York in 1945. J. Econ. Entomol., 39:208–219.

Harris, C. R., and Lichtenstein, E. P. (1961). Factors affecting the volatilization of insecticidal residues from soils. J. Econ. Entomol., 54:1038–1045.

Hartley, G. S. (1969). Evaporation of pesticides. In: *Pesticidal Formulations Research*, edited by R. F. Gould, pp. 115–134. Adv. Chem. Ser. 86, American Chemical Society, Washington, DC.

Hayes, W. J., Jr. (1959). Pharmacology and toxicology of DDT. In: *DDT, the Insecticide Dichlorodipenyltrichloroethane and its Significance*, edited by P. Muller, Vol. 2, pp. 9–247. Birkhauser Verlag, Basel.

Hayes, W. J., Jr. (1966). Monitoring food and people for pesticide content. In: *Scientific Aspects of Pest Control*, pp. 314–342. Publ. 1402, National Academy of Sciences-National Research Council, Washington, DC.

Hayes, W. J., Jr., Dale, W. E., and Pirkle, C. I. (1971). Evidence of safety of long-term, high, oral doses of DDT for man. Arch. Environ. Health, 22:119–135.

Hayes, W. J., Jr., Durham, W. F., and Cueto, C., Jr. (1956). The effect of known repeated oral doses of chlorophenothane (DDT) in man. J. A. M. A., 162:890–897.

Hayes, W. J., Jr., Quinby, G. E., Walker, K. C., Elliott, J. W., and Upholt, W. M. (1958). Storage of DDT and DDE in people with different degrees of exposure to DDT. Arch. Ind. Health, 18:398–406.

Helling, C. S., and Turner, B. C. (1968). Pesticide mobility: determination by soil thin-layer chromatography. Science, 162:562–563.

Henderson, C., Inglis, A., and Johnson, W. L. (1971). Residues in fish, wildlife, and estuaries. Pestic. Monit. J., 5:1–11.

Hess, A. D., and Keener, G. G., Jr. (1947). Effect of airplane-distributed DDT thermal aerosols on fish and fish food organisms. J. Wildl. Manage., 11:1–10.

Hoffman, C. H., and Merkel, E. P. (1948). Fluctuations in insect populations associated with aerial applications of DDT to forests. J. Econ. Entomol., 41:464–473.

Hoffman, C. H., and Surber, E. W. (1948). Effects of an aerial application of wettable DDT on fish and fish-food organisms in Back Creek, West Virginia. Trans. Am. Fish. Soc., 75:48–58.

Hunter, C. G., Robinson, J., and Roberts, M. (1969). Pharmacodynamics of dieldrin (HEOD). Arch. Environ. Health, 18:12–21.

Ivie, G. W., and Casida, J. E. (1970). Enhancement of photoalteration of cyclodiene insecticide chemical residues by rotenone. Science, 167:1620–1622.

Jegier, Z. (1964a). Exposure to guthion during spraying and formulating. Arch. Environ. Health, 8:565–569.

Jegier, Z. (1964b). Health hazards in insecticide spraying of crops. Arch. Environ. Health, 8:670–674.

Kallman, B. J., and Andrews, A. K. (1963). Reductive dechlorination of DDT to DDE by yeast. Science, 141:1050–1051.

Keil, J. E., Finklea, J. F., Pietxch, R. L., and Gadsden, R. H. (1969). A pesticide use survey of urban households. J. Agric. Chem., 24:10–12.

Laubscher, J. A., Dutt, G. R., and Roan, C. C. (1971). Chlorinated insecticide residues in wildlife and soil as a function of distance from application. Pestic. Monit. J., 5:251–258.

Lichtenberg, J. L., Eichelberger, J. W., Dressman, R. C., and Longbottom, J. E. (1970). Pesticides in surface waters of the United States—a 5-year summary, 1964–68. Pestic. Monit. J., 4:71–86.

Lichtenstein, E. P. (1957). DDT accumulation in midwestern orchard and crop soils treated since 1945. J. Econ. Entomol., 50:545–547.

Lichtenstein, E. P. (1958). Movement of insecticides in soils under leaching and non-leaching conditions. J. Econ. Entomol., 51:380–383.

Lichtenstein, E. P. (1959). Absorption of some chlorinated hydrocarbon insecticides from soils into crops. J. Agric. Food Chem., 7:430–433.

Lichtenstein, E. P. (1966). Persistence and degradation of pesticides in the environment. Sci. Asp. Pest Control, 221–229.

Lichtenstein, E. P., and Corbett, J. R. (1969). Enzymatic conversion of aldrin to dieldrin with subcellular components of pea plants. J. Agric. Food Chem., 17:589–594.

Lichtenstein, E. P., DePew, L. J., Eshbaugh, E. L., and Sleesman, J. P. (1960). Persistence of DDT, aldrin, and lindane in some midwestern soils. J. Econ. Entomol., 53:136–142.

Lichtenstein, E. P., Fuhremann, T. W., and Schulz, K. R. (1971c). Persistence and vertical distribution of DDT, lindane, and aldrin residues, 10 and 15 years after a single soil application. J. Agric. Food Chem., 19:718–721.

Lichtenstein, E. P., Mueller, C. H., Myrdal, G. R., and Schulz, K. R. (1962). Vertical distribution and persistence of insecticidal residues in soils as influenced by mode of application and a cover crop. J. Econ. Entomol., 55:215–219.

Lichtenstein, E. P., Myrdal, G. R., and Schulz, K. R. (1965a). Absorption of insecticidal residues from contaminated soils into five carrot varieties. J. Agric. Food Chem., 13:126–131.

Lichtenstein, E. P., and Polivka, J. B. (1959). Persistence of some chlorinated hydrocarbon insecticides in turf soils. J. Econ. Entomol., 52:289–293.

Lichtenstein, E. P., and Schulz, K. R. (1959a). Breakdown of lindane and aldrin in soils. J. Econ. Entomol., 52:118–124.

Lichtenstein, E. P., and Schulz, K. R. (1959b). Persistence of some chlorinated hydrocarbon insecticides as influenced by soil types, rate of application and temperature. J. Econ. Entomol., 52:124–131.

Lichtenstein, E. P., and Schulz, K. R. (1960). Epoxidation of aldrin and heptachlor in soils as influenced by autoclaving, moisture, and soil types, J. Econ. Entomol., 53:192–197.

Lichtenstein, E. P., and Schulz, K. R. (1961). Effect of soil cultivation, soil surface and water on the persistence of insecticidal residues in soils. J. Econ. Entomol., 54:517–522.

Lichtenstein, E. P., and Schulz, K. R. (1964). The effects of moisture and microorganisms on the persistence and metabolism of some organophosphorus insecticides in soils, with special emphasis on parathion. J. Econ. Entomol., 57:618–627.

Lichtenstein, E. P., and Schulz, K. R. (1965). Residues of aldrin and heptachlor in soils and their translocation into various crops. J. Agric. Food Chem., 13:57–63.

Lichtenstein, E. P., and Schulz, K. R. (1970). Volatilization of insecticides from various substrates. J. Agric. Food Chem., 18:814–818.

Lichtenstein, E. P., Schulz, K. R., and Fuhremann, T. W. (1971a). Long-term effects of carbon in reducing uptake of insecticidal soil residues by crops. J. Econ. Entomol., 64:585–588.

Lichtenstein, E. P., Schulz, K. R., and Fuhremann, T. W. (1971b). Pesticides in soil. Effects of a cover crop versus soil cultivation on the fate and vertical distribution of insecticide residues in soil 7 to 11 years after soil treatment. Pestic. Monit. J., 5:218–222.

Lichtenstein, E. P., Schulz, K. R., Fuhremann, T. W., and Liang, T. T. (1970). Degradation of aldrin and heptachlor in field soils during a ten-year period. J. Agric. Food Chem., 18:100–106.

Lichtenstein, E. P., Schulz, K. R., Skrentny, R. F., and Stitt, P. A. (1965b). Insecticidal residues in cucumbers and alfalfa grown on aldrin- or heptachlor-treated soils. J. Econ. Entomol., 58:742–746.

Lichtenstein, E. P., Schulz, K. R., Skrentny, R. F., and Tsukano, Y. (1966). Toxicity and fate of insecticidal residues in water. Arch. Environ. Health, 12:199–212.

Lipscomb, G. Q. (1968). Residues in food and feed—pesticide residues in prepared baby foods in the United States. Pestic. Monit. J., 2:104–108.

MacRitchie, F. (1969). Evaporation retarded by monolayers. Science, 163:929–930.

McGill, A. E. J., and Robinson, J. (1968). Organochlorine insecticide residues in complete prepared meals: a 12-month survey in S.E. England. Food Cosmet. Toxicol., 6:45–57.

McGill, A. E. J., Robinson, J., and Stein, M. (1969). Residues of dieldrin (HEOD) in complete prepared meals in Great Britain during 1967. Nature, 221:761–762.

McKinney, L. L., Eldridge, A. C., and Cowan, J. C. (1959). Cysteine Thioesters from chloroethylene. J. Am. Chem. Soc., 81:1423–1427.

Mauney, J. R. (1973). Personal communication.

Merck Index: An Encyclopedia of Chemicals and Drugs (1968), edited by P. G. Stetcher, Ed. 8. Merck Publishing Company, Rahway, NJ.

Middleton, F. M., and Lichtenberg, J. J. (1960). Measurements of organic contaminants in the Nation's rivers. Ind. Eng. Chem., 52:99A–102A.

Miles, J. W. (1969). Personal communication.

Miles, J. W., and Pearce, G. W. (1957). Rapid method for measurement of rate of sorption of DDT by mud surfaces. Science, 126:169–170.

Miles, J. W., and Sedlak, V. (1960). Cited in: Safe Use of Pesticides in Public Health. WHO Expert Committee on Pesticides. WHO Tech. Rep. Ser. No. 356, 1967.

Miller, L. L., and Narang, R. S. (1970). Induced photolysis of DDT. Science, 169:368–370.

Mills, P. A. (1963). Section C: Pesticide residue content, J. Assoc. Off. Anal. Chem., 46:749–767.

Mitchell, J. W., Hodgson, R. E., and Gaetjens, C. F. (1946). Tolerance of farm animals to food containing 2,4-dichlorophenoxyacetic acid. J. Anim. Sci., 5:226–232.

Moeller, H. C., and Rider, J. A. (1962). Plasma and red blood cell cholinesterase activity as indications of the threshold of incipient toxicity of ethyl-p-nitrophenyl thiobenzenephosphate (EPN) and malathion in human beings. Toxicol. Appl. Pharmacol., 4:123–130.

Morgan, D. P., and Roan, C. C. (1970). Chlorinated hydrocarbon pesticide residue in human tissues. Arch. Environ. Health, 20:452–457.

Mosier, A. R., Guenzi, W. D., and Miller, L. L. (1969). Photochemical decomposition of DDT by a free-radical mechanism. Science, 164:1083–1085.

Moubry, R. J., Myrdal, G. R., and Sturges, A. (1968). Residues in food and feed: rate of decline of chlorinated hydrocarbon pesticides in dairy milk. Pestic. Monit. J., 2:72–79.

Munro, I. C., and Morrison, A. B. (1967). Factors influencing the nutritional value of fish flour. V. Chlorocholine chloride, a toxic material in samples extracted with 1,2-dichloroethane. Can. J. Biochem., 45:1049–1053.

Murphy, R. T., Barthel, W. F., and Lofgren, C. S. (1962). Insecticide residues: residual studies in connection with successive applications of heptachlor for imported fire ant eradication. J. Agric. Food Chem., 10:5–7.

Nash, R. G., and Beall, M. L., Jr. (1970). Chlorinated hydrocarbon insecticides: root uptake versus vapor contamination of soybean foliage. Science, 168:1109–1111.

Nash, R. G., and Woolson, E. A. (1967). Persistence of chlorinated hydrocarbon insecticides in soils. Science, 157:924–927.

National Academy of Sciences (1972). Degradation of Synthetic Organic Molecules in the Biosphere. Washington, DC.

Nicholson, H. P., Grzenda, A. R., Lauer, G. J., Cox, W. S., and Teasley, J. I. (1964). Water pollution by insecticides in river and treated municipal water. Limnol. Oceanogr., 9:310–317.

Nishimoto, T., Uyeta, M., and Taue, S. (1966). Studies on the pesticide residues in food: Analysis of organochlorine pesticide residues by electron capture gas chromatography. J. Food Hyg. Soc. Japan, 7:152–162.

Norton, L. B., Bigelow, C. R., and Vincent, W. B. (1940). Partial vapor pressures from nicotine solutions at 25æ. J. Am. Chem. Soc., 62:261–264.

Pal, R., and Sharma, M. I. D. (1952). Rapid loss of biological effectiveness of DDT applied to mud surfaces. Indian J. Malariol., 6:251–263.

Peterle, T. J. (1969). DDT in Antarctic snow. Nature, 224:620.

Phillips, F. T., and Gillham, E. M. (1971). Persistence to rainwashing of DDT wettable powders. Pestic. Sci., 2:97–100.

Plimmer, J. R., Klingebiel, U. I., and Hummer, B. E. (1970). Photooxidation of DDT and DDE. Science, 167:67–69.

Quinby, G. E., Walker, K. C., and Durham, W. F. (1958). Public Health hazards involved in the use of organic phosphorus insecticides in cotton culture in the delta area of Mississippi. J. Econ. Entomol., 51:831–838.

Quinby, G. E., Loomis, T. A., and Brown, H. W. (1963). Oral occupational parathion poisoning treated with 2-PAM iodide (2-pyridine aldoxime methiodide). N. Engl. J. Med., 268:639–643.

Radomski, J. L., Deichmann, W. B., and Clizer, E. E. (1968). Pesticide concentrations in the liver, brain and adipose tissue of terminal hospital patients. Food Cosmet. Toxicol., 6:209–220.

Risebrough, R. W., Huggett, R. J., Griffin, J. J., and Goldberg, E. D. (1968). Pesticides: transatlantic movements in the Northeast trades. Science, 159:1233–1235.

Robeck, G. G., Dostal, K. A., Cohen, J. M., and Kreissl, J. F. (1965). Effectiveness of water treatment process in pesticide removal. J. Am. Water Works Assoc., 57:181–200.

Rosen, A. A., and Middleton, F. M. (1959). Chlorinated

insecticides in surface waters. J. Anal. Chem., 31:1729–1732.

Rowe, D. R., Canter, L. W., Snyder, P. J., and Mason, J. W. (1971). Dieldrin and endrin concentrations in a Louisiana estuary. Pestic. Monit. J., 4:177–183.

Scudder, H. I., and Tarzwell, C. M. (1950). Effects of DDT mosquito larviciding on wildlife. IV. The effects on terrestrial insect population of routine larviciding by airplane. Public Health Rep., 65:71–87.

Seabury, J. H. (1963). Toxicity of 2,4-dichlorophenoxyacetic acid for man and dog. Arch. Environ. Health, 7:202–209.

Seal, W. L., Dawsey, L. H., and Calvin, G. E. (1967). Pesticides in soil. Pestic. Monit. J., 1:22–25.

Sharangapani, M. V., and Pingale, S. V. (1954). The hazards of DDT-treatment of potatoes. Bull. Cent. Food Tech. Res. Inst. Mysore, 4(3):57.

Shepard, H. H. (1951). *The Chemistry and Action of Chemosterilants.* McGraw-Hill, New York.

Simpson, G. R. (1965). Exposure to orchard residues, dermal and inhalation exposures. Arch. Environ. Health, 10:884–885.

Simpson, G. R., and Beck, A. (1965). Exposure to parathion. Arch. Environ. Health, 11:784–786.

Smith, V. K. (1968). Pesticides in soil: long-term movement of DDT applied to soil for termite control. Pestic. Monit. J., 2:55–57.

Smith, V. K. (1973). Personal communication.

Spencer, W. F., and Cliath, M. M. (1969). Vapor density of dieldrin. Environ. Sci. Technol., 3:670–674.

Stanley, C. W., Barney II, J. E., Helton, M. R., and Yobs, A. R. (1971). Measurement of atmospheric levels of pesticides. Environ. Sci. Technol., 5:430–435.

Stein, A. A., Serrone, D. M., and Coulston, F. (1965). Safety evaluation of methoxychlor in human volunteers. Toxicol. Appl. Pharmacol., 7:499.

Stern, A. C. (ed.) (1968). *Air Pollution,* Vols. 1–3. Academic Press, Inc., New York.

Sumner, A. K., Saha, J. G., and Lee, Y. W. (1972). Mercury residues in fish from Saskatchewan waters with and without known sources of pollution in 1970. Pestic. Monit. J., 6:122–125.

Surber, E. W., and Friddle, D. D. (1949). Relative toxicity of suspension and oil formulations of DDT to native fishes in Black Creek, West Virginia. Trans. Am. Fish. Soc., 76:315–321.

Swackhamer, A. B. (1965). Report on pesticide residues in restaurant meals in Canada. Pestic. Prog., 3:108–114.

Tabor, E. C. (1965). Pesticides in urban atmospheres. J. Air Pollut. Control Assoc., 15:415. [Republished (1966). Contamination of urban air through the use of insecticides. Trans. NY Acad. Sci., 28:569–578.]

Talekar, N. S., and Lichtenstein, E. P. (1971). Influence of plant nutrition on lindane penetration and its translocation within pea plants. J. Agric. Food. Chem., 19:846–850.

Tarrant, K. R., and Tatton, J. O'G. (1968). Organochlorine pesticides in rainwater in the British Isles. Nature, 219:725–727.

Tarrant, R. F., Moore, D. G., Bollen, W. B., and Loper,B. R. (1972). Pesticides in soil. Pestic. Monit. J., 6:65–72.

Tarzwell, C. M. (1950). Effects of DDT mosquito larviciding on wildlife. V. Effects of fishes of the routine manual and airplane application of DDT and other mosquito larvicides. Public Health Rep., 65:231–255.

Trautmann, W. L., Chesters, G., and Pionke, H. B. (1968). Pesticides in soil: organochlorine insecticide composition of randomly selected soils from nine states–1967. Pestic. Monit. J., 2:93–96.

US Department of Agriculture, Agricultural Research Service (1966). *Monitoring Agricultural Pesticide Residues. A Preliminary Report of Studies on Soil, Sediment, and Water in Mississippi River Delta.* US Government Printing Office, Washington, DC.

Walker, K. C., Goette, M. B., and Batchelor, G. S. (1954). Pesticide residues in foods: dichlorodiphenyltrichloroethane and dichlorodiphenyldichloroethylene content of prepared meals. J. Agric. Food Chem., 2:1034–1037.

Ware, G. W., Estesen, B. J., and Cahill, W. P. (1971). DDT moratorium in Arizona—agricultural residues after 2 years. Pestic. Monit. J., 5:276–280.

Warnick, S. L. (1972). Organochlorine pesticide levels in hu·nan serum and adipose tissue, Utah—Fiscal years 1967–71. Pestic. Monit. J., 6:9–13.

Wassermann, M., Iliescu, S., Mandric, G., and Horvath, P. (1960). Toxic hazards during DDT- and BHC-spraying of forests against Lymantria Monacha. Arch. Ind. Health, 21:503–508.

Wassermann, M., Zellermayer, L., and Gon, M. (1963). L'étude de la toxicologie des pesticides en climat subtropical: I. L'intensité de l'exposition toxique pendant l'application de pesticides. In: *Proceedings of the 14th International Congress on Occupational Health,* Madrid. Excerpta Med. Int. Congr. Ser. No. 62:1728–1733.

Weaver, L., Gunnerson, C. G., Breidenbach, A. W., and Lichtenberg, J. J. (1965). Chlorinated hydrocarbon pesticides in major U. S. river basins. Public Health Rep., 80:481–493.

Wheatley, G. A., and Hardman, J. A. (1965). Indications of the presence of organochlorine insecticides in rainwater in Central England. Nature, 207:486–487.

Wiegand, C. L., Heilman, M. D., and Gerbermann, A. H. (1968). Detailed plant and soil thermal regime in agronomy. In: *Proceedings of the 5th Symposium on Remote Sensing of Environment,* pp. 325–342. University of Michigan, Ann Arbor.

Wiersma, G. B., Tai, H., and Sand, P. F. (1972a). Pesticide residues in soil from eight cities—1969. Pestic. Monit. J., 6:126–129.

Wiersma, G. B., Tai, H., and Sand, P. F. (1972b). Pesticide residue levels in soils, FY 1969—National Soils Monitoring Program. Pestic. Monit. J., 6:194–228.

Williams, S. (1964). Total diet study: pesticide residues in total diet samples, J. Assoc., Off. Anal. Chem., 47:815–821.

Willis, G. H., Parr, J. F., and Smith, S. (1971). Volatilization of soil-applied DDT and DDD from flooded and nonflooded plots. Pestic. Monit. J., 4:204–208.

Wilson, H. F., Allen, N. N., Bohstedt, G., Betheil, J., and Lardy, H. A. (1946a). Feeding experiments with DDT-treated pea vine silage with special reference to dairy cows, sheep, and laboratory animals. J. Econ. Entomol., 39(6):801–806.

Wilson, H. F., Srivastava, A. S., Hull, W. B., Betheil, J., and Lardy, H. A. (1946b). DDT residues on pea vines and canned peas from fields treated with DDT dusts. J. Econ. Entomol., 39:806–809.

Wolfe, H. R., Armstrong, J. F., and Durham, W. F. (1966). Pesticide exposure from concentrate spraying. Arch. Environ. Health, 13:340–344.

Wolfe, H. R., Armstrong, J. F., Staiff, D. C., and Comer,S. W. (1972). Exposure of spraymen to pesticides. Arch. Environ. Health, 25:29–31.

Wolfe, H. R., Durham, W. F., and Armstrong, J. F. (1963). Health hazards of the pesticides endrin and dieldrin: Hazards in some agricultural uses in the Pacific Northwest. Arch. Environ. Health, 6:458–464.

Wolfe, H. R., Durham, W. F., and Armstrong, J. F. (1967). Exposure of workers to pesticides. Arch. Environ. Health, 14:622–633.

Wolfe, H. R., Durham, W. F., and Batchelor, G. S. (1961). Health hazards of some dinitro compounds: effects associated with agricultural usage in Washington state. Arch. Environ. Health, 3:468–475.

Wolfe, H. R., Walker, K. C., Elliott, J. W., and Durham,W. F. (1959). Evaluation of the health hazards involved in house-spraying with DDT. Bull. WHO, 20:1–14.

7

RECOGNIZED AND POSSIBLE EFFECTS OF PESTICIDES IN MAN

The recognized harmful effects of pesticides in man are mortality and morbidity. Another recognized effect that may or may not be associated with injury is storage. Information on these matters may be obtained from official mortality statistics, reports of poison control centers and workers' compensation boards, and the results of special studies. In addition to these effects known to be caused by pesticides, it has been suspected that they cause certain other pharmacologically predictable effects.

It has been alleged that pesticides contribute to diseases or conditions that existed before the compounds were invented. It is the duty of the toxicologist to investigate quantitatively not only the epidemiology of recognized effects of toxicants, but also to explore even the most unlikely suggestion that toxicants contribute to illness other than recognized poisoning.

7.1 Incidence of Poisoning

7.1.1 Poisoning Generally

7.1.1.1 Mortality.

Relative Importance of Poisoning as a Cause of Mortality. Table 7-1 permits a comparison of the mortality rates (a) associated directly or indirectly with chemical poisoning; (b) associated with the major causes of death; and (c) associated with all causes combined. Deaths caused directly by chemicals are recorded, according to the Eighth Revision of International Classification of Diseases (National Center for Health Statistics, 1967), under at least 40 separate, three-digit classifications including one for food poisoning, two for alcoholism, one for other drug dependence, 10 for drugs, 10 for accidental poisoning by other solid and liquid substances (including separate headings for alcohol, pesticides, and noxious foods), eight for accidental poisoning by gases and vapors, one for accidents caused by bites and stings of venomous animals, three for suicide by chemicals, one for homicide by chemicals, and three for deaths by poisoning where it could not be determined whether they were accidental or purposely inflicted. Some of these categories are divided into subgroups (four-digit classifications) so that at least 153 separate classes are recognized. All of these 40 three-digit classifications are summarized by groups in Table 7-1.

Chemicals may cause deaths recorded under classifications other than those just listed. This is recognized to be true in connection with the contribution of alcohol to motor vehicle accidents and the contribution of cigarette smoking to several diseases, notably carcinoma of the lung. Death rates for some of these diseases secondary to poisoning also are shown in Table 7-1. More than half of fatal automobile accidents are associated with persons whose blood alcohol levels indicate intoxication. More than half of deaths from carcinoma of the lung occur in persons who were heavy smokers of cigarettes. As a minimum, there are 3 times as many deaths secondary to excessive use of alcohol and tobacco, as there are deaths caused directly by accidental, suicidal, and homicidal poisoning combined.

A few classes of poisoning were omitted intentionally from Table 7-1 because their occurrence depends to such a large degree on unrelated, pre-existing factors. These classes, which involve only a few deaths, include poisoning associated with therapeutic, diagnostic, and prophylactic misadventures with anesthetics and other drugs and legal intervention with gas. Late effects of accidental poisoning (12 cases in 1968) also were omitted from the table because comparable cases are not listed separately for suicides, or for those instances where it could not be determined whether they were accidental or purposely inflicted.

Deaths attributed to accidental acute poisoning by drugs, solids and liquids, and by gases and vapors constitute less than 4% of all accidental deaths. The number of deaths caused each year by accidental poisoning is about the same as the number recognized as being caused directly by alcoholism and other drug addiction, and substantially less than the number of suicides associated with chemicals. In addition, as already noted, alcohol contributes to many motor vehicle accidents and it may contribute to some suicides, not only those accomplished with chemicals but also those carried out with firearms and other physical means.

Mortality Associated with Accidental Poisoning in General. The death rate associated with solids and liquids has remained remarkably stable since 1939 when the present method of recording was instituted. On the contrary, there was a significant decrease in the death rate associated with gases and vapors beginning about 1945 and leveling off about 1955. The improvement was associated with increasing substitution of natural gas for manufactured gas during the decade after World War II. Carbon monoxide is by far the most important single cause of strictly accidental poisoning. It may be formed by incomplete combustion of any carbonaceous material, including natural gas. However, natural gas, unlike manufactured fuel gases, does not contain preformed carbon monoxide, and, therefore, simple leaks of natural gas offer far less toxic hazard. Carbon monoxide ranks second only to alcohol as a direct cause of fatal intoxication.

The introduction of modern pesticides in the United States of America—symbolized in Fig. 7-1 by arrows indicating the introduction of DDT on an experimental basis in 1942 and on

Table 7-1

Deaths from All Causes and from Selected Causes and Groups of Causes, United States of America, 1956, 1961, and 1968[a]

Class number[b]	Cause of death	1956		1961		1968	
		No. of deaths	Rate[c]	No. of deaths	Rate[c]	No. of deaths	Rate[c]
	All Causes	1,564,476	935.4	1,701,522	930.0	1,930,082	965.7
	I. Infective and Parasitic Diseases	25,378	15.1	20,078	11.0	23,968	12.0
E 005	food poisoning (infection and intoxication)	75	0.0	44	0.0	10	0.0
	II. Neoplasms	252,244	150.9	278,253	152.1	323,495	161.9
E 162	malignant neoplasm of trachea, bronchus, and lung	29,181	17.5	38,929	21.2	59,367	29.7
	V. Mental, Psychoneurotic, and Personality Disorders	3,384	2.0	4,465	3.0	6,628	3.3
E 291	alcoholic psychosis	242	0.1	470	0.3	637	0.3
E 303	alcoholism	2,066	1.2	2,247	1.2	3,904	2.0
E 304	other drug dependence	95	0.1	332	0.2	219 [d]	0.1 [d]
	VII. Diseases of the Circulatory System	661,003	395.2	731,671	399.8	1,040,292 [d]	520.6 [d]
	XVII. Accidents, Poisonings, and Violence	119,179	71.3	119,863	65.5	155,237	77.7
E 810-819	motor-vehicle traffic accidents	38,740	23.2	37,025	20.2	53,801	26.9
E 850-869	accidental poisoning by solid and liquid substances[e]	1,422	0.9	1,804	1.0	2,583	1.2
E 865	accidental poisoning by pesticides, fertilizers, or plant foods	152 [f]	0.1	111 [f]	0.1	72	0.0
E 870-877	accidental poisoning by gases and vapors	1,213	0.7	1,192	0.7	1,526	0.8
E 905	accidents caused by bites and stings of venomous animals and insects	36	0.0	54	0.0	69	0.0
E 950-959	suicide (total)	16,720	10.0	18,997	10.4	21,372	10.7
E 950	suicide by solid and liquid poisons	1,582	0.9	2,388	1.3	3,276	1.6
E 951-952	suicide by gases	1,785	0.9	2,113	1.2	2,408	1.2
E 962	homicide assault by poisoning	32	0.0	24	0.0	28	0.0
E 980	poisoning by solid or liquid substances[g]	--	--	--	--	911	0.5
E 981-982	poisoning by gases[g]	--	--	--	--	182	0.0

a.   U.S. Public Health Service. Vital Statistics of the United States, 1956, 1961, 1968.
b.   Class number in the Eighth Revision International Classification of Diseases. These numbers apply only to 1968; other numbers from earlier revisions were used in 1956 and 1961.
c.   Per 100,000 population.
d.   The large change in number of deaths and rate in this category is due to revision in the International Classification of Diseases.
e.   Includes drugs.
f.   Values based on special studies (see Section 7.1.2.2).
g.   Undetermined whether accidental or purposely inflicted. This category was not recognized before 1968.

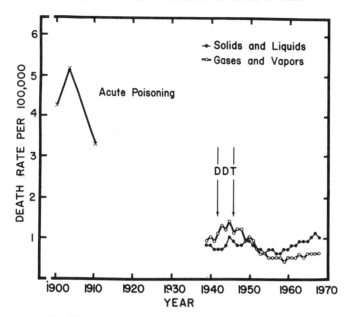

Fig. 7-1. Death rates in the United States of America associated with accidental poisoning. The first arrow indicates the year (1942) in which DDT was introduced experimentally, and the second one indicates the year (1946) of its commercial introduction. From US Public Health Service *Vital Statistics of the United States.*

a commercial basis in 1946—failed to increase the mortality rates associated with accidental poisoning generally.

The classification "Other acute poisonings" used around the turn of the century was comparable to a combination of several classifications used today: "Accidental poisoning by drugs and medicaments" (E850–E859), "Accidental poisoning by other solid and liquid substances" (E860–E869) (including "Accidental poisoning by noxious foodstuffs" (E868), and "Accidents caused by bites and stings of venomous animals and insects" (E905). In 1968 these categories carried a combined rate of 1.5 per 100,000 population; the rate for the former classification for the death registration states of 1900 was 4.2 per 100,000. During the following decade, this figure rose to 5.2 in 1903 and then declined to 3.4 in 1909. Thus, it appears that the rate of accidental poisoning decreased during a period from 1910 to 1939 in which the use of chemicals increased greatly.

Although the mortality rate associated with accidental poisoning by solids and liquids has remained relatively stable for the last 30 years, there have been marked changes in the relative importance of different materials that contribute to this rate. Examples are illustrated in Fig. 7-2, which shows the slowly decreasing importance of arsenic and strychnine, and the great but highly variable impor-

tance of barbiturates as causes of fatal accidental poisoning.

Accidental intoxication is not a major cause of mortality, but it is of special interest because it is potentially preventable.

7.1.1.2 Morbidity. Information on morbidity is not gathered and recorded as systematically as that on mortality. The number of cases of nonfatal poisoning must be estimated from the ratio of nonfatal to fatal cases in special studies. Among a total of 2,407 hospitalized poisoning cases reported by the American Red Cross for one important city, the ratio of nonfatal to fatal cases varied from 25:1 to 115:1 and averaged 50:1 for the separate years 1951 through 1958. By contrast, among cases reported to poison control centers, the rate of hospitalization was less than 10%, and the ratio of nonfatal to fatal cases was 750:1. Approximately 70% of cases reported to poison control centers were asymptomatic (Cann *et al.,* 1958).

Severity of illness is obviously the chief variable leading to the very different estimates of the ratio of nonfatal to fatal cases; some investigators count every report as a case while others count only cases of significant illness. There may be other unrecognized variables, the importance of which may differ according to the age, ethnic group, occupational status, or other conditions of a particu-

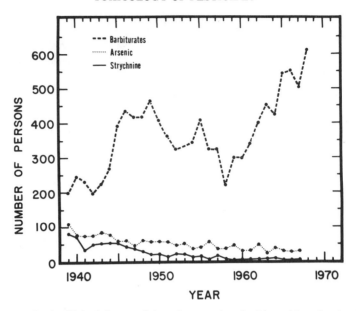

Fig. 7-2. Death rates in the United States of America associated with accidental poisoning by arsenic, strychnine, and barbiturates. From US Public Health Service *Vital Statistics of the United States.*

lar population. However, at the present time it appears that a ratio of 100:1 for the entire population is the most accurate estimate possible, taking into account even mild cases of illness, but excluding cases of exposure without illness.

Information from Poison Control Centers. A note on the origin and distribution of poison control centers is in Section 9.4.1.2.

In 1971, the last year for which complete reports are available, the National Clearinghouse for Poison Control Centers (1971) received 136,051 individual case reports. Of these reports, 6,446 or 4.7% involved exposure to pesticides. In the same year, the total number of reported cases in children under 5 years of age was 84,370, of which 4,513 or 5.3% involved pesticides (see Table 7-2).

The fact that the majority of cases reported to poison control centers do not involve symptoms reflects the high degree of concern that both parents and physicians feel about the possibility of poisoning. This concern is especially marked in connection with children. Inevitably, some of the reports are associated with contact too trivial to permit significant absorption of the suspect material. Only 9.8% of all cases in children less than 5 years of age involve symptoms. The proportion (7.0%) is about the same for cases involving pesticides in these same young children. The picture is distinctly different for the older age groups. For persons of all ages, the proportion of cases involving symptoms is higher, being 22.7% for

all reports and 14.1% for pesticides. Separate values for adults are not available. The difference is certainly related to the greater accuracy with which one can determine whether an older child or an adult has really ingested a material or had some other dangerous contact with it. The difference is related also to the greater average toxicity of compounds encountered by adults, and to the greater dosage rate associated with suicide attempts as compared to accidents. During 1971, 49 suicide attempts involving pesticides were reported to the Clearinghouse, and there were in addition 170 self-poisonings, 19 "gestures," and 102 cases of unknown intent.

The difference in the incidence of symptoms in young children and in the total reported population is not uniform for different classes of pesticides. For example, the incidence is about the same for mothballs regardless of age, but the incidence for other categories is distinctly higher in the total reported population than in children under 5 years of age. Mothballs present a uniform hazard, but pesticides as a class vary greatly in toxicity. It may be that adults who report contact with pesticides are more likely than young children to contact the most dangerous ones.

Although the proportion of young children who have symptoms after exposure to pesticides is small, the proportion of those with symptoms who are hospitalized is high, being 93.7% for pesticides generally. The proportion is 309% for rodenticides, reflecting the hospi-

Table 7-2

Cases of Ingestion During 1971 Reported to the National Clearinghouse for Poison Control Centers [a]

Classes of products	Cases, under 5 years					Cases, all ages				
	Total (No.)	Symptoms [b] (No.)	(%) [b]	Hospitalized (No.)	(%) [c]	Total (No.)	Symptoms (No.)	(%) [b]	Fatal (No.)	(%) [c]
insecticides	1,886	181	9.6	154	85.1	3,035	561	18.4	10	1.7
rodenticides	1,274	34	2.7	105	308.8	1,535	67	4.4	0	0
fungicides	81	3	3.7	3	100.0	119	13	10.9	1	7.7
herbicides	126	16	12.7	5	31.3	267	74	27.7	2	2.7
moth balls	892	33	3.7	26	78.8	1,023	45	4.4	0	0
animal repellents	85	33	38.8	1	3.0	198	101	51.0	0	0
insect repellents	164	16	9.7	4	25.0	236	36	15.2	0	0
pesticide combinations	5	2	40.0	0	0	33	14	42.4	1	7.1
total pesticides	4,513	318	7.0	298	93.7	6,446	911	14.1	14	1.5
total all reports	84,370	8,321	9.8	4,909	59.0	136,051	30,963	22.7	285	0.9
pesticides (as % of total)	5.3	3.8		6.0		4.7	2.9		4.9	

a.   Based on data from the National Clearinghouse for Poison Centers Bulletin, September-October 1972.

b.   Percent of total cases in class.

c.   Percent of cases with symptoms.

talization of some children who remain asymptomatic after exposure to these compounds, some of which are extremely dangerous.

Of the 911 persons reported to poison control centers in 1971 who had symptoms following exposure to pesticides, 14 (1.5%) died. This proportion is nearly twice that (0.9%) for symptomatic cases generally.

The statistics gathered by poison control centers in 1971 are similar to those for the preceding several years in most respects. There does seem to have been a real increase in reported suicides, self-poisonings, and "gestures." Whether the reported decrease in mortality among persons with symptoms following exposure to pesticides represents a trend or random variation is probably too early to say. On the contrary, the decrease in cases of aspirin poisoning (see below) is real.

Reports from poison control centers constitute an important source of information on strictly accidental poisoning, especially in children. However, it is necessary to recognize the limitations of these statistics. The collection of information is voluntary and may be irregular both in time and space. The centers are most frequent and most active in cities. Thus, cases in many areas may be missed because there is no convenient center. Although young children are especially liable to

ingest poisons, it also is true that the poison control centers have been a special interest of pediatricians and have given special attention to children. Certain situations associated with poisoning, especially suicide and murder, are unlikely to come to the attention of poison control centers, although some of them eventually are recorded as accidents. Occupational cases often are missed by the centers. Even active centers may fail to receive reports of the majority of fatal intoxications in their areas (Reich et al., 1968b). Nationally, between 10 and 15% of deaths due to accidental poisoning by solid and liquid substances are brought to the attention of poison control centers. In 1971, 285 deaths were reported to centers, compared to an annual total of over 2,000 deaths from this cause in recent years. An even much smaller proportion of accidental deaths due to gases and vapors are reported to the centers. In 1971, 21 of these deaths were reported, compared to an annual total of over 1,500 from gases and vapors in recent years.

Because of their special emphasis, poison control centers almost certainly have been able to reduce the incidence of poisoning among children. Paradoxically, much of the progress is reflected by official mortality statistics, not by the records of the centers themselves. The number of centers has increased and, in many instances, the coverage achieved by individual centers has enlarged. As might be anticipated from these increases, the total number of cases reported to the National Clearinghouse became larger for a number of years after the center movement started.

The official national record shows that deaths caused by accidental poisoning by solid and liquid substances among children under 5 years of age oscillated irregularly between 422 and 456 during 1958 through 1962. After that, the number declined steadily from 454 in 1963 to 284 in 1868. This decline was not due to poorer reporting or any overall decline in poisoning, for the number of deaths from this cause among persons of all ages increased without interruption from 1,429 in 1958 to 2,506 in 1967. In 1968 the number was essentially the same (2,483) or (if one includes the new category of injuries undetermined whether accidental or purposely inflicted) continued to increase, primarily due to poisoning by barbiturates (US Public Health Service, 1960–1972).

The number of reports to poison control centers is now relatively steady, having varied irregularly from 72,661 to 84,370 during the period 1967 to 1971. During this same period, the number of cases involving aspirin decreased steadily from 16,887 to 8,529, that is from 23.2 to 10.1% of all reports. This notable improvement regarding aspirin has been accompanied by an essentially steady state regarding pesticides, the number of reports decreasing only slightly from 4,087 in 1967 and then increasing later to 4,513 in 1971.

7.1.2 Poisoning by Pesticides

7.1.2.1 Compounds That Have Caused Poisoning.
Pesticides that have caused significant poisoning, either fatal or otherwise, are listed in Table 7-3.

7.1.2.2 Endemic Mortality.
Accidental Poisoning. Nearly all mortality associated with pesticides in the United States of America has been endemic in character. That is, it has been scattered in time and space, each case usually being unrelated to the others.

Chronic poisoning by certain pesticides (especially the fungicides, hexachlorobenzene, and several alkyl mercury compounds) is easily diagnosed and has been the cause of major outbreaks in other countries. Except for the effects of arsenic (often administered with homicidal intent), chronic poisoning by pesticides has not been a problem in the United

States of America, partly because use of compounds likely to cause chronic poisoning has been limited.

Table 7-4 shows the categories in which deaths from pesticides were classified prior to 1968, the last year for which complete data are available; it also shows the number of cases in each class in a typical year. It may be seen that the majority of cases fell in classification E888 (other and unspecified liquids and solids). This was not because the identity of the offending poison usually was omitted from the death certificate, but because no single poison in this category was sufficiently important to justify a separate category. Furthermore, a variable percentage of cases in other categories were actually caused by pesticides. Thus, in 1961, 91% of cases associated with arsenic and 75% of those associated with fluorides were caused by pesticides. On the contrary, none of the cases associated with lead were caused by pesticides, although some pesticides contain lead.

In 1968 a revised system of classification was used and a separate category (E865, accidental poisoning by pesticides, fertilizers, or plant foods) was introduced. Before 1968, the number of deaths caused by pesticides in the United States of America had to be determined from special studies such as those carried out in 1956 and 1961 (Hayes, 1960; Hayes and Pirkle, 1966) or had to be estimated. A reasonable estimate of the total number of deaths from pesticides in a given year could be obtained by adding the total number in selected categories to the number in category E888 actually caused by pesticides in such a way that the excess of cases in the selected categories compensates for the omission of other categories. Thus, one author (Cann, 1963) estimated the total number of deaths in 1956 as 141 by adding all cases caused by fluorides (E887) and by arsenic and antimony (E886) to those in category E888, in which a pesticide was named in the death certificate. Later Hayes and Pirkle (1966) estimated the total for the same year as 147 by adding cases caused by strychnine (E876) and by arsenic and antimony to those attributed to pesticides under E888. The dotted line at the top of Fig. 7-3 shows the estimated number of deaths caused by pesticides in the United States in different years. The value of 147 shown in the figure for 1956 agrees well with 152, the number of cases found by special study in that year. Good agreement was also found in 1961, when there was another special study.

Thus, from 1950 through 1961, the number of deaths caused by pesticides varied from 100 to 152, and showed no clear trend, although a

Table 7-3

List of Pesticides that Have Caused Poisoning in Man[a]

Kind of Pesticide	Compound
Inorganic and organometal pesticides:	arsenic trioxide, barium carbonate, copper sulfate, lead arsenate, mercuric chloride, phosphorus, sodium arsenate, sodium chlorate, sodium fluoride, thallium sulfate, zinc phosphide, several methyl and ethyl mercury compounds
Pesticides derived from plants and other organisms:	anabasine, nicotine, pyrethrum, rotenone, sabadilla, strychnine
Solvents, propellants, and oil insecticides:	dichlorodifluoromethane, kerosene, Tetralin®, xylene
Fumigants and nematocides:	acrylonitrite, aluminum phosphide, carbon tetrachloride, chloropicrin, 1,2-dibromoethane, p-dichlorobenzene, 1,2-dichloroethane, hydrogen cyanide, hydrogen phosphide, Lethane 384, methyl bromide, methylene chloride, naphthalene, Nemagon®, sulfuryl fluoride, tetrachloroethylene, trichloroethane
Chlorinated hydrocarbon insecticides:	aldrin, BHC, chlordane, DDT, dieldrin, DMC, endosulfan, endrin, isobenzan, lindane, methoxychlor, TDE, toxaphene
Organic phosphorus insecticides:	azinphosmethyl, carbophenothion, demeton-O-methyl, demeton-S-methyl, diazinon, dichlorvos, dicrotophos, dimethoate, endothion, EPN, fensulfothion, fenthion, Hinosan®, methyl demeton, methyl parathion, mevinphos, mipafox, monocrotophos, naled, parathion, phorate, phosphamidon, Phostex®, tepp, thiometon, trichlorfon
Carbamates and related pesticides:	aldicarb, 4-benzothienyl-N-methyl carbamate, BUX®, carbaryl, carbofuran, isolan, 2-isopropyl phenyl-N-methyl carbamate, 3-isopropyl phenyl-N-methyl carbamate, maneb, propoxur, thiram, Zectran®, zineb, ziram
Phenolic and nitrophenolic pesticides:	dinitrobutylphenol, 2,4-dinitrophenol, dinocap, DNOC, pentachlorophenol
Miscellaneous pesticides:	chlorfenson
Synthetic organic rodenticides:	coumafuryl, fluoroacetamide, sodium fluoroacetate, warfarin
Molluscicides:	metaldehyde
Herbicides and related compounds:	acrolein, 2,4-D, dalapon, dicamba[b], dichlorprop, diquat, MCPA, paraquat, propazine, simazine, 2,4,5-T, TCA
Fungicides and related compounds:	captafol, diphenyl, hexachlorobenzene, sodium azide, thiabendazole
Repellents and attractants:	chloralose, deet

a. Cases of ingestion or other exposure without subsequent illness are omitted, but illness is recorded regardless of whether the particular formulation that caused it was intended as a pesticide or not.

b. Attempted suicide by ingestion of a mixture of 2,4-D and dicamba.

Table 7-4

Classes of Accidental Poisoning (United States of America, 1961)
to Which Cases of Poisoning by Pesticides
Could Have Been Assigned

Cause of death[a]	Total cases	Pesticide cases No.	%
E876 (strychnine)	6	1	16.7
E884 (mercury)	8	1	12.5
E885 (lead)	77	0	0
E 886 (arsenic, antimony)	32	29	90.6
E887 (fluorides)	8	6	75.0
E888 (other and unspecified liquids and solids)	239	68	28.5
subtotal E870-E888 (solids and liquids)	1,804	105	5.8
E893 (cyanide)	4	3	75.0
E894 (other specified gases and vapors)	122	3	2.5
subtotal E890-E895 (gases, vapors)	1,192	6	0.5.
total - all accidental poisoning	2,996[b]	111	3.7

a.   Categories which are used in the United States of America and many other countries are from the International Classification of Disease.

b.   The total for those categories which contain any pesticide cases was 496.

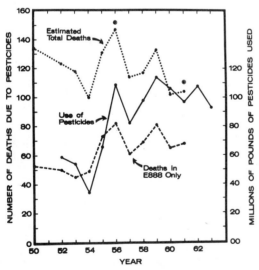

Fig. 7-3. Comparison of the use of pesticides in the United States of America and the number of related deaths. The total mortality measured by special studies in 1956 and 1961 stands slightly above the corresponding points estimated from less complete data. From Hayes and Pirkle (1966) by permission of the American Medical Association.

slight decrease was suggested. There was an interesting, partial correspondence between the number of deaths caused by pesticides and the use of pesticides during the same years (Fig. 7-3). The values for use of pesticides plotted in Fig. 7-3 represent an index based on totals for the aldrin-toxaphene group, benzene hexachloride (gamma basis), DDT, 2,4-D, 2,-4,5-T, calcium arsenate, and lead arsenate.

Under the new system of recording introduced in 1968, the number of deaths attributed to pesticides and other agricultural chemicals was 72, offering more convincing evidence of a decrease in mortality associated with these compounds.

Table 7-5 lists pesticides that either were the cause of death in 1956 or 1961, or for which this possibility could not be excluded clearly. (The report of the 1961 study (Hayes and Pirkle, 1966) pointed out that in only about 90% of deaths attributed to pesticides was the diagnosis supported by evidence of adequate exposure, a consistent clinical course, or appropriate laboratory or autopsy findings.)

Pesticides have accounted for a decreasing proportion of accidental deaths caused by solid

Table 7-5

Identity of Pesticides Responsible for Accidental
Deaths in 1956 and 1961

From Hayes and Pirkle (1966) by permission of the American Medical
Association.

Pesticide	1961	1956
arsenic	29	54
thallium	2	8
mercury	1 [a/]	--
phosphorus	12	21
fluorides	6	--
sodium chlorate	--	1
calcium polysulfide	1	--
boric acid	--	1
cyanide (solid)	3	--
copper oleate mixed with tetrahydronaphthalene	--	1
strychnine	1	3
nicotine	3	4
pyrethrum	--	1
camphor	--	1
rotenone, copper, and sulfur	--	1
subtotal - inorganic and botanical solid and liquid pesticides	58	96
diazinon	1	2
demeton	--	1
malathion	3	3
methyl parathion	3	--
parathion	15	11
mevinphos	1	--
unspecified organic phosphorus insecticides	1	1
subtotal - organic phosphorus insecticides	24	20
aldrin	--	1
BHC (including lindane)	1	2
chlordane	--	3
DDT	--	1
dieldrin	1 [a/]	1
endrin	1	3
toxaphene	2	1
combination of chlorinated hydrocarbon insecticides	1	1
subtotal - chlorinated hydrocarbon insecticides	6	13
formaldehyde	--	1
combination of specified insecticides	4 [a/]	--
2, 4-D	1	--
warfarin	1 [b/]	1
coumarin	1 [b/]	--
isobornyl thiocyanoacetate	1	1
unspecified insecticides	6 [a/]	7
unspecified rodenticides	3	6
subtotal - solids and liquids (E870-E888) (pesticides only)	105	145
carboxide gas	1	--
cyanide gas	3 [a/]	1
ethylene dibromide	1	--
mercury	--	2
methyl bromide	--	3
sulfur dioxide	1	1
subtotal - gases and vapors (E890-E895) (pesticides only)	6	7
grand total	111	152

a.   Diagnosis of pesticide poisoning open to serious question.

b.   Diagnosis of pesticide poisoning open to some question.

and liquid substances. In 1946 and 1947 the fractions were 12.8 and 10.2%, respectively, and from 1949 through 1955, the fractions were 9.6, 9.6, 9.2, 9.6, 7.8, and 9.8%, respectively (Conley, 1958). The two special studies that have been made showed that solid and liquid pesticides accounted for 9.8 and 5.8% of accidental deaths caused by solids and liquids in 1956 and 1961, respectively. In 1968, the proportion had dropped to 2.5%. Pesticides accounted for only 0.6 and 0.5% of deaths caused by gases and vapors in 1956 and 1961, respectively.

Thus, the mortality rate associated with accidental poisoning by pesticides in the United States has been reduced to less than 1 per million population. In 1968, the rate was 0.36 per million.

In Europe, the incidence of poisoning by pesticides is low and constitutes only a small proportion of poisoning as a whole (Anonymous, 1972a).

The number of accidental deaths caused by pesticides in the United States of America is greater than the number caused by food poisoning (see Table 7-1). In the USA, what is called food poisoning consists largely of the effect of bacterial toxins, including botulinum toxins. The situation may be very different in other places and at other times. In some situations, fungal toxins may be of tremendous importance. For example, during the years 1942 to 1947, "alimentary aleukia," an intoxication caused by certain cereal fungi, caused great suffering in the Orenburg district of the USSR, an area north of the Caspian Sea, east of the Volga River, and west of the Ural Mountains. Other districts were affected also. Only three of the 50 counties of the Orenburg district were spared during 1944, the peak year; mortality reached 10% of the entire population of 16 counties and exceeded 10% in nine additional counties (Joffe, 1965). Internationally, this kind of thing must be taken into account in evaluating the safety of fungicides in particular, and pesticides in general.

Intentional Poisoning. Deaths resulting from suicide or murder are classified and recorded in official statistics, as are deaths from other causes. Some of these intentional deaths are accomplished with poisons, including pesticides. Much less has been written about the part pesticides play in intentional deaths as compared to accidental deaths. Studies of accidental poisoning are made in the hope of ultimately preventing such accidents. The primary problem in accidents is improper contact with poisons. The record shows that real progress has been made in accident prevention through education regarding safe storage and application. However, otherwise safe storage may be entirely inadequate to prevent a person bent on suicide or murder from obtaining a poison. Furthermore, the primary problem here is not the poison but the social and mental state of the person, and those interested in prevention must focus their attention on the primary problem.

One of the best studies of endemic suicide with pesticides is that of Reich *et al.* (1968b). Very briefly, they found that in south Florida, suicides constituted from 51 to 72% of deaths from all poisons in each of the 12 years, 1956 to 1967. During the entire period, pesticides accounted for 121 deaths, of which 69 (57%) involved suicide and 12 (10%) involved murder. The epidemiology of the suicides differed from that of the accidents in connection with age, race, sex, and agent. The average age of the suicides was 46 years, while the majority of accidents involved children under 5 years of age. The proportion of Negroes among the suicides (20%) was slightly greather than their proportion in the total population (13.7 to 17% in different years); their proportion among the accidents (72%) was even more disproportionate. Almost as many women as men committed suicide with pesticides, but only half as many girls as boys were involved in accidents. Organic phosphorus compounds were less involved in suicides (39%) than in accidents (64%). The authors noted that, during the period of study, the rate for fatal poisoning by all agents in south Florida was more than twice the national average and that, like the national average, it increased substantially during the period 1956 to 1965, due entirely to an increase in the rate of suicide.

Because of the stigma associated with suicide, there is some tendency to report these deaths as accidents. Such errors of recording probably are greatest in connection with sedative drugs, because of the importance of these drugs as suicidal agents. However, mistakes can be made in connection with pesticides also. Of 111 deaths in the United States of America in 1961 ascribed to accidental poisoning by an identifiable pesticide, there was strong indication that eight deaths among adults were suicides, and that a ninth death involved murder (Hayes and Pirkle, 1966).

7.1.2.3 Endemic Morbidity. What was said in Section 7.1.1.2 about poisoning in general applies with equal force to morbidity associated with pesticides. In the absence of systematic reporting, it is impossible to be certain about the number of nonfatal cases or the proportion of fatal ones. However, some information is available.

Reports to Poison Control Centers. Over a period of years, pesticides have contributed a decreasing proportion of the total cases reported to poison control centers. During 1956 to 1958 the proportion was 8% (Cann *et al.*, 1958). During a 4-year period, the percentage of cases involving pesticides in children under 5 years of age decreased annually as follows: 6.1% in 1965, 5.8% in 1966, 5.6% in 1967, and 5.5% in 1968 (National Clearinghouse, 1969). The improvement is progressive and undoubtedly real. There is reason to think that the decrease reflects the special emphasis that has been placed on the safe use of all pesticides, and on restrictions that the Department of Agriculture placed on home use of thallium and some of the other most dangerous pesticides.

Special emphasis should continue to be placed on safety in the use of pesticides because, although they were associated with only 5.4% of all cases reported to poison control centers in 1968, they were the cause of 11.7% of the mortality reported to these centers during the same year. Of course, emphasis on pesticides should not detract from attention to other causes of death. Medicines continue to be the main cause of mortality reported to poison control centers, having been responsible for over 59% of it in 1968.

Reports of Occupational Disease within the United States of America. The best reporting scheme for occupational disease associated with pesticides and other agricultural chemicals has been, for many years, the one in California. The thoroughness of the reporting system, which probably depends in part on its relation to compensation, is remarkable. The range of disability reported is indicated by the fact that in 1967, when the total number of complaints associated with agricultural chemicals was 1,400, the number associated with poison oak was 3,724 (California, 1967).

When an injured employee requires medical attention other than ordinary first aid treatment, the attending physician must file a report (the "Doctor's First Report of Work Injury") with the California Department of Industrial Relations (State of California Labor Code, 1967, Section 6407). Through an interagency agreement, these reports also are analyzed in connection with a selected list of diseases by the California Department of Public Health. In 1968, workmen required to file the reports constituted 80% of the 7.7 million employed persons in California covered under the California Workmen's Compensation Law. Self-employed persons and persons in certain minor categories are not required to file the reports but apparently sometimes do. Reports of occupational disease gathered in this way and attributed to pesticides and other agricultural chemicals during the years 1954 through 1970 are shown in Table 7-6. It may be seen that the number of cases increased slightly during the first few years of record and then remained essentially steady, with the exception of a possible decrease in 1968 and 1969, but not 1970. Agricultural chemicals were considered responsible for 5% of the 33,085 reports of all occupational disease tabulated in 1970. In the same year, the incidence of all occupational disease, excluding eye conditions and chemical burns, was 0.26% among farm laborers, 0.67% among loaders, flagmen, agricultural pest control operators, and others engaged in agricultural services, 0.57% among structural pest control operators, and about 0.1% among the workers of mosquito abatement districts. Of the reports of occupational disease attributed to pesticides and other agricultural chemicals, excluding eye conditions and chemicals burns, 17% of the reports involved illness affecting two or more systems, 27% involved skin conditions, 5% involved respiratory symptoms only, and most of the remaining reports were confined to the gastrointestinal system or some other single system other than the respiratory system or skin. As part of the first report, the physicians estimated that 37.6% of the cases would involve time lost from work (12.0% not reported), but only 8.5% were ill enough to require hospitalization. Organic phosphorus pesticides were implicated in 22% of the tabulated reports, herbicides in 14%, halogenated hydrocarbon pesticides in 6%, and fertilizers in 11%; other specified chemicals (sulfur, phenols, lead, mercurials, other fungicides, carbamates, and others) accounted for 17% of the cases (California, 1970).

The situation was essentially unchanged in 1969, except that was a year in which there were several outbreaks of cropworkers' poisoning, this time associated with a combination of azinphosethyl and ethion. In spite of these outbreaks, the total number of reports was slightly less than in the preceding year (California, 1969).

Unfortunately, the California reports either do not include nonchemical farm accidents or such information is so segregated that no comparison is readily available. Studies focused on human health rather than on chemi-

Table 7-6

Reports of Occupational Disease Attributed to
Pesticides and Other Agricultural Chemicals
California, 1954 - 1970

From State of California, Department of Public Health, Occupational
Disease in California Attributed to Pesticides and Other Agricultural
Chemicals, Annual Reports.

| Year | Nonfatal injuries | | | Deaths in all industries |
	All industries	Agriculture	Other	
excluding eye conditions and chemical burns				
1954	391	248	143	2
1955	531	326	205	1
1956	789	464	325	4
1957	749	434	315	2
1958	910	599	311	3
1959	1,093	782	311	5
1960	975	668	307	0
1961	911	578	333	3
1962	827	545	282	1
1963	1,013	746	267	1
1964	844	539	305	1
1965	779	520	259	1
1966	869	565	304	3
1967	921	571	350	2
1968	834	499	335	0
1969	727	454	273	1
1970	957	634	323	0
including eye conditions and chemical burns				
1964	1,328	821	507	
1965	1,340	836	504	
1966	1,347	820	527	
1967	1,400	838	562	
1970	1,493	938	552	

cals have revealed that chemicals, including pesticides, play a relatively small part in the accidental injury of agricultural workers.

In a study in New York State, Hoff (1970) found that only 1.2% of farm accidents involved contact with pesticides during application, and only 2.4% involved chemicals under any condition. This percentage was slightly less than that associated with chain saws (2.8%) or power shop tools (2.8%). The highest proportion of agricultural accidents were caused by some farm machinery excluding tractors (20.9%), tractors (8.5%), animals (16.6%), and slips and falls (10.2%). The accident rate for males was higher than that for females, and the rate for employees was higher than that for family members. These results are similar to those in compensation cases closed by the New York State Workmen's Compensation Board during the last decade (New York, 1961, 1969), and not unlike those in Hungary and other countries (Volkov, 1973).

7.1.2.4 Epidemics of Poisoning by Pesticides. There have been a number of outbreaks of accidental poisoning by pesticides

that deserve special mention. Almost every outbreak draws attention to hazards different from those contributing to what we have called endemic mortality and morbidity. Many of the recognized outbreaks have occurred in countries that make no orderly collection of mortality statistics, not to mention morbidity statistics.

The main sources of epidemics of accidental poisoning by pesticides have been the contamination of food by pesticide formulations during transport or storage and the use of pesticide-treated grain as food. Another source of epidemics, not all of which have been reported, has been the use of parathion to treat human lice. The recorded mortality in some single outbreaks of food poisoning by pesticides has been over half the endemic mortality associated with all pesticides each year in a country as large as the United States of America. It is fair to mention, however, that, whereas the reporting of poisoning by pesticides may be imperfect, there is reason to think it is more complete than reporting of poisoning by fungal and other naturally occurring toxins. The most dramatic reported endemic and epidemic poisoning by fungal toxins occurred in the USSR (see Section 7.1.2.2) but the situation may be worse on the average in some tropical areas.

Contamination of Food or Clothing During Transport or Storage. The major reported

outbreaks of poisoning associated with the contamination of food or clothing by pesticides during transport or storage are listed in the first portion of Table 7-7.

In an outbreak of poisoning by endrin (Da-

Table 7-7

Epidemics of Poisoning by Pesticides

Kind of accident	Pesticide involved	Material contaminated	Number of cases	Number of deaths	Location	Reference
	endrin	flour	159	0	Wales	Davies and Lewis, 1956
	endrin	flour	3	0	Egypt	Coble et al., 1967
	endrin	flour	691	24	Qatar	Weeks, 1967; Curley et al., 1970
	endrin	flour	183	2	Saudi Arabia	Weeks, 1967; Curley et al., 1970
spillage	dieldrin	food	21	0	shipboard	Przyborowski et al., 1962
during	carbophenothion	flour	7	0	USA	Older and Hatcher, 1969
transport	diazinon	doughnut mix	20	0	USA	West, 1965
or	parathion	wheat	360 [a/]	102 [a/]	India	Karunakaran, 1958
storage	parathion	barley	38	9	Malaya	Kanagaratnam et al., 1960
	parathion	flour	200	8	Egypt	Wishahi et al., 1958
	parathion	flour	26	0	Yugoslavia	Maver and Belamaric, 1961
	parathion	flour	600	88	Colombia	Gomez Ulloa et al., 1967-1968
	parathion	flour and sugar	559	16	Mexico	Marquez Mayaudon et al., 1968
	parathion	sheets	3	0	Canada	Anderson et al., 1965
	mevinphos	pants	6	0	USA	Warren et al., 1963
	organic mercury	seed-grain	34	4	W. Pakistan	Haq, 1963
	ethyl mercury	seed-grain	321	35	Iraq	Jalili and Abbasi, 1961
	methylmercury	seed-grain	6530	459	Iraq	Bakir et al., 1973
	organic mercury	seed-grain	45	20	Guatemala	Ordonez et al., 1966
	ethyl mercury	seed-grain	70	2	USSR	Shustoz and Tsyganova, 1970
	thallium sulfate	bait	>31	6	USA	Munch et al., 1933
eating	sodium fluoride	roach powder	260	47	USA	Lidbeck et al., 1943
formulation	barium carbonate	flour	85	0	Iran	Morton, 1945
	barium carbonate [b/]	sausage	100	0	Israel	Lewi and Bar-Khayim, 1964
	DDT	meatballs	11	0	Taiwan	Hsieh, 1954
	lindane	sugar	11	0	Bulgaria	Bambou et al., 1966
	hexachlorobenzene	seed-grain	>3000	3-11% [c/]	Turkey	Cam and Nigogosyan, 1963; Schmid, 1960
	warfarin	bait	14	2	Korea	Lange and Terveer, 1954

Table 7-7 (continued)

Kind of accident	Pesticide involved	Material contaminated	Number of cases	Number of deaths	Location	Reference
	organic mercury	pork[d/]	3	0	USA	Curley et al., 1971b
	toxaphene	collards	4	0	USA	McGee et al., 1952
improper	toxaphene	chard	3	0	USA	McGee et al., 1952
application	nicotine	mustard	11	0	USA	Lemmon, 1956
	parathion	[e/]	>17	15	Iran	Amin ol Achrafi, 1963
	pentachlorophenol	clothing	20	2	USA	Robson et al., 1969; Armstrong et al., 1969; Barthel et al., 1969
miscellaneous	parathion	crops	400	0	USA	Quinby and Lemmon, 1958 Milby et al., 1964

a.　The cause was unclear but may have been parathion in 40 additional cases including 4 deaths.

b.　Barium carbonate mistaken for potato flour.

c.　3% to 11% annually in different years.

d.　Treated seed-grain was fed to hogs, one of which later was eaten.

e.　Used as a treatment for lice.

vies and Lewis, 1956), 150 people who ate rolls or bread made from contaminated flour were made sick and about 30 of them had fits. This outbreak was especially instructive because apparently it demonstrated that contamination of food by a pesticide during shipment can occur, even though the two are not shipped together. Briefly, it was shown that bags of flour had been contaminated by endrin during shipment in a railroad car in which the insecticide has been shipped—and spilled—2 months earlier. According to a personal communication from Dr. Ieuan Lewis, the Chief Public Health Inspector, the endrin was in xylene solution. Some sacks of contaminated flour were not used by the baker, and it was possible to distinguish two of them from hundreds of uncontamined ones merely by odor. Examination of these two unused, contaminated sacks showed that, at the time of loading, they must have been placed on liquid insecticide, which was absorbed into the flour at the bottom of the sacks. Agglomeration of the flour in the lower several inches of each sack indicated prior saturation by a liquid and could not have been the result of contamination by crystalline material. On the contrary, it was never explained how liquid persisted, for 2 months on the floor, or what solvent was introduced when the flour was shipped. When the car was found and examined over 4 months after the recorded spillage, the floor was divided into six equal parts, each of which was thoroughly scraped, and the scrapings were analyzed separately. Only a trace of endrin was found in five of the sections, but the concentration of endrin in the scrapings from the sixth section was 11%. Any effort to sweep or clean the car probably would have resulted in a more equal distribution of the poison.

The outbreak in Singapore (Kanagaratnam et al., 1960) was notable in two ways. It was one of the few episodes in which the source of contamination was never discovered. In spite of this, it remains the outstanding example of alert and effective public health action in connection with the contamination of food by a chemical. Had it not been for prompt recognition of poisoning, warning of the people, and seizure of suspect grain, the death toll almost certainly would have been much higher.

Contamination of boys' pants by mevinphos (Warren et al., 1963) and of flannelette sheets by parathion (Anderson et al., 1965) led to illnesses requiring hospitalization. Contamination of clothing and other fabric by pesticides is a potential source of serious injury, although contamination of food has caused more illness and death.

Most spillage of pesticides on food or fabric has occurred during transport. Ships, trains, and trucks have been involved. Spillage or contamination by contact has also occurred during storage. In one instance where the source of contamination was not established, the possibility of direct application at a disinfection station along the highway was not excluded (Marquez Mayaudon et al., 1968).

The problem of preventing poisoning caused by the contamination of food or fabric during transport is considered in Section 9.1.2.

Use of Pesticide-Treated Seed or Meal as Food. Epidemics of poisoning associated with the eating of treated grain or other pesticidal formulations are shown in a portion of Table 7-7.

Peasants driven by starvation were the victims of the major outbreaks under discussion. The fact that the treated grain was poisonous and not intended as food was generally known. In several of the outbreaks some of the grain was washed to rid it of poison and warning color. Physicians investigating the outbreak in Guatemala had great difficulty at first in getting the peasants to reveal the source of trouble because the peasants feared that, if they told, they would not receive treated grain the next year. They fully recognized the agricultural value of the treated seed; they ate it because they were hungry (Ordóñez et al., 1966). In another instance, people washed mercury-treated grain with confidence because they knew that, in a similar situation, DDT could be removed well enough to prevent illness (Derban, 1974).

At least in some instances (Wray et al., 1962) the basic difficulty was administrative. Genetically select seed protected by pesticides was supplied to the peasants too late for the planting season. The people had already been forced to use their own supplies of relatively inferior grain for planting and then were left with inadequate food.

Although most of the epidemics involving treated grain have not been strictly accidental, the magnitude of the disasters serves as a warning of what accidents might involve. Although complete statistics are not available, it is certain that far more tons of treated seed are used in economically and agriculturally advanced countries than in the developing countries where the use of such seed has led to tragedy.

The family epidemic of poisoning by warfarin involved prolonged eating of a rodenticidal formulation, which the family had acquired accidentally (Lange and Terveer, 1954). The outbreak differs from those just discussed in that seed grain was not involved and the victims were not aware at first of the poisonous nature of the prepared bait. Labeling was the problem. The rodenticide, intended for military use, was fully labeled in English, but this was of no help to the Koreans who ate it.

Poisoning from Grossly Improper Application of Pesticides Directly to Food or Feed. There has not been a case of poisoning traced to eating food treated with pesticides and harvested according to good agricultural practice (Edson, 1957).

As recorded in Table 7-7, both old and new pesticides have caused poisoning when they were applied to growing vegetables in complete violation of label directions. An episode involving toxaphene is typical. The insecticide was sprayed on collards, a kind of leafy vegetable, even though the label prohibited such use (McGee et al., 1952). Some of the collard leaves were gathered and cooked only 3 days after spraying, with the result that four of seven members of the family were made sick. After the accident, it was found that the residue on the collards averaged 3,315 ppm, and 3,126 ppm remained after the leaves were washed three times. The permissible residue at the time was zero.

Nicotine sulfate residues caused illness in 11 persons who ate mustard greens which a farmer had sprayed with an unusually high dosage and then sold the next day. Even 2 weeks after spraying, the residues on this particular crop were as high as 69 to 123 ppm; the official tolerance was 2 ppm (Lemmon, 1956). The report, which was part of the Annual Report of the Bureau of Chemistry of the Department of Agriculture of the State of California, mentioned that this was the most outstanding episode encountered in 30 years of investigation. It also noted that nicotine sulfate had been on the market for 40 years at the time.

At least in other countries, a few cases of poisoning have been traced to direct but unintentional application of pesticides to food.

Consumption of Meat from Contaminated Animals. Consumption of meat from a hog that had been fed for 2 to 6 weeks on grain, some of which had been treated with alkyl mercury fungicides, led to the poisoning of four persons in a family of 10 who were exposed directly or indirectly. The family continued to eat meat from this hog even though the 14 remaining hogs on the same diet became blind, ataxic, and partially paralyzed, and 12 of them died during a period of 4 to 7 weeks after the first hog was slaughtered. Three children (ages 8 to 20) became ill from almost 3 to almost 4 months after first exposure. Illness involved ataxia, dysarthria, blindness, purposeless movements, and eventually coma. Treatment with BAL was followed by partial recovery after some delay. Illness did not occur in other members of the family, including the mother, who was 3 months pregnant when she began eating contaminated pork. She ate no more of the pork after her 6th month, but her urinary mercury levels were markedly elevated during the 7th and 8th months. One minute after birth her son became dusky. Intermittent gross movements of his extremities developed and persisted for several days. His urinary mercury levels were high. His EEG was considered normal at 1 month, slightly abnormal after 3 months, and severely abnormal at 6 months. The infant grew normally but was hypotonic and irritable and suffered nystagmus. The concentration of mercury in the remaining grain was 32.8 ppm, and that in the remaining pork was 29.4 ppm. Analysis of urine, serum, and spinal fluid from the victims established beyond question that their illnesses were caused by alkyl mercury (Curley et al., 1971b; Snyder, 1971; Pierce et al., 1972).

Cropworker Poisoning. Poisoning of cropworkers by residues of parathion is a poorly understood form of occupational poisoning. It is epidemiologically and even clinically different from poisoning of formulators and applicators who work directly with parathion. To indicate its separate status, it has been called "cropworker poisoning" and "reentry poisoning." The distribution and severity of cases involving direct exposure to formulations of parathion are proportional to the degree of exposure. Poisoning of cropworkers has shown a marked, unexplained clustering of cases. Of many fields or orchards in the same area treated in essentially the same way during the same season, only a few produced cases of poisoning, but those that produced any cases led to poisoning of a high proportion of exposed workers. Furthermore, the cases have had a peculiar distribution in time. There were few or no cases in some years and many cases in others. Clinically, the cases conformed to the picture of poisoning by organic phosphorus compounds, but they differed from the spectrum of cases caused by parathion in other circumstances in that no cropworkers were seriously sick. Some were hospitalized, but their survival was never in doubt (Quinby and Lemmon, 1958; Milby et al., 1964). It has been suggested that the peculiar circumstances leading to the poisoning of some cropworkers involved the conversion of parathion residues on the crops to some more toxic com-

pound. Some support for this suggestion was offered by the finding of slightly more paraoxon (3.0 ppm) than parathion (2.8 ppm) in the only leaf residue sample clearly associated with poisoning and analyzed for both compounds.

The cause of poisoning among cropworkers exposed to residues of parathion remains uncertain. The unpredictability of outbreaks of such poisoning makes their study difficult. It is supposed that some peculiar combination of environmental conditions permits a more rapid than normal conversion of parathion to paraoxon (or some other toxic derivative), or a greater persistence of the new toxicant after it is formed. However, it has not been possible so far to produce under experimental field conditions a residue such as that reported by Milby et al. (1964).

Other Occupational Poisoning. For any given country, occupational poisoning is a part of endemic morbidity and mortality. Thus, occupational poisoning by pesticides in the United States of America was included in the statistics for endemic poisoning presented in Sections 7.1.2.2 and 7.1.2.3. It was noted that occupational exposure was associated with only a small fraction of deaths caused by pesticides. However, the situation has been entirely different in some developing countries, where the introduction of a new pesticide sometimes led to serious outbreaks of poisoning. In some of these instances, there were no local morbidity or mortality statistics against which the outbreak could be compared. However, it was clear that there were enough recorded cases of occupational poisoning that the outbreak would have been viewed as completely unusual and extremely serious if it had occurred in one of the more developed countries.

The greatest difficulty has involved parathion under a variety of trade names. Ninety-six cases of parathion poisoning with 13 deaths were reported in a single year and as early as 1950 from a small portion of the cotton-raising section of Brazil (Planet, 1950). Parathion remained an important cause of occupational poisoning in Brazil until 1963, after which there was some improvement. Methyl parathion and methyl demeton were involved also (Almeida and Pereira, 1963; Almeida, 1967).

According to reports of the Secretariat of Health and Welfare of Mexico reviewed by Almeida (1966), parathion was the most common agricultural pesticide in Mexico in 1964 and 1965, and the main one responsible for poisoning of rural workers. Among these men, there were about 1,150 to 1,500 cases per year. The morbidity was 13 to 15% among those directly exposed, and 0.2% for the total population of the cotton-growing region. The mortality rate was 0.8 to 2.9% among the directly exposed workers. For the general population, the mortality rate was 100 to 380 per million, compared to a rate of about 1 per million in the United States of America during the same period.

There were over 1,500 cases and hundreds of deaths from parathion per year in Japan during 1953 and 1954 (Horasawa, 1956; Hayes, 1960). In 1955, legislation concerning parathion was made stricter. The number of accidents was reduced immediately to about one-half, and by 1960 to about one-third. There was no corresponding decrease in suicides with parathion, which averaged about 500 annually, from 1955 through 1960. Although the figures for suicide seem high, it was pointed out by Juhl (1971) that the rate in Japan was only somewhat more than half that in Denmark, while the rate for fatal accidents was 2 to 3 times that in Denmark during the same period.

Cases of occupational poisoning by dieldrin in Venezuela, Ecuador, Nigeria, India, and Indonesia have been reviewed (Hayes, 1957, 1959a), and cases from several other countries including Kenya and Tanganyika have been recognized but not reported in publication. At least 90 persons showed full epileptoid convulsions, and 11 suffered recurrence of illness several months after last exposure to the compound. The occurrence of illness among the spraymen on different projects apparently was proportional to the intensity and duration of occupational exposure.

Direct Dermal Application. Of the epidemics of dermal poisoning by organic phosphorus compounds listed in Table 7-7, one involved direct application of parathion to combat head lice. Other epidemics of this kind have occurred but apparently were not reported in medical journals. Related sporadic cases of poisoning by the dermal route are discussed in Section 7.1.4.3.

Apparently parathion is the only pesticide whose misuse as a shampoo for louse control had led to death. There are a number of other highly toxic organic phosphorus compounds capable of the same effect. Fortunately, the rarity of lice and the very careful regulation of the labeling of pesticides make this kind of poisoning unlikely in developed countries.

Suicides and Homicides. Historically, poisons have been a recognized method for both suicide and homicide. Many of the inorganic pesticides have been used for these purposes, but arsenic has remained a favorite for centuries.

Some of the newer pesticides have been used for both suicide and murder in the United States of America, but such use is unusual, and the cases have been endemic in distribution (see Section 7.1.2.2). On the contrary, new pesticides have been associated with virtual epidemics of suicide and murder in certain countries. At least 75 suicides and murders with parathion occurred in Germany in 1954 (reported in articles in the European edition of *Stars and Stripes,* July 1954, and in *Newsweek,* July 19, 1954). For the years 1955–1957, 219 suicides with parathion were reported for Finland (Toivonen *et al.,* 1959).

7.1.2.5 Experience of Special Groups.

Special groups such as formulators, spraymen, or the residents of sprayed houses have been studied for a variety of reasons. Some studies were simply a part of good occupational medicine in the plant where the group worked. Some of these are listed in Table 5-2. Other studies were made by outside specialists because of some local complaint, often involving the unexposed population as well as groups with relatively heavy exposure, and other studies were made by outside specialists on their own initiative to learn the effects of persistent and often intense exposure to pesticides. So far, no study of a special group has revealed an epidemic not already recognized when the study began. Studies of special groups have given a great deal of information on the health status of the groups involved. Probably their major contribution, however, is toward evaluation of the safety of pesticides in general.

Studies in Response to Local Complaints of Whatever Origin. Outbreaks of poisoning, such as those resulting from the contamination of food during transport, have required intensive work at the time to discover the cause of illness and extent of the trouble and to care for the patients and their families. However, these tragedies, sometimes involving hundreds of cases and many deaths, have not required any studies once the epidemics themselves were dealt with. The situations that did require special study involved fear and apprehension more than illness. In some instances there was underlying illness; for example, Ganelin and his co-workers (1964) investigated the claim that the symptoms of known asthmatics were made worse and more frequent by environmental exposure to organic phosphorus insecticides. In other instances, no single disease or special group of patients was involved. Sometimes the alarm could be traced to one person in the community. This was apparently true of the rural area studied by Fowler (1953).

This area of the Mississippi Delta included one small city where questions similar to those raised by Biskind (1949a, b, c, 1953), Biskind and Bieber (1949), Merking (1954), and Scott (1954) had been asked by one physician. It was suggested that insecticides might be at least the contributing cause of fungus infection, hay fever, asthma, sinusitis, gastrointestinal upsets, dehydration, alkalosis, malnutrition, pneumonitis, cancer, poliomyelitis, arteriosclerosis, heart disease, and insanity.

All physicians in the study area were urged through their medical societies to report cases of suspected insecticide poisoning. Other groups, including hospital staffs, county agricultural agents, and civic clubs, were approached for the same purpose. As was anticipated, a few cases of acute poisoning by parathion and several chlorinated hydrocarbon insecticides were reported, and a few other cases were uncovered by Fowler himself in an epidemiological survey of 83 farm laborers and a survey of 639 unselected persons living on a large plantation. The cases of poisoning were all caused by excessive exposure to the insecticides and were frequently associated with gross carelessness on the part of workers.

In addition to direct clinical studies, Fowler (1953) reviewed school attendance records, mortality records of the Delta and of the state as a whole, and morbidity records of a plantation hospital. He also sought the expert judgment of county health officers. He compared the incidence of disease in these areas during the periods before and after the introduction of the newer agricultural chemicals. He also compared the incidence of disease in the regions of the State of Mississippi where insecticides are little used with the disease incidence in the Delta, where cotton culture necessitates the extensive use of agricultural chemicals. In all of the studies, no evidence could be found that pesticides were the direct or indirect cause of any chronic disease, or a contributing factor in diseases generally recognized as having other etiologies.

One community reached near hysteria largely because it was suspected that the deaths of two infants were caused by incidental exposure to organic phosphorous insecticides. Spraying and dusting of trees had been done in the neighborhood and the odor of insecticides was evident. Epidemiological and clinical studies by the US Public Health Ser-

vice failed to show evidence that incidental exposure was the cause of disease. Alarm was dispelled, although the study did reveal cases of poisoning associated with occupational exposure, and investigation was made of several cases in which children swallowed poison with fatal or near-fatal results (Johnston, 1953; Sumerford et al., 1953).

The direct requests of state and federal agricultural agencies were responsible for a study carried out by Quinby et al. (1958) in the Mississippi Delta area of Mississippi. Both a responsible professional attitude regarding the introduction of organic phosphorus insecticides and the presence of some apprehension in the community contributed to the requests. However, during the course of the study one local physician attributed many cases of respiratory infection to poisoning and this mistaken diagnosis, which received widespread publicity by newspapers and radio, caused considerable alarm. As might have been predicted, about half of the persons with the epidemic infection had some occupational exposure to pesticides, but the others were essentially unexposed. As part of a thorough epidemiological and clinical investigation, some cases of poisoning were confirmed, but only in persons with extensive exposure. The valid cases were associated with some nine observed violations of safety regulations enumerated in the report.

The potential hazards from incidental exposure to pesticides require special consideration. By incidental exposure is meant any exposure that is neither voluntary nor strictly accidental. Thus, incidental to treating a crop, some pesticides may fall in neighboring fields or in suburbs without there being any intent to treat those areas and without there being any accident in the usual sense.

Evidence has been presented by Fowler (1953), Sumerford and his associates (1953), Barnes (1953), Hayes et al. (1957), Quinby et al. (1958), and others that under ordinary conditions persons exposed incidentally to pesticides do not contact enough of the materials to cause any injury. Complaints continue to be heard occasionally, but they are much less frequent. Furthermore, these complaints have shown striking variation from one locality to another, and they appear to bear no strict relationship to the amount of pesticides used in the area or, in fact, whether pesticides are used at all.

Responsible toxicologists must investigate each new suspicion of injury as it arises. However, no further attention is required when claims that have been disproved are renewed as they sometimes are (Biskind and Mobbs, 1972) without additional evidence of a causal relationship between illness and one or more chemicals. Although the studies done so far have revealed cases of poisoning in workers or other persons who were heavily exposed, not a single study uncovered any evidence that pesticides contribute to diseases other than poisoning, or that even mild poisoning occurred in persons without occupational or other substantial, direct contact with these compounds.

Community Studies. Acute local anxiety about the danger of pesticides was relieved in part by special studies and in part by the passage of time bringing realization that the compounds were safe for persons with only incidental exposure. More recently, additional studies of persons with moderate to heavy exposure have been carried out, even though no local concern was expressed. Some of these investigations were specially designed to learn more about storage, enzyme induction, or some other specific effect; discussions of them are integrated into appropriate sections of this and other chapters. However, one set of administratively unified studies carried out in over one-fourth of the states requires discussion at this point.

The Community Studies on Pesticides were established by the US Public Health Service. By 1967 the Pesticides Program was well organized; the Community Studies portion of it was carried out through contracts. It involved laboratories in state and local departments of health or in universities in 16 states (Simmons, 1968).

Although the programs of these 16 laboratories were varied somewhat depending on local problems and local interest, the core programs are the same. A profile of the use of pesticides in each state is kept current and confirmed by analysis of pesticides in environmental samples. Persons who had worked with pesticides and might be expected to continue to do so were selected for continuing study. Controls who differed as little as possible, except in their exposure to pesticides, were selected also. At quarter-year intervals, each subject provides a detailed exposure history and a medical history, undergoes a physical examination, and provides samples for the analysis of pesticides and for a battery of about 50 clinical laboratory tests. The chemical and biochemical tests are done by methods set forth in manuals designed for the studies. Adherence to these methods and participation in periodic interlaboratory quality control tests ensure a greater degree of comparability of data from the Community Studies laboratories than could be anticipated from an equal number of unrelated laboratories.

As opportunity permitted, each state laboratory reported cases of accidental poisoning, epidemiological studies of recognized cases, improvements in analytical methods, and monitoring of chlorinated hydrocarbon insecticides in people and in environmental samples. One of the laboratories did an outstanding study of the storage and excretion of DDT and its metabolites in volunteers, and one reported the reduction of such storage by antiepileptic drugs. These kinds of studies are discussed in other, appropriate sections.

No general summary of the results of all the laboratories has been issued. Until this is done, the possibility of regional trends (over and above those noted in the general literature) cannot be excluded. Even some of the individual laboratories have been slow to report the results of their surveillance of workers. This may be related in part to the fact that few if any of the groups under surveillance were so heavily exposed to pesticides as was true of special groups selected by others for investigation of storage, enzyme induction, and other specific effects.

Results from studies of volunteers and highly exposed workers indicated even when the Community Pesticides Studies were begun that dramatic findings were unlikely. However, it is reassuring that continuing, meticulous study (Long *et al.*, 1969; Morgan and Roan, 1969; Warnick and Carter, 1972; Sandifer *et al.*, 1972; Embry *et al.*, 1972) has failed to reveal effects of clinical significance among workers with prolonged, moderate exposure to a wide variety of pesticides.

As might have been predicted, measurement of blood levels of some chlorinated hydrocarbon insecticides and their metabolites and measurement of blood cholinesterase levels have served to confirm the workers' known degree of occupational exposure. Inevitably, small but statistically significant differences have appeared in the medical history or clinical laboratory results of an occasional group of workers, as compared with controls. However, in no instance have the differences been of any medical importance, and dosage-response relationships have been unclear or absent. In several instances, the statistically significant differences were opposite in different groups of workers; for example, creatine phosphokinase activity lower than that of controls in applicators but higher in operators. Seasonal variations that seemed to be present in one year were lacking the following year. It cannot be said that the studies exclude the possibility that pesticides are associated with small, real differences in the parameters measured. The studies do prove that if such differences exist they are small and clinically unimportant. The possibility of adaptive change has been mentioned (Tocci et al., 1969) but this, like the reality of differences, is unproved.

WHO Program for Testing Pesticides. Some of the most instructive studies of the safety of groups exposed to pesticides are those connected with the collaborative, long-range program started by the World Health Organization a little before 1960 for the evaluation of insecticides for vector control. As mentioned in Section 1.4.1.2, this program was instituted in the hope of overcoming or at least minimizing the effects of resistance of some vectors to DDT. In spite of intensive research to find biological means of pest control, the use of alternative insecticides remains the only solution generally available (Wright et al., 1969).

Candidate materials are contributed by industry, governments, and university scientists. Evaluation is carried out by a number of laboratories throughout the world in a program of seven stages. The first several stages are concerned with entomological testing and with tests for safety in laboratory animals. Compounds that still seem promising for malaria control (having not been excluded either because of ineffectiveness or danger) are submitted successively to one or more village-scale tests (Stage V), operational field trials (Stage VI), and finally, an epidemiological study (Stage VII) to determine their ability to stop transmission of malaria (Wright et al., 1969).

Only compounds considered safe on the basis of animal tests are ever studied for vector control in the field. However, those responsible for the collaborative study were aware from the beginning that field tests would have to involve not only a careful evaluation of entomological effectiveness, but an equally careful evaluation of the safety of each compound for spraymen and for the inhabitants of sprayed houses. Both effectiveness for disease control and safety for people must be judged against the outstanding record of DDT (see especially Sections 1.4.1.2 and 7.5). So far more than 1,300 compounds have been tested. Of these, only 12 had been recommended by 1969 for village-scale trials (Wright et al., 1969). The following paragraphs illustrate that some substitutes for DDT have proved truly safe; some present certain problems and must be used with precaution. Other potential substitutes proved too dangerous for use under the specific conditions required for malaria control. No attempt has been made to discuss every compound that has reached the stage of village testing.

The major defects of dieldrin as a means of vector control (Carrillo, 1954; Hayes, 1957, 1959a) were apparent when the WHO collaborative program was set up. Under the circumstances, greatest attention was turned to organic phosphorus and carbamate insecticides. It was hoped that the cross-resistance associated with some chlorinated hydrocarbon insecticides could be avoided. There was also some hope that resistance would be less a problem in connection with compounds that are less persistent in the environment. Finally, provision was made that no compound would be introduced for vector control without toxicological surveillance.

Because organic phosphorus and carbamate compounds are known to act by inhibition of cholinesterases, activity of these enzymes in the blood of exposed persons was monitored carefully. Where possible, measurement of a compound or its metabolites in urine was used as another index of absorption. Finally, exposed persons were examined and questioned regarding any clinical effects. It was recognized from the beginning that a trial in a single, small village might reveal an essentially complete picture of injury to occupants of sprayed houses as well as any acute effects in spraymen, but an extensive field trial would be required to learn whether injury would be detectable in workers only after they had been exposed more or less continuously for weeks or months.

In the collaborative program for evaluation of insecticides for vector control, every effort was made to take advantage of what was already known about the relative safety of compounds and their use for control of agricultural pests. The first compound tested was malathion. A village-scale trial of it was conducted in 1960–1961 (Elliot and Barnes, 1963). The compound reached Stage VII of testing in 1963–1964. One test in southern Uganda involved a population of about 26,000 (Najera et al., 1967), and the compound was used routinely in 29,000 houses in Central America (WHO, 1968). Even though no precautions were taken beyond those commonly used for DDT, no evidence of illness was seen or reported, except in three spraymen who for several days without interruption wore work clothes wet with kerosene solution of malathion. Two of them were moderately ill for 3 days and one of them for 1 day; the symptoms were characteristic of anticholinesterase poisoning. Reports of these studies led the WHO Expert Committee on Insecticides (1967) to approve the use of malathion in public health programs when required, provided the same precautions recommended for DDT were observed.

Greater precautions were used when carbaryl was first tested. Spraymen were dressed in overalls, impervious hats, and gumboots. They were instructed to wear face masks while spraying indoors, but failed to do so. No clinical signs of poisonong were reported. Very slight, transient falls in plasma cholinesterase were noted among spraymen, but none among residents. One case of pronounced skin eruption was observed in an African sprayman whose back was splashed with the insecticide (Vandekar, 1965). In the opinion of the WHO Expert Committee on Insecticides (1967), carbaryl is safe provided general precautions are taken. Unfortunately, carbaryl is ineffective on dried mud (Wright et al., 1969), which probably constitutes the walls of more homes than any other material in the world.

Propoxur has been tested under field conditions in Haiti, El Salvador, Nigeria, and Iran. In these countries it has proved effective for control of at least five species of malaria mosquitoes. It probably has been studied more extensively in connection with vector control than any other carbamate, and its successful passage through the first six stages of the seven-stage evaluation program has been summarized in an unusually thorough way (Wright et al., 1969). From the standpoint of mosquito control, propoxur is unique because it is applied as a spray but has more extensive vapor action than any other compound, including dichlorovos, the action extending for some distance out of doors. The practical effect from an entomological standpoint is that results varied between localities, between well ventilated and poorly ventilated houses, between villages with houses close together and those with isolated houses, and between dry and rainy seasons. In some compact villages, the entire vector population disappeared for up to 14 weeks. There is no evidence, however, that the vapor has any effect on human health.

Observations on the safety of propoxur as a residual insecticide have been carried out in three different parts of the world with a total of more than 4,000 man-days of spraying and the use of over 30 metric tons of water-dispersible powder. There were minor symptoms among some spraymen and a few inhabitants in two trial areas. All patients recovered within a very short time, usually without treatment. However, a few drops of tincture of belladonna speeded recovery.

Operators who complained of symptoms were mainly those who lacked experience and care in avoiding mist and who washed insufficiently during and after work. Inhabitants who complained usually had direct contact with the spray. A few cases of skin eruptions in Africans have been observed.

The excretion of phenols in the urine falls off promptly after exposure to propoxur is stopped. The concentration may be high in persons who are well and low in those who are sick, apparently depending on when the samples are taken. However, somewhat higher excretion was noted on the second day of wearing an unwashed uniform. Frequent washing of the hands markedly reduced absorption of propoxur. No additional protection was demonstrated in persons who wore respirators. Thus, there are objective reasons for the precautions that are recommended.

Unfortunately, the measurement of phenolic metabolites apparently was not made so that the rates of excretion and corresponding absorption could be stated quantitatively. It is clear, however, that the rates under conditions of work are small. In studies on volunteers, it was found that, when taken at half-hour intervals, 5 oral doses each at the rate of 0.20 mg/kg produced a symptomless inhibition of erythrocyte cholinesterase, down to about 60% of normal (approximately the same as the average depression seen in spraymen (Vandekar et al., 1968). A single dose at the rate of 0.36 mg/kg produced essentially the same depression of cholinesterase, but also produced stomach discomfort and moderate redness and sweating of the face lasting about 5 minutes. A single dose of 1.5 mg/kg reduced erythrocyte cholinesterase to 27% of normal 15 minutes after ingestion. At that time the volunteer felt "pressure in the head;" a few minutes later he developed blurred vision, profound perspiration, and vomiting, all of which lasted less than 1 hour. No significant depression of plasma cholinesterase could be detected throughout the investigation (Pleština, 1968; Wright et al., 1969).

A pronounced fall in whole blood cholinesterase activity occurred in operators soon after exposure started, and a distinct recovery took place within 3 hours after exposure stopped. When there was no possibility of futher exposure, recovery of cholinesterase was complete the morning after work was finished. There was no progression of inhibition as exposure continued day after day and week after week. In view of the very marked symptomless daily fluctuation in cholinesterase activity and the lack of cumulative inhibition, routine cholines-terase determination is of little, if any, practical value in indicating whether a worker should be withdrawn from further exposure to propoxur. Essentially the same is true of the measurement of phenolic metabolites in the urine. On the contrary, minor complaints, from which recovery is spontaneous and rapid, cause the operator to stop work and thus prevent further exposure (Vandekar et al., 1968).

Propoxur is suitable for wide-scale epidemiological evaluation (Wright et al., 1969). Protective measures should include clean overalls daily, an impervious broad-brimmed hat, impervious shoes, rubber gloves (for mixer only), washing of the hands and face following each pump charge, and bathing at the end of each day's work.

When fenthion was tested with precautions and medical supervision in single villages, no signs or symptoms were observed or reported; depression of cholinesterase was confined to the plasma enzyme and was significant but not alarming. When, through misunderstanding, the compound was used with hardly any precautions and without toxicological supervision in a single large test involving 50 villages and 5,000 people, 21 of the 28 spraymen had signs and symptoms of poisoning, some of them severe. There were 9 certain and at least 11 probable cases of poisoning in the villages. Whole blood cholinesterase activity was markedly reduced both in spraymen and in many residents. A second, smaller round of spraying was carried out by 12 new, properly trained applicators using protective clothing and appropriate precautions. Only three cases of mild poisoning were recorded, one in a mixer and two in residents. Such depressions of whole blood cholinesterase activity as occurred were not marked, except in the three cases of poisoning and in another sprayman who remained well. In view of these results, especially those involving no special supervision, the WHO Expert Committee on Insecticides (1967) considered that fenthion is not suitable for routine residual indoor spraying. However, it is both safe and effective as a mosquito larvicide (Wright et al., 1969).

A full account of the toxicological observations made during the village-scale trial of 3-isopropylphenyl N-methylcarbamate have been published (Vandekar, 1965). Briefly, a mild to moderate degree of poisoning occurred in all spraymen within 2 to 3 hours after spraying began, even though the men had worn protective clothing and masks while they worked. A consultant who sprayed only about half an hour vomited and was otherwise mildly poisoned. Of 70 villagers exposed to 3-isopropylphenyl N-methylcarbamate, three were mildly poisoned, five vomited, and a 14-month-old child was severely poisoned and was hospitalized. An itching macular rash occurred in 17 of 34 exposed male villagers, all of whom were Africans. The rash was largely confined to unclothed areas, and this was true in a girl who was the only one of 36 females who developed a rash. The lesion lasted 2 to 3 weeks in most cases, but persisted more than a month in three persons. Soon after spraying, plasma cholinesterase activity was markedly depressed in all spraymen; recovery was incomplete the next morning but complete 3 days later. Increased excretion of phenols persisted several days in villagers. In some of them, excretion of phenolic metabolites remained high for 8 days after spraying, and in one man, who was confined to his room by illness, this excretion persisted until he was taken to hospital 14 days after application of the insecticide.

The WHO Expert Committee on Insecticides (1967) concluded that 3-isopropylphenyl N-methylcarbamate is too toxic to recommend as a house spray by conventional methods of application.

Even this brief review serves to show those familiar with agricultural use of pesticides that the hazards associated with indoor application of residual sprays are different from those in agriculture. It was demonstrated many years ago that spraymen receive about 7 times as much exposure per unit time in indoor spraying as they receive outdoors (see Section 6.2.3.1). Furthermore, the range of persons exposed is much greater when an entire community is sprayed than when a crop is treated. Another point illustrated is that not all injuries produced by chemicals can be related to their main mode of action. Examples include the rashes produced by several carbamates. The fact that the rashes so far have occurred only in Africans even though others have been exposed suggests the possibility of genetic differences in susceptibility. Thus, there is no choice but to test each promising compound under the conditions of intended use.

It must be concluded that the human safety of DDT for vector control was due to good fortune in the original choice, while the safety of the small number of alternatives now available for malaria control is due to careful testing and cautious appraisal.

In a discussion of the direct effects on human health of pesticides used to control vectors of disease, it is important to recognize how minor these effects are, both in absolute terms and relative to their tremendous indirect benefit to health through control of disease and increased availability of food. It also must be recognized that DDT is the safest compound used for vector control. Its clinical record is unbelievably good. It has caused serious illness very rarely and only following the ingestion of large amounts. According to experience in the western world, occupational injury has been confined to irritation of the skin, eyes, and throat of no greater frequency or severity than would be expected from the same exposure to inert dust. No injury to residents of sprayed houses has been confirmed. Storage of DDT and DDE is increased among spraymen, but without injury to health; storage among residents of sprayed houses is not increased above the traces caused by dietary intake in the same country.

7.1.3 Record of Different Countries

The very unequal national distribution and epidemic character of poisoning associated with accidents and sometimes with occupational exposure and with suicide and homicide was described in separate paragraphs of Section 7.1.2.4. The following remarks are concerned with endemic poisoning.

The proportion of recorded poisoning associated with pesticides differs from country to country. As already mentioned (Section 7.1.2.2), the proportion of accidental poisoning by solids and liquids in the United States associated with pesticides decreased from values around 10% in the 1950's to 2.5% in 1968. Corresponding values for some other countries are: 1.5% or less in England and Wales (Hayes and Pirkle, 1966), 23% in Australia (Clements et al., 1963), and 39% in Israel (based on data of Wislicki, 1961). In 1961, the mortality in England and Wales associated with acute poisoning by chemicals that can be used as pesticides was at the rate of 0.15 per million population (Anonymous, 1963). All of the victims were adults. In five of the seven instances the compound involved could be used for a purpose other than pest control, and there was no way to determine with certainty whether a pesticide was involved or not. As already mentioned, the corresponding mortality rate for the United States of America was 0.65 per million (Hayes and Pirkle, 1966).

The limited use of pesticides in England and Wales may more than account for their relatively good safety record there. In 1961, the number of deaths associated with all pesticides in England and Wales and in the United States of America, respectively, was 2.6 and 1.1 per thousand metric tons of selected pesticides. The compounds included the major organic phosphorus compounds, aldrin and related compounds, benzene hexachloride, DDT, nicotine, lead arsenate, mercurials, and the phenoxyacetic acid herbicides. These compounds were selected because they are important and because information was available on the weight of each used in the two countries (Farm Chemicals Handbook, 1965; Strickland, 1965). The weakness of the comparison is that of the seven deaths associated with pesticides in England and Wales in 1961, only two were caused by compounds (malathion and 2,4-D) which have no use except as pesticides, and the other compounds (strychnine, trichloroethylene, arsenic, cyanide, and a mercurial) may have been intended for some other purpose. However, even on the basis of only two deaths, the mortality was 0.8 per thousand metric tons. Thus, the British safety record for pesticides is good in relation to population at risk, but of questionable difference from that in the United States of America in relation to tonnage of pesticides used. The annual per capita use of the compounds mentioned above was 58 g in England and Wales, but 564 g in the United States of America.

However, as suggested by Table 7-8, other factors may be more important in determining safety than the amount of pesticide used. The mortality rate from pesticides in different countries does not correspond with the degree of their use. To be sure, the high mortality rates reported in Israel (Wislicki, 1961) were associated with high rates of use and the same probably was true of the high mortality rate reported in Japan (Namba, 1961).

The relatively limited use of pesticides in England and Wales is an important factor in the good safety record there, but this factor cannot account for the reported fact that children in England are spared almost entirely from severe injury by these compounds. Uniformity of language, education, and tradition must be contributing factors, but it is difficult to evaluate their importance or to determine whether they represent an adequate explanation. There may be other factors. Records of the poison control center for England and Wales show that children are not spared completely from contacts with poisonous materials; in fact, children contribute 59% of the morbidity that is reported (Goulding and Watkin, 1965). In the United States of America, children are involved in even a higher proportion (88%) of reports from poison control centers, and each year over half of those killed by

Table 7-8

Relation of Use of Insecticides to
Mortality Caused by Them

	Annual mortality (deaths per million)	Annual use (grams per capita)
USA, 1956	1.11	--
1961	0.65	564
England and Wales, 1961	0.15	58
R.V., 1960-1962	2.08-2.67	36
Japan, 1950-1958	>5 [a]	--
Israel, 1957-1960	3.11-5.16	435-627

a.   Parathion only but includes suicides.

pesticides are children under 10 years of age (Hayes and Pirkle, 1966). The predominance of fatal poisoning in children has been noted in Israel (Arnan, 1962), Australia (Clements et al., 1963; Isbister, 1963; Phelan, 1963), and Switzerland (Nouhen-Lang, 1964), and it appears to be the usual pattern.

Apparently, no survey has been made of the relative importance of different circumstances of poisoning in different countries, but the pattern found in the United States of America is distributed widely. For example, in Casablanca, Morocco, during the period 1963–1969, 1,397 cases were self-poisoning, 480 were accidental, 40 were occupational, and 19 criminal, with an overall mortality of 3% (Dezoteux and Vinceneux, 1971).

7.1.4 Factors in Poisoning

Section 2.4 contains a discussion of the basic factors influencing toxicity. The present section is concerned with those factors that may be recognized as contributing to poisoning by pesticides in man. So far only a portion of the basic factors have been found to be of practical significance in the limited environment in which man moves. However, other factors such as labeling and availability to children, which really involve dosage but are peculiar to the human situation, are of great importance in determining the incidence of cases.

7.1.4.1 Compound. Table 7-3 lists pesticides known to have caused poisoning in man at one time or another. Table 7-5 lists pesticides that produced poisoning in the United States of America in two selected years.

If absorption is an established fact, the possibility that the absorbed dosage of a toxicant will be sufficient to cause death depends on the inherent toxicity of the compound. Thus, the number of deaths caused by rodenticides is entirely disproportionate to the tonnage of these materials used (Table 7-9). This circumstance is due entirely to the high toxicity of the older rat poisons. Deaths or even illnesses caused by anticoagulant rodenticides are rare (McLeod, 1970).

Although the factor of "complacency" cannot be measured objectively, it is clear to those familiar with the field that some compounds, especially older ones, are taken for granted more than others. In 1956 and 1961, more than 68 and 58%, respectively, of deaths caused by pesticides were associated with compounds older than DDT (Hayes and Pirkle, 1966). Both complacency and inherent toxicity seem to play a part in the poor safety record of the arsenicals, especially arsenical herbicides (Table 7-9).

An important shift in the use of compounds may be expected to produce a corresponding change in the occurrence of poisoning. The recent action to limit severely the use of DDT may be expected to increase the use of other insecticides, including the organic phosphorus compounds. Some of the latter are only a little more dangerous than DDT. However, some of the most inexpensive and versatile organic phosphorus insecticides are highly dangerous. The safety record of DDT for people has always been remarkably good; the amount that found its way into food was always small, and, through regulation, these residues actually

Table 7-9

Number of Deaths in a Typical Year According
to Intended Use of Pesticide

From Hayes and Pirkle (1966) by permission of the American
Medical Association.

	All pesticides	Arsenicals
insecticides	62	4
herbicides	15	14
rodenticides	25	7
fungicides	2	0
unspecified	7	4
total	111	29

were reduced over a period of years. Unfortunately, DDT has the property of building up in some food chains so that a few predaceous animals, especially hawks and large fish, received prolonged heavy exposure, and some were killed. Unlike the food of man, there was no practical way to regulate the DDT content of food eaten by hawks and fish. The effort to protect these forms of wildlife by essentially stopping the use of DDT may lead to increased poisoning of children.

The indoor spraying of houses for malaria control does not contribute significantly to environmental contamination; therefore, there is no need to restrict this form of malaria control in order to protect wildlife. As pointed out by the Director General of the World Health Organization (World Health Organization, 1969, 1971), DDT remains crucial for malaria control. Any restriction of it for this use would lead to sickness and death of millions of people.

7.1.4.2 Dosage. In the last analysis it is dosage that determines poisoning and other pharmacological effects. The relation of storage to dosage in man is neatly demonstrated (see, for example Fig. 7-7, p. 355). It is often difficult to demonstrate the relation of mortality and morbidity to dosage in man in any refined sense because of the difficulty of measuring dosage in the erratically occurring situations leading to injury. It is this very difficulty that makes it so necessary to use every opportunity to determine both harmful and harmless dosage levels. Methods for this

measurement are discussed in Sections 5.5 and 3.2.2.2.

It is unusual that the human situation permits a demonstration of the importance of dosage schedule in determining outcome. There are a few exceptions. Heavy smokers inhale enough nicotine in one day to cause severe illness or death if it were all absorbed rapidly from a single dose.

There are some industrial situations, notably exposure to silica dust and some mercury compounds, in which the duration of exposure is of great importance. However, with rare exceptions—including again some compounds of mercury—pesticides are metabolized efficiently enough that they do not cause any recognized chronic illness. Acute illness follows excessive exposure and is often more likely in new employees than in those who, through experience, have learned to minimize their exposure.

7.1.4.3 Route of Exposure. The great majority of deaths caused by pesticides follow ingestion of the poison. A few deaths, caused almost exclusively by fumigants, follow respiratory exposure. An approximately equal proportion are associated with dermal exposure to some of the chlorinated hydrocarbon and organic phosphorus insecticides. In many instances of occupational poisoning, it is clear that exposure is both respiratory and dermal, and it is often difficult to assess the contribution of each to the outcome if the compound can be absorbed dermally (Hayes and Pirkle,

1966). However, measurement of exposure and absorption by these two routes (see Sections 6.2.3.1 and 7.2.4.1) emphasizes the importance of dermal exposure in many instances where fumigants are not involved. Some epidemiological studies also have emphasized the importance of dermal absorption (Reich et al., 1968a).

In addition to the epidemics of dermal poisoning mentioned in Section 7.1.2.4, there have been a number of scattered cases. Some of these have involved the use of parathion for combatting lice (Koeffler, 1958; Introna, 1959; Nameche and Bartman, 1964), scabies (Hristic and Milenkovic, 1961), or pruritus of unknown cause (Prinz, 1969). Others involved occupational contact (Lindbjerg, 1960) or accidental exposure (Chamberlin and Cooke, 1953; Dixon, 1957; Pilat et al., 1961; Rosen, 1960; Meneses de Almeida and Peroso de Lima, 1964; Hayes, 1963).

Although parathion has been the most common cause of dermal poisoning, mevinphos, diazinon, chlorophos, and chlordane also have been the cause of serious, sometimes fatal poisoning by the dermal route. Undoubtedly some other compounds have had the same effect.

7.1.4.4 Interaction of Compounds. Clear examples of effects of the interaction of compounds on poisoning in man are unusual. Some examples are discussed in Section 2.4.6.1. Effects of interaction on storage or excretion are more common (see Section 7.2.4.1).

7.1.4.5 Race and Ethnic Group. In the 1961 study of fatal accidental poisoning by pesticides in the United States of America, it was found that 30.6% of the deaths involved nonwhite persons although these persons constituted only 11.5% of the total population in that year (Hayes and Pirkle, 1966). In addition, five of the 77 white victims had distinctly Spanish surnames, a proportion probably higher than that in the general population.

In certain areas, the proportion of poisoning by pesticides that involves nonwhites may be very high (McLeod, 1970). In south Florida it averaged 72% (Reich et al., 1968b), and in studies of children reached 84 to 93% (Davies et al., 1969b; Davies et al., 1970).

A higher rate of poisoning in general has been observed in nonwhites (Cann, 1963).

It seems likely that the distribution of cases by race or ethnic group is associated in some instances with (a) inability to read labels (either because the victim is illiterate or the label is in the wrong language), or (b) a high rate of occupational exposure.

There is no evidence that race influences inherent susceptibility to any pesticide, except possibly susceptibility among Africans to dermatitis associated with certain anticholinesterase carbamates.

7.1.4.6 Sex. The predominance of poisoning among males has been noted repeatedly (Cann, 1963; Cann et al., 1960; Isbister, 1963; Nouhen-Lang, 1964; Reich et al., 1968b, McLeod, 1970). In England and Wales this predominance applies to pesticides but does not, in fact, apply to poisons generally (Anonymous, 1962, 1963).

In the 1961 study, the predominance of fatal poisoning in males was evident among children (63%) as well as adults (69%) (Hayes and Pirkle, 1966). The distribution apparently reflects a greater tendency to exploration among boys and certainly represents a greater occupational exposure of men to pesticides.

7.1.4.7 Age and Competency.

Poisoning in Children. In the United States of America, more than half of the cases of fatal poisoning caused by pesticides are in children under 10 years (Hayes and Pirkle, 1966). Figure 7-4 shows the distribution of accidental deaths caused by pesticides in 1961, according to age and sex. Poisoning was most frequent among children 1 to 3 years of age.

The predominance in children of accidental poisoning by solids and liquids in general has been noted in the USA (Cann, 1963; Cann et al., 1960; Wehrle et al., 1960; McLeod, 1970), Australia (Clements et al., 1963; Isbister, 1963; Phelan, 1963), Switzerland (Nouhen-Lang, 1964), and Israel (Arnan, 1962). However, the records for England and Wales and for Sweden constitute a marked exception. In England and Wales children under 15 years of age contributed only 5.8 and 7.7% of the total deaths caused by solids and liquids in 1960 and 1961, respectively (Anonymous, 1962, 1963), and records for nonfatal poisoning (Goulding and Watkin, 1965) confirm the relatively small involvement of children. In the United Kingdom, only 59% of inquiries to the National Poisons Information Service involved children (Goulding and Watkin, 1965), whereas in the United States of Americia such calls constituted 88% of the total (Cann, 1963). Data from statistical abstracts of Sweden show that children contribute less than 10% of fatal cases of accidental poisoning in that country.

In the context just discussed, the liability of

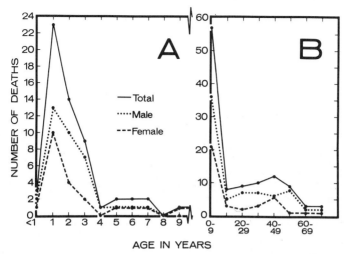

Fig. 7-4. Distribution of accidental deaths caused by pesticides in 1961 according to age and sex. A, Children under 10 years of age; B, all ages. From Hayes and Pirkle (1966) by permission of the American Medical Association.

children to poisoning depends on their greater exposure more than on any difference in susceptibility. However, a few differences in susceptibility are known to exist. The most striking example involves susceptibility to poisoning by parathion. In situations in which food contaminated with parathion was eaten by adults and children approximately in proportion to their weights, the children were affected more frequently and more severely (Kanagaratnam *et al.*, 1960).

Poisoning of the Incompetent. Incompetents other than children are also relatively frequent victims of poisoning. Although only 111 cases of fatal poisoning by pesticides were revealed by the 1961 study, three cases involved persons more than 70 years old, who may have been senile; two involved persons (one a child) recognized as mentally deficient; and five involved persons stated to have been under the influence of alcohol at the time they ingested a pesticide (Hayes and Pirkle, 1966). Thus, about 8% of the cases were associated with incompetency other than that of childhood.

7.1.4.8 Accessibility.

Urban-Rural Distribution of Poisoning. Since the greatest tonnage of pesticides is used in agriculture and since the number of deaths caused by them appears to correspond with the tonnage used in different years, one might suppose that most of these deaths would occur in rural areas. However, no evidence of this was found in the 1961 study of deaths caused by pesticides. The proportion of deaths in rural areas was almost exactly the

same as the proportion of population living in these areas (Hayes and Pirkle, 1966).

Data from poison control centers tend to reflect urban experience. They are not a good source of information on the urban-rural incidence of poisoning.

Regional Differences in Poisoning. In the 1961 study, the percentage of cases exceeded the percentage of population for the four regions that constitute the southern United States of America as far west as Arizona (Hayes and Pirkle, 1966). The high proportion of cases in this area probably reflects: (*a*) the growth of cotton, a crop requiring extensive use of insecticides; (*b*) higher temperatures leading to greater problems with pests generally; and (*c*) the relatively high proportion of nonwhite or migrant agricultural workers. This argument fails to explain why pesticides have caused somewhat fewer deaths in California than would be predicted on the basis of population. California produces cotton and employs many migrant laborers. They do record many cases of nonfatal poisoning (see Section 7.1.2.3). In fact, more than 1,300 cases of nonfatal occupational injury from pesticides were reported in California each year during the period 1964–1970 (see Table 7-6). It may be that the relatively good record of California so far as mortality is concerned can be credited to greater alertness to the problem and more extensive regulation of pesticides there than in other states (Section 9.1.2.2).

Petroleum products as well as pesticides cause a relatively higher incidence of poisoning in the southeastern United States of

America than in other areas of the same country (Cann *et al.*, 1960). By contrast, cases associated with medicines, paints and varnishes, and other materials were relatively more frequent in other regions (Cann *et al.*, 1960).

National Differences in Poisoning. The marked national differences that exist in mortality and morbidity from pesticides (see Section 7.1.3) depend on: (*a*) climatic differences leading to inherent differences in the need to use pesticides; (*b*) variation in literacy; (*c*) variation in the degree and dispersion of information on the handling of chemicals in general, and pesticides in particular; (*d*) degree of mechanization of formulation and application; (*e*) fashions in murder and suicide; and (*f*) perhaps other unrecognized factors.

Location of Container. Although misplacement of poison containers can lead to disaster for anyone, this factor is of greatest importance for children and the incompetent. This is particularly true in and around the home, where placement of containers determines the availability of poison to children. Placement of containers is of somewhat less importance in work places only because few if any children are present.

In connection with over 82,000 cases of accidental ingestion among children under 5 years of age, Verhulst and Crotty (1964) reported that the substances were not in their customary storage places in 46 to 72% of instances classified by place of accident. Most ingestions occur in the kitchen, followed by the bedroom, bath, and living room, in decreasing order. However, children may find access to poisons, including pesticides, in the basement, garage, and out of doors. When classified by type of compound, it was found that, when pesticides were ingested, the poison was not in its customary place of storage in 75% of instances.

Season. The seasonal distribution of fatal cases of accidental poisoning in 1961 is shown in Fig. 7-5. Pesticides cause slightly more deaths in summer than in winter. This distribution is similar to that for accidental poisoning by solids and liquids generally, and is what one would expect since most pesticides are solid or liquid. The seasonal distribution undoubtedly reflects the greater average availability of pesticidal formulations in summer when their use is greatest. However, there is no way to exclude the possibility that more rapid absorption of pesticides by the skin at higher ambient temperatures is not a factor in some instances (see Section 3.2.2.5).

The seasonal distribution of nonfatal poisoning associated with solids and liquids in

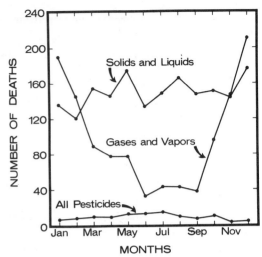

Fig. 7-5. Seasonal distribution of fatal accidental poisoning in 1961 caused by solids and liquids, by gases and vapors, and by all pesticides from both groups. From Hayes and Pirkle (1966) by permission of the American Medical Association.

general is similar to that just described for fatal poisoning (Cann, 1963; Cann *et al.*, 1960).

The seasonal distribution of deaths caused by fumigants does not follow that for total gases and vapors, because the general rate really is determined by carbon monoxide.

7.1.4.9 Containers and Labeling.

Among the 111 deaths caused by pesticides in the USA during 1961, seven were associated with storage of the poison in an unlabeled food or beverage container, two were caused by pesticides packaged in such a way that they were mistaken for medicine, and four were associated with "empty" containers that had not been properly discarded (Hayes and Pirkle, 1966). Thus, at least 11% of the deaths were associated with some misuse of containers.

The proportion of misuse of containers is even higher in connection with ingestion among children under 5 years of age. Verhulst and Crotty (1964) found that in 52% of instances of ingestion of pesticides, the material was not in its original container.

Although mislabeling of pesticides by the formulator is unusual, it has occurred. This kind of mislabeling apparently has not caused human illness. It has led to severe loss of livestock.

It often happens that improper containers are also mislabeled and misplaced. Carelessness is a way of life and a way to death.

7.1.4.10 Occupation. Most deaths caused by fumigants are occupational in origin. With this exception, only a small proportion of fatalities caused by pesticides are occupational. Hayes and Pirkle (1966) reported 3.3 and 15% of the accidental fatalities in the United States associated with all pesticides in 1956 and 1961, respectively, were connected with the work situation in the broadest sense. In California during the years 1951 through 1968, there were 155 accidental deaths attributed to pesticides and other agricultural chemicals; of these 34 (22%) were occupational accidents (California, 1968). In south Florida during the period 1956 through 1967, there were 121 deaths from pesticides, of which 36 were nonoccupational accidents and only 3 (8%) were occupational accidents (Reich et al., 1968b).

Since half or more of deaths associated with pesticides are suicides, considerably lower values are obtained if occupational deaths are reported as a percentage of all deaths associated with pesticides, rather than as a percentage of accidental deaths. In California during 1968, 28 (85%) of the 33 deaths associated with pesticides were suicides, and there were no occupational deaths. In Florida during the period 1956 through 1967, occupational deaths constituted only 2.5% of all deaths associated with pesticides.

7.2 Incidence of Storage or Excretion

The storage of materials in the body is not new, nor is it limited, as some suppose, to the chlorinated hydrocarbon insecticides. Some storage of heavy metals and metalloids is inevitable because of their wide, natural distribution in soil and water and, consequently, in food and drink. Storage above a minimal level may be a direct or indirect result of one or more uses of the metal. Potentially, increased storage of lead, mercury, or arsenic may be associated with their use as pesticides; however, this relationship is unusual, being confined to some workers and rare cases of accident.

The widespread use of some synthetic compounds has led to their storage in many or all persons in the general population. Compounds known to be stored include the polychlorinated biphenyls (PCB's) (Widmark, 1967; Biros et al., 1970; Yobs, 1972; Price and Welch, 1972; Curley et al., 1973), butylated hydroxytoluene (BHT) (Collings and Sharratt, 1970), and hexachlorophene (Curley et al., 1971a).

Measurable amounts of PCB's were found in 31.1% of 637 samples of fat from people in the general population of the United States of America, and trace amounts (< 1 ppm) were found in an additional 19.6% of the samples. Positive samples were found in each of the 18 states and the District of Columbia where collections were made (Yobs, 1972). PCB's were found in all analyzed samples from Japan, in concentrations ranging from 0.30 to 1.48 (Curley et al., 1973). The identity of some PCB's was confirmed by combined gas chromatography-mass spectrometry.

Hexachlorophene was found in all samples of blood tested (Curley et al., 1971a). The toxicity of this compound was reviewed recently by Kimbrough (1971).

Of the chlorinated insecticides, DDT and one of its metabolites, DDE, are stored in far greatest concentration. However, the concentration of lead in the blood of the general population is approximately as great as the concentration of DDT and all its metabolites combined, and the concentration of hexachlorophene is approximately twice as great. In addition to the materials that are stored as a result of environmental exposure, one must add a wide range of therapeutic, diagnostic, or habituating drugs that are stored at least briefly by those who take them.

Undoubtedly, many compounds are stored that either have not been looked for by modern analytical techniques or, once found, were not identified. In fact, a few papers (Hayes et al., 1963; Kanitz and Castello, 1966) have mentioned, in connection with tissue analyses in special groups of people, the finding of definite gas chromatographic peaks that did not correspond with known compounds.

Over 40 compounds are known to be excreted in human milk. Many of these are therapeutic materials, including not only minerals, vitamins, hormones, and antibodies, but also antihormones, antibiotics, analgesics, antihistamines, sedatives, tranquilizers, anticonvulsants, cathartics, and miscellaneous drugs. Some excreted materials are antigens. Among the compounds known to occur in human milk are alcohol, caffein, nicotine, and some narcotics (Knowles, 1965).

Although not all chlorinated hydrocarbon insecticides are stored even at dosage levels encountered by workers who make or use them, six chlorinated hydrocarbon insecticides or their metabolites are found in the tissues of many people in the general population and are excreted by them. These compounds are: DDT, DDD, BHC, heptachlor, aldrin, and dieldrin. (In several instances, measurable storage or excretion is in the form of metabolites.) In addition, pentachlorophenol and hexachlorobenzene have been found in many persons without occupational exposure living in areas where the compounds are used extensively. Finally, a number of other chlorinated hydrocarbon insecticides and other pesticides including endrin, unmetabolized aldrin, toxaphene, paradichlorobenzene, 2,4-D, DNOC, parathion, methyl parathion, EPN, malathion, and carbaryl have been measured in persons with direct occupational or accidental exposure. Storage and excretion of some of these "miscellaneous" compounds is discussed in Section 7.2.3.

The relevant samples and tests useful for differential diagnosis of suspected poisoning are described in Section 8.1.4.1. The value of the same tests as a part of general medical surveillance of workers to prevent their injury by pesticides is described in Section 9.3.1.8. The following paragraphs are concerned with what has been learned about the concentrations of pesticides in the tissues and excreta of persons with different degrees of exposure to the compounds, especially persons of the general population with no special exposure. Emphasis is placed on DDT because it was the first of the newer pesticides to be found stored in man, and because it is the compound about which there has been greatest concern.

7.2.1 Storage of Certain Chlorinated Hydrocarbon Pesticides

7.2.1.1 Storage in Bone. Bone is not an important site for the storage of any commonly used pesticide. It is important for the storage of lead, strontium, fluorine, and, to a lesser extent, barium.

7.2.1.2 Storage in Fat.
DDT and Related Compounds. The storage of DDT in one man first was reported in 1948 (Howell, 1948). Storage undoubtedly was present in the general population even earlier. However, samples taken from people before DDT was manufactured did not contain the compound or anything else giving a similar reaction on analysis (Hayes *et al.*, 1958). The first general survey for DDT was carried out by Laug and his colleagues in Washington, DC, in 1950 and was reported the following year (Laug *et al.*, 1951). This and some more recent studies in the United States of America are listed in Table 7-10. Similar studies have been made in South America, Europe, Africa, Asia, and Oceania; details and references are shown in Table 7-11. The results show that DDT is found in virtually everyone in the general population of the USA and other countries.

Figure 7-6 shows the average concentration of DDT and of all DDT-related material in the body fat of people in the United States of America as revealed by samples collected from 1950 onward. Since the insecticide in the samples collected in 1950 was reported as DDT, and since the concentrations reported were, with minor exception, as great as those found later, a number of investigators (Hayes *et al.*, 1958; Hoffman *et al.*, 1964; Quinby *et al.*, 1965a) concluded that there has been no increase in the storage of DDT by the general population since the first measurement was made in 1950. However, it was pointed out (Quaife *et al.*, 1967) that the method used in the 1950 study was based on the conversion of DDT to DDE, which was then quantitated. Thus, the 1950 study probably measured the sum of both compounds, even though the existence of DDE as a metabolite was not recognized at that time. If this is true and the samples were representative, one must conclude that there was a substantial increase in storage of DDT-related material between 1950 and 1955.

Some caution must be exercised in interpreting the results since 1955 because the early sets of samples were small and the method of chemical analysis changed about 1962. Perhaps just as important, the samples were taken without any plan regarding geographical distribution. It became apparent only gradually that the values obtained tended to increase from north to south. However, an astonishingly accurate estimate of DDT storage in human population may be obtained by examining a small subset (Quinby *et al.*, 1965a). Furthermore, the shift from the Schechter-Haller to the gas chromatographic method of analysis made little difference in the overall results. To be sure, in some series of paired samples, slightly less or more DDT or total DDT-related material is found by gas chromatography than by the colorimetric method (see Table 7-12), probably because of a certain inherent inaccuracy of the older procedure (Dale and Quinby, 1963; Hayes *et al.*, 1963). However, the difference is small and not detectable at all in some sets of samples (Dale *et al.*, 1965). The observed decrease in the concentration of DDT in food (Walker *et al.*, 1954; Durham *et al.*, 1965b; Duggan, 1968) offers an adequate reason for the decrease in stoage in people. The average intake of p,p'-DDT and of total DDT-derived material was 0.178 and 0.280 mg/man/day, respectively, in 1954, but only 0.028 and 0.063 mg/man/day, respectively, during the period 1964–1967. Finally, the apparent rate of decrease from an average storage level of about

Table 7-10

Concentration of DDT-Derived Material in Body Fat
of the General Population of the United States of America

Year	Location	No. of samples	Method of analysis	DDT[a] (ppm)	DDE as DDT (ppm)	Total as DDT (ppm)	DDE as DDT (% of total)	Reference
<1942	Louisville, Ky.	10	color	ND[b]	ND[b]	ND[b]	--	Hayes et al., 1958
1950	Washington, D. C.	75	color	5.3	--	5.3	--	Laug et al., 1951
1955	Tallahassee, Fla.	49	color	7.4	12.5	19.9	63	Hayes et al., 1956
1954-1956	Savannah, Ga. and Wenatchee, Wash.	61	color	4.9	6.8	11.7	58	Hayes et al., 1958
1956	Atlanta, Ga.	36	color	5.5	10.1	15.6	65	Hayes et al., 1971
1961-1962	Atlanta, Ga., Louisville, Ky., Phoenix, Ariz., and Wenatchee, Wash.	130	color	4.0	8.7	12.7	69	Quinby et al., 1965a
1961-1962	Wenatchee, Wash.	28[c]	GLC[d]	2.4	4.3	6.7	64	Dale and Quinby, 1963
1962-1963	Chicago, Ill.	282	GLC	2.9	8.2	11.1	74	Hoffman et al., 1964
1964	Northeast, Midwest, Deep South, and Far West	64	GLC	2.5	5.1	7.6	67	Zavon et al., 1965
1964	New Orleans, La.	25	GLC	2.3	8.0	10.3	77	Hayes et al., 1965
1964-1965	Ohio	18	GLC			9.0		Schafer and Campbell, 1966
1964-1965	Florida	42	GLC	3.1	7.5	10.6	71	Radomski et al., 1968
1962-1966	Chicago, Ill.	994	GLC	2.6	7.8	10.4	75	Hoffman et al., 1967
1964-1965	Florida	12	GLC	3.79	7.7	11.5	67	Davies et al., 1965
1965-1967	Florida	17	GLC		3.1	5.5	56	Davies et al., 1968
		90	GLC		6.1	8.4	73	Davies et al., 1968
		17	GLC		4.6	7.8	59	Davies et al., 1968
		35	GLC		12.0	16.7	72	Davies et al., 1968
--	Florida	42	GLC	3.13[e]	7.43	10.56	70	Fiserova-Bergerova et al.,
--	Hawaii	30[e]	GLC	1.33	5.17	6.51	79	Casarett et al., 1968
		29[f]	GLC	1.35	4.91	6.31	78	Casarett et al., 1968
		30[g]	GLC	1.16	4.99	6.17	81	Casarett et al., 1968
1966-1968	Arizona	70	GLC	1.54	5.15	6.69	77	Morgan and Roan, 1970
1967	11 states	733	GLC	1.34	4.74	6.22	77	Yobs, 1969
1968	20 states	3104	GLC	1.56	5.96	7.67	77	Yobs, 1969
1967-1971	Utah	103	GLC	1.5	5.6	7.1	79	Warnick, 1972
1970	Idaho	200	GLC	1.9	8.0	9.9	81	Wyllie et al., 1972

a. p,p'-DDT and o,p'-DDT only. Total as DDT includes DDD and other forms when given which are not shown in this table.
b. Not detected.
c. These 28 samples also were tested for DDT and DDE content by a colorimetric method (see Table 7-12). These results are included in the 130 samples listed above.
d. Gas-liquid chromatography.
e. Perirenal fat.
f. Mesenteric fat.
g. Panniculus fat.

6 ppm of p,p'-DDT and about 16 ppm of total DDT-related compounds in 1955 was considerably slower than the rate of decrease from about 300 ppm observed experimentally in man (Hayes et al., 1971). The slower rate of decrease at a lower rate of storage is exactly what would be predicted on the basis of animal experiments. Therefore, there is reason to believe that the observed decrease in storage of DDT in the general population of the United States of America since 1955 is real.

In Great Britain, the concentrations of BHC

Table 7-11

Concentration of DDT-Derived Material in Body Fat of the General Population
of Countries Other Than the United States of America

Country	Year	No. of samples	Method of analysis	DDT (ppm)	DDE as DDT (ppm)	Total as DDT (ppm)	DDE as DDT (% of total)	Reference
North America								
Canada	1959-1960	62	color	1.6	3.3	4.9	67	Read and McKinley, 1961
Canada	1966	47	GLC and ELC	1.09	2.96	4.39	67	Brown, 1967
Canada	1967-1968	51	GLC	1.56	4.16	5.86	71	Kadis et al., 1970
South America								
Argentina	1967	37	GLC	5.5	6.5	13.2	--	Wassermann et al., 1968b
Venezuela	1964	38	GLC	2.9	7.4	10.3	72	Dale, 1971
Europe								
Belgium		20	GLC	1.2	2.1	3.3	64	Maes and Heyndrickx, 1966
Czechoslovakia	1963-1964	229	color	5.5	4.1	9.6	43	Halacka et al., 1965
Denmark	1965	18	GLC	0.6	2.7	3.3	82	Weihe, 1966
England	1961-1962	131	color	--	--	2.2	--	Hunter et al., 1963
England	1963-1964	66	GLC[a/]	1.1	2.2	3.3	67	Egan et al., 1965
England	1964	100	GLC[a/]	--	--	3.9	--	Robinson et al., 1965
England	1964	44	GLC[a/]	--	--	4.0[a/]	--	Robinson and Hunter, 1966
England	1965	101	GLC	1.13	1.72	2,85	60	Cassidy et al., 1967
England	1965-1967	248	GLC	0.78	2.22	3.00	74	Abbott et al., 1968
United Kingdom	1969-1971	201	GLC	0.5	1.8	2.5	72	Abbott et al., 1972
France	1961	10	color	1.7	3.5	5.2	67	Hayes et al., 1963
Germany (East)	1966-1967	100	GLC and TLC	3.7	9.47	13.1	71	Engst et al., 1967
Germany (West)	1958-1959	60	color	1.0	1.3	2.3	57	Maier-Bode, 1960
Germany (West)	1970	20	GLC	1.1	2.5	3.6	69	Acker and Schulte, 1970
Hungary	1960	48	color	5.7	6.0	12.4	48	Denes, 1962
Italy	1965	9	GLC	1.8	3.2	5.0	63	Kanitz and Castello, 1966
Italy	1965-1966	18	GLC	2.58	8.28	10.86	76	Paccagnella et al., 1967
Italy	1966	22	GLC and TLC	4.69	10.69	15.48	68	DelVecchio and Leoni, 1967
Netherlands	1964	20	color	1.6	6.1	7.7	79	Wit, 1964
Netherlands	--	11	GLC	0.32	1.89	2.22	86	deVlieger et al., 1968
Poland	1965	72	color			13.4		Bronisz et al., 1967
Poland	1970	70[b/]	GLC			11.4		Juszkiewicz and Stec, 1971
Rumania	1965	137	--	13.4	8.3	21.7	39	Aizicovici et al.
Spain	1966	41	--	6.5	9.2	15.7	59	Llinares and Wassermann, 1968

Table 7-11 (continued)

Country	Year	No. of samples	Method of analysis	DDT (ppm)	DDE as DDT (ppm)	Total as DDT (ppm)	DDE as DDT (% of total)	Reference
Africa								
Nigeria	1967	43	GLC	5.4	3.1	8.8	57	Wassermann et al., 1968b
Asia								
India (Delhi area, civilian)	1964	67	color	17	10	26	39	Dale et al., 1965
India (other cities, military)	1964	16	color	8	5	13	37	Dale et al., 1965
Israel	1963-1964	254	color	8.5	10.7	19.2	56	Wassermann et al., 1965
Israel	1965-1966	71	color	4.6				Wassermann et al., 1967
Israel	1965-1966	133	color	8.2				Wassermann et al., 1967
Japan	1968-1969	241	GLC	0.6	1.8	2.4	75	Curley et al., 1973
Oceania								
Australia	1965	53	GLC	0.77[a/]	1.03[a/]	1.81[a/]	57	Bick, 1967
Australia	1965-1966	46	color	3.6	6.6	10.2	64	Wassermann et al., 1968a
Australia	1965-1966	12	GLC	3.0	7.1	10.5	68	Wassermann et al., 1968a
New Zealand	1966	52	GLC	1.6	4.2	5.8	72	Brewerton and McGrath, 1967
New Zealand	1965-1969	254	GLC	3.6	11.0	14.6	75	Copplestone et al., 1973

a.   Geometric means.
b.   Among 70 samples, BHC was found in 45, (<0.5 in 42 samples), DDD in 8, and hexachlorobenzene in 2; aldrin, dieldrin, and methoxychlor were not found.

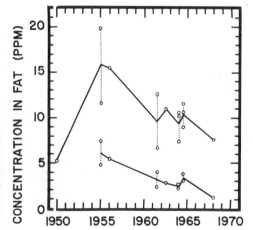

Fig. 7-6. Reported storage of DDT and of all DDT-related materials in the body fat of ordinary people of the United States of America. Each point represents the mean for one study. When more than one study was made in a particular year, the curve has been drawn through the mean of means. References are listed in Table 7-10.

and dieldrin as well as those of DDT decreased also (Abbott *et al.*, 1968).

The storage of DDT in people with occupa-

tional, special environmental, or other special exposure to the insecticide is summarized in Table 7-13. Meat abstainers and Eskimos, whose diet is relatively free of DDT, store significantly less of it than most people do. On the other hand, people with occupational exposure to the compound store more of it. Apparently, the highest recorded storage in a healthy man was 648 ppm DDT, or 1131 ppm total DDT-related material measured in the fat of a formulator (Hayes *et al.*, 1956). Based on DDT alone, this value is 162 or more times the average storage found in the general population in separate investigations since 1960 (Table 7-10).

Other Chlorinated Hydrocarbon Insecticides. Several chlorinated hydrocarbon insecticides in addition to DDT were measured quite early in the tissues of people with heavy occupational exposure to the compounds or in people who had ingested formulations accidentally. These include aldrin (Bell, 1960), dieldrin (Paul, 1959), and lindane (Joslin *et al.*, 1960). However, it was not until the introduction of gas-liquid chromatography that it became possible to measure the small traces of chlorinated hydrocarbon insecticides, other than DDT and DDE, that occur in the general

Table 7-12

Comparison of Results of the Schecter-Haller Colorimetric and the Gas-Liquid
Chromatographic Methods for Measuring DDT-Derived
Material in Body Fat

From Hayes (1966) by permission of the National Academy of Sciences.

Country	Year	No. of samples	Analysis method	DDT [a] (ppm)	DDE as DDT (ppm)	Total [b] as DDT (ppm)	DDE as DDT (% of total)	Reference
United States of America	1961-1962	28	colorimetric	3.7	6.9	10.6	65	Dale and Quinby, 1963
			GLC [c]	2.4	4.3	6.7	64	
France	1962-1963	5	colorimetric	3.1	6.5	9.6	68	Hayes et al., 1963
			GLC [c]	3.5	5.3	8.8	60	
India (Delhi area, civilian)	1964	24	colorimetric	18	12	30	40	Dale et al., 1965
			GLC [c]	14.3	12.9	27.2	47	
India (other cities, military)	1964	11	colorimetric	7	4	11	36	Dale et al., 1965
			GLC [c]	4.7	7.1	11.8	60	

a.   Includes p,p'- and o,p'-DDT.

b.   Includes all detected isomers of DDT and DDE, but not DDD.

c.   Gas-liquid chromatography.

Table 7-13

Concentration of DDT-Derived Material in Body Fat of People in the United States of
America with Special Exposure (Environmental, Occupational, or Dietary) to DDT [a]

Slightly modified from Hayes (1966) by permission of the National Academy of Sciences.

Exposure	Year	No. of samples	DDT (ppm)	DDE as DDT (ppm)	Total as DDT (ppm)	DDE as DDT (% of total)	Reference
died before DDT	< 1942	10	ND [b]	ND [b]	ND [b]	--	Hayes et al., 1958
environmental [c]	1954-1956	110	6.0	9.6	15.6	62	Hayes et al., 1958
environmental [c]	1961-1962	28	4.3	8.6	12.9	67	Quinby et al., 1965a
applicators	1954-1956	30	14.0	21.1	35.1	60	Hayes et al., 1958
applicators	1961-1962	14	10.7	24.1	34.8	69	Quinby et al., 1965
formulator	1951	1	122	141	263	54	Mattson et al., 1953
formulator	1954	1	648	483	1131	43	Hayes et al., 1956
meat abstainers	1955-1956	16	2.3	3.6	5.9	61	Hayes et al., 1958
Eskimos [d]	1960	20	0.8	2.2	3.0	73	Durham et al., 1961
volunteers given 3.5 mg/day orally [e]	1953-1954	2	30	3.9	34	11	Hayes et al., 1956
volunteers given 3.5 mg/day orally [f]	1957-1958	6	50	21	71	30	Hayes et al., 1971
volunteers given 35 mg/day orally [e]	1953-1954	6	234	24	258	9	Hayes et al., 1956
volunteers given 35 mg/day orally [f]	1957-1958	6	281	40	321	12	Hayes et al., 1971

a.   All analyses were done using a colorimetric method.
b.   Not detected.
c.   Residents of the Wentachee, Wash. area living within 500 ft. of agricultural application.
d.   Alaskan Eskimos who ate predominately a native diet shown to contain little or no DDT.
e.   Based on samples taken after 11 months or more of dosage.
f.   Based on samples taken after 21.5 months of dosage.

Table 7-14

Average Concentration of Chlorinated Hydrocarbon Pesticides
(Other than Those Derived from DDT) in Body Fat of the General Population of Various
Countries as Measured by Gas Chromatography

Country	Year	No. of positive samples	Storage level in body fat (ppm) BHC isomers	Dieldrin	Heptachlor epoxide	Reference
North America						
Canada	1966	35		0.22		Brown, 1967
Canada		42	0.07			Brown, 1967
Canada		22			0.14	Brown, 1967
USA	1961-1962	28	0.20	0.15		Dale and Quinby, 1963
USA	1962-1963	282	0.57	0.11		Hoffman et al., 1964
USA	1964	64		0.31	0.10	Zavon et al., 1965
USA	1964	25	0.60	0.29	0.24	Hayes et al., 1965
USA	1964-1965	19		0.002 - 0.8		Schafer and Campbell, 1966
USA (Florida)		42		0.215		Fiserova-Bergerova et al., 1967
USA (Chicago)	1962-1966	221		0.14		Hoffman et al., 1967
USA (Chicago)	1962-1966	505			0.16	Hoffman et al., 1967
USA (Chicago)	1962-1966	994	0.48			Hoffman et al., 1967
USA	1965-1967	146		0.22		Edmundson et al., 1968
USA		42		0.21		Radomski et al., 1968
USA (Hawaii)		30		0.0300	0.0220	Casarett et al., 1968
USA (Hawaii)		29		0.630	0.0320	Casarett et al., 1968
USA (Hawaii)		30		0.0270	0.0270	Casarett et al., 1968
USA (11 states)		733	0.29	0.15	0.05	Yobs, 1969
USA (20 states)		3,104	0.24	0.10	0.05	Yobs, 1969
USA (Arizona)	1966-1968	70		0.14		Morgan and Roan, 1970
USA (Idaho)	1970	200	0.3 ppm	0.2	0.1	Wyllie et al., 1972
South America						
Argentina	1967	37	2.44	0.38	0.192	Wasserman et al., 1968a
Venezuela	1964	38	0.16	0.60		Dale, personal communication 1971
Europe						
Denmark	1965	18		0.20		Weihe, 1966
England	1961-1962	131		0.21		Hunter et al., 1963
England	1963-1964	65	0.42	0.26	0.1	Egan et al., 1965
England	1964	100	0.02	0.21	0.01	Robinson et al., 1965
England	1964	44		0.22		Robinson and Hunter, 1966
England	1965-1967	248	0.31	0.21	0.04	Abbott et al., 1968
England		101	0.19	0.34		Cassidy et al., 1967

population (Table 7-14). The first report of this kind came from England (Hunter *et al.*, 1963). The finding was soon confirmed, and it was shown that people in other countries, including the USA, store DDD, BHC, heptachlor epoxide, and dieldrin. Details and references are given in Table 7-14.

Since DDD is an insecticide in its own right, as well as a metabolite of DDT, and since dieldrin in the tissues may be derived from aldrin as well as from preformed dieldrin, it follows that six insecticides or their metabolites have now been demonstrated in the adipose tissue of people from the United States of America without special exposure. The forms in which these six insecticides have been reported in fat from people of the general population of this or other countries are: p,p'-DDT, o,p'-DDT, p,p'-DDE, o,p'-DDE, p,p'-DDD, α-BHC, β-BHC, γ-BHC, heptachlor epoxide, and dieldrin.

Since only one chlorinated hydrocarbon insecticide, DDT, has been measured for more than a few years, it is not yet possible to state whether people have reached a steady or decreasing state of storage for the other five

compounds. However, there is growing evidence this is true. Undoubtedly the apparent decline in storage of dieldrin reflects the fact that the dietary intake of dieldrin in Britain began to decline in 1965 (Robinson and Roberts, 1969).

Apparently hexachlorobenzene has not been detected in the tissues of anyone in the United States of America. It has been reported in human fat in Germany (Acker and Schulte, 1970), Australia and its territories (Brady and Siyali, 1972), and Japan (Curley *et al.*, 1973). It also has been found in human milk (Acker and Schulte, 1970) and serum (Zeman *et al.*, 1971), both in Germany. In Germany, the concentration found tended to be slightly greater than the concentration of total DDT-related material in the same tissue. Concentrations in Australia and especially Japan were lower.

7.2.1.3 Storage in Blood. Robinson made a great forward step when he introduced a method capable of measuring dieldrin and the sum of DDT-related materials in human blood (Robinson, 1963). Early measurements of

Table 7-14 (continued)

Country	Year	No. of positive samples	Storage level in body fat (ppm)			Reference
			BHC isomers	Dieldrin	Heptachlor epoxide	
Europe (cont.)						
United Kingdom	1969-1971	201	0.29	0.16	0.03	Abbott et al., 1972
France	1961	10	1.19			Hayes et al., 1963
Germany (East)	1966-1967	100	0.16			Engst et al., 1967
Germany (West)	1970	20	0.45			Acker and Schulte, 1970
Hungary	1964	15		Traces-0.16		Denes, 1966
Italy	1965	9		0.594		Kanitz and Castello, 1966
Italy	1966	22	0.08	0.68	0.23	Del Vecchio and Leoni, 1967
Italy		18	2.25	0.84	0.46	Paccagnella et al., 1967
Netherlands		11	0.11	0.20	0.01	de Vlieger et al., 1968
Asia						
India	1964	35	1.43	0.04		Dale et al., 1965
Japan		241	0.12-1.28	0.13	0.02	Curley et al., 1973
Oceania						
Australia	1965	53		0.05		Bick, 1967
Australia	1965-1966	12	0.68	0.67	0.02	Wassermann et al., 1968a
New Zealand		52		0.27		Brewerton and McGrath, 1967
New Zealand	1965-1969	254		0.35		Copplestone et al., 1973

dieldrin in the blood of the general population were reported by Brown et al. (1964) and by Kazantzis and his colleagues (1964). A further improvement in the analysis of insecticides in blood was introduced by Dale and his colleagues (1966). The new method gave results in good agreement with those of Kazantzis et al. (1964) and Brown et al. (1964), but it also permitted the separate measurement of DDT and DDE, dieldrin, heptachlor epoxide and β-BHC in the blood of people in the general population. In fact, the method is capable of measuring any of the chlorinated hydrocarbon insecticides in human blood provided they reach a concentration of 0.0001 ppm or greater.

Dale et al. (1966) showed that there was no significant difference in the concentrations of chlorinated hydrocarbon insecticides in plasma and serum. However, the compounds are not always evenly distributed between the red cells and the plasma. Although some compounds, especially DDD, are more concentrated in the red cells, most of the compounds are more concentrated in the plasma. Because of this distribution and the convenience of sample preparation, plasma or serum is the preferred sample. It must be recalled that other compounds—notably organic and inorganic lead—show much greater differences in distribution between red cells and plasma or serum. For compounds of unknown behavior, it is necessary to confine the study to whole blood or to sample both red cells and plasma.

Typical results on the occurrence of chlorinated hydrocarbon insecticides in the blood of people in the general population of the United States of America are shown in Table 7-15. Later papers not shown in this table are those of Radomski et al. (1971), Wyllie et al. (1972), Keil et al. (1972), and Warnick (1972). The values reported in these later papers are not systematically different from those reported earlier.

Table 7-15

Average Concentrations (ppm) of Chlorinated Hydrocarbon Insecticides in the Blood of People in the General Population of the United States of America

Compound	Atlanta, USA 1965 10 plasma Dale et al., 1966	Louisiana 1966-1967 53 [a] whole blood Selby et al., 1969b	4 States, USA 1967 64 serum Yobs, 1969	3 States, USA 1968 106 serum Yobs, 1969	Idaho 1967-1968 1,000 serum Watson et al., 1970	Atlanta, USA 1969 30 [b] blood [c] Curley et al., 1969
p,p'-DDT	0.0119	0.00182	0.00335	0.00342	0.0047	0.0046
o,p'-DDT	0.0013		0.00044	0.00006		0.0011
p,p'-DDE	0.0257	0.00265	0.00837	0.00927	0.0220	0.0062
o,p'-DDE			0.00096	0.00000		0.0003
p,p'-DDD		0.00062	0.00032	0.00004		0.0014
o,p'-DDD			0.00000	0.00009	0.0002	
total DDT equiv.	0.0418	0.00501	0.01425	0.01397	0.0294	0.0144
DDE as % total DDT	68.6	59.0	78.0	73.4	83.5	50.0
α-BHC			0.00000	0.00000	0.00007	0.0004
β-BHC	0.0034		0.00144	0.00000	0.00007	0.0026
γ-BHC		0.00039	0.00006	0.00000	0.00007	0.0000
δ-BHC			0.00000	0.00000		
total BHC	0.0034	0.00048				
heptachlor		0.00013	0.00050	0.00000		
heptachlor epoxide	0.0011	0.00021	0.00000	0.00000	0.00007	0.0011
aldrin		0.00041				
dieldrin	0.0019	0.00026	0.00069	0.00014	0.0005	0.0007

a.   Geometric mean.

b.   Mean of positive values only

c.   Cord blood from live, term infants.

During 1964, people in England (Robinson and Hunter, 1966) had (compared to values reported by Dale *et al.*, 1966) somewhat lower blood levels of DDT but almost equal levels of dieldrin. However, the difference in blood levels reported by different investigators in the USA indicates caution in concluding either that minor differences are real or that similarity of results excludes minor real differences. Furthermore, problems of analytical chemistry are not the only factor contributing to the lack of certainty. No single survey has covered adequately all the factors that may influence storage and excretion and that are discussed in Section 7.2.4. This is not meant as a criticism of the surveys but as a realistic statement of the difficulty of obtaining a single range and a single average value for the storage of a compound in a population that is not fully homogeneous.

It is important, however, while recognizing the variation from one survey to another, to realize that the degree of variation in the storage of chlorinated hydrocarbon insecticides within the general population of the USA is small and without toxicological significance.

Whereas the differences in blood levels among countries may not be clinically significant, there can be no doubt of their reality in some instances. For example, Radomski *et al.* (1971) found about 16 times as much β-BHC in blood from unexposed people in Argentina as they found in comparable samples from the USA. The concentration of γ-BHC also was much higher in Argentina. In contrast, values for dieldrin and DDT-related compounds were similar in the two countries.

In addition to the compounds found commonly in the blood of the general population, *o,p'*-DDE, *p,p'*-DDE, *p,p'*-DDD, *o,p'*-DDT, *p,p'*-DDT, α-BHC, β-BHC, γ-BHC, chlordane, aldrin, dieldrin, endrin, heptachlor epoxide, and toxaphene have been demonstrated in the blood of people with occupational or accidental exposure to these materials.

The introduction of a method sufficiently sensitive to measure the traces of insecticide present in blood represents a marked advance over methods useful only for analysis of pesticides in fat because: (*a*) it permits selection of samples from persons who should be studied because of the special conditions of their exposure to pesticides; and (*b*) there is some evidence that there is a greater correlation between the concentrations of chlorinated hydrocarbon insecticides in blood and brain than there is between their concentrations in fat and brain (Dale *et al.*, 1963). This latter distinction is not important in connection with studies on the general population. In this group, the concentrations of pesticides in the fat are higher than those in any other tissue, and storage of the materials in fat shows an

Table 7-16

Average Concentration of Chlorinated Hydrocarbon Insecticides in Various Tissues from Autopsies of 44 People in the General Population

From Casarett et al. (1968) by permission of the American Medical Association.

Tissue	No. analyzed	Lipid content (%)	DDT (ppm)	DDE (ppm)	DDD (ppm)	Heptachlor epoxide (ppm)	Dieldrin (ppm)	Total ± SD[a] (ppm)	
perirenal fat	30	55.7	1.33	4.64	0.0110	0.0220	0.0300	6.03 ±	5.30
mesenteric fat	29	54.2	1.35	4.40	0.0470	0.0320	0.0630	5.89 ±	4.98
panniculus fat	30	60.6	1.16	4.48	0.0180	0.0270	0.0270	5.71 ±	5.25
bone marrow	19	20.6	0.411	2.08	0.0760	0.0040	0.0620	2.63 ±	2.21
lymph node[b]	11	8.6	0.892	1.38	0.0100	0.0001	0.0190	2.30 ±	4.52
adrenal	18	10.5	0.125	0.875	0.0570	0.0012	0.0060	1.06 ±	1.31
kidney	38	3.2	0.0827	0.209	0.0022	0.0009	0.0056	0.300 ±	0.651
liver	42	2.1	0.0467	0.200	0.0326	0.0019	0.0037	0.285 ±	0.369
brain	32	7.9	0.0105	0.0831	0.0020	0.0002	0.0031	0.0989 ±	0.171
gonad	36	1.3	0.0150	0.0688	0.0015	0.0001	0.0021	0.0875 ±	0.103
lung	25	0.7	0.0147	0.0585	0.0009	0.0003	0.0022	0.0766 ±	0.125
spleen	27	0.6	0.0112	0.0305	0.0031	trace	0.0021	0.0469 ±	0.074

a. SD = standard deviation.

b. Tracheobronchial lymph nodes.

excellent correlation with dosage. However, in persons whose history of exposure to pesticides is imperfectly known and may include accidental exposure, blood samples should be analyzed, because the results may be valuable for differential diagnosis.

7.2.1.4 Storage in Organs. So far, only a few measurements have been made of pesticides in human organs, and many of them were made in connection with recognized cases of fatal poisoning. Thus, high concentrations of DDT in the liver, kidneys, and heart of a poisoned person were observed as early as 1952 (Luis, 1952). Lindane at concentrations of 83 to 343 ppm was reported in the tissues of a child who died after eating one or more vaporizer tablets (Joslin et al., 1960), but much lower concentrations of 2.4 to 30.6 ppm were found in another child who died in the same way (Coulson and McCarthy, 1963). Endrin has been found at concentrations up to 10 ppm in the tissues of people poisoned by it (Hayes, 1963).

Only recently it has become possible to detect chlorinated hydrocarbon insecticides in the organs of people who were presumably unaffected by them. The first such report was that of Radomski and Fiserova-Bergerova (1965), who found DDT, DDE, and dieldrin in most samples of brain, kidney, liver, and gonads that they analyzed. They also reported aldrin and lindane in a few of the samples. If one may judge from results on blood (Dale et al., 1966), the finding of aldrin and γ-BHC, and the failure to find β-BHC in tissue, indicated that Radomski's subjects may have had some special exposure to pesticides and certainly were not typical of the general population.

Typical findings regarding the concentration of chlorinated hydrocarbon insecticides in the organs of people of the general population are shown in Table 7-16.

7.2.1.5 Storage in the Fetus. The transfer of foreign compounds to the fetus is discussed in Section 3.2.3.3. The early observation (Denes, 1962) that DDT is transferred to and stored in the human fetus has been confirmed (Zavon et al., 1969; Curley et al., 1969; O'Leary et al., 1970c). As shown in Table 7-17, at least 10 isomers or metabolites of six chlorinated hydrocarbon insecticides have been measured in various fetal tissues. It seems likely that we do not begin to reach a steady state of pesticide storage after birth but rather are born—and probably conceived—with it.

The placenta may be partially protective; for example, the concentrations of DDT and DDE are less in cord blood than in maternal blood (O'Leary et al., 1970b).

7.2.2 Excretion of Certain Chlorinated Hydrocarbon Pesticides

7.2.2.1 Excretion in Milk. Chlorinated hydrocarbon insecticides and fumigants are excreted in the milk of cows that ingest them (Hayes, 1959b). Until recently, DDT was the only chlorinated pesticide reported in human milk (Table 7-18), but Egan et al. (1965) and other investigators reported that traces of BHC and dieldrin also are present.

It is of interest that human milk contains more DDT than does cows' milk (Egan et al., 1965; Quinby et al., 1965b; Ritcey et al., 1972; Olszyna-Marzys et al., 1973) and that the mother is apparently in negative DDT balance during lactation (Quinby et al., 1965b). However, it is of far greater importance that the concentrations in the United States of America and in Western Europe are small and, at least in the USA, have not increased since they were first measured in 1950. Much higher concentrations have been reported in the milk of Guatemalan women (see Table 7-19), and to a lesser degree in milk of Russian, Rumanian, and Polish women. There is nothing new about the presence of DDT in human milk; it is just the relationship of its concentrations in human and cows' milk that was noted in 1965 and completely misinterpreted recently by persons without training in medicine.

The medical importance of DDT in human milk depends entirely on the dosage of the compound received by babies, and the relative concentrations in human and cows' milk is irrelevant. Any calculation should be made in terms of DDT, because DDE and other related materials present in milk are much less toxic. An infant consumes about 0.6 liter of milk per day. Taking this value and a DDT concentration of 0.08 ppm, a daily intake of 0.048 mg/infant may be calculated. If this is divided by 3.36 kg, the average weight of babies at birth, one obtains a value of 0.014 mg/kg/day. As the infant grows, the intake on a per kilogram basis probably decreases slightly. Therefore, the average daily intake of breast-fed infants in this country is little, if any, greater than the permissible rate originally set by the World Health Organization and the Food and Agriculture Organization (0.01 mg/kg). Furthermore, this "permissible rate" is highly conservative. It offers a safety factor of about 25, compared with what workers in a DDT manufacturing plant have tolerated for 19 years without any detectable clinical effect

Table 7-17

The Range and Mean of Measurable Concentrations of Various Chlorinated Hydrocarbons
(ppm) in Different Tissues From Stillborn Infants

From Curley et al. (1969) by permission of the American Medical Association.

Tissues received		p,p'-DDT	o,p'-DDT	p,p'-DDE	o,p'-DDE	p,p'-DDD	α-BHC	β-BHC	γ-BHC	Heptachlor epoxide	Dieldrin
10 adipose	measurable concentration	3	4	8	0	6	3	6	3	4	3
	range	0.16 to 2.15	0.35 to 11.47	0.16 to 3.19	--	0.23 to 14.17	0.09 to 0.24	0.14 to 0.44	0.09 to 0.14	0.07 to 0.51	0.09 to 0.
	mean	0.88	3.39	1.22	--	3.17	0.14	0.26	0.11	0.32	0.24
	SE ±	0.63	2.70	0.38	--	2.22	0.05	0.05	0.02	0.10	0.08
3 spinal cord	measurable concentration	1	1	2	0	2	0	1	1	0	1
	range	0.47	0.47	0.30 to 1.16	--	0.31 to 0.70	--	0.17	0.10	--	0.09
	mean	--	--	0.73	--	0.51	--	--	--	--	--
	SE ±	--	--	0.43	--	0.20	--	--	--	--	--
8 brain	measurable concentration	3	1	4	0	3	3	1	1	1	2
	range	0.28 to 0.99	0.84	0.25 to 1.47	--	0.20 to 1.22	0.04 to 0.49	3.81	0.06	0.13	0.84 to 0.
	mean	0.56	--	0.65	--	0.64	0.19	--	--	--	0.05
	SE ±	0.22	--	0.28	--	0.30	0.15	--	--	--	0.01
9 adrenals	measurable concentration	3	2	6	0	3	2	3	3	2	1
	range	1.28 to 1.65	0.36 to 1.05	0.13 to 1.96	--	0.91 to 1.45	0.40 to 0.57	0.12 to 0.71	0.20 to 0.53	0.46 to 1.00	0.92
	mean	1.48	0.71	1.05	--	1.11	0.49	0.37	0.33	0.73	--
	SE ±	0.11	0.35	0.28	--	0.17	0.09	0.18	0.10	0.27	--
10 lungs	measurable concentration	4	0	6	0	5	5	3	3	3	2
	range	0.57 to 1.01	--	0.25 to 1.35	--	0.31 to 1.05	0.07 to 0.69	0.05 to 0.18	0.05 to 0.25	0.08 to 0.31	0.27 to 0.
	mean	0.79	--	0.85	--	0.75	0.25	0.12	0.12	0.17	0.50
	SE ±	0.11	--	0.22	--	0.13	0.11	0.04	0.07	0.07	0.23
10 heart	measurable concentration	4	2	4	0	4	3	3	3	4	3
	range	1.04 to 4.17	0.57 to 0.68	1.27 to 4.79	--	1.02 to 5.82	0.23 to 0.52	0.15 to 0.31	0.19 to 0.27	0.30 to 1.56	0.08 to 1
	mean	2.17	0.63	2.74	--	3.27	0.33	0.22	0.22	0.80	0.49
	SE ±	0.69	0.06	0.74	--	1.10	0.09	0.05	0.03	0.30	0.28
10 liver	measurable concentration	5	3	6	0	6	3	4	4	3	2
	range	0.15 to 1.59	0.22 to 3.42	0.22 to 2.45	--	0.19 to 2.14	0.21 to 0.32	0.03 to 0.20	0.05 to 0.36	0.03 to 1.67	0.16 to 0
	mean	0.79	1.32	0.98	--	1.01	0.25	0.11	0.24	0.68	0.19
	SE ±	0.24	1.05	0.34	--	0.29	0.04	0.04	0.07	0.50	0.03
9 kidney	measurable concentration	4	3	6	0	5	4	5	4	3	3
	range	0.62 to 7.60	0.29 to 2.07	0.11 to 9.78	--	0.48 to 9.12	0.11 to 1.45	0.06 to 0.61	0.11 to 0.69	0.19 to 1.14	0.06 to 0
	mean	3.71	1.38	3.57	--	3.84	0.82	0.29	0.39	0.70	0.34
	SE ±	1.70	0.55	1.72	--	1.87	0.32	0.12	0.14	0.28	0.14
8 spleen	measurable concentration	3	2	3	1	3	1	1	3	5	3
	range	0.48 to 1.04	0.45 to 2.94	0.60 to 1.05	0.29	0.18 to 0.91	0.21	0.16	0.17 to 0.18	0.10 to 0.52	0.18 to 0
	mean	0.80	1.70	0.86	--	0.56	--	--	0.18	0.35	0.31
	SE ±	0.17	1.25	0.13	--	0.21	--	--	0.005	0.08	0.10
3 pancreas	measurable concentration	1	0	1	1	0	0	0	0	0	0
	range	0.49	--	0.23	0.08	--	--	--	--	--	--
	mean	--	--	--	--	--	--	--	--	--	--
	SE ±	--	--	--	--	--	--	--	--	--	--

(Laws et al., 1967). It offers a safety factor of about 150 compared to the dosage of DDT given daily for 6 months to a patient with congenital unconjugated jaundice without producing any side effects (Thompson et al., 1969). In the absence of any new information indicating a hazard, no justification is apparent for changing the permissible rate from 0.01 to 0.005 mg/kg (see Section 9.1.4.2).

The highest concentration of p,p'-DDT in a single sample of human milk (5.94 ppm) and the highest average concentration in samples collected in one locality (1.78 ppm) were reported from Guatemala (Olszyna-Marzys et al., 1973). Calculations based on these values indicate that babies in that town would have a maximal intake of 1.06 mg/kg/day and an average intake of 0.32 mg/kg/day. This average value is of the same order of magnitude as that encountered by workers who make and formulate DDT. The corresponding maximal and average intakes of total DDT-related material for infants in Guatemala would be 2.18 and 0.73 mg/kg/day.

Infants are more susceptible than adults to some compounds, but the difference is seldom great (see Section 2.4.10). Although there is no information on the relative susceptibility of human infants and adults to DDT, it was shown by Lu et al. (1965) that weanling rats are slightly more resistant than adult rats to this compound, and that preweanling rats are more than twice as resistant and newborn rats are over 20 times more resistant than adults. The results obtained by Henderson and Woolley (1969) were similar.

The health of breast-fed infants in Guatemala, who receive a high intake of DDT, apparently has not been the subject of a special study, but available information is insuf-

Table 7-18

Concentration of DDT-Derived Material in Human Milk

Country	Year	No. of samples	Analytical method	DDT (ppm)	DDE as DDT (ppm)	Total as DDT	DDE as DDT (% of total)	Reference
North America								
Canada	1967-1968	147	GLC	0.032[a/]	0.097	0.139	--	Ritcey et al., 1972
USA	1950	32	color		--	0.13	--	Laug et al., 1951
USA	1960-61	10	color	0.08	0.04	0.12	33	Quinby et al., 1965b
USA	1962	6	color	0-0.12 [b/]	0.025[b/]	0.37[c/]	--	West. 1964
USA	1968	?	GLC	0.026	0.047	0.078	60	Curley and Kimbrough, 1969
USA	1970	53[d/]	GLC	0.022	0.083	0.101	80	Kroger, 1972
USA	1970-71	101	CLC	--	--	0.17		Wilson et al., 1973
Europe								
Belgium	1968	20	GLC	0.05	--	--	--	Heyndrickx and Maes, 1969
Czechoslovakia	1968	--	--	0.101	--	--	--	Hruska, 1969
England	1963-64	19[e/]	GLC	0.05	0.08	0.13	62	Egan et al., 1965
Germany(West)	1970?	43	GLC	0.031	0.090	0.121	74	Acker and Schulte, 1970
Hungary	1963	10	color	0.13-0.26[b/]	--	--	--	Denes, 1964
Italy	1965?	2[f/]	GLC	0.001	0.055	0.056		Tuinstra, 1971
Netherlands	1969	50	GLC	0.9[g/]	1.8[g/]	2.7[g/]	66	
Poland	1966	26	color	0.27	--	--	62	Bronisz and Ochynski 1968
Poland	1967	25	color	0.40	--	--	58	Bronisz and Ochynski, 1968
Poland	1970?	40[h/]	GLC	0.08	0.19	0.28	71	Kontek et al., 1971
Rumania	1968?	100	color	0.054-0.749	0.026-8.30	0.080-9.05	--	Unterman and Sirghie, 1969
Russia	1964	16	color	1.22-4.88	--	--	--	Damaskin, 1965
Russia	1968?	4,505	--	0.1-1.0	--	--	--	Gracheva, 1969
Russia	1969?	--	--	0.09	--	0.14	--	Gracheva, 1970
Russia	1967?	370	GLC	0.1	--	--	--	Komarova, 1970
Sweden	1967?	--	--	--	--	0.117	--	Löfroth, 1968
Sweden	1967-1969	22 [i/]	GLC	0.039	0.076	0.115	63	Westöö, et al., 1970
Asia								
Japan	1971-1972	398	--	0.0562	--	--	--	Anonymous, 1972b
Japan	1971	43	GLC	0.095	0.084	0.179	47	Hidaka et al., 1972
Oceania								
Australia	1970	67	GLC	--	--	0.014 [j/] 0.007 [k/] 0.066 [l/]	--	Newton and Greene, 1972
New Guinea (Kar Kar Island)	1972	16	GLC	0.002	0.002	0.004	50	Hornabrook et al., 1972
New Guinea (Sepik district)	1972	19	GLC	0.008	0.007	0.015	47	Hornabrook et al., 1972

a. Average concentration of lindane, 0.003 ppm; of heptachlor epoxide, 0.003; and of dieldrin, 0.005.
b. Range of values for milk containing 4% fat containing 3.3 to 6.6 ppm.
c. Maximal value.
d. Average concentration of lindane, 0.0034 ppm and of heptachlor epoxide, 0.0066 ppm.
e. These samples also contained an average of 0.013 ppm BHC and 0.006 ppm dieldrin.
f. Samples reported to contain 0.001 ppm aldrin, an unlikely finding.
g. Concentration in milk fat.
h. All samples contained γ-BHC with an average concentration of 0.006 ppm.
i. A few samples contained traces of p,p'-DDD, α-BHC, and γ-BHC, and many contained dieldrin with an average concentration of 0.001 ppm.
j. At beginning of feeding, 1.8% fat.
k. At middle of feeding, 1.2% fat.
l. At end of feeding, 5.1% fat.

ficient to establish any correlation between child morbidity and mortality in the area and DDT in mothers' milk (Olszyna-Marzys, 1973). Signs of DDT poisoning are so striking they would be noticed easily by mothers, and yet the paper reporting high DDT intake (Olszyna-Marzys et al., 1973) makes no mention of unusual illness of babies in the towns where samples of milk were collected. This is direct evidence of the very conservative na-

Table 7-19

Ranges, Means, and Standard Errors of the Concentrations
of Chlorinated Hydrocarbon Insecticides in the Milk of Women
in Three Towns in Guatemala

After Olszyna-Marzys et al. (1973).

Compound	La Bomba 1970 n=10	El Rosario 1970 n=27	Cerro Colorado 1971 n=9
p, p'-DDT (ppm)	0.23 - 4.95 (1.00 ± 0.38)	0.16 - 2.24 (0.77 ± 0.10)	0.49 - 5.94 (1.78 ± 0.56)
p, p'-DDE (ppm)	0.12 - 6.36 (1.02 ± 0.58)	0.28 - 3.10 (0.99 ± 0.14)	0.60 - 6.13 (2.10 ± 0.61)
p, p'-DDD (ppm)	tr[a] - 0.16 (0.03 ± 0.02)	0.01 - 0.09 (0.02 ± 0.004)	0.05 - 0.11 (0.07 ± 0.01)
o, p'-DDT (ppm)	tr - 0.29 (0.09 ± 0.03)	0.01 - 0.18 (0.06 ± 0.01)	0.06 - 0.22 (0.12 ± 0.02)
total as DDT (ppm)	0.41 - 11.50 (2.15 ± 1.05)	0.34 - 4.97 (1.84 ± 0.24)	1.57 - 12.21 (4.07 ± 1.11)
total BHC (ppm)	0.01 - 0.10 (0.03 ± 0.01)	tr - 0.07 0.007 ± 0.003	0 - 0.06 0.02 ± 0.01
heptachlor epoxide (ppm)	0 - 0.02 (0.003 ± 0.002)	tr - 0.01 (0.007 ± 0.0004)	tr
dieldrin (ppm)	tr	tr - 0.01 0.002 ± 0.0005	

a. tr = trace.

ture of the WHO/FAO "permissible rate." On the other hand, the maximal or even the average rate of intake of p,p'-DDT by infants in Guatemala approaches the tolerance of adults, which, as shown in Table 7-24, lies somewhere between 1.5 mg/kg/day (the highest dosage administered therapeutically for several months) and 6.0 mg/kg (the lowest dosage to cause recognized toxicity). This fact constitutes no test of whether babies, like infant rats, are more tolerant than adults, but there can be no justification for testing this academic point on a national scale. It is clear that DDT exposure of people in Guatemala ought to be reduced.

7.2.2.2 Excretion in Urine. DDA, a metabolite of DDT, was the first excretory product of one of the newer pesticides to be detected. It was first identified in the urine of a volunteer (Neal et al., 1946).

Until recently, the methods for measuring DDA were not sufficiently sensitive to detect it in the majority of samples of urine from the general population (Durham et al., 1965b). It has been known for a long time that its excretion is dosage-related in situations in which it can be measured (see Table 7-20). Later, Cranmer et al. (1969) showed that the average concentration of DDA in the urine of people in the general population is only slightly less than the lower limit of sensitivity of the old, colorimetric method.

The urinary excretion of dieldrin in highly exposed workers was reported in 1962 (Cueto and Hayes, 1962). Cueto and Biros (1967) were first to show that excretory products of a wide range of chlorinated hydrocarbon insecticides are detectable in the urine of people in the general population. They regularly found two isomers of DDT, one each of DDE and DDD, as well as α-BHC and dieldrin. Some samples contained γ-BHC, δ-BHC, o,p'-DDE, and heptachlor epoxide.

7.2.2.3 Excretion in Feces. Although stud-

Table 7-20

Urinary Excretion of DDA by People in the United States of America with Varying Degrees of Exposure to DDT

Slightly modified from Hayes (1966) by permission of the National Academy of Sciences.

Exposure	Year	No. of samples	DDA excretion (ppm)		Reference
			Range	Mean	
general population	1954	8	<0.05	--	Hayes et al., 1956
general population	1957	8	<0.02-0.07	--	Hayes et al., 1971
general population	1962	23	<0.02-0.18	--	Durham et al., 1965b
general population	1968	11	0.008-0.019	0.014	Cranmer et al., 1969
environmental[a]	1962	13	<0.02-0.11	--	Durham et al., 1965
applicators	1962	11	<0.02-0.17	--	Durham et al., 1965
formulators	1957	40	0.12-7.56	1.71	Ortelee, 1958
makers and formulators	1966	35	<0.01-2.67	0.97	Laws et al., 1967
volunteers given 3.5 mg/day orally	1953-1954	2	0.10-0.42[b]	0.21[b]	Hayes et al., 1956
volunteers given 3.5 mg/day orally	1957-1958	6	0.06-1.98[c]	0.23[c]	Hayes et al., 1971
volunteers given 35 mg/day orally	1953-1954	6	0.69-9.67[b]	2.46[b]	Hayes et al., 1956
volunteers given 35 mg/day orally	1957-1958	6	0.18-9.21[c]	3.09[c]	Hayes et al., 1971

a. Residents living within 500 ft. of agricultural application.

b. Based on all samples after 35th week of dosage.

c. Based on all samples from the 35th through the 93rd week after dosage started.

ies in animals show that chlorinated hydrocarbon insecticides are excreted mainly in the feces, this has not been shown to be true in man. Few studies have been made, and isolated reports of fecal excretion of these compounds in man have not been confirmed (see Section 3.2.4.2). It is recognized, however, that many of the heavy metals are excreted in human feces, even predominantly so.

7.2.2.4 Excretion in Expired Air. Although no chlorinated hydrocarbon residual insecticide is known to be excreted by way of the lungs, chlorinated hydrocarbon and other solvents and fumigants, and some other compounds such as styrene, regularly are excreted by this route. Data are available on the excretion of at least 20 of these materials in man, and at least 16 others have been studied in animals. It seems likely that breath analysis would work for nematocides as well as for fumigants used in closed spaces. Some of the compounds are retained in the body for days or even weeks following occupational or other substantial exposure, and decreasing concentrations of them may be measured by breath analysis during this time. In spite of this considerable degree of retention, these compounds have not been detected in the general population, who are exposed to traces of the compounds or none at all. The exceptions that prove the rule involve the detection of acetone associated with diabetes and certain other conditions, and the detection of alcohol following its ingestion.

The use of breath analysis in diagnosis is mentioned in Section 8.1.4.1.

7.2.3 Storage and Excretion of Other Pesticides

The foregoing sections discuss in some detail the storage and excretion of certain chlorinated hydrocarbon pesticides and solvents that are not only of great interest in themselves, but also serve to illustrate important principles, including dosage-response relationships, tissue distribution, and others. It remains to document briefly the storage and excretion of other compounds. Some of these compounds found in the general population of large areas if not the entire world are listed in Table 7-21. Some chlorinated hydrocarbon insecticides, notably methoxychlor, chlordane, endrin, and toxaphene, are metabolized and excreted so efficiently that they are found only in persons with occupational exposure, or only in those who received large doses accidentally or with suicidal intent (see Tables 8-1, 8-2, and 8-3).

Excretion of Organic Phosphorus Insecticides. Shafik and Enos (1969) developed a gas chromatographic method capable of measuring two metabolites of organic phosphorus insecticides at concentrations found in the urine of ordinary people and in the blood serum of heavily exposed workers. The method also detects at least four other metabolites at concentrations found in the urine of

Table 7-21

Storage and Excretion of Miscellaneous Pesticides and Some Other
Compounds in the General Population of Various Countries

Compound	Sample	Concentration (ppm)	Reference
Inorganic and organo-metal pesticides			
arsenic	blood or serum	0.001-0.500	Based on recent papers; early papers gave values as high as 5.25 ppm
lead	blood or serum	0.000-0.100	Goldwater and Hoover, 1967
mercury	blood or serum	<0.005-0.070	Goldwater et al., 1964
Phenolic and nitro-phenolic pesticides			
hexachlorophene	blood or serum	<0.01-0.089	Curley et al., 1971a
pentachlorophenol	blood or serum	0.000-0.018	Armstrong et al., 1969
"	urine	.0022-.0108	Cranmer and Freal, 1970
"	urine	0.040-0.044	Bevenue et al., 1967
Fungicides and related compounds			
hexachlorobenzene	body fat	6.3	Acker and Schulte, 1970
"	body fat	1.25	Brady and Siyali, 1972
"	body fat	<0.003-0.77	Curley et al., 1973

heavily exposed workers. The metabolites found most commonly are diethylphosphate and dimethyldithiophosphate. The first might be derived from tepp, from several little used insecticides, and from the =O metabolite of a number of phosphorothioates, notably metabolites of parathion and demeton. The second metabolite might be derived from malathion, dimethoate, and a number of less used compounds. The method has not been used sufficiently to evaluate it from anything but a chemical standpoint. It is of interest, however, that the average concentration of dimethyldithiophosphate (0.25 ppm) found in the urine of people without special exposure would be equivalent to a malathion intake of 0.7 mg/man/day (see Table 7-22). This value is about 100 times greater than the rate of intake of malathion from food as determined by analysis of representative food samples (Duggan, 1968). However, the metabolite in urine may be absorbed as breakdown products and not as the original pesticide. Such products have not been measured in the total diet. Furthermore,

food may not be the most important source of exposure, whether to malathion or its derivatives. Finally, there may be other environmental sources of alkyl phosphates. In any event, the values reported in urine are not unreasonable. The average concentration found in samples from ordinary people is about half that found in samples from men who served as controls in a study of malathion (and thereby received some exposure from association with other volunteers). The average concentration found in "heavily exposed" workers (Table 7-22) is only a little over half the average in volunteers thoroughly treated with 1% malathion dust (Hayes et al., 1960).

The concentrations of metabolites in urine indicate far less excretion of ethyl than of methyl compounds. If all of the diethylphosphate found in the urine of the most heavily exposed worker were derived from parathion the dosage would be easily tolerated but, if continued for several weeks, would be expected to produce some inhibition of plasma cholinesterase.

Table 7-22

Mean Concentration of Dimethyldithiophosphate
(DMDTP) and of Diethylphosphate (DEP)
in the Urine of People with Different Degrees of
Exposure to Organic Phosphorus Insecticides

From data of Shafik and Enos (1969).

Degree of exposure	Mean in urine (ppm)	
	DMDTP	DEP
heavy	1.52	0.68
moderate	1.00	0.04
light	0.25 [a]	0.03

a.   Equivalent to malathion excretion of 0.7 mg/man/day.

7.2.4 Factors Involved in Storage and Excretion

7.2.4.1 Identity of Factors.

Dosage. The degree of storage of any given compound in man is a function of dosage, as is true in other animals (see Fig. 7-7, which presents the findings for DDT and dieldrin). Similar observations have been made in connection with the excretion of several compounds studied in volunteers. Additional information on the storage and excretion of pesticides in persons with occupational or other heavier than ordinary exposure is given in Tables 7-13, 7-20, 8-1, 8-2, and 8-3.

Whereas there is abundant evidence that both storage and excretion are dosage-related in man, it has not been possible to achieve a single successful balance study in man. This is almost certainly because of the inadequacy of present chemical methods, since some of these studies in animals have been successful when radioactive isotopes were used.

Storage of a material may be modified by drug-metabolizing enzymes induced by the material itself. This is probably true of DDT, as illustrated by the flexure of the curve in Fig. 7-7. However, the importance of dosage remains paramount. Modification of the storage of a pesticide through interaction with drugs is discussed in a separate paragraph below.

Any decrease in the storage of DDT and related compounds that has occurred in the USA since 1955 (see Section 7.2.1.2) can easily be explained by decreased dosage associated with decreased residues of DDT in food (see Section 6.1.5.1).

Route of Exposure. The route of exposure can make a great difference in the proportion

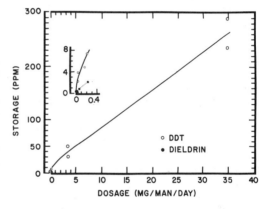

Fig. 7-7. Storage of DDT and dieldrin in people receiving different dosage rates. The graph is based on data of Durham *et al.* (1965c), Hayes *et al.* (1956, 1958, 1971), Quinby *et al.* (1965a), and Walker *et al.* (1954) for DDT and of Hunter *et al.* (1969), Zavon *et al.* (1965), Duggan *et al.* (1966), Robinson and Hunter (1966), and Robinson and McGill (1966) for dieldrin.

of any particular dose that is absorbed. The proportion has been measured in connection with the dermal exposure of orchard spraymen to parathion. In one study it was found to constitute only 0.1 to 2.8% (mean 0.9%) of the compound on the skin available for absorption (Durham and Wolfe, 1963). In a later study the corresponding values ranged from 0.40 to 1.95%, with a mean of 1.23% (Durham *et al.,* 1972). A higher proportion of malathion was absorbed when it was applied experimentally to simulate its use as an antilouse powder. The absorption averaged 1.8 to 3.3% for different groups, but one man absorbed an average of 7.7% and reached a peak of 18.0%. This is not intended to suggest that malathion is absorbed any more readily than parathion because the conditions of study were different; malathion was applied in higher concentration to the entire body except the head and hands, and it was left in place about 23 hours each day (Hayes *et al.*, 1960).

The importance of a given rate of absorption is determined, of course, by the dosage available to be absorbed. In spite of the small proportion of parathion absorbed by the skin, this route may be of critical importance because exposure of this kind may be so much greater than that by other routes. Using the Smyth technique (see Section 5.5.4.1), Durham *et al.* (1972) found that dermal exposure accounted for a minimum of 80.4 to 90.7% of the absorption of parathion experienced by men who sprayed orchards with that compound. An entirely similar result was obtained by use of the complete differential protection technique described in Section 5.5.4.2. The results are shown in Table 7-23. Men with only respiratory exposure excreted no more than 20% as much metabolite as the men who had either dermal exposure or combined respiratory and dermal exposure. In other words, dermal exposure accounted for a minimum of 80% of their absorption. This was true even though (as indicated by measurements with absorptive pads) the immediate environment of one man with only respiratory exposure was somewhat more contaminated than the environments in which the other men worked.

The relative importance of food and respiratory exposure to household insecticides as sources of residues in the general population is considered in Section 6.4.1.

Compound. As discussed in Section 3.2.3.3, compounds show a wide range in their tendency to be stored in tissues. To a large degree, compounds that are stored significantly in mammals are broken down only slowly by plants and soil organisms (some chlorinated hydrocarbon compounds) or not broken down at all (heavy metals). It follows that the very compounds man is likely to store most avidly may be ones most likely to remain as residues in his food or in other situations that permit their absorption. The storage of a wide range of materials in people of the general population already has been mentioned in the introduction (Section 7.2).

Interaction of Compounds. One of the most fascinating examples of antagonism, probably based on induction of drug-metabolizing enzyme (see Section 7.3), involves DDT and certain drugs used for the treatment of epilepsy. The relationship was detected when it was noted that patients who received phenobarbital or, especially, diphenylhydantoin, stored little or no DDT or DDE in their fat or blood (Davies *et al.*, 1969a; Edmundson *et al.*, 1970; Watson *et al.*, 1972). The relationship was established experimentally by Davies *et al.* (1971) who reported that nonepileptic volunteers given diphenylhydantoin at a rate of 300 mg/man/day for 9 months had at the end of that period an average of only 25% of the

Table 7-23

Potential Skin Contamination and Total p-Nitrophenol Excretion for Orchard Spraymen Exposed to Parathion Spray Mist While Wearing Various Protective Equipment From Durham et al. (1972) by permission of the American Medical Association.

Subject	Protective equipment	Route of exposure	Potential skin contamination (mg parathion/sq in)		Total p-nitrophenol excretion (mg)	
			Test 1	Test 2	Test 1	Test 2
1	plastic and rubber clothing	respiratory only	0.031 [a]	0.020 [a]	0.088	0.006
2	pure air supply	dermal only	0.029	0.019	0.666	0.497
3	none	respiratory and dermal	0.017	-----	0.433	-----

a. Since this subject's skin was covered by the plastic and rubber clothing, he could not absorb any of this potential dosage. The quantity was measured and is shown to illustrat the similarity in exposure conditions for the various subjects.

DDT, 39% of the DDE, and 27% of the dieldrin concentration found in their body fat before administration of the drug was begun. Ordinary maintenance doses of phenobarbital, diphenylhydantoin, or a combination of them serve to keep the storage levels of several chlorinated hydrocarbon insecticides as low or lower in exposed, epileptic workers as in the general population (Schoor, 1970; Kwalick, 1971).

Race. It has been reported that Negroes in Illinois (Hoffman *et al.*, 1967), Hawaii (Casarett *et al.*, 1968), Florida (Davies *et al.*, 1968, 1969b), and South Carolina (Keil *et al.*, 1972) store more DDT and DDE than white people in the same states. However, the opposite relationship was found in South Africa (Wassermann *et al.*, 1970). Some authors have found no racial difference in the storage of DDT (Selby *et al.*, 1969b).

Under controlled conditions no difference was found between Negroes and white persons in the storage of DDT (Hayes *et al.*, 1956, 1971). What is known about racial differences in exposure is discussed in Section 6.4.1. It seems likely that the higher storage of DDT and DDE by Negroes in certain geographical areas is environmental rather than physiological in origin. Davies has emphasized this possibility.

The largest reported racial difference in the storage of DDT-related compounds is about two-fold.

No racial difference has been found in the storage of dieldrin (Edmundson *et al.*, 1968).

Individual Differences. Individual differences can be demonstrated among members of inbred strains of laboratory animals (see Section 2.4.8). It is little wonder then that individual differences occur among human individuals who differ widely in genetic background. Individual differences in storage and excretion are so great that there was only partial success when an effort was made to predict storage levels among formulating plant workers by classifying them into high, medium, and low exposure groups according to their duties in the plant (Laws *et al.*, 1967). Storage groups that show little or no overlapping can be expected only when the underlying differences in exposure are large. Of course, distinctly different average storage values may be found for the general population, agricultural applicators, and formulators, respectively, but the ranges overlap (Hayes, 1966). The attempt to predict high and low storage groups within the general population by some index of exposure is almost certain to fail, and the recorded efforts were failures (Selby *et al.*, 1969a). On the

contrary, a prediction of exposure differences based on storage differences may be possible, especially when groups are involved. Thus, Edmundson *et al.* (1970) record the successful prediction of DDT dust in a home where several members of the family showed high blood levels of DDT.

It is only when the dosage is controlled, as in studies of volunteers, that most can be learned about individual differences among people. Considering the equilibrium period from the 38th through the 94th week of receiving DDT orally at the rate of 35 mg/man/day, the average DDA excretion of two volunteers differed by a factor of 30 times. The highest rate ever reached by the lowest excreter during more than a year was almost the same as the lowest rate reached by the highest excreter. The excretion of four other men in the same dosage group fell somewhere between the extremes of 0.089 and 0.269 mg/hr. Obviously there was no statistical difference between the rates of certain men. However, the rate for one of the intermediate ones was statistically different from both the high ($P < 0.05$) and the low ($P < 0.001$) extremes (Hayes *et al.*, 1971).

Although a relatively constant steady-state excretion rate was characteristic of each individual in this study, a few samples revealed an increase or decrease in excretion rate ranging from 2- to 10-fold or more. Some of these changes persisted for 2 or 3 weeks, as revealed by repeated sampling. Thus, the expected differences between individuals may be complicated by temporary differences in the performance of some of them.

Far less variation was found in the excretion of malathion than of DDT. For malathion, the greatest observed differences between average excretion rates of volunteers in the same dosage group ranged only from 1.5- to 3.1-fold for different groups. Furthermore, part of the observed difference in excretion could be accounted for by difference in body surface area available for absorption of the dermally applied malathion (Hayes *et al.*, 1960).

Sex. Most studies have revealed no difference in the storage of DDT-related material in the adipose tissues of men and women (Laug *et al.*, 1951; Hayes *et al.*, 1958; Dale *et al.*, 1965; Wassermann *et al.*, 1965; Robinson *et al.*, 1965; de Vlieger *et al.*, 1968; Maier-Bode, 1960; Read and McKinley, 1961; Egan *et al.*, 1965). Significantly higher storage in men was reported by Hunter *et al.* (1963) in England. Higher storage of DDT was found in Negro men, but not in white men, in Florida (Davies *et al.*, 1968, 1969b); among both white and Negro men in Chicago (Hoffman et al., 1967) and South Africa (Wassermann et al., 1970); among men of unspecified race in California and Idaho (Rappolt, 1970; Watson et al., 1970; Wyllie et al., 1972); and among women of unspecified race in New Orleans (Hayes et al., 1965). In these same studies, men and women stored BHC equally in Chicago, but women stored more of it in New Orleans.

The largest sex-related difference found in the average storage of DDT and its metabolites has been less than two-fold.

Some investigators found that dieldrin is stored in slightly higher concentration in men than in women (Hunter et al., 1963; Robinson et al., 1965; Zavon et al., 1965; Egan et al., 1965; Abbott et al., 1968), but Edmundson et al. (1968) and de Vlieger et al. (1968) found no difference in this regard between men and women.

Pregnancy and Parturition. There is a small but statistically significant decrease in the plasma concentration of p,p'-DDT, p,p'-DDE, o,p'-DDE, p,p'-DDD, and total BHC 1 to 6 days postpartum as compared to the same women early in pregnancy. Most of the decrease appears to occur during about the last 10 days before delivery (Curley and Kimbrough, 1969). The concentrations of p,p'-DDT, o,p'-DDT, p,p'-DDD, o,p'-DDD, dieldrin, and several isomers of BHC are lower in various tissues of women at the time of cesarean section or normal delivery, than in nonpregnant women in the same community (Polishuk et al., 1970). The negative balance continues into the period of lactation (see Section 7.2.2.1).

Age. The storage of DDT, BHC, heptachlor epoxide, and dieldrin in the human fetus is recorded in Table 7-17. There is some tendency for the concentration of organic chlorine insecticides to decrease during the first few months after birth (Abbott et al., 1968; Wassermann et al., 1967), although not all babies follow the trend. When a decrease occurs, it probably can be explained by a more rapid deposition of fat than of insecticide.

The initial decline in storage is followed by an increase, so that approximately the adult level is reached at about 10 years of age (Hayes et al., 1958; Hunter et al., 1963; Wassermann et al., 1965; Robinson et al., 1965; Wassermann et al., 1967; Davies et al., 1968, 1969a; Watson et al., 1970). Some studies have indicated that storage of DDT and DDE is slightly higher in persons over 20 or over 40 years old (Egan et al., 1965; Hoffman et al., 1967; Abbott et al., 1968; Davies et al., 1968, 1969b; Watson et al., 1970; Juszkiewicz and

Stec, 1971; Wassermann et al., 1970; Wyllie et al., 1972; Keil et al., 1972; Warnick, 1972). The difference may involve only one sex (Davies et al., 1968, 1969b). No corresponding increase in storage in older people was found in connection with BHC (Juszkiewicz and Stec, 1971; Wyllie et al., 1972).

In spite of what has just been said, it is questionable whether any dependable pattern exists. Results of the same laboratory for different population groups within a single small country may reveal entirely different curves when storage is plotted against age (Wassermann et al., 1965). In no instance has a biologically important difference in storage of chlorinated hydrocarbon insecticides in people been associated primarily with a difference in age. The largest observed difference was about seven-fold from birth on (Davies et al., 1968, 1969b). This particular difference involved Negro men and probably was related mainly to environmental factors rather than to age *per se.* The same may be true of all observed variation in storage in relation to age.

Diet. The general correspondence of national dietary levels of insecticides and storage of the compounds in people without occupational exposure is recognized. Also reported occasionally is the presence of high concentrations of pesticides in certain foods grown under unusual local conditions that made contamination almost inevitable (see Section 6.1.5.2). However, there have been few studies linking high levels of a pesticide in local food with high levels of storage in the native population. An exception is a report by Kolmodin-Hedman et al. (1973) pointing out that fish from the Baltic Sea are known to contain high levels of DDT and that fishermen from the Island of Gothland in the middle of the Baltic, who ate 2 to 3 times more fish than most Swedes, had average serum levels of 0.034 ppm for DDT and 0.088 ppm for DDE. These levels are 4 to 5 times higher than those of most Swedes, and are even high in comparison with average values in the USA (see Table 7-15).

Nutrition. It is easily possible to precipitate poisoning by starving rats previously fed large doses of DDT (see Section 3.2.3.3). No such test has been carried out in man, and, in fact, it would be impossible because people cannot starve so rapidly, their metabolic rate being much lower than that of rats. Hunter and Robinson (1968) found no increase in the concentration of dieldrin in whole blood during surgical stress or during periods of complete fasting. Whereas DDT might show some increase during marked loss of weight because it is less efficiently excreted, it constitutes no danger of intoxication.

It has been reported that the storage of dieldrin by volunteers given daily doses of it is inversely proportional to their fatness (Hunter and Robinson, 1968), and a similar conclusion was reached regarding dogs that also received daily doses of dieldrin (Keane and Zavon, 1969).

Differences Associated with State of Health. Experimental studies make it clear that certain defects of the skin greatly increase its permeability to chemicals (see Section 3.2.2.5). An apparent example of such an increase under occupational conditions involves a pesticide formulator whose skin exhibited for 14 years or more the atrophy, ulceration, and crusting characteristic of scleroderma. Although his exposure to chlorinated hydrocarbon insecticides was not greater than that of his occupational associates, and although he used protective clothing, his blood levels of dieldrin, β-BHC, heptachlor epoxide, and chlordane (but not DDT and DDE) exceeded those found in any other worker involved in the same survey. When the man died at the age of 64 of causes unrelated to pesticides, samples of fat, liver, and kidney were obtained, and these, too, showed higher than expected concentrations of chlorinated hydrocarbon insecticides other than DDT and DDE (Starr and Clifford, 1971).

There is no agreement in the literature regarding the effect of general health on the storage of chlorinated hydrocarbon insecticides. Some investigators have found no difference in the concentration of DDT in the fat of persons undergoing minor, elective surgery and in those who had died in the USA (Hayes *et al.*, 1958). A similar conclusion was reached in connection with specimens from India (Dale *et al.*, 1965), Israel (Wassermann *et al.*, 1965), and England (Robinson *et al.*, 1965), although the variability of concentration of both DDT and dieldrin was greater in autopsy than in biopsy specimens in the latter country. Considering autopsy specimens only, some investigators have found no relationship between storage of chlorinated hydrocarbon insecticides and cause of death (Hunter *et al.*, 1963; Robinson *et al.*, 1965; Hoffman *et al.*, 1967; Hoffman, 1968; Morgan and Roan, 1970).

By contrast, Deichmann and his colleagues (Deichmann and Radomski, 1968; Radomski *et al.*, 1968) reported that the storage of some chlorinated hydrocarbon insecticides in body fat of persons dying of certain diseases was increased. Compared to the average for persons of unstated age and race dying of un-

stated causes, the average storage of DDE was increased by the following factors in persons dying of the diseases listed: carcinoma including primary and metastatic neoplasm of the liver, 2.0 to 2.9; portal cirrhosis, 1.7; atherosclerosis, 1.8; hypertension, 2.7; and idiopathic amyloidosis, 7.6. The storage of DDT and of several other chlorinated hydrocarbon insecticides was increased to approximately the same small degree.

A similar result has been reported in connection with the storage of DDT and dieldrin in the lungs of persons known to have died of lung cancer (Dacre and Jennings, 1970).

Casarett *et al.* (1968) found no correlation when the cause of death and the wet-weight concentration of total organochlorine residues in tissues were compared. However, they found a marked correlation when the comparison was made on the basis of the concentration of pesticides in extractable lipids. In the latter instance, the five persons with the highest total levels had three characteristics in common: emaciation, cancer, and widespread focal or generalized abnormality of the liver. Other persons who died of carcinoma did not show high levels of total organochlorines.

The diseases in which some increase of insecticide storage has been reported are those that are chronic, often characterized by a protracted, downhill course. They are the wasting diseases. Although evidence is given in Section 3.2.3.3 that the mobilization of DDT from fat through starvation is unlikely to produce poisoning in people, it does not follow that such mobilization will not lead to measurably higher residues in every tissue. This most likely cause of slightly increased storage has not been investigated in the cases under discussion. Duration of hospitalization is not a measure of nutritional status. Furthermore, increased storage may have more than one cause, or different causes in different instances. There is a suggestion that rates of biotransformation are reduced in some conditions, notably amyloidosis, thus increasing storage.

Those who have raised the possibility that the insecticides may cause, or at least aggravate, the diseases in which storage sometimes is slightly increased have failed to emphasize: (*a*) how unlikely it is that a single cause would have such diverse effects; (*b*) that persons with occupational exposure may average 10 times more storage and 25 times more absorption than the highest values reported in connection with disease, but without any predisposition to the diseases in question; and (*c*) that the diseases in question have not shown an increase in age-specific incidence related to the introduction and use of insecticides.

Geographical Differences. DDT has been found in all human populations when it was sought. There is some tendency for the storage levels to be higher in warm countries where insects present a greater problem in agriculture (see Table 7-11). A similar trend may be observed in connection with the warmer and cooler parts of the United States of America. Whether the difference reflects the degree of household use of pesticides, the use of locally raised food, a physiological difference in absorption secondary to temperature, or a combination of factors is not known. Furthermore, not all regional differences in storage are secondary to temperature. Levels of DDT in human adipose tissue or milk from Russia and countries under Russian influence are relatively high. There is considerable reason to think that the difference between the storage observed in civilian and military populations in India were associated with direct application of DDT to stored food—especially that eaten by civilians—and had no relationship to temperature.

Although it may not be possible to explain the exact degree of storage of DDT observed in each country, there is nothing in the observed facts to suggest that the differences do not correspond with differences in exposure. This basic conclusion is reinforced by a study of storage in people with occupational, special environmental, or other special exposure to the insecticide, as summarized in Table 7-13.

Seasonal Differences and Other Changes in Time. In a community where DDT was used extensively in agriculture and used as a thermal fog for municipal mosquito control, the concentrations of DDT and DDE in the sera of three groups of 28 or more men were measured bimonthly during all of 1968. At each sampling period, applicators tended to have the highest storage levels, and the controls the lowest levels. Storage in applicators was about 4 times greater than in the controls. However, all three groups showed a six-fold increase in serum level of total DDT equivalent between April and August. This large increase for all groups overshadowed the smaller differences between groups. From relatively high levels in January and February, average concentrations of total DDT declined sharply in all three groups during March and April. Thereafter, serum levels in all three groups rose rapidly at first and then more slowly. The rises were in effect as early as May, when the use of thermal insecticide began, and well before applications of DDT to

cotton were started. The increases became maximal in August, 2 months before application of DDT to cotton was finished, and about 3 months before fogging was finished. During these 2 or 3 months, the levels remained steady or declined slightly. Between April and August, levels of DDE increased, but not so rapidly as those for total DDT equivalent, so that DDE constituted a progressively smaller percentage of the total during this period. It was estimated that the community use of DDT consumed only about 0.2% the amount used on farms. In addition to these uses, DDT was used extensively for indoor spraying. The possibility that temperature was a factor in the seasonal differences was considered less likely than the possibility that differences depended on dosage derived mainly from nonagricultural uses of the compound (Perron and Barrentine, 1970). That this conclusion probably is correct is indicated by the failure of others to observe seasonal variation in storage values in areas where there is little or no use of DDT for municipal and household control of insects.

Changes in storage from year to year based on corresponding changes in exposure are discussed in Section 7.2.1.2

The urinary excretion of *p*-nitrophenol following exposure to parathion shows diurnal variation after occupational, mainly dermal exposure ends. *p*-Nitrophenol levels are low late at night and early in the morning, and reach higher levels during the afternoon and evening. Excretion usually becomes insignificant 5 to 8 days after exposure, but occasionally lasts only 2 days. The excretion of DDA following exposure to DDT shows a similar but less striking diurnal pattern. In many workers, the excretion of DDA continues at a low level from one exposure to the next (Wolfe *et al.,* 1970).

The cause of the diurnal variation in excretion for a period of several days after exposure is unknown. It may be a result of variation in absorption, rather than a variation in excretion *per se.* Absorption from the skin is known to be increased by increased ambient temperature. Under the occupational conditions observed by Wolfe and his colleagues, there was an average delay of 8.7 hours from the beginning of exposure until the peak of excretion of *p*-nitrophenol was reached. The interaction of ambient temperature and this lag period may explain the diurnal pattern.

Tissue. What has been said in the preceding paragraphs concerns storage in the entire body, or in blood or fat chosen as representative of the entire body.

The general principles of the distribution and storage of compounds in relation to different tissue in the same animal, discussed in Sections 3.2.3.1 and 3.2.3.3, apply to man also. In fact, certain points have been illustrated more neatly for man than for animals. Figure 7-8 shows that there is a close correspondence between the lipid content of the organs and the concentration of DDE, DDT, and dieldrin in blood, kidney, liver, and adipose tissue. The correspondence does not apply to the brain, an organ that includes almost no neutral fat, although its lipid content is relatively high.

7.2.4.2 Evaluation of Factors Influencing Storage of Pesticides in Man.

Important Factors. Clearly, the only two important factors influencing the storage of pesticides in man are compound and dosage. Some materials, such as the organic phosphorus compounds, are little stored even in situations where excretion of the compounds or their metabolites proves that substantial absorption has occurred. By contrast, some but not all of the chlorinated hydrocarbon insecticides are effectively stored. The storage of all compounds is related to dosage, regardless of the efficiency of the storage compared to that of other compounds. For a given compound, high exposure, especially occupational exposure, can produce many times the storage found in the general population.

Minor Factors. The universal importance of dosage in determining storage and excretion must be distinguished from practical but restricted questions regarding the relative importance of different sources of exposure in separate instances. Further investigation of persons whose storage or excretion of a compound is unexpected often will reveal an unexpected source of dosage. In connection with their study of the storage of DDT in people who do not eat meat, Hayes *et al.* (1958) noted but did not publish a value that would have been exceptionally high for the general population and was even more extraordinary when compared to the low values for meat abstainers. Reinvestigation of the exposure history confirmed the meat-free diet, but revealed that the person worked part time in a DDT formulating plant. She was promptly reclassified from "meat abstainer" to "formulator."

Although the possibility of real physiological differences cannot be excluded entirely, there is considerable evidence that differences in storage and excretion sometimes associated with race, sex, and age really depend on differences in dosage. Background information on exposure is discussed in Section 6.4.1. Dif-

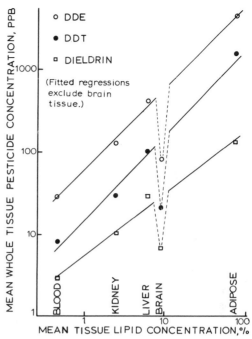

Fig. 7-8. Mean pesticide concentration in five human tissues in relation to their mean lipid content. The values for the brain were excluded in fitting the regression lines. After Morgan and Roan (1970) by permission of the American Medical Association.

ferences in storage in different geographical regions also probably depend on dosage (see Section 6.1.5.1), and the same may be true of seasonal differences in storage.

A number of factors (other than compound and dosage) have been shown clearly to influence storage of foreign compounds in experimental animals (see Section 3.2.3.3). Although man certainly is not immune to these factors, it does not follow that their influence is important or even measurable under practical conditions.

Under controlled conditions, no difference was found in the storage of DDT in Negro and white men (Hayes *et al.*, 1956, 1971). The differences in storage among Negro and white populations in Florida and South Africa were opposite, a phenomenon most easily explained by differences in relative exposure of the two races in these places. Apparently the Negroes of South Africa are less able to purchase household insecticides than are those in Florida.

In connection with reports that increased storage of chlorinated hydrocarbon insecticides is associated with certain diseases, at least three logical possibilities must be considered: (a) one or more of the compounds involved causes or aggravates the disease; (b) the disease predisposes the observed increase in storage in some specific way; and (c) the disease predisposes the observed increase in a nonspecific way.

Of these possibilities, the first is ruled out by epidemiology and especially by studies in workers. If the minor increases in storage reported in persons from the general population who have the disease can aggravate the disease, then the tremendous increases of storage that result from prolonged, intense occupational exposure would cause the condition to occur universally and severely among workers. However, in fact, the diseases involved are not increased among workers.

The possibility that one or more diseases predispose the storage of one or more compounds cannot be excluded categorically. Each combination of a compound and a disease must be considered separately for each tissue. Actually, only a few combinations have been explored. It must be noted, however, that it is unlikely that two or more diseases of very different natures will have the same effect on storage on a specific basis.

It is far more likely that diseases of different natures will have a common effect based on some nonspecific characteristic shared by the diseases. All of the illnesses reported to be associated with increased storage of chlorinated hydrocarbon insecticides are chronic conditions, such that many patients killed by them undergo a terminal phase of weight loss that varies greatly in duration and degree. It is well known that the concentration of DDT and DDE can be increased in experimental animals by weight loss (see Sections 2.4.11 and 2.4.14). The weight losses suffered by patients in the terminal phase of chronic disease often are more severe than any in persons whose pesticide storage levels have been followed systematically (see Section 7.2.4.1). It is, therefore, entirely reasonable that marked weight loss will cause some increase in DDT storage in man. Although some authors have claimed that weight loss has been excluded as a cause of increased storage associated with disease, the evidence is unconvincing. Change of weight during final hospitalization has no necessary bearing on the question. In chronic disease, final hospitalization is often brief and for terminal care of a condition that caused great weight loss before the final admission.

7.3 Other Effects of Pesticides

Besides mortality, morbidity, and storage and excretion, a few other effects of pesticides in man are recognized clearly. They are mainly biochemical in character and, when moderate in degree, are without any known clinical importance in themselves. However, some of them serve as convenient indices of exposure, and they may have other practical applications. Some even represent the biochemical lesion of the compound involved and, if sufficiently severe, are the direct cause of injury.

Enzyme Inhibition. The best known and most commonly measured effect of the kind under discussion is the inhibition of blood cholinesterase by organic phosphorus and carbamate insecticides (see Section 4.1.2.1). Inhibition of this enzyme is commonly seen not only in cases of poisoning but also in workers exposed to the more toxic anticholinesterases. Inhibition is rarely if ever encountered in workers using the less toxic compounds, or in persons whose exposure is environmental only. Measurement of blood cholinesterase is of considerable value both in diagnosis and in monitoring workers to maintain good occupational hygiene.

Changes have been reported in certain other serum enzymes of workers exposed to organic phosphorus insecticides and of other workers exposed to chlorinated hydrocarbon insecticides (Bogusz, 1968). The significance of these changes is not clear, for the men were asymptomatic, and their exposure to or absorption of the compounds involved was unknown.

Enzyme Induction. Another scientifically interesting effect of pesticides is the induction of microsomal enzymes of the liver. This effect is well known in experimental animals (see Section 3.1.2.2) and in people treated with certain drugs. However, it was not until 1969 that this effect was demonstrated in workers exposed to a variety of pesticides, notably DDT (Kolmodin et al., 1969). The result was confirmed the next year in connection with workers exposed to DDT alone at an average rate of 0.25 mg/kg/day (Poland et al., 1970). The dosage of the workers may be compared to 0.0004 mg/kg/day, which is approximately the intake of people in the general population. Occupational exposure increases the drug-metabolizing ability of some workers, so that all of them metabolize test drugs with the efficiency of those persons in the general population who are most efficient in this respect. Poland concluded that, because the effect seen in workers is limited, an effect, if any, in the general population must be small. The induction of microsomal enzymes was demonstrated in a different way by Thompson et al. (1969), who administered DDT orally at a dosage of

1.5 mg/kg/day for 6 months in the successful treatment of unconjugated hyperbilirubinemia.

Since Poland showed that the urinary excretion of 6β-hydroxycortisol was increased by 57% in workers with average serum p,p'-DDT levels of 0.573 ppm, it is of interest to note that at least in workers with lesser exposure to DDT (average serum level, 0.022 ppm), but with some exposure to a wide range of pesticides, adrenal function responded normally to a test dose of dexamethasone (Clifford and Weil, 1972).

Although piperonyl butoxide is a potent inhibitor of microsomal enzyme activity in mice, it is far less active in rats, and a dosage of 0.71 mg/kg was without effect in man (Conney et al., 1972).

7.4 Possible Effects of Pesticides

The clinical picture of poisoning by all the major pesticides is well established. The same is true for basic information on storage and certain other effects. All of these effects are dosage-related. These facts do not exclude the possibility that individual pesticides or groups of pesticides may have effects not yet detected. It is the responsibility of the professional toxicologist to explore objectively any possibility of this sort, no matter how remote. At the same time, the toxicologist has an equal responsibility to reserve judgment on each possibility until there is firm evidence to support a conclusion. Once a causal relation of pesticides to a harmful effect is established firmly, the effect becomes merely one aspect of recognized morbidity.

At any given time, the effects whose possible relation to pesticides are under study are likely to fall into two classes: (a) marginal effects, and (b) speculative effects. These classes are defined and illustrated in the following sections.

7.4.1 Marginal Effects

Marginal effects are those that are not fully established by evidence but that might be predicted from existing knowledge of toxicology. Their importance or even existence must be measured under practical conditions.

For example, it is well known that serious poisoning by organic phosphorus compounds may be accompanied by mental derangement. Furthermore, there are individual case histories suggesting that some pilots who apply various organic phosphorus insecticides by aircraft have suffered lapses of attention or judgment leading to accidents. Obviously, no conclusion can be reached from the individual

cases because of their small number, the inherent danger of flying cropdusting aircraft, the factor of fatigue, etc. This is true even though a substantial proportion of 12 tested cropduster pilots whose planes had wrecked showed decreased blood cholinesterase levels or other laboratory evidence of excessive exposure to organic phosphorus insecticides. The same study emphasized that aerial applicator accidents are complex, involving principally certain geographical areas, certain aircraft makes and models, and certain categories of pilots (Reich and Berner, 1968). However, if these compounds do lead to lapses of attention or judgment, these effects should be dosage-related and subject to objective study. It is possible, too, that apparent lack of judgment might be related to a lack of attention at a critical moment. It is now well known that sleep deprivation and many sedative drugs, as well as petit mal epilepsy, lead to lapses of attention, while proper doses of certain stimulants improve attention. Standard methods for studying attention are available. Some of these methods were used by Durham and his colleagues (1965a) to study people with different degrees of exposure to organic phosphorus insecticides. They found that lapses of attention do occur, but apparently increase in rate only in persons who have absorbed enough poison to show other ill effects at the same time. The experimental results suggest that pilots should stop flying at the slightest hint of illness. Apparently, this is done to some degree, for the rate of accidents associated with cropdusting did not increase from 1951 to 1959, although the use of organic phosphorus compounds and the use of aircraft for cropdusting did increase during the same period (Fig. 7-9).

Blood dyscrasias provide another example of marginal effects. It is well known that both myelogenic and hemolytic dyscrasias can be caused by chemicals. For the worst offenders, it is even possible to measure the chance of adverse reaction. It is known that persons with a genetic defect in glucose 6-phosphate dehydrogenase are abnormally susceptible to hemolytic anemia caused by primaquine and a number of other drugs and naturally occurring compounds. This defect is especially common among the Mediterranean races (see Section 3.1.3.3).

Since blood dyscrasias are known to be caused by some chemicals, it is only reasonable that one or more pesticides might have this effect. Individual reports have been reviewed in connection with DDT (Hayes, 1959b) and BHC (West, 1967). Not enough cases have been associated with any one pesti-

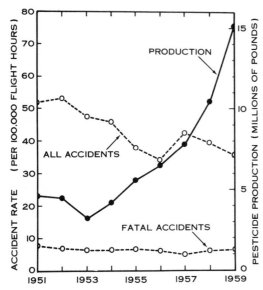

Fig. 7-9. Total and fatal aircraft accidents rates for applicators in relation to production of organic phosphorus pesticides in the United States of America. From Durham *et al.* (1965a) by permission of the American Medical Association.

cide to constitute convincing epidemiological evidence.

Although several tests have been proposed (see Section 8.1.4.1), there is no generally recognized, safe procedure to prove the causative relation of a chemical to an individual case of blood dyscrasia. It follows that no pesticide has been proved to be the cause of a case of blood dyscrasia. The mortality rates associated with blood dyscrasias in the USA are shown in Fig. 7-10. (The curves cannot be extended meaningfully any further to the left because of changes in the way in which the different entities were recorded.) It is clear that there has been no systematic change in the incidence of blood dyscrasias during a period in which the use of pesticides increased. In fact, aplastic anemia was found to have consistently a slightly lower incidence in Kern County, an area of heavy pesticide use, than in California as a whole (Rappolt, 1970). This means that pesticides are not important causes of blood dyscrasias; it does not exclude the possibility that a few compounds may cause an occasional case.

Apparently the only pesticide that has been studied in man as a possible cause of blood dyscrasia is lindane, which previously had been alleged to be the cause of a few cases of aplastic anemia. It was shown clearly that the concentration of lindane in the blood is a measure of recent exposure (Milby *et al.*, 1968). In a study of 79 persons known to be

exposed to lindane for periods of several weeks to several years, aplastic or hypoplastic anemia was not encountered, and no change was found that correlated with blood levels of lindane or with duration of exposure. Certain isolated hematological abnormalities were seen occasionally, and the effects of lindane in these instances could not be excluded totally (Milby and Samuels, 1971).

Some effects that have not been demonstrated in animals have been searched for actively in people. For example, when the relation of DDT and DDE to abortion was explored, it was found that the concentration of these compounds was slightly less in the blood of both white and Negro women who spontaneously aborted than in comparable ones who did not, although the difference was not statistically significant (O'Leary *et al.*, 1970c). On the contrary, the average concentration of DDE in the blood of premature babies (those weighing less than 2,500 g) was significantly greater than that of infants of higher birth weight (O'Leary *et al.*, 1970a). Findings of the same investigators may explain the observation if it is confirmed. The normal placenta is partially protective (see Section 7.2.1.5); it may be that prematurity and increased concentration of DDE in fetal blood both reflect placental abnormality in women whose DDE blood values do not differ from those of women who carry to term.

Some reported actions of pesticides fall on

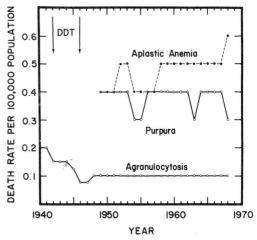

Fig. 7-10. Death rates in the United States of America in different years associated with aplastic anemia, purpura, and agranulocytosis. From US Public Health Service, *Vital Statistics of the United States.* The first arrow indicates the year (1942) in which DDT was introduced experimentally and the second one indicates the year (1946) of its commercial introduction.

the borderline between what we have called "marginal" and "speculative" effects. In the absence of evidence, it is unwise to conclude that any particular effect cannot be caused by a particular compound. For example, a material that acts as a central nervous system depressant in laboratory animals might act as an irritant stimulant in some organism. On the other hand, it is unlikely that the same cluster of effects will be caused by all drugs or by all pesticides. Some specificity of effect is a pharmacological necessity. When this principle appears to be violated, the presence of an unrecognized causative factor can be inferred.

An example of a cluster of effects attributed to pesticides is the report by Tocci *et al.* (1969) that heavy exposure to pesticides causes changes in kidney and liver function and in the concentrations of some circulating amino acids in about 30% of the people studied. The exposed group tended to have higher serum glutamic oxaloacetic transaminase, alkaline phosphatase, serum osmolality, and creatinine values than were found in a control population, and 16% of the group were thought to have specific renal tubular transport defects. It was considered that the changes might be adaptive. It was recognized that poisoning by organic phosphorus insecticides did not raise the levels of amino acids in plasma, thus ruling this out as an acute toxic effect of these compounds.

Such a report raises a question of whether the apparent clustering of effects is real, or whether the individual effects were due to individual compounds (or groups of closely related compounds) or, perhaps, to some unrecognized, nonchemical variable. No definitive answer seems possible at this time. In an attempt to explore the various possibilities, some investigators have studied workers exposed to pesticides in other geographical areas, and others have conducted studies in animals.

Gombart *et al.* (1970) failed to find relevant changes associated with exposure to pesticides, but they did find that the ratio between urinary α-amino acid nitrogen to osmolality changed from summer to winter both in men with high and in those with low exposure to pesticides. Morgan and Roan (1969) found no difference between high and low exposure groups in their glomerular function, tubular reabsorption of phosphate, or total urinary α-amino acid nitrogen. The average plasma concentration of uric acid and the average plasma clearance of uric acid was higher in one group of pesticide workers than in controls, but lower in another group of workers.

Hassan and Cueto (1970) found normal blood and urine levels of amino acids and normal tubular phosphorus resorption in rabbits that received DDT, carbaryl, and parathion concurrently at dosage levels of 5, 5, and 0.5 mg/kg/day, respectively, for 222 days.

Another example of a borderline relationship involves a generally well designed study of blood pressure and serum lipids in pesticide formulators and paired controls matched by age, race, sex, and physical activity (Sandifer and Keil, 1972). Exposure was to a wide range of unnamed pestcides, but blood levels of p,p'-DDT were used as an index of exposure for statistical purposes. No significant differences in systolic or diastolic blood pressure or in blood cholesterol levels were found in white formulators. The authors recognized that the presence of significant differences in these parameters among nonwhite formulators did not prove a causal relation between pesticides and cardiovascular risk factors, even in this group. They speculated that the psychic strain of working with toxic materials might increase blood pressure. What they failed to note was the unusual susceptibility of Negroes to hypertension, and the fact that the correlation with body weight was as high for systolic blood pressure and higher for diastolic blood pressure than the corresponding correlations with blood levels of DDT. Since subclinical levels of pesticides have not been shown to cause hypertension in animals and did not cause it in the white formulators, the relationship observed in the nonwhite formulators may have been circumstantial. The correlation with DDT *per se* (in contrast to DDT as an index of exposure to other pesticides) was certainly misleading in view of the fact that five-fold higher blood levels of DDT in men exposed about 20 years were not associated with an increased incidence of hypertension (Laws *et al.*, 1967).

Certain changes were found in patients with myasthenia gravis who had received what proved to be excessive dosages of neostigmine or pyridostigmine, and whose conditions were studied by electromyography (EMG), namely: (a) some degree of repetitive activity in response to each stimulus; (b) depression of the first potential after voluntary activity; and (c) lower than normal amplitude potentials (Roberts and Wilson, 1969). Later, similar changes were reported in about 50% of factory workers whose predominant exposure was to organic phosphorus insecticides, and in all of six persons following brief, accidental, but subclinical exposure, chiefly to organic phosphorus compounds. The changes were found in only 4% of persons whose exposure was predominantly to chlorinated hydrocarbon insecticides. The changes showed little or no correlation with cholinesterase inhibition, being as frequent in persons whose whole blood enzyme activity was in the high normal range as in those whose activity was slightly below the normal range. As indicated by this and other relationships, it may be that the EMG changes were not a direct result of cholinesterase inhibition. The changes were almost entirely reversible in 48 hours following a single, slight exposure, and partially reversible during the week-end following occupational exposure during the week (Jager *et al.*, 1970).

Later, abnormal EMG patterns were reported in approximately 40% of 102 male agricultural workers who used a wide range of pesticides. Two months later, the records of 25 of 53 who were reexamined were found to have changed from normal to abnormal or *vice versa*. Concurrent measurements of blood cholinesterase activities (all of which were within normal limits) showed no difference between men with normal and those with abnormal EMG records. No special causal relationship was identified and no dosage-response relationship was established (Drenth *et al.*, 1972).

Whether the reported EMG changes have any clinical significance is unknown, and the frequency of their occurrence in healthy, unexposed persons in different physiological states is unclear. The observed lack of a dosage-response relationship leaves a serious question whether the changes really are related to one or more pesticides. Certainly, it will be interesting to see whether the EMG changes will be of similar character but more severe in connection with clinical poisoning. It will also be interesting to determine whether there is any relationship between the EMG changes and the changes in mechanical response of skeletal muscle produced in rats by several insecticides administered at about half their LD 50 values (Santolucito and Whitcomb, 1971). It is already clear that the mechanical changes are not confined to anticholinesterases nor caused by all of them.

It is also unknown whether the hyporeflexia reported by Rayner *et al.* (1972) among workers exposed mainly to organic phosphorus insecticides is of any clinical significance. It is of interest that the reflex force tended to return to control values immediately after exposure and was not associated with any abnormality of muscle strength, EMG spike potential, or nerve conduction velocity.

7.4.2 Speculative Effects

Speculative effects of pesticides are those not supported by any substantial evidence and not predictable from existing toxicological knowledge. An astonishing array of diseases has been linked to pesticides in this way only. Of course, such speculation usually involves diseases or conditions whose causes are unknown or at least unproved. Occasionally, speculation has been inspired by such striking circumstantial evidence that no one could avoid wondering whether there was a causal relation between one or more pesticides and a particular disease. Usually, however, the kind of speculation under discussion has no real foundation. It can be traced to a very small number of persons whose statements often betray ignorance of epidemiology, commitment to organic gardening, or a thinly disguised political motivation.

Regardless of its nature, each speculation must be considered on its merits. The possibility that one or more pesticides contribute to a disease can always be examined epidemiologically. If the disease existed before a particular pesticide was introduced and showed no increase of incidence related to the introduction, it may be concluded that the pesticide is causally related to few if any cases. This kind of evidence cannot exclude the possibility that a pesticide contributes to a few cases of the disease in question. Such exclusion must await proof of the true cause of the disease. Progress is slow in explaining diseases of unknown cause. If the explanation were easy, it would have been found long ago. However, at least one of the diseases once attributed to pesticides is now fully explained. Biskind (1953) claimed 20 years ago that DDT increased susceptibility to poliomyelitis, even though the suggestion was contrary to epidemiological evidence. Apparently poliomyelitis has not been attributed to a pesticide since the success of vaccines proved even to laymen that the disease is infectious and subject to control. Biskind (1953) also attributed hepatitis to DDT, even though epidemics of the disease ("camp jaundice") had been recognized at least as early as the American Civil War. It is generally believed that the disease is of viral origin. Viruses have been isolated from cases, but investigators are not agreed that the etiological relationship has been proved. It seems only a matter of time until such a relationship is established and one more speculation about pesticides is brought to an end.

However, speculation is easy and scientific study difficult. It will be a very long time before the true cause can be discovered for most of the age-old diseases that have been linked to pesticides by speculation. Some of the diseases linked in this way are of enough importance that their epidemiology should be reviewed.

The incidence of both leukemia and Hodgkin's disease was increasing when it was claimed (Biskind, 1953) that cancer was influenced by DDT. However, inspection of Fig. 7-11 shows that both diseases had been on the increase in the United States of America since at least about 1930. The rate of increase was not influenced in the slightest degree by the experimental introduction of DDT in 1942 or its commercial introduction in 1946. Finally, in spite of extensive use of DDT and expanding use of many newer pesticides, the trend of leukemia in the USA began to decrease between 1961 and 1965 when considered on a cohort basis (Fraumeni and Miller, 1967). The improvement was attributed to more restricted use of ionizing radiation.

These diseases are not more common in agricultural communities subject to large inputs of agricultural chemicals. In fact, investigation during the period of 1954 to 1963 revealed consistently slightly lower age-adjusted mortality rates in Kern County (which is said to have the third highest input of pesticides per area in the world) than in California as a whole (Rappolt, 1970). Thus, all epidemiological evidence contradicts a relationship between pesticides and either leukemia or Hodgkin's disease.

The possibility that pesticides might contribute to the incidence of brain tumors was suggested by an episode in which three men who worked in close association died of brain tumors. The men were a county agent, his replacement, and his adopted son. They were not genetically related, but all had some contact with pesticides. The rapid onset and progression of illness in these men and the apparent identity of their uncommon diseases made it almost inevitable that the diseases would be attributed to pesticides. However, the tumors (a glioblastoma multiforme, a subependymal glomerate astrocytoma, and a protoplasmic astrocytoma) were as different from one another as is possible among tumors arising from brain tissue. It is true that the recorded mortality rate associated with malignant neoplasms of the brain and other parts of the nervous system increased from 0.7 (per 100,000) in 1930 to 3.8 in 1968. However, the trend of increase was well established before DDT and all the newer pesticides were introduced. There was little, if any, increase after 1963. Some think that the increase was explained completely by improved diagnosis. In any event, there is no evidence that pesticides are causally related to the condition in man.

7.5 Criteria of Safety

The toxicity of a substance is its capacity for causing injury, whereas the hazard of a substance is the probability that such injury will occur. In other words, hazard may be regarded as the product of toxicity multiplied by a factor expressing both the probability that dosing will occur and the magnitude of dosage. Much more progress has been made in measuring toxicity than in measuring hazard. However, some information is available on the relative importance of factors that influence the observed occurrence of poisoning. Quantitation is most advanced in connection with storage and excretion. Since storage and excretion are dosage-related, their measurement permits an evaluation of the hazard of other effects in any group whose exposure is relatively constant, no matter whether all of the factors influencing this exposure can be identified or not.

It is only through due regard for the critical importance of the dosage-response relationship, and thorough knowledge of the limited degree of difference that may be produced by other factors when the dosage is constant, that we can have assurance of the safety of any pesticide, drug, food, or other chemical when used under specified conditions.

The circumstances surrounding illnesses and deaths caused by pesticides are described earlier in this chapter. Knowledge of these injuries and their circumstances indicates practices that must be avoided and permits selection of protective measures (Chapter 9) to minimize injuries.

However, most concern is expressed not about the obvious hazards from pesticides, but

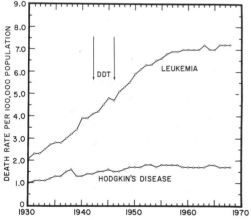

Fig. 7-11. Death rates in the United States of America in different years associated with leukemia and Hodgkins disease. From US Public Health Service, *Vital Statistics of the United States.* The first arrow indicates the year (1942) in which DDT was introduced experimentally and the second one indicates the year (1946) of its commercial introduction.

about the possibility that repeated absorption of traces of a single compound or some combination of compounds will lead eventually to serious illness. It is sometimes implied that if such illness occurred, it would necessarily be chronic and would probably be obscure and difficult to diagnose. The lack of any necessary correspondence between the chronicity of injury and that of dosage has already been pointed out (Section 2.1.2). As a matter of fact, when workers have become sick following repeated, heavy, occupational exposure to a pesticide, the illness has been very similar to that produced by a single dose of the same compound. The same relationship is observed in experimental animals.

Criteria of safety in relation to the traces of pesticides that result from good agricultural practice and are ingested by people of the general population usually are based on similarity—albeit imperfect—in the reactions of experimental animals and man and on long-term tests which produce no effect considered significant, or perhaps no detectable effect at all. In some instances, the potentially major factor of species is eliminated by direct observations on workers or volunteers.

As reviewed at some length in Section 2.3, all of the various kinds of toxicity follow dosage-response relationships. Thus, if a certain daily dosage of a compound produces an injury, one can expect a larger dosage to produce the same injury in a shorter time and often more severely. It is certainly true, as statisticians point out, that the number of observations necessary to detect a phenomenon dependably increases in inverse proportion to the frequency of the phenomenon. For rare phenomena, the necessary number of observations may exceed practicality. However, the difficulty can be overcome by observing the effects of high dosages. In experimental animals the dosage should be carried to the point of causing death. Even in volunteers or workers, it is frequently feasible to search for possible effects of dosages from 100 to 1,000 times those encountered by the general population. If such dosages produce no detectable injury to the volunteers or workers, the chance that some injury to the general population will ultimately occur is extremely small, and, in fact, statistically negligible. Table 2-13 shows that in one instance injury was produced in rats fed for their lifetime at a dosage only one-twentieth of the dosage required to produce the same injury in other rats fed for only about 90 days, ie, about one-eighth of their life-span. This factor of 20 was the largest found for any set of conditions involving a particular species dosed by a particular route. No example is available of any drug or any other chemical that has produced illness in the course of a lifetime when given at a dosage one-twentieth of that which produced no effect when given for one-eighth or more of the life-span of the species.

Time slips by so rapidly we tend to forget that DDT has now been commercially available for over 25 years, and its military use is even longer. Twenty-five years is far more than one-eighth of the human life-span; in fact, it is about one-third of the average lifetime. In many parts of the world, including some sectors of Naples where DDT was used so effectively to combat typhus in 1943 and 1944 (Simmons, 1959), 25 years is more than a human generation.

Records are available for workers who have been employed in the formulation of DDT since 1945 or even earlier. These people remain well while absorbing dosages that for some are equivalent to 35 mg/man/day taken by mouth in solution (Ortelee, 1958). Laws et al. (1967) reported on a group of workers who had been exposed to DDT for 11 to 19 years and whose average intake was estimated to be 17.5 mg/man/day. A thorough study of the liver function of these same workers after they had been exposed for 16 to 25 years (average of 21 years) revealed no evidence of hepatic disease or abnormality of liver function (Laws et al., 1973).

Examinations of workers with more moderate exposure to DDT, but with exposure to a far wider range of pesticides, also have failed to reveal effects of clinical significance (Warnick and Carter, 1972).

Although one can find some reassurance in the fact that experimental animals tolerate even higher dosages without injury, the effect of high occupational dosages in man cannot be known with complete assurance until workers have spent their entire active lives in such employment. However, very substantial assurance about the prospects of the general population can be gained from consideration of these same workers. Exposure of different groups of workers (Ortelee, 1958; Laws et al., 1967, 1973) is approximately 100 to 200 times greater than the exposure of people who ate ordinary restaurant meals in the United States of America in 1953 and 1954. Because of the decrease of DDT in our food (see Section 6.1.5.1), the factor is now in the order of 500 to 1,000 in the United States of America. Of course, the safety factor is greater or less in different countries, depending on the average concentration of DDT in their food. Based on storage reported by Egan *et al.* (1965) and Robinson *et al.* (1965), the average intake of DDT in England and Wales was estimated at slightly less than 0.02 mg/man/day (Hayes, 1967). Thus, the safety factor there is in the order of 1,750.

In a few instances, the storage of a pesticide in the general population of one area may be used as a criterion of the safety of the population of some other area. The factor of safety obtained in this way is, of course, smaller than factors obtained by comparing workers with the general population. However, comparison of two or more populations has the advantage of considering both sexes and all ages and conditions of people at the higher as well as at the lower dosage. As an example, it may be estimated from Fig. 7-7 and from the storage values reported by Dale *et al.* (1965), that the inhabitants of one Indian city have an average absorption of DDT about 20 times greater than in the USA, and about 40 times that in England and Wales.

For DDT and some other compounds studied in volunteers, it is possible to estimate dosage rates from measurements of storage, and thus compare the dosage received by the general population with the dosages tolerated by volunteers and workers, and the even higher dosages that have produced symptoms. Table 7-24 shows this range of dosages for DDT. Table 7-25 shows comparable information for dieldrin.

There is considerable advantage in approaching the question of safety through measurement of the storage or excretion of a compound or its metabolites, as was done in Section 7.2 above. The reason is that either storage or excretion reflects total absorption. This approach avoids the error that might result from basing estimates of safety on measurement of exposure to materials which are actually never adsorbed, or a different error that might result from measuring exposure by a single route when one or more other routes were actually of importance. Measurement of storage or excretion also may have the advantage of being more sensitive than any other available measurements. Of course, the value of measurements of storage or excretion is increased when it is possible to learn the relationship between one of them and dosage in man, as has been done for DDT and dieldrin in Fig. 7-7.

Another approach to measuring the dosage of pesticides which people receive is to measure these compounds in food, particularly representative whole meals, as reviewed in Sec-

Table 7-24

Dosage-Response to DDT in Man

Dosage (mg/kg/day)	Remarks	Reference
unknown[a]	fatal	Hayes, 1959b[b]
16-286[a]	prompt vomiting at higher doses (all poisoned, convulsions in some)	Hayes, 1959b[b]
10[a]	moderate poisoning in some	Hayes, 1959b[b]
6[a]	moderate poisoning in one man	Hsieh, 1954
1.5	tolerated therapy for 6 months	Thompson et al., 1969
0.5	tolerated by volunteers for 21 months	Hayes et al., 1971
0.5	tolerated by workers for 6.5 years	Ortelee, 1958
0.25	tolerated by workers for 19 years	Laws et al., 1967
0.0025	dosage of general population 1953-54	Walker et al., 1954
0.0004	current dosage of general population	Duggan, 1968

a.   One dose only.

b.   Review of many relevant papers.

Table 7-25

Dosage-Response to Dieldrin in Man

Dosage (mg/kg/day)	Remarks	Reference
70 [a/]	estimated fatal single dose	Hodge et al., 1967
26-44 [a/]	convulsions and recovery	Princi, 1954; Spiotta, 1951 [b/]
>0.0332	daily intakes of this order for long periods of time may cause signs and symptoms of convulsive or nonconvulsive intoxication in some men intakes of up to twice this dose are known not to cause signs and symptoms of intoxication in some men	Jager, 1970
0.0332	tolerated by workers for up to 15 years	Jager, 1970
0.0175	long-term occupational exposure with no detectable increase in hepatic microsomal enzyme activity	Jager, 1970
0.0084-0.0170	tolerated by workers for 3-12 years	Hunter et al., 1967; Robinson and Roberts, 1969a; Hayes and Curley, 1968
0.0031	tolerated by volunteers for 2 years without indication of enzyme induction	Hunter and Robinson, 1967 Hunter et al., 1969 Jager, 1970
0.00008-0.00030	dosage of general population of U.K. during 1961-1968	Robinson and Roberts, 1969a
0.00004-0.00024	dosage of general population of USA during 1961-1967	Robinson and Roberts, 1969a

a.   One dose only.

b.   Compound was aldrin, which is metabolized to dieldrin.

tion 6.1.5. The use of meals rather than raw produce has the advantage that whatever cleaning, discarding of outer leaves, or cooking that might affect chemical residues will have been carried out. Therefore, measurements on prepared meals are more typical of true intake than are measurements carried out on food as sold in stores.

The direct or indirect regulation of residues in food and water in terms of tolerances, acceptable daily intake values, and other standards and regulations is discussed in Section 9.1. The same section discusses regulation of the concentration of pesticides and other industrial chemicals in the air of work places. Section 9.1.4.1 treats statistical considerations in the setting of safety factors.

The discussion in this section has concentrated on DDT and dieldrin because they have been widely used in agriculture and public health and have been studied more extensively in animals and man than the other cholorinated hydrocarbon insecticides, some of which are also causes of public concern. The

other compounds of ths class have been monitored, and traces of some of them have been found in human food (Table 6-4). Traces of some of them have been found in human tissues also (Tables 7-14 to 7-17, inclusive). However, the concentrations of other chlorinated hydrocarbon insecticides generally are lower than those of DDT and dieldrin, both in food and in man. It is already clear that the same general conclusions will apply to other chlorinated hydrocarbon insecticides as apply to DDT and dieldrin, although the exact factors of safety may be even greater.

The safety of the chlorinated hydrocarbon insecticides seems especially great if it is compared to that of lead, which we seem to accept without concern. Kehoe (1961) showed that daily ingestion of 2 mg of lead per day (only about 6 times as much as occurs in the ordinary diet) produced a distinct, continuing increase in the concentration of lead in the blood, and only 3 mg per day produced a more rapid rise in the blood lead concentration and the onset of mild symptoms of intoxication. In fact, the safety factors for several heavy metals are small, even if one considers remote areas where the natural occurrence of the metals is not augmented by industrial use or any other human agency.

The majority of modern pesticides are not stored to a significant degree and, therefore, for them this property need not be considered.

Taking all criteria of safety into account, pesticides as encountered by the general population are remarkably safe. As already discussed, the safety factor for the general population as compared with workers who are exposed directly to DDT and dieldrin is very great. It is likely to be even greater in connection with any compound that is readily biodegradable, for the simple reason that such compounds do not persist. The general population encounters only traces of them, or none at all.

Countries interested in human health would do well to minimize the time and talent they expend on monitoring and regulating the traces of pesticides encountered by the average person and to concentrate on achieving practices that will avoid accidental ingestion by young children or excessive exposure of those who use these and other industrial chemicals.

REFERENCES

Abbott, D. C., Collins, G. B., and Goulding, R. (1972). Organochlorine pesticide residues in human fat in the United Kingdom 1969–71. Br. Med. J., 2:553–556.

Abbott, D. C., Goulding, R., and Tatton, J. O'G. (1968). Organochlorine pesticide residues in human fat in Great Britain. Br. Med. J., 3:146–149.

Acker, L., and Schulte, E. (1970). Über das vorkommen von chlorierten biphenylen und hexachlorbenzol neben chlorierten insektiziden humanmilch und menschlichem Fettgewebe. Naturwissenschaften, 57:497.

Aizicovici, et al. Travaux Scientifiques de l'Institut d'Hygiene de Jassy, 1960–1966, p. 142. (Crede: Wassermann, M., Sofoluwe, G. O., Wassermann, D., Groner, Y., and Lazarovitch, S. (1968). Storage of organochlorine insecticides in the body fat of people in Nigeria. Proceedings of the Lagos International Seminar on Occupational Health for Developing Countries, Nigeria, April 1–6).

Almeida, W. F. (1966). Epidemiological aspects of pesticide poisoning in the United States and Latin America. Mimeographed report of the Food and Agriculture Organization of the United Nations.

Almeida, W. F. (1967). Intoxicacões Acidentais Humanas por Inseticidas. Instituto Biologico Publ. No. 120, São Paulo, Brazil.

Almeida, W. F., and Pereira, A. P. (1963). Parations como principais responsáveis pelos casos acidentais de intoxicacão por inseticidas de uso agrícola. Biológico, 29:245–257.

Amin ol Achrafi, T. (1963). Sur douze décès dûs à l'emploi d'un insecticide anticholinestérase: parathion. Description pharmacologique, symptômes et traitement. Rev. Med. Moyen Orient, 20:429–436.

Anderson, L. S., Warner, D. L., Parker, J. E., Bluman, N., and Page, B. D. (1965). Parathion poisoning from flannelette sheets. Can. Med. Assoc. J., 92:809–813.

Anonymous (1962). Poisoning cases in 1960. Pharm. J., 189:453–455.

Anonymous (1963). Poisoning cases in 1961. Pharm. J. 190:177–179.

Anonymous (1972a). Prevention of pesticide poisoning. WHO Chron., 26:156–159.

Anonymous (1972b). BHC and DDT residues in human milk on the decline in Japan. Noyaku Bijin, 56:458.

Armstrong, R. W., Eichner, E. R., Klein, D. E., Barthel,W. F., Bennett, J. V., Jonsson, V., Beuce, H., and Loveless, L. E. (1969). Pentachlorophenol poisoning in a nursery for newborn infants. II. Epidemiologic and toxicologic studies. J. Pediatr., 75:317–325.

Arnan, A. (1962). Accidental poisoning from agricultural pesticides. Bull. WHO, 26:109–120.

Bakir, F., Damluji, S. F., Amin-Zaki, L., Murtadha, M., Khalidi, A., Al-Rawi, N. Y., Tikriti, S., Dhahir, H. I., Clarkson, T. W., Smith, J. C., and Doherty, R. A. (1973). Methylmercury poisoning in Iraq. Science, 181:230–240.

Bambou, H., Comakou, M., and Dimitrova, N. (1966). Group intoxications with lindane. Savr. Med., 17:477–481.

Barnes, J. M. (1953). Toxic hazards of certain pesticides to man. Bull. WHO, 8:419–490, 535–589. (Reprinted WHO Monogr. Ser. No. 16).

Barthel, W. F., Curley, A., Thrasher, C. L., Sedlak, V. A., and Armstrong, R. (1969). Determination of pentachlorophenol in blood, urine, tissue, and clothing. J. Assoc. Off. Anal. Chem., 52:294–298.

Bell, A. (1960). Aldrin poisoning: a case report. Med. J. Aust., 2:698–670.

Bevenue, A., Wilson, J., Casarett, L. J., and Klemmer,H. W. (1967). A survey of pentachlorophenol content in human urine. Bull. Environ. Contam. Toxicol., 2:319–332.

Bick, M. (1967). Chlorinated hydrocarbon residues in human body fat. Med. J. Aust., 1:127–129.

Biros, F. J., Walker, A. C., and Medbery, A. (1970). Polychlorinated biphenyls in human adipose tissue. Bull. Environ. Contam. Toxicol., 5:317–323.

Biskind, M. S. (1949a). DDT poisoning and X-disease in cattle. J. Am. Vet. Med. Assoc., 114:20.

Biskind, M. S. (1949b). DDT poisoning a serious public health hazard. Am. J. Dig. Dis., 16:73.

Biskind, M. S. (1949c). DDT poisoning and the elusive "virus X": a new cause for gastro-enteritis. Am. J. Dig. Dis., 16:79–84.

Biskind, M. S. (1953). Public health aspects of the new insecticides. Am. J. Dig. Dis., 20:331–341.

Biskind, M. S., and Bieber, I. (1949). DDT poisoning—a new syndrome with neuropsychiatric manifestations. Am. J. Psychother., 3:261–270.

Biskind, M. S., and Mobbs, R. F. (1972). Psychiatric manifestations from insecticide exposure. J. A. M. A., 220:1248.

Bogusz, M. (1968). Influence of insecticides on the activity of some enzymes contained in human serum. Clin. Chim. Acta, 19:367–369.

Brady, M. N., and Siyali, D. S. (1972). Hexachlorobenzene in human body fat. Med. J. Aust., 1:158–161.

Brewerton, H. V., and McGrath, H. J. W. (1967). Insecticides in human fat in New Zealand. N. Z. J. Sci., 10:486–492.

Bronisz, H., and Ochýnski, J. (1968). Zawartosc DDT I DDE W Mleku Kobiecym. Biul. Inst. Ochrony Róslin, 41:99–102.

Bronisz, H., Rusiecki, W., Ochýnski, J., and Bernhard, E. (1967). DDT in adipose tissue of Polish population. Diss. Pharm. Pharmacol., 19:309–314.

Brown, J. R. (1967). Organo-chlorine pesticide residues in human depot fat. Can. Med. Assoc. J., 97:367–373.

Brown, V. K. H., Hunter, C. G., and Richardson, A. (1964). A blood test diagnostic of exposure to aldrin and dieldrin. Br. J. Ind. Med., 21:283–286.

California, State of (1967). Occupational Disease in Califor-

nia. Department of Public Health, Bureau of Occupational Health and Environmental Epidemiology.

California, State of (see appropriate years, 1968–1970). *Occupational Disease in California Attributed to Pesticides and Other Agricultural Chemicals.* Department of Public Health, Bureau of Occupational Health and Environmental Epidemiology.

Cam, C., and Nigogosyan, G. (1963). Acquired toxic porphyria cutanea tarda due to hexachlorobenzene, J. A. M. A., 183:88–91.

Cann, H. M. (1963). Pesticide poisoning accidents among young children. Am. J. Public Health, 53:1418–1426.

Cann, H. M., Iskrant, A. P., and Neyman, D. S. (1960). Epidemiologic aspects of poisoning accidents. Am. J. Public Health, 50:1914–1924.

Cann, H. M., Neyman, D. S., and Verhulst, H. L. (1958). Control of accidental poisoning—a progress report. J. A. M. A., 168:717–724.

Carrillo, S. J. (1954). El empleo del dieldrin en Venezuela. Bol. Of. Sanit. Panam., 37:76–81.

Casarett, L. J., Fryer, G. C., Yauger, W. L., and Klemmer, H. W. (1968). Organochlorine pesticide residues in human tissue—Hawaii. Arch. Environ. Health, 17:306–311.

Cassidy, W., Fisher, A. J., Peden, J. D., and Parry-Jones, A. (1967). Organo-chlorine pesticide residues in human fats from Somerset. Mon. Bull. Minist. Health (London), 26(1):2–6.

Chamberlin, H. R., and Cooke, R. E. (1953). Organic phosphate insecticide poisoning. Am. J. Dis. Child., 85:164–172.

Clements, F. W., Southby, R., Rowlands, J. B., and Veuthey, P. (1963). An analysis of deaths from accidental poisonings in children aged under five years. Med. J. Aust., 2:649–652.

Clifford, N. J., and Weil, J. (1972). Cortisol metabolism in persons occupationally exposed to DDT. Arch. Environ. Health, 24:145–147.

Coble, Y., Hildebrandt, P., Davis, J., Raasch, F., and Curley, A. (1967). Acute endrin poisoning. J. A. M. A., 202:489–493.

Collings, A. J., and Sharratt, M. (1970). The BHT content of human adipose tissue. Food Cosmet. Toxicol., 8:409–412.

Conley, B. E. (1958). Morbidity and mortality from economic poisons in the United States. A. M. A. Arch. Ind. Health, 18:126–133.

Conney, A. H., Chang, R., Levin, W. M., Garbut, A., Munro-Faure, A. D., Peck, A. W., and Bye, A. (1972). Effects of piperonyl butoxide on drug metabolism in rodents and man. Arch. Environ. Health, 24:97–106.

Copplestone, J. F., Hunnego, J. N., and Harrison, D. L. (1973). Insecticides in adult New Zealanders—a five year study. N. Z. J. Sci., 16:27–39.

Coulson, D. M., and McCarthy, E. M. (1963). *Effects of Pesticides on Animals and Human Beings.* Stanford Res. Inst. Tech. Rep. 6.

Cranmer, M. F., Carroll, J. J., and Copeland, M. F. (1969). Determination of DDT and metabolites, including DDA, in human urine by gas chromatography. Bull. Environ. Contam. Toxicol., 4:214–223.

Cranmer, M. F., and Freal, J. (1970). Gas chromatographic analysis of pentachlorophenol in human urine by formation of alkyl ethers. Life Sci., 9:121–128.

Cueto, C., Jr., and Biros, F. J. (1967). Chlorinated insecticides and related materials in human urine. Toxicol. Appl. Pharmacol., 10:261–269.

Cueto, C., Jr., and Hayes, W. J., Jr. (1962). The detection of dieldrin metabolites in human urine. J. Agric. Food Chem., 10:366–369.

Curley, A., Burse, W. W., Jennings, R. W., Villanueva,E. C. (1973). Chlorinated hydrocarbon pesticides and related compounds in adipose tissue from people of Japan. Nature, 242:338–340.

Curley, A., Copeland, M. F., and Kimbrough, R. D. (1969).

Chlorinated hydrocarbon insecticides in organs of stillborn and blood of newborn babies. Arch. Environ. Health, 19:628–632.

Curley, A., Hawk, R. E., Kimbrough, R. D., Nathenson, G., and Finberg, L. (1971a). Dermal absorption of hexachlorophene in infants. Lancet, 2:296–297.

Curley, A., Jennings, R. W., Mann, H. T., and Sedlak, V. (1970). Measurement of endrin following epidemics of poisoning. Bull. Environ. Contam. Toxicol., 5:24–29.

Curley, A., and Kimbrough, R. (1969). Chlorinated hydrocarbon insecticides in plasma and milk of pregnant and lactating women. Arch. Environ. Health, 18:156–164.

Curley, A., Sedlak, V. A., Girling, E. F., Hawk, R. E., Barthel, W. F., Pierce, P. E., and Likosky, W. H. (1971b). Organic mercury identified as the cause of poisoning in humans and hogs. Am. Assoc. Adv. Sci., 172:65–67.

Dacre, J. C., and Jennings, R. W. (1970). Organochlorine insecticides in normal and carcinogenic human lung tissues. Toxicol. Appl. Pharmacol., 17:277.

Dale, W. E. (1971). Personal communication.

Dale, W. E., Copeland, M. F., and Hayes, W. J., Jr. (1965). Chlorinated insecticides in the body fat of people in India. Bull. WHO, 33:471–477.

Dale, W. E., Curley, A., and Cueto, C., Jr. (1966). Hexane extractable chlorinated pesticides in human blood. Life Sci., 5:47–54.

Dale, W. E., Gaines, T. B., Hayes, W. J., Jr., and Pearce, G. W. (1963). Poisoning by DDT: relation between clinical signs and concentration in rat brain. Science, 142:1474–1476.

Dale, W. E., and Quinby, G. E. (1963). Chlorinated insecticides in the body fat of people in the United States. Science, 142:593–595.

Damaskin, V. I. (1965). The extent of the accumulation of DDT in the human body in connection with its assimilation with food, and its toxic effect. Gig. Sanit., 30:109–111.

Davies, G. M., and Lewis, I. (1956). Outbreak of foodpoisoning from bread made of chemically contaminated flour. Br. Med. J., 2:393–398.

Davies, J. E., Edmundson, W. F., Carter, C. H., and Barquet, A. (1969a). Effect of anticonvulsant drugs on dicophane (D.D.T.) residues in man. Lancet, 2:7–9.

Davies, J. E., Edmundson, W. F., Maceo, A., Barquet, A., and Cassady, J. (1969b). An epidemiologic application of the study of DDE levels in whole blood. Am. J. Public Health, 59:435–441.

Davies, J. E., Edmundson, W. F., Maceo, A., Irvin, G. L., III, Cassady, J., and Barquet, A. (1971). Reduction of pesticide residues in human adipose tissue with diphenylhydantoin. Food Cosmet. Toxicol., 9:413–423.

Davies, J. E., Edmundson, W. F., Schneider, N. J., and Cassady, J. C. (1968). Problems of prevalence of pesticide residues in humans. Pestic. Monit. J., 2(2):80–85.

Davies, J. E., Jewett, J. S., Welke, J. O., Barquet, A., and Freal, J. J., III (1970). Epidemiology and chemical diagnosis of organophosphate poisoning. Pesticides Symposia, Inter-American Conference on Toxicology and Occupational Medicine, August 1970.

Davies, J. E., Welke, J. O., and Radomski, J. L. (1965). Epidemiological aspects of the use of pesticides in the South. J. Occup. Med., 7:612–618.

Deichmann, W. B., and Radomski, J. L. (1968). Retention of pesticides in human adipose tissue—preliminary report. Ind. Med. Surg., 37:218–219.

Del Vecchio, V., and Leoni, V. (1967). La ricerca ed il dosaggio degl: Insetticidi clorurati in materiale biologico. Nota II. G1: Insetticide clorurati nei tessuti adiposi di alcuni gruppi della popolazione italiana. Nuovi Ann. Ig. Microbiol., 18:107–128.

Denés, A. (1962). Lebensmittelchemische Probleme von Ruckstanden chlorierter Kohlenwasserstoffe. Nahrung, 6:48–56.

Denés, A. (1964). Investigation of chlorinated hydrocarbon

residues in animal and vegetable fats. In: *1963 Year Book*. Institute of Nutrition, Budapest, Hungary.

Denés, A. (1966). Dieldrin residues in foodstuffs and biological material. In: *1965 Year Book*. Institute of Nutrition, pp. 47–49. Budapest, Hungary.

Derban, L. K. A. (1974). Outbreak of food poisoning due to alkyl-mercury fungicide. Arch. Environ. Health, 28:49–52.

de Vlieger, M., Robinson, J., Baldwin, M. K., Crabtree,A. N., and van Dijk, M. C. (1968). The organochlorine insecticide content of human tissue. Arch. Environ. Health, 17:759–767.

Dezoteux, H., and Vinceneux, P. (1971). Acute intoxications in Casablanca. Bull. Méd. Lég. Toxicol. Méd., 14:30–37.

Dixon, E. M. (1957). Dilation of the pupils in parathion poisoning. J. A. M. A., 163:444–445.

Drenth, H. J., Ensberg, I. F. G., Roberts, D. V., and Wilson, A. (1972). Neuromuscular function in agricultural workers using pesticides. Arch. Environ. Health, 25:395–398.

Duggan, R. E. (1968). Residues in food and feed. Pesticide residue levels in foods in the United States from July 1, 1963 to June 30, 1967. Pestic. Monit. J., 2:2–46.

Duggan, R. E., Barry, H. C., and Johnson, L. Y. (1966). Pesticide residues in total-diet samples. Science, 151:101–104.

Durham, W. F., Armstrong, J. F., and Quinby, G. E. (1965b). DDA excretion levels. Arch. Environ. Health, 11:76–79.

Durham, W. F., Armstrong, J. F., and Quinby, G. E. (1965c). DDT and DDE content of complete prepared meals. Arch. Environ. Health, 11:641–647.

Durham, W. F., Armstrong, J. F., Upholt, W. M., and Heller, C. (1961). Insecticide content of diet and body fat of Alaskan natives. Science, 134:1880–1881.

Durham, W. F., and Wolfe, H. R. (1963). An additional note regarding measurement of the exposure of workers to pesticides. Bull. WHO, 29:279–281.

Durham, W. F., Wolfe, H. R., and Elliott, J. W. (1972). Absorption and excretion of parathion by spraymen. Arch. Environ. Health, 24:381–387.

Durham, W. F., Wolfe, H. R., and Quinby, G. E. (1965a). Organophosphorus insecticides and mental alertness. Arch. Environ. Health, 10:55–66.

Edmundson, W. F., Davies, J. E., and Hull, W. (1968). Dieldrin storage levels in necropsy adipose tissue from a South Florida population. Pestic. Monit. J., 2:86–89.

Edmundson, W. F., Davies, J. E., Maceo, A., and Morgade, C. (1970). Drug and environmental effects on DDT residues in human blood. J. South. Med. Assoc., 63:1440–1441.

Edson, E. F. (1957). Occupational health aspects of pesticides in Britain. Trans. Assoc. Ind. Med. Off., 8:24–30.

Egan, H., Goulding, R., Roburn, J., and Tatton, J. O'G. (1965). Organo-chlorine pesticide residues in human fat and human milk. Br. Med. J., 2:66–69.

Elliot, R., and Barnes, J. M. (1963). Organophosphorus insecticides for the control of mosquitos in Nigeria. Bull. WHO, 28:35–54.

Embry, T. L., Morgan, D. P., and Roan, C. C. (1972). Search for abnormalities of heme synthesis and sympathoadrenal activity—in workers regularly exposed to pesticides. J. Occup. Med., 14:918–921.

Engst, R., Knoll, R., and Nickel, B. (1967). Über die Anreicherung von chlorierten Kohlenwasserstoffen, insbesondere von DDT und seinem metaboliten DDE, im menschlichen Fett. Pharmazie, 22:654–661.

Farm Chemicals Handbook (1965). Meister Publishing Company, Willoughby, Ohio.

Fiserova-Bergerova, V., Radomski, J. L., Davies, J. E., and Davies, J. H. (1967). Levels of chlorinated hydrocarbon pesticides in human tissues. Ind. Med. Surg., 36:65–70.

Fowler, R. E. L. (1953). Insecticide toxicology. Manifestations of cottonfield insecticides in the Mississippi Delta. J. Agric. Food Chem., 1:469–473.

Fraumeni, J. F., and Miller, R. W. (1967). Leukemia mortality: downturn rates in the United States. Science, 155:1126–1128.

Ganelin, R. S., Cueto, C., Jr., and Mail, G. A. (1964). Exposure to parathion: effect on general population and asthmatics. J. A. M. A., 188:807–810.

Goldwater, L. J., and Hoover, A. W. (1967). An international study of "normal" levels of lead in blood and urine. Arch. Environ. Health, 15:60–63.

Goldwater, L. J., Ladd, A. R., and Jacobs, M. B. (1964). Absorption and excretion of mercury in man. VII. Significance of mercury in blood. Arch. Environ. Health, 9:735–741.

Gombart, A. K., Veat, V. B., Bonderman, P., and Long,K. R. (1970). Seasonal pesticide exposure relationships. Arch. Environ. Health, 21:128–132.

Gómez Ulloa, M., Velasco, F., Laverde de Fandino, H., and Guerrero, E. (1967–1968). Epidemiological investigation of the food poisoning which occurred in the municipality of Chiquinquira. Ministry of Public Health, Colombia, South America.

Goulding, R., and Watkin, R. R. (1965). National Poisons Information Service. Mon. Bull. Minist. Health (London), 24:26–32.

Gracheva, G. V. (1969). The possibility of DDT accumulation in the organism of persons not having occupational contact with it. Faktory Vneshn. Sredy i ikh Znachen, 1:125–129.

Gracheva, G. V. (1970). DDT excretion with the milk of nursing mothers occupationally unexposed to the effect of this insecticide. Vopr. Pitan., 29:75–78.

Halacka, K., Hakl, J., and Vymetal, F. (1965). Odraz masivne pouzivaneho DDT v lidske tukove tkani. Cs. Hyg., 10:188–192.

Haq, I. U. (1963). Agrosan poisoning in man. Br. Med. J., 1:1579–1582.

Hassan, A., and Cueto, C., Jr. (1970). Biochemical effects in the rabbit of repeated administration of a mixture of DDT, carbaryl, and parathion. Z. Naturforsch., 25b:521–525.

Hayes, W. J., Jr. (1957). Dieldrin poisoning in man. Public Health Rep., 72:1087–1091.

Hayes, W. J., Jr. (1959a). The toxicity of dieldrin to man: report of a survey. Bull. WHO, 20:891–912.

Hayes, W. J., Jr. (1959b). Pharmacology and toxicology of DDT. In: *DDT, The Insecticide Dichlorodiphenyltrichloroethane and its Significance*, edited by P. Müller, Vol. 2, pp. 9–247. Birkhäuser Verlag, Basel.

Hayes, W. J., Jr. (1960). Pesticides in relation to public health. Annu. Rev. Entomol., 5:379–404.

Hayes, W. J., Jr. (1963). *Clinical Handbook on Economic Poisons. Emergency Information for Treating Poisoning*. Public Health Service Publ. 476, US Government Printing Office, Washington, DC.

Hayes, W. J., Jr. (1966). Monitoring food and people for pesticide content. In: *Scientific Aspects of Pest Control*, pp. 314–342, Publ. 1402, National Academy of Sciences-National Research Council, Washington, DC.

Hayes, W. J., Jr. (1964). Toxicological problems associated with use of pesticides. Ind. Trop. Health, 5:118–132.

Hayes, W. J., Jr. (1967). Toxicity of pesticides in man: risks from present levels. Proc. R. Soc. B, 167:101–127.

Hayes, W. J., Jr., and Curley, A. (1968). Storage and excretion of dieldrin and related compounds. Effect of occupational exposure. Arch. Environ. Health, 16:155–162.

Hayes, W. J., Jr., Dale, W. E., and Burse, V. W. (1965). Chlorinated hydrocarbon pesticides in the fat of people in New Orleans. Life Sci., 4:1611–1615.

Hayes, W. J., Jr., Dale, W. E., and LeBreton, R. (1963). Storage of insecticides in French people. Nature, 199:1189–1191.

Hayes, W. J., Jr., Dale, W. E., and Pirkle, C. I. (1971). Evidence of safety of long-term, high, oral doses of DDT for man. Arch. Environ. Health, 22:119–135.

Hayes, W. J., Jr., Dixon, E. M., Batchelor, G. S., and Upholt, W. M. (1957). Exposure to organic phosphorus sprays and occurrence of selected symptoms. Public Health Rep., 72:787–794.

Hayes, W. J., Jr., Durham, W. F., and Cueto, C., Jr. (1956). The effect of known repeated oral doses of chlorophenothane (DDT) in man. J. A. M. A., 162:890–897.

Hayes, W. J., Jr., Mattson, A. M., Short, J. G., and Witter, R. F. (1960). Safety of malathion dusting powder for louse control. Bull. WHO, 22:503–514.

Hayes, W. J., Jr., and Pirkle, C. I. (1966). Mortality from pesticides in 1961. Arch. Environ. Health, 12:43–55.

Hayes, W. J., Jr., Quinby, G. E., Walker, K. C., Elliott,J. W., and Upholt, W. M. (1958). Storage of DDT and DDE in people with different degrees of exposure to DDT.A. M. A. Arch. Ind. Health, 18:398–406.

Henderson, G. L., and Woolley, D. E. (1969). Tissue concentrations of DDT: correlation with neurotoxicity in young and adult rats. Proc. West. Pharmacol. Soc., 12:58–62.

Heyndrickx, A., and Maes, R. (1969). The excretion of chlorinated hydrocarbon insecticides in human mother milk. J. Pharm. Belg., 9–10:459–463.

Hidaka, K., Ohe, T., Fujiwara, K. (1972). PCB and organochlorine pesticides in mother's milk. Igakuno Ayumi, 82:519–520.

Hodge, H. C., Boyce, A. M., Deichmann, W. B., and Kraybill, H. F. (1967). Toxicology and no-effect levels of aldrin and dieldrin. Toxicol. Appl. Pharmacol., 10:613–675.

Hoff, P. R. (1970). Accidents in agriculture. A survey of their causes and prevention. Information Bulletin 1. New York State College of Agriculture, Ithaca, NY.

Hoffman, W. S. (1968). Clinical evaluation of the effects of pesticides in man. Ind. Med. Surg., 37:289–292.

Hoffman, W. S., Adler, H., Fishbein, W. I., and Bauer,F. C. (1967). Relation of pesticide concentrations in fat to pathological changes in tissues. Arch. Environ. Health, 15:758–765.

Hoffman, W. S., Fishbein, W. I., and Andelman, M. B. (1964). The pesticide content of human fat tissue. Arch. Environ. Health, 9:387–394.

Horasawa, I. (1956). Personal communication.

Hornabrook, R. W., Dyment, P. G., Gomes, E. D., and Wiseman, J. S. (1972). DDT residues in human milk from New Guinea natives. Med. J. Aust., 1:1297–1300.

Howell, D. E. (1948). A case of DDT in human fat. Proc. Okla. Acad. Sci., 29:31–32.

Hristic, B., and Milenkovic, D. (1961). Les empoisonnements accidentels par le parathion introduit par la voie cutanee. Arh. Hig. Rada, 12:185–189.

Hruska, J. (1969). DDT residues in the milk, butter, and fat of cattle. Veterinarstvi, 19:493–498.

Hsieh, H. C. (1954). DDT intoxication in a family in Southern Taiwan. Arch. Ind. Hyg., 10:334–346.

Hunter, C. G., and Robinson, J. (1967). Pharmacodynamics of dieldrin (HEOD). I. Ingestion by human subjects for 18 months. Arch. Environ. Health, 15:614–626.

Hunter, C. G., and Robinson, J. (1968). Aldrin, dieldrin, and man. Food Cosmet. Toxicol., 6:253–260.

Hunter, C. G., Robinson, J., and Jager, K. W. (1967). Aldrin and dieldrin—the safety of present exposures of the general populations of the United Kingdom and the United States. Food Cosmet. Toxicol., 5:781–787.

Hunter, C. G., Robinson, J., and Richardson, A. (1963). Chlorinated insecticide content of human body fat in southern England. Br. Med. J., 1:221–224.

Hunter, C. G., Robinson, J., and Roberts, M. (1969). Pharmacodynamics of dieldrin (HEOD). Arch. Environ. Health, 18:12–21.

Introna, F. (1959). Acute poisoning by percutaneous absorption of E605. Riv. Infort. Mal. Prof., 46:1222–1231.

Isbister, C. (1963). Poisoning in childhood, with particular reference to kerosene poisoning. Med. J. Aust., 2:652–656.

Jager, K. W. (1970). Aldrin, Dieldrin, Endrin, and Telodrin: An Epidemiological and Toxicological Study of Long-term Occupational Exposure. American Elsevier Publishing Co., Inc., New York.

Jager, K. W., Roberts, D. V., and Wilson, A. (1970). Neuromuscular function in pesticide workers. Br. J. Ind. Med., 27:273–278.

Jalili, M. A., and Abbasi, A. H. (1961). Poisoning by ethyl mercury toluene sulphonanilide. Br. J. Ind. Med., 18:303–308.

Joffe, A. Z. (1965). Toxin production by cereal fungi causing toxic alimentary aleukia in man. In: Mycotoxins in Foodstuffs, edited by G. N. Wogan, pp. 77–85. The M.I.T. Press, Cambridge, Mass.

Johnston, J. M. (1953). Parathion poisoning in children. J. Pediatr., 42:286–291.

Joslin, E. F., Forney, R. L., Huntington, R. W., Jr., and Hayes, W. J., Jr. (1960). A fatal case of lindane poisoning. Proc. Natl. Assoc. Coroners, Seminars, pp. 53–57.

Juhl, E. (1971). Deaths from phosphostigmine poisoning in Denmark. An analysis of the medico-social and medico-legal aspects. Dan. Med. Bull., 18(Suppl. 1):1–112.

Juszkiewicz, T., and Stec, J. (1971). Polichlorinated insecticide residues in adipose tissue of farmers in the Lublin Province (Poland). Pol. Tyg. Lek., 26:462.

Kadis, V. W., Breitkreitz, W. E., and Jonasson, O. J. (1970). Insecticide levels in human tissues of Alberta residents. Can. J. Public Health, 61:413–416.

Kanagaratnam, K., Boon, W. H., and Hoh, T. K. (1960). Parathion poisoning from contaminated barley. Lancet, 1:538–542.

Kanitz, S., and Castello, G. (1966). Sulla presenza di residui di alcuni disinfestanti nel tessuto adiposo umano ed in alcuni alimenti. G. Ig. Med. Prev., 7:1–19.

Karunakaran, C. O. (1958). The Kerala food poisoning. J. Indian Med. Assoc., 31:204–207.

Kazantzis, G., McLaughlin, A. I. G., and Prior, P. F. (1964). Poisoning in industrial workers by the insecticide aldrin. Br. J. Ind. Med., 21:46–51.

Keane, W. T., and Zavon, M. R. (1969). The total body burden of dieldrin. Bull. Environ. Contam. Toxicol., 4:1–16.

Kehoe, R. A. (1961). The metabolism of lead in man in health and disease. II. The metabolism of lead under abnormal conditions. J. R. Inst. Public Health, 24:129–143.

Keil, J. S., Weston, W., III, Loadholt, C. B., Sandifer, S. H., and Colcolough, J. J. (1972). DDT and DDE residues in blood from children, South Carolina—1970. Pestic. Monit. J., 6:1–3.

Kimbrough, R. D. (1971). Review of the toxicity of hexachlorophene. Arch. Environ. Health, 23:119–122.

Knowles, J. A. (1965). Excretion of drugs in milk—a review. J. Pediatr., 66:1068–1082.

Koeffler, H. (1958). Acute E605 poisoning by percutaneous absorption of the poison. Med. Klin., 53:749–751.

Kolmodin, B., Azarnoff, D. L., and Sjoqvist, F. (1969). Effect of environmental factors on drug metabolism: decreased plasma half-life of antipyrine in workers exposed to chlorinated hydrocarbon insecticides. Clin. Pharmacol. Ther., 10:638–642.

Kolmodin-Hedman, B., Palmér, L., Götell, P., and Skerfving, S. (1973). Plasma levels of lindane, p,p'-DDE and p,p'-DDT in occupationally exposed persons in Sweden. Work. Environ. Health, 10:100–106.

Komarova, L. I. (1970). The excretion of DDT in mother's milk and its effect on the organism of mother and child. Pediatr. Akush. Ginekol., 1:19–20.

Kontek, M., Kubacki, S., Paradowski, S., and Wierzchowiecka, B. (1971). Chlorinated insecticides in human milk. Pediatr. Pol., 46:183–188.

Kroger, M. (1972). Insecticide residues in human milk. J. Pediatr., 80:401–405.

Kwalick, D. S. (1971). Anticonvulsants and DDT residues. J. A. M. A., 215:120–121.

Lange, P. F., and Terveer, J. (1954). Warfarin poisoning. Report of fourteen cases. U.S. Armed Forces Med. J., 5:872–877.

Laug, E. P., Kunze, F. M., and Prickett, C. S. (1951). Occurrence of DDT in human fat and milk. A. M. A. Arch. Ind. Hyg. Occup. Med., 3:245–246.

Laws, E. R., Jr., Curley, A., and Biros, F. J. (1967). Men with intensive occupational exposure to DDT. A clinical and chemical study. Arch. Environ. Health, 15:766–775.

Laws, E. R., Jr., Maddrey, W. C., Curley, A., and Burse,V. W. (1973). Long-term occupational exposure to DDT. Arch. Environ. Health, 27:318–321.

Lemmon, A. B. (1956). Bureau of Chemistry Annual Report for the Calendar Year 1955, Department of Agriculture, State of California. 45:128–142.

Lewi, Z. and Bar-Khayim, Y. (1964). Food-poisoning from barium carbonate. Lancet, 2:342–343.

Lidbeck, W. L., Hill, I. B., and Beeman, J. A. (1943). Acute sodium fluoride poisoning. J. A. M. A., 121:826–827.

Lindbjerg, I. F. (1960). Parathion poisoning treated with 2-PAM and complicated by subcutaneous emphysema. Ugeskr. Laeger, 122:1788–1790.

Llinares, V. M., and Wasserman, M. (1968). Storage of DDT in the body fat of the people of Spain. Unpublished data. Cited by Wasserman et al., 1968b.

Löfroth, G. (1968). Pesticides and catastrophe. New Scientist, 40:567–568.

Long, K. L., Beat, V. B., Gombart, A. K., Sheets, R. F., Hamilton, H. E., Falabella, F., Bonderman, D. P., and Choi, U. Y. (1969). The epidemiology of pesticides in a rural area. Am. Ind. Hyg. Assoc. J., 30:298–304.

Luis, P. (1952). Plasma levels and urinary excretion of three barbituric acids after oral administration to man. Acta Pharmacol., 10:147–165.

Lu, F. C., Jessup, D. C., and Lavallee, A. (1965). Toxicity of pesticides in young versus adult rats. Food Cosmet. Toxicol., 3:591–596.

McGee, L. C., Reed, H. L., and Fleming, J. P. (1952). Accidental poisoning by toxaphene. Review of toxicology and case reports. J. A. M. A., 149:1124–1126.

McLeod, A. R. (1970). An epidemiological study of pesticide poisoning in patients admitted to Charity Hospital, New Orleans. J. La. Med. Soc., 122:337–343.

Maes, R., and Heyndrickx, A. (1966). Distribution of organic chlorinated insecticides in human tissues. Meded. Rijksfac. Landb. Wetensch. Gent., 31:1021–1025.

Maier-Bode, H. (1960). DDT im Körperfett des Menschen. Med. Exp., 1:146–152.

Marquez Mayaudón, E., Fujigaki Lechuga, A., Moguel,C. A., and Aranda Reyes, B. (1968). Problemas de contaminación de alimentos con pesticidas. Caso Tijuana (1967). Salud Publica Mex., 10:293–300.

Mattson, A. M., Spillane, J. T., Baker, C., and Pearce, C. W.(1953). Determination of DDT and related substances in human fat. J. Anal. Chem., 25:1065–1070.

Maver, H., and Belamaric, T. (1961). Alimentary parathion poisoning. Arh. Hig. Rada, 12:231–233.

Merkin, S. (1954). Warning: poison in milk. Natl. Police Gaz, 159:8–9.

Meneses de Almeida, L., and Pedroso de Lima, A. (1964). A proposito da intoxicacio de uma crianca pelo parathion. O Médico, 31:306–317.

Milby, T. H., Ottoboni, F., and Mitchell, H. W. (1964). Parathion residue poisoning among orchard workers.J. A. M. A., 189:351–356.

Milby, T. H., and Samuels, A. J. (1971). Human exposure to lindane. Comparison of an exposed and unexposed population. J. Occup. Mfd., 13:256–258.

Milby, T. H., Samuels, A. J., and Ottoboni, F. (1968). Human exposure to lindane. J. Occup. Med., 10:584–587.

Morgan, D. P., and Roan, C. C. (1969). Renal function in persons occupationally exposed to pesticides. Arch. Environ. Health, 19:633–636.

Morgan, D. P., and Roan, C. C. (1970). Chlorinated hydrocarbon pesticide residue in human tissues. Arch. Environ. Health, 20:452–457.

Morton, W. (1945). Poisoning by barium carbonate. Lancet, 2:738–739.

Munch, J. C., Ginsburg, H. M., and Nixon, C. E. (1933). The thallotoxicosis outbreak in California. J. A. M. A., 100:1315–1319.

Najera, J. A., Shirdawi, G. R., Gibson, F. D., and Stafford, J. S. (1967). A large-scale field trial of malathion as an insecticide for antimalarial work in Southern Uganda. Bull. WHO, 36:913–935.

Namba, T. (1961). Oxime therapy for poisoning by alkyl-phosphate-insecticides. In: Proceedings of the 13th International Congress of Occupational Health, pp. 757–758. Book Craftsmen Associates, Inc., New York.

Nameche, J., and Bartman, J. (1964). Intoxication au parathion. Acta. Pediatr. Belg., 18:41–45.

National Academy of Sciences-National Research Council (1966). Monitoring food and people for pesticide content. Scientific Aspects of Pest Control. Publ. No. 1402, pp. 314–342.

National Center for Health Statistics (1967). Eighth Revision International Classification of Diseases, Adapted for Use in the United States, Vol. 1, Tabular List. Public Health Publ. No. 1693, US Government Printing Office, Washington, DC.

National Clearinghouse for Poison Control Centers (1969). Tabulations of 1968 reports. September–October.

National Clearinghouse for Poison Control Centers (1971). Tabulations of 1970 reports. September–October.

Neal, P. A., Sweeney, T. R., Spicer, S. S., and von Oettingen, W. F. (1946). The excretion of DDT 2,2-bis p-chlorophenyl-1,1,1-trichloroethane) in man, together with clinical observations. Public Health Rep., 61:403–409.

Newton, K. G., and Greene, N. C. (1972). Organochlorine pesticide residue levels in human milk—Victoria, Australia—1970. Pestic. Monit. J., 6:4–8.

New York State Department of Labor (1961). Work injuries in New York State agriculture; characteristics of accidents and workmen's compensation coverage and permium rates. Division of Research and Statistics, Publ. No. B–123.

New York State Department of Labor (1969). Work injuries in New York State agriculture. Division of Research and Statistics, Publ. No. B–173.

Nouhen-Lang, M. (1964). Vergiftungsunfälle im Kindesalter. Ann. Paediatr., 202:379–397.

Older, J. J., and Hatcher, R. L. (1969). Food poisoning caused by carbophenothion. J. A. M. A., 209:1328–1330.

O'Leary, J. A., Davies, J. E., Edmundson, W. F., and Feldman, M. (1970a). Correlation of prematurity and DDE levels in fetal whole blood. Am. J. Obstet. Gynecol., 106:939.

O'Leary, J. A., Davies, J. E., Edmundson, W. F., and Reich, G. A. (1970b). Transplacental passage of pesticides. J. Obstet. Gynecol., 107:65–68.

O'Leary, J. A., Davies, J. E., and Feldman, M. (1970c). Spontaneous abortion and human pesticide residues of DDT and DDE. Am. J. Obstet. Gynecol., 108:1291–1292.

Olszyna-Marzys, A. E. (1973). Personal communication.

Olszyna-Marzys, A. E., de Campos, M., Farvar, M. T., Thomas, M. (1973). Residuos de plaguicidas clorados en la leche humana en Guatemala. Bol. Of. Sanit. Panam., 74:93–107.

Ordóñez, J. V., Carrillo, J. A., Miranda, M., and Gale, J. L. (1966). Estudio epidemiologico de una enfermedad considerada como encefalitis en la region de los altos de Guatemala. Bol. Of. Sanit. Panam., 55:510–517.

Ortelee, M. F. (1958). Study of men with prolonged intensive occupational exposure to DDT. A. M. A. Arch. Ind. Health, 18:433–440.

Paccagnella, B., Prati, L., and Cavazzini, G. (1967). Insetticidi cloroderovat; organici nel tessuto adiposo di persone resident: nella provincia di Ferrara. Nuovi Ann. Ig. Microbiol., 18:17–26.

Paul, A. H. (1959). Dieldrin poisoning. Report of a case. N. Z. Med. J., 58:393–396.

Perron, R. C., and Barrentine, B. F. (1970). Human serum DDT concentration related to environmental DDT exposure. Arch. Environ. Health, 20:368–376.

Phelan, P. D. (1963). Accidental poisoning in childhood. Med. J. Aust., 2:656–658.

Pierce, P. E., Thompson, J. F., Likoksky, W. H., Nickey, L. N., Barthel, W. F., Hinman, A. R. (1972). Alkyl mercury poisoning in humans: Report of an outbreak. J. A. M. A., 220:1439–1442.

Pilat, L., Moscovici, B., and Georgescu, A. M. (1961). Parathion poisoning (clinical observations). Med. Interna. (Bucur.), 13:1567–1573.

Planet, N. (1950). Envenenamentos produzidos pelos insecticidas fosforados em operarios rurais empregados no combate as pragas do algodao (nota previa). Rev. Paul. Med., 37:83–84.

Pleština, R. (1968). Prilog poznavanju toksičnih svojstava o-izopropoksifenilmetilkarbamata. Zagreb (M.Sc. Thesis).

Poland, A., Smith, D., Kuntzman, R., Jacobson, M., and Conney, A. H. (1970). Effect of intensive occupational exposure to DDT on phenylbutazone and cortisol metabolism in human subjects. Clin. Pharmacol. Ther., 11:724–732.

Polishuk, Z. W., Wassermann, M., Wassermann, D., Groner, Y., Lazarovici, S., and Tomatis, L. (1970). Effects of pregnancy on storage of organochlorine insecticides. Arch. Environ. Health, 20:215–217.

Price, H. A., and Welch, R. L. (1972). Occurrence of polychlorinated biphenyls in humans. Environ. Health Perspect., 1:73–78.

Princi, F. (1954). Toxicity of the chlorinated hydrocarbon insecticides. In: Atti dell'xi Cong. Int. Med. Labor., pp. 253–272. Napoli.

Prinz, H. J. (1969). A severe percutaneous poisoning with parathion (E 605ᵉ). Arch. Toxikol., 25:318–328.

Przyborowski, T., Rychard, J., and Tyrakowski, M. (1962). Mass poisoning on a ship caused by the insecticide dieldrin. Bull. Inst. Mar. Med. Gdansk, 13:185–188.

Quaife, M. L., Winbush, J. S., and Fitzhugh, O. G. (1967). Survey of quantitative relationships between ingestion and storage of aldrin and dieldrin in animals and man. Food Cosmet. Toxicol., 5:39–50.

Quinby, G. E., Armstrong, J. F., and Durham, W. F. (1965b). DDT in human milk. Nature, 207: 726–728.

Quinby, G. E., Hayes, W. J., Jr., Armstrong, J. F., and Durham, W. F. (1965a). DDT storage in the US population. J. A. M. A., 191:175–179.

Quinby, G. E., and Lemmon, A. B. (1958). Parathion residues as a cause of poisoning in crop workers. J. A. M. A., 166:740–746.

Quinby, G. E., Walker, K. C., and Durham, W. F. (1958). Public health hazards involved in the use of organic phosphorus insecticides in cotton culture in the Delta area of Mississippi. J. Econ. Entomol., 51:831–838.

Radomski, J. L., Astolfi, E., Deichmann, W. B., and Rey, A. A. (1971). Blood levels of organochlorine pesticides in Argentina: occupationally and nonoccupationally exposed adults, children, and newborn infants. Toxicol. Appl. Pharmacol., 20:186–193.

Radomski, J. L., Deichmann, W. B., and Clizer, E. E. (1968). Pesticide concentrations in the liver, brain, and adipose tissue of terminal hospital patients. Food Cosmet. Toxicol., 6:209–220.

Radomski, J. L., Deichman, W. B., Rey, A. A., and Merkin, T. (1971). Human pesticide blood levels as a measure of body burden and pesticide exposure. Toxicol. Appl. Pharmacol., 20:175–185.

Radomski, J. L., and Fiserova-Bergerova, V. (1965). The determination of pesticides in tissues with the electron capture detector without prior clean-up. Ind. Med. Surg., 34:934–939.

Rappolt, R. T. (1970). Kern County pesticide study. Ind.

Med. Surg., 39:351–355.

Rayner, M. D., Popper, J. S., Carvalho, E. W., and Hurov, R. (1972). Hyporeflexia in workers chronically exposed to organophosphate insecticides. Res. Commun. Chem. Pathol. Pharmacol., 4:595–606.

Read, S. T., and McKinley, W. P. (1961). DDT and DDE content of human fat. A survey. Arch. Environ. Health, 3:209–211.

Reich, G. A., and Berner, W. H. (1968). Aerial application accidents 1963 to 1966. Arch. Environ. Health, 17:776–784.

Reich, G. A., Davis, J. H., and Davies, J. E. (1968b). Pesticide poisoning in South Florida. Arch. Environ. Health, 17:768–775.

Reich, G. A., Gallaher, G. L., Wiseman, J. S. (1968a). Characteristics of pesticide poisoning in South Texas. Tex. Med. 64:1–3.

Ritcey, W. R., Savary, G., and McCully, J. A. (1972). Organochlorine insecticide residues in human milk, evaporated milk, and some milk substitutes in Canada. Can. J. Public Health, 63:125–132.

Roberts, D. V., and Wilson, A. (1969). Electromyography in diagnosis and treatment. In: Myasthenia Gravis, edited by R. Greene, pp. 29–42. Heinemann, London.

Robinson, J. (1963). The determination of dieldrin in the blood by gas liquid chromatography. Presented at the 3rd International Meeting in Forensic Immunology, Medicine, Pathology, and Toxicology. London, April 16–24.

Robinson, J., and Hunter, C. G. (1966). Organochlorine insecticides: concentrations in human blood and adipose tissue. Arch. Environ. Health, 13:558–563.

Robinson, J., and McGill, A. E. J. (1965). Organochlorine insecticide residues in complete prepared meals in Great Britain during 1965. Nature, 212:1037–1038.

Robinson, J., and Roberts, M. (1969). Estimation of the exposure of the general population to dieldrin (HEOD). Food Cosmet. Toxicol., 7:501–514.

Robinson, J., Richardson, A., Hunter, C. G., Crabtree, A. N., and Rees, H. J. (1965). Organo-chlorine insecticide content of human adipose tissue in Southeastern England. Br. J. Ind. Med., 22:220–229.

Robson, A. M., Kissane, J. M., Elvick, H. N., and Pundavela, L. (1969). Pentachlorophenol poisoning in a nursery for newborn infants. I. Clinical features and treatment. J. Pediatr., 75:309–316.

Rosen, F. S. (1960). Toxic hazards, parathion. N. Engl. J. Med., 262:1243–1244.

Sandifer, S. H., and Keil, J. E. (1972). Pesticide exposure: association with cardiovascular risk factors. In: Trace Substance in Environmental Health, edited by D. D. Hemphill, pp. 329–334. University of Missouri, Columbia, Missouri.

Sandifer, S. H., Keil, J. E., Finklea, J. F., and Gadsden, R. H. (1972). Pesticide effects on occupationally exposed workers: a summary of four years observation of industry and farm volunteers in South Carolina. Ind. Med., 41:7–12.

Santolucito, J. A., and Whitcomb, E. (1971). Mechanical response of skeletal muscle following oral administration of pesticides. Toxicol. Appl. Pharmacol., 20:66–72.

Schafer, M. L., and Campbell, J. E. (1966). Distribution of Pesticide Residues in Human Body Tissues from Montgomery County, Ohio. Adv. Chem. Ser. 60, pp. 89–98, American Chemical Society, Washington, DC.

Schmid, R. (1960). Cutaneous porphyria in Turkey. N. Engl. J. Med., 263:397–398.

Schoor, W. P. (1970). Effect of anticonvulsant drugs on insecticide residues. Lancet, 2:520–521.

Scott, A. E. (1954). Health foods doorway to death. Sir 11:44–45, 62–64.

Selby, L. A., Newell, K. W., Hauser, G. A., and Junker, J. (1969b). Comparison of chlorinated hydrocarbon pesticides in maternal blood and placental tissues. Environ. Res., 2:247–255.

Selby, L. A., Newell, K. W., Waggenspack, C., Hauser, G. A., and Junker, G. (1969a). Estimating pesticide exposure in man as related to measurable intake; environmental versus chemical index. Am. J. Epidemiol., 89:241–253.

Shafik, M. T., and Enos, H. F. (1969). Determination of metabolic and hydrolytic products of organophosphorus pesticide chemicals in human blood and urine. J. Agric. Food Chem., 17:1186–1189.

Shustov, V. I. A., and Tsyganova, S. I. (1970). Clinical aspects of sub-acute intoxication with Granosan. Kazan. Med. Zh., 2:78–79.

Simmons, S. W. (1959). The use of DDT insecticides in human medicine. In: *DDT, The Insecticide Dichlorodiphenyltrichloroethane and Its Significance*, edited by P. Müller, Vol. 2, pp. 251–502. Birkhäuser Verlag, Basel.

Simmons, S. W. (1968). The pesticides program activities of the Public Health Service. Public Health Rep., 83:967–974.

Snyder, R. D. (1971). Congenital mercury poisoning. N. Engl. J. Med., 284:1014–1016.

Spiotta, E. J. (1951). Aldrin poisoning in man. Arch. Ind. Hyg. Occup. Med. 4:560–566.

Starr, H. G., Jr., and Clifford, N. J. (1971). Absorption of pesticides in a chronic skin disease. Arch. Environ. Health, 22:396–400.

Strickland, A. H. (1965). Amounts of organochlorine insecticides used annually on agricultural, and some horticultural crops in England and Wales. Ann. Appl. Biol., 55:319–343.

Sumerford, W. T., Hayes, W. J., Jr., Johnston, J. M., Walker, K., and Spillane, J. (1953). Cholinesterase response and symptomatology from exposure to organic phosphorus insecticides. A. M. A. Arch. Ind. Hyg. Occup. Med., 7:383–398.

Thompson, R. P. H., Pilcher, C. W. T., Robinson, J., Stathers, G. M., McLean, A. E. M., and Williams, R. (1969). Treatment of unconjugated jaundice with dicophane. Lancet, 2:4–6.

Tocci, P. M., Mann, J. B., Davies, J. E., and Edmundson, W. F. (1969). Biochemical differences found in persons chronically exposed to high levels of pesticides. Ind. Med., 38:188–195.

Toivonen, T., Ohela, K., and Kaipainen, W. J. (1959). Parathion poisoning increasing frequency in Finland. Lancet, 2:175–176.

Tuinstra, L. G. M. T. (1971). Organochlorine insecticide residues in human milk in the Leiden Region. Ned. Melk-Zuiveltijdschr., 25:24–32.

Unterman, H. W., and Sirghie, E. (1969). Impregarea organismului uman cu organoclorate. Igiena, 18:221–226.

US Public Health Service (See appropriate years). *Vital Statistics of the United States.* US Government Printing Office, Washington, DC.

Vandekar, M. (1965). Observations on the toxicity of carbaryl, folithion and 3-isopropylphenyl N-methylcarbamate in a village-scale trial in Southern Nigeria. Bull. WHO, 33:107–115.

Vandekar, M., Hedayat, S., Plestina, R., and Ahmady, G. (1968). Study of the safety of o-isoproproxyphenyl-methylcarbamate in an operational field trial in Iran. Bull. WHO, 38:609–623.

Verhulst, H. L., and Crotty, J. J. (1964). *Poisoning Report Data for Children Under 5 Years of Age*, pp. 1–9. National Clearinghouse for Poison Control Centers, September–October.

Volkov, M. V. (1973). Accidents in the social context: their prevention and treatment as a social and medical problem. WHO Chron., 27:290–300.

Walker, K. C., Goette, M. B., and Batchelor, G. S. (1954). Pesticide residues in foods. Dichlorodiphenyltrichloroethane and dichlorodiphenyldichloroethylene content of prepared meals. J. Agric. Food Chem., 2:1034–1037.

Warnick, S. L. (1972). Organochlorine pesticide levels in human serum and adipose tissue, Utah—fiscal years 1967–71. Pestic. Monit. J., 6:9–13.

Warnick, S. L., and Carter, J. E. (1972). Some findings in a study of workers occupationally exposed to pesticides. Arch. Environ. Health, 25:265–270.

Warren, M. C., Conrad, J. P., Jr., Bocian, J. J., and Hayes, M. (1963). Clothing-borne epidemic. Organic phosphate poisoning in children. J. A. M. A., 184:266–268.

Wassermann, M., Curnow, D. H., Forte, P. N., and Groner, Y. (1968a). Storage of organochlorine pesticide in the body fat of people in Western Australia. Ind. Med. Surg., 37:295–300.

Wassermann, M., Gon, M., Wassermann, D., and Zellermayer, L. (1965). DDT and DDE in the body fat of people in Israel. Arch. Environ. Health, 11:375–379.

Wassermann, M., Sofoluwe, G. I., Wassermann, D., Groner, Y., and Lazarovitch, S. (1968b). Storage of organochlorine insecticides in the body fat of people in Nigeria. Proceedings of the Lagos International Seminar on Occupational Health for Developing Countries, Lagos, Nigeria, April 1–6.

Wassermann, M., Wassermann, D., Lazarovici, S., Coetzee, A. M., and Tomatis, L. (1970). Present state of the organochlorine insecticides in the general populations of South Africa. S. Afr. Med. J., 44:646–648.

Wassermann, M., Wassermann, D., Zellermayer, L., and Gon, M. (1967). Pesticides in people. Storage of DDT in the people of Israel. Pestic. Monit. J., 1:15–20.

Watson, M., Benson, W. W., and Gabica, J. (1970). Serum organochlorine pesticide levels in people in Southern Idaho. Pestic. Monit. J., 4:47–50.

Watson, M., Gabica, J., and Benson, W. W. (1972). Serum organochlorine pesticides in mentally retarded patients on differing drug regimens. Clin. Pharmacol. Ther., 13:186–192.

Weeks, D. E. (1967). Endrin food-poisoning. A report of four outbreaks caused by two separate shipments of endrin-contaminated flour. Bull. WHO, 37:499–512.

Wehrle, P. F., Day, P. A., Whalen, J. P., Fitzgerald, J. W., and Harris, V. G. (1960). The epidemiology of accidental poisoning in an urban population. II. Prevalence and distribution of poisoning. Am. J. Public Health, 50:1925–1933.

Weihe, M. (1966). Chlorinated insecticides in the body fat of people in Denmark. Ugeskr. Laeger., 128:881–882.

West, I. (1964). Pesticides as contaminants. Arch. Environ. Health, 9:626–631.

West, I. (1965). Public health problems are created by pesticides. Calif. Health, July, pp. 11–18.

West, I. (1967). Lindane and hematologic reactions. Arch. Environ. Health, 15:97–101.

Westöö, G., Noren, K., and Andersson, M. (1970). Levels of organochlorine pesticides and polychlorinated biphenyls in margarine, vegetable oils, and some foods of animal origin on the Swedish market in 1967–1969. Var föda, 22:9–31.

Widmark, G. J. (1967). Organochlorine pesticide residue analysis: possible interference by chlorinated biphenyls. J. Assoc. Off. Anal. Chem., 50:1069.

Wilson, D. J., Locker, D. J., Ritzen, C. A., Watson, J. T., and Schaffner, W. (1973). DDT concentrations in human milk. Am. J. Dis. Child., 125:814–817.

Wishahi, A., Aboul-Dahab, Y. W., Sherif, Y., and El-Darawy, Z. (1958). Parathion poisoning (phosphorus compound). A report on 22 children in an outbreak. Arch. Pediatr., 75:387–396.

Wislicki, L. (1961). Accidental poisoning in Israel. Isr. Med. J., 20:299–303.

Wit, S. L. (1964). Aspects of toxicology and chemical analysis of insecticide residues. Voeding, 25:609–628.

Wolfe, H. R., Durham, W. F., and Armstrong, J. F. (1970). Urinary excretion of insecticide metabolites. Arch. Environ. Health, 21:711–716.

World Health Organization, Expert Committee on Insecticides. (1967). Safe use of pesticides in public health.

WHO Tech. Rep. Ser. No. 356.

World Health Organization (1968). Evaluation of insecticides for vector control. Part I. WHO/VEC/68.66, p. 110.

World Health Organization (1969). Twenty-second World Health Assembly-1. WHO Chron., 23:389–493.

World Health Organization (1971). The place of DDT in operations against malaria and other vector-borne diseases. Official Records of WHO, No. 190, Geneva.

Wray, J. D., Müftü, Y., and Döğramaci. I. (1962). Hexachlorobenzene as a cause of porphyria turcica. Turk. J. Pediatr., 4:132–137.

Wright, J. W., Fritz, R. F., Hocking, K. S., Babione, R., Gratz, N. G., Pal, R., Stiles, A. R., and Vandekar, M. (1969). Ortho-isopropoxyphenyl methylcarbamate (OMS–33) as a residual spray for control of anopheline mosquitos. Bull. WHO, 40:67–90.

Wyllie, J., Gabica, J., and Benson, W. W. (1972). Comparative organochlorine pesticide residues in serum and biopsied lipoid tissue: a survey of 200 persons in Southern Idaho—1970. Pestic. Monit. J., 6:84–88.

Yobs, A. (1969) Personal communication.

Yobs, A. (1972). Levels of polychlorinated biphenyls in adipose tissue of the general population of the nation. Environ. Health Perspect., 1:79–81.

Zavon, M. R., Hine, C. H., and Parker, K. D. (1965). Chlorinated hydrocarbon insecticides in human body fat in the United States. J. A. M. A., 193:837–839.

Zavon, M. R., Tye, R., and Latorre, L. (1969). Chlorinated hydrocarbon insecticide content of the neonate. Ann. NY Acad. Sci., 160:196–200.

Zeman, A., Wolfram, G., and Zollner, N. (1971). Über das vorkommen von hexachlorbenzol im menschlichen serum. Naturwissenschaften, 58:276.

8

DIAGNOSIS AND TREATMENT OF POISONING

8.1 Diagnosis

The main reason for missing the diagnosis of poisoning by a particular compound is failure to consider the possibility of poisoning of any kind. The main reason for making the diagnosis of poisoning incorrectly is failure to require positive evidence. Every physician should have a high index of suspicion that a chemical may be the cause of any illness not otherwise fully explained. On the other hand, both the patient and the physician will be better off if the illness is treated symptomatically and a diagnosis is announced only after it has been proved. The recommendation of symptomatic treatment is not meant to exclude the prudent use of certain antidotes. Some of them are both safe and effective enough to be regarded as diagnostic agents. For example, atropine may be used symptomatically, but favorable response to it and tolerance for relatively large repeated doses of it are, in themselves, evidence for poisoning by an anticholinesterase compound. Marked improvement following a single dose of 2-PAM is diagnostic of poisoning by an organic phosphorus compound.

The problem of misdiagnosis is more serious than one might suppose. About 10% of all deaths in the United States during 1961 diagnosed as poisoning by pesticides probably had some other cause (Hayes and Pirkle, 1966). Not only could no proof be found that pesticides were involved in these cases, but there was proof ranging from circumstantial to final

that a completely different etiology was involved. In most instances, the mistake apparently depended on the physician's too ready acceptance of an easy but entirely unproved diagnosis. In some instances, it was clear the physician had accepted uncritically the patient's self-diagnosis. In at least one instance, a claim had been made for compensation based on the incorrect diagnosis.

How, then, is a correct diagnosis to be reached? First, by viewing every unexplained illness as a possible example of poisoning. Second, by seeking evidence of adequate dosage, consistent clinical findings, and analytical proof before making a final decision.

8.1.1 Chemical Epidemiology

In most cases of poisoning, the facts are all too evident. If recognized exposure is followed by illness typical of poisoning, establishment of the diagnosis usually is only a matter of orderly documentation.

However, in some instances the real cause of illness is not evident. Even though poisoning is suspected, there may be no clear proof. In these situations an epidemiological study is indicated. Even a single case of unexplained illness may constitute an epidemic, which is simply an unusual incidence of disease. Of course, the occurrence of multiple, similar cases during a relatively brief period increases the certainty that one is dealing with an unusual situation and has not merely failed to recognize what should have been an obvious explanation of a single case.

The only essential difference between the epidemiology of infection and intoxication is that infectious agents reproduce, but toxicants do not. The phenomenon of dosage is relatively unimportant in relation to infectious disease, simply because the harmful organisms do multiply. Several infectious diseases have been transmitted, at least in animals, by a single microorganism. Administering a larger number of organisms may increase the incidence of infection, hasten the onset, and even increase the severity, but it will rarely if ever change the basic character of illness. Furthermore, many kinds of infection may spread from a single case to many members of the susceptible population.

By contrast, dosage is of paramount importance in poisoning. A certain minimal dose of even the most toxic material is required to injure a particular subject, and the degree of injury is proportional to the dosage. The existence of a case of poisoning does not, in itself, influence the occurrence of any other case. For poisoning, there is no such thing as a secondary case in the sense used in infectious disease. So-called "secondary poisoning" in animals and rarely in man usually is the result of eating a poisoned animal. It depends on essentially mechanical dispersion of the toxicant and involves no increase whatever in its quantity.

The importance of dosage often is evident in the course of an individual case. It often happens that patients who have been poisoned through continuous or repeated exposure will begin to recover soon after they are removed from exposure. Any such time relationship is exceptional in connection with infectious disease, where clinical progress usually is independent of further exposure, once infection has occurred.

A secondary difference between the epidemiology of infection and intoxication depends on the relative importance of immunity in the two processes. Recovery from many infections leads to immunity. Some infections produce imperfect immunity, but some degree of protection is the rule, and complete protection under practical conditions is frequent. By contrast, acquired tolerance to chemicals is the exception. Of course, tolerance to certain chemicals such as nicotine and morphine is well known. However, even in these instances, the degree of protection is relatively small. Thus, the entire population is susceptible to any poison; the minor, individual differences that exist can be overcome easily by differences in dosage. Only a portion of the population is really susceptible to many infections; the immunity of others cannot be overcome under practical conditions.

It follows that no case of poisoning is explained fully until the source of poison is found. This is true even when a diagnosis is reached by chemical analysis of the tissues of a person found dead. The case remains something of a mystery until it can be determined how the dose was acquired. Except for certain exotic infections, firm proof that a person is affected leaves no mystery, because the disease is known to be constantly present in the community.

Ordinarily, deficiency, metabolic, and genetic diseases need not be confused with poisoning because their onset is usually gradual, and they rarely have any special association with a particular occupation or other source of environmental exposure. There are exceptions, notably acute intermittent porphyria, which is characterized by sudden onset, often triggered by absorption of a small amount of drug or other chemical that would be harmless to a normal person. The signs and symptoms are not dictated in this instance by the particular chemical, but by the underlying defect. This exception serves to emphasize the importance of establishing the dosage as well as the identity of any compound that seems to have initiated an illness.

Until poisoning is proved, it must be regarded as merely one of several hypotheses. Illnesses reasonably assumed to be infectious or metabolic have been found to be toxic and *vice versa*. For example, widely separated outbreaks of a neurological disorder, for which an infectious origin was considered seriously at first, eventually were shown to be caused by triorthocresylphosphate (Harris, 1930; Smith and Spalding, 1959). An outbreak of febrile illness in a nursery for newborns that resembled infection and initially was treated as such was shown to be caused by poisoning from pentachlorophenol (Smith *et al.*, 1967; Robson *et al.*, 1969). Conversely, it required years of study to show that kuru is not an intoxication or a metabolic disorder of genetic origin, but the result of infection (Gajdusek *et al.*, 1966; 1967). The final accounts of outbreaks tend to neglect early hypotheses, no matter how reasonable they were in the light of information available at the time. Thus, the final accounts disguise the genuine diffculty of such epidemiological studes.

No matter what the type of disease, the epidemiological study should be much the same. Toxins as well as infections may be carried by food, water, or air. The exact time and place of onset of each case, and the age, sex, dwelling place, occupation, food and beverage intake, and clinical course of each victim should be recorded. All of this information may reveal a pattern offering a clue to the source of the injury.

During the entire course of such an epidemiological study, consideration of poisoning means search for a source of poison, and eventually demonstration of a dosage-response relationship. Some details of this search and demonstration are discussed in Sections 8.1.2, 8.1.3, and 8.1.4. However, before going on to these matters, it is necessary to discuss retrospective and prospective studies.

8.1.1.1 Retrospective Study.

What has just been said was concerned almost entirely with retrospective study; that is, study made by looking back over information already available but usually not previously assembled for the purpose. Such study may be instituted because of one or more cases of illness and with the aim of placing them in epidemiological perspective. Retrospective study also may be made in the absence of any recognized illness. The work attendance and clinical records of workers may be reviewed systematically to learn whether the introduction of a new compound or process has produced a change in their health. Depending on circumstances, official vital statistics, hospital records, school attendance records, and medical examination of selected groups may be used to explore the possibility that some new factor (for example, the introduction of a pesticide in agriculture) had produced a change in the health of the general population (for example, the population of a farming community). Thus, some retrospective studies seek the epidemiological background of recognized illness, while others seek to use epidemiological principles to learn whether illness—or some other change of specific etiology—has occurred.

Any thoroughly investigated case history is a retrospective epidemiological study. A good example of a more complex, almost exclusively retrospective study is that of Fowler (1953), who reviewed mortality records, hospital admissions, and school attendance records for equal periods before and after the introduction of modern pesticides, and who conducted health surveys of exposed and unexposed persons in order to learn whether pesticides cause chronic illness or contribute to diseases of other etiology.

Retrospective study suffers from weaknesses that are unlikely to be important in connection with recently introduced kinds of illness or events that are obviously distinct from others affecting the same group of people. On the other hand, if a kind of illness is known to have been present before the factor under study was introduced, or if the illness is difficult to distinguish from those to which the group is subject, it may be hard to prove retrospectively that introduction of the factor altered the frequency of the disease; the observed change may have another cause.

8.1.1.2 Prospective Study.

A prospective study is simply one based on events that occur after the study is planned and set in motion. Like the retrospective study, the prospective one may be concerned with recognized illness, or it may attempt only to establish whether a selected factor changes the frequency of a specific illness or other event.

The prospective study is based on a hypothesis. If the study involves recognized illness, the hypothesis usually will have been the result of a more or less formal and complete retrospective study. If no specific change is recognized, the hypothesis simply may be that the exposure, age, sex, and other circumstances of one group (called a "cohort" by epidemiologists) make them different from another group. Whether the prospective study involves recognized illness or merely exploration, groups of people and kinds of tests will be selected that can be expected to prove or disprove the hypothesis.

The presence of a clear plan often makes it possible to collect more accurate data. Each subject will be more likely to recall his symptoms if he knows that he will be questioned about them at regular intervals, rather than if he is asked out of the blue to recall how he has felt for the last 6 months. Partly because of the accuracy of data, the opportunity to identify a real but subtle change may be increased.

A good example of a prospective study lasting only one season is that of Ganelin *et al.* (1964), in which they found that the effect of incidental or environmental exposure to parathion was negligible among the general population, including those who had asthma. A very large investigation of the potential effects of pesticides that continues year after year is the Community Studies initiated by the US Public Health Service and continued by the Environmental Protection Agency (see Section 7.1.2.5).

Disadvantages of prospective studies include their often longer duration and their inflexibility. It is possible to scan 30 years of recorded vital statistics in a few hours, but to make a prospective study of 30 years requires the entire period. Prolongation of study may be associated with a corresponding increase in expense. Perhaps more important is the inflexibility of prospective studies. There are examples of single or successive retrospective studies that started with the hypothesis that the cause of illness was infection but eventually proved it was intoxication and *vice versa,* as discussed above. Prospective studies are so highly structured that it is unlikely one designed to investigate infection will gather data on toxicity, or the reverse.

8.1.2 History of Exposure

If contact with a particular chemical is virtually part of the patient's chief complaint, there is usually little difficulty in establishing a satisfactory history of exposure. The container and remaining chemical should be obtained. If the material is still in the original package, the label almost always will provide information regarding identity. However, as a precaution, a sample should be submitted to the laboratory to confirm that the nature and concentration of the contents are the same as represented by the label. Examples of mislabeling are rare, but have occurred. A further reason for saving a sample of the formulation for analysis is that solvents generally are not identified on the label but may be important in poisoning.

An effort should be made to learn whether contact with the chemical is certain or is merely suspected. The route or routes of exposure should be learned. If possible, the actual dosage should be determined by history and later investigated independently by laboratory means. Both history and laboratory examination may help in learning the type, duration, and frequency of exposure and the period from last exposure to onset. Not only is the most recent exposure important, but all preceding known instances should be listed.

If contact with a particular chemical is not part of the initial history but some other feature of the illness suggests poisoning, then a search must be made for the material that may be responsible. Depending on circumstances, the search may really be for a source of poison rather than for the compound itself. For example, in many instances of poisoning by carbon monoxide, little or none of the gas remains even at the time the victim is discovered, much less at the time the toxicologist reaches the scene. Under these conditions it is necessary to demonstrate how carbon monoxide could have been formed. Frequently it will be discovered that the room in which the victim was found was poorly ventilated and

provided with a defective heater. The matter of proving that carbon monoxide was present and was absorbed is not really different from the problem of proving that any other compound was absorbed. There should always be a double check on the history of exposure by means of suitable laboratory analyses of tissues or excreta.

Although it is usually simple to identify the compound leading to accidental poisoning, the task can sometimes be extremely difficult. The mere finding of a poison in the patient's environment can be misleading rather than helpful. This may be especially true when the patient or his representatives are mistaken but, nonetheless, certain about the relationship between a chemical and an illness. This is one kind of situation leading to false claims for compensation, and it is one of the most difficult problems faced by the clinical toxicologist. However, mistakes about the etiology are not confined to situations in which compensation may be a factor. For example, in an episode in which babies were poisoned by pentachlorophenol, the epidemiological investigation led first to a disinfectant composed of a mixture of other substituted phenols. The mistake was not suspected until an additional case occurred after use of the disinfectant was omitted completely. Further checking revealed the previously unsuspected and prohibited use of pentachlorophenol in the last rinse during laundering of the babies' diapers and other linens. Chemical analyses of blood and other tissues eventually not only proved that pentachlorophenol was responsible, but excluded any contribution from the other phenols (Armstrong *et al.,* 1969).

8.1.3 Clinical Findings

It must be emphasized that the effects of chemicals are predictable. The variation in symptomatology among individual cases of poisoning by a particular chemical is no greater than the variation observed among the same number of cases of a specific infection. Of course, both kinds of illness may show an entire spectrum of severity, ranging from subclinical to fatal. In the case of intoxication, dosage is the preponderant factor in determining the severity of illness. The nature of the chemical is more important in determining the interval from exposure to onset, the systems involved, the characteristic signs and symptoms, the duration of illness, and the likelihood that there will be any sequelae. This does not mean, of course, that all cases caused by the same compound exhibit exactly the same signs and symptoms. It does mean that practically all cases exhibit a sufficient number of the same signs and symptoms arranged in a characteristic pattern or syndrome to permit a diagnosis specific for the chemical group, if not for the individual compound.

The more the clinical course of a particular case differs from the picture previously observed in confirmed cases of poisoning by the same compound, the more cautious the physician must be in reaching this diagnosis.

It is entirely unreasonable to expect the average physician to be familiar with the clinical pictures of poisoning induced by the wide range of pesticides now available. It is even less reasonable to expect him to be familiar with the clinical pictures produced by a far wider range of industrial chemicals, drugs, and toxic plants. However, since the physician encounters occasional cases of poisoning, some solution of the problem is needed. Books on symptom diagnosis may constitute a partial solution. Several books (Yater and Oliver, 1961; MacBryde, 1964) devoted exclusively to this subject are available. In addition, von Oettingen (1958) and Moeschlin (1965) have supplied detailed lists of signs, symptoms, and laboratory findings encountered in cases of poisoning by different compounds. No such list is attempted in this book, because it seems too likely that its use would prove misleading in connection with a restricted group of compounds such as pesticides. After all, lists of symptoms are generally consulted only when the diagnosis is completely in doubt and the physician is searching for possibilities to consider. If the diagnosis is apparently clear, but the clinical picture presents one or more features that may present a problem, the best procedure is to consult a description of the toxicology of the compound in question. For example, if the diagnosis appears to involve carbon monoxde, but the physician is in doubt whether this compound could explain the presence of fever observed in his patient, he has only to read in order to learn that poisoning by carbon monoxide can, in fact, cause fever.

If physicians are in doubt about diagnosis and wish to use lists of symptoms, it is suggested that they begin with the more general lists just cited, and continue if necessary with the lists provided by von Oettingen and by Moeschlin. It will seldom occur that one has no specific lead and, at the same time, has dependable evidence restricting the diagnosis to poisoning by a pesticide.

The possibility of doubt makes it especially important that the physical examination be done with particular care and recorded in detail. A careful neurological examination is essential because the syndromes associated with many pesticides are predominantly neurological. Signs that are seen infrequently in ordinary practice ought to be described in full and not merely referred to by name. Confusion has arisen when a physician used a technical term (eg, fasciculation) in a general or literary sense, rather than in its restricted medical definition. Confusion (and embarrassment) can be avoided by writing down just what was seen, felt, heard, and smelled. Wherever possible, the examination ought to be quantitative. For example, in recording the results of the Romberg test, state how well and for how many seconds the patient can maintain his balance on one foot after he has shut his eyes.

8.1.4 Laboratory Findings

Proof of diagnosis usually is established by analysis of the poison or one or more of its metabolites. In a few instances, diagnosis can be established by measuring a change in an enzyme or some other parameter known to undergo specific change in response to the poison. In addition, there is a wide range of laboratory tests that might be called supportive because they may throw light on the patient's condition and help greatly in guiding his treatment.

Of course, the physician will perform only those tests and administer only those treatments that he believes are indicated. On the other hand, to learn more about poisoning and treatment, it is desirable to collect comparable data from a number of patients.

Tests that are abnormal should be rechecked to rule out laboratory error. Confirmed abnormalities should be studied in detail. Reports of all tests should include a statement of the method and of the normal range for that test in the laboratory where it was made.

8.1.4.1 Diagnostic Tests.

Tests for Toxicants or Their Metabolites. The concentrations of some pesticides or their metabolites found in the general population, in workers, in patients, and in persons killed by the compounds are summarized in Tables 8-1, 8-2, and 8-3. It may be seen from these tables that a number of pesticides and some other materials commonly are found in people with no special exposure to them. It sometimes happens that people with potential occupational exposure to these materials have no more of them or their metabolites in their tissues than do some people in the general population. The reason is two-fold. First, some of the values reported for the general popula-

Table 8-1

Storage of Selected Materials in the Body Fat or in Certain Specified Organs[a] of the General
Population of the United States of America, of Exposed Workers, and of Patients
who Survived Poisoning or Failed to Do So

Compound	General population[b] (ppm)	Workers (ppm)	Patients (ppm)	Dead (ppm)
DDT	0.09 - 48.8	18.12 - 283.83[c]		19 - 36 (H,K,L)[a,d]
DDE	0.48 - 97.9	16.48 - 319.32[c]		
total DDT	0.49 - 110.45	38.45 - 646.63[c]		
BHC	N.D.[e] (<0.03)			343; 89 (L)[f]
dieldrin	0.002 - 4.62	0.60 - 31.96[g]	48[h]	
aldrin	N.D.[e] (<0.01)	N.D.[e] (<0.01)[g]	45 as dieldrin[h]	
endrin	N.D.[e] (<0.03)	N.D.[e] (<0.03)[g]		0.6 - 0.7 (K,B); 7.2 (L)[h]; 0.11 - 0.69 (K,L)[h]
heptachlor epoxide	0.02 - 1.82			
toxaphene	N.D.[e] (<0.03)			78.0 (L)[h]
chlordane			3.5[i]	
2,4,5-T				8 - 109 (K,L,B,H)[h]
hexachlorobenzene	1.25 - 6.3			

a. H = heart; L = liver; K = kidney; B = brain.
b. Values in this column indicate the ranges reported in papers listed in Tables 7-10, 7-14, and 7-21.
c. Laws et al., 1967.
d. Luis, 1952
e. Searched for but not detected. (The sensitivity is shown in parentheses. Because of the sample size, the limit is not always the same even for the same compound.)
f. Joslin et al., 1960.
g. Hayes and Curley, 1968.
h. Unpublished result.
i. Haun and Cueto, 1967.
j. Curley and Garrettson, 1969.

tion may not be representative. This is especially true of the larger surveys where it has not been possible to obtain an exposure history from thousands of subjects, a few of whom may have had occupational exposure. Second, some of the persons who have been studied as workers really had only light and occasional exposure. Some of the workers were clerical employees of formulating plants whose total exposure may not have been increased by their employment. However, many workers do have substantial and prolonged exposure to one or more pesticides, and the levels of these materials found in their tissues give some indication of the amount that may be tolerated.

Although the overlapping between the ranges of values for ordinary people and for workers is very broad in some instances, the great majority of the values for these two groups do not overlap at all in connection with the chlorinated hydrocarbon insecticides. Unfortunately, serious overlapping does exist in connection with heavy metals.

In some instances, the tissue levels of some workers have overlapped with those of patients. Theoretically, this could be caused by variations in individual susceptibility to the compound in question. Actually, some of the high values under discussion were observed in workers in plants where cases had occurred, indicating a serious need for improved occupational hygiene and reduction of exposure.

It is somewhat astonishing to see how little overlap has been observed between tissue levels from patients who survived and those who died. One would expect occasional overlapping as a result of individual variation in susceptibility. The fact that little overlapping is seen is evidence for the importance of dosage—especially dosage at the tissue level—in determining the outcome of poisoning.

The number of doses may have to be taken into account in interpreting tissue levels (see Section 3.2.3). This is particularly true of those compounds that are excreted relatively slowly and of those tissues in which they are preferentially stored. For example, the amount of a chlorinated hydrocarbon insecticide stored in fat following poisoning by a

Table 8-2

Storage of Selected Materials in the Blood or Serum of the General Population
of the United States of America, of Exposed Workers, and of
Patients who Survived or Failed to Do So

Compound	General population[a] (ppm)	Workers (ppm)	Patients (ppm)	Dead (ppm)
p,p'-DDT	0.0002-0.0800	0.0271-0.9955[b]		
p,p'-DDE	0.0003-0.3830	0.0315-0.8546[b]		
total DDT	0.0008-0.4630	0.1089-2.2017[b]		
BHC	0.0001-0.0240[c]	0.0010-0.0930[d]	0.468 - 0.84 [e]	
dieldrin	0.0001-0.0250	<0.0007-0.1370[f] 0.182[g]	0.28[h]	0.65[h]
aldrin	N.D.[i] (<0.0001)	<0.0001-0.0039[f] 0.029[g]	0.036 as aldrin[h] 0.28 as dieldrin	
chlordane	N.D.[i] (<0.0001)		2.7 - 3.4[j]	
endrin	N.D.[i] (<0.0001)	N.D.[i] (<0.004)	<0.004 - 0.053[k]	
heptachlor epoxide	<0.0001-0.0051			
toxaphene	N.D.[i] (<0.0001)		0.156[h]	10[h]
2,4,5-T				506[h]
dinitro-o-sec-butylphenol				72.5[h]
pentachlorophenol	0.000-0.018	0.06 - 20 [l]	118.0[m]	
hexachlorophene	<0.001 - 0.089			
lead	0.000 - 0.100	0.010 - 0.070[n]		
mercury	0.005 - 0.070	0.033 - 0.550[o]	0.264[o]	
arsenic	0.001 - 0.500			

a. Except as otherwise noted, the values in this column indicate the ranges given in papers cited in Tables 7-15 or 7-21.
b. Laws et al., 1967.
c. The range in general population with exposure from home vaporizer only was 0.0009 - 0.0052 ppm.
d. Milby et al., 1968.
e. Harris et al., 1969; Starr and Clifford (1972) list five metabolites.
f. Hayes and Curley, 1968.
g. Mick et al., 1972.
h. Unpublished results.
i. Searched for but not detected. (The sensitivity is shown in parentheses. Because of sample size, the limit is not always the same even for the same compound.)
j. Curley and Garrettson, 1969; Aldrich and Holmes, 1969.
k. Coble et al., 1967; Curley et al., 1970.
l. Casarett et al., 1969.
m. Armstrong et al., 1969.
n. Fleming, 1964.
o. Goldwater et al., 1964.

single dose may be less than the amount stored in the same tissue without any injury following repeated intake at a low daily rate.

The concentrations of chemicals in blood and urine reflect recent intake to a far greater extent than is true of the levels in depots such as adipose tissue. The concentrations in blood or serum tend to parallel those in critical organs such as the brain. In spite of some overlapping between the various tissue levels of groups with different degrees of exposure, the measurement of these concentrations usually serves to establish or exclude the diagnosis of poisoning by a chlorinated hydrocarbon insecticide or by a phenol.

Use of Chelating Agents to Mobilize Lead. Lead may be the only toxicant whose diagnosis is dependably helped by using a drug to mobilize it from storage and increase its excretion in the urine. The diagnostic use of calcium disodium EDTA was proposed by Bastenier et al. (1957), although the ability of the chelating agent to mobilize lead in persons with no special exposure to the metal had been noted earlier (Hardy et al., 1954). As it is now commonly used, the test involves the infusion of 2 g of calcium disodium EDTA during a period of 6 hours (Hernberg and Laamanen, 1964). Another test employs calcium trisodium pentetate (DTPA) (Brugsch et

Table 8-3

Excretion of Selected Materials in the Urine of the General Population of the
United States of America, of Exposed Workers, and of Patients
Who Survived or Failed to Do So

Compound	General population[a] (ppm)	Workers[a] (ppm)	Patients (ppm)	Dead (ppm)
p,p'-DDT	0.0005 - 0.0138[a,b]	0.0023 - 0.0238		
p,p'-DDE	0.0004 - 0.0285[a,b]	0.0133 - 0.0371		
p,p'-DDA	0.008 - 0.180[a]	<0.01 - 2.67		
total DDT		0.0505 - 3 3727		
BHC	<0.0001 - 0.0004[b]		0.01 - 0.74[c]	
dieldrin	0.0005 - 0.0019[b]	0.0013 - 0.0660[d]	0.081[e]	
aldrin	N.D. (<0.0001)[b]	N.D. (<0.0002)[d]		
chlordane			0.309 -193 [f]	
endrin	N.D. (<0.0001)[b]	N.D. (<0.004)[d]	<0.004 - 0.039[g]	
heptachlor	< 0.0001 - 0.0009[b]			
toxaphene	N.D. (<0.0001)[b]			
pentachlorophenol	.0022 - .0108	0.01 - 20 [h]		

a. Except as noted otherwise, the values in this column indicate the ranges given in papers cited in Tables 7-20 or 7-21.
b. Cueto and Biros, 1967.
c. Harris et al., 1969; Starr and Clifford, 1972.
d. Hayes and Curley, 1968.
e. Unpublished result.
f. Curley and Garrettson, 1969; Aldrich and Holmes, 1969.
g. Coble et al., 1967; Curley et al., 1970.
h. Cranmer and Freal, 1970; Casarett et al., 1969.

al., 1965). Evidence has been presented that, taking dosage into account, orally administered penicillamine is more effective than calcium disodium EDTA (Ohlsson, 1963). A specimen of urine is collected just before the person goes to bed at night, and immediately afterward he swallows 450 mg of DL-penicillamine hydrochloride. The first urine voided in the morning is also analyzed for lead. The maximal permissible concentrations, proposed for workers (0.1 ppm before penicillamine and 0.3 ppm the following morning) are very conservative; higher levels have been found in unexposed adults and children by other investigators. Incidentally, a marked increase in excretion of lead is established within 2 hours after a dose of penicillamine, and the effect is maintained through the 8th hour, after which it decreases sharply.

The test in whatever form is of special value in persons suffering some illness from excessive lead intake, even though their urinary excretion of lead is within the normal limits and, therefore, less than 0.08 ppm. Following administration of a chelating agent, persons with a history of excessive exposure to lead usually will show a 10-fold or greater increase in urinary lead excretion, so that the concentration is at least 0.8 ppm and often much

more (Hernberg and Laamanen, 1964; Sandstead et al., 1969). Persons without special exposure to lead may also show a 10-fold or slightly greater increase in lead excretion (Hardy et al., 1954; Whitaker et al., 1962), but the maximal concentration reached seldom if ever exceeds 0.5 ppm.

Tests for Pharmacological Effects. Significant absorption of any of the organic phosphorus or carbamate insecticides may be indicated by decrease in blood cholinesterase level. Normal values as measured by the two most popular methods are shown in Tables 8-4 and 8-5. There is a certain inherent difficulty in accurately measuring cholinesterase activity depressed by carbamates. For these compounds, measurement of the compound or a metabolite may be a more practical means for diagnosing patients or monitoring workers. The same is true even of some organic phosphorus compounds, notably parathion (Elliott et al., 1960).

More recently it has been shown that exposure to parathion can be measured in a more sensitive as well as more direct way by gas chromatographic analysis of parathion in serum than by analysis of *p*-nitrophenol in urine (Roan et al., 1969).

Selection of Samples. The basic samples

Table 8-4

Cholinesterase Activity (Δ pH/hr) of Normal Human Blood as
Measured by the Method of Michel.

Simplified from Rider et al. (1957) by permission of C. V. Mosby Co.

		men			women		
red cells	range	0.39	-	1.02	0.34	-	1.10
	mean $\pm$ s.e.	0.766	$\pm$	0.081	0.750	$\pm$	0.082
plasma	range	0.44	-	1.63	0.24	-	1.54
	mean $\pm$ s.e.	0.953	$\pm$	0.187	0.817	$\pm$	0.187

Table 8-5

Cholinesterase Activity (μM/min/ml) of Normal Human Blood
as Measured by the Recording Titrimetric Method

From data of Nabb and Whitfield (1967).

red cells	range	11.1	-	16.0
	mean $\pm$ s.d.	13.2	$\pm$	0.31
plasma	range	3.6	-	6.8
	mean $\pm$ s.d.	4.9	$\pm$	0.02

should be collected with the idea of determining the identity of the toxicant and the rate of dosage. For example, if there is evidence that poisoning has occurred through the contamination of flour used to make bread, then primary samples would consist not only of suitable samples from patients, but also of samples of the particular formulation, flour, and bread suspected of causing poisoning. There might be good reason to collect other ingredients of the bread as well as other food and water in order to rule out the possibility of multiple contamination or even an initial mistake. However, analysis of secondary samples that probably contain no poison should be postponed until the identity and approximate concentration of the poison in primary samples has been established. This procedure will increase greatly the efficiency of chemical analysis. The primary set of samples, therefore, should consist of the following as may be appropriate: (a) the suspect formulation (this sample should be sent to the laboratory under completely separate cover from the remaining samples, because of the possibility of cross-contamination); (b) remnants of the specific food, water, or other material assumed to have been the direct cause of poisoning; (c) vomitus or lavage fluid; (d) blood; (e) urine; (f) stool specimens; (g) skin washings; (h) expired air; (i) bile (especially for narcotics); (j) various tissues (especially liver, kidney, brain, and the storage tissue peculiar to the suspect compound), provided death has occurred and an autopsy has been performed (samples of fat sufficient for analysis may be taken from living patients by needle biopsy without danger, see below); and (k) other specimens as required.

Poison may have been spilled on the clothes. Vomitus may have contaminated clothing or sheets or it may have been mopped up with a towel or other cloth. Any fabric known or suspected to contain poison, vomitus, or even urine should be sent to the laboratory.

It is most important that formulations and any other specimens suspected of heavy contamination be sent to the laboratory under separate cover. Otherwise, it may be difficult to exclude the possibility that a trace of poison found in a tissue sample may have entered the sample as a contaminant during shipment.

A number of plastics and rubbers contain extractable impurities that may be difficult to distinguish from pesticides in the very likely event that the specimens are analyzed by gas chromatography. The impurities can be separated and identified, but the procedure complicates and delays analysis. It is better to have imperfect specimens than none at all; however, if a choice is available, all solid and liquid specimens should be collected in glass bottles or jars with ground glass stoppers or with screw caps lined with aluminum foil.

All samples should be labeled carefully. The following information generally is required: (a) name of patient; (b) weight of sample; (c) date sample taken; (d) place sample taken; and (e) name of referring physician. Samples that remain under the same administrative control may be labeled by code number.

If there is any possibility that a sample will be of medicolegal importance, it must be sealed and transmitted in such a way that its identity and validity can be established in court. Lids and corks may be secured by adhesive tape and then labeled in India ink or some other suitable writing material in such a way that the writing crosses two or more strips of tape. The closure cannot be removed without removing the tape, and the tape cannot be removed and then replaced without the tampering being obvious.

Some samples such as flour, hair, and other dry materials require no preservation. Other samples such as blood, tissues, excreta, and many foods must be preserved unless they can be transferred to the laboratory immediately. Unpreserved samples may undergo chemical change, the importance of which in relation to diagnosis depends on the compound. Furthermore, putrid samples may be refused by the laboratory. Refrigeration is always an acceptable means for preserving samples. It may be achieved by shipping the material in an insulated container with "refreezents," or with crushed ice in plastic bags to prevent leakage. It may be technically easier to use dry ice, but freezing destroys red blood corpuscles and prevents their separation from plasma. Separate measurements of plasma and red cells are valuable in connection with several heavy metals and with cho-

linesterase activity. Dry ice will last much longer if it is shipped in an insulated container.

It usually is satisfactory to preserve urine with a few drops of 10% formalin without refrigeration. Tissues also may be preserved with an equal or greater volume of 10% formalin if chlorinated hydrocarbon insecticides are the only compounds to be analyzed.

Regardless of the type of preservation, shipment to the laboratory should be by the most rapid means available.

Adjustment of Urine Samples. The concentration of each normal excretory product in the urine varies greatly, depending on water intake, ability of the kidney to concentrate, and other causes. This factor of dilution also influences the concentration of foreign compounds in the urine and may be confounded with variation associated with dosage and interval since last exposure.

If exposure to a foreign compound is essentially constant (eg, dietary exposure), it may be desirable to collect a series of 24-hour samples and to express excretion in terms of milligrams per day. If the amount of material excreted changes rapidly (eg, following one or a few doses), the use of 24-hour samples will obscure many important details. The rate at which excretion declines may be of interest; if so, timed samples are the only solution for the problem. However, some refinement may be gained in connection with both grab samples and timed samples by making an adjustment for their dilution when voided. This may be done by relating excretion of the foreign compound to the concentration of a component such as creatinine known to be excreted at a very constant rate. Another and more common approach is to correct the samples to a standard specific gravity. This is equivalent to relating the concentration of the foreign compound to the concentration of total solids in the same sample. A standard value of 1.024 has been suggested (Elkins *et al.*, 1966), in which case the correction formula is:

adjusted concentration (ppm) =

$$\frac{\text{observed concentration in ppm} \times 0.024}{(\text{observed specific gravity}) - 1.000}$$

Technique for Fat Biopsy. Analysis of chlorinated hydrocarbon insecticides in fat by the older methods required samples of a gram or more and, therefore, required surgical biopsy. Much smaller samples can be used if analysis is by gas chromatography. A special biopsy needle has been described by Hunter and Kendrick (1968); it consists of an outer cannula and an inner trochar. The sample of fat is cut off by the trochar and retained within its lumen when it is turned within the cannula. The sample obtained averages 15.5 mg. The outer dimension of the entire assembly is 4.5 mm, and it is inserted under local anesthesia.

Satisfactory samples of fat also can be obtained using an ordinary 10- or 20-ml hypodermic syringe and a large needle (eg, Nos. 13 to 18). The pain involved is no greater than that involved in taking a blood sample, and anesthesia is unnecessary. In this instance, fat is cut off by the sharp edge of the needle itself and pulled into the lumen of the needle or even into the syringe by strong suction. The needle is inserted through the skin and aimed along the course it will follow through the fat tissue. Full suction is then applied to the syringe; the needle is jabbed through the tissue; the plunger is allowed to return gently to its resting poistion; the needle is withdrawn; and firm pressure is applied to the biopsy site for 5 minutes. Samples obtained with an 18-gauge needle weigh 3 to 10 mg (Garrettson and Curley, 1969).

Breath Analysis. The use of expired air for practical toxicological monitoring and diagnosis has been developed more recently than use of other kinds of samples. To be sure, for a long time physicians have smelled acetone on the breath of diabetics and alcohol on the breath of drunks and guided their treatment accordingly. However, since the advent of infrared spectrophotometry and gas chromatography, it has become routine in some laboratories to distinguish at least 36 gas and solvent vapors in breath samples, to measure their concentrations, and to determine the body load of them. Practical directions for the collection of breath samples and illustrations of the interpretation of data have been given by Stewart (1974).

Limitations of Present Tests for Hypersensitivity. Many of the tests now available for diagnosing poisoning are remarkably good from the standpoint of specificity, sensitivity, and accuracy. Unfortunately, most of them are complex and completely beyond the scope of the ordinary hospital laboratory. It seems unlikely that the tests will be simplified to a significant degree in the foreseeable future.

A completely different kind of limitation concerns tests intended to prove that a particular chemical is the cause of hypersensitivity in general or of myelogenic blood dyscrasias in particular. It is recognized on the basis of epidemiological evidence that some drugs produce agranulocytosis (aminopyrine), thrombocytopenic purpura (neoarsphena-mine, quinine, quinidine, apronal, potassium iodide, and phenylbutazone), or aplastic anemia (chloramphenicol) in a small proportion of persons treated with them (Carr, 1954). In the present state of knowledge, there is no way to exclude the possibility that any chemical will produce one of these myelogenic blood dyscrasias in an occasional person. Therefore, it is not astonishing that a few cases have been linked circumstantially to pesticides; however, most cases apparently are caused by drugs.

According to some investigators, the only way to prove that a particular chemical—even a known offender like chloramphenicol—is the cause of trouble in a specific case is to give the recovered patient a challenge dose of the suspected material and precipitate a second attack. Obviously, this approach is both dangerous and impractical. Some dependence has been placed on patch tests, but these tests carry some danger and are not conclusive. Not only are drugs the worst offenders, but it often happens that a patient who develops a myelogenic blood dyscrasia is being treated with more than one. What is needed is an effective *in vitro* test that can be carried out on samples withdrawn from the patient both as soon as illness is detected and later during the recovery period. Such a test would permit prompt withdrawal of the offending drug or other chemical and would allow patients to be continued on those needed drugs that were not a source of trouble. Any test applicable to a wide range of drugs undoubtedly could be applied to the relatively small number of cases in which a pesticide or other industrial chemical is suspected of causing a myelogenic blood dyscrasia.

A number of *in vitro* tests have been proposed, but none has found general favor. It sometimes happens that a test appears to be diagnostic for a condition produced by one drug but not useful for diagnosing what seems to be the same condition produced by another drug. Some of the procedures are obviously tedious. Apparently the various tests have not been compared in a single laboratory. The fact that any success whatever has been achieved in this kind of testing should serve as a stimulus for further work to develop a really useful test.

The tests attempted so far may be divided into: (*a*) those employing a type of cell involved in the clinical disease (eg, platelets in connection with thrombocytopenic purpura); (*b*) those employing a type of cell selected because of some special or even fundamental relationship to hypersensitivity (eg, the basophilic granulocyte, because it releases histamine presumably involved in most or all allergic processes); and (c) those using a specially treated cell (eg, tanned sheep red blood cells treated with a hapten conjugate).

Tests with platelets were used in connection with thrombocytopenic purpura associated with a drug, apronal (Ackroyd, 1949a, 1949b, 1949c, 1951, 1952, 1953, 1954, 1955). It appears that apronal combines with a protein in the platelets and probably in the endothelial cells of all patients to whom the drug is administered. Certain persons develop antibodies to the apronal-protein complex and thus become sensitive to the drug. If platelets from the sensitive person or from a normal person are exposed to apronal in saline and then brought in contact with the antibody from the patient's serum, the platelets will be agglutinated, and, if complement is present, it will be fixed and the platelets will be lysed. Various aspects of the reaction may be demonstrated through complement fixation, through platelet agglutination, or through direct observation of imperfect clot retraction in blood in which the platelets have been destroyed through lysis. It is believed that the injury to the endothelial cells occurs through a mechanism similar to that responsible for platelet destruction. Purpura of this etiology is thought to be dependent upon injury to the endothelial cells but to be accentuated by thrombocytopenia.

The work with apronal has been confirmed to a considerable degree for thrombocytopenic purpura associated with guinine (Grandjean, 1948) and with quinidine (Bigelow and Desforges, 1952; Larson, 1953; Barkham and Tocantins, 1954).

The results with agranulocytosis (Moeschlin and Wagner, 1952; Dausset *et al.*, 1954) do not agree closely with those for thrombocytopenia, but even in the study of agranulocytosis *in vitro* methods hold some promise. Furthermore, a complement fixation method has been explored with some success in connection with dermatosis caused by nickel (Wendlberger and Frohlich, 1954).

Another approach involves the use of basophils from the circulating blood to study a wide variety of allergic reactions to drugs and other chemicals. Most of the histamine in the blood stream is carried by these cells (Graham *et al.*, 1955). In a person with recognized allergy, exposure to the antigen to which he is sensitive may cause a striking reduction in the number of circulating basophils and degranulation of many of the remaining ones, without any significant effect on other types of circulating cells (Juhlin and Westphal, 1962). Shelley (1963) has described six variants of the baso-

phil test, but he considers the one involving the study of stained living cells from rabbits to offer the greatest overall clinical value (Shelley, 1962, 1963). This three-drop test requires only one drop (0.003 to 0.005 ml) of the patient's serum, a similar drop of a dilute solution of the chemical under study, and a drop of the buffy coat from 1 ml of fresh, heparinized rabbit blood. The mixture is prepared on the surface of a slide carrying a dry residue of neutral red vital stain. The mixture is covered by a vaseline-rimmed cover glass and examined with an oil immersion lens. Readings for control as well as test slides should be completed in 10 minutes, since nonspecific degranulation may occur simply on standing. The entire procedure requires less than 1 hour. Chemicals insoluble in water may be dissolved in alcohol, ether, or acetone, placed on the test slide, allowed to dry, and then used; in this event only two drops (serum and cells) are added to the slide. In a positive test, a majority of the basophils show a loss of sphericity; distortion and swelling of the cell; swelling, lysis, and loss of granules; brownian movement of the granules; clearing the nucleus; formation of blebs in the cell wall; and streaming of granules from the cell. Degranulation may be explosive in highly sensitive individuals. The test was found useful in confirming reactions to both foods and chemicals and in connection with anaphylaxis, purpura, asthma, hay fever, and dermatitis, including contact dermatitis (Shelley, 1962, 1963). The test was positive in a case of purpura caused by paradichlorobenzene (Nalbandian and Pearce, 1965).

The three-drop test may be carried out with either fresh or frozen serum. Plasma may be used also if the anticoagulant is heparin; however, oxalate interferes with the test by removing free calcium. Fillers, buffers, or flavoring in drug formulations often interfere with the test. Pure chemicals should be used for testing.

The three-drop test is quantitative. The difference between the reactivity of different patients or the same patient at different times may be expressed in terms of the greatest dilution of patient's serum capable of giving a positive reaction in a properly controlled test. Controls must include: (a) tests with serum from nonsensitized people, and (b) tests with patient's serum and rabbit basophils, but no test chemical. These tests will help to detect and eliminate degranulation caused by: (a) nonspecific toxic effects from an excessive concentration of chemical (a dilution of 1:100 is suggested for initial trails); (b) unsuitable basophils requiring a change of rabbits; or (c) sensitivity of the patient to rabbit serum, in which event human cells may be tried. A negative test indicates a lack of circulating antibody and not necessarily a lack of allergy. The test is usually negative for a week or two following an anaphylactic reaction.

A third kind of test (Halpern et al., 1967) involves the transformation of small lymphocytes to lymphoblasts in culture. It is reasoned that the lymphocytes contain some "immunological information" that permits them to recognize an antigen. Thus, they are regarded as having a special relation to hypersensitivity, but the chemical nature of this relation is not so neatly defined as is that of basophils. The lymphoblastic transformation test was found useful in confirming reactions to a variety of drugs and in connections with anaphylaxis, asthma, hay fever, dermatitis including contact dermatitis, and certain other allergies. Briefly, 60 ml of heparinized blood from the patient are filtered through glass wool to isolate the small lymphocytes. These lymphocytes are dispersed at the rate of 1×10^6 cells/ml in a culture medium composed in part of the patient's serum. The entire process must be carried out under aseptic conditions, even though the culture is protected by an antibiotic. The proper concentration of antigen to add to the culture must be determined separately for each chemical. Cultures with chemicals and a control culture with no chemical are incubated at 37°C for 96 hours and then examined to determine the percentage of cells that have transformed to lymphoblasts. Transformation rates ranging from 1.5 to 45% were considered positive. Most control values were less than 1.0% (Halpern et al., 1967).

A fourth approach involves the indirect hemagglutination technique using tanned sheep red blood cells treated with hapten conjugate. Such a test for sensitivity to aspirin was described by Weiner et al. (1963). The fact that the chemicals to be studied may have to be converted to a derivative and certainly must be combined with a foreign protein (eg, albumin or bovine γ-globulin) prior to impregnation on red cells and testing with the patient's serum, may limit application to the test.

8.1.4.2 Supportive Tests. By supportive tests are meant those tests of body condition or function that are of little or no use for diagnosing poisoning by a particular compound but may be of tremendous value: (a) in exploring certain findings of the neurological and general physical examinations; and (b) in guiding supportive treatment of the patient. A list of such tests constitutes Table 8-6; use of the tests must be determined by the condition of

the patient. Usually only a few tests are required in a given case, but any questionable or positive findings ought to be explored adequately. The selection of tests need not be limited to those in the table, which has been restricted to those most commonly found abnormal in one or more kinds or poisoning.

8.2 Treatment

Removal of the toxic agent and supportive treatment may be equally as important as antidotes in the care of patients suffering from poisoning. The choice of what to do first must be determined by the condition of the individual patient at the moment. The judgment must be based at first entirely on clinical findings. Later laboratory measurements, such as those listed in Table 8-6 and most especially measurements of blood electrolytes, may be of real value in guiding treatment. Chemical identification and quantitation of the poison usually are delayed, and only in rare instances contribute importantly to care of the patient.

Respiration should be relieved first if it is embarrassed. If the airway is obstructed, it must be cleared. If breathing has stopped, artificial respiration must be prompt. If the patient is in shock, treatment for it should be started at once. When these conditions do not exist or have been corrected, the poison should be removed as quickly and thoroughly as possible. Often one can remove poison and administer specific treatment without significant delay in either process. However, with rare exceptions, of which treatment of cyanide poisoning is one, administration of specific treatment and antidotes other than those that detoxify or neutralize should not take precedence over removal of poison. Details and certain precautions are given in the following sections.

In these sections, greater emphasis and documentation has been alloted to specific antidotes, not because they have any inherently greater importance in treatment, but because, in comparison with information on pharmacological antidotes and preparations used in supportive treatment, information on specific antidotes (a) permits an understanding of the poison against which they are used, but (b) is less easily accessible to the physician.

Much additional information on treatment of common acute poisonings may be found in a book by Matthew and Lawson (1970) that deserves to be better known.

8.2.1 Removal of Poison

It is of great importance to remove unabsorbed poison as rapidly and completely as possible from whatever part of the body it has reached. However, even in the absence of symptoms, a dangerous dose may have been absorbed before decontamination can be started. Furthermore, decontamination is never complete even under optimal conditions. This has been demonstrated experimentally for some compounds in connection with induced vomiting (Arnold et al., 1959; Goldstein et al., 1963),

Table 8-6

Clinical Tests Frequently of Value in Guiding Supportive Treatment

Organ or system	Test	Normal values
blood	complete blood count including:	
	red cell count	$4.5-6$ million/mm^3 (M)[a]
		$4.5-5$ million/mm^3 (F)[b]
	reticulocytes	$0\% - 2\%$
	white cell count	$5,000-10,000/mm^3$
	differential count	
	platelet count	$100,000-300,000/mm^3$
	hemoglobin	$13 - 18$ g% (M)
		$11 - 16$ g% (F)
	methemaglobin	up to 3%
	hematocrit	$40 - 54$ (M)
		$37 - 47$ (F)
	prothrombin time	$70 - 100\%$
	CO_2 content	$22 - 32$ mM/l
cardiovascular	blood pressure	
	electrocardiogram	
respiratory	chest x-ray	
kidney	24-hour urinary output	
	urinalysis	
	urea nitrogen (serum)	$5-25$ mg%
	creatinine (serum)	$0.7 - 1.5$ mg%
	creatinine clearance	$85 - 125$ ml/min (M) $75 - 115$ ml/min (F)
	phenosulfophthalein (inject 1.0 ml (6 mg) of dye intravenously and collect specimens of urine every 15 minutes for 2 hours)	
liver	icterus index	$2 - 8$ units
	bilirubin (serum)	
	conjugated	$0 - 0.3$ mg%
	total	to 1.0 mg%
	total serum protein	$6.0 - 8.0$ g%
	bromsulfalein (inject 5 mg/kg; retention less than 5% at 45 minutes and less than 2% at 60 minutes)	

Table 8-6 (continued)

Organ or system	Test	Normal values
	SGOT (serum glutamic oxalic transaminase)	12 - 40 units/ml
	SGPT (serum glutamic pyruvic transaminase)	$\begin{cases} 11 - 66 \text{ units/ml (M)} \\ 5 - 53 \text{ units/ml (F)} \end{cases}$
	LDH (serum lactic dehydrogenase)	90-200 units/l
	urinary porphyrins	
	urinary δ-aminolevulinic acid	0.003 - 1.02 mg%
neurological	lumbar puncture and spinal fluid	
	electroencephalogram	

a. Males

b. Females

and even washing of the skin (Fredriksson, 1961). Therefore, after poison has been removed as thoroughly as possible, the patient should be followed carefully for signs of increasing intoxication and treated as required.

8.2.1.1 Emesis. Vomiting is a complex reflex mechanism for emptying the stomach and upper intestine. The mechanism is similar and well developed in man and the dog, poorly developed in the cat, and essentially absent in the rat. The reflex involves not only peripheral or central excitation but central coordination. The physiology and pharmacology of vomiting were reviewed by Borison and Wang (1953).

The act of vomiting is complex. It usually is preceded by nausea and often accompanied by salivation, lacrimation, and deep breathing. Vomiting involves contraction of the pylorus, relaxation of the stomach cardiac sphincter, reverse peristalsis in the esophagus, closure of the glottis, raising of the soft palate to seal off the nasopharynx, extension of the neck, opening of the mouth, and finally, almost simultaneous contraction of the abdominal muscles leading to ejection of the gastric contents. Preceding vomiting or between bouts of it, there may be relaxation of the pylorus and reverse peristalsis of the upper intestine, leading to the presence of bile in the stomach contents and eventually in the vomitus. Vomiting produces a considerable increase in intraabdominal pressure and blood pressure, usually leading to reflex slowing of the heart. Following vomiting, there is some degree of faintness, pallor, sweating, and a fall in blood pressure.

The stimulus to vomiting may come not only from irritation of the pharynx (gagging), the stomach, or intestines, but also from stimulation of the semicircular canals and labyrinth (motion sickness and certain other conditions), a special chemoreceptor zone in the medulla (apomorphine), the mesentery and peritoneum (peritonitis), and various viscera (eg, cardiac and menstrual vomiting). Finally, vomiting may be induced by certain odors—notably that of vomitus—or even the thought of odor.

According to Wang and Borison (1952) the medullary emetic mechanism consists of two anatomically close but anatomically and functionally separable units. There is an emetic center in the region of the fasciculus solitarius and the underlying reticular formation, which is excited by afferent stimuli from the gastrointestinal tract and elsewhere. Electrical stimulation of this area produces vomiting. Destruction of it in dogs made them highly refractory to the emetic action of both stomach irritants and centrally acting compounds. Passage of emetic stimuli through the vomiting center is influenced by a number of factors, including a sudden fall in blood pressure.

Separate from the vomiting center but very near it is a chemoreceptor trigger zone. It lies in the area on the lateral postrema surface of the caudal end of the fourth ventricle. This vascular zone contains many nerve endings connected with the nucleus of the fasciculus solitarius. Destruction of this zone with little or no injury to the vomiting center made dogs refractory to apormophine, but left them fully susceptible to the action of stomach irritants. There is some evidence that different sites or mechanisms within the vascular zone are distinguishably sensitive to stimuli by different emetic drugs.

Contraindications to Induction of Vomiting. Vomiting cannot occur in persons whose central nervous system is sufficiently depressed by an anesthetic, narcotic, hypnotic, or sedative. However, the mere fact of coma does not ensure against vomiting, but may interfere with it and lead to aspiration of the vomitus. Therefore, no attempt should be made to induce vomiting in a semiconscious or unconscious person. By the same token, if a stuporous person seems about to vomit, he should be rolled onto his side and his neck should be extended to minimize the chance of aspiration.

Serious erosion of the gastrointestinal tract, whether by a caustic poison or by a peptic ulcer, is another contraindication to the induction of vomiting. Increased abdominal pressure may be dangerous in the presence of pregnancy or hernia. The ingestion of kerosene is also considered a contraindication to vomiting, lest it lead to aspiration of the oil and thus to chemical pneumonitis. Vomiting should not be induced in persons with cardiac decompensation, serious hypertension, or pulmonary tuberculosis because of the danger of increasing the blood pressure. On the contrary, the fall in blood pressure following vomiting may be dangerous to very young children, debilitated persons, or those already in shock.

Selection of Method for Emptying the Stomach. Although it is sometimes stated that gastric lavage is more efficient than vomiting in emptying the stomach, actual study apparently reveals the opposite (Arnold *et al.,* 1959; Abdallah and Tye, 1967). Furthermore, all studies (Arnold *et al.,* 1959; Matthew *et al.,* 1966; Abdallah and Tye, 1967) show that, regardless of the method used, the degree of success decreases with delay. Vomiting has the great advantage that it can sometimes be induced very rapidly and long before the patient is brought to hospital where gastric lavage can be started. Thus, vomiting has the advantage of both efficiency and speed. Gastric lavage should be reserved for situations in which vomiting is contraindicated or its induction has failed. Unconsciousness is the most common contraindication to vomiting. The selection of a method for emptying the stomach depends largely on the type of practice. Most poisoning in young children is accidental; most acute poisoning in adults is self-induced. Children who may have ingested a toxic substance often are fully conscious when their treatment begins. For them, induction of vomiting usually is indicated. By contrast, adults who are self-poisoned often are unconscious when their treatment begins, and aspiration and lavage is the only safe method.

Gagging. Gagging has the advantage over other methods for inducing emesis that it can be done at once. Admittedly, the method is relatively ineffective when used alone. Dabbous *et al.* (1965) found that gagging worked in only four of 30 children and that the volume of vomitus obtained in this way was small compared with the amount obtained later by administering syrup of ipecac to the same children. However, the efficiency can be increased by giving the patient either salt solution or a suspension of mustard if the first attempt at gagging is not immediately successful. Furthermore, vomiting can be promoted by volition. Some patients are very cooperative in gagging themselves. In treating another person, it is well to use the first two fingers of the left hand to force the patient's left cheek between his teeth to ensure that he does not bite the index finger of the right hand used to gag him. Finally, gagging can be reinforced by unpleasant odors or even by suggesting to the patient that he think of such odors. Use Anglo-Saxon.

Table Salt. Concentrated salt is sufficiently irritating to the stomach that some healthy people vomit if they attempt to take the ordinary salt tablets frequently recommended to replace salt lost through sweating. Advantage may be taken of this irritating property by administering a strong solution of salt (2 to 4 tablespoonfuls of salt in a glass of warm water) before gagging the patient and then repeating the process after he has vomited. One difficulty in clearing the stomach may be that there is not enough liquid to mobilize the toxicant, whether solid or liquid. Although plain water or some antidotal fluid may be used, there is something to be said for using a harmless irritant, especially during early treatment.

Other Salts. Cupric sulfate, potassium antimony tartrate, and zinc sulfate have long been recommended as local emetics. Cupric sulfate was used by the Arab physician Rhazes in the 9th century. The difficulty is that these compounds are so toxic that they must be removed by lavage if they fail to work. Their use should be discouraged.

Dry Powdered Mustard. When dry powdered mustard is added to water, one of the glycosides is hydrolyzed enzymatically to liberate a volatile, emetic oil, allyl isothiocyanate, which is completely lost from prepared mustards. The dose is 1 to 3 teaspoonsful of powder in warm water. Black mustard is said to be better than the yellow kind.

Syrup of Ipecac, USP. Following the reports by Gyllens-wärd (1960) and Robertson (1962), syrup of ipecac gradually came to be recommended as an emetic by most poison control centers in the United States of America. When indicated, it is now used routinely in the emergency rooms of many hospitals.

The emetic action of ipecac is caused by the combined local and central action of two alkaloids, emetine and cephaeline, which, with other soluble alkaloids, constitute about 2% of powdered ipecac or about 0.14% of syrup of ipecac. Fluid extract of ipecac is about 14 times more concentrated than the syrup. Its use must be avoided because of the serious danger of overdosage it it were confused with the syrup. The extract is not suitable for use even at a reduced dose, because its bitter taste makes it unacceptable.

In a systematic study of 250 children, Robertson (1962) found that 56% vomited in 15 minutes or less after receiving 20 ml of syrup of ipecac, and 88% vomited within 30 minutes or less. The remaining children took longer to vomit, failed to respond, or left the clinic when it was learned that the foreign material they had swallowed was not toxic. In that study, the delay in reaching treatment facilities accounted, on the average, for almost 80% of the total delay in evacuating accidentally ingested substances from children's stomachs. Thus, Robertson suggested that an effort be made to reduce the time necessary for recognizing the danger of ingestion and for bringing the patient to treatment. Others suggested instead that syrup of ipecac be placed in home medicine chests and used as an emergency aid measure. This suggestion is consistent with the safety record of syrup of ipecac. After using the preparation in several thousand children over a period of several years, Robertson (1962) reported no evidence of toxicity attributable to it. The experience of Spector (1958) was similar. However, some cases of poisoning and a few deaths have resulted from unintentional substitution of fluid extract for syrup of ipecac (Allport, 1959; Robertson, 1962). The fairly frequent but usually not serious toxicity associated chiefly with the cumulative effect of repeated doses of emetine (a derivative of ipecac) used to combat amebiasis has no real bearing on the safety of syrup of ipecac when used as an emetic.

Syrup of ipecac is available for over-the-counter sale in 30-ml containers. The syrup should be kept in home medicine cabinets for use in emergencies. A dose of 15 ml followed by 200 to 300 ml of water is recommended officially. It ought to be repeated in 20 minutes if the first dose is not effective before that time. Following Robertson's lead many pediatricians prefer to administer 20 ml initially.

Apomorphine Hydrochloride, NF. The action of apomorphine is entirely central and depends on the presence of an intact chemoreceptor trigger zone (Wang and Borison, 1952). The drug usually is administered subcutaneously at a rate of 0.1 mg/kg. The dose may be repeated in 15 minutes if vomiting does not occur. The response is said to be greater if the patient is seated rather than lying down (Isaacs, 1957). Its action usually occurs in 2 to 3 minutes and is more rapid than that of ipecac, but there may be more delay in its administration because, if used in the ordinary way, it is not adapted for emergency aid. A few people are hypersusceptible to the drug and react with far more nausea and vomiting than would be expected. After vomiting caused by apomorphine, most patients feel sleepy. This is of therapeutic value in treating those who are overactive, especially perhaps as the result of acute alcoholic intoxication. In a few people the depression is excessive but rarely to the point of collapse. If nausea persists, it often is followed by weakness, pallor, rapid breathing and rapid pulse, and a fall of blood pressure. Chlorpromazine hydrochloride will prevent vomiting in dogs injected with apomorphine (Boyd et al., 1954), but narcotic antagonists (levallorphan at 0.02 mg/kg or nalorphine hydrochloride at 0.1 mg/kg) are generally preferred to stop excessive action of apomorphine. In fact, a narcotic antagonist often is administered routinely to terminate vomiting and alleviate drowsiness (AMA Drug Evaluations, 1971).

Abdallah and Tye (1967) found that equal dosages of apomorphine hydrochloride were equally effective in dogs whether injected subcutaneously or placed in the conjunctival sac as eye drops. This method apparently has not been used in man, but it would appear to offer an opportunity for the most rapid emergency aid treatment. This drug acts quickly enough that it is of value for combating poisoning by antiemetic or depressant drugs, provided it is administered promptly after they have been ingested and before they have an opportunity to take effect.

Wang and Borison (1952) showed that intravenous dosages of 0.01 to 0.03 mg/kg produced in dogs almost immediate vomiting lasting only 1 to 2 minutes and without untoward effect. Gosselin and Smith (1966) suggested a controlled study of this method of treatment in man. The suggested dose would be 0.7 to 2.0 mg for a 70-kg man.

8.2.1.2 Gastric Aspiration and Lavage.

Advantage of Lavage. Gastric lavage is less efficient than induced vomiting (Arnold *et al.*, 1959; Abdallah and Tye, 1967), but it has the advantage that it can be used with care in patients who have swallowed a petroleum distillate (which would be dangerous to vomit), or in patients who are unconscious or have absorbed an excessive dose of an antiemetic and, therefore, cannot vomit. Press *et al.* (1962) reported a careful study of 299 patients who had swallowed petroleum distallates. Use of gastric lavage was alternated with its omission on even and odd dates according to protocol. It was found that gastric lavage was not harmful, although there was no conclusive proof that it was beneficial in this kind of poisoning.

There is no doubt that dangerous amounts of toxicant may be recovered from the stomach of some patients by aspiration and lavage (Caro and Kawerau, 1965; Matthew *et al.*, 1966). Slightly over 5 g of barbiturate and over 20 g of salicylate have been recovered in this way from patients (Matthew *et al.*, 1966).

Time of Lavage. Some authors have recommended that gastric lavage not be done on patients admitted more than an hour after ingestion. However, it is perfectly clear that some compounds remain in the stomach much longer than others. Matthew *et al.* (1966) recovered significant amounts of barbiturate up to but not exceeding 4 hours after ingestion. They recommended that gastric lavage not be attempted in patients who have swallowed a barbiturate if the time of ingestion is known to be over 4 hours. They suggested that no time limit be set if a salicylate has been swallowed. Since nothing is known about how long different pesticides are retained in the stomach, no rule can be laid down, but careful observation of patients may eventually provide information on the point.

Aspiration and Lavage of the Unconscious Patient. There has been disagreement particularly about the merits of attempting gastric aspiration and lavage in unconscious patients—and, as discussed above, it appears that induced vomiting is more beneficial for most conscious patients. Marriott (1933) pointed out that gastric lavage could be fatal if the cough reflex were absent. He recommended that lavage be done in the operating room with the patient in the Trendelenburg position to prevent aspiration. Harstad and her colleagues (1942) concluded that lavage was never beneficial to the unconscious patient or even the conscious one. By adding radiopaque material to the lavage fluid, they showed that much of the fluid passed into the small intestine. By adding charcoal to the fluid, they showed at autopsy how much fluid had entered the lungs. They considered aspiration pneumonia an important cause of death associated with poisoning. In 1964 Mys-

chetzky (quoted by Caro and Kawerau, 1965) recommended against the use of lavage except in conscious patients who had ingested poison less than an hour before admission. On the other hand, those who have stated that they used strict precautions to protect the lungs have either advocated (Matthew *et al.*, 1966) or not opposed (Caro and Kawerau, 1965) aspiration and lavage of completely unconscious patients.

Technique of Gastric Lavage. If the patient has a poor cough reflex, protect the lungs and the patency of the airway by inserting a cuffed endotracheal tube before passing a stomach tube. In conscious patients and even unconscious patients with intact cough and gag reflexes, a large bore stomach tube may be passed at once. Place the patient so that his mouth is lower than his trachea. Remove any dentures and keep the mouth open with a gag. Lubricate the tube with glycerine or a suitable jelly, and ease it over the tongue and down the esophagus to a distance of about 50 cm in adults. Suck out the stomach contents using gentle mechanical suction if available. If a source of continuous suction is not available, a large syringe fitted with an adaptor will help. It little or nothing is obtained, it may be that the tube is not correctly located. Proper positioning of the tube can be checked by forcing a little air down it and listening with a stethoscope over the stomach for bubbling sounds. After making a reasonable effort to remove any stomach contents and being quite certain that the end of the tube is in the stomach, attach a large evacuator or funnel to the oral end of the tube. Add 300 ml or less of water or physiological saline heated to about body temperature. If a funnel is used, elevate the oral end of the tube and allow the water to enter the stomach by gravity. For this purpose, it may be necessary to use an adaptor and add a length of tubing between the funnel and the stomach tube so as to increase the overall length and make it easier to regulate the height of the column of water. Before all the water has passed into the stomach, lower the tube into a basin or jar and allow the stomach contents to siphon off. Save the first sample separate from later ones for chemical analysis. Do not use more than 300 ml for each washing, because a larger volume would have more tendency to cause emptying of the stomach contents into the duodenum. Repeat the lavage until the returning fluid is clear. Save all the washings because it may become desirable to measure the total amount of poison recovered. Before removing the tube, it is usually desirable to add about 300 ml of fluid containing a cathartic or one of the detoxicating or neutralizing antidotes discussed in Sections 8.2.1.3 and 8.2.3.1.

A tube used for evacuating the stomach must have a rounded, solid end to facilitate passage through the esophagus. It must have at least one large opening in the side just behind the tip and is better if it has several large holes placed at intervals back from the tip. The outer wall must be very smooth. Stomach evacuator tubes commonly sold for use in children have an outside diameter of 7.33 mm (No. 22 Charrière scale). Those for adults commonly measure 10 mm (No. 30 Charrière scale). It is only reasonable that soft food and the remains of pills and other solid formulations can be removed most easily by the largest tube that can be passed safely through the esophagus. Based on their extensive experience, Matthew and Lawson (1970) recommend a tube of 16 mm outside diameter (30 English gauge) for adults.

8.2.1.3 Evacuation of the Gut.

It is well known that substantial portions of some absorbable compounds may pass unabsorbed through the intestine. Furthermore, some compounds or their metabolites are excreted in part in the feces. Apparently no systematic study has been made of a series of cases of poisoning in which an effort was made to measure the amount of different toxicants evacuated either unaltered or metabolized in the feces. Of course, unchanged toxicant has been analyzed in the feces in individual cases. Conversely, dangerous amounts of poison often remain in the intestine after death. This is sometimes true in patients who survive long enough that one would have supposed the entire gastrointestinal tract would have been evacuated. For example, unabsorbed malathion was found in the stools and at autopsy in the stomach contents of a woman who survived 46 hours after drinking a solution of the insecticide; peristalsis, ordinarily stimulated by malathion, may have been suppressed by drugs used in treatment. Such cases and common sense suggest that every effort should be made to reduce the duration and degree of absorption, and detoxifying or neutralizing antidotes may reduce the rate of absorption per unit time.

Classification and Choice of Cathartics. The action of cathartics is often attributed to their emollient or irritant properties, or to their ability to increase the bulk of the intestinal contents. The presence of bulk is a stimulant of peristalsis and evacuation. Cathartics differ in their rate of action, tendency to cause colic, and incidental effects. The ideal one would be dependable and rapid, but would produce no colic and no undesirable side effects; if possible, it should benefit the patient through incidental action. In general, saline cathartics are best for dispelling poisons because they are dependable and rapid, and produce little colic. In selected patients, magnesium salts may have the desirable incidental effect of mild sedation and diuresis. The selection of other cathartics in the treatment of poisoning is often based largely on their incidental effects, especially the possible effect of mineral oil in dissolving some toxicants and thus preventing their absorption from the intestine.

The following paragraphs are confined to drugs of special value in treating poisoning or to common ones that may be contraindicated.

Liquid Petrolatum Emulsion, NF. This material has little effect on the emptying time of the intestine. It acts by lubrication and by interfering with the reabsorption of water. The possibility that it might be able to dissolve fat-soluble poisons, even in competition with other intestinal contents, makes it of interest in treating poisoning by these materials. Presumably, an emulsion of the oil would be more quickly and finely dispersed than the oil itself in the intestinal contents. Unfortunately, no objective test seems to have been made to determine how efficient the oil or the emulsion is in protecting patients or experimental animals. The dose of emulsion is 30 ml; that of the oil is 15 ml.

Castor Oil, USP, BP, NF. Castor oil is the triglyceride of ricinoleic acid. It is nonirritant but is hydrolyzed by intestinal lipases to form the irritant ricinoleic acid, which promotes intestinal peristalsis. There is less stimulation of the large intestine, but its normal antiperistalsis and, therefore, reabsorption of water are inhibited. The net effect is evacuation of the intestine about 2 to 6 hours after dosing; the dose is 15 ml. Castor oil might dissolve fat-soluble poisons in the same way that mineral oil may do. However, the action of castor oil depends on its digestion, which would tend to release any compound dissolved in the oil. It is true that purgation tends to remove any undigested oil, but some absorption of its intestinal metabolites occurs before the intestine is cleared (Watson *et al.,* 1963). Thus, castor oil has no special advantage in the treatment of poisoning and it is probably inferior to the saline cathartics, or especially to a combination of one of these with liquid petrolatum emulsion.

Saline Cathartics. Table 8-7 is a list of some saline cathartics and their recommended doses. The proper amount of any one of them may be dissolved in about 300 ml of water and

Table 8-7

Saline Cathartics and Their Doses

Compound	Usual dose for adults (g$\underline{a}$)
magnesium sulfate USP, BP (Epsom salt)	15
magnesium oxide USP, BP	4
magnesium citrate solution NF (1.55 to 1.9 g/100 ml magnesium oxide with citric acid and sodium bicarbonate for effervescence)	200 ml
magnesium carbonate USP, BP	8
magnesium hydroxide NF (milk of magnesia tablets)	0.3
magnesia magma (milk of magnesia) USP 7.5% to 8.5 suspension of magnesium hydroxide BP	15 ml
sodium sulfate NF, BP (Glauber's salt)	15
sodium phosphate NF, BP	4
potassium sodium tartrate NF, BP (Rochelle salt)	10

a. Grams unless otherwise stated.

placed in the stomach when gastric lavage is complete and before the tube is removed. Saline cathartics work because they are absorbed slowly. By osmotic action, the ions tend to hold water in the intestine or draw it from the tissues to maintain an isotonic state. The resulting bulk stimulates peristalsis, and the highly liquid state of the intestinal contents facilitates a flushing out of the small and large intestine 0.5 to 3 hours after dosing. The salts are less effective when given on a full stomach, but in poisoning a cathartic usually should not be given until the stomach has been emptied as thoroughly as possible. Use of a hypertonic solution causes closure of the pylorus and delays passage of the fluid until it has been made isotonic by diffusion of fluid into the stomach. Some absorption of the ions of saline cathartics does occur, but there is no toxic accumulation if kidney function is normal. In fact, magnesium ions are diuretic. Magnesium ion is a depressant of the central nervous system and once had limited use for this purpose (Sollmann, 1957). Any absorptim of magnesium ion that may occur following use of a cathartic is likely to have no effect in connection with most kinds of poison, but would be beneficial to a patient poisoned by a stimulant (eg, a chlorinated hydrocarbon insecticide) and injurious to a patient poisoned by a depressant (eg, a barbiturate). Serious side effects from a saline cathartic are rare.

8.2.1.4 Removal of External Poison.

Washing the Eyes. The eyes should be washed if they are contaminated by any material. Mechanical irritation from a gritty powder or chemical irritant can cause damage and increase the chance of infection. A toxic material may produce local injury. For example, chlorates may burn the cornea and organic phosphorus compounds may produce severe miosis. Furthermore, many poisons may be rapidly absorbed from the conjunctiva or from the mucosae of the lacrimal duct and the nose to which they may drain from the eye.

Wash the eyes with lots of water. If a faucet is available, wash the face and eyelids quickly and then hold the head so cold water washes across the eye while the lids are held open and the eye is moved first in one direction and then in another. Do not permit any but the most gentle stream to flow directly against the eye. Wash both eyes thoroughly. Contamination may be more general than the patient supposes. If no suitable faucet is available, use an eye cup or pour on water from a bottle or pan or use well washed hands. Normal saline is less irritating than water and should be used if available. At least two flasks of it should be kept in every emergency aid station.

Washing the Skin. If a poison has been dusted or splashed on the skin, remove all contaminated clothing and flood the area with water. If the spillage is at all extensive, and the contaminated person is near a stream, pond, or tank, he should jump in. If water is available for mixing spray, it may be used for washing. The fact that many pesticides are generally employed as emulsion concentrates or water-wettable powders makes washing with plain water an effective procedure. If there is any soap or especially detergent at hand, use that, too. However, speed is more important than soap. Remove as much poison as possible as near the place of the accident as possible. Depending on the person's condition, he may take a proper bath as soon as he reaches home or hospital.

If water is not immediately available, liquid formulations should be gently blotted from the skin. Never rub the skin in order to remove poison. It is impossible to get off all of the chemical in this way, and the damage done to the superficial layers of the skin by rubbing may promote absorption (see Section 3.2.2.5).

If washing is quick and thorough, it may prevent illness. However, if the poison was one likely to cause serious illness through dermal absorption, it is best for the contaminated person to contact his physician.

Depending on his condition, every hospitalized patient who may have had dermal contact with a pesticide should be bathed even though he may have washed as an emergency aid measure. Most pesticides are absorbed through the skin to some degree. Ordinary detergents are more effective than soap in mobilizing a wide range of materials. Detergent bars are available in almost every store where soap is sold. Use detergents and water liberally but avoid harsh scrubbing, which may injure the skin and promote absorption. Don't forget the hair.

Whether any further cleaning is to be done after bathing with detergent and water apparently depends on the compound. Some toxicologists have expressed the fear that organic solvents would injure the skin. This fear may be justified in connection with irritants such as xylene; it is not justified in connection with alcohol used as a final rinse after ordinary washing.

Effectiveness of Washing. There has been at least one instance in which washing appeared to be lifesaving. In an industrial accident in which two men seemed to be splashed about equally with parathion, one of them, a foreman, ordered the other to bathe and change clothes, but he did not do so himself. The foreman died in less than 24 hours; the workman did not get sick (Hamblin and Marchand, 1951). Dramatic as this example appears, it does not constitute proof, for other factors may have been involved in the outcome.

In a few instances, objective benefits of cleanliness have been noted under practical conditions. For example, when propoxur was applied to villages under toxicological supervision, it was reported that the frequency of reactions was less when personal hygiene was good and clean protective clothing was worn (Wright *et al.*, 1969).

Measurements of the dermal exposure of workers based on washing their skin (Section 5.5.2.3) or studies of the rate of dermal absorption in volunteers (Section 3.2.2.5) give no direct evidence of whether washing can be therapeutic. These studies do show that substantial amounts of pesticides can be washed from the skin of exposed persons.

Experiments with animals have shown that some may be saved by washing without any additional treatment, even though they initially received a dermal dose sufficient to kill all control animals. Protection is greatest if washing is prompt, but the experiments showed that in some instances washing may be still be lifesaving after symptoms of poisoning have appeared. Using dermal doses of parathion that killed all unwashed rats, it was shown that a higher proportion of animals was saved by washing with 70% alcohol after washing with either soap or detergent than by ordinary washing alone. Thus, bathing with 70% alcohol appears to be indicated *after* ordinary washing.

8.2.1.5 Removal to Fresh Air. If a person has been made ill by breathing a gas or vapor, he should be rushed to fresh air. A number of respiratory poisons may produce so much confusion that the victim is not aware of his condition nor alert enough to seek relief even though he is conscious. Of course, some poisons act so quickly that the victim may lose consciousness before he has time to escape. In an atmosphere of this sort, the rescuer must have full respiratory protection.

As soon as the victim has reached fresh air, he should be watched carefully for the onset of respiratory difficulty. Be ready to give articifical respiration if it is needed while the person is being moved to hospital. Be sure he is kept as quiet as possible and that he is warm but not hot.

8.2.2 Supportive Treatment

8.2.2.1 Maintenance of Airway and Artificial Respiration. Unless the apneic victim is in a toxic atmosphere, do not waste time moving him. Check his airway and start artificial respiration at once.

Maintenance of Airway. When a person is unconscious and stops breathing, the base of the tongue tends to press against the back of the pharynx and block the passage of air from either the nose or mouth into the lungs. To clear the upper airway, wipe out the mouth with your finger covered by your handkerchief or your shirt. Roll the victim onto his back. Place both your hands at the angles of his lower jaw and lift it so it juts out and the head tilts back. You may do the same thing by putting your thumb in his mouth, grasping the jaw, and pulling it forward or you may raise the neck and press the forehead back (Fig. 8-1A). What has been said about maintenance of an airway assumes an emergency situation and a lack of special equipment; there is no possibility of bringing the complete equipment of an emergency room to such situations. However, the physician might do well routinely to carry in his bag oropharyngeal and cuffed endotracheal tubes suitable

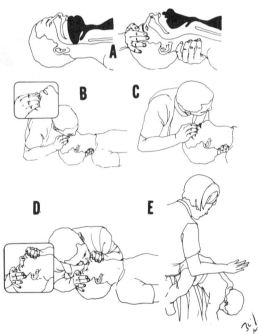

Fig. 8-1. Artificial respiration. (A) One method of opening the airway. (B) Position of victim and operator for mouth to mouth artificial respiration. (C) Method for looking and listening for expiration. (D) Position of victim and operator for mouth to nose artificial respiration. (E) One way of holding a child to dislodge something caught in his windpipe. Drawings reproduced with permission of the American National Red Cross.

for 1- to 2-year-old infants and for average sized adults. The choice between the oropharyngeal and the endotracheal tube depends on the level of consciousness of the patient. Since it is impractical to carry a full range of sizes, the choice of sizes suggested corresponds to the size of the two main groups of persons subject to poisoning.

The lives of a few people have been saved by tracheostomy performed with an ordinary knife and a reed or tube intended for some other purpose. Except for such completely emergency situations, tracheostomy seldom is indicated unless endotracheal intubation otherwise could be required for more than 48 hours.

Having cleared the airway and inserted an appropriate tube if available, pinch the victim's finger so that your fingernail is driven in hard enough to cause sharp pain in a normal person. This may cause the victim to gasp and start breathing again. If this maneuver fails, start artificial respiration at once.

Artificial Respiration. The mouth-to-mouth (or mouth-to-nose) technique of artificial respiration is the only one that requires no equipment and will still overcome the airway resistance that may be present in poisoning by some compounds, notably the organic phosphorus insecticides, which produce both bronchial constriction and excessive secretion. No matter why breathing has stopped, this technique allows the rescuer to get a better idea of the volume and pressure needed to inflate the victim's lungs than can be gotten by other methods. Timing tends to be correct automatically with the mouth-to-mouth method, because the nonbreathing adult needs about the same volume of air as the rescuer breathes at the normal rate (12 to 16 per minute), while the infant or very young child requires a smaller volume per breath, delivered at a slightly higher rate (about 20 per minute).

If the victim is adult, place your mouth over either his mouth (Fig. 8-1B) or nose (Fig. 8-1D) and pinch the other opening closed with the fingers of one hand. (You can blow between his teeth even though his jaws are closed.) Watch the victim's chest; when you see it rise, stop inflation. Then, while watching to see the chest fall, turn your head and listen for exhalation (Fig. 8-1C). When exhalation is finished, inflate again, keeping a rhythm of about 12 to 16 per minute. You will have to blow fairly hard to get enough air into an adult, especially a heavily muscled one. Insofar as possible, keep the jaw jutting out while artificial respiration progresses.

If the victim is a child, place your mouth

over his mouth and nose and blow into him gently so that the chest is inflated to about the normal degree. Remove your mouth to take fresh air and to let the victim breath out. As you remove your mouth, turn your ear to listen for air being passively exhaled by the victim. Repeat the active inflation and passive deflation of the victim 20 times per minute.

If there seems to be resistance to your blowing, recheck the position of the jaw. A child may be held up by the ankles or hung with his abdomen over one of your arms (Fig. 8-1E) while you pat him sharply on the back in the hope of dislodging any obstructing matter. This effort should last only a moment. Wipe out the mouth again and continue artificial respiration.

If obstruction is still present after the jaw has been rechecked and if the victim is too heavy to lift, he may be rolled onto his side and struck several times between the shoulder blades in the hope of disloding foreign matter. Clean out the mouth and continue artificial respiration.

If the victim vomits, turn the head quickly to the side. Clear out the mouth and continue artificial respiration as soon as possible. Those who do not wish to contact the victim directly may cover his mouth with a cloth. This will not interfere very much with the exchange of air.

If someone comes to help, send him to call the police for an ambulance equipped for mechanical artifical respiration.

If the victim begins to breathe for himself, try to time your blowing to match his rate of breathing and help his natural inspiration. As his breathing becomes stronger, stop helping but watch very closely lest he stop again. Keep the person as quiet as possible.

If the victim does not start to breathe promptly, do not despair. Remember that some poisoned people who required artificial respiration for many hours survived without permanent injury. A parathion patient, who had to be maintained on artificial respiration for 60 hours, recovered completely (Milthers *et al.*, 1963).

Summary and Note. (*a*) Don't waste time moving the victim unless he is actually in a toxic atmosphere. (*b*) Quickly clear the mouth and throat. (*c*) Tilt the head back as far as possible. (*d*) Lift the lower jaw forward. (*e*) Pinch the patient sharply to see if he will gasp and breathe. If this fails, (*f*) open your mouth wide and blow into the victim's mouth and nose (or one of them with the other squeezed shut) until you see the chest rise. (*g*) Listen for exhalation. (*h*) Repeat the active inflation and passive exhalation 12 to 16 times per minute for adults or 20 per minute for small children. (*i*) Don't give up.

Frequently, the physician is in telephone contact with the patient's family or associates quite early. The physician should inquire about the victim's breathing and color. If anoxia seems to be present or imminent, a warning should be given against moving the patient, and someone trained and equipped for giving emergency mechanical artificial respiration (either the police or fire department) should be called. If necessary, the person initiating the telephone call should be instructed in artificial mouth-to-mouth respiration to be carried out while the physician goes to the patient.

8.2.2.2 Oxygen Therapy. Oxygen is necessary for respiration. Therapeutic oxygen is valuable in any situation in which it can help restore to normal the concentration of oxygen available at the tissue level. Therapeutic oxygen may also be valuable if it reduces the amount of work the patient must expend in breathing air. If the oxygen tension in the alveoli is increased, the gradient between the concentration in the alveolus and the concentration dissolved in plasma in the pulmonary capillaries is increased. Thus, the opportunity is set up for increasing the saturation of oxygen in the arterial blood and, step by step, eventually in the tissues. This is true regardless of the cause of tissue hypoxia.

In a normal person breathing air at sea level, the oxygen tension of the arterial blood is 94 mm Hg and that of the venous blood is 46 mm Hg; the carbon dioxide tensions of arterial and venous blood are 40 and 46 mm Hg, respectively. Respiration is compromised if the arterial oxygen is less than normal but more than 60 mm Hg, or if carbon dioxide tension is more than normal but less than 50 mm Hg. Under these circumstances, treatment with oxygen is indicated.

Respiratory failure is present if the arterial oxygen tension is less than 60 mm Hg or the carbon dioxide tension exceeds 50 mm Hg. Under these circumstances, oxygen and assisted respiration are indicated.

The most common condition associated with poisoning and benefited by oxygen is (*a*) pulmonary edema or pneumonitis caused, for example, by irritant gases or kerosene. Other conditions benefited by oxygen include (*b*) obstruction of the respiratory tract, for example obstruction caused by bronchoconstriction and excessive secretions resulting from organic phosphorus insecticides, (*c*) paresis of the respiratory muscles, as in poisoning by organic phosphorus insecticides or in any severe muscular weakness, (d) lack of functional hemoglobin, as in hemolytic anemias, methemoglobinemia associated with the treatment of cyanide poisoning, or carboxyhemoglobinemia resulting from poisoning by carbon monoxide, and (e) circulatory failure, as in toxic shock.

Pure oxygen is so irritant that it is difficult to breathe for more than about 7 hours at atmospheric pressure. At pressure of 3 to 4 atmospheres, signs of systemic toxicity of oxygen appear after 3 to 4 hours.

Oxygen, USP. USP oxygen is prepared from the fractional distillation of liquid air. It is supplied in green cylinders at a pressure of 2,000 psi.

It is only when oxygen needs to be given by a tight fitting mask or in a hyperbaric chamber that care must be taken to avoid its toxicity. If prolonged use of 100% oxygen is required, it should be interrupted by the use of air or 50% oxygen for 1 hour, four times daily. When oxygen is delivered by catheter, tent, face tent, or loosely fitting mask, the concentrations ordinarily obtained are safe and sufficient for most therapeutic uses. Since oxygen as it comes from the cylinder is free of water, it should be humidified before delivery to the patient to avoid drying of the mucous membranes with consequent irritation and interference with ciliary action.

8.2.2.3 Infusions and Transfusions. Many kinds of poisoning may disrupt the water-electrolyte balance either through vomiting diarrhea, excessive secretion, or a disturbance of excretion or of fluid distribution. A smaller number of kinds of poisoning produce anemia through destruction of the corpuscles, or by interference with their formation. All of these injuries may be identified through examination of the patient and without identification of the poison. Treatment of each condition must be based much more on the condition of the patient than on the cause of the trouble. Thus, fluid replacement should be postponed or attempted with great moderation as long as there are signs of excessive fluid in the lungs and bronchi, even though the patient may have lost considerable fluid through vomiting, diarrhea, and sweating. Unconsciousness is not, in itself, an indication for infusion. Even deeply unconscious patients, in the absence of dehydration, do not require parenteral fluid for the first 12 hours, and they may be able to take liquids by mouth before that time has elapsed.

Even an outline of the treatment of fluid and electrolyte imbalance or of the physiology and pathophysiology underlying this treatment is beyond the scope of this book. Valuable information may be found in textbooks on pharmacology and in more specialized books, for example that by Weisberg (1962). Fortunately, many patients may be benefited by the simplest procedures.

Physical Regulation of Fluid Balance. The condition of patients in hypovolemic or neurogenic shock (see Section 8.2.2.5) may be benefited almost instantaneously by physical measures. Of these, the simplest procedure is to raise the foot of the bed or in some other way lower the patient's head in relation to his body. Some good is done by raising the patient's legs on a board or on pillows, even when it is not practical to put him on an inclined plane. A more complicated procedure is to put the patient's legs in inflatable pressure splints, such as those used for athletes injured on ski slopes and other places difficult to reach. Of course, such a splint must merely compress the legs without restricting venous return; otherwise the effect will be opposite of the one desired.

Balanced Electrolyte Injection. The use of normal saline and of 5% glucose infusions largely has been replaced by use of balanced electrolyte infusions. The latter are better than solutions of sodium chloride alone, because their composition is much more nearly identical to the electrolyte composition of normal plasma. They are better than 5% glucose alone because they avoid water intoxication.

Balanced electrolyte formulations contain not only sodium chloride, but also potassium, magnesium, and sources of bicarbonate. Some contain 5% glucose in addition to the electrolytes. The formulations are either (a) hypotonic and used to supply the normal water and electrolyte requirements of patients who cannot drink, or (b) isotonic and used to restore acute losses of plasma fluid.

Adults should receive the hypotonic solution as the daily rate of 1,500 ml/m^2 of body surface, or about 3 liters per day. Children should receive 1,000 to 1,500 ml/m^2. Use of the isotonic solutions must be according to the needs of the patient.

Dextrose Injection, USP. A 5% solution of dextrose in water is the preferred vehicle for administering water without electrolytes. It also may be used as an isotonic vehicle for normal human serum albumin. Each liter of 5% dextrose provides about 200 calories. In children it is best to use balanced saline injection, for they rarely have a relative excess of electrolyte.

Solutions containing 10% or more of dextrose are irritating to the veins. In fact, 50% dextrose with sodium chloride formerly was used as a sclerosing agent.

Dextrose is supplied in concentrations of 2.5, 5, 10, 20, and 50%.

Citrated Whole Human Blood, USP. Citrated whole human blood, identified according to the donor's blood group and Rh type, is available from hospital blood banks. In addition to its usual uses, which are dictated by the condition of the patient, whole blood exchange transfusions are of great value in treating a few forms of poisoning, notably poisoning by certain phenols. This is possible because these compounds reach considerably greater concentrations in the blood than in other tissues and because excretion is almost adequate to prevent poisoning in many instances. Thus, exchange transfusion is far more likely to be effective in treating poisoning by these phenols than would be true of most poisons.

The amount of blood given to an adult usually is 500 to 1,000 ml, repeated as necessary. Exchange transfusion seldom is attempted except in infants or young children. For them, a two-volume exchange [2 × (85 ml/kg)] often is used and is calculated to remove 85% of the blood originally present. Blood is removed and injected via a single vein. In the newborn, a polyethylene tube generally is inserted through the umbilical vein into a great vein. Blood is removed and added alternately in small volumes. The volume in the body must be kept almost the same throughout. This is accomplished by carefully measuring and recording the subtractions and additions or by carrying out the entire procedure with the baby on a sufficiently sensitive scale. Detailed directions are given in textbooks of pediatrics (eg, Nelson *et al.,* 1969; Barnett and Einhorn, 1968).

Normal Human Plasma, USP. This is the cell-free portion of uncoagulated blood obtained from pooling about equal portions from eight or more healthy adults. When fresh, it contains all blood constituents except the corpuscles. Its major contribution (beyond that of isotonic balanced electrolyte injection) in nearly all forms of poisoning requiring fluid replacement is protein. It would, of course, contribute prothrombin to anyone sufficiently poisoned by an anticoagulant rodenticide to require replacement of prothrombin, but in most of these patients treatment with vitamin K is sufficient.

No effective way has been found to sterilize plasma, and its use carries a certain danger of serum hepatitis. The danger is reduced but not eliminated by storage in liquid form, but this entails loss of some of the more labile constituents.

Normal human plasma is available from hospital blood banks in liquid form or as a powder that can be reconstituted with sterile, pyogen-free water. The usual intravenous dose for both adults and children is 500 ml. As much as 1,500 ml may be given.

Because plasma carries the danger of hepatitis, its use ought to be restricted. Fluid loss of many poisoned persons can be replaced adequately by balanced electrolyte injection. In the majority of remaining cases, adequate replacement can be achieved by supplementing the balanced electrolyte injection with normal human serum albumin or by use of plasma protein fraction.

Normal Human Serum Albumin, USP. This is a sterile preparation of plasma protein. It is prepared by fractionation of whole blood from healthy donors, and it is pasteurized at 60°C for 10 hours to remove the danger of homologous serum hepatitis. It is safer than normal human plasma as a replacement for protein in hypovolemic shock. It may be of value in combatting edema in the absence of shock, unless the edema is secondary to severe cardiac failure.

Normal human serum albumin is supplied as 5% solution in 250- and 500-ml containers, and as 25% solution in 20-, 50-, and 100-ml containers. The larger containers are supplied with sets for intravenous injection. A 5% solution may be given undiluted; a 25% solution may be given undiluted provided it is injected slowly, or it may be diluted with balanced electrolyte injection or with 5% dextrose.

The initial dose for adults or children in shock is 25 g (500 ml of 5% solution). The 25% solution either undiluted or diluted in 5% dextrose is indicated in treatment of edema. The preparations contain no preservative and must not be used except promptly after opening. They should not be used if turbid when viewed in transmitted light.

Plasma Protein Fraction, USP. This 5% solution of stabilized human plasma proteins may be used in place of plasma as a source of protein and electrolyte in the treatment of hypovolemic shock. Its major advantage is its failure to transmit serum hepatitis. It is supplied as a 5% solution in 250- and 500-ml containers. The dosage is similar to that of plasma.

8.2.2.4 Sedatives. Several kinds of pesticides may cause convulsions. If the convulsions are the direct result of the poison on the nervous system, as in the case of the chlorinated hydrocarbon insecticides, then anticonvulsant drugs reasonably may be regarded as pharmacological antidotes and, on this basis, these drugs are discussed in Section 8.2.3.2. If the cause of convulsions is largely anoxia, as is often true in connection with the organic phosphorus insecticides, sedatives may be used cautiously at the same time that every effort is made to improve delivery of oxygen to the tissues.

8.2.2.5 Stimulants. The term, stimulant, can be used to cover drugs used to combat shock and those used to combat nervous system depression, especially depression of respiration.

Shock is any of a variety of conditions in which the circulation of blood is inadequate to perfuse the tissues. At least four kinds sometimes associated with foreign chemicals may be recognized; (a) *Hypovolemic shock* involves external or internal loss of blood, plasma, or electrolyte solution. Most commonly this loss is the result of hemorrhage or burns, loss may follow corrosion or vesication of epithelium or protracted vomiting or diarrhea caused by some poisons, including heavy metal pesticides. (b) *Neurogenic shock* involves interference with the neurohormonal integration of circulation. This interference often is caused by chemicals, including large doses of anesthetics and other depressant drugs. (c) *Anaphylactic shock* involves peripheral vasodilatation and increased capillary permeability in response to an antigen. The most common and powerful antigens are of biological origin; pyrethrum is a rare but possible cause of anaphylactic shock. (d) *Cardiogenic shock* involves inadequate ejection of blood by the heart, whether caused by infarction, arrhythmia, or failure of ventricular filling. Of these disorders, certain arrhythmias may be caused by the sensitization of the myocardium to epinephrine by certain solvents, especially those inhaled in high concentration by thrill-seeking youths. Usually the condition is self-correcting, or the victim dies before help is available. Treatment by electric countershock would be indicated if treatment were possible.

There are at least two other kinds of shock not associated with foreign chemicals, namely, (e) bacteremic shock and (f) shock associated with removal of pheochromocytoma.

In hypovolemic shock, there is no vasomotor collapse; on the contrary, peripheral resistance generally is increased as a compensatory mechanism. The only effective treatment is replacement of the lost fluid volume, preferably in as nearly as possible the form in which it is lost (ie, plasma for plasma, etc.). Vasopressor drugs are of no proven benefit in this kind of shock and may be harmful if used for an extended period.

Vasopressor drugs often are used in treating shock caused by depressants (mainly barbiturates), but their value is in doubt.

In anaphylactic shock, epinephrine is the drug of choice. It constricts the dilated peripheral vessels, relieves bronchial constriction, and may be lifesaving. As soon as a clear airway has been assured and measures taken to correct possible loss of circulating blood volume, adequate blood pressure may be maintained by slow infusion of levarterenol or metaraminol.

Epinephrine Hydrochloride, NF, pINN. Epinephrine is the neurohormone produced by the adrenal medulla that serves to maintain and raise blood pressure. Used as a drug, it increases blood pressure chiefly by increasing cardiac output, but it also constricts arterioles in the skin, mucosae, and splanchnic areas, dilates those of skeletal muscle, and constricts the venous capacitance bed. It also dilates the bronchioles. Its action is rapid in onset but brief in duration. Used in excess it causes a dangerous increase of blood pressure.

Epinephrine hydrochloride is supplied as an aqueous solution at a concentration of 1 mg/ml (1:1,000) in 1- and 30-ml containers.

Epinephrine is best given intramuscularly or subcutaneously in an initial dose of 0.5 mg (0.5 ml of 1:1,000 solution) to adults and 0.3 mg to children. Only in a severe emergency should it be given intravenously. The same amount or half as much may be given at intervals of about 15 minutes if required. If more than three or four doses are needed, maintenance of blood pressure should be continued with levarterenol or metaraminol.

Levarterenol Bitartrate, USP, pINN. Norepinephrine is the compound responsible for transmission of impulses from postganglionic fibers of the sympathetic nerves to their effector organs (except sweat glands) and at some synapses within the central nervous system. When used as a drug, the compound is called levarterenol. The compound has essentially the same range of actions as epinephrine, but differs in that the major action is to increase peripheral resistance rather than to stimulate the heart. In anaphylactic shock, levarterenol is used to maintain blood pressure after it has been raised from shock levels by epinephrine.

Levarterenol bitartrate is supplied as a 0.2% solution (1 mg of base/ml) in 2- and 4-ml containers.

Usually 4 to 8 ml of the 0.2% solution is administered to adults in 500 ml of 5% glucose by continuous intravenous infusion at a rate required to keep the blood pressure up to 20 or 30 mm Hg below normal. For children, 1 ml of 0.2% solution is added to 250 ml of 5% glucose and given at the rate of about 0.5 ml/minute. Extravasation of the drug may cause necrosis, which can be prevented by prompt infiltration of the tissue with 0.5 to 1 mg of phentolamine in 10 ml of water or by adding 5 to 10 mg of phentolamine to each liter of infusion fluid prophylactically. Another prophylactic measure is the addition of heparin to the infusion solution at a rate necessary to supply 100 to 200 units of heparin per hour to reduce the incidence of venous thrombosis.

Metaraminol Bitartrate, USP, recINN. The actions of this drug are similar to those of levarterenol but of longer duration.

Metaraminol bitartrate is supplied as a 10 mg/ml solution in 10-ml containers.

Following the use of epinephrine to control anaphylactic shock, 100 to 250 mg of metaraminol bitartrate is given to adults in 500 ml of 5% glucose by continuous intravenous infusion, at a rate necessary to keep the blood pressure up to 20 or 30 mm Hg below normal. For children, 10 mg is added to 250 ml of 5% glucose and administered in the same way. Some authors recommend 100 mm Hg as the upper limit of systolic blood pressure stimulated by metaraminol because of a net reduction of cardiac output and a danger of kidney damage secondary to intense vasoconstriction if the blood pressure goes higher (Matthew and Lawson, 1970).

In the treatment of neurogenic shock not adequately corrected by elevation of the legs, metaraminol may be the first vasopressor drug administered. Under these circumstances, 5.0 mg (0.5 ml) may be given intramuscularly and repeated every 20 minutes as required for two or perhaps three doses. If this is inadequate, then plasma or a plasma substitute must be used.

Analeptics. Drugs used to stimulate the central nervous system, especially the respiratory center, are called analeptics. With the exception of levallorphan, nalorphine, and other narcotic antagonists used exclusively to combat the effect of morphine and related compounds, analeptics are nonspecific. The margin of safety of the nonspecific analeptics is small. They may cause nausea, violent vomiting, cardiac arrhythmias, convulsions, and other overstimulation of the central nervous system, as well as delayed psychotic reactions. They should never be used in an attempt to restore full consciousness. Except perhaps in the presence of ideal support of respiration, respiratory depression is always accompanied by some degree of hypoxia and hypercapnia, both of which are stimulants of respiration. Because of this fact and the characteristics of available drugs, use of analeptic drugs has been almost abandoned and emphasis is placed on maintenance of airway, supply of oxygen, artifical respiration, restoration of

fluid balance, and maintenance of blood pressure.

Use of an analeptic may be indicated when depression of respiration is marked and entirely of central origin. This picture is seen in severe poisoning by barbiturates and morphine. In these instances, the intravenous injection of 2 ml (500 mg) of nikethamide may be required while safer and more permanent means of respiratory assistance are being readied (Matthew and Lawson, 1970).

8.2.2.6 Antiemetics. An outline of the nature and causes of vomiting is given in Section 8.2.1.1. It also is mentioned in Section 8.2.1.1 that narcotic antagonists often are used after apomorphine hydrochloride to terminate its action.

If poisoning is suspected but its existence is unproved, antiemetics of any kind ought to be used with caution, for they may mask effects other than vomiting and increase the difficulty of diagnosis. Antiemetics ought to be used with caution even if the fact of poisoning is established. With few exceptions, vomiting following ingestion of noxious substances is protective, and it ought not to be stopped until it has done whatever good may be possible. Although gagging associated with vomiting in the first few moments after ingestion of kerosene and some other solvents commonly leads to severe pneumonitis, there is little evidence that delayed vomiting of these materials, after they have been mixed with stomach contents and mucus, carries a significant threat.

In poisoning, nausea and vomiting occasionally persist after there is no further chance of removing additional poison. If such vomiting is profuse and frequent, it contributes to dehydration and electrolyte imbalance as well as to the patient's discomfort. In these relatively rare instances, control of vomiting is justified. Unfortunately, the selection of a drug is difficult. None is without some danger, and none has been subjected to controlled study in connection with vomiting of this kind. Scopolamine hydrobromide and the antihistaminic compounds are used mainly in connection with motion sickness, vestibular disorders, postoperative nausea, and nausea and vomiting of pregnancy. Barbiturates and phenothiazines are more likely to be effective in vomiting of toxic origin. The barbiturates may be indicated for other reasons. The phenothiazines probably are the most effective antiemetics. However, they show additive effects with central nervous system depressants (including alcohol), and they may cause extrapyramidal reactions (especially in children and young adults), as well as hypotension, jaundice, granulocytopenia, thrombocytopenia, cutaneous eruptions, and other toxic reactions. They should not be administered to patients with coma or hypotension or to those given other drugs likely to cause hypotension. Their use in poisoning by organic phosphorus compounds has been considered specifically contraindicated (Arterberry *et al.*, 1962), although others have used them extensively without difficulty either for their tranquilizing or antiemetic action.

Chlorpromazine Hydrochloride, USP. Chlorpromazine is the prototype of phenothiazine compounds. Except for hypotension, the more serious untoward reactions occur only after prolonged use.

Injectable solution containing 25 mg/ml is supplied in 1-, 2-, and 10-ml containers. The drug is also supplied in tablets, capsules, syrup, and suppositories.

To combat vomiting, chlorpromazine hydrochloride is given intramuscularly to adults in doses of 25 to 50 mg every 3 or 4 hours until vomiting is controlled. For children, the dosage is 0.5 mg/kg every 4 to 6 hours. Alternatively, the drug may be given rectally to adults at a dose of 100 mg every 6 to 8 hours, or to children at a rate of 1 mg/kg every 6 to 8 hours. After vomiting has stopped, dosing may be continued orally at a rate of 0.5 mg/kg or slightly less every 4 to 6 hours.

8.2.2.7 Steroids. Glucocorticoids do not cure disease, but their use may prevent complications of inflammation or alter other cellular reaction in such a way that there is time for natural body defenses or therapeutic measures to become effective. The numerous and sometimes serious toxic effects of glucocorticoids are direct extensions of their pharmacological properties and are the result of overdosage. The possibility of uncomplicated beneficial effects are greatest in transient conditions in which the patient may be expected to recover if he survives a crisis. In general, glucocorticoids with little or no sodium-retaining activity are most useful in treating effects of toxic compounds, and these drugs may be used interchangeably in equivalent anti-inflammatory doses. If steroids are used, the dosage should be reduced gradually after a desired effect has been obtained; otherwise withdrawal effects may appear.

The conditions associated with poisoning, for which treatment with steroids is recommended, include: (*a*) shock that does not respond to elevation of the legs, oxygen, correction of acidemia, and (if required) no more than three intramuscular 5.0-mg doses of metaraminol, (*b*) marked and prolonged hypothermia, and (*c*) pulmonary edema.

Hydrocortisone, USP. Hydrocortisone is the compound recommended by Matthew and Lawson (1970) for those toxic conditions benefited by steroids. The recommended dose is 100 mg intravenously, repeated at intervals of 6 hours. Hydrocortisone solution for injection is available in concentrations of 100 mg per 20 ml and 250 mg per 5 ml.

Catatoxic Steroids. The first part of the word "catatoxic" is derived from the Greek word *kata* meaning down or against. Thus, catatoxic steroids are those that oppose poisoning. Pretreatment of rats with these compounds, including spironolactone, ethylestrenol, and norbolethone protected rats against otherwise fatal doses of several organic phosphorus compounds (Selye, 1970a). Spironolactone and ethylestrenol also protected against the fungicide, cycloheximide (Selye, 1970b). The same steroids had been shown earlier to protect against a great variety of compounds, but not against all. It is Selye's view that the detoxicating effect is independent of the classical hormonal properties of the steroids examined and that in many if not all instances the antidotal effect is due to the induction of hepatic, microsomal, drug-metabolizing enzymes. Be that as it may, these steroids deserve study to see whether they have any therapeutic effect when given after various poisonous materials have been absorbed. Of the more active catatoxic steroids, at least spironolactone is already in limited use in medicine (but as a diuretic based on its antagonism toward aldosterone). Spironolactone is safe enough to use if it is, in fact, therapeutic. However, the diuretic dosage in man (1.4 mg/kg/day) is very much smaller than the catatoxic dosage in rats (about 200 mg/kg/day).

8.2.2.8 Antibiotics. Antibiotics ought not to be given prophylactically to poisoned people. They ought to be given if there is clear clinical or X-ray evidence of infection. It must be admitted that two situations offer special difficulty and may justify the use of an antibiotic as a precaution. Fever usually is the result of infection. It may be entirely of toxic origin, either through uncoupling of oxidative phosphorylation, or through injury to temperature control centers in the brain. Although acute opacities of the lung suggest infection, they may reflect uncomplicated pulmonary edema.

8.2.2.9 Nursing Care. Just as there is reason to begin a discussion of supportive treatment with maintenance of an airway and artificial respiration, so there is reason to conclude with nursing care. Nothing is gained by saving the patient dramatically only to let him die from neglect. Constant care is required, particularly if the patient is unconscious or if he may be subject to respiratory failure.

Monitoring. Persons seriously poisoned by an organic phosphorus insecticide ought to be under constant surveillance lest respiratory failure occur suddenly. Persons who are seriously poisoned by any agent ought to have their pulse, respiratory rate, blood pressure, temperature, and level of consciousness recorded every half hour. Constant monitoring of the heart and respiration of seriously ill patients is highly desirable.

Care of Unconscious Patients. Patients suffering respiratory difficulty in addition to unconsciousness (eg, those poisoned by an organic phosphorus compound) require constant attention. Patients suffering unconsciousness only (eg, some poisoned by an overdose of a sedative) may require attention no more often than every half hour. At least that often, the chest must be examined by percussion and auscultation, and the upper respiratory tract and endotracheal tube must be cleared thoroughly by suction. In the process of examining the chest, the patient is turned to his other side. Before he is rolled over, the top arm and leg must be passively, but fully, flexed and extended. After he is turned, the other arm and leg are moved. The movements and repositioning help to prevent pressure sores and respiratory blockage, including pockets of atelectasis.

Temperature Control. Poisoning involves the possibility of hypothermia as well as fever. Therefore, the measurement of temperature must be done with a thermometer capable of recording as low as about 25°C. The danger of hypothermia occurring is less if the patient is kept in a room somewhat warmer than the ordinary level for comfort. Moderate hypothermia requires no use of external heat, but the patient should be kept well covered by blankets. A rectal temperature of 29.5°C may be taken as the threshold at which active heating must be started. Heating may be accomplished most conveniently and safely with an ordinary electric blanket. These blankets are thermostated lower than heating pads, and, therefore, the danger of burning an unconscious patient is much less. Heating also may be accomplished by other means such as immersing a forearm in a water bath held at 43°C.

Patients poisoned by nitrophenols and other uncouplers of oxidative phosphorylation are subject to hyperthermia. If it is certain that poisoning is of this nature, preparation to reduce the temperature ought to be taken before it begins to rise, for the rise to a dangerous level may be rapid. Such patients should be kept in a cool room with little cover. More active measures should be started as soon as the temperature exceeds normal, provided, of course, that the cause is known with certainty. Even if the cause of fever is unknown, a temperature above 40.5°C is an indication for active cooling. Moderate cooling may be achieved by covering the patient with a wet sheet and directing the current of air from a fan over him. Greater cooling will occur if he is laid on a bed of crushed ice.

8.2.3 Antidotes

In spite of some overlapping, antidotes may be divided usefully into three classes, namely: (*a*) detoxifying or neutralizing antidotes, which interact with unabsorbed poison to prevent its absorption; (*b*) pharmacological antidotes, which counteract the pharmacological effects of absorbed poison without altering the biochemical lesion; and (*c*) specific antidotes, which interact directly with absorbed poison or some product of it to correct the biochemical lesion. These classes of antidotes are discussed in the following sections. There are few specific antidotes, but they are of such great interest that a separate section is devoted to each group of them.

8.2.3.1 Detoxifying or Neutralizing Antidotes.

This group of antidotes offers only imperfect protection against the poisons they help to combat. The compounds or complexes they form with the poisons may be slowly absorbed or they may break down, slowly permitting renewed absorption of the toxicant. Therefore, this group of antidotes generally should be used in combination with one or more maneuvers to remove the toxic agent.

Activated Charcoal, NF, USP. Activated charcoal presents a tremendous surface area capable of adsorbing a variety of compounds, including gases and dissolved materials. To be effective, the charcoal must be fresh. If it is stored unsealed, it gradually adsorbs vapors from the air and becomes worthless. The practical capacity of charcoal is illustrated by its use for the purification of drinking water or for the quantitative removal of organic material from water for chemical study (see Section 6.1.4.2). According to Andersen (1946), its value for treating poisoning was discovered about 1830 but largely forgotten until it was rediscovered by Lichtwitz in 1908 . Since then it has been advocated in standard texts, eg, Starkenstein *et al.* (1929).

Not all compounds are adsorbed by charcoal to the same extent. Only 35 mg of potassium cyanide is taken up from simple aqueous solution by 1 g of charcoal. However, activated charcoal will adsorb significant quantities of some pesticides, including mercury, strychnine, and nicotine (Andersen, 1946), as well as arsenic, phosphorus, and parathion (Gosselin and Smith, 1966). No doubt many pesticides that have not been tested can be adsorbed.

The adsorption of ionized chemicals by charcoal is influenced by pH; changes in pH that decrease dissociation of the chemical increase its adsorption. However, loss of adsorptive power may be compensated by increasing the proportion of charcoal in the mixture (Andersen, 1947). Adsorption of toxicants by a given amount of charcoal *in vitro* is reduced to about one-half or one-third if they are first mixed with either gastric contents or intestinal contents (Andersen, 1948a). Although the same reduction of adsorption undoubtedly occurs *in vivo*, there is no indication that, once adsorbed, toxicants are released in the lower gastrointestinal tract (Chin *et al.*, 1970). In spite of the lesser adsorption *in vivo*, the depth of narcosis produced by a standard dose of a barbiturate was markedly reduced (Andersen, 1948b) and the blood levels of several drugs were controlled (Andersen, 1948c; Chin *et al.*, 1970) when charcoal was given to intact animals. The drugs were given in a form most favorable for absorption, and of course it was found that charcoal was useless if it was given after absorption was complete. However, accidental poisoning frequently involves ingestion of tablets or some other formulation that tends to delay absorption by the gastrointestinal tract, and thus there is an opportunity for the poison to be adsorbed by charcoal.

Another kind of objective evidence for the value of charcoal was given by Gosselin and Smith (1966), who reported that charcoal-treated rats survived an oral dose of bichloride of mercury that killed all control rats, even though no attempt was made to accelerate passage of the poison through the intestine or to carry out any other treatment.

It is important that enough charcoal be used. Andersen (1948c) estimated that it required 4 g of charcoal to adsorb 1 g of sulfanilamide in dogs and 6 g to do the same thing in rabbits, even though he had shown earlier that only 1 g of charcoal was required to adsorb 1 g of the drug from water. Fortunately, charcoal is harmless in the gastrointestinal tract, and whatever action it has is all to the good.

"Universal Antidote." This mixture usually consisted of two parts activated charcoal, one part magnesium oxide, and one part tannic acid. The charcoal was supposed to act as a general adsorbent; the magnesium oxide was supposed to neutralize acids and act as a cathartic; and the tannic acid was supposed to precipitate some—but not all—metals and alkaloids. The difficulty is that the different parts of the mixture interfere with one another. Picchoni *et al.* (1965) reported that when the amount of charcoal was equal, activated charcoal alone was more effective than the "universal antidote" in protecting rats against strychnine, malathion, or pentobarbital. Thus, the ingredients of the "universal antidote," especially the charcoal, may be of value separately, but the mixture is not recommended.

Egg White and Milk. Proteins react with metals, especially mercury. Egg white, milk, and other demulcents hinder absorption less effectively than charcoal, but may be of some value if charcoal is not available promptly. Because of their amphoteric nature, proteins may be used to neutralize both acids and bases.

Acids and Alkalis. Within limits, acids may be used to neutralize alkalis and *vice versa*. Acids suitable for neutralizing alkalis that have been swallowed are dilute vinegar and dilute lemon juice. To about 100 ml of vinegar or juice add about 300 ml of water.

Alkalis suitable for neutralizing ingested acids include milk of magnesia and magnesium oxide. The dose of milk of magnesia for this purpose is 3 to 4 tablespoonsful. The dose of magnesium oxide is 20 g administered as a slurry in milk or in a mixture of egg white and milk. As already mentioned, the milk and egg white are active by themselves.

Baking soda or other carbonates should not be given by mouth to neutralize acids because they produce carbon dioxide, which may cause distension and perforation.

No acid or base should be put in the eye in the hope of neutralizing an accidental contamination. Instead, emphasis should be placed on thorough irrigation with water or with isotonic saline, if that is available.

Neutralizing solutions may be used on the skin, but they seldom are desirable. It is much better to flood the area with water than to wait even a few moments to prepare a neutralizing solution.

Tannic Acid, NF. A teaspoonful of tannic acid in water or very strong warm tea tends to precipitate strychnine, lead, and copper, as well as some other alkaloids and metals that are not pesticides. Tannic acid is of little use against nicotine, arsenic, or mercury (Sollmann, 1902).

Iodine Solution. Tincture of iodine, 15 drops in a half glass of water, is of some value in precipitating alkaloids (Sollmann, 1957).

Potassium Permanganate, USP. Potassium permanganate is a powerful oxidizing agent capable of destroying alkaloids, glycosides, cyanide, and some other organic poisons. Unfortunately, its efficiency in the presence of stomach contents or other organic matter is limited. A 1:2,000 solution may be given by mouth between bouts of vomiting or it may be used for lavage. The solution is irritant and must be filtered to be certain that no undissolved crystals are administered (Sollmann, 1957).

Dialysis Fluids. Dialysis is of two kinds, peritoneal and blood. In peritoneal dialysis, an essentially isotonic solution is introduced into the peritoneal cavity and later withdrawn. The peritoneum itself serves as the dialysis membrane. In hemodialysis, blood from an artery is passed through a tubular membrane, which is bathed in the dialysis fluid, before being returned to the body via a vein. Here, a plastic membrane serves for removal of toxic substances.

Both kinds of dialysis are used far more often for removing ordinary waste products or helping to restore water-electrolyte balance in persons with kidney failure that they are used for removal of foreign compounds. Either kind of dialysis may be used to remove water-soluble poisons. However, these are the very poisons that are effectively excreted by the intact kidney. Efforts have been made to develop dialysis fluids capable of accepting oil-soluble compounds. So far no system suitable for general use is available, but the dialysis of foreign compounds against activated charcoal is promising (Decker *et al.,* 1971). At present, dialysis is of greatest use in persons with kidney failure resulting from water-soluble toxicants.

Solutions for peritoneal dialysis and for hemodialysis are available commercially.

8.2.3.2 Pharmacological Antidotes. Drugs that have opposite actions to poisons but no direct interaction with them or with enzymes inhibited by them are generally spoken of as pharmacological or physiological antidotes. There is no doubt that by opposing the action of absorbed toxicants they can make the difference between life and death in some cases of poisoning.

Many of the drugs described in Section 8.2.2 on supportive treatment might be regarded as pharmacological antidotes. The distinction—which is academic—concerns the somewhat greater specificity of pharmacological antidotes. For example, a variety of sedatives and

hypnotics are valuable for treating patients who are overexcited, no matter whether the cause is severe fright or poisoning. However, because of their anticonvulsant and microsomal enzyme-stimulating properties, barbiturates act as pharmacological or even specific antidotes in connection with poisoning by chlorinated hydrocarbon insecticides. The detoxication effect may extend to other poisons, for example the anticoagulant rodenticides.

Atropine Sulfate, USP. Atropine is used to block the pharmacological effect of anticholinesterases, including organic phosphorus compounds and carbamate insecticides. Suffice it to say here that inhibition of cholinesterase at certain nerve endings permits an abnormal persistence and accumulation of acetylcholine normally produced by these endings. A small excess of acetylcholine produces excessive function of the end organ, which may be followed by cessation of function as the concentration of acetylcholine increases even further. Atropine makes some of these end organs insensitive to acetylcholine. Specifically, it helps to relieve excessive secretions of the respiratory tract, bronchospasm, and spasm of other smooth muscle. It is not effective in treating the effects of anticholinesterases on skeletal muscle.

Patients poisoned by organic phosphorus compounds or carbamates are tolerant to atropine and can receive large doses of it without experiencing rapid pulse (over 140 per minute), dryness of the mouth, and hot flushed skin that constitute atropinization when mild, and side effects when severe. In fact, tolerance to repeated doses of atropine is a useful sign of poisoning by anticholinesterases and justifies maintenances of atropinization and the addition of an oxime (see Section 8.2.3.3) to the regimen of treatment. Thus, the dosage of atropine for treating poisoning by an anticholinesterase is entirely different from those for other purposes. Under these circumstances, atropine sulfate has been given by intravenous infusion for hours at the rate of 10 mg every half hour, with great benefit to the patient. A total dose of 453 mg was required by a patient who recovered except for a mild paresis of the right arm unrelated to atropine (Milthers *et al.,* 1963).

Having made sure that the patient severely poisoned by an anticholinesterase has a clear airway and is not cyanotic, he should receive 2 to 4 mg of atropine sulfate intravenously. This dose should be repeated at intervals of 5 to 10 minutes until signs of mild atropinization appear and at less frequent intervals thereafter to maintain atropinization. The patient should be kept on the verge of atropine intoxication.

Smaller doses are indicated if poisoning is less severe. Atropinization needs to be maintained for only one or a few hours in case of poisoning by carbamates.

Atropine sulfate for injection is available in concentrations of 0.3, 0.4, 0.5, 0.6, and 1.2 mg/ml in 1-, 20-, and 30-ml ampules. It is also available to the military in automatic injectors which permit intramuscular injection under field conditions.

Anticonvulsants. Studies in animals have shown that barbiturates not only may be lifesaving, but that an animal poisoned by some convulsant compounds is tolerant to these drugs, requiring a dosage level for moderate sedation that would cause surgical anesthesia in a normal animal of the same species. In animals poisoned by dieldrin, successful treatment requires a high rate of administration for 2 weeks or more. The benefit of barbiturates in treating poisoning by chlorinated hydrocarbon insecticides is two-fold. Not only are they effective and relatively safe anticonvulsants, but some of them, notably phenobarbital (see below), are powerful inducers of microsomal enzymes.

Barbiturates are virtually nontoxic if their use is confined to periods of acute poisoning and if they are used in dosages that leave the patient conscious and able to respond. Higher dosages may produce respiratory depression.

Of the many excellent barbiturates available, two may be mentioned.

Pentobarbital Sodium, USP. Pentobarbital is classed as a short-acting barbiturate. Its effects last long enough to treat most cases of poisoning by chlorinated hydrocarbon insecticides. This is not true of the ultrashort-acting compounds such as thiopental.

Pentobarbital sodium for injection is supplied as a 50-mg/ml solution in 2-, 5-, 20-, and 50-ml containers. For oral administration it is supplied as 30-, 50-, and 100-mg capsules. For rectal administration it is supplied as 30-, 60-, 120-, and 200-mg suppositories.

Intravenous injection must be slow. The usual intravenous dose is 100 mg initially for adults and 50 mg for children. After at least 1 minute to determine the effect, additional doses may be given, up to a total of 500 mg (about 7 mg/kg) in adults. A dosage greater than the maximal one for ordinary purposes may be required in poisoning by aldrin, dieldrin, and perhaps other chlorinated hydrocarbon insecticides. An initial dosage of 20 mg/kg followed by a maintenance dosage of 5 mg/kg twice daily was optimal for this purpose in dogs. Man might not require so much, but the dosage should be increased until some degree of sedation is achieved.

The initial dose may be injected deeply into a large muscle. Deep injection helps to avoid intra-arterial injection, pain, sterile abscesses, or sloughs.

Phenobarbital, USP. Phenobarbital is a long-acting barbiturate. As such, it is rather too long lasting for initial use in poisoning but ideal if sedation or enzyme induction is required for several days or weeks.

Phenobarbital sodium for injection is available as 130-mg/ml solution in 1-ml containers and 160-mg/ml solution in 2- or 10-ml containers or as powder (120, 130, and 320 mg for making solutions). Phenobarbital for oral administration is available in various forms including 16-, 32-, 50-, 64-, and 100-mg tablets.

The usual dose as a hypnotic in adults is 100 to 200 mg. Ordinarily, total daily dosage in adults or children does not exceed 6 mg/kg. However, in persons poisoned by chlorinated hydrocarbon insecticides, a much higher dosage may be required to produce the desired degree of sedation.

Phenobarbital has been studied more than other barbiturates in connection with the induction of microsomal enzymes of the liver (see Section 3.1.2). Cueto and Hayes (1967) showed that repeated doses of phenobarbital reduce the storage of dieldrin that otherwise results from daily intake. There is some evidence from the same laboratory that phenobarbital can hasten the excretion of dieldrin already in the tissues. Although the action is indirect, the net effect is similar to that of some chelating agents toward heavy metals. Patients who receive large dosages of phenobarbital [or diphenylhydantoin (phenytoin, recINN)] in the treatment of epilepsy store less DDT, DDE, and dieldrin (see Section 7.2.4.1).

The dosage of phenobarbital known to cause induction of liver enzymes in man is 1 mg/kg/day (Thompson *et al.,* 1969). Higher dosages also are effective.

The use of barbiturates and perhaps other inducers of liver enzymes as pharmacological antidotes deserves more extensive study.

8.2.3.3 Oximes. Except for vitamins and other nutrients, few classes of drugs are known that correct a biochemical lesion directly. Even fewer classes of drugs have been developed as the result of a planned effort based on pharmacological theory, but the oximes fulfill these requirements (Nachmansohn and Wilson, 1956). Oximes release the enzyme acetylcholinesterase from combination with most organic phosphorus insecticides and thus restore the enzyme to normal function, sometimes with dramatic benefit to the patient

Specifically, the biochemical lesion corrected by oximes is the phosphorylation of acetylcholinesterase.

Because the phosphorylation is firm, the organic phosphorus compounds act as inhibitors of the enzyme rather than as substrates. Although the combination of enzyme and inhibitor is often spoken of as "irreversible," the term is justified only in contrast with the combination formed between the enzyme and its normal substrate, acetylcholine,.or even that between the enzyme and various carbamates. In fact, the prophylactic use of the carbamates physostigmine (eserine) and neostigmine (Comroe et al., 1946; Grob et al., 1947) probably represented the first experimental effort to interfere with the combination between an organic phosphorus compound and the enzyme. These carbamates almost certainly act by forming a relatively unstable bond, which serves to protect the enzyme during a limited period when the organic phosphorus compound is available in the circulation. The carbamates have no antidotal action when given after the poison, but have an additive action instead (Koster, 1946; Salerno and Coon, 1950).

Success in preventing the combination of organic phosphorus compounds with acetylcholinesterase was followed by attempts to disrupt the combination after it was formed. That disruption might be possible was indicated by the fact that, when the enzyme is inhibited by tepp, it recovers some of its activity if permitted to stand in water for a sufficiently long time. It is more difficult to reactivate an enzyme inhibited by DFP. Although some success in disrupting the bond between enzyme and inhibitor was achieved with choline, hydroxylamine (Wilson, 1951, 1952), and certain metal salts and chelates (Wagner-Jauregg et al., 1955), the greatest success was achieved with hydroxamic acids (Epstein and Freeman, 1955), and especially oximes (O'Leary et al., 1961). This development occurred essentially simultaneously on both sides of the Atlantic (Wilson and Ginsburg, 1955; Davies and Green, 1955).

The oximes and their action in reactivating phosphorylated acetylcholinesterase have been reviewed at length by Heath (1961), Hobbiger (1963), and Ellin and Wills (1964a, 1964b). The following paragraphs outline the findings considered important in the therapeutic use of oximes.

Mechanism of Action. It was expected that reagents (such as esters or acids) capable of making a nucleophilic attack on the phosphorus atom of phosphorylated cholinesterase would regenerate the enzyme. Theory further predicted that the presence within the reactivating molecule of a cationic structure, such as the ammonium radical, would facilitate this reaction by acting, as does the nitrogen atom in acetylcholine, to position the molecule properly for its reaction with the enzyme. The hydroxamic acids and oximes fulfilled these requirements imposed by theory by having both nucleophilic and cationic ammonium groupings in the molecule.

The mechanism of action of oximes in regenerating freshly inhibited cholinesterase is thought to consist of an initial direct combination between the organic phosphorus-inhibited enzyme and the hydroxamic acid, followed by a reaction in which the organic phosphorus moiety is split off and hydrolyzed. The hydroxamic acid residue is then released to regenerate the active enzyme. the important thing from a practical standpoint is that the hydroxamic acid has a greater affinity for the phosphorus moiety than does the enzyme.

Table 8-8 shows the chemical names, common names, and structural formulae of hydroxylamine and selected oximes. Those that have received most extensive clinical trial are discussed in separate paragraphs below. Some of their common pharmacological properties may now be reviewed briefly.

In addition to their desirable properties of (a) reactivating inactivated cholinesterase, (b) reacting directly with organic phosphorus molecules and thus detoxifying them, and (c) possibly having an anticholinergic effect similar to that of atropine, they also (d) depolarize the neuromuscular junction, (e) produce a sympathomimetic effect and potentiate the pressor effect of epinephrine, and (f) inhibit cholinesterase.

The clearly desirable properties just mentioned were taken into account by Green (1958) in constructing a mathematical model of the pharmacology of poisoning and treatment. In most instances, agreement between the experimental and calculated relative efficiencies of different therapeutic processes were in good quantitative agreement.

Reactivation of Cholinesterase. The reactivation of inhibited cholinesterase is the dominant effect of oximes in poisoned animals. *In vitro*, 2-PAM is a very powerful reactivator. At a concentration of 10^{-5} M, 2-PAM iodide reactivates as much as 80% of alkyl phosphate-inhibited enzyme within 1 minute (Wilson and Ginsburg, 1955; Davies and Green, 1955; Childs et al., 1955). The efficiency of reactivation differs greatly for enzyme inactivated by different classes of organic phosphorus insecticides. The fact that these differences are parallel *in vivo* and *in vitro* is good

Table 8-8

Chemical Name, Common Name, and Structural Formula
of Hydroxyl Amine and of Selected Oximes Used as Antidotes
in Poisoning by Organic Phosphorus Compounds

Chemical name	Common name	Structural formula
hydroxyl amine	--	(structure)
pyridine-2-aldoxime [a]	pralidoxime chloride [a]	(structure)
diacetylmonoxime	DAM	(structure)
monoisonitrosoacetone	MINA	(structure)
1,1'-trimethylene bis(4-formyl-pyridinium)	Trimedoxime (recINN) TMB-4 dibromide	(structure)
bis-(4-hydroxy-imino-methyl-pyridinium-(1)-methyl) ether dichloride	obidoxime chloride (pINN) BH-6 dichloride Lu H6, Toxogonin, Dimedoxodoxime	(structure)

a. Salts with the following anions have been studied: 2-PAM iodide (-I⁻); 2-PAM chloride, pralidoxime chloride or Protopam Chloride® (-Cl⁻); 2-PAM methanesulfonate or P2S (-SO₃CH₃⁻); 2-PAM-methylsulfate, 7676R.P., or Contrathion (-SO₄CH₃⁻).

evidence that the antidotal properties of oximes depend upon reactivation of inhibited cholinesterase.

In a comparative *in vitro* study of 2-PAM iodide, DAM, and monoisonitrosoacetone (MINA), Cohen and Wiersinga (1959) found that 2-PAM iodide was the most efficient reactivator, followed closely by MINA. The reactivation by DAM was slow when compared with those of the two other oximes. In a later paper, Cohen and Wiersinga (1960) theorized that the antidotal efficacy of DAM was primarily due to its ability to inactivate the organic phosphorus molecule, rather than its capacity to regenerate inhibited cholinesterase.

Direct Detoxication. Direct reaction between 2-PAM and organic phosphorus molecules has been shown to occur (Wagner-Jauregg and Hackley, 1953; Hobbiger, 1956). The importance of this reaction in either the prevention of dermal absorption or local effects of anticholinesterase compounds, or both, has been discussed by Summerson (1955). Kewitz *et al.* (1956) have, however, pointed out that it is unlikely that the direct reaction is an important factor in the antidotal action on systemic effects *in vivo*, inasmuch as *in vitro* experiments have shown that this direct reaction is very slow at concentrations obtainable under physiological conditions. These authors note that even with a 10^{-3} M concentration of 2-PAM iodide at 25°C, pH 7.8, only about 1% of paraoxon (10^{-4} M) reacts per hour. By contrast, Cohen and Wiersinga (1960) found that both DAM and MINA detoxified sarin during *in vitro* incubation. These authors suggested that DAM acts mainly by virtue of direct reaction with the toxicant, that 2-PAM acts primarily by reactivating inhibited enzyme, and that MINA shows both types of activity.

Atropine-like Effect. Lindgren and Sundwall (1960) found that the therapeutic effect of TMB-4 on bradycardia resembled that of atropine. Even in unpoisoned animals, TMB-4 strongly blocked the bradycardia and pressure waves caused by vagal stimulation without interfering with peristalsis; 2-PAM methane-sulfonate and DAM showed less vagolytic effect. Other evidence that oximes have some degree of anticholinergic action was established by Rajapurkar and Panjwani (1961) in studies of ciliary movement in the frog esophagus. This preparation has been shown to contain the acetylcholine-cholinesterase-choline acetylase system, but no nervous tissue. DAM produced slowing of the ciliary movement similar to that produced by atropine or curare. The action was the same in eserinized or normal cilia. Thus, apparently neither a central mechanism nor a reactivation of inhibited enzyme was responsible for the effect of DAM in this instance. Lehman (1962) reviewed a number of reports, some affirming and others refuting the finding that the oximes have an anticholinergic action similar to that of atropine. His own investigation showed that a concentration of 2-PAM chloride or TMB-4 too small to cause detectable reactivation of cholinesterase would, nevertheless, restore normal function of intestinal muscle. Lehman (1962) interpreted this finding as indicating that this atropine-like action "may be the initial event which saves the life of a poisoned animal by restoring the activity of the respiratory muscles and providing the period of grace during which cholinesterase reactivation can occur as a result of oxime action, other mechanisms, or both."

It appears impossible to determine at this time whether oximes exert a significant anticholinergic effect in poisoned mammals when given at therapeutic doses. However, the fact that a combination of atropine and oxime usually is superior to either drug alone in the treatment of poisoning is evidence that they have different mechanisms of action and that any anticholinergic action of oximes is of secondary importance under practical conditions.

Depolarization of the Neuromuscular Junction. Probably related to their atropine-like effect is the action of oximes in depolarizing the neuromuscular junction. Although the actions of both postganglionic, parasympathetic fibers and somatic motor nerves are mediated by acetylcholine, the first is blocked by atropine and the second by curare and related drugs. Wills *et al.* (1959) described experiments in anesthetized cats strongly suggesting that intravenous injection of 2-PAM iodide at less than the therapeutic rate led to depolarization of the neuromuscular junction; the treatment antagonized blocks produced by the competitive blocker d-tubocurarine and intensified those produced by depolarizing blockers

succinylcholine and decamethonium. A related finding is that lipid-soluble quaternary ammonium ions reduce the resting potential of nerve fibers (Dettbarn, 1959). It appears that depolarization of membranes is a general property of quaternary ammonium ions, limited only by their ability to reach the membrane.

It is not clear what importance oxime-induced depolarization of the neuromuscular junction may have in the treatment of poisoning by organic phosphorus compounds under practical conditions. It undoubtedly is involved in prolonging the effect of succinylcholine in a patient poisoned by parathion and treated with both 2-PAM-iodide and succinylcholine (Quinby *et al.*, 1963).

Ganglionic and Sympathomimetic Effects. Zarro and DiPalma (1965) reviewed earlier studies and reported extensive investigations of the sympathomimetic effects of 2-PAM chloride. They found that when given at a dosage of 10 mg/kg or more intravenously to dogs, this oxime caused a biphasic elevation of blood pressure characterized by an immediate spike followed by a sustained rise, maximal about 2 minutes after injection. The oxime also caused a rise in blood catecholamine levels in dogs receiving a constant infusion of norepinephrine. Studies of the normal and chronically denervated nictitating membrane of cats indicated that the action of 2-PAM chloride on this structure is mainly indirect and mediated by release of norepinephrine. It was concluded that both the direct ganglionic effect and the norepinephrine-mediated sympathomimetic effect paralleled the effect of nicotine. No measurement was made of cholinesterase, but (because some of the dosage rates caused muscle twitching and salivation) the possibility is not excluded that inhibition occurred. Thus, the possibility exists that the ganglionic and sympathomimetic effects of oximes are nicotinic effects secondary to inhibition of cholinesterase.

Inhibition of Cholinesterase. At sufficiently high dosages, 2-PAM iodide is capable of inhibiting both serum and erythrocyte cholinesterase *in vitro* (Holmes and Robins, 1955; Hobbiger, 1956; Grob and Johns, 1958). The same is true of motor end-plate cholinesterase previously inactivated by tepp; 2-PAM iodide reactivates the enzyme but inhibits it again if permitted to stay in contact too long (Bergner and Wagley, 1958). Although the antidotal dosages that have generally been used are below the toxic level, there would seem to be, on the basis of studies reported by Loomis (1956), a definite possibility of lessened antidotal effect if greater than the optimal dose of

2-PAM were given. This author noted that dogs given an intravenous dose of 0.06 mg of sarin per kilogram required more than 340 minutes to recover spontaneously their normal response to injected acetylcholine. Following intravenous administration of 10, 25, or 250 mg/kg of 2-PAM iodine to normal dogs, 2, 3, and 120 minutes, respectively, were required for return of the normal acetylcholine response. The same dosage levels of 2-PAM iodide, when given to sarin-poisoned dogs, produced return to normal acetylcholine response after 40 to 45, 80 to 100, and 120 minutes, respectively. These results indicate that 2-PAM iodide is a cholinesterase inhibitor, that 10 mg/kg was the optimal antidotal dosage under the condition of the test, and that larger doses were less effective.

It is important to note that in poisoned people given therapeutic doses, the inhibition of cholinesterase by 2-PAM is trivial, whereas the release of enzyme inhibited by the organic phosphorus compound is highly significant.

Other Factors Influencing the Action of Oximes. Both organic phosphorus compounds and oximes differ in their ability to pass the blood-brain barrier. In contrast to the quaternary oximes (2-PAM, TMB-4, and obidoxime), which are mainly peripheral in action, the nonquaternary oximes have a predominantly central action (Wills and Borison, 1959; Brown, 1960). DAM, a compound known to have its predominant effect on the central nervous system, has been shown to penetrate the blood-brain barrier and affect some reactivation of brain cholinesterase (Jager *et al.,* 1958; Edery, 1959). In fact, there is a possibility of excessive transfer, for DAM in large doses has produced coma in man (Jager and Stagg, 1958).

On the basis of its structure, 2-PAM would not be expected to cross the blood-brain barrier. Early studies in animals (Kewitz and Nachmansohn, 1957; Loomis, 1963) indicated it does not. However, it was frequently observed that certain patients treated with 2-PAM showed a rapid return of consciousness, which (in the absence of serious respiratory or circulatory difficulty in these particular cases) could not be explained by improved oxygen supply to the brain (Quinby and Clappison, 1961). The apparent contradiction of experience with animals and man was resolved by more refined measurements that detected traces of 2-PAM in the brains of animals (Firemark *et al.,* 1964). Furthermore, the concentration of oxime reaching the brain was increased by trichlorfon. It is not known whether other organic phosphorus compounds have the same effect.

Another important variable influencing the effectiveness of reactivation of inhibited cholinesterase is the phenomenon of "aging" of the enzyme-inhibitor complex. The combination becomes truly irreversible on standing and no longer susceptible to the action of oximes.

There are a few organic phosphorus insecticides, for example schradan, whose combination with cholinesterase is not influenced by known oximes. Apparently all these compounds are bisdiamids.

Side Effects of Oximes. As discussed above, very high doses of oximes produce undesirable side effects, the pharmacological basis of which is understood. Very high doses also have certain effects not yet explained. Thus, both 2-PAM iodide and DAM, when injected intravenously in large doses, have a direct depressant action on the respiratory center (Wislicki, 1960). However, when administered in therapeutic doses, oximes give few side effects and those that do occur are seldom severe enough to require discontinuation of therapy. As would be expected, side effects are less severe in poisoned persons than in volunteers involved in tests of safety, because in patients the poison may be thought of as "inactivating" the drug. Whether the side effects that do occur at therapeutic levels are caused by inhibition of cholinesterase is not clear, although this possibility must be considered, for many of the signs and symptoms closely resemble those of cholinesterase inhibition.

Furthermore, many distressing conditions seen in patients treated with oximes undoubtedly are caused by the poison and not by the drug. As long as any treatment prolongs life but does not produce recovery immediately, it can be expected to increase the incidence and severity of "side effects." With modern treatment, patients who formerly would have died in a few hours now survive for days, and some of them eventually go on to complete recovery. It is no wonder that such patients often exhibit findings that were—and are—rare in patients who were initially less seriously poisoned.

Rapid intravenous injection of 2-PAM iodide has produced transient mild weakness, diplopia, blurred vision, and dizziness in a high percentage of normal volunteers, and impairment of accommodation, headache, nausea, and tachycardia in some of them (Jager and Stagg, 1958; Jager *et al.,* 1958). There was no irritation at the point of injection even when extravasation occurred. There was no effect on blood pressure, respiration, or electrocardiogram at the dosage used. Laboratory study revealed no change in the formed elements of the blood, bleeding or clotting time, clot retraction, urinalysis, endogenous creatinine clearance, urinary urobilinogen, or bromosulfophthalein retention.

A few patients given 2-PAM iodide have complained of a bitter taste that no doubt resulted from the iodine moiety of the molecule; 2-PAM has also produced rhinitis and a feeling of fatigue in the jaws (Namba, unpublished data). Studies in volunteers indicated that iodine was responsible for the difficulty. Seven of nine normal men who took oral doses of 1 to 10 gm of 2-PAM iodide experienced pharyngeal pain and two had enlarged parotid glands. A similar group of volunteers who took oral, intravenous, or intramuscular doses of 2-PAM chloride did not experience these or any other toxic effects. Twenty-nine normal women took 2-PAM chloride by mouth at the rate of 1 to 4 g/day for 2 to 8 months. No significant toxic effects were revealed by repeated laboratory tests of the blood, urine, liver, and heart.

Temporary pain at the site of injection was the only significant side effect of automatic intramuscular injection of 2-PAM methane sulfonate into volunteers at the rate of 10 mg/kg. A therapeutically effective level (4 ppm) was achieved within 6 minutes and maintained about 90 minutes (Barkman et al., 1963).

Intravenous injection of DAM has caused a burning sensation at the site of injection radiating up the vein, giddiness, drowsiness, a sensation of warmth and tingling in the abdomen and chest, tachycardia, mild postural hypotension (Grob and Johns, 1958), and occasionally bitter taste, paresthesias and decreased position sense in the extremities, decreased sweating, transient loss of consciousness, clonic movements of the head, and decreased amplitude of the electroencephalogram and of the T-wave segment of the electrocardiogram (Jager and Stagg, 1958).

Many of the oximes liberate cyanide in the body and also on long standing in vitro (Askew et al., 1956; Brown, 1960). When there is doubt concerning the integrity of a 2-PAM preparation, particularly solutions of old or uncertain age, a simple test for free cyanide should be carried out.

Relative Worth of Different Oximes. It is clear that oximes differ in their properties, notably in their ability to pass the blood-brain barrier. Some oximes are distinctly more valuable than others for treating poisoning by specific organic phosphorus compounds of widely different type. In some tests in experimental animals, mixtures of oximes were more effective than either compound alone (O'Leary et al., 1961; Edery and Schatzberg-Porath, 1958; Shein, 1967). However, most organic phosphorus insecticides belong to a few closely related types, and poisoning by almost all of them is susceptible to treatment by the oximes available for prescription in different countries. All of these available drugs are effective. No systematic, comparative study has been made of their relative value for treating human, systemic poisoning by organic phosphorus insecticides. The value of 2-PAM, TMB-4, and obidoxime chloride (all at concentrations between 1 and 2 mg/drop) for correcting mioses caused by paraoxon was investigated in volunteers by Graupner and Wiezorek (1966). Although the authors drew certain distinctions, the actual record indicated no important difference in the value of the three drugs.

The only important difference among the salts of 2-PAM is their solubility. Of course, in comparing these salts, it is necessary to consider the amount of free base derived from the dose administered. For example, 1.0 g of 2-PAM chloride is equivalent to 1.53 g of the iodide, 1.43 g of the methylsulfate, or 1.34 g of the methanesulfonate. The first one developed was 2-PAM iodide, which is less soluble and less convenient to use than the others. A person receiving it may taste the iodine dissociated from it after injection. The use of 2-PAM iodide was abandoned as soon as other salts of 2-PAM became available.

Interaction of Oximes with Atropine. A matter of tremendous practical importance is the synergism of oximes and atropine in the treatment of poisoning by most organic phosphorus compounds (O'Leary et al., 1961). The synergism of oximes and atropine is especially evident in animals supported when necessary by artificial respiration; with such combined treatment, Bethe et al. (1957) were able to protect animals against 20 lethal doses of DFP, 70 of parathion, and 160 of paraoxon, even though any one of these treatments protected against no more than six lethal doses of any of the three poisons. Although numerical factors cannot be given in connection with poisoning in man, the fact of synergism is evident.

Pralidoxime Chloride, ND. Pralidoxime chloride (Table 8-8), generally referred to as 2-PAM chloride, is sold under the trade name Protopam Chloride. It is a white, nonhygroscopic, crystalline powder, which is soluble in water to the extent of 1 g in less than 1 ml.

The compound is absorbed from the gastrointestinal tract. Although absorption from an isolated intestinal loop of rats is complete in a few hours, the blood levels of drug achieved by oral dosage are relatively low because of the efficiency of metabolism and excretion (Levine and Steinberg, 1966). In many persons, less than half of an oral dose can be accounted for by excretion in 24 hours. However, animal experiments show that the drug may be highly effective if given by mouth in sufficient dosage. Of course, the toxic dose is increased also, and it is claimed that the therapeutic index of oral doses is greater (Lehman and Nicholls, 1960).

Pralidoxime chloride may be administered subcutaneously or intramuscularly, but in the early treatment of acute poisoning it is best given slowly, intravenously. When given in this way, it is immediately dispersed throughout the extracellular water. It does not enter the erythrocyte to a measurable degree and is not bound by plasma protein. The blood level falls rapidly due to excretion by the kidney. The halflife in man is about 0.9 hour. In a patient with chronic nephrosis and azotemia, the plasma level fell slowly. In a normal person, most of an intravenous dose is excreted within 6 hours. The rate of elimination in dogs is greater than the rate of glomerular filtration; active tubular secretion is the principal transport mechanism, but an element of nonionic diffusion cannot be excluded. Excretion is promoted by acidosis and inhibited by alkalosis (Jager et al., 1958; Berglund et al., 1962). Pralidoxime penetrates the eye to some extent following topical application, but it is usually injected subconjunctivally or directly into the anterior chamber when treatment of the eye is required (Mamo and Leopold, 1958; Byron and Posner, 1964; Dekking, 1964; Byron, 1963).

The mode of action and side effects of pralidoximes are described above in connection with oximes in general. Careful studies in volunteers and experience with patients indicate that side effects following therapy are infrequent and almost always mild. In fact, no serious side effects have ever been reported in patients that might not have been the result of poisoning alone. The serious effects that have been reported are as follows: a 16-month-old child poisoned by parathion developed acute laryngospasm 3 minutes after rapid intravenous injection of pralidoxime at the excessive rate of 50 mg/kg. Fatal cardiac arrest occurred at the moment of passage of an endotracheal tube (Prater, 1964). The same author mentioned transient muscle rigidity approaching opisthotonos, marked tachycardia, and priapism in another patient following injection of 2-PAM chloride that was considered too rapid. A number of treated patients

have exhibited "great excitement," mania, or "wild" behavior, apparently accompanied by hallucinations (Simon, 1963; Brachfeld and Zavon, 1965). It must be emphasized that similar disturbances have occurred in untreated cases or cases treated with atropine alone. Compounds producing this effect in the absence of oximes include parathion (Holmes et al., 1957), malathion (Wenzl and Burke, 1962), dichlorvos (Hayes, 1963), and certain mixtures (Arterberry et al., 1962).

There is an unpublished report of two cases of narcolepsy in persons who had earlier been treated with 2-PAM chloride. In the absence of similar reports, it is not clear that the narcolepsy was related to either poisoning or therapy.

Pralidoxime chloride is available in vials containing 1 g of sterile powder and also in the form of 500-mg tablets. A solution of the powder may be prepared by adding 20 ml of sterile water. Intravenous injection should occupy at least 5 minutes, and if feasible the drug should be added to a small infusion of glucose or saline and given by slow intravenous drip. The intravenous dose for adults is 1 g. Children should receive a proportional dosage no higher than 15 mg/kg. If required, the dose should be repeated in 1 hour. In very serious cases, the drug may be given by continuous drip at the rate of 0.5 g/hour, being careful not to overload the patient with fluid. Doses as high as 24 g in 6 days have been given to patients who survived without complications (Gitelson et al., 1966).

Although the practice apparently has not been reported, consideration might be given to administering the first dose intravenously and later doses by mouth, if vomiting caused by poisoning has been controlled sufficiently, and if additional treatment is required.

The oral therapeutic dose is 2 g for an adult; this dose may be repeated at about twice the rate used for intravenous therapy. As the patient improves, the dosage should be reduced gradually.

Kidney damage is not a contraindication to a single dose of 2-PAM but, if such damage is present, additional doses should be given with caution lest blood levels of the drug increase.

Obidoxime Chloride, pINN. Obidoxime chloride has the trade name Toxogonin as well as other names and code designations (see Table 8-8). The crystals are freely soluble in water, and the compound is stable in 1 to 10% aqueous solution.

In slightly atropinized dogs, obidoxime is efficient in increasing the activity of erythrocyte cholinesterase inhibited by a diethoxy organic phosphorus insecticide (parathion), less effective in reversing inhibition caused by several dimethoxy compounds, and ineffective in reversing inhibition caused by a bis-di-methylamid (triamphos) (Hahn and Henschler, 1969).

Obidoxime generally is administered to people intramuscularly. It is absorbed rapidly. Following intramuscular injection of 12 volunteers at a rate of about 3 mg/kg, a maximal blood level of almost 6 ppm was reached in 20 minutes. Within 2 hours, 52% of the injected dose was recovered in the urine, and 87% was recovered in 8 hours (Erdmann et al., 1965). Entirely similar results were reported by Sidell and Groff (1970) in a study involving 10 volunteers and dosages of 2.5 to 10 mg/kg. The average plasma halflife was found to be 83 minutes.

Side effects of obidoxime chloride include pain at the site of injection, a sensation of heat and tension in the upper part of the body, especially the facial area, and a menthol taste in the nasopharynx (Erdmann et al., 1965; Sidell and Groff, 1970). A sensation that the eyes are enlarged, dryness of the mouth, paresthesia in the arms and fingers, and objective warmth and reddening of the affected area around the mouth may occur. Dosages of 5 mg/kg or higher produce an increase in heart rate and a moderate increase in systolic and diastolic blood pressure (Sidell and Groff, 1970).

Based on a review of various studies in animals, Sidell and Groff concluded that obidoxime is generally more effective and also more toxic than pralidoxime. In animals the therapeutic advantage appears to lie with obidoxime. However, there are so few reports of treatment of patients with obidoxime that its real value in man is less clear than the value of pralidoxime. This is true even though it has been employed in the successful treatment of poisoning by large doses of parathion taken with suicidal intent. In one case, 16 doses of obidoxime chloride (250 mg each or a total of 58 mg/kg) were given during the first day of illness with somewhat smaller dosages on subsequent days. No side effects of the kind listed above were reported in patients (Barckow et al., 1969).

Some patients treated with obidoxime did exhibit a disturbance of liver function as indicated by abnormal SGOT and similar tests (Barckow et al., 1969). A review of cases showed that liver injury had been reported prior to the introduction of oximes, indicating that intoxication itself can be responsible for the damage (Boelcke et al., 1970). Furthermore, tests in dogs showed that parathion, but not obidoxime, resulted in abnormal SGOT

and similar tests; in fact, obidoxime prevented change in the test results when given to dogs that received parathion also (Boelcke and Gaaz, 1970). In a similar way, obidoxime or atropine prevented to a large degree the decrease in secretion of bile and bilirubin produced in rats by parathion (Boelcke and Kamphenkel, 1970). However, in rats, but not in rabbits, obidoxime showed a tendency to cause the same effect as organic phosphorus compounds on the elimination of bromosulfophthalein (Boelcke et al., 1970).

8.2.3.4 Chelating Agents. Chelation and related terms are derived from the Greek word *chele*, a claw. Chelation is sometimes called sequestration. A chelating agent is any compound capable of forming a complex with a polyvalent metal whereby the metal is held by one or more ligands, often to form one or more five- or six-membered rings. Such compounds are called chelates. A ligand is any atom, ion, or molecule capable of functioning as a donor partner in one or more coordinate bonds. In living systems, ligands are usually sulfur, nitrogen, or oxygen, often in the form of —SH, —NH_2, —OH, —COO, and —$PO_4\overline{H}_2$ groups. A natural chelating agent is protoporphyrin III; combined with ferrous ion it forms the chelate, heme. Other natural chelates include vitamin B_{12} (cobalt), cytochrome oxidase (iron and copper), and chlorophyll (magnesium). Extensive basic information on chelation is contained in a book edited by Dwyer and Mellor (1964).

The toxic effects of heavy metals are explained, at least in part, by their combination with the ligands (eg, —SH groups) of enzymes and other critical compounds in the tissues. Chelating agents may capture heavy metal ions before they combine with the tissues or extract them from combinations already formed with tissues. Once captured by a chelating agent, the heavy metal may be excreted more readily and with less tissue damage than if it were not chelated. Increased excretion may be of therapeutic value or it may serve as a diagnostic test. In other instances, increased excretion has not been demonstrated, and it is speculated that the beneficial effect observed is associated with redistribution of the metal in the body.

Each chelating compound has distinctive pharmacological properties depending on the ligands it provides, its distribution in the tissues, its rate of metabolism (if any), and its rate of excretion. These properties not only establish the usefulness of each compound but also its toxicity. By necessity, therapeutic chelating agents act in competition with a variety of ligands of the tissues. Metals normally found in the body may act as interfering substances. For example, EDTA reacts with calcium about 1000 times more readily than with zinc.

Other limits on the value of chelating agents arise from the fact that they are always partially dissociated and some of them are readily broken down in the body. The possibility that molecules of heavy metal produce some injury even when chelated is difficult to prove but has not been excluded. What has been proved is that BAL reacted with inorganic mercury *in vitro* is highly toxic when injected, presumably because the BAL is oxidized *in vivo*, thus releasing ionic mercury (Gilman *et al.*, 1946). Even chelating agents that are more stable must be used in adequate dosage or some degree of characteristic injury may be detected in survivors. This has been illustrated clearly for kidney damage caused by inorganic mercury and treated with different dosages of penicillamine (Aposhian and Aposhian, 1959). On a molar basis, it may always be necessary to have an excess of chelating agent to compensate for decomposition of the chelator and dissociation of the complex.

Table 8-9 shows chelating agents that are recognized or proposed for treating poisoning by one or more pesticides. One of them is the calcium disodium salt of EDTA. Some hint of the variety of known chelating agents may be gained from Table 8-10, which shows the structure of several derivatives of EDTA and the metals they are known to bind. Although the value of some chelating agents is known, they present so many variables that, like other drugs, they eventually must be tested empirically in man. The value of some of them, including BAL to combat arsenic and calcium disodium edetate to combat lead, is well established. It is entirely too early, however, to say that better chelating agents cannot be found for these old uses and too early for an answer on the real value of many other uses to which chelating agents might be put as antidotes. The mere fact that a chelating agent is effective in promoting the excretion of a metal does not ensure that it will be useful for therapy. BAL promotes the excretion of lead but is of little or no value in treating poisoning by lead. On the contrary, dithizon is a chelating agent which, according to Chamberlain *et al.* (1958), is definitely beneficial in the treatment of poisoning by thallium in animals and man, even though there is no evidence that it promotes excretion of thal-

Table 8-9

Some Chelating Agents and the Metals They Bind

Compound	Formula[a]	Metal chelated
dimercaprol (BAL)[b] pINN	H_2-C-SH $H\ \ -C-SH$ H_2-C-OH	As[c], Hg[c], Au[c], Sb, Ca, Cr, Bi, Ni, Cu
calcium disodium edetate (sodium calcium edetate, recINN)	$O=C-O\diagdown\quad\diagup O-C=O$ $\qquad\quad Ca$ $H_2-C-N\diagdown\qquad\diagup N-CH_2$ $H_2-C\quad CH_2-CH_2\quad CH_2$ $O=C-O^-\quad O^--C=O$ $\qquad Na^+\ Na^+$	Pb[c], Cr, Cd, Ni, Cu, Mn, Zn
penicillamine recINN	$\qquad CH_3\quad\ \ O$ $CH_3-C-CH-C-OH$ $\qquad SH\quad NH_2$	Cu[c], Pb, Hg, Fe
dithizon	$\bigcirc-N=N-C-NH-N-\bigcirc$ $\qquad\qquad\ \ S\qquad\ \ H$	Tl[c], Co, Cu, Pb, Hg
deferoxamine pINN	$NH_2-(CH_2)_5-N-C-\left[(CH_2)_2-C-NH-(CH_2)_5-N-C-\right]CH_3$ $\qquad\qquad OH\ O\qquad\qquad O\qquad\qquad\qquad OH\ O\ \ ]_2$	Fe^{3+}[c]

a. Ligands are underlined.
b. The reaction between British antilewisite (BAL) and the war gas lewisite is as follows:

$$BAL + Cl_2-As-CH\!\equiv\!CHCl \longrightarrow \begin{matrix} H_2-C-S \\ H\ -C-S \\ H_2-C-OH \end{matrix}\!\!\diagup\!\!As-CH\!\equiv\!CHCl + 2HCl$$

c. Indicates a toxic metal the chelation of which, clearly, is therapeutic.

Table 8-10

Derivatives of Ethylenediaminetetraacetic Acid (EDTA) or of
Some of its Analogs, All of Which Have the General Formula:

$$O=\overset{|}{C}-\underline{O}-R' \quad R'-\underline{O}-\overset{|}{C}=O$$
$$H_2C \qquad\qquad CH_2$$
$$N-R-N$$
$$H_2C \qquad\qquad CH_2$$
$$O=\overset{|}{C}-\underline{O}-R' \quad R'-\underline{O}-\overset{|}{C}=O$$

Compound	R	R'	Metals chelated
EDTA recINN	$-CH_2-CH_2-$	$-H$	Ca, Zn, Mn, Pb, V
CaNa$_2$EDTA recINN	$-CH_2-CH_2-$	Ca, Na$_2$[a]	Pb, Cr, Ni, Cu, M
BAETA	$-CH_2-CH_2-\underline{O}-CH-CH-$	$-H$	Sr^{90}
ACTA	$-CH_2-CH_2-\underline{O}-CH-CH-$ $H_2C \quad CH_2$ H_2C-CH_2	$-H$	Fe
DCTA	$-CH-CH-$ $H_2C \quad CH_2$ H_2C-CH_2	$-H$	Fe
DTPA	$-CH_2-CH_2-N-CH_2-CH_2-$ CH_2 $C=O$ $\underline{O}H$	$-H$	Pu, Th, Fe
DTPA-E	same as DTPA	$-C_2H_5$	Pu

a. See Table 8-9.

lium. Chelating agents may, of course, have actions not directly related to chelation. For example, BAL is a reducing agent and converts methemoglobin to hemoglobin.

It is of interest in passing that a number of drugs with hormonal action (epinephrine and cortisone), antibiotic action (penicillin, streptomycin, terramycin, isoniazide), or other actions (aspirin and Antabuse) are chelating agents. It has been speculated, or in some instances proved, that these drugs function by transporting trace metals to or from the tissues or microorganisms.

Dimercaprol, USP, BP, pINN. Dimercaprol is dimercaptopropanol, more commonly known as BAL even to pharmacologists (see Table 8-9). BAL is an abbreviation for British anti-lewisite. It was developed by Peters *et al.* (1945) for treatment of poisoning by the vesicant war gas, β-chlorethyldichloroarsine (Cl—CH—CH—As—Cl$_2$) called lewisite. BAL constitutes one of the best examples of a compound capable of repairing a biochemical lesion. In fact, the term, first introduced in connection with thiamine deficiency (see Section 4.1.2), may have been first applied to poisoning by a foreign chemical in connection

with the research leading to the discovery of BAL. The antidote was developed logically rather than by screening. It was known that monothiol compounds such as cysteine and glutathione give some protection against arsenoxide by forming thioarsenites. It was found that lewisite forms highly dissociable combinations of the form —S—As—S— with the sulfhydryl groups of keratin. It was reasoned that simple dithiols might form more stable compounds with trivalent arsenic than monothiols do. BAL was one of the first of the simple dithiols synthesized and tested.

BAL acts by reversing the action of some metals (calcium, arsenic, mercury, gold, antimony, chromium, bismuth, nickel, and copper), which react with sulfhydryl groups of enzymes to form mercaptides. It is ineffective against a metal (selenium), which inhibits sulfhydryl enzymes by oxidation. BAL is actually injurious to patients poisoned by selenium, cadmium, and iron, because the complexes formed are more toxic than each metal alone, especially to the kidneys.

Not only does BAL react with some toxic metals, but also with trace metals in the prosthetic groups of some enzymes such as catalase, carbonic anhydrase, and peroxidase. BAL also inactivates insulin.

The intramuscular LD 50 of BAL in experimental animals varies from 50 to 100 mg/kg. Fatal doses cause severe metabolic acidosis with a fall in the pH and CO_2-combining power of the blood. There is an initial rise of blood sugar with a terminal fall as the liver glycogen is exhausted. Blood lactic acid is increased, probably as the result of marked inhibition of cellular respiration, especially the cytochrome system. In animals large doses cause ataxia, urination, and stimulation of external respiration. Fatal doses cause respiratory depression, pulmonary edema, convulsions, and a fall of blood pressure to shock levels.

A dosage of 2.5 mg/kg can be injected intramuscularly without side effects and repeated at 4-hour intervals without cumulation. In fact, doses as high as 5 mg/kg have been given every 3 hours without evidence of cumulative effect. However, individual doses at rates as low as 3.0 mg/kg often produce paresthesias of the eyes, nose, mouth, and skin; tearing and blinking of the eyes; perspiration; salivation; vomiting; pain of any part; apprehension; weakness; fatigue; and an increase in heart rate and blood pressure. All these effects appear soon after an intramuscular injection but last only an hour or two, even after a large dose. Judging from the character and intensity of signs following therapeutic doses, man is no more susceptible than experimental animals to poisoning by BAL. Thus, the drug appears to be safe. If the side effects are excessive they may be diminished by either ephedrine sulfate (50 mg) or diphenhydramine hydrochloride (50 mg).

BAL is valuable for treating poisoning by all pentavalent compounds of arsenic and all trivalent compounds of it except arsine (AsH_3), for which the oxygen ethyl ether of BAL is effective. It is also useful for treatment of poisoning by compounds of antimony, bismuth, chromium, nickel, polonium, tungstate, and gold, and for early treatment of poisoning by mercury. It is ineffective for most other metals.

BAL is an oily liquid with the offensive odor of a mercaptan. It is soluble in water to the extent of 8.7% but aqueous solutions are unstable. BAL is soluble and stable in vegetable oils and is supplied as a 10% solution (100 mg/ml) in peanut oil with 20% benzyl benzoate as a stabilizer in 3-ml containers.

Dimercaprol is injected intramuscularly except when used for treating skin injured by lewisite or similar materials. Ten times the intramuscular dose may be applied to the skin without producing systemic toxicity. It is important to continue the treatment until the patient has recovered and to renew the treatment if signs and symptoms of metal poisoning recur.

It is recommended that in systemic poisoning by arsenic BAL be given intramuscularly at a rate of 2.5 mg/kg every 4 hours for 2 days, every 6 hours on the 3rd day, and every 12 hours for 10 additional days. In poisoning by inorganic mercury, it is desirable to clear as much mercury as possible at the earliest moment to avoid kidney damage. Therefore, in this condition, it is recommended that the initial dosage be 5 mg/kg, followed by 2.5 mg/kg every 12 hours for a total of 10 days.

Calcium Disodium Edetate, USP (*Sodium Calcium Edetate* recINN). This material, also called calcium disodim versenate, is the monocalcium disodium salt of ethylenediaminetetraacetic acid or EDTA (Tables 8-9 and 8-10). It is a white, crystalline, slightly hygroscopic powder. It is freely soluble in water.

EDTA was used as an analytical reagent and as a chemical in the manufacture of dyes as early as 1935. Later, the proposal to use the acid as a food additive led to its thorough toxicological study. It was found that it produced lowered serum calcium levels, if administered rapidly to animals. The change in serum calcium was small or absent following gradual dosing, which nevertheless caused an overall loss of calcium. The disodium salt without calcium (disodium edetate) is used investigationally in situations in which reduction of blood calcium levels is desired (American Medical Association, 1971).

Calcium disodium edetate has little or no effect on the level of calcium in the blood or on its storage. This drug was first introduced for medical use in 1951 when Bessman *et al.* (1952) employed it to treat encephalopathy caused by lead.

The side effects of disodium edetate are those of hypocalcemia, including tetany, convulsions, and respiratory and cardiovascular collapse. $CaNa_2$ EDTA lacks these serious effects. Its side effect resembles fume fever. This begins within 8 hours after infusion and is characterized by malaise, fatigue, thirst, fever, chills, myalgia, headache, anorexia, and occasionally nausea and vomiting. Side effects may also resemble a histaminic reaction characterized by sneezing, nasal congestion, and lacrimation. In rare instances, $CaNa_2$ EDTA produces glycosuria, anemia, or dermatitis. The drug should be used cautiously if renal disease is present.

$CaNa_2$ EDTA is of great value in treating

most cases of acute and chronic poisoning by lead. The excretion of lead may be increased as much as 40 times. However, the drug may make lead encephalopathy worse, presumably by increasing the concentration of available lead within the central nervous system. The drug may be of value in poisoning by cadmium, chromium, copper, manganese, nickel, and zinc.

The use of $CaNa_2$ EDTA in the diagnosis of lead poisoning is described in Section 8.1.4.1.

Calcium disodium edetate suitable for intravenous injection is available in the form of a 20% solution (200 mg/ml) in 5-ml containers. It usually is given intravenously as an infusion in either 5% glucose or isotonic sodium chloride, so that the concentration of $CaNa_2$ EDTA does not exceed 0.5%. Higher concentrations may lead to thrombophlebitis. For adults, the usual dose is 1 g dissolved in 250 ml or more of fluid, and injected intravenously over a period of 1 hour. Usually two such doses are given daily for 3 to 5 days. The maximal intravenous dosage for adults or children is 37.5 mg/kg/hour, 75 mg/kg/day, and 375 mg/kg/week. If a second course of injections is required, there should be a rest period of at least 1 week. More than two courses are generally inadvisable. Ordinarily, the total dosage should not exceed 550 mg/kg.

Dithizon. Dithizon is diphenylthiocarbazone (Table 8-9). It is a sensitive reagent for several heavy metals, including cobalt, copper, lead, and mercury. It is much used in measuring traces of lead. It apparently has not been placed in any official list of drugs. Lund (1956) showed that oral doses of dithizon at a rate of 20 mg/kg/day for 5 days completely protected rats that had received an otherwise fatal dose of thallium sulfate (30 mg/kg, subcutaneously). This dosage did not affect blood sugar, but larger doses given intravenously cause diabetes and other serious permanent injury in some species (see Sections 4.2.9.7 and 4.2.8.1). Chamberlain *et al.* (1958) used the analytical grade of dithizon to treat children poisoned by thallium. They found it clinically beneficial in five of six cases, and noted no side effects even though they made a special search for any diabetogenic action. Even though the patients were made better by dithizon, they showed no increase in urinary excretion of thallium. Action of the drug may involve some redistribution of the poison in the body. It seems at least as likely, however, that fecal excretion is increased, for the element is secreted in the bile and from the wall of the upper gastrointestinal tract.

Reagent grade dithizon is a bluish black crystalline powder. It is insoluble in water and sparingly soluble but unstable in alcohol. In order to treat children, Chamberlain ground it with guar gum and a little water in a mortar. The resulting thick, gelatinous suspension was administered immediately through a nasogastric tube by means of a large syringe. This method need not be used in older patients able to swallow dithizon in capsules.

Penicillamine, USP, recINN. Although systemic poisoning of normal persons by copper is unusual, it can occur. Penicillamine is the drug of choice for removing excess copper from the body. Of course, it finds its main use in treatment of hepatolenticular degeneration (Wilson's disease) associated with an inborn error of metabolism.

The most common side effects from penicillamine involve rash and other signs of hypersensitivity. Although the side effects generally are not severe enough to require that treatment be stopped, the skin should be examined carefully, and urinalysis, differential blood counts, direct platelet counts, and measurements of hemoglobin should be done every 3 days for the first 2 weeks and every 10 days for 3 or 4 months after treatment.

The use of penicillamine in the diagnosis of overexposure to lead is described in Section 8.1.4.1. Its use in the treatment of lead poisoning in man has been suggested (Ohlsson, 1962).

Penicillamine is furnished in 250-mg capsules. The usual dosage for adults is 250 mg four times daily and increased gradually up to a maximum of 4 to 5 g/day. The effect can be followed by measuring urinary copper.

8.2.3.5 Antidotes for Poisoning by Cyanide.

Poisoning by cyanide is one of the few kinds of intoxication in which two entirely different types of drugs are used in a specific antidotal system. Each makes its own contribution to resolution of the biochemical lesion, which is inhibition of cytochrome oxidase. Although cyanide inhibits some 40 enzymes, it is the inhibition of cytochrome oxidase that blocks tissue respiration and is critical to survival. Treatment consists of (*a*) displacing cyanide from cytochrome oxidase by converting about 20 to 25% of the hemoglobin of the blood to methemoglobin (which, unlike hemoglobin, has a tremendous affinity for cyanide), and (*b*) ensuring an adequate supply of sulfur to permit conversion of cyanide ion to the relatively nontoxic thiocyanate ion under the influence of rhodanese (transsulfurase) in the plasma. Methemoglobin is formed by means of amyl nitrite and sodium nitrite. Sodium thiosulfate serves as a source of sulfur.

It must be emphasized that supportive treatment (clearing of the airway; oxygen, preferably under pressure; and artificial respiration) may be at least as important as the specific treatment in determining survival.

Amyl Nitrite, NF. Amyl nitrite is a clear yellowish liquid which is volatile even at low temperatures. Like other nitrites, it causes relaxation of smooth muscles and the conversion of hemoglobin to methemoglobin. In the treatment of cyanide poisoning, the fall in blood pressure, acceleration of the heart, and flushing of the face, resulting from a reduction of arteriolar tension, are undesirable but unavoidable side effects.

Amyl nitrite is supplied in easily breakable 0.18- and 0.3-ml containers. The material is administered by crushing one of these "pearls" in a handkerchief, which is held over the patient's nose until his face flushes. The handkerchief is then returned to the nose for about a quarter to a half of every minute until sodium nitrite can be readied for intravenous injection. The advantage of the amyl nitrite is the speed with which it can be administered. Its disadvantage is the variability of the dosage of a vapor.

Sodium Nitrite, USP. The actions of sodium nitrite are the same as those of amyl nitrite, but its administration is much more easily controlled. In use, 300 mg of sodium nitrite (10 ml of a 3% solution) is injected intravenously at a rate of 2.5 to 5 ml per minute. Then, through the same needle one injects 50 ml of a 25% solution of sodium thiosulfate over a period of 10 minutes.

Sodium Thiosulfate, USP. Cyanide is detoxicated mainly by conversion to thiocyanate. Although the amount of sulfur in the tissues available for this conversion is entirely adequate for metabolism of the small amounts of cyanide encountered by everyone daily, it is inadequate for rapid detoxication of injurious doses of cyanide. Thiosulfate ion constitutes a ready source of sulfur for the formation of thiocyanate ion. Following the administration of sodium nitrite, 50 ml of a 25% solution of sodium thiosulfate should be injected intravenously at the rate of about 5 ml per minute. At least 0.9 g of sodium nitrite and 37.5 g of sodium thiosulfate have been administered in a case with full recovery (Hirsch, 1964). These doses are much larger than those listed in the US Pharmacopeia (1970), but may be required if cyanide poisoning is severe.

8.2.3.6 Oxygen. Because of the tremendous value of oxygen in the supportive treatment of a variety of conditions, oxygen therapy is described in Section 8.2.2.2. However, it must be pointed out here that oxygen qualifies as a specific antidote in poisoning by carbon monoxide and cyanide.

The rate of displacement of carbon monoxide from hemoglobin is increased by increasing the concentration of oxygen in the plasma. Furthermore, an increased level of plasma oxygen is a valid, pharmacological way of providing oxygen to the tissues. This latter action may reach an effective level soon after oxygen is administered, whereas repair of the biochemical lesion progresses more slowly. The oxygen tension in the red cells and in the tissues is in equilibrium with that in the plasma at the same anatomical site. In the lung, the oxygen tension in the plasma is only slightly less than that in the alveolar air, which corresponds to a normal oxygen concentration there of 14.2% by volume and is, therefore, 100 mm of mercury (at standard atmospheric pressure, body temperature, and saturation as regards water vapor). Under normal conditions, the concentration of oxygen dissolved in the water of the arterial blood is 0.3 volumes per 100 ml (vol %). By contrast, if the concentration of oxygen is increased to 100% by therapy using a suitable mask, the oxygen tension in the arterial blood becomes 673 mm Hg, and the concentration that is physically dissolved becomes 2.0 vol %. Since the hemoglobin of arterial blood is almost completely saturated with oxygen under normal conditions, the breathing of 100% oxygen by a normal person does not significantly increase the amount of oxygen carried in that way, but it does increase the total oxygen content of the arterial blood by about 10% by increasing the physically dissolved oxygen. Because only a part of the hemoglobin of a person poisoned by carbon monoxide can carry oxygen, the same increase in dissolved oxygen constitutes a greater percentage increase in the total oxygen content of the arterial blood, for example, about a 20% increase in a person of whose hemoglobin half is rendered useless by carbon monoxide. The physically dissolved oxygen is transferred to the tissues with unusual efficiency because of the great difference in its tension in the arterial—and even the capillary—blood as compared with the tissues. At the higher partial pressure, oxygen can compete against carbon monoxide more effectively for hemoglobin and, by mass action, speed the elimination of the poison.

The exact mechanism or mechanisms by which oxygen is beneficial in the treatment of poisoning by cyanide is unknown, but the reality of the benefit has been demonstrated experimentally as well as clinically. It is assumed that at least one effect is the displacement of cyanide from cytochrome oxidase by mass action.

8.2.3.7 Calcium. Calcium is a specific corrective for hypocalcemia of whatever cause, including poisoning by oxalic acid and oxalates. Furthermore, animal experiments show that calcium is both prophylactic and antidotal in poisoning by DDT. Even though blood calcium ordinarily is not depressed in poisoning by DDT, recent discoveries about the mode of action of this compound suggest that calcium may act to stabilize the surface membrane of nerve axons and thus help to correct the biochemical lesion. To what extent calcium is effective in treating poisoning by other chlorinated hydrocarbon insecticides and other convulsant poisons is not known. Presumably, it would benefit only conditions involving a disturbance of axonal transmission.

Calcium Gluconate, USP. This is the compound of choice for intravenous administration of calcium. It is not recommended for intramuscular use because the dose must be large and the danger of sterile abscess formation is too great. This compound or calcium lactate may be used for oral maintenance, but initial treatment of poisoning must be intravenous.

Calcium gluconate is supplied as a 10% solution in 10-ml containers and as 300-, 500-, 600-, and 1,000-mg tablets. Initial treatment should be the slow intravenous injection of 10 ml of 10% solution (1,000 mg). For a person weighing 70 kg, this represents a dosage of 14.3 mg/kg. A dosage of 40 mg/kg is effective in treating animals poisoned by DDT. Moeschlin (1965) recommends an initial dosage of about 57 mg/kg in the treatment of poisoning by oxalates. Once tetany or convulsions are controlled, adequate calcium levels may be maintained by a slow intravenous drip of a 0.3% solution (30 ml of a 10% solution in 1 liter of balanced saline injection).

8.2.3.8 Vitamin K. Although the complete details of how warfarin and related anticoagulants act at a molecular level is not known, it is clear that they are competitive antagonists of vitamin K in the formation of prothrombin. Whether experimental animals will develop hemorrhage when given a moderate daily dose of anticoagulant can be regulated by the dosage of vitamin K they receive concurrently. Clinically, low levels of prothrombin may be returned to normal by doses of the vitamin sufficient to counteract the poison. Although vitamin K is a specific antidote for poisoning by dicoumarin and indandione anticoagulants,

some time is required for the formation of new prothrombin after the drug is administered. If hemorrhage is actually present, preformed prothrombin should be supplied at once by a small transfusion of carefully matched, fresh, whole blood. If hemorrhage is only potential, treatment with vitamin K is sufficient. Any form of the vitamin is effective, but phytonadione (vitamin K_1) has the advantages that its action is more prompt, potent, and prolonged than that of other forms, and it does not hemolyze the red cells of persons deficient in glucose-6-phosphate dehydrogenase (see Section 3.1.3.3).

Vitamin K must be administered with great care to patients to whom anticoagulants have been given purposely to combat intravascular clotting. Here, the vitamin must be "titrated" against the anticoagulant, lest the patient be reexposed to the same threat of clotting that led to anticoagulant therapy in the first place. No such problem exists in treating persons poisoned accidentally or suicidally by anticoagulant rodenticides. There is no evidence that an oversupply of vitamin K produces in normal persons any excessive tendency of the blood to clot.

Phytonadione, USP (*Phytomenadione,* recINN). This is the naturally occurring form of vitamin K. It not only is a specific antagonist against coumarin and indandione compounds, but it is useful in treating the hemorrhagic effects of some other drugs, including salicylates, phenylbutazone, quinine, quinidine, sulfonamides, and barbiturates.

Intravenous injection can cause flushing of the face, a feeling of constriction in the chest, peripheral vascular collapse, sweating, and cyanosis. Subcutaneous and intrauscular injection may cause pain and the delayed formation of a nodule at the point of injection.

Phytonadione for injection is supplied as a solution containing 2 mg/ml in 0.5-ml containers, and as a solution containing 10 mg/ml in 1-, 2.5-, and 5-ml containers. It is also supplied in tablets and capsules containing 5 mg. For poisoning by anticoagulant rodenticides, phytonadione should be given intravenously in a dose of 10 to 50 mg at a rate of not over 5 mg/minute, best administered as a drip following dilution in 5% dextrose or isotonic saline. This treatment should be given three times in the first 24 hours. Smaller doses should be continued until the prothrombin level is normal.

REFERENCES

Abdallah, A. H., and Tye, A. (1967). A comparison of the efficacy of emetic drugs and stomach lavage. Am. J. Dis. Child., 113:571–575.

Ackroyd, J. F. (1949a). The pathogenesis of thrombocytopenic purpura due to hypersensitivity to sedormid. Clin. Sci., 7:249–283.

Ackroyd, J. F. (1949b). The mechanism of the reduction of clot retraction by sedormid in the blood of patients who have recovered from sedormid purpura. Clin. Sci., 8:235–267.

Ackroyd, J. F. (1949c). The cause of thrombocytopenia in sedormid purpura. Clin. Sci., 8:269–289.

Ackroyd, J. F. (1951). The role of complement in sedormid purpura. Clin. Sci., 10:185–207.

Ackroyd, J. F. (1952). Sedormid purpura: an immunological study of a form of drug hypersensitivity. Prog. Allergy, 3:531–572.

Ackroyd, J. F. (1953). Allergic purpura including purpura to foods, drugs and infections. Am. J. Med., 14:605–632.

Ackroyd, J. F. (1954). The role of sedormid in the immunological reaction that results in platelet lysis in sedormid purpura. Clin. Sci., 13:409–423.

Ackroyd, J. F. (1955). Thrombocytopenic purpura due to hypersensitivity to the antihistaminic drug antazoline (2(N-phenyl-N-benzyl-aminomethyl)imidazoline). Sang, 26:115–117.

Aldrich, F. D., and Holmes, J. H. (1969). Acute chlordane intoxication in a child. Arch. Environ. Health, 19:129–132.

Allport, R. B. (1959). Ipecac is not innocuous. Am. J. Dis. Child., 98:786–787.

American Medical Association (1971). AMA Drug Evaluations, Ed. 1. American Medical Association, Chicago.

Andersen, A. H. (1946). Experimental studies on the pharmacology of activated charcoal. I. Adsorption power of charcoal in aqueous solution. Acta Pharmacol., 2:69–78.

Andersen, A. H. (1947). Experimental studies on the pharmacology of activated charcoal. II. The effect of pH on the adsorption by charcoal from aqueous solutions. Acta Pharmacol., 3:199–218.

Andersen, A. H. (1948a). Experimental studies on the pharmacology of activated charcoal. III. Adsorption from gastro-intestinal contents. Acta Pharmacol., 4:275–284.

Andersen, A. H. (1948b). Experimental studies on the pharmacology of activated charcoal. IV. Adsorption of allyl-isopropyl-barbituric acid) in vivo. Acta Pharmacol., 4:379–388.

Andersen, A. H. (1948c). Experimental studies on the pharmacology of activated charcoal. V. Absorption of sulphanilamide in vivo. Acta Pharmacol., 4:389–400.

Aposhian, H. V., and Aposhian, M. M. (1959). N-acetyl-DL-penicillamine, a new oral protective agent against the lethal effects of mercuric chloride. J. Pharmacol. Exp. Ther., 126:131–135.

Armstrong, R. W., Eichner, E. R., Klein, D. E., Barthel, W. F., Bennett, J. V., Jonsson, V., Bruce, H., and Loveless, L. E. (1969). Pentachlorophenol poisoning in a nursery for newborn infants. II. Epidemiologic and toxicologic studies. J. Pediatr., 75:317–325.

Arnold, F. J., Jr., Hodges, J. B., Jr., and Barta, R. A., Jr. (1959). Evaluation of the efficacy of lavage and induced emesis in treatment of salicylate poisoning. Pediatrics, 23:286–301.

Arterberry, J. C., Bonifaci, R. W., Nash, E. W., and Quinby, G. E. (1962). Potentiation of phosphorus insecticides by phenothiazine derivatives. J. A. M. A., 182:848–850.

Askew, B. M., Davies, D. R., Green, A. L., and Holmes, R. (1956). The nature of the toxicity of 2-oxo-oximes. Br. J. Pharmacol., 11:424–427.

Barckow, D., Neuhaus, G., and Erdmann, W. D. (1969). Zur behandlung de schweren parathion-(E 605®)-vergiftung mit dem cholinesterase-reaktivator obidoxim (Toxogonin®). Arch. Toxikol., 24:133–146.

Barkham, P., and Tocantins, L. M. (1954). Observations on the thrombocytopenia due to hypersensitivity to quinidine. Blood, 9:134–143.

Barkman, R., Edgren, B., and Sundwall, A. (1963). Self-administration of pralidoxime in nerve gas poisoning with a note on the stability of the drug. J. Pharm. Pharmacol., 15:671–677.

Barnett, H. L., and Einhorn, A. H. (1968). Pediatrics. Ed. 4, Appleton-Century-Crofts, New York.

Bastenier, H., Deslypere, P., and Mme. de Graef-Millet (1957). Un test utile pour le diagnostic du saturnisme. XII. Conf. Ind. Med., Helsinki, 3:243–345.

Berglund, F., Elwin, C. E., and Sundwall, A. (1962). Studies on the renal elimination of N-methylpyridinium-2-aldoxime. Biochem. Pharmacol., 11:383–388.

Bergner, A. D., and Wagley, P. F. (1958). An effect of pyridine-2-aldoxime methiodide (2-PAM) on cholinesterase at motor end-plates. Proc. Soc. Exp. Biol. Med., 97:90–92.

Bessman, S. P., Ried, H., and Rubin, M. (1952). Treatment of lead encephalopathy with calcium disodium versenate. Report of a case. Med. Ann. DC, 21:312–315.

Bethe, K., Erdmann, W. D., Lendle, L., and Schmidt, G. (1957). Spezifische Antidot-Behandlung bei protrahierter Vergiftung mit Alkylphosphaten (Paraoxon, Parathion, DFP) und Eserin und Meerschweinchen. Naunyn-Schmiedebergs Arch. Exp. Pathol., 231:3–22.

Bigelow, F. S., and Desforges, J. F. (1952). Platelet agglutiation by an abnormal plasma factor in thrombocytopenic purpura associated with quinidine ingestion. Am. J. Med. Sci., 224:274–280.

Boelcke, G., Feise, G., de Cassan, K., and Keyser, E. (1970). Der einfluss der vergiftung durch alkylphosphate und der spezifischen antidot-rapie auf die leberfunktion von ratten und kaninchen. Arzneim. Forsch., 20:770–774.

Boelcke, G., and Gaaz, J. W. (1970). Zur frage von lebertoxicitat von nitrostigmin (E 605 forte®) und obidoxim (Toxogonin®) an hunden. Arch. Toxikol., 26:93–101.

Boelcke, G., and Kamphenkel, L. (1970). Der einfluss der nitrostigminvergiftung und der spezifischen antidottherapie mit obidoxim auf die bilirubin-clearance und den gallefluss der ratte. Arch. Toxikol., 26:210–219.

Borison, H. L., and Wang, S. C. (1953). Physiology and pharmacology of vomiting. Pharmacol. Rev., 5:193–230.

Boyd, E.M., Boyd, C. E., and Cassell, W. A. (1954). The antiemetic action of chlorpromazine hydrochloride. Can. Med. Assoc. J., 70:276–280.

Brachfeld, J., and Zavon, M. R. (1965). Organic phosphate (Phosdrin) intoxication. Report of a case and the results of treatment with 2-PAM. Arch. Environ. Health, 11:859–862.

Brown, R. V. (1960). The effects of intracisternal sarin and pyridine-2-aldoxime methyl methane-sulfonate in anaesthetized dogs. Br. J. Pharmacol., 15:170–174.

Brugsch, H. G., Colombo, N. J., and Pagnotto, L. D. (1965). Chelation by calcium trisodium pentetate in workers exposed to lead. N. Engl. J. Med., 272:993–996.

Byron, H. M. (1963). Ocular trauma. Eye, Ear, Nose Throat Mon., 42:48–56.

Byron, H. M., and Posner, I. (1964). Clinical evaluation of Protopam. Am. J. Ophthalmol., 57:409–418.

Caro, D., and Kawerau, E. (1965). Need for gastric lavage. Br. Med. J., 1:189–190.

Carr, E. A., Jr. (1954). Drug allergy. Pharmacol. Rev., 6:365–424.

Casarett, L. J., Bevenue, A., Yauger, W. L., and Whalen, S. A. (1969). Observations on pentachlorophenol in human blood and urine. Am. Ind. Hyg. Assoc. J., 30:360–366.

Chamberlain, P. H., Stavinoha, W. B., Davis, H., Kniker, W. T., and Panos, T. C. (1958). Thallium poisoning. Pediatrics, 22:1170–1182.

Childs, A. F., Davies, D. R., Green, A. L., and Rutland, J. P. (1955). Reactivation by oximes and hydroxamic acids of cholinesterase inhibited by organo-phosphorus compounds. Br. J. Pharmacol., 10:462–465.

Chin, L., Picchioni, A. L., and Duplisse, B. R. (1970). The action of activated charcoal on poisons in the digestive tract. Toxicol. Appl. Pharmacol., 16:786–799.

Coble, Y., Hildebrandt, P., Davis, J., Raasch, F., and Curley, A. (1967). Acute endrin poisoning. J. A. M. A., 202:489–493.

Cohen, E. M., and Wiersinga, H. (1959). Oximes in the treatment of nerve gas poisoning: I. Acta Physiol. Pharmacol. Neerl., 8:40–51.

Cohen, E. M., and Wiersinga, H. (1960). Oximes in the treatment of nerve gas poisoning: II. Acta Physiol. Pharmacol. Neerl., 9:276–302.

Comroe, J. H., Jr., Todd, J., and Koelle, G. B. (1946). The pharmacology of di-isopropyl fluorophosphate (DFP) in man. J. Pharmacol. Exp. Ther., 87:281–290.

Cranmer, M., and Freal, J. (1970). Gas chromatographic analysis of pentachlorophenol in human urine by formation of alkyl ethers. Life Sci., 9:121–128.

Cueto, C., Jr., and Biros, F. J. (1967). Chlorinated insecticides and related materials in human urine. Toxicol. Appl. Pharmacol., 10:261–269.

Cueto, C., Jr., and Hayes, W. J., Jr. (1967). Effect of repeated administration of phenobarbital on the metabolism of dieldrin. Ind. Med. Surg., 36:546–551.

Curley, A., and Garrettson, L. (1969). Acute chlordane poisoning: clinical and chemical studies. Arch. Environ. Health, 18:211–215.

Curley, A., Jennings, R. W., Mann, H. T., and Sedlak, V. (1970). Measurement of endrin following epidemics of poisoning. Bull. Environ. Contam. Toxicol., 5:24–29.

Dabbous, I. A., Bergman, A. B., and Robertson, W. O. (1965). The ineffectiveness of mechanically induced vomiting. J. Pediatr., 66:952–954.

Dausset, J., Nenna, A., and Brecy, H. (1954). Leuko-agglutinins. V. Leuko-agglutinins in chronic idiopathic or symptomatic pancytopenia and in paroxysmal nocturnal hemoglobinuria. Blood, 9:696–720.

Davies, D. R., and Green, A. L. (1955). The physical chemistry of enzymes: general discussion. Discuss. Faraday Soc., 20:269.

Decker, W. J., Combs, H. F., Treuting, J. J., and Banez, R. J. (1971). Dialysis of drugs against activated charcoal. Toxicol. Appl. Pharmacol., 18:573–578.

Dekking, H. (1964). Stopping the action of strong miotics. Ophthalmologica, 148:428–430.

Dettbarn, W. D. (1959). Action of lipid-soluble quaternary ammonium ions on the resting potential of myelinated nerve fibers of the frog. Biochim. Biophys. Acta, 32:381–386.

Dwyer, F. P., and Mellor, D. P. (eds.) (1964). Chelating Agents and Metal Chelates. Academic Press, Inc., New York.

Edery, H. (1959). Effects of diacetyl monoxime on neuromuscular transmission. Br. J. Pharmacol., 14:317–322.

Edery, H., and Schatzberg-Porath, G. (1958). Pyridine-2-aldoxime methiodide and diacetyl monoxime against organophosphorus poisoning. Science, 128:1137–1138.

Elkins, H. B., Pagnotto, L. D., and Richmond, M. (1966). The osmolality adjustment in urinalysis. J. Occup. Med., 8:528–531.

Ellin, R. I., and Wills, J. H. (1964a). Oximes antagonistic to inhibitors of cholinesterase. Part I. J. Pharm. Sci., 53:995–1007.

Ellin, R. I., and Wills, J. H. (1964b). Oximes antagonistic to inhibitors of cholinesterase. Part II. J. Pharm. Sci., 53:1143–1150.

Elliott, J. W., Walker, K. C., Penick, A. E., and Durham, W. F. (1960). A sensitive procedure for urinary p-nitrophenol determination as a measure of exposure to parathion. J. Agric. Food Chem., 8:111–113.

Epstein, M. A., and Freeman, G. (1955). Toxicity of hydroxamic acid analogues and their prophylactic and therapeutic efficacy against nerve gas poisoning in mice. Medical Laboratories Research Rep. No. 346, Army Chemical Center, Maryland.

Erdmann, W. D., Bosse, I., and Franke, P. (1965). Zur resorption und ausscheidung von toxogonin nach intramuskularer injektion am menschen. Dtsch. Med. Wochenschr., 33:1–9.

Firemark, H., Barlow, C. F., and Roth, L. J. (1964). The penetration of 2-PAM-C^{14} into brain and the effect of cholinesterase inhibitors on its transport. J. Pharmacol. Exp. Ther., 145:252–265.

Fleming, A. J. (1964). Industrial hygiene and medical control procedures. Arch. Environ. Health, 8:226–270.

Fowler, E. L. (1953). Insecticide toxicology: manifestations of cottonfield insecticides in the Mississippi Delta. J. Agric. Food Chem., 1:469–473.

Fredriksson, T. (1961). Percutaneous absorption of parathion and paraoxon. IV. Decontamination of human skin from parathion. Arch. Environ. Health, 3:185–188.

Gajdusek, D. C., Gibbs, C. J., Jr., and Alpers, M. (1966). Experimental transmission of a Kuru-like syndrome to chimpanzees. Nature, 209:794–796.

Gajdusek, D. C., Gibbs, C. J., Jr., and Alpers, M. (1967). Transmission and passage of experimental "Kuru" to chimpanzees. Science, 155:212–214.

Ganelin, R. S., Cueto, C., Jr., and Mail, G. A. (1964). Exposure to parathion: effect on general population and asthmatics. J. A. M. A., 188:807–810.

Garrettson, L. K., and Curley, A. (1969). Dieldrin—studies in a poisoned child. Arch. Environ. Health, 19:814–822.

Gilman, A., Allen, R. P., Philips, F. S., and St. John, E. (1946). Clinical uses of 2 , 4-dimercaptopropanol (BAL). X. The treatment of acute systemic mercury poisoning in experimental animals with BAL thiosorbital and BAL glucoside. J. Clin. Invest., 25:549–556.

Gitelson, S., Aladjemoff, L., Hador, Ben, S., and Katznelson, R. (1966). Poisoning by a malathion-xylene mixture. J. A. M. A., 197:819–821.

Goldstein, M. I., Robertson, W. O., and Harlor, A. D. (1963). Evaluating methods for emptying the stomach. Bull. Natl. Clearinghouse Poison Control Centers, March–April, p. 3.

Goldwater, L. J., Ladd, A. R., and Jacobs, M. B. (1964). Absorption and excretion of mercury in man. VII. Significance of mercury in blood. Arch. Environ. Health, 9:735–741.

Gosselin, R. E, and Smith, R. P. (1966). Trends in the therapy of acute poisonings. Clin. Pharmacol. Ther., 7:279–299.

Graham, H. T., Lowry, O. H., Wheelwright, F., Lenz, M. A., and Parish, H. H., Jr. (1955). Distribution of histamine among leucocytes and platelets. Blood, 10:467–481.

Grandjean, L. C. (1948). A case of purpura haemorrhagica after administration of quinine with specific thrombocytolysis demonstrated in vitro. Acta Med. Scand. [Suppl.], 213:165–170.

Graupner, K., and Wiezorek, W.-D. (1966). Zur Wirksamkeit verschiedener Oxime auf die Ruckbildung der Miosis nach lokaler Applikation von Cholinesterase-Inhibitoren. Graefe. Arch. Ophthal., 169:94–101.

Green, A. L. (1958). The kinetic basis of organophosphate poisoning and its treatment. Biochem. Pharmacol., 1:115–128.

Grob, D., and Johns, F. J. (1958). Use of oximes in the treatment of intoxication by anticholinesterase compounds in normal subjects. Am. J. Med., 24:497–511.

Grob, D., Lilienthal, J. L., Harvey, A. M., and Jones, B. F. (1947). The administration of di-isopropyl fluorophosphate (DFP) to man. Bull. Johns Hopkins Hosp., 81:217–244.

Gyllensward, A. (1960). Inducerad kräkning i stället för magsköljning vid hotande förgiftning hos barn. Sven. Läk.-Tidn., 57:3364–3367.

Hahn, H. L., and Henschler, D. (1969). Zur reaktivierbarkit phosphorylierter cholinesterasen durch obidoximchlorid (Toxogonin) *in vivo*. Arch. Toxikol., 24:147–163.

Halpern, B., Ky, N. T., Amache, N., LaGrue, G., and Hazard, J. (1967). Diagnostic de l'allergie médicamenteuse "in vitro" par l'utilisation du test de transformation lymphoblastique (T.T.L.). Presse Med., 75:461–465.

Hamblin, D. O., and Marchand, J. F. (1951). Parathion poisoning. Am. Pract. Digest Treat., 2:1–12.

Hardy, H. L., Elkins, H. B., Ruotolo, B. P. W., Quinby, J., and Baker, W. H. (1954). Use of monocalcium disodium ethylene diamine tetra-acetate in lead poisoning. J. A. M. A., 154:1171–1175.

Harris, C. J., Williford, E. A., Kemberling, S. R., and Morgan, D. P. (1969). Pesticide intoxications in Arizona. Ariz. Med., 26:872–876.

Harris, S., Jr. (1930). Jamaica ginger paralysis (a peripheral polyneuritis). South. Med. J., 23:375–380.

Harstad, E., Møller, K. O., and Simesen, M. H. (1942). Uber den Wert der Magenspülung bei der Behandlung von akuton Vergiftungen. Acta Med. Scand., 112:478–514.

Haun, E. C., and Cueto, C., Jr. (1967). Fatal toxaphene poisoning in a 9-month-old infant. Am. J. Dis. Child., 113:616–618.

Hayes, W. J., Jr. (1963). *Clinical Handbook on Economic Poisons. Emergency Information for Treating Poisoning.* US Government Printing Office, Washington, DC. PHS Publ. 476.

Hayes, W. J., Jr., and Curley, A. (1968). Storage and excretion of dieldrin and related compounds. Effect of occupational exposure. Arch. Environ. Health, 16:155–162.

Hayes, W. J., Jr., and Pirkle, C. I. (1966). Mortality from pesticides in 1961. Arch. Environ. Health, 12:43–55.

Heath, D. F. (1961). *Organophosphorus Poisons.* Pergamon Press, Elmsford, NY.

Hernberg, S., and Laamanen, A. (1964). Results of diagnostic lead mobilisation tests in a Finnish series. Ann. Med. Intern. Fenn., 53:123–128.

Hirsch, F. G. (1964). Cyanide poisoning. Arch. Environ. Health, 8:622–624.

Hobbiger, F. (1956). Chemical reactivation of phosphorylated human and bovine true cholinesterases. Br. J. Pharmacol., 11:295–303.

Hobbiger, F. (1963). Reactivation of phosphorylated acetylcholinesterase. In: *Handbuch der Experimentellen Pharmakologie.* Vol. 15, pp. 921–988. Springer-Verlag, Berlin.

Holmes, J. H., Kinzer, E. J., and Hibbert, R. W. (1957). Parathion poisoning case report. Rocky Mt. Med. J., 54:1022–1031.

Holmes, R., and Robins, E. L. (1955). The reversal by oximes of neuromuscular block produced by anticholinesterases. Br. J. Pharmacol., 10:490–495.

Hunter, C. G., and Kendrick, R. R. (1968). Repeated samples of fat obtained with a biopsy needle. Postgrad. Med. J., 44:851–852.

Isaacs, B. (1957). The influence of head and body position on the emetic action of apomorphine in man. Clin. Sci., 16:215–221.

Jager, B. V., and Stagg, G. N. (1958). Toxicity of diacetyl monoxime and of pyridine-2-aldoxime methiodide in man. Bull. Johns Hopkins Hosp., 102:203–211.

Jager, B. V., Stagg, G. N., Green, N., and Jager, L. (1958). Studies on distribution and disappearance of pyridine-2-aldoxime methiodide (PAM) and of diacetyl monoxime (DAM) in man and in experimental animals. Bull. Johns Hopkins Hosp., 102:225–234.

Joslin, E. F., Forney, R. L., Huntington, R. W., Jr., and Hayes, W. J., Jr. (1960). A fatal case of lindane poisoning. Proc. Natl. Assoc. Coroners, Seminars. pp. 53–57.

Juhlin, L., and Westphal, D. (1962). Degranulation of basophil leukocytes in a case of milk allergy. Acta Dermatol., 42:273–279.

Kewitz, H., and Nachmansohn, D. (1957). A specific anti-

dote against lethal alkylphosphate intoxication: IV. Effects in brain. Arch. Biochem., 66:271–283.

Kewitz, H., Wilson, I. B., and Nachmansohn, D. (1956). A specific antidote against lethal alkyl phosphate intoxication: II. Antidotal properties. Arch. Biochem., 64:456–465.

Koster, R. (1946). Synergisms and antagonisms between physostigmine and di-isopropyl fluorophosphate in cats. J. Pharmacol. Exp. Ther., 88:39–46.

Larson, R. K. (1953). The mechanism of quinidine purpura. Blood, 8:16–25.

Laws, E. R., Jr., Curley, A., and Biros, F. J. (1967). Men with intensive occupational exposure to DDT. A clinical and chemical study. Arch. Environ. Health, 15:766–775.

Lehman, R. A. (1962). Mechanism of the antagonism by pralidoxime and 1, 1-trimethylenebis(4-hydroxyiminomethylpyredinium) of the action of echothiophate on the intestine. Br. J. Pharmacol., 18:287–298.

Lehman, R. A., and Nicholls, M. E. (1960). Antagonism of phospholine (echothiophate) iodide by certain quaternary oximes. Proc. Soc. Exp. Biol. Med., 104:550–554.

Levine, R. R., and Steinberg, G. M. (1966). Intestinal absorption of pralidoxime and other aldoximes. Nature, 209:269–271.

Lindgren, P., and Sundwall, A. (1960). Parasympatholytic effects of TMB-4 (1, 1-trimethylene-bis(4-formylpyridinium bromide)-diorime) and some related oximes in the cat. Acta Pharmacol. Toxicol., 17:69–83.

Loomis, T. A. (1956). The effect of an aldoxime on acute sarin poisoning. J. Pharmacol. Exp. Ther., 118:123–128.

Loomis, T. A. (1963). Distribution and excretion of pyridine-2-aldoxime methiodide (PAM), atropine, and PAM in sarin poisoning. Toxicol. Appl. Pharmacol., 5:489–499.

Lund, A. (1956). The effect of various substances on the excretion and the toxicity of thallium in the rat. Acta Pharmacol., 12:260–268.

Luis, P. (1952). A case of detection of DDT in viscera. Rev. Assoc. Bioquim. Arg., 17:334–338.

MacBryde, C. M. (1964). *Signs and Symptoms: Applied Pathologic Physiology and Their Clinical Interpretation,* Ed. 4. J. B. Lippincott Co., Philadelphia.

Mamo, J. G., and Leopold, I. H. (1958). Evaluation and use of oximes in ophthalmology. Am. J. Ophthalmol., 46:724–731.

Marriott, H. L. (1933). On washing out the stomach in comatose doses of poisoning. Lancet, 1:962.

Matthew, H., and Lawson, A. A. H. (1970). *Treatment of Common Acute Poisonings.* E. & S. Livingstone Ltd., Edinburgh, Scotland.

Matthew, H., Mackintosh, T. F., Tompsett, S. L., and Cameron, J. C. (1966). Gastric aspiration and lavage in acute poisoning. Br. Med. J., 1:1333–1337.

Mick, D. L., Long, K. R., and Bonderman, D. P. (1972). Aldrin and dieldrin in the blood of pesticide formulators. Am. Ind. Hyg. Assoc. J., 33:94–99.

Milby, T. H., Samuels, A. J., and Ottoboni, F. (1968). Human exposure to lindane: Blood lindane levels as a function of exposure. J. Occup. Med., 10:584–587.

Milthers, E., Clemmsen, C., and Nimb, M. (1963). Poisoning with phosphostigmines treated with atropine, pralidoxime methiodide and diacetyl monoxime. Dan. Med. Bull., 10:122–129.

Moeschlin, S. (1965). *Poisoning. Diagnosis and Treatment.* Grune & Stratton, Inc., New York.

Moeschlin, S., and Wagner, K. (1952). Agranulocytosis due to occurrence of leukocyte agglutinins (pyramidon and cold agglutinins). Acta Haematol., 8:29–41.

Nabb, D. P., and Whitfield, F. (1967). Determination of cholinesterase by an automated pH stat method. Arch. Environ. Health, 5:147–154.

Nachmansohn, D., and Wilson, I. B. (1956). Trends in the biochemistry of nerve activity. In: *Currents in Biochemical Research,* edited by D. E. Green. Interscience Publishers, Inc., New York.

Nalbandian, R. M., and Pearce, J. F. (1965). Confirmation by indirect basophil degranulation test. J. A. M. A., 194:238–239.

Nelson, W. E., Vaughan, V. C., and McKay, R. J. (1969). *Textbook of Pediatrics,* Ed. 9. W. B. Saunders Company, Philadelphia.

Ohlsson, W. T. L. (1962). Penicillamine as lead-chelating substance in man. Br. Med. J., 1:1454–1456.

Ohlsson, W. T. L. (1963). Detection of exposure to lead by a mobilization test with peroral penicillamine. Occup. Health Rev., 13:14–18.

O'Leary, J. F., Kunkel, A. M., and Jones, B. H. (1961). Efficacy and limitations of oxime-atropine treatment of organophosphorus anticholinesterase poisoning. J. Pharmacol. Exp. Ther., 132:50–57.

Peters, R. A., Stocken, L. A., and Thompson, R. H. S. (1945). British anti-lewisite (BAL). Nature, 156:616–619.

Picchioni, A. L., Chin, L., and Verhulst, H. L. (1965). A preliminary investigation involving the relative efficacy of activated charcoal and the "universal antidote." Bull. Natl. Clearinghouse Poison Control Centers, Jan.–Feb.

Prater, H. W. (1964). Organic phosphate insecticide poisoning. Bull. Tulane Univ. Med. Fac., 23:175–185.

Press, E., Adams, W. C., Chittenden, R. F., Christian, J. R., Grayson, R., Stewart, C. C., and Everist, B. W. (1962). Evaluation of gastric lavage and other factors in the treatment of accidental ingestion of petroleum distillate products. Pediatrics, 29:648–674.

Quinby, G. E., and Clappison, G. B. (1961). Parathion poisoning: a near-fatal pediatric case treated with pyridine aldoxime methiodide (2-PAM). Arch. Environ. Health, 3:538–542.

Quinby, G. E., Loomis, T. A., and Brown, H. W. (1963). Oral occupational parathion poisoning treated with 2-PAM iodide (2-pyridine aldoxime methiodide). N. Engl. J. Med., 268:639–643.

Rajapurkar, M. V., and Panjwani, M. H. (1961). The action of diacetylmonoxime (DAM) on ciliary activity. Arch. Int. Pharmacodyn. Ther., 131:107–115.

Rider, J. A., Hodges, J. L., Swader, J., and Wiggins, A. D. (1957). Plasma and red cell cholinesterase in 800 "healthy" blood donors. J. Lab. Clin. Med., 50:376–383.

Roan, C. C., Morgan, D. P., Cook, N., and Paschal, E. H. (1969). Blood cholinesterases, serum parathion concentrations and urine p-nitrophenol concentrations in exposed individuals. Bull. Environ. Contam. Toxicol., 4:362–369.

Robertson, W. O. (1962). Syrup of ipecac—a slow or fast emetic? Am. J. Dis. Child., 103:136–139.

Robson, A. M., Kissane, J. M., Elvick, N. H, and Pundavela, L. (1969). Pentachlorophenol poisoning in a nursery for newborn infants. I. Clinical features and treatment. Pediatr. Pharmacol. Ther., 75:309–316.

Salerno, P. R., and Coon, J. M. (1950). Drug protection against the lethal action of parathion. Arch. Int. Pharmacodyn. Ther., 84:227–236.

Sandstead, H. H., Stant, E. G., Brill, A. B., Arias, L. I., and Terry, R. T. (1969). Lead intoxication and the thyroid. Arch. Intern. Med., 123:632–635.

Selye, H. (1970a). Resistance to various pesticides. Arch. Environ. Health, 21:706–710.

Selye, H. (1970b). Protection by catatoxic steroids against cycloheximide intoxication. Toxicol. Appl. Pharmacol., 17:721–725.

Shein, G. K. (1967). Combined use of isonitrosine and TMV-4 in the poisoning of animals with organic phosphorus compounds. Farmakol. Toksikol., 4:491–494.

Shelley, W. B. (1962). New serological test for allergy in man. Nature, 195:1181–1183.

Shelley, W. B. (1963). Indirect basophil degranulation test for allergy to penicillin and other drugs. J. A. M. A., 184:105–112.

Sidell, F. R., and Groff, W. A. (1970). Toxogonin: blood levels and side effects after intramuscular administration in man. J. Pharm. Sci., 59:793–797.

Simon, R. D. (1963). Parathion: a case report. Am. J. Dis. Child., 105:527.

Smith, H. V., and Spalding, J. M. K. (1959). Outbreak of paralysis due to ortho-cresyl phosphate poisoning. Lancet, 2:1019–1021.

Smith, J. E., Loveless, L. E., and Belden, E. A. (1967). Pentachlorophenol poisoning in newborn infants. Morbidity and Mortality Weekly Report, NCDC, 16(40):334–335.

Sollman, T. (1902). Coffee and tea as precipitants for poisons. J. Med. Res., 7:43–53.

Sollman, T. (1957). *A Manual of Pharmacology,* Ed. 8. W. B. Saunders Company, Philadelphia.

Spector, S. (1958). Management of acute aspirin poisoning in children. Q. Rev. Pediatr., 13:179–187.

Starkenstein, E., Rost, E., and Pohl, J. (1929). *Toxikologie, Ein Lehbuch für Ärzte, Medizinalbeamte und Medizinstudierende.* Urban & Schwarzenberg, Munich.

Starr, H. G., and Clifford, N. J. (1972). Acute lindane intoxication. Arch. Environ. Health, 25:374–375.

Stewart, R. D. (1974). The use of breath analysis in clinical toxicology. Essays Toxicol., 5:121–147.

Summerson, W. H. (1955). Progress in the biochemical treatment of nerve gas poisoning. Armed Forces Chem. J., Jan.–Feb.

Thompson, R. P. H., Pilcher, C. W. T., Robinson, J., Stathers, G. M., McLean, A. E. M., and Williams, R. (1969). Treatment of unconjugated jaundice with dicophane. Lancet, 2:4–6.

US Pharmacopeia, Ed. 18 (1970). Mack Publishing Company, Easton, Pa.

von Oettingen, W. F. (1958). *Poisoning.* W. B. Saunders Company, Philadelphia.

Wagner-Jauregg, T., and Hackley, B. E., Jr. (1953). Model reactions of phosphorus-containing enzyme inactivators; III. Interaction of imidazole, pyridine, and some of their derivatives with dialkyl halogeno-phosphates. J. Am. Chem. Soc., 75:2125–2130.

Wagner-Jauregg, T., Hackley, B. E., Jr., Lies, T. A., Owens, O. O., and Proper, R. (1955). Model reactions of phosphorus-containing enzyme inactivators: IV. The catalytic activity of certain metal salts and chelates in the hydrolysis of diisopropyl fluorophosphate. J. Am. Chem. Soc., 77:922–929.

Wang, S. C., and Borison, H. L. (1952). A new concept of organization of the central emetic mechanism: recent studies on the sites of action of apomorphine, copper sulfate, and cardiac glycosides. Gastroenterology, 22:1–12.

Watson, W. C., Gordon, R. S., Jr., Karmen, A., and Jover, A. (1963). The absorption and excretion of castor oil in man. J. Pharm. Pharmacol., 15:183–188.

Weiner, L. M., Rosenblatt, M., and Howes, H. A. (1963). The detection of humoral antibodies directed against salicylates in hypersensitive states. J. Immunol., 90:788–792.

Weisberg, H. F. (1962). *Water, Electrolyte, and Acid Base Balance. Normal and Pathological Physiology as a Basis for Therapy.* The Williams & Wilkins Company, Baltimore.

Wendlberger, J., and Frohlich, E. (1954). Uber Komplemenbidungsversuche zur Erweiterung der Diagnostik beim Nickelekzem. Arch. Hyg. Bakteriol., 138:430–435.

Wenzl, J. E., and Burke, E. C. (1962). Poisoning from a malathion-aerosol mixture. A case report. J. A. M. A., 182:495–497.

Whitaker, J. A., Austin, W., and Nelson, J. D. (1962). Edathamil calcium disodium (Versenate) diagnostic test for lead poisoning. Pediatrics, 29:384–388.

Wills, J. H., and Borison, H. L. (1959). Modification by sarin and antagonists of medullary respiratory activities. Fed. Proc., 18:459.

Wills, J. H., Kunkel, A. M., O'Leary, J. F., and Oikemus, A. H. (1959). Effect of 2-PAM on neuromuscular blockade induced by certain chemicals. Proc. Soc. Exp. Biol. Med., 101:196–197.

Wilson, I. B. (1951). Acetylcholinesterase: XI. Reversibility of tetraethyl pyrophosphate inhibition. J. Biol. Chem., 190:111–117.

Wilson, I. B. (1952). Acetylcholinesterase: XIII. Reactivation of alkyl phosphate-inhibited enzyme. J. Biol. Chem., 199:113–120.

Wilson, I. B., and Ginsburg, S. (1955). A powerful reactivator of alkylphosphate-inhibited acetylcholinesterase. Biochim. Biophys. Acta, 18:168–170.

Wislicki, L. (1960). Differences in the effect of oximes on striated muscle and respiratory centre. Arch. Int. Pharmacodyn. Ther., 129:1–19.

Wright, J. W., Fritz, R. F., Hocking, K. S., Babione, R., Gratz, N. G., Pal, R., Stiles, A. R., and Vandekar, M. (1969). Ortho-isopropoxyphenyl methyl carbamate (OMS-33) as a residual spray for control of anopheline mosquitos. Bull. WHO, 40:67–90.

Yater, W. M., and Oliver, W. F. (1961). Symptom Diagnosis, Ed. 5. Appleton-Century-Crofts, New York.

Zarro, V. J., and DiPalma, J. R. (1965). The sympathomimetic effects of 2-pyridine aldoxime methylchloride (2-PAM Cl). J. Pharmacol. Exp. Ther., 147:153–160.

9

PREVENTION OF INJURY BY PESTICIDES

We live in an age of responsibility as well as in an age of chemistry. Self-discipline in the use of chemicals has paralleled their introduction into industry and agriculture; if this had not been true, the safety record of chemicals would have deteriorated rapidly instead of improving during the early part of the century and then either remaining essentially stable for the last 30 years or, in some instances, showing some further improvement.

Measures for preventing injury by pesticides must be based on a firm knowledge of their physical, chemical, and biological properties. Once the research has been done, certain appropriate safety measures may be enforced under law, while other measures and a proper attitude toward safety may be better communicated by education. There is no substitute for proper care by all persons having any contact whatsoever with poisons. Choice of compound, method and timing of application, and other practices associated with pest control in its broadest sense are always important. It may be found that protective clothing, respirators, masks, air-conditioned cabs, special factory ventilation, or a wide variety of other devices may be applicable to particular problems. In addition to regulations, appropriate practices, protective devices, and education, a cooperative working relationship between those who apply pesticides and those who may receive incidental exposure as a result of the application will do much to promote the welfare of all in the community.

Partly because of the need to limit the length of this text and partly because of the relative accessibility of illustrative material for it, the following discussion of the prevention of injury by pesticides is presented mainly in terms of laws and practices in the United States of America. Specific laws and practices in other countries usually are mentioned only when they appear to offer a real improvement in protection and saving to the community, and not merely a difference in administrative approach.

However, the problems of protection are the same in every country. Comparison of the remainder of this chapter with a review of practical experience in controlling the application of agricultural poisons in the Moldavian SSR (Rusnak *et al.,* 1968) shows that even the distribution of responsibility for medical, environmental, and agricultural aspects of protection may be remarkably similar in countries with different forms of government.

A valuable discussion of modern trends in the prevention of intoxication by pesticides is the report of a regional conference of the World Health Organization (1972).

9.1 Regulations

In the United States of America, economic poisons are subject to extensive state and federal regulations. In a few instances, specific poisons are subject to local regulations also. Whether in this country or elsewhere, there are four main kinds of laws, those regulating: (a) labeling; (b) transportation; (c) use; and (d) residues in food, water, or air. One might add a fifth category, (e) laws to regulate storage, but only minor legislative attention has been given to this matter.

A useful review of legislative control of pesticides in different countries was published by the World Health Organization (WHO, 1970). A different kind of publication, directed to developing countries that may wish guidance in formulating their own legislation, was issued jointly by this Organization and the Food and Agriculture Organization (FAO) (FAO/WHO, 1969a).

9.1.1 Regulation of Labeling

Of the four kinds of regulations, the one concerned with labeling is by far the most important. This conclusion is indicated by a review of the safety record of pesticides in different countries. Thus, the United States of America and the United Kingdom have effective provisions for the labeling of pesticides and both have good safety records, although their regulations regarding residues and use are very different. On the contrary, certain other countries with advanced technology—not to mention developing countries—have inadequate regulation of pesticide labels and a poor safety record. No matter whether labeling is enforced by law, as in the USA, or by less formal agreement between government and industry, as in England (Edson, 1958), good labeling is the most important single means of educating people in the proper procedures and precautions for using pesticides.

Good labels provide essential information on proper application and necessary precautions, and thus offer an indirect control of use. By the same token, overlabeling is self-defeating. For example, if all pesticides were labeled "Poison" or made to bear the skull and crossbones, there would be no way to distinguish the highly toxic ones from those that are relatively safe.

Illiteracy is an obstacle to realizing the benefits of good labeling. However, even if farm workers cannot read, good labeling is the best way of getting information on pesticides to them through the farm owner or foreman. Furthermore, much good can be accomplished by graphic warning labels.

Limitation of Sale Through Labeling. Any law that makes it illegal to offer a product for sale, unless its labeling is approved, is a powerful tool to regulate use. Acting under the law discussed in the following section, this device was used by the US Department of Agriculture to eliminate the use of certain pesticides, especially rodenticides, that were known to be the causes of a disproportionate number of accidental deaths. These actions met with extensive opposition from the manufacturers, even though the volume of trade was small. Formulations successfully restricted were certain arsenicals (40 CFR 162.123) and phosphorus paste (40 CFR 162.124). Later, the Environmental Protection Agency became responsible for administration of labeling and was successful in eliminating the use of thallium sulfate as a rodenticide (Fed. Reg. 37:5719–5720, 1972), and the use of all alkyl mercury pesticides. All mercury pesticides were eliminated for use on rice seed, in laundry, or in marine paint, and the use of all mercury pesticides for any purpose was restricted (Fed. Reg. 37:6419–6420, 1972). These changes were intended mainly for the prevention of human poisoning. Unfortunately, restrictions on the use of certain arsenicals was relaxed (Fed. Reg. 38:23010, 1973). With the objective of protecting wildlife rather than man, the use of sodium cyanide, strychnine, and sodium fluoroacetate for predator control was cancelled and suspended (Fed. Reg. 37:5718–5720, 1972). This latter action left unchanged the uses of calcium cyanide, strychnine, and sodium fluoroacetate for rodent control, and the use of strychnine for control of pigeons and sparrows. More recently, sale of several other pesticides has been stopped or restricted, not because of danger to man but because of danger to wildlife.

9.1.1.1 Labeling in the United States of America. The federal labeling act for pesticides in the USA is entitled "The Federal Insecticide, Fungicide, and Rodenticide Act" (7 USC 135-135k), often referred to as FIFRA. It was approved 25 June 1947, replacing the Federal Insecticide Act of 1910. Following a number of minor revisions, the law underwent major revision in 1972 (7 USC 136-136y). Laws similar to the FIFRA exist in most of the states. These state laws have been reprinted and are easily available (Chemical Specialties Manufacturers Association, 1967; National Agricultural Chemicals Association, 1967). The full text, regulations, and interpretations of the regulations of the federal law prior to revision were available from the Department of Agriculture (USDA, 1964a, 1964b, 1965). The principal features of the Act were briefly reviewed by Perry (1948) and Rohrman (1968). Ward (1965) traced the development of this legislation and its early administration in relation to the whole field of pest control.

Before a label is approved under the federal law, research must be carried out and data presented which show that, if used according to directions, the pesticide will produce the biological result claimed and will be safe. Dangers are cited and precautions are clearly stated in the label before it is approved. Much research usually is necessary for label approval. Labels are written in terms of specific uses only, and, when a label is first issued, the poison may be restricted to a single use. Other uses may be permitted later if additional research justifies them in accordance with the same criteria. Good labeling also applies to the residue problem, because labels are not accepted for uses involving crops until residues have been determined, proper intervals from treatment to harvest have been set, and tolerance limits have been established.

In keeping with good labeling practice, the federal act and regulations made under it (40 CFR 162) require with few exceptions the following information to appear on each label:

(a) Name and address of the manufacturer.

(b) Name of the product.

(c) Name and concentration (by weight) of each active ingredient and the concentration of the inactive ingredients. (The manufacturer must submit for record the complete composition, including the name and concentration of each inert ingredient.)

(d) Net content of the container.

(e) Adequate direction for the control of each pest for which the manufacturer claims control. When appropriate, the directions must specify the rate of dilution, the rate of application, the time of applications and, in the case of food crops, the limitations necessary to avoid excessive residues. Limitations may include the required interval between application and harvest in terms of days or the development of the plant (eg, "when the fruit begins to form").

(f) Adequate precautionary labeling to prevent injury to persons applying the product or injury to persons, animals, or plants coming in contact with it. Highly toxic products must bear the skull and crossbones, the word "Poison" (prominently in red on a background of distinctly contrasting color), a statement "Keep out of the reach of children," and information on treatment of poisoning. The definition of highly toxic as used in the Act is given in Table 9-1. By interpretation (40 CFR 162.116) the labels of highly toxic products

Table 9-1

Comparison of the Criteria of Toxicity Under Two Laws

Experimental conditions	Highly toxic substance as defined by the Regulations for the enforcement of the Federal Insecticide, Fungicide and Rodenticide Act (40 CFR 162.8)[a]			Class B poison as defined by Rules and Regulations Governing Hazardous Materials, Department of Transportation. (49 CFR 73.343)		
	Oral	Dermal	Respiratory	Oral	Dermal	Respiratory
test animal	rat[b]	rabbit	rat	rat	rabbit	rat
sex	m and f	-	m and f	-	-	-
body weight	-	-	-	200-300 g	-	200-300 g
maximal period of exposure	-	24 hr	1 hr	-	24 hr	1 hr
period of observation	14 days	14 days	14 days	48 hr	48 hr	48 hr
maximal dosage for positive test[c]	50 mg/kg	200 mg/kg	2 mg/1 air or 200 ppm	50 mg/kg	200 mg/kg	2 mg/1 of air

a. Human experience takes precedence if in conflict with animal data.

b. Requires 24 hr fasting period before dosing.

c. Requires death of half or more of ten or more test animals.

must carry the signal word "Warning." Three other classes or degrees of toxicity are recognized. The second is the class immediately below highly toxic, and in general includes formulations having toxicities down to one-tenth of those in the highly toxic class. Labels for these materials are required to carry the same signal word as highly toxic materials, but they do not need to bear the skull and cross-bones, the word "Poison," or an antidote statement. The third group embraces products having hazards and toxicities down to about one-tenth of those in Class 2. Use of the signal word "Caution" and statements indicating the means for avoiding the principal hazards of use are required for Class 3 formulations. The fourth class is comparatively free of danger, no warning, caution, or antidote statements are required for this category, although unqualified claims for safety are usually not justified (40 CFR 162.122).

(g)   Registration number [40 CFR 162.6(f)].

(h)   Use classification.

The coloring or discoloring of certain pesticides also is required by the Act and constitutes a sort of graphic labeling (40 CFR 162.12).

The Act contains appropriate sections on enforcement, exemptions, penalties, seizures and condemnations, imports, delegation of duties, authorization for appropriations, and co-operation necessary for its successful administration.

Prior to 1972, most states had similar or identical basic legislation, which served to control products manufactured and sold within their own borders, and thus not subject to the federal law. For the guidance of states, the Association of American Pesticide Control Officials (1972–1973) has prepared a Suggested State Pesticide Control Act. It has been adopted by the Council of State Governments and it is revised at intervals to keep it up-to-date.

In some states additional controls have been added. For example, the licensing of manufacturers and importers has been required for several years by the California Agricultural Code (Chap. 2, Art. 4).

The most important single change in the Federal Insecticide, Fungicide, and Rodenticide Act made by the 1972 amendments (the "Federal Environmental Pesticide Control Act of 1972") was the introduction of two interrelated procedures: classification of pesticides and certification of applicators. As a part of the registration process, each specific use of a pesticide is to be classified as either general or restricted. Designation for general use indi-

cates that the material will not generally cause unreasonable adverse effects on the environment when applied according to label directions and warnings. Designation for restricted use indicates that the material may generally cause unreasonable adverse effects on persons or the environment, unless it is used by or under the direct supervision of a certified applicator. The assigned classification will be an inherent part of the labeling. The certification of applicators is discussed in Section 9.1.3.3. Some other important changes in the Act are mentioned in Section 9.1.3.5.

Items that generally have not been specified in labeling but ought to be specified when appropriate include: (a) protective clothing to be worn; (b) the interval that should be allowed to elapse from application until anyone is permitted to have substantial, direct contact with the treated crops (see Section 7.1.2.4); (c) any required restriction of the working hours of applicators; and (d) proper disposal of the container.

9.1.1.2 Labeling in Great Britain.

Labeling in Great Britain is regulated by three closely related arrangements, which, although voluntary, are almost universally observed. The first of these, the Agricultural Chemicals Approval Scheme, was adopted in its present form in 1960 to replace an earlier scheme initiated in 1942; it is concerned with the effectiveness of pesticides used in agriculture, horticulture, and the home garden. The Pesticides Safety Precautions Scheme adopted in 1964 is a revised form of the Notification of Pesticides Scheme initiated informally in 1954 and formally in 1957. Both the efficiency and safety aspects of labeling are agreed on between the government departments involved and the manufacturer (efficiency), or the industrial associations concerned (safety). The Schemes are interrelated; approval of the efficiency of a pesticide product containing a new active ingredient or involving a new use of an existing active ingredient cannot be given until the use of that ingredient has first been considered and cleared for safety under the Pesticides Safety Precautions Scheme. The safety scheme is closely related to the Veterinary Products Safety Precautions Scheme concerned with products for the treatment of animals. The three Schemes were described by Miller (1965) and in greater detail by the Advisory Committee on Pesticides and Other Toxic Chemicals (1967). These three Schemes and the Agriculture Poisonous Substances Act (see Section 9.1.3.2) have resulted in a most enviable safety record.

While recognizing the good record, the Advisory Committee (1967) noted the possibility of incomplete coverage and other deficiencies under any voluntary system. The Advisory Committee recommended that legislation should be enacted to require the licensing of pesticides and veterinary products. Although many of their detailed recommendations are administrative in nature, some of them are of particular toxicological interest. Special emphasis is placed on the exposure of workers and their protection. Although conventional tests involving continued administration of different doses over long periods are recognized, it is also suggested that 10 to 20 animals that have survived an LD 50 dose of a new compound be observed for a lifetime. This is an important test for truly chronic effects. A proposed requirement for reporting of all suspected poisoning by pesticides or veterinary products is important, and its successful implementation would be a great step forward.

9.1.1.3 International Proposals for Labeling. A review of international proposals for labeling or a review of rules adopted by the countries of continental Europe is beyond the scope of this book. It is equally impossible to undertake a description of the methods the developing countries have adopted in view of their differing requirements. It is necessary, however, to point out the excellent guidance offered by the Council of Europe (1968) in a book entitled "Dangerous Chemical Substances and Proposals Concerning Their Labeling." The volume contains sections in French, English, German, Dutch, and Italian. The work, generally known as "The Yellow Book," deals with the danger symbols applicable to over 500 dangerous chemical substances and groups classed under various headings, the risks they represent, and the safety advice that should be given to all who handle them.

It was prepared over a number of years by the Sub-Committee on Industrial Safety and Health (Chemical Questions), a subsidiary body of the Social Committee (Partial Agreement) of the Council of Europe. (The term "Partial Agreement" arises from the fact that only some of the Council of Europe Member Countries participate in the work of this Committee, which is comprised of government experts from the following countries: Belgium, France, the Federal Republic of Germany, Italy, Luxembourg, the Netherlands, and the United Kingdom.)

The regulations proposed do not all carry the force of law in the seven countries signatory to the Partial Agreement, but government authorities, industrialists, and dealers in these countries are strongly urged to take them into consideration.

Dangerous chemicals are divided into six classes according to the major hazard they offer. The classes are as follows: (I) explosive substances, (II) oxidizing substances, (III) flammable substances, (IV) toxic substances, (V) corrosive substances, and (VI) radioactive substances. Each of the six kinds of danger is symbolized by a graphic warning label as described in the following section. Two minor dangers are recognized as subdivisions of two of the major classes; thus "harmful" substances are recognized as those in Class IV that present a minor but, nonetheless, real toxic hazard. In a similar way, irritant substances are recognized as a subdivision of Class V. Although this classification represents the limits of graphic labeling, the book provides a great deal more detail by listing 72 specific risks and 109 separate items of safety advice. Among the recognized risks is "danger of cumulative effects." It is pointed out that this warning covers danger to human health involving either actual retention of the substance in the body or disturbance of body function as a result of repeated exposure without retention.

Each chemical listed in the book is identified by structural formula and complete chemical name. Its major dangers, whether explosive, toxic, or other, are pointed out. In addition, the specific risks and safety precautions are identified by numbers so that a complete label for the material can be prepared in any of the five languages in which the book is written. A typical precautionary label for the fumigant carbon disulfide is reproduced as Fig. 9-1. Although the book under discussion is not restricted to pesticides, it does contain information on the majority of the important ones.

9.1.1.4 Graphic Warning Labels. Easy visibility and instant comprehensibility are advantages of graphic warning labels even for literate workers. In addition, graphic labels help to overcome differences in language and the problem of illiteracy. There is extensive international trade in pesticides. For all these reasons, the graphic warning labels required by regulation (49 CFR 173.405 et seq.), under appropriate circumstances in the USA and advocated by the International Labour Office, the Council of Europe (1968), and other international organizations should be adopted as standard in every country.

Fig. 9-2 shows the more important graphic warning labels.

CARBON DISULPHIDE			
		Gives off very poisonous vapour	R 67
		Highly flammable	R 23
		Vapour - air mixture explosive	R 33

Keep this product locked up and out of reach of children.	S 3
Keep container sealed, in a cool place, away from living quarters.	S 14
When using, do not eat or smoke.	S 21
Do not empty into drains.	S 23
Take precautionary measures against static discharges.	S 27
Keep away from heat and sources of ignition.	S 36
Take off immediately all contaminated clothing.	S 71
When using, ventilate room well or wear an efficient respirator.	S 76
In case of fire, avoid breathing fumes.	S 101
In case of fire, use the equipment provided.	S 104
If you feel unwell call the doctor and show him this label.	S 108

Fig. 9-1. Sample of precautionary label as recommended by the Council of Europe (1968).

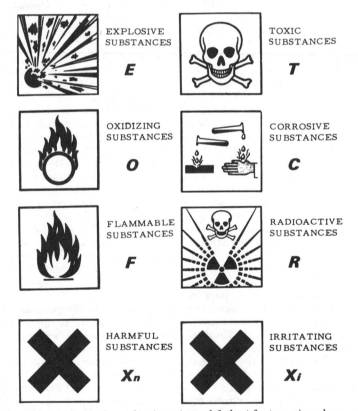

EXPLOSIVE SUBSTANCES *E*

TOXIC SUBSTANCES *T*

OXIDIZING SUBSTANCES *O*

CORROSIVE SUBSTANCES *C*

FLAMMABLE SUBSTANCES *F*

RADIOACTIVE SUBSTANCES *R*

HARMFUL SUBSTANCES X_n

IRRITATING SUBSTANCES X_i

Fig. 9–2. Graphic warning labels (above) for six major and (below) for two minor dangers offered by some chemical substances. The letters are the codes used in the list of substances to indicate important dangers of each compound. From the Council of Europe (1968).

9.1.2 Regulation of Transport and Storage

9.1.2.1 Regulation of Transport in the United States of America. Regulations for the transport of dangerous goods apply sepa-rately and not necessarily equally to the four major kinds of carriers: marine, rail, automo-tive, and aircraft. The regulations for the different carriers have evolved separately as the need arose. This helps to explain why the regulations for the transport of chemicals are so repetitious and complex.

In the United States of America, a very few pesticides are classified as Class A poisons. Of the remaining pesticides, the more toxic ones are classified as Class B poisons. The transportation of both Class A and Class B poisons is regulated.

Class A poisons are defined (49 CFR 173.326) as: "poisonous gases or liquids of such nature that a very small amount of the gas, or vapor of the liquid, mixed with air is dangerous to life." This class includes hydrogen cyanide and several highly toxic industrial chemicals and war gases, as well as some pesticides in compressed gas containers (49 CFR 173.334).

Class B poisons are defined (49 CFR 173.343) as liquids or solids, including pastes and semisolids, other than Classes A, C, or D poisons that are known to be so toxic to man as to afford a hazard to health during transportation or that, in the absence of adequate data on human toxicity, are presumed to be toxic to man because they kill half or more of the test animals when administered by either the oral, dermal, or respiratory route under conditions defined in the appropriate part of Table 9-1.

It may be seen that the definition of Class B poisons for purposes of transportation is essentially the same as that for highly toxic compounds for purposes of registration and labeling (see Section 9.1.1.1), and it is consistent with other toxicity ratings (see Section 9.1.4.7). Compounds of lesser toxicity and even sufficiently dilute formulations of Class B poisons are not subject to any regulation associated with transportation.

Most of the USA federal regulations of the transportation of poisons are concerned with packaging. The requirements are appropriate and very detailed. However, it seems unlikely that any container or combination of containers can be made at a price that is economically feasible and yet strong enough to be unbreakable, both in the course of ordinary (careless) handling and even during wrecks and collisions that inevitably occur. Certainly, there have been accidents in which pesticides were spilled, sometimes onto food or clothing with disastrous results (see Section 7.1.2.4). It was, therefore, a tremendous step forward when new regulations were issued (Fed. Reg. 32:20816–20817; Fed. Reg. 32:20982–20983) prohibiting the transportation of Class B poisons in the same rail car or vehicle (49 CFR 174.532 [m]), aircraft (14 CFR 103.35 [W]), or ship's hold (46 CFR 146.25–45[j]), with food or feed that is not packaged in airtight, non-permeable containers.

The new regulations do not protect against the contamination of clothing and other fabric. Such contamination has been a real but relatively unimportant source of poisoning. The regulations fail to protect against the contamination of food by chemicals less toxic than Class B poisons. Contamination of food by some of these compounds such as DDT or triorthocresyl phosphate have caused poisoning. However, in most and perhaps all of these instances, the contamination was the result of using a formulation as food, or of the direct addition of a formulation to food. Apparently, no poisoning has been reported in connection with food contamination resulting from improper transportation of a compound not toxic enough to fall in Class B. Even so, there is no way to exclude the possibility entirely. Finally, the regulations fail to protect against the contamination of food resulting from spillage of poison during an earlier shipment. Such contamination between separate shipments has occurred (Section 7.1.2.4), but it is rare.

More certain protection would be given by regulations requiring that, with certain exceptions, all industrial chemicals, including fertilizers and pesticides, be shipped in rail cars, vehicles, aircraft, or the holds of ships reserved for them. Reasonable exceptions might include (a) shipment of samples and other suitably packaged single containers not to exceed 500 ml in volume, and (b) shipment of machinery, building materials, and other specified things, contamination of which would involve a minimal hazard. In summary, there is some question whether the present regulations are adequate, but no question that the new regulations represent a great improvement over the old ones.

The different kinds of carriers are responsible for observing the regulations on the transportation of poisons. Although there is little or no inspection by governmental authorities to ensure compliance, the rules apparently are adhered to strictly, probably more because of insurance implications than because of the legal sanctions. The law does provide a fine of not more than $1,000 or imprisonment for not more than 1 year or both for violations involving no personal injury, and a fine of not more than $10,000 and imprisonment for not more than 10 years or both for violations leading to injury of persons (18 USC 832). Of great importance, however, is the fact that generally no insurance company will pay claims resulting from an accident involving direct violation of law. Under the circumstances, the carriers, especially trucking firms, have tended to restrict cargoes including poisons to nothing but poisons, thus offering greater protection than the law requires.

Regulations now in effect regarding hazardous cargo have evolved piecemeal since the turn of the century. Separate regulation of the different modes of transportation is traditional and has been retained. At the request of the US Department of Transportation, a special group of the National Research Council made recommendations contained in "A Study of Transportation of Hazardous Materials: A Report to the Office of Hazardous Materials of the US Department of Transportation." Briefly, the group found need for a unified regulatory system, encompassing all modes of transportation and based on standard criteria (Anonymous, 1969).

9.1.2.2 International Regulation of Transportation.

It is an interesting fact that the international regulations of transportation, like those in the United States of America, are largely separate for the four major modes of transport.

International agreements regarding the marine carriage of dangerous goods form part of the International Convention for Safety of Life at Sea. Some 86 nations subscribe to this Convention.

Concern of the United Nations for safety at sea, including the safe carriage of dangerous goods, is expressed through the International Maritime Consultive Organization (IMCO) with headquarters in London. As might be expected, international agreements regarding poisons now emphasize packaging rather than the segregation of chemicals from foods. The Organization is examining the international code to see whether it offers sufficient protection against the contamination of food in transit. Obviously, greater protection would be offered if chemicals were carried entirely separately from food.

9.1.2.3 Regulation of Storage.

Although some serious accidents have involved the contamination of food during storage (Section 7.1.2.4), there are few regulations of the storage of poisons. Any such regulation would have to be local. It is interesting to speculate whether the principle of insurance liability could contribute to greater safety in the storage of poisons. In the United Kingdom, the Advisory Committee on Pesticides and Other Toxic Chemicals (1967) has suggested that commercial users be required under law to store all regulated pesticide and veterinary products in separate accommodations under lock and key.

9.1.3 Regulation of Use

Labeling offers an indirect control of the use of pesticides, and it is the most important single factor promoting their safety. The use of pesticides is regulated directly in a number of ways including (a) regulation of sale, (b) regulation of application, and (c) licensing of operators.

9.1.3.1 Regulation of Importation or Sale.

Some countries forbid the importation and sale of certain pesticides either through specific regulations or through exercise of their registration laws. Parathion is probably the compound most commonly forbidden, but other highly toxic organic phosphorus and chlorinated hydrocarbon insecticides may be included. In some instances, developing countries have employed this method to protect agricultural workers and others who lack experience with the safe use of toxic compounds and frequently lack access to equipment that would help to make safe use of such materials possible. Under these circumstances, prohibition is justified.

In other instances, countries may use the same kind of regulation to channel specific products to users found qualified to receive them.

In the United States of America, the interstate sale of thallium intended for use as a rodenticide except by government agencies has been prevented by nonregistration (40 CFR 162.120). The interstate sale of products containing more than 2% sodium arsenite or more than 1.5% arsenic trioxide (40 CFR 162.123), and the sale of phosphorus paste (40 CFR 162.124) for home use have been limited through somewhat the same mechanism. The poor safety record of these materials is discussed in Section 7.1.2.2.

Some local governments have forbidden or curtailed the sales of materials or devices that were registered at the national level. For example, some cities regulated the sale of thermal vaporizers for lindane.

9.1.3.2 Regulation of Application.

Direct regulation of the use of pesticides is generally limited to specified compounds that offer some clearly recognized hazard. The hazards that have required attention are poisoning of applicators and damage to crops. The compounds most commonly specified in relation to human health are arsenicals, the more toxic organic phosphorus and chlorinated hydrocarbon insecticides, and certain rodenticides. The compounds most commonly specified in relation to crop damage are the chlorophenoxy herbicides.

Laws regulating application of pesticides may involve one or more of the following:

(a) Requirement that a permit be obtained for each use of a specified compound. The applicant must satisfy the designated authority (often the county commissioner of agriculture) that the pesticide is needed and that he is qualified to use it safely.

(b) Prohibition of sale of specified pesticides except to holders of permits.

(c) Requirement that employers furnish approved instructions and protective equipment to workers who apply a specified compound.

(d) Requirement that applicators follow safety instructions and use approved equipment.

(e) Requirement that workers who are to apply specified compounds have medical surveillance.

(f) Provision of punishment for violation.

By necessity, regulations of application are written in terms of compounds considered dangerous in any of several ways. Such regulations may help to prevent damage to crops or excessive residues at harvest, as well as injury of applicators. Regulations with the single objective of ensuring occupational safety are discussed in Section 9.1.3.4.

Probably the most complete and effective law regulating the use of pesticides is that in the United Kingdom (Great Britain, 1952). The most notable feature of the law is the responsibility it imposes on workers as well as on employers. In enforcement of the act, fines are levied against workers who fail to use protective equipment issued to them. Fines are also imposed on employers who fail to acquaint their employees with hazards or fail to provide the protective equipment specified by regulation. The legislation also covers hygienic practices, hours of work, minimal age of persons who may use regulated poisons, notification of sickness, and the keeping of records. This and other legislation regarding the safety of pesticides was reviewed by Papworth (1965) and by Miller (1965).

In the United States of America, California for many years has had the most extensive direct regulation of the use of pesticides. These regulations are authorized under the California Agricultural Code (Chap. 7, Art. 4).

Until recently, the federal government did not regulate the application of pesticides directly, inasmuch as application is always carried on locally. A partial exception was and remains the regulating of use through federal licensing of pilots. The 1972 amendments of the Federal Insecticide, Fungicide, and Rodenticide Act include two provisions that impose federal control on local use. One, the provision for setting standards for certifying applicators, is similar in many ways to other statutes permitting the setting of national standards, including those for pilots. However, a new requirement [7 USC 136j (G)], which makes it illegal "to use any registered pesticides in a manner inconsistent with its labeling," would appear to make it a federal crime for a housewife to apply a formulation for home garden use to a species of ornamental plant for which it was not labeled.

9.1.3.3 Licensing of Operators. Any requirement for the licensing of operators limits the number of persons who may be applicators and makes it possible to establish minimal standards for their qualifications and performance. Applicants in some states are required to take and pass an examination covering, among other things: (a) the identity and toxicity of important pesticides; (b) the compounds to be used for specific pests of crops or of structures; (c) the proper use and maintenance of equipment, including protective equipment; (d) proper disposal of containers; (e) signs and symptoms of poisoning; and (f) simple emergency measures. The examination also usually covers other matters less directly related to health including, for agricultural custom applicators, (g) injuries to crops, livestock, pollinating insects, wildlife, or aquatic life that may result from improper application of pesticides.

The operators most commonly licensed to use pesticides are pest control operators, pilots, and custom applicators. By convention, the term *pest control operator* designates a commercial applicator concerned with household or structural pests, including termites; pests in vehicles, ships, and aircraft; and other domestic and institutional pest problems. A *custom applicator* is one concerned with the control of pests of crops, livestock, or forests. Under California's law, custom applicators are called agricultural pest control operators.

The Association of American Pesticide Control Officials (1972–1973) has prepared a "Suggested State Pesticide Use and Application Act." The Act is available in the Official Publication of the Association. In addition to the examination discussed above, the Act provides for the right of inspection of equipment, the requirement of a bond or insurance, and the necessity for pilots covered by the Act to comply with the requirements of the Federal Aviation Agency and the Aeronautics Commission of the state before being issued a license. The administrator of the Act is authorized to promulgate regulations requiring applicators to maintain records and submit reports. The administrator may also require that notice of proposed applications be given to the owners of property near that to be treated. After public hearings and due notice, the administrator may issue a list of restricted pesticides and, in general, carry out all the regulations of application discussed in Section 9.1.3.2.

A number of states license pest control operators. The important feature of such laws from a toxicological standpoint is the requirement that successful applicants pass an examination on pesticides, use and maintenance of equipment, symptoms of poisoning, and emergency measures. An example of this kind of law is the Florida Structural Pest Control Act (482 Florida Statutes) and rules made under it (Chapter 170I–2).

In addition to regulations that may be imposed by the states, pilots are subject to federal aviation regulations issued under authority of the Federal Aviation Act of 1958 [49 USC 1348(c), 1354(a), 1421, and 1427]. The regulations (14 CFR 137) require that (a) agricultural aircraft operators must be licensed, (b) an applicant must pass a test of his knowledge of economic poisons and their application and a test of his flying skill, and (c) operators must not dispense any economic poison for a use other than one for which it is registered or contrary to any safety instruction on its label.

The 1972 amendments to the Federal Insecticide, Fungicide, and Rodenticide Act (see Section 9.1.1.1) require the Administrator to establish separate standards for licensing certified private applicators and certified commercial applicators. Under the Act, private applicators shall not be required to maintain any records or file any reports or other documents. A private applicator will be permitted to use or supervise the use of restricted pesticides for producing agricultural commodities on property owned or rented by him or his employer or (if applied without compensation other than exchange of personal services) on the property of another producer of agricultural commodities. A certified commercial applicator will be permitted to use or supervise the use of restricted pesticides for a fee. It is understood that classification for general use or for restricted use does not apply to a pesticide *per se* but to specific uses of each compound. Thus, some compounds will be restricted for no uses, some for only part of their uses, and some for all uses.

As a part of the registration process, the Administrator of the Environmental Protection Agency is required to designate each permitted use of each pesticide as general or restricted. The Administrator is also required to set federal standards for certified applicators of pesticides for restricted use. However, the actual certification is to be carried out by the states after each has submitted a plan for this purpose to the Administrator and he has approved it. It seems likely that this control will take forms similar to those already in use in some states. However, the necessary regulations and administrative details remain to be worked out. The requirement that a pesticide be registered for use only by a certified applicator shall not be effective until 4 years from the date of enactment (21 October 1972), and a period of 4 years from date of enactment shall be provided for certification of applicators.

9.1.3.4 Regulation of Working Conditions. The Occupational Safety and Health Act of 1970 (29 USC 651 *et seq.*) is designed to ensure each worker conditions of work free from recognized hazards likely to cause death or serious physical harm. The law applies to dangers from fire, falls and other mechanical injury, electric shock, excessive heat, excessive noise, inadequate lighting, and other causes, as well as chemical injury. It provides for the inspection of work places, and an employee who believes that a violation of standards exists in his place of work or that an imminent danger exists may request an inspection. The law also requires employers to record and report to the Secretary of Labor or the Secretary of Health, Education, and Welfare (a) work-related deaths, injuries, and illnesses, and (b) exposures of employees to potentially toxic materials. Administration of the law is based on standards promulgated by the Secretary of Labor. The standards not only set acceptable levels of exposure but, as applicable, may prescribe suitable labels and other warnings, protective equipment and practices, monitoring of the work place, and monitoring or more complete, specified medical examination of employees. Penalties are provided for employers who fail to follow the law and regulations made under it. The Occupational Safety and Health Act apparently has a serious defect in that no penalty is provided for an employee who fails to use protective equipment provided, or fails to follow recommended procedures, and in this way endangers his own safety or the safety of his associates.

An annotated list of state laws dealing with occupational safety is available (Trasko, 1970).

9.1.3.5 Inspection. Inspection is an integral part of several protective regulations, notably the law regulating the use of pesticides in the United Kingdom and the Occupational Safety and Health Act of 1970.

The 1972 amendments of the Federal Insecticide, Fungicide, and Rodenticide Act (see Section 9.1.1.1) require registration of all establishments that produce pesticides and permit inspection not only of such registered establishments but also of any distributor, carrier, or dealer. The inspection in this instance is mainly for examining records on the shipment and distribution of pesticides or for sampling or even seizing pesticides, devices, or labels that may be in violation of the Act.

9.1.4 Regulation of Residues

9.1.4.1 The Bases for Safety Factors. Although all tolerances and other limits designed to help regulate residues in food, water, and air are based in part on toxicity data, none of them is a measure of toxicity. There are two basic reasons for this: (a) a series of limits may be based on different criteria and different safety factors for different compounds, and (b) the limits for chemicals in different media and sometimes the limits for different chemicals in the same medium (eg, water) are based on fundamentally different philosophies regarding the role of the safety factor. This difference in philosophy may lead to the practice of adjusting each limit to the conditions of use of the compoud involved.

Philosophical and Practical Considerations. The criteria for threshold limit values designed to guide industrial hygienists in regulating the exposure of workers to industrial chemicals must involve irritancy for some compounds but not for others. Obviously, only a small safety factor has to be allowed for compounds that are highly irritating but cause no injury lasting beyond exposure, unless the concentration is extremely high. Such compounds involve a built-in warning system. Some industrial chemicals are not significantly irritating or toxic, but limits may be placed on them as "nuisance dusts." At the opposite extreme are those compounds known to cause cancer. Compounds that cause malignancy in animals when given by the oral route are not permitted to be used as food additives, even though they are not strong carcinogens and there is little correlation between the carcinogenicity of different compounds for different species. Of course, an even stricter approach is taken with the small number of compounds known to cause cancer in man. Usually no attempt is made to set a safety factor—no matter how large—for these

compounds, and many governments have prohibited their manufacture even as industrial chemicals.

Thus, differences in the criteria for judging the safety of different compounds often are required by the properties of the compounds themselves. In addition, there are some curious differences in criteria explainable only in terms of custom. For example, at any given level of toxicity, there is a strong tendency to accept smaller safety factors for materials that (a) occur naturally, (b) have been known for generations, or (c) are invisible. If they are equally harmless, vapors are permitted at a higher concentration than dusts in industrial atmospheres.

All systems for the regulation of residues in food, water, and air involve the concept that exposure to non-nutrients will be held to the lowest practical level. However, the systems differ sharply in basic philosophy regarding the magnitude of safety factors. Limits for industrial chemicals involve safety factors considered sufficient to protect workers in connection with exposure during full employment (ie, 8 hours a day for 45 or 50 years) and to permit them to retire in good health to enjoy a normal old age. However, the safety factors applied to industrial chemicals are small compared to those applied to chemicals, especially synthetic ones, in food. Threshold limit values are premised on the idea that industry should be required to undertake the expense of reducing residues in the air of working places only if this is required for safety or comfort. A threshold limit is never reduced merely because the industry (or a major segment of it) can and does limit the concentration of a particular chemical to levels far below those considered safe. On the contrary, the tolerances for pesticides in food are based on much larger safety factors and, in addition, are limited to the concentrations actually requited by good agricultural practice when such concentrations are smaller than those considered safe.

Summarizing some of the points discussed above, the degree of protection we require from real toxic danger depends on (a) the nature of the danger, (b) the nature of the population to be protected, and (c) the quality of our knowledge of the danger. A safety factor of only 2 to 5 may be sufficient if the danger is merely one of irritation, if only few informed workers rather than a large segment of the general population may be exposed, and if assurance of safety is based on extensive occupational experience. On the contrary, a larger safety factor is required if the kind of danger involves any serious or chronic disease, if the general population may be exposed, or if information on safety must be extrapolated from tests on experimental animals.

Mathematical Considerations. Safety factors of whatever character are based on the effects of small dosages, a matter discussed in Section 2.2.7.4. The small dosages involved may be studied directly in experimental animals or man or, as discussed below, they may be extrapolated from the results of studies carried out at high dosage levels in animals.

The first statistical approach to safety factors was the definition of "maximum tolerated dose" proposed by Gray and his colleagues (1931), including Trevan, who was first to define the dosage-response relationship in a modern way. These authors noted that the term had implied a dosage that killed very rarely, but that no attempt had been made to state quantitatively what was meant by "very rarely." They proposed that the term be defined as a dosage 3 standard deviations less than the LD 50. This defines "very rarely" statistically as occurring in approximately 1 of 742 subjects under conditions used in the test. The suggestion is based on the workable assumption that response to different dosage levels (expressed as logarithms) is normally distributed, in other words that 15.866% of deviations are less than the mean minus 1 standard deviation. It is implicit in the theory of probits that the magnitude of the standard deviation is related to the slope of the log-probit curve, approaching zero as the curve approaches vertical and approaching infinity as the curve approaches horizontal. It follows that the LD 50 and LD 15.866 (rounded to LD 16) can be read from any LD 50 curve and used to calculate a dosage 3 standard deviations less than the LD 50 according to the following relationship:

log safe dosage
= log LD 50 − [3 (log LD 50 − log LD 16)]

The same result may be obtained entirely graphically by measuring off to the left from the LD 50 intercept 3 times the horizontal distance between the LD 50 and LD 16 intercepts. Of course, the same kind of extrapolation can be made from any ED 50 curve.

Gaddum (1956) extended the statistical concept of safety by suggesting that a safe dosage be considered (*a*) a dosage 6 standard deviations less than the LD 50 or, more conservatively, (*b*) a dosage 6 standard deviations less than a threshold dosage presumed to be harmless. Finally, he suggested that a safe dosage might be considered one 4 standard deviations

less than one producing no effect. (The difficulty of rigorously defining no effect is discussed in Section 2.2.7.4.) Gaddum used the term "threshold effect" in connection with measurements of body weight, food and water consumption, blood pressure, blood counts, and other parameters for which control animals demonstrate variability, and he defined such an effect as one exceeded about once in every 20 control animals. A threshold dosage, then, is one that produces a threshold effect, which is presumed to be harmless.

A dosage reduced by 6 standard deviations is one that may be expected to produce the effect on which it is based (whether death, increase in blood pressure above threshold level, or whatever) in only 1 in 1,000,000,000 subjects under the conditions of the test. In spite of this very conservative approach, the "safety factor" (that is the factor by which the dosage is decreased below LD 50 or threshold level) usually is not great. In nine examples discussed by Gaddum this factor varied from 1.6 to 6.3 with the exception of a factor of 139 for thiourea, which has an unusually flat dosage-response curve. Certainly, one of the main reasons for a statistical approach to safety is that it permits a scientific evaluation of the behavior of each compound.

However, as Gaddum observed, the statistical approach takes no account of possible differences between the responses of experimental animals and those of man. The same point has been emphasized by Weil (1972). Although these differences between species are small on the average, they may be large in individual cases (see Section 2.4.7.2). Finally, a statistical approach offers no help in choosing the most critical test to be made in animals. Considerations of this kind undoubtedly permit or even recommend the continued use of numerical safety factors as a method of estimating safe dosage levels.

The *numerical safety factor* most commonly used in connection with food additives and pesticides in foods is 100. Lehman and Fitzhugh (1954) discussed and endorsed this factor although they made no claim to have originated it. They expressed the view that man is about 40 times more sensitive to poisoning than the rat, and that some persons may be as much as 10 times more susceptible than others. It was implied but not stated that the factor of 100 was obtained by multiplying these two factors for interspecific and intraspecific variation. They recognized that the 100-fold margin of safety is not an absolute yardstick of safety, but they considered it high enough to reduce the hazard of food additives to a minimum and at the same time low enough to permit the use of some chemicals that are necessary in food production or processing.

Both the factor of 100 (for estimating human safety from animal experiments) and the factor of 10 (for estimating safety of the general population from information on safety of a limited number of persons) have been widely adopted in connection with food safety. Apparently no example is known in which these factors failed to offer protection. This good record is hardly astonishing when one considers that, for many compounds, safety factors varying from 1.6 to 6.3 are sufficient to reduce the risk in the species tested to one in one thousand million. Furthermore, on the average, species differ little in susceptibility to poisons (see Section 2.4.7.2). To be sure, one must be alert for the small number of compounds that show striking differences in toxicity to different species. Comparative studies of biotransformation may offer great help in predicting whether man will react about the same as other animals or very differently.

Further evidence that a factor of 100 really is not required is the good safety record of the chemical industry where much smaller factors commonly are employed, even when all critical data are from animals. On the other hand, it seems desirable to make greater use of statistical methods for setting safety factors. The occasional compound (such as thiourea) that requires a safety factor greater than 100 just to protect experimental animals ought to be recognized. Use of a compound that needs only a small safety factor ought not needlessly to be restricted.

Druckrey (1967), who demonstrated dosage-response relations of many carcinogens, proposed a safety factor somewhat less conservative than the one of 100 based on a no-effect level. Specifically, he suggested that 1% of the lowest dosage that produces cancer in susceptible animals only at the end of their life-span following daily intake for life can be considered the maximal tolerable dosage for people, and then only when complete exclusion of the compound from the human environment is not feasible.

For any carcinogenic compound, the use of which in food is considered important, Weil (1972) proposed a safety factor based on the lowest dosage producing a measurable increase in the incidence of cancer in a properly designed experiment in animals. The factor of 5,000 was arrived at by accepting the conventional factor of 100 and introducing a factor of 10 for carcinogenesis and a factor of 5 for use of the minimal-effect level (in contrast to the no-effect level).

It seems clear that Druckrey meant his factor of 100 to apply to aflatoxin and other carcinogens that occur naturally in food and therefore cannot be excluded completely. The factor of 5,000 applies to a wider range of compounds and is 50 times more conservative than that proposed by Druckrey.

Toxicologically Insignificant Levels. The concept of toxicologically insgnificant levels usually is discussed in connection with food packaging materials (Frawley, 1967) and food additives (National Academy of Sciences, 1969). Briefly, it is proposed that concentrations of < 0.1 ppm of compounds suitable for these purposes are toxicologically insignificant, inasmuch as the no-effect dietary level is greater than 40 ppm for all of them that have been tested in lifetime feeding studies. Compounds not suitable for these purposes include: (*a*) certain impurities or contaminants of natural origin, (*b*) certain essential nutrients and hormones, (*c*) certain heavy metals and their compounds, and (*d*) certain organic compounds employed for their biological activity (National Academy of Sciences, 1969).

It is generally accepted by toxicologists that the amount of attention given to investigation (and, if necessary, to control) ought to be determined by relative hazard in connection with the vast array of naturally occurring chemicals to which people are exposed. However, not all administrators seem willing to extend this principle to all matters of environmental health, as suggested by Frawley (1967). Failure to do so leads, as Frawley said, to wasted money and wasted skill of trained personnel in testing materials for uses that offer no hazard, and thus to apathy regarding regulations requiring such testing.

As already mentioned, pesticides, drugs, and other "organic compounds employed for their biological activity" are excluded as a class from materials for which toxicologically insignificant levels may be considered without testing. Some pesticides, for example difenphos, are less toxic by objective measurement than some food additives. The reason then for excluding biologically active compounds from the possibility of assigning toxicological insignificance without prior test is not any necessary danger, but the impossibility of excluding danger without test.

Whereas some oncologists have objected strongly to the idea that a very limited concentration of any compound can be judged toxicologically insignificant, some of them have reached essentially the same conclusion for practical purposes. Specifically, it has been suggested that, since laboratory and manpower resources are not available for testing all compounds to which people are exposed, priority for testing ought to be assigned on the basis of (a) the degree of exposure of the greatest number of people, and (b) the likelihood of hazard as judged by chemical similarity to compounds considered dangerous.

9.1.4.2 Acceptable Daily Intake. From a scientific standpoint, avoidance of injury from chemicals must be based on regulation of dosage. As long as the route and schedule of intake remain essentially constant, it makes little difference whether this dosage comes from one or many sources. It was partly a realization of these facts and partly the great variety of dietary habits in different parts of the world that led the World Health Organization Expert Committee on Pesticide Residues and the Food and Agriculture Organization Panel of Experts on the Use of Pesticides in Agriculture to propose at their first joint meeting (FAO/WHO, 1962) the concept of acceptable daily intake in connection with residues of pesticides in food.

The joint meeting defined *acceptable daily intake* as: "The daily dosage of a chemical which, during an entire lifetime, appears to be without appreciable risk on the basis of all the facts known at the time. 'Without appreciable risk' is taken to mean the practical certainty that injury will not result even after a lifetime of exposure. The *acceptable daily intake* is expressed in milligrams of the chemical, as it appears in the food, per kilogram of body weight (mg/kg/day)."

The joint meeting proposed that a *permissible level* of residue for a person's intake could be calculated from the acceptable daily intake and information on the average fraction of his total diet made up of the food or class of foods under discussion. Thus, if a certain insecticide were applied to rice only, the permissible level for it would be much lower in a country where rice is the most important food than in a country where people eat rice only occasionally. The joint meeting defined *tolerance* in the usual way, namely: "The permitted concentration of a residue in or on a food, derived by taking into account both the range of residues actually remaining when the food is first offered for consumption (following good agricultural practice) and the permissible level."

The meeting noted that the tolerance must never be greater than the permissible level for the food in question and would usually be smaller.

The joint meetings of the two committees led to a series of reports which contained careful reviews of toxicology and, when the available information permitted, set values for acceptable daily intake of individual pesticides. The first of these reports (FAO/WHO, 1964) contained information on 37 compounds and set acceptable values for 16 of them. Later reports (FAO/WHO, 1965a, 1965b, 1965c, 1969b, 1970a, 1970b, 1971a, 1971b, 1972a, 1972b, 1973a, 1973b, 1974) brought the total number of compounds reviewed to more than 110 and set acceptable values for more than 75. Not only were new values added but some of the old ones were revised as more information was acquired. Values published in 1973 are shown in Table 9-2. These ADI's tend to be conservative, as may be illustrated for DDT and dieldrin by comparing the values in Table 9-2 with those in Table 7-24 and 7-25, or by considering evidence presented by Hunted (1968).

Because of practical considerations of world trade in food and feed, the joint meetings have tended to give decreasing attention to acceptable daily intakes and increasing attention to standardized tolerances. The conservatism of these standard tolerances makes them safe even though they fail to take into account possible differences in the consumption of different foods in different countries.

9.1.4.3 Tolerances. Tolerances for pesticides are legal limits for the concentration of specific compounds on or in specific foods. In the United States of America, interstate tolerances are established under authority of the Federal Food, Drug, and Cosmetic Act as amended. This law (21 USC 301) was approved 25 June 1938 to replace legislation enacted in 1906. The major relevant amendments of the 1938 law are the Miller Amendment, approved 22 July 1954 (21 USC 346a), and the Food Additives Amendment, approved 6 September 1958 (21 USC 348). States have similar laws, but with a few exceptions the states adopt the interstate tolerances for intrastate use. An example of such a state law is the California Agricultural Code (Chap. 7, Art. 1).

In connection with pesticides, the Federal Food, Drug, and Cosmetic Act and the Federal Insecticide, Fungicide, and Rodenticide Act were directly interrelated by regulations made under them. No registration was granted for use of any pesticide on a crop or in any other way that would lead to a residue on food until a tolerance or exemption from tolerance has been granted for the particular pesticide on the particular food. Conversely, no tolerance was granted for a pesticide on a food unless the Secretary of Agriculture certified that the particular pesticide was necessary for protecting the specific crop or other specific

Table 9-2

Maximal Acceptable Daily Intake (ADI) Of Certain Pesticides

From FAO/WHO (1973).

Compounds arranged by groups	ADI (mg/kg)
Inorganic and organometal pesticides	
fentin	0.0005
tricyclohexyltin hydroxide	0.0075
Pesticides derived from plants and other organisms	
pyrethrins	0.04
Synergists	
piperonyl butoxide	0.03
Fumigants and nematocides	
bromide	1.0
hydrogen cyanide	0.05
Chlorinated hydrocarbon insecticides	
DDT and related compounds	
chlorobenzilate	0.02
DDT, DDE and DDD	0.005
dicofol	0.025
methoxychlor	0.1
cyclodienes and related compounds	
aldrin	0.0001
chlordane	0.001
dieldrin	0.0001
endosulfan	0.0075
endrin	0.0002
heptachlor	0.0005
lindane	0.0125
Organic phosphorus insecticides	
dimethoxy compounds	
azinphosmethyl	0.0025
bromophos	0.006 [a/]
carbophenothion	0.005 [a/]
chlorfenvinphos	0.002
dichlorvos	0.004
dimethoate	0.02

Table 9-2 (continued)

Compounds arranged by groups	ADI (mg/kg)
Organic phosphorus insecticides (cont'd)	
fenitrothion	0.001
fenthion	0.0005 [a]
malathion	0.02
methidathion	0.005
mevinphos	0.0015
parathion methyl	0.001
phosphamidon	0.001
ronnel	0.01
trichlorfon	0.01 [a]
diethoxy compounds	
bromophos-ethyl	0.003
carbophenothion	0.005
coumaphos	0.0005
crufomate	0.1
demeton	0.0025
diazinon	0.002
dioxathion	0.0015
ethion	0.005
fensulfothion	0.0003
monocrotophos	0.0003
parathion	0.005
phosalone	0.006
Carbamates and related pesticides	
carbaryl	0.01 [a]
dithiocarbamates	
ferbam	0.025 [a]
mancozeb	0.025 [a]
maneb	0.025 [a]
nabam	0.025 [a]
thiram	0.025 [a]
zineb	0.025 [a]
ziram	0.025 [a]
Phenolic and nitrophenolic pesticides	
binapacryl	0.0025
o-phenylphenol	1.0

Table 9-2 (continued)

Compounds arranged by groups	ADI (mg/kg)
Miscellaneous pesticides	
chlorbenside	0.01
chlorfenson	0.01
Herbicides and related compounds	
chlormequat	0.05
2, 4-D	0.3
diquat	0.005
ethoxyquin	0.06
paraquat	0.002
Fungicides and related compounds	
captafol	0.05[a]
captan	0.125[a]
diphenyl	0.125
folpet	0.16[a]
hexachlorobenzene	0.0006[a]
quintozene	0.001[a]
thiabendazole	0.05
Repellants and attractants	
diphenylamine	0.025

a. Temporary value

food. These legal requirements for coordination formalized administrative arrangements in effect long before the regulations were issued. Now, there is no need for special coordination because registration, the setting of tolerances, and the establishment of efficacy are all the responsibility of the Environmental Protection Agency.

The most important monitoring of our food in regard to pesticides is that carried out each year by the Food and Drug Administration and the Department of Agriculture in connection with food shipped in interstate commerce and by comparable agencies in different states in regard to food brought to market within their own jurisdictions. The federal government alone analyzes over 26,000 samples per year, which constitutes approximately 1% of the total food shipped in interstate commerce (Monfore, 1965). The samples involve (a) the Market Basket Program to measure pesticides in 117 items of food constituting the total diet, (b) the Rational Monitoring Program aimed at surveillance and enforcement at the point of origin (10,000 to 12,000 samples per year), and (c) the Consumer Protection Program for sampling meats and poultry (Duggan and Cook, 1971).

Approximately half of the samples contain detectable residues, and about one-third contain more than one residue. However, 95% of the residues are below 0.51 ppm. Most of the foods sampled in the surveillance program undergo further processing or preparation prior to consumption, and the concentration of pesticides in the edible portion is substantially less (Duggan, 1968).

Among the states, California apparently carries out the most extensive program of testing food products for pesticide residues. During 1964, the California State Department of Agriculture tested 14,596 samples of foods and feeds for pesticide residues (Rollins, 1965). Of these, 537 samples (3.7%) were found to contain residues in excess of the tolerance level. The biggest problem associated with illegal residues was encountered not with food intended directly for man, but with hay and fodder crops. Of 3,253 samples of these commodities analyzed, 405 samples (12.5%) contained residues in excess of the low tolerance level set for them. Many of the samples, both federal and state, are taken from shipments suspected of containing excessive residues. Suspicion is based on information regarding use of pesticides, which tend to be heavier in certain places and in certain seasons where conditions are particularly favorable for crop pests.

Analyses carried out for the purpose of enforcement occasionally reveal violations. An example may be found in the seizures of large shipments of potatoes and carrots in the Pacific Northwest in 1962 because they contained excessive residues of aldrin and dieldrin (Monfore, 1965). Aldrin had been applied not to the vegetables but to the soil in which they were grown. Corrective measures were taken, and excessive residues were not found during the following year (Monfore, 1965). This episode is typical of recent experience in that the small number of residues found to be at or above tolerance limits are often the result of drift or some other environmental factor, rather than direct misuse of pesticide on the crop involved (Duggan, 1968).

Monitoring for the purpose of enforcement tends to give information on maximal potential intake of pesticides rather than on typical intake. Enforcement of the law, which is an integral part of the monitoring, is a powerful force to prevent illegal residues of pesticides from reaching the consumer market.

A different kind of monitoring has been carried out to learn the extent of the average daily intake of a wide range of pesticides. In this instance, an effort is made to get samples that are representative of the total diet, rather than to seek out samples likely to be in violation. A description of these total diet studies and their findings is given in Section 6.1.5.1.

When established, tolerances are published in the Federal Register. Official compilations of current values are available (40 CFR 180.101 et seq.). In addition to legally established tolerances, it always has been necessary for the Food and Drug Administration to set action levels or criteria for legal action. These action levels concern toxicants that occur naturally in food, compounds used for a purpose but for which no tolerance has been set, and compounds that may find their way into food through drift or in some other way not directly related to their intended use. The action levels apply essentially to inadvertent residues, and the existence of these action levels does not prevent legal action on lower residue levels if there is evidence of misuse of pesticides, or some other factor appears to warrant action. Action levels for a number of common pesticides were released by the Food and Drug Administration on May 5, 1972.

Recent joint meetings of the World Health Organization Expert Committee on Pesticide Residues and the Food and Agriculture Organization Panel of Experts on the Use of Pesticides in Agriculture have used the term "practical residue limit" to signify an action level for unintentional residues, and a number of these limits have been published (FAO/WHO, 1970b, 1971b, 1972b, 1973b).

9.1.4.4 Water Standards. In the United States of America, drinking water standards (42 CFR 72.201 et seq.) are established by the Public Health Service under authority of the Public Health Service Act. These standards apply directly only to interstate carriers and those subject to federal quarantine regulations. However, the standards are generally accepted and form the basis of state and local regulation and practice.

At first, the Public Health Service standards (Treasury Department, 1914) involved bacteriological contaminants only. Limits for some chemicals were added in 1925 (Advisory Committee on Official Water Standards, 1925). In 1962 the standards were extended to include radioactive materials (US Public Health Service, 1962). The 1962 revision contained no entry for pesticides as such; arsenic, cyanide, and fluoride were specified, but there is no reason to expect that an important source of these ions in water would be pesticides. The 1962 revision also placed a limit (0.2 mg/liter) on carbon chloroform extract [42 CFR 72.205 b(l)]. Although many pesticides are adsorbed by charcoal and can be eluted from it by chloroform, according to the technique described by Ettinger (1960), the standard was established for organic residues in general and not for pesticides, which constitute only a small fraction of organic residues in water.

The Manual for Evaluating Public Drinking Water Supplies issued by the Public Health Service (1969) to supplement the 1962 standards did set limits on several pesticides listed in Table 9-3. Although not stated, the standards for chlorinated hydrocarbon insecticides were based mainly on the susceptibility of fish, and they offer much larger human safety factors than do the standards for materials that are not pesticides.

9.1.4.5 Threshold Limit Values or Maximal

Table 9-3

Upper Limits for Pesticides in Drinking Water

Compounds arranged by groups	Concentration[a] (mg/liter)
Chlorinated hydrocarbon insecticides	
DDT and related compounds	
DDT	0.042
methoxychlor	0.035
cyclodienes and related compounds	
aldrin	0.017
chlordane	0.003
dieldrin	0.017
endrin	0.001
heptachlor	0.018
heptachlor epoxide	0.018
toxaphene	0.005
lindane	0.056
Total organophosphorus and carbamate compounds[b]	0.1
Herbicides	
2,4-D	0.1[c]
2,4,5-T	0.1[c]
2,4,5-TP	0.1[c]

a. For long term exposure unless otherwise stated.

b. Expressed in terms of parathion-equivalent cholinesterase inhibition.

c. Short period limit only: 2 to 3 days, no more than once or twice a year for individual compound or any combination of chlorinated phenoxy alkyl pesticides.

Allowable Concentrations. Standards for permissible concentrations of industrial chemicals in air are intended for the protection of workers. Unlike the acceptable daily intakes, tolerances, and water standards discussed above, these standards for air are not meant to apply to the general population. Recently, there has been some effort to develop community air standards that would apply to the continuous exposure of everyone, but no such values have been proposed for pesticides.

Standards for permissible concentrations of materials in air were first stated as *maximal allowable concentrations* (MAC). Some countries still use this form of standard. However, injury from the majority of industrial chemicals depends on excessive average daily intake and not on brief exposure to exceptionally high concentrations. An accurate estimate of the effective concentration of a compound in the air of a work place can be obtained only by systematic sampling and the calculation of a time-weighted average concentration. An understanding of these facts led to the replacement of maximal allowable concentrations by *threshold limit values* (TLV) as standards for respiratory exposure in work situations.

Both MAC and TLV values must be regarded as guidelines rather than as rigid limits or exact thresholds. The term "maximal allowable" has an administrative rather than a pharmacological connotation. The term "threshold" does not refer to the zone within which some specific, undesirable response begins but rather the zone within which experienced industrial hygienists will establish an alert. The threshold for minimal pharmacological response may correspond with the guideline values for harmless irritants, but are higher than the guidelines for materials injurious to health.

The same units are used to express either a

MAC or a TLV. It is conventional to express the limits for gases and vapors in terms of parts per million (ppm) of air at 25°C and a pressure of 760 mm of mercury. Limits for most particulates are expressed in terms of **milligrams per cubic meter (mg/m³)**. These units are interchangeable for any given compound according to the equation:

$$ppm = \frac{\text{observed concentration (mg/l)} \times 24,450}{\text{molecular weight of compound}}$$

or:

$$ppm = \frac{mg/m^3 \times 24.45}{\text{molecular weight of compound}}$$

The figure, 24,450 ml, is the gram molecular volume of a gas at a temperature of 25°C and a pressure of 760 mm of mercury.

Limits for some particulates, especially silica, silicates, graphite, and "inert" or nuisance dusts are expressed in terms of number of particles per unit volume. The most common unit, million particles per cubic foot (mppcf), may be converted as follows:

$$mppcf \times 35 = \text{million particles per m}^3$$
$$= \text{particles per cc.}$$

A TLV is a permissible time-weighted average for the concentration of a material in the air breathed by workers. In general, an excursion above the average is permitted if balanced by an equal excursion below the average. The actual magnitude of the excursion permitted depends on the magnitude of the TLV itself. The permissible variation is 3-fold for compounds with TLV's ranging from 0 to 1, 2-fold for those with limits from 1.1 to 10, 1.5-fold for those with limits from 10.1 to 100, and 1.25-fold for those with limits from 100.1 to 1000. For some compounds (principally irritants) that are most likely to cause injury or discomfort by reaching a relatively high although brief peak, it is necessary to set a *ceiling value* (C-value). The only distinction between a C-value and a MAC is the conceptual distinction based on recognition of the advantage of using systematic sampling and daily, time-weighted averages even for the purpose of predicting and avoiding excessive peak values.

In the United States of America, threshold limit values are set by the American Conference of Governmental Industrial Hygienists (ACGIH). The values are reviewed and published annually. A book presenting background information and references justifying each TLV and a booklet of current values may be purchased from the Secretary of ACGIH (American Conference of Governmental Industrial Hygienists, 1971, 1973). Problems in the development and use of TLV's have been discussed by Stokinger (1969), who has long been chairman of the ACGIH Committee on Threshold Limits.

TLV values for pesticides published in 1973 are shown in Table 9-4.

If the threshold limits of pesticides are plotted against their LD 50 values (Fig. 9-3) it may be seen that an apparently greater safety margin has been provided for the chlorinated hydrocarbon insecticides than for the organic phosphorus and some other pesticides. This action is meant to take into account the tendency of the chlorinated compounds to be more cumulative than the other compounds, both chemically and clinically.

Comparison of the TLV's for pesticides (other than those generally thought of as industrial chemicals) with those for other industrial chemicals shows that the TLV values for pesticides often are more conservative. No scientific justification for this distinction is apparent. There may be a tendency to be more cautious in dealing with compounds manufactured as poisons than in dealing with other compounds of identical toxicity.

It has been pointed out frequently that the standards set for the concentration of chemicals in the air of work places are more conservative in the Soviet Union than in Western Europe and North and South America. The difference is associated with differences in the kinds of tests and the philosophical bases for setting standards. One method emphasizes physiological, biochemical, and other preclinical tests, in the belief that permissible limits can be set safely within the compensatory zone of reaction; the Eastern European method emphasizes behavioral tests in the belief that limits ought to be established well within the region of homeostasis at a dosage level that produces no effect whatever (Hatch, 1972).

Table 9-5 summarizes a comparison made by Elkins (1961) of the standards used in the United States of America and in the Soviet Union. The two sets of standards do not vary much for most mineral and inert dusts or, in fact, for dusts and fumes generally. The standards show great divergence for many other materials, especially chlorinated hydrocarbon solvents. Elkins pointed out that industrial exposures to some chemicals have never occurred in the United States of America at the

Table 9-4 (continued)

Threshold Limit Values for Certain Pesticides

From American Conference of Governmental Industrial Hygienists
(1973) by permission of the American Conference of Governmental
Industrial Hygienists.

Compounds Arranged by Groups	TLV (mg/m^3)
Inorganic and organometal pesticides	
arsenic	
calcium arsenate	1
lead arsenate	0.15
mercury	
alkyl compounds	0.01
all other compounds	0.05
phosphorus	0.1
thallium	0.1
tin	2
tricyclohexyltin hydroxide	5
Pesticides derived from plants and other organisms	
nicotine	0.5
pyrethrum	5
rotenone	5
strychnine	0.15
Fumigants and nematocides	
acrylonitrile	45
carbon disulfide	60
carbon tetrachloride	65
chloroform	120[a]/
chloropicrin	0.7
cyanide	5
hydrogen cyanide	11
1, 2-dibromoethane	145[a]/
o-dichlorobenzene	300
p-dichlorobenzene	450
1, 1-dichloroethane	820[a]/
1, 2-dichloroethane	200
1, 2-dichloropropane	350
1, 2-epoxyethane	90
hexachlorocyclopentadiene	0.1
methyl bromide	60[a]/
methylene chloride	870

(handwritten annotation: mg / cubic meter)

Table 9-4 (continued)

Compounds arranged by groups	T L V (mg/m^3)
Fumigants and nematocides (cont'd)	
naphthalene	50
sulfur dioxide	13
tetrachloroethylene	670
1, 1, 1-trichloroethane	1,900
trichloroethylene	535
Chlorinated hydrocarbon insecticides	
DDT and related compounds	
DDT	1
methoxychlor	10
cyclodienes and related compounds	
aldrin	0.25
chlordane	0.5
dieldrin	0.25
endosulfan	0.1
endrin	0.1
heptachlor	0.5
toxaphene	0.5
lindane	0.5
Organic phosphorus insecticides	
dimethoxy compounds	
azinphosmethyl	0.2
dichlorovos	1
difenphos	10
malathion	10
methyl demeton	0.5
mevinphos	0.1
ronnel	10
diethoxy compounds	
demeton	0.1
diazinon	0.1
disulfoton	0.1
Dursban ®	0.2
parathion	0.1
phorate	0.05
tepp	0.05
EPN	0.5
Ruelene ®	5

Table 9-4 (continued)

Compounds arranged by groups	T L V (mg/m^3)
Carbamates and related compounds	
N-methyl carbamates	
carbaryl	5
carbofuran	0.05
propoxur	0.5
dithiocarbamates	
ferbam	10
thiram	5
Phenolic and nitrophenolic pesticides	
DNOC	0.2
pentachlorophenol	0.5
Synthetic organic rodenticides	
antu	0.3
sodium fluoroacetate	0.05
warfarin	0.1
Herbicides and related compounds	
acrolein	0.25
ammonium sulfamate	10
2, 4 - D	10
paraquat	0.5
picloram	10
2, 4, 5 - T	10
Fungicides and related compounds	
diphenyl	1
Repellants and attractants	
diphenylamine	10

a.   Trial limit

levels set by their standards except for brief periods; it must be recalled that the USA standards are supposed to be based on safety without reference to the ease with which each standard can be followed. On the other hand Elkins expressed doubt that conventional control methods can meet the Soviet standards in all processes. What is needed is a quantitative study of air concentrations of materials in the air of work places in different countries.

In its Sixth Report, the Joint International Labor Organization/World Health Organization Committee on Occupational Health (ILO/WHO, 1969) recommended safe concentration zones for 24 compounds about which there already was general, international agreement.

The Committee used the term "safe concentration zone" to cover both maximal allowable concentrations and time-weighted averages, implying that the practical difference may be unimportant. (Although precision in measuring toxic effect may not justify the distinction between MAC's and TLV's, the distinction may be justified on a conceptual basis.)

Biological Index.   The Committee also discussed at some length the possibility of developing biological indices of occupational exposure. They considered that the primary practical means of protecting exposed persons is the sampling and analysis of environmental air. The great value of biological indices is in the establishment of maximal permissible limits,

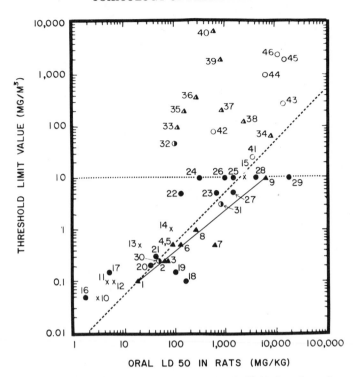

Fig. 9-3. Relationship between acute oral toxicity and threshold limit values for certain classes of compounds, namely: *chlorinated hydrocarbon insecticides* (▲) (endrin, 1; aldrin, 2; dieldrin, 3; heptachlor, 4; toxaphene, 5; lindane, 6; chlordane, 7; DDT, 8; methoxychlor, 9), *organic phosphorus insecticides* (×) (tepp, 10; parathion, 11; demeton, 12; EPN, 13; dichlorvos, 14; malathion, 15), *miscellaneous pesticides* (●) (sodium fluoroacetate, 16; strychnine, 17; warfarin, 18; lead arsenate, 19; DNOC, 20; antu, 21; rotenone, 22; thiram, 23; 2,4,5-T, 24; 2,4-D, 25; sesone, 26; pyrethrum, 27; AMS, 28; ferbam, 29) *chlorinated hydrocarbon solvents* (△) *and other industrial chemicals* (◑) *used as pesticides but generally thought of as industrial chemicals* (acrolein, 30; formaldehyde, 31; acrylonitrile, 32; dichloroethylether, 33; carbon tetrachloride, 34; ethylenedibromide, 35; propylenedibromide, 36; ethylenedichloride, 37; chloroform, 38; methylchloroform, 39; trichloroethylene, 40), and *typical industrial chemicals* (O) *not used as pesticides* (acetic acid, 41; diethylamine, 42; methanol, 43; isopropyl alcohol, 44; ethanol, 45; and acetone, 46). The dotted, horizontal line corresponds to the highest TLV permitted for particulates including some of low toxicity thought to constitute a nuisance only. The solid, oblique line shows the trend for the TLV's of chlorinated hydrocarbon insecticides. The dashed, oblique line is the locus of points with a ratio of LD 50 values to TLV values identical to that of endrin.

and in the subsequent diagnosis of overexposure in individuals. Storage and excretion of pesticides in people and other relevant changes that have been measured in the laboratory and might be made the basis of biological indices or biological threshold limits are discussed in Sections 7.2 and 7.3. The relative value of biological indices for evaluating exposure to different classes of compounds is discussed in Section 9.3.1.8 in connection with monitoring of workers.

9.1.4.6 Other Standards. Standards of a more comprehensive kind that eventually may involve some pesticides are those promulgated under terms of the Occupational Safety and Health Act of 1970 (29 USC 651 *et seq.*).

So far, such standards have been developed only for important industrial chemicals or other factors known to constitute potential problems for hundreds and often thousands of workers. These standards for the regulation of occupational hazards are based on research carried out and criteria proposed by the National Institute for Occupational Safety and Health (NIOSH) of the Public Health Service, Department of Health, Education, and Welfare. The final regulation and enforcement program is determined by the Occupational Safety and Health Administration (OSHA) of the Department of Labor. In line with the growing tendency to set standards by consensus of those with varying interests, OSHA assembles an advisory committee to review

Table 9-5

Factors by Which Limits Set for Substances in the Air of Work Places
in the United States of America Exceed Those in the Soviet Union

Class of substance	Number of substances	Factor	
		range	mean
irritant gases and vapors	19	0. 7 - 80	11. 7
hydrocarbon solvents	8	2. 0 - 22	10. 4
chlorinated hydrocarbon solvents	9	7. 0 - 42	25. 4
miscellaneous solvents and organic vapors	25	1. 5 - 40	8. 0
miscellaneous gases and vapors	7	0. 5 - 40	12. 9
organic dusts and fumes	12	1. 0 - 20	4. 7
inorganic dusts, fumes, and mists	23	1. 0 - 20	4. 0
mineral and inert dusts	10	2. 0 - 9	4. 6

the standards for related kinds of hazards or problems (for example, toxic metals, radiation, health care, and heat stress and noise). Each committee consists of no more than 15 members. The suggested distribution of representatives is: employees, 4; employers, 4; state officials, 2; federal officials, 2; and experts associated with neither employees nor employers, 3.

9.1.4.7 Toxicity Rating or Class. The toxicity rating or toxicity classification of all materials from botulinum toxins to food and water seldom is considered in discussions of standards. Yet this classification is of great practical importance in regulating labeling and the transportation of dangerous goods. Toxicity classification is also important in guiding physicians regarding the danger of foreign substances and proper symptomatic medical management of poisoning. Standards for toxicity rating are inherently arbitrary in their details, for they consist of marking off intervals on what clearly is a continuous spectrum of toxicity from the greatest known to the least. By contrast, standards for acceptable daily intake of individual compounds or for the concentration of substances in food, water, or air can be and are tailor-made to fit each compound and the occupational or other circumstances in which it is encountered.

Whereas the exact breakpoints in toxicity rating are arbitrary, the necessity of having breakpoints is obvious. The correspondence of response to the logarithm of dosage indicates that the intervals ought to be logarithmic, except that a ceiling (eg, 15,000 mg/kg for ingestion) may be set for compounds that are practically nontoxic. Since the opportunity for exposure by one route may be far greater than

that by another, it is only reasonable to take a conservative approach by setting the cutoff point for the most toxic category at a higher dosage level for a route of heavy exposure (the skin, for example) than that for another route.

In the United States of America, there is general agreement about where the cutoff points ought to be. As already mentioned, the criteria for toxicity are consistent for labeling (Section 9.1.1.1) and for the regulation of the transportation of dangerous goods (Section 9.1.2.1). This agreement permits great economies for manufacturers and shippers and favors the greatest possible degree of understanding and benefit on the part of the public generally. The regulatory criteria are also consistent with the toxicity ratings commonly used in evaluating the danger of accidental poisoning through ingestion. This may be seen by comparing Table 9-1 and the associated text with Table 9-6, taken with slight modification from the deservedly popular book *Clinical Toxicology of Commercial Products* (Gleason et al., 1969).

Unfortunately, agreement about the details of toxicity rating or classification is not worldwide. A uniform system would be a convenience for trade, inasmuch as regulations governing labeling and transportation are built around toxicity classes. Information on the classification used for the toxicological assessment of pesticides in the Soviet Union and the one proposed by the Council of Europe was published by WHO (1972).

9.1.5 Cost of Regulations

The direct cost of regulating pesticides includes the salaries and office costs of the administrators, lawyers, analysts, technicians,

Table 9-6

Toxicity Classification Commonly Used in Evaluating
the Danger of Accidental Poisoning Through Ingestion

Slightly modified from Gleason et al. (1969) and reproduced
by permission of the Williams and Wilkins Company.

Toxicity rating	Probable lethality for people	
	Dosage (mg/kg)	Dose for 70-kg man
6 super toxic	less than 5	a taste (less than 7 drops)
5 extremely toxic	5-50	between 7 drops and 1 teaspoonful
4 very toxic	50-500	between 1 teaspoonful and 1 ounce
3 moderately toxic	500-5,000	between 1 ounce and 1 pint (or 1 pound)
2 slightly toxic	5,000-15,000	between 1 pint and 1 quart
1 practically nontoxic	above 15,000	more than 1 quart

clerks, and inspectors who regulate labels, residues, transportation, or use of these compounds. It is difficult to estimate this regulatory cost because the agencies involved regulate other materials too, and they have non-regulatory duties.

In addition to administrative costs, a portion of the preregistration cost of measuring residues and determining toxicity must be counted as part of the cost of regulation. Considerable research would have to be done even if no regulations existed, but much of the research done is specifically designed to satisfy regulations. As shown in Table 9-7, the average cost per compound for developing a pesticide to the point of sale has increased more than 3 times since 1956. This increase is partly because of inflation but also because the amount and quality of required information have increased, requiring an increase in the number of man-years of work per compound.

By 1970 the average estimated cost of bringing a new pesticide to market was $5.49 million. This cost covered several thousand compounds screened in the process of finding a successful one. Of the total cost, approximately 12 to 13%, or about $688,000 per successful compound, was devoted to safety evaluation.

The cost of regulating pesticides has serious implications for many developing nations. On the one hand, some countries are in special need of pesticides either to combat malaria and other vector-borne diseases or to increase agricultural efficiency, or both. On the other hand, these same nations can ill afford the direct cost of regulation or the hidden cost of diverting trained chemists and other professional people to nonproductive work. Some compromise must be reached.

Evidence indicates that regulation of labeling is of greatest importance. Therefore, every government must have a staff with enough training and independence to question in a meaningful way the data and claims submitted by manufacturers in support of their products. However, each nation need not have facilities for checking the wide range of data that will be submitted; they can get unbiased, expert opinion on these technical matters from other nations, and especially from the World Health Organization. As already suggested, it may be best to exclude the most toxic pesticides from countries without a labor force accustomed to using industrial chemicals.

It appears that, after labeling, regulation of use is next, both in importance and economy. Not only is the regulation of use relatively inexpensive, but the staff required is the kind a developing country can best afford. Such a country is less likely to spare an analytical chemist than an entomologist or agronomist who can help farmers with production as well as safety.

Finally, in regard to residues, more that is

really relevant to health can be learned from analysis of a limited number of samples of human blood, tissue, and excreta than from analysis of an extensive series of food samples. If the intake of a particular pesticide is considered excessive, its source can be found and corrected. However, as Barnes (1967) said, "It is better that a population has some tissue fat in which the chemist can find high levels of chlorinated hydrocarbon insecticides than undernourished people die of diseases like tuberculosis but with tissue levels of DDT no greater than their wealthier neighbours."

9.1.6 Liability

Laws regulating pesticides are intended to protect the user or the public generally. Violations lead to seizures and condemnations, fines, and more rarely imprisonments, as provided by the laws. In spite of wise regulation and energetic enforcement, there remains the possibility of injury and, therefore, of civil suit under common law. Such suits usually involve third party actions or products liability. Even an outline of these matters is beyond the scope of this book. However, two points are worth noting. First, Turner (1968), in a review of trends in pesticide usage liability, concluded that a disclaimer of liability on a warranty is no bar to recovery of damages. In fact, the US Department of Agriculture has rendered an advisory opinion to this effect in regard to its labeling jurisdiction. Contractual disclaimers, while at one time validated in regard to all warranty obligations, have fallen into disfavor in the courts. Second, in many jurisdictions, detailed and cumbersome substantive prerequisites have been streamlined in products liability cases involving faulty, ineffective, or injurious pesticides. Although it is difficult to evaluate the importance of liability in regulating the use of pesticides, its influence for good is obviously considerable—and its misuse, whether innocent or intentional, also is considerable.

9.2 Choice of Compound and Formulation

In order to achieve control of a particular pest, the choices of compounds, formulations, and application rates are limited or even fixed by the susceptibility of the pest, the cost of different compounds, and other practical considerations. The fact that hazardous chemicals remain in use is proof that safer but equally effective materials are not available at an economical cost. However, considerable progress regarding both compounds and formulations has been made during the period since World War II, which has witnessed such an increase in the use of pesticides.

9.2.1 Choice of Compound

The use of inherently less toxic active ingredients is the most obvious improvement that can be made in the formulation of a pesticide, and frequently this is the only change mentioned in discussions involving safety. One should not overlook the possibility that highly toxic compounds may be practical, especially if they lend themselves to safe formulation. In fact, the substitution of a relatively poisonous compound with little cumulative effect for a material having less acute but more residual toxicity may be desirable in some instances. The hazard of using the former type of compounds on food products involves only the

Table 9-7

Average Cost of Developing a Pesticide
to the Point of Sale

Year	Estimated overall cost per compound	Reference
1956	$1,196,000	Field, 1964
1963	2,000,000	Golz, 1963
1964	2,918,000	Field, 1964
1969	4,060,436	von Rümker et al., 1970

workers concerned, while the latter potentially involves the whole population.

The substitution of DDT for lead arsenate and other arsenicals is the change that has contributed most to human safety. Instances of chronic lead poisoning associated with orchard spraying were reported (Farner *et al.,* 1949). Acute poisoning by arsenicals continues to constitute an important proportion of all fatal accidental poisoning by pesticides (see Section 7.1.2.2). By contrast, there are no confirmed cases of chronic poisoning by DDT. Even in regard to acute poisoning, DDT has maintained a good safety record during more than 25 years of extensive use. The record of DDT has been so good that it has been necessary to emphasize at every turn that the compound is not harmless and should be used with appropriate precaution.

Another striking example of the use of inherently less toxic active ingredients is the extensive substitution of warfarin and other anticoagulant rodenticides for a number of highly toxic, quick-acting rodenticides, including sodium fluoroacetate. It has been clearly demonstrated that warfarin is at least equal, if not superior, to any of the old rodenticides from the standpoint of control. By contrast, it has an excellent safety record.

Other examples include the partial substitution of malathion or even methyl parathion and azinphosmethyl for parathion or tepp.

The substitution of so-called nonchemical methods of control in place of pesticides may be considered as the ultimate extension of the "choice of compound." So far, research that might lead to such substitution has been prompted chiefly by the need for better control or by a desire to protect wildlife. The development of new methods does not exclude consideration of improved human safety. However, as pointed out in Section 9.5, the use of alternate methods of control offers no automatic guarantee of safety.

9.2.2 Choice of Formulation

A chemical retains its inherent toxicity regardless of how it is formulated. However, even when the kind and extent of use remain constant, proper formulation can minimize the chance that the active ingredient will be absorbed or that a pesticidally inert ingredient will be harmful.

The safety records of individual pesticides are sufficiently distinct that it is frequently possible to compare them under practical conditions of use. The same is seldom true of different formulations of the same pesticide. By necessity, evidence on the relative safety of different formulations usually must be drawn from environmental monitoring or animal experiments.

9.2.2.1 Liquid and Paste Formulations.

Solvents. In developing formulations with a maximal safety factor for any particular active ingredient, the solvent is of great importance. One or more solvents frequently constitute the bulk of liquid preparations. As pointed out by Jacobziner (1966), the pesticidally inert ingredient in some formulations actually constitutes their major hazard to human health.

The avoidance of solvents with high inherent toxicity is of major importance. Benzene may cause a severe depression of the bone marrow activity with consequent anemia, and should never be used as a solvent for pesticides.

Another danger inherent in many solvents is their flammability. In this regard, the chlorinated hydrocarbon solvents are relatively safe, and this property must be kept in mind in evaluating their overall applicability. The conditions of use also must be considered. Formulations that would be entirely too flammable for use in aircraft can be used safely in certain other situations.

Sudden deaths from cardiac arrythmias following exposure to hydrocarbon solvents used as anaesthetics or for a variety of purposes in industry have been recognized for many years. Deaths also have followed use of aerosols intended to relieve asthma or willful misuse (sniffing) of various aerosols to produce a thrill. Recent, unpublished cases are consistent with the conclusion that sufficient inhalation of the propellants released from the discharge of otherwise harmless insecticide aerosols can cause death, even though there is no intentional misuse and no attempt to seek a thrill.

Danger from solvents can be minimized by using paste or mayonnaise-type concentrates, or essentially eliminated by using water-wettable powders, dusts, or granules.

Paste and Other Special Liquid Concentrates. Some semisolid formulations have been prepared to reduce absorption either by reducing the possibility of contamination or in some more subtle fashion. For example, the same dermal dosage of dieldrin (100 mg/kg) produced only 20 to 30% mortality when applied in the form of paste or mayonnaise-type formulations instead of 95% mortality that followed application of solutions (Hayes and Pearce, 1953). This was true even though in the experimental procedure the thick materials at the prescribed dosage were rather laboriously rubbed into the skin. The true safety factor is much greater than the figures indicate because, if contamination does occur with the paste or mayonnaise-type preparations, the material does not spread on the skin but tends to stand up in a mound. Unlike a liquid preparation, most of it can be quickly wiped from the skin without the use of soap and water.

It may be possible to reduce the toxicity of a pesticide to mammals by formulating it with one or more active ingredients. For example, parathion was formulated with DDT and rosin in an effort to get a longer residual action and in the hope of finding some synergistic action against resistant houseflies. The effectiveness of the combination as a residual, when tested in the laboratory against DDT-resistant houseflies, was found greatly superior to equivalent dosages of DDT or parathion alone. On the contrary, the combination was less toxic to mammals. When the concentration of parathion in xylene (2.5%) and its rate of application (40 mg/kg) were both held constant, the mortality of white rats averaged only 15% for the mixture but was constantly 100% for parathion alone (Hayes and Pearce, 1953).

The use of special emulsifiers to increase the safety of demeton formulations has been reported (Deichmann *et al.*, 1952).

9.2.2.2 Dry Formulations.

Dusts and Water-Wettable Powders. Dusts serve as a vehicle or diluent in dry formulations and should be selected for nontoxicity, just as liquid solvents are selected. In particular, this means holding the percentage of free silica to a minimum and avoiding the use of talc, one of the few silicates known to cause pneumoconiosis. There is little danger of silicosis to the person who uses dusts occasionally, but the exposure of the commercial applicator or mixing plant worker may be significant.

Over and above the threat of silicosis, all dusts are somewhat irritating to the respiratory tract. For this reason, and because of the toxicity of the active ingredient in the dust or powder, the development of antidusting formulations is a marked improvement. Their use in water-wettable powders allows the worker who mixes suspensions in the field to encounter significantly smaller concentrations in the air. In a study involving measurements during two spray seasons, the concentration of parathion in the air at the level of workers' faces during the mixing process in apple orchards averaged 2.21 mg/m³ with ordinary wettable powder, and 0.37 mg/m³ with antidusting powder. The highest value found (1.68 mg/m³) with antidusting powder was smaller than the mean for the unimproved formulation (Hayes and Pearce, 1953).

In the same study, the average concentration of parathion in the air associated with the mixing of sprays from liquid concentrates was less than 0.04 mg/m³. Several other studies confirm that liquid concentrates of the same compound and concentration offer less hazard so far as respiratory exposure is concerned. Considerations of this kind have led to the adoption of liquid concentrates in some countries. In the United States of America, it has been thought that the advantage of liquid formulations in regard to respiratory exposure will be overbalanced by their supposedly greater hazard in regard to skin exposure. Actually, the dermal toxicity of xylene solutions of some compounds is only slightly greater than the toxicity of water-wettable powders. For example, the LD 50 of technical parathion in xylene solution was 10.9 mg/kg, while those of aqueous suspensions of plain and antidusting water-wettable powder were 15.0 and 18.0 mg/kg when all were measured in female white rats in the same laboratory. It is argued that the hazard of powders is less because they are less likely than liquids to adhere to the skin. The conditions of use in England and in the United States of America are not sufficiently similar to permit a comparison. It must be recorded, however, that no fatal accidents with parathion have been reported from England. The possibility that liquid formulations may have more overall safety than any kind of dust or powder formulation of the same concentration is worth considering. This is true not only of concentrates, but also of formulations ready for use, including those dispersed by aircraft.

Granules. Granular preparations of insecticides have long been used for the control of malaria mosquito larvae or soil insects, where the cover is too dense to permit direct treatment of the water or soil. The granules reach places that sprays or ordinary dusts cannot penetrate, and also reduce somewhat the hazard of respiratory exposure. More recently, granular formulations have been used for the sole purpose of minimizing respiratory—and to some degree dermal—exposure to a highly toxic compound.

Various clays, sand, coal, and finely chopped plant fiber have been used as granules. The active ingredient may be applied to the outside of a preformed granule, sometimes with a dust suppressant. In other instances, the active material may be formulated with an adhesive and a powder, which is then pelleted. The pesticide tends to be concentrated on the surface of preformed granules but distributed evenly in pelletized granules. All granule formulations are relatively free of fine particles as compared with dusts, water-wettable powders, or aerosols, which dry out moments after the spraying of any liquid formulations. Some pelletized granules are virtually dust-free.

9.2.2.3 Protective Additives.

Emetics. Emetics have been used with rodenticides but their value is not clear. Antimony potassium tartrate has been combined with either zinc phosphide, thallium sulfate, or arsenic trioxide. Combination of the tartrate with anticoagulants and some other rodenticides is unnecessary because of their low toxicity to man, and combination with sodium fluoroacetate is useless, because the latter poison acts too rapidly. Red squill has an inherent emetic property attributed to the toxic glycoside itself and not to contaminants. Unfortunately, the acceptability to rats of red squill and of other emetic rodenticide formulations is poor. Furthermore, tartar emetic has considerable toxicity of its own. Apparently no effort has been made to study the effectiveness and safety of zinc phosphide or similar rodenticides combined with ipecac.

Color. Color has been used to make treated seed or rodenticidal formulations distinct from desirable food or potable water. In addition to precautions required by the Federal Seed Act (7 USC 1551 *et seq.*), the Food and Drug Administration has ruled that treated seed will be considered adulterated and the shipper subject to penalties unless they are adequately colored to prevent subsequent use as food or feed (Fed. Reg. 28:11925, 1963).

Sodium fluoroacetate was used only after the addition of nigrosine black.

Undoubtedly some protection is given by coloring poisons. However, such protection is far from complete. Children may even be attracted by color. Color does not always dissuade adults from eating treated seed. In several instances, peasants attempted to remove color by washing before they ate grain, which they were aware was not meant to be eaten (Section 7.1.2.4).

9.3 Protective Practices and Devices

It is possible to supply only an outline of selected protective practices and devices in this book. Further details may be found in leading tests in industrial hygiene (eg, Patty, 1958), or especially books devoted exclusively to safety and accident prevention in chemical operations (Fawcett and Wood, 1965).

The United Nations Industrial Development Organization (1972) has prepared a two-volume work, *Industrial Production and Formulation of Pesticides in Developing Countries*. It contains chapters on safety related to exposure of workers in pesticide formulation plants and related to transportation and storage of toxic pesticides.

Valuable, current information on good work practices and other aspects of safety may be obtained from trade associations. Whereas this information is prepared for members of the associations, many of the groups are very public spirited about distribution of their safety brochures. For example, such statements of the National Pest Control Association regularly are abstracted by the World Health Organization in the Information Circular on the Toxicity of Pesticides to Man and sent to health authorities in all parts of the world.

No strict separation should be made between protective practices and devices. Either one or the other may be of predominant importance in a given situation. The fact that protective or hygienic practices are often simple and represent little more than common sense does not detract from their value. Finally, the improper use of protective devices may cancel their potential benefit.

9.3.1 Protective Practices

9.3.1.1 Avoidance of Exposure.

It often happens that a great deal of exposure can be avoided by such simple procedures as spraying downwind or using a paddle instead of a hand to mix formulations. Because circumstances vary, it is difficult to lay down precise rules for avoiding exposure. However, the worker can find many ways to minimize contact with chemicals if he is constantly alert to the problem.

Maintenance of Equipment. Proper maintenance of equipment may minimize day-to-day exposure or prevent a gross accident. For example, maintenance of the shut-off valve of a sprayer will reduce leakage of the formulation onto the sprayman's hand and arm. Maintenance of pressure hoses may prevent rupture of a hose and gross contamination of a worker.

It is of great importance that foremen of spray teams be trained to carry out maintenance both effectively and safely. The same is true of farmers who do their own pest control. Such practices as using the mouth to blow out nozzles have led to serious poisoning.

The maintenance engineers of pesticide manufacturing and formulating plants must not only be fully trained, but they require the cooperation of both management and the operating staff.

9.3.1.2 Removal of Contamination.

This section is devoted to the protection of persons who work directly with pesticides. The protection of a much larger population through the removal of residues from food and water is discussed in Section 6.1.4.

Some degree of contamination is inevitable when pesticides are used. It is important that the degree and duration of exposure be limited as much as possible by washing and bathing. If there has been a recognized splash or spillage, work must stop immediately and washing must begin just as soon as possible. Even though there has been no unusual contamination, washing should precede smoking, drinking, or eating, and there should be a complete bath at the end of the work day.

Provision of Water and "Soap." Water and a detergent bar should be provided at any place where a pesticide is to be made, mixed, or used. It may not be practical to have enough water on a truck or spray rig for routine use, but there should be enough for an emergency. In the case of field operations, enough water for routine washing before smoking or drinking may be provided at the mixing or loading point. Facilities for washing before meals may be where the meals are served and facilities for bathing where the workers sleep.

Detergent bars or soap should be available for all routine washing and bathing. Detergent is considerably more efficient than soap for mobilizing oil-soluble materials from the skin.

Personal Decontamination after an Accident. Decontamination after an accident is of the greatest importance in preventing poisoning. First aid measures and some discussion of their effectiveness are given in Section 8.2.1.4.

9.3.1.3 Working in Pairs. The lone worker is in special danger. Whenever possible, men making, mixing, or using highly dangerous pesticides should work in pairs so they can check on one another and give help as needed. This does not mean that they should have identical tasks, but that they should work together closely enough to be able to communicate easily. This use of the "buddy system" has long been recognized as good practice in applying fumigants. It should be universal practice with all very hazardous materials. Even when men work in groups of four or more, they should be divided into pairs lest one man become ill or confused and wander off unnoticed.

9.3.1.4 Storage for Safety.
Prevention of Misuse. More than half of the injury to human health caused by isolated accidents with pesticides would be prevented if the chemicals were always kept in their original labeled containers and stored under lock and key. Section 7.1.4 gives information justifying this statement. It is understood that some applicators, notably pest control opera-tors, must transfer pesticides from drums and other original, large containers to containers suitable for the place of use. However, the spirit of this safety requirement is fulfilled if the new containers are made for the purpose and labeled properly. The National Pest Control Association has prepared blank labels for this purpose. In no instance should a beverage bottle or any other container that might be associated with food or drink be used for storing pesticides.

Not only should pesticides be stored in locked cabinets or separate locked sheds, but individual bottles should be provided with tamper-proof caps. This is especially true of liquid formulations intended for home or garden use. Bottle and jar caps that infants find virtually impossible to open are now available in several countries. The best ones involve an inner and outer cap so arranged that the outer one must be pressed against the pressure of a spring in order to contact and turn the inner cap. It would be a great step forward if all pesticide formulators used closures of this kind for all bottles and jars sold to the public. Pesticide operators would do well to use these closures on all containers on their service trucks.

One very popular form of child-resistant closure was the result of a contest held in 1964 by a Canadian pharmaceutical association. The closure is inexpensive. In a test of 300 children, it was found that those under 3 years could not open the closure even after being shown how. Few children under 8 years could open it without demonstration (Stracener *et al.*, 1967).

The Poison Prevention Packaging Act of 1970 (15 USC 1471 *et seq.*) requires the Secretary of Health, Education, and Welfare to establish standards for the packaging of materials that may cause poisoning, and to require the use of approved packaging under certain conditions. Application of the law has been slow. However, safety closures now are required for aspirin, and these closures undoubtedly will be required more generally in the future. One of the 1972 amendments to the Federal Insecticide, Fungicide, and Rodenticide Act authorizes the Administrator to establish standards for packaging of pesticides consistent with standards established under the Poison Prevention Packaging Act.

Most outbreaks of poisoning caused by gross accidental contamination of food by pesticides have involved spillage during transportation. However, gross contamination of food may occur during storage. Transportation is subject to regulation (Sections 9.1.2.1 and 9.1.2.2). So far, no way has been found to regulate warehouses or the way in which things are stored. It is hoped that the greatly improved new rules regulating transportation will lead to improvement in storage practices. Specifically, it is hoped that warehousemen will realize that if food and poisons should not be shipped together, they should not be stored together.

Prevention of Fire. It is now clearly established that perthane undergoes decomposition with the evolution of heat. Under certain circumstances, this property can lead to spontaneous combustion and probably has been the cause of warehouse fires. Chlorates are strong oxidizing agents and must be stored separately from other pesticides.

Quite aside from compounds that are oxidizing agents or that may undergo spontaneous combustion, some attention should be given to the possibility of fire and to fire-fighting problems in connection with the storage of any considerable quantity of pesticide. Most solutions and solution-concentrates of pesticides contain flammable solvents. It is common practice to store gasoline, fuel oil, and similar materials in tanks surrounded by a dike of such size that all of the fluid in the tank would be held by the dike if the tank breaks. Would it not be reasonable to store the more flammable pesticides in small separate warehouses surrounded by dikes?

Compatibility of Pesticides. Care must be taken how pesticides are stored in relation to one another, especially in warehouses where relatively large amounts are kept. The problem of chlorates has already been mentioned. In addition, herbicides may cause severe damage to crops if they become mixed with insecticides or fungicides. Such mixture may occur without spillage in the case of highly volatile herbicides. Severe damage to people or animals could occur if preparations of low toxicity, for example those intended for home use or for the treatment of domestic animals, were contaminated by spillage of highly toxic compounds.

9.3.1.5 Disposal of Empty Containers.

Disposal of Containers. Containers of pesticides sold for household or garden use are generally best disposed of through regular municipal trash collection. If the label includes any special instructions about disposal, they should be followed. Empty containers must never be used to store anything else, and they must be guarded just as carefully as full ones to prevent their ever being accessible to children or pets.

Especially on the farm, bags, paper or wooden boxes, fiber drums or boxes, and plastic liners for pesticides are, with few exceptions, best disposed of by incineration or by burning in an isolated place. The limitations are explained in Section 9.3.1.6. For formulating plants or other operations near a town, a supervised municipal dump may be a good place for burning pesticide containers. The operator of the dump must, of course, be told what is to be burned and what precautions he should take.

Containers that cannot be burned but are small enough to crush or break should be rinsed and then buried. The rinsings should be poured into a pit dug at least 18 inches deep, which is refilled after the operation. The containers themselves should be punctured or crushed to prevent reuse. Depending on the size and number of containers, it may be more convenient to put them into the same pit with the rinse water or to hold them in storage for transport to a sanitary landfill.

Containers that cannot be destroyed by burning and are too large to crush may present a serious disposal problem. They should be rinsed inside and out in much the same way as smaller containers. After rinsing, those that can be salvaged should have all bungs and closures tightened. Some drums are valuable enough that it is economically feasible to store them and later return groups of them to the manufacturer for reuse. Also, under certain conditions, formulators may arrange with the manufacturer to relabel containers and use them for formulations. It may also be possible to send drums to a cooperage firm for reconditioning. The head of each drum is removed, the drum is heated hot and long enough to volatilize or destroy any remaining chemical. Finally, the drum is sand- or shotblasted to remove all traces of foreign matter. The National Agricultural Chemicals Association can furnish a current list of companies that do this sort of work.

Under no conditions should pesticide containers—reconditioned or otherwise—be used for food or feed. Drums used for poisons should be embossed with a skull and cross bones or other suitable marking so that repainting or relabeling cannot disguise its original use.

If reuse or reconditioning of drums is impossible, they should be punctured or otherwise mutilated to prevent reuse and either burned out under supervision or buried in an isolated area, preferably in a sanitary landfill.

Cleaning of Drums. Empty drums should be handled with just as much caution as full ones. Workers should use the protective devices appropriate to the compound involved.

Equipment for holding and emptying large drums will save work and help prevent accidents.

Regardless of the contents, the first step in cleaning a drum is to drain it as completely as possible. The drainage and the later rinsings should be added to the spray mix being prepared or, if that is impossible, they should be emptied into a pit, described in Section 9.3.1.6. Another general point is that it is important to clean the outside of drums, as well as the inside.

Drums that have contained solutions must be rinsed with solvent or with water and an adequate amount of a suitable detergent.

Fresh emulsion concentrates and water-wettable powders can be rinsed from containers with water alone. Cleaning is done most efficiently by repeated rinsing with small volumes rather than by a single rinse with a large volume. Of course, the rinsing is especially effective if a stream of fresh water from a hose can be directed upward against the inner walls of a drum held in such a way that the contaminated water drains continuously during the rinsing process. Cleaning should be done promptly. It can only become more difficult if the remaining formulation is permitted to dry and perhaps undergo chemical change.

It is commonly suggested that detergent and lye be added to water in an appropriate ratio of 1:4:16 for the purpose of rinsing containers that have held organic phosphorus insecticides. This is a satisfactory recommendation. The detergent will help to mobilize the formulation, especially if it is a solution or technical material. They lye eventually will help to hydrolyze the insecticide after the rinsings have been added to the soil. However, it should not be expected that the reaction will progress far during the cleaning process. Except for dilution, the rinsings must be considered just as poisonous as the original material (Wolfe *et al.*, 1961).

Other Safety Measures Involving Containers. It has been suggested that pesticides be sold by formulators in unit packages, such that one or more whole units would be used to charge a spray tank. It has also been suggested that the inner hermetically sealed container might be made of some material soluble in water so that there would be no possibility of dusting or splashing of the pesticide at the moment the unit package was placed in water. The practicality of these suggestions is not established.

9.3.1.6 Disposal of Unwanted Pesti-

cide. The most economical, efficient, and safe way to dispose of a pesticide chemical is to use it for one of the purposes indicated on its legally approved label, and in accordance with the precautions and limitations specified thereon. The following paragraphs are concerned with means of disposal that may be employed when proper application cannot be carried out.

Decontamination of Vehicles after an Accident. In several instances, containers of pesticides have broken during transit and the contents grossly soiled the vehicle. By chance, no food was contaminated in the best studied of these episodes. A pesticide sometimes leaked through a wooden floor or between the floor and side of a vehicle, spreading to the underside of the floor and any supports, axles, or other parts that happened to be below. This latter contamination could be removed in a reasonably satisfactory way by steam cleaning in an isolated place. However, it has proved impossible to really clean the wooden floor of a vehicle well enough that it could be safely used for carrying food. Such floors and occasionally the sides of trucks must be replaced and the removed parts destroyed.

Collection of Spillage. The most common form of unwanted pesticide, except the rinsings from "empty" containers, is material that has been spilled. No matter how or where the spillage occurred, an effort should be made to limit its extent. As much as possible should be collected for reuse or disposal, and as little as possible should be washed away. If a single dust or granular formulation is involved, it may be possible to collect much of it and return it to use. If the spillage occured in a building, an industrial vacuum cleaner may help in the collection. Even if the spillage occurred in the wreck of a vehicle or in some other situation where no special equipment is available, it may still be possible to recover much of the spilled material, thus reducing both the waste and the amount of poison that contaminates either soil or water. If a vacuum cleaner is not available, the portion that cannot be shoveled up should be swept up for reuse or for later disposal in a suitable place.

Liquid spills should be covered with sawdust, loose dry soil, or some other absorbent material, and then swept up for disposal in a suitable place. Of course, the broom should be disposed of along with the sweepings.

In at least one instance, a trailer fully equipped for decontaminating spills of pesticides has been designed and constructed cooperatively by industry and various local and state government agencies at a cost of

$1,165.00. The trailer is available through the County Commissioner of Agriculture (Smith, 1969).

Commercial Disposal. Pesticide that is unwanted, for whatever reason, may be disposed of by burial, by incineration, or, in a few instances, by burning in the open or adding to city sewage. In addition, the industry uses specialized methods, including trickling filters, activated sludge, and related biological methods; precipitation, ion exchange, coagulation, oxidation, and a variety of other chemical methods; and deep well disposal. Disposal at sea has been used to a limited extent but is now discouraged because of its possible effect on wildlife. The various industrial methods for pesticide disposal are beyond the scope of this book. Information about them can be obtained by formulators from the National Agricultural Chemicals Association or from the manufacturers of specific compounds. Deep well disposal was the subject of a recent review (Anonymous, 1968).

Individual users of pesticides or those responsible for disposing of waste after a mishap in transportation may be able to make arrangements with a local formulator to use his commercial facilities for disposal.

Burial. Burial of pesticides should be at least 18 inches deep and at least 25 feet from a stream, pond, or well. By far the best and most convenient way is to add the pesticide to a properly operated sanitary landfill. This will involve a deeper burial and also ensure that the land will not be disturbed for a sufficient number of years to permit decomposition of all except the heavy metal poisons. The operator of the landfill should be told what the waste is and what precautions he should take. Mail *et al.* (1960) reported that an operator who compacted and buried containers for parathion, mevinphos, and phorate in a sanitary landfill received exposure that was barely measurable and showed no inhibition of blood cholinesterase. They gave no evidence that similar disposal of waste pesticides would constitute any danger to operators.

Incineration. All organic pesticides, whether of botanical or synthetic origin, can be destroyed by incineration. On the contrary, the heavy metals remain toxic no matter what their chemical combination. If an arsenical, for example, is burned, the toxic material is merely divided between the smoke and ash. This difficulty does not involve organic poisons, but the possibilities exist that (*a*) unaltered compound will be vaporized and lost before it has had time to reach a destructive temperature, or (*b*) one of the combustion products (eg, HCl) will be objectionable.

The danger of vaporization is especially serious in connection with the chlorophenoxy herbicides because only traces of them in the air can injure plants. For these compounds, the combustion temperature must be 1,800°F with 1 sec detention time for a straight combustion process. A temperature of only about 900°F is required if catalytic combustion is used.

No significant amount of hydrochloric acid should be produced in an incinerator that lacks a scrubbing device to remove this vapor from the stack gas. Thus, chlorinated hydrocarbon insecticides and the chlorophenoxy herbicides cannot be burned in many incinerators because they lack scrubbers.

Keeping these limitations in mind, it may be possible for the individual pesticide user or others who may need to dispose of pesticides to make arrangements with the operator of a nearby municipal incinerator. Manufacturers or formulators of very large amounts of pesticides may find it advantageous to build incinerators adequate to destroy all organic pesticides and equipped with scrubbers to remove acid wastes.

Burning in the Open. A portion of even the most flammable materials is likely to be lost by vaporization when they are burned in the open. Thus, the smoke from an open fire used to destroy pesticides will contain some of the poison. Burning should be attempted only in an isolated place. Inhalation of smoke must be avoided. Chlorophenoxy herbicides should not be burned in the open because such small traces of them injure crops and other plants.

Because burning in the open is likely to be incomplete, it is well to kindle the fire in a pit that is later filled in to cover the ashes.

Formulations and compounds that lend themselves to burning in the open are (*a*) all petroleum solvent solutions and emulsion concentrates, except those containing chlorophenoxy herbicides, (*b*) perthane, and (*c*) chlorates.

Addition to Sewage. Care must be taken not to contaminate surface or ground water with pesticides. However, some cities have sewage disposal systems adequate to degrade certain pesticides biologically. Persons with a continuing disposal problem should consult the authorities about the kinds of compounds and—just as important—the daily load of them the disposal system is able to handle.

For the very small quantities of pesticides that the householder may need to destroy occasionally, no safer method of disposal exists than flushing the material into the sewer.

9.3.1.7 Environmental Surveillance. The use of threshold limit values as standards by plant industrial hygienists and by regulatory authorities was described in Section 9.1.4.5. It remains to discuss the use of air monitoring and other environmental surveillance as one aspect of good industrial hygiene.

The importance of environmental surveillance is universally accepted. Although illness and discomfort among workers has been the primary motivation for improving industrial safety over a period of many decades, air monitoring has been the primary tool for locating foci and measuring contamination. Air monitoring is generally supervised by the same engineers who, directly or indirectly, are responsible for plant ventilation. They are in the best possible position to take corrective measures, either by adjusting existing equipment or by installing new safety equipment.

Monitoring of food and water extends the protection of workers and of persons with far less exposure.

9.3.1.8 Medical Surveillance. Medical surveillance of workers is of great importance to their health. The practice of industrial medicine may be divided usefully into: (a) those examinations and corrective measures directed toward the worker's general health, regardless of his particular job or even the kind of industry; (b) those examinations and corrective measures directed to the specific hazards to which the individual may be subject; and (c) education. In spite of the importance of general measures, the following remarks are limited to specific surveillance and education.

Monitoring of Workers. Traditionally, regulation of the occupational environment has depended more on sampling air than on sampling workers. This is partly because some of the classical occupational diseases can be followed poorly if at all by clinical laboratory tests. For example, silicosis, a disease of tremendous importance involving a surprising range of industries, cannot be followed by clinical laboratory tests, or, in fact, by any test specifically related to silica. No compound of silicon has been found in the blood and urine. By the time the physical examination or the X-ray findings are abnormal, injury already has occurred.

The heavy metals, a continuing source of trouble, can be measured in blood and urine, but the correspondence between these tests and exposure and illness is not as satisfactory as that for some of the newer industrial chemicals and pesticides.

On the contrary, there are compounds for which air measurements supply less adequate information than can be gained by monitoring the worker. For example, over a decade ago Dutkiewicz and Piotrowski (1961) concluded that because of its considerable absorption through the skin, the exposure of workers to aniline cannot be assessed adequately by air measurements, but can be evaluated for prophylactic purposes by measuring *p*-aminophenol in the urine.

There is a growing tendency to supplement monitoring of the work environment (especially air) by specific tests on each worker's blood and urine. In some instances, it has already been found practical to monitor workers to learn whether any are receiving excessive exposure, which, although not immediately harmful, should be reduced either through improved hygiene or through transfer of the worker to an entirely different job. Individual monitoring has been prompted by astonishing advances in analytical chemistry. It has become clear that the worker—or, in fact, anyone—may be the best sampler of his own environment. Such measurements (a) indicate absorption from all portals without distinction, (b) ignore exposure that does not lead to absorption, and (c) have the potential to indicate absorption for an entire day or a selected part of a day.

Known levels of several pesticides in tissue, blood, and urine useful for diagnosis are summarized in Tables 8-1, 8-2, and 8-3. In most instances, formal biological standards, or biological threshold limits as they are sometimes called, have not been set even for those compounds for which chemical analysis is useful not only for diagnosis but also as a herald of impending danger.

Legal Requirement for Surveillance. It is now commonplace to use specific tests for monitoring workers exposed to a few pesticides. California requires that agricultural workers who apply the more toxic organic phosphorus insecticides must be under medical supervision. In effect, this regulation has led to preexposure and periodic testing of blood cholinesterase as a routine practice for monitoring these workers. Those whose results fall below a critical level are not permitted to have further exposure until the test has returned to normal. Similar practice prevails on a voluntary basis in relation to many other applicators, formulators, and manufacturers exposed to highly toxic organic phosphorus compounds in California and elsewhere.

The value of monitoring people exposed to highly toxic organic phosphorus insecticides has led some to suppose, erroneously, that there is something to be gained from monitoring blood cholinesterase of persons exposed to carbamates or to organic phosphorus compounds of low toxicity.

Since many specific tests for pesticides in blood, urine, or tissue have been developed by research, it seems likely that the use of some of them for monitoring exposed workers will become a routine of industrial hygiene.

The Occupational Safety and Health Act (see Section 9.1.3.4) requires the employer to ensure ". . . the ready availability of medical personnel for advice and consultation on matters of plant health." This language makes no specific reference to monitoring but may include that concept where appropriate.

Education. The physician is in a particularly good position to carry out effective safety education. Pediatricians should warn parents of the danger of storing drugs and household chemicals where children can reach them. Physicians who care for chemical workers should use every opportunity to encourage the workers in safe practices. Any instance of poisoning should be investigated thoroughly to learn its cause so that similar episodes may be prevented. Every office visit should serve as an occasion for training suitable for the individual patient. The first step in the safe use of a chemical is the realization of its danger. However, the physician may find that his patient has learned this lesson in relation to his own work but failed to apply it in relation to empty containers, which he neglects in such a way that they are a hazard to others. In any event, all subjects mentioned in this chapter may become, at one time or another, the proper content of a physician's safety message.

On occasion, the occupational health physician may prove just as valuable to the employer as he more frequently is to the employees. The physician familiar with occupational disease is in the best possible position to recognize the mistake and defend his own diagnosis if someone else alleges that a completely unrelated condition is caused or aggravated by occupational conditions. A physician with special training in occupational medicine obviously has an advantage in dealing with many problems of workers and managers. However, beyond basic medical training and experience, intimate familiarity with the work situation is of greatest importance. In connection with pesticides, this includes thorough knowledge of the toxicology of both solvents and active ingredients.

9.3.2 Protective Devices

In spite of some overlapping, protective devices may be divided conveniently into industrial ones that are permanently installed in relation to some specific operation and those that are more or less portable and intended for personal protection, whether in industry or under field conditions.

9.3.2.1 Industrial Protective Equipment. Even an outline of industrial protective equipment is beyond the scope of this book. Those interested should consult the manual on industrial ventilation published by the American Conference of Governmental Industrial Hygienists (1968) and other manuals issued by the same organization.

The construction of cropdusting planes is important to the safety of pilots who apply pesticides. When recognized principles of safety design were observed in making planes, the safety record was improved (Bruggink *et al.,* 1964).

9.3.2.2 Personal Respiratory Protection. Extensive information on personal respiratory protective devices may be found in a manual published by the American Industrial Hygiene Association and the American Conference of Governmental Industrial Hygienists (1963). Manufacturers of protective equipment also can supply information.

Personal respiratory protection requires a source of pure air and a system for delivering this air to the worker. Theoretically, any source of pure air could be used with any delivery system, but only certain combinations are common in practice.

Sources of Pure Air for the Worker. There are three basic ways of supplying clean air to a worker whose surroundings may be contaminated. Air may be pumped from a distance, it may be compressed and furnished in cylinders, or it may be purified on the spot.

The simplest way, at least in theory, is to pump air from a completely uncontaminated area. This necessitates a blower or compressor of some kind and a tube long enough to extend from the source of clean air to the worker. Since drift and diffusion may be extensive, the tube may have to be long. The pumping equipment may be movable or completely stationary. The system is ideal for protection of men who do not have to move about much, such as those cleaning the inside of tanks, attending grinding machines, or operating package fillers.

For temporary jobs, such as cleaning out tanks, the blower may be hand-operated or driven by a portable gasoline engine. For continuing operations, such as grinding or packaging, the blower or compressor should be installed permanently and driven by an electric motor. If a piston-type compressor is employed, it should be provided with a device to prevent it from accidentally overheating and producing carbon monoxide through partial oxidation of the lubricant. In no event should the pump, tank, or airline supplying air to workers be used for any other purpose. A separate system is required because there is too much chance of cross-contamination (Hartwell and Hayes, 1965). Some formulating plants in hot areas refrigerate the air supplied to hoods worn by workers to make it more pleasant than ambient air. This practice leads to essentially universal acceptance of the protective equipment.

Another source of pure air is cylinders filled with compressed air or oxygen, or cannisters from which oxygen can be generated. The cylinders are made in sizes to last 0.5, 1, and 2 hours. Use of compressed gas combined with an appropriate system of delivery permits complete respiratory protection and offers essentially unlimited mobility to the worker, but it strictly limits the duration of protection. The cannisters contain potassium tetroxide from which oxygen is generated through the action of water and carbon dioxide from the breath. The rate of evolution of oxygen is regulated by the rate of breathing.

Whether obtained by pumping or bought in cylinders or cannisters, air that requires no chemical cleanup has the advantage that it always contains enough oxygen. Men who clean large tanks or fumigate closed spaces may be in danger of oxygen deprivation as well as poisoning by chemical vapors.

A basically different approach in obtaining pure air is to clean air drawn from the worker's immediate environment. This method tends to favor mobility but raises questions about the completeness of cleaning. In general, a more thorough job can be done by heavy equipment, but such equipment has only limited mobility. The most mobile equipment may offer protection against only low concentrations of chemical and only for a relatively brief period.

Centrifugal filter-blowers are available for mounting on tractors and other heavy equipment, whether mobile or stationary. A high speed, 6-, 12-, or 24-volt DC motor or a 115-volt AC motor drives an impeller that accelerates air into a circular path. Centrifugal force throws particles to the outside of the stream where they are "skimmed off" by slots and continuously discharged. If such a blower and centrifugal filter is protected by a screen to exclude large particles and followed by a fine filter (eg, a pleated paper or fiber glass filter), it is possible to remove 99.8% by weight of particles larger than 1 μm. Particles of smaller size and also vapor may then be removed by a suitable chemical cannister. The complete apparatus may be large, inasmuch as the worker does not have to carry it. Limited mobility for the worker is achieved by using a long flexible tube from the cleaning device to the worker. Since the air is under positive pressure, there is no problem of dead space or of leakage of contaminated air into the facepiece or hood used to deliver the air. Because the equipment is mounted and already depends on external power, it may be combined with heaters or refrigerating devices to make their air comfortable for the worker.

By the use of smaller filters and smaller chemical cannisters, it is possible to make a self-contained device that a man can carry while he works. This gain in mobility is accompanied by a potential loss of protection arising from either physical or chemical inadequacy of the system. If the worker's breathing supplies the energy necessary to force air through a filter and cannister, then the air he receives must be under negative pressure, and any leak in the system will permit unpurified air to be inhaled. Furthermore, filters and cannisters light enough to carry may offer protection for a relatively brief period.

Veils (discussed in a separate paragraph below) and face shields constitute a kind of filter for selective removal of large aerosol particles. Their efficiency is greater than might be supposed and they are the ultimate in simplicity. A veil may be considered as a way for cleaning air without any necessity for a special system to deliver it to the wearer.

Systems for Delivering Air to Workers. These systems include: (*a*) suits, which cover the head, hands, and sometimes feet; (*b*) hoods, which cover the entire head and neck or even extend over the shoulders; (*c*) masks, which cover the nose, mouth and eyes; and (*d*) half masks, which cover the nose and mouth but not the eyes. Some of these systems and the sources of pure air used with them are discussed in some detail in separate paragraphs below.

Hoods. Hoods suitable for use with pesticides consist of a helmet, a face shield, and a shroud to cover the neck and sometimes the shoulders. A hood may be considered a combination of a mask, a hard hat, goggles, and complete dermal protection of the head and neck. The shroud is designed so that the lower part of it fits closely against the clothing. Hoods are always used in connection with air supplied under positive pressure and either obtained from a completely uncontaminated source or purified by relatively heavy equipment not carried by the worker. The incoming air is usually delivered to the hood through many small holes in a circular hollow tube beneath the helmet and above the worker's head. Since the air is under positive pressure, some unbreathed air, as well as exhaled air, leaks out constantly from the lower margin of the hood. Back mixing is prevented by the positive pressure and by the close contact of the shroud with the clothing of the upper part of the body.

Air should be supplied to hoods at a rate of at least 170 liters per minute (6 ft³/min). No valve should be supplied to permit the wearer to adjust the flow to less than the safe amount. The airflow should be checked periodically to be sure that it does not fall below the minimum. Refrigeration of the air supplied to hoods is virtually a necessity in hot places and certainly promotes acceptance by workers.

Masks. Masks, which cover the mouth, nose, and eyes, involve a facepiece made of rubber in such a way that it can form an airtight seal when held firmly against the face by straps passed over the head and around the neck. The windows (or lenses as they are called) of masks are an integral part of the equipment and they are hermetically sealed into the facepiece. Masks may have holders for filters and cannisters as an integral part of their construction, but usually masks are connected to a source of pure air by a flexible hose.

Half Masks. Half masks are similar to masks in construction but cover only the mouth and nose. They usually have holders for filters and cannisters integrated into their structure, but they may be connected to a source of pure air by a flexible hose. Half masks are often called respirators, but there is a tendency to restrict this term to its most general meaning, namely, any device used to provide respirable air.

Supplied-Air Respirators. A *hose mask without blower* is a combination of a mask and a hose of large diameter through which the wearer draws air from an uncontaminated source by his own breathing effort. A *hose mask with blower* is similar, except that the large hose is connected to a hand- or motor-operated blower. However, the wearer can inhale through the hose whether or not the blower is operated. Masks of this kind are generally made with a harness that not only supports the necessary hose connections, but is strong enough to be used for pulling the wearer from a tank or other area of heavy exposure in the event he collapses. The hose for such equipment should be at least 7.5 m and no more than 45 m long.

The term *air-line respirator* is used for either half-masks, masks, or hoods used in connection with a supply of pure, compressed air. Depending on the nature of the air supply, an airflow control valve or critical orifice may be needed to limit the rate of airflow into the facepiece; however, it is important that it be impossible to reduce the flow below the minimal requirement. Although air-line respirators give the best and most dependable protection available in many situations, they should not be used in atmospheres that are an immediate hazard to life, because there is no provision for protection if the air supply fails.

Self-Contained, Supplied-Air Respirators. The usefulness of self-contained air—or oxygen—supplying respirators or masks is limited by their weight and complexity. They are necessary in a few situations requiring mobility in an oxygen-deficient atmosphere. These masks should not be used by a person without special training regarding the mechanism. The mechanism of a self-contained breathing apparatus may be of three types: demand flow, recirculating, and oxygen generating.

Briefly, a *demand, atmosphere-supplying respirator* is one in which air or oxygen is admitted to the facepiece only when the wearer inhales, and in quantities governed automatically by his breathing. Oxygen not absorbed after it has been inspired is wasted.

The *recirculating, atmosphere-supplying respirator* overcomes the wastage of oxygen by use of a breathing bag. When the vaule of the oxygen cylinder is opened, oxygen flows through a pressure-reducing valve, and then into a breathing bag through an admission valve that opens only when the bag is insufficiently full. Air is inhaled directly from the bag but exhaled back into the bag after passing through an adsorbent for removing carbon dioxide and through a radiator to permit loss of heat.

Closely related to the latter respirator is the *oxygen-generating, self-contained breathing apparatus* in which oxygen is obtained not from a cylinder, but from potassium tetroxide by carbon dioxide and water from the breath. The rate of evolution of oxygen is regulated by the rate of breathing of the wearer.

Air-Purifying Respirators. As the name implies, an air-purifying respirator is one that removes contaminants from the air inhaled by the wearer. For most of them, the wearer must furnish the energy to move air through the air-purifying mechanism. However, a few supplied-air respirators are provided not only with an electric blower but also with a centrifugal filter, a fiber filter, and sometimes a chemical cannister, all of which purify air. Thus, there is some overlapping between the conventional categories of respirators.

All air-purifying respirators powered by the wearer involve masks or half masks. All air-purifying respirators with electric blowers involve hoods.

Air-purifying respirators are commonly

classified as: (a) *gas and vapor removing respirators,* (b) *particulate removing respirators,* and (c) *combination respirators.* However, these distinctions apply only to a particular assembly. In most instances, air-purifying respirators are designed so that the filters and chemical cannisters are replaceable, and in some instances a variety of filters and cannisters are available. Thus, a single facepiece may form part of any type of respirator, depending on how it is assembled.

Apparently all air-purifying half masks have holders for filters and cannisters as an integral part of their structure. Some full masks (*chin-type masks*) are designed the same way. However, air-purifying masks usually involve cannisters too large to be supported by the facepiece; consequently, the cannister is strapped to the body by a special harness and is connected to the facepiece by a flexible hose. The total volume of cannisters for a half mask ranges from 50 to 100 ml. Because of the small size of the cannisters, the duration of protection given by them is limited. The cannister for a chin-type mask may vary from 180 to 500 ml in capacity. A separately supported cannister may range from 750 to 1500 ml in capacity. The filter that precedes each cannister is of corresponding size. Regardless of the size of the cannister, it is separated from the interior of the facepiece by a one-way valve placed at the level of the mask, to reduce the deadspace in the mask and to protect the cannister from moisture of the breath. Another one-way valve permits exhaled air to leave the mask.

Selection and Care of Cannisters. Cannisters are made for protection against a number of different types of chemicals or combinations of chemicals. A cannister for one compound may be useless for another. For example, activated charcoal is valuable for adsorption of organic vapors but entirely useless against carbon monoxide, which requires hopcalite, a porous granular mixture of manganese and copper oxides. Basically different cannisters are made to protect against organic vapors, acid gases, ammonia, hydrogen cyanide, and chlorine. Some cannisters are made to protect against various combinations, while others protect against these materials or their combinations in the presence of dust or smoke.

Only large cannisters for use with masks should be used for protection against fumigants.

Because different manufacturers do not use identical nomenclature for cannisters, it is important to be certain that the cannister selected has been approved for protection against the toxicant to be used. Approval should be by the US Department of Agricul-

ture, the US Bureau of Mines, the National Institute for Occupational Safety and Health (NIOSH), or appropriate authorities in other countries. It may be noted that the US Department of Agriculture tested and approved respirators, masks, and hoods from the time of World War II through 1966 (Fulton *et al.,* 1951; 1955; 1962; 1963; 1964; Fulton and McClellan, 1957; Fulton and Smith, 1958; Yeomans *et al.,* 1966). At the request of the Department of Agriculture, this task was undertaken in 1967 by the Bureau of Mines. Later the task was shared with NIOSH.

Selection, Use, and Maintenance of Personal Respiratory Equipment. As already indicated, supplied-air hoods and masks offer the most complete protection against respiratory exposure. Masks and respirators with chemical cannisters offer proportionally less protection and for a shorter period. Respirators are not adequate for protection against respiratory exposure in greenhouses, buildings, or other inadequately ventilated spaces where highly toxic chemicals are applied. Appropriate air-purifying half mask respirators are generally adequate for protection of operators out-of-doors during the loading of sprayers or the disposal of containers, or whenever dust or mist is visible intermittently. Such respirators are also adequate for protection of pilots during the normal dusting or spraying operations with most pesticides. However, pilots have a special need for eye protection and should either wear masks or be sure their respirators and goggles are compatible.

Face shields are recommended to avoid splashing of the eyes or face while concentrates of pesticides of negligible vapor toxicity are being handled. In some other situations, such as indoor spraying for malaria control, face shields are impractical because so much spray is deposited on them that the sprayman's vision is obscured. Veils have sometimes been acceptable to workers under the same conditions; veils offer partial protection without interfering with vision.

It is important when using a pesticide to employ the respiratory protection recommended by the manufacturer of the chemical. Of course, greater protection may be substituted. For example, a mask with appropriate cannister may be substituted for an approved half mask with its smaller cannister.

It is of the greatest importance that the facepieces of all cannister-type masks and half masks fit properly. The negative pressure inside such facepieces during inhalation varies from about 64 to 89 mm of water. It follows, that, if there is any leak between the facepiece and the face, contaminated air will be drawn through the opening rather than through the cannister which offers some obstruction, albeit small. The facepiece should be drawn snugly but not too tight against the face. Intake of air should be completely obstructed if the air intake of the cannister is sealed momentarily to test the fit. Manufacturers can supply special facepieces if standard ones do not fit, but eyeglasses, long sideburns, or a beard may make an airtight seal of any mask impossible.

Regardless of the equipment used, added protection may be achieved by good practice. For example, when the source of contamination is obviously in front of the operator—as in the addition of fumigants to grain—the cannister of his mask should be mounted on his back. If work is being done outdoors, the operator should stand upwind so that most of the contamination drifts away from him. A given cannister can react with only a certain amount of toxicant. If the concentration of the chemical in the intake air is higher, the useful life of the cannister will be correspondingly less.

High humidity shortens the life of chemical cannisters whether during use or storage. Rain or aqueous mists or sprays reduce the effective period. The ingredients of cannisters from which the seal has been removed gradually react with moisture and, in some instances, other gases in the air, and they must be replaced.

When a half mask is used, the filters must be changed at least twice a day, or more often if breathing becomes difficult. Half mask cartridges should be changed after 8 hours of actual use or just as soon as the odor of insecticide is detected. Cannisters for masks should be used according to the manufacturer's directions, but in no case after an odor of chemical is detectable.

After use, the filter and cannister should be removed and the facepiece should be washed with detergent and water. After washing, the facepiece should be rinsed thoroughly, dried with clean cloth, air-dried in a completely uncontaminated area, and stored in a tightly closed paper or plastic bag or in a special case if one is available.

9.3.2.3 Protective Clothing. As discussed in Section 3.2.2.5, some pesticides are easily absorbed by the skin. Furthermore, as described in Section 6.2.3.1, the contamination received by parts of the body that are frequently unclothed is substantial. Considerable protection is given to covered areas by ordinary clothing. Of course, additional protection is given by waterproof clothing, but workers in warm, moist climates may not be able to tolerate such covering. It is not only necessary to use precautions adequate to meet any likely hazard, but also to ensure that the precautions will allow work to be carried out effectively.

Spray teams responsible for malaria control and similar public health measures have to meet the public as a part of their work. The same is true of pest control operators. It might be supposed that use of protective devices by these workers would cause the householders whom they meet to consider them strange, or to suppose they are unwilling to face without protection the spray they leave with the householder. On the contrary, where they have been used, special work clothes, hats, and other equipment have added to the prestige of workers, marking them as a special group properly equipped and trained to do a special job.

Gloves. Ordinary cotton gloves offer protection against direct contact with granules or wax formulations of pesticides. If used for this purpose, they must not be used for any other work and they must be laundered at least once a day during a period of use.

Completely impermeable gloves may give protection against any type of formulation. Unfortunately, as often as not, gloves are more a hazard than a help. If pesticide is permitted to reach the inside of a glove, it remains there under conditions that encourage dermal absorption. The moisture accumulated inside a glove as a result of sweating tends to macerate the skin and thus promote the absorption of foreign chemicals.

Gloves should be worn for handling concentrates but should be avoided for continuous wear, except with the most hazardous compounds. Care must be taken to prevent the spillage of pesticidal concentrates into gloves or the drifting of dust into them. If significant contamination of the inside of the glove is observed, the glove should be destroyed to prevent further use. Under ordinary conditions, gloves should be washed on the outside before they are removed, and later washed with just as much care both inside and outside.

Impermeable gloves for repeated use are made of natural rubber, synthetic rubber, and a variety of other plastics. It is well established that no material is best. One may be least permeable to one compound but quite permeable to another. No source of systematic information on the permeability of "rubbers" by a wide range of pesticides has been found. A chemical glove selection chart in Best's Safety Directory (1973) evaluates the protection offered by five basic glove materials against more than 400 industrial chemicals, including several used as solvents, fumigants, or nematocides; the chart lists only a very few pesticides of other classifications. Manufacturers commonly evaluate their own products and do not hesitate to state that some "rubbers" offer poor resistance to a particular industrial chemical. Manufacturers may be the best source of information on the degree of impermeability of their products to specific pesticides or pesticide formulations.

Although apparently no test of their effectiveness has been made with pesticides, it seems possible that the disposable gloves now available for many laboratory uses would offer good protection against contamination by pesticides. In making this suggestion it is understood that each pair of gloves would be used only once and then discarded. Under these conditions the major protection would be mechanical; chemical penetration would be minimal if only because the duration of exposure was brief.

Hats. Hats should be of an impervious material with a broad brim to protect the face and neck. They should be able to withstand regular cleaning unless they are made from cheap, locally available material, so that they may be replaced frequently. Some antimalarial spray teams have been provided with hats in the form of a tropical helmet but made of polished aluminum. They proved to be light and cool and added considerably to the prestige of the wearers. In other situations, workers have used sou'westers, especially in connection with fully waterproof clothing.

Veils. An astonishing degree of protection is provided by a veil of plastic netting attached all the way around the brim of a tropical helmet, as described in detail by Wolfe *et al.* (1959). The veil is tolerated well by workers because it allows free passage of air, interferes little with vision, and is easy to clean. Large particles impinge on the netting as they fall through the air, whereas small ones may miss the netting as they are carried horizontally by eddy currents. Therefore, the veil offers greater protection (50 to 80%) against larger particles that otherwise would deposit on the skin of the face, neck, and shoulders and lesser protection (about 30%) against particles small enough to inhale. Since, in the absence of any protection, the amount of material reaching the skin is much greater than that inhaled, the degree of protection offered by the veil is well worth the minor inconvenience caused by the device.

Body Clothing. Measurements made under the conditions of actual work have shown that a single layer of cloth such as that used for making shirts is remarkably effective in protecting the skin from contamination by pesticides. In one study, the undershirts of men who wore no shirt while spraying orchards absorbed parathion at a rate of 7.40 mg/hour, but the identical undershirts of men who wore ordinary shirts while doing the same work absorbed at a rate of only 0.34 mg/hour. Of course, ordinary clothing offers little or no protection against spillage, and by holding the pesticide in contact with the skin may even aggravate absorption.

Waterproof clothing is protective but entirely impractical in many climates where pesticides are needed.

It follows that spraymen should wear coveralls buttoned at the neck, or at least wear clothing covering as high a proportion of the body as the climate will permit. It also follows that the clothing should be removed at the end of each day's work and should be laundered daily. In general, ordinary laundry procedures are adequate to remove pesticides from clothing. The use of washing soda will promote the hydrolysis as well as physical removal of organic phosphorus compounds. Dry cleaning or rinsing in mineral spirits or light kerosene may be needed for the clothing of workers exposed day after day to the more toxic chlorinated hydrocarbon insecticides. The clothing should be laundered in the usual way after it has been rinsed in solvent.

Capes or Ponchos. A cape or poncho of light plastic may be used to protect the shoulders and body of a workman, especially one involved in overhead spraying. This kind of protection may be tolerated in situations that are too hot and humid to permit the use of completely waterproof clothing.

Aprons. Rubber or polyvinyl chloride aprons will help to protect from spills of liquid concentrates. They also protect against the penetration of dust if it is necessary to lift heavy bags against the body in order to raise them to the level of a truck bed. If an apron is provided, it may be put on conveniently, even for brief intervals of potentially great exposure. For this reason, aprons may be very practical in climates that do not permit use of fully waterproof clothing.

Boots. Rubber boots will protect the feet and legs from pesticides. Great care must be taken that the inside of boots does not become contaminated. As an added protection, trousers and socks should be changed and laundered just as if no additional protection were available. This practice will discourage absorption of any small residue that may reach the inside of the boot.

9.3.2.4 Other Prophylactic Devices.

Prophylactic Creams. It may be possible to develop skin creams that would partially protect workers from dermal exposure to certain chemicals. Theoretically, this protection could operate through chemical inactivation of the toxin or through preventing its absorption. Skin treatments must be tested rigidly before any confidence is placed in them. Research on skin protective creams might be rewarding, but no cream can be recommended now.

Backflow Preventers. Water from city mains or from wells is subject to contamination in connection with mixing or application of pesticides. Accidents of this kind can occur if liquid is siphoned back into water pipes due to a sudden. temporary loss of pressure in the system or if liquid is forced into water pipes by an external pump. These accidents may be prevented if (*a*) water hoses are never allowed to touch contaminated water, (*b*) pumps are always primed by pouring water into them (ie, never connecting the outflow side to a water system), and (*c*) backflow preventers are used routinely. Some equipment such as proportionators used in the application of chemicals must be connected directly to a water system. Especially when this kind of equipment is used, a backflow preventer is required. These devices incorporate a spring-loaded valve that prevents reverse flow into the pipe to which they are attached. The device selected should meet the appropriate standard of the American Society of Sanitary Engineers or an equivalent standard. Such devices are available from large plumbing supply distributors and from some pest control equipment distributors.

Automatic Flagman. When pesticides are applied by aircraft, it is common practice to station one or two men on the field to hold flags and mark the swaths. One flagman (or swamper) marks where the plane is to enter the airspace over the field; between each pass of the plane he paces off the width of another swath and is then ready to guide the pilot for the next pass. If the plane flies parallel to the rows, only one flagman may be required, but if the flight is not parallel to the rows at least two flagmen are needed, one where the plane enters and one where it leaves the airspace. It often happens that flagmen receive more exposure to a pesticide than any other member of the application team. Mechanical devices called "automatic flagmen" have been developed to meet this problem and perhaps to save labor costs. The device itself is merely a strip of fabric that the pilot can see on the ground as he approaches a field. A weight on one end of the strip makes it fall from plane to ground in a predictable way. Equipment installed on the plane for the purpose makes it possible for the pilot to release 160 of these strips, one by one, at will; thus, he marks his own path and spaces each succeeding swath in reference to the last one.

9.4 Education and Cooperative Community Relations

9.4.1 Education

Training and experience in the use of industrial chemicals generally, and of pesticides in particular, is of tremendous importance for safety. Such training is much easier to conduct among a literate, stable population. However, illiterate migrant workers may achieve a good safety record if their training is thorough.

The first requirement of safety training is recognition of danger. The need for appropriate care then becomes a corollary. All pesticides are toxic to some degree, and care in handling all types should be routine practice. Nothing is gained in the long run by misrepresenting the danger. Underestimating a particular danger leads to carelessness and thus to "accidents." Unqualified overestimation of a danger leads to nothing more serious than unnecessary inconvenience at first, but later it leads to a general disregard for all precautions when it is found that the warnings were without basis.

Since the object of safety training is avoidance of injury, it is difficult to evaluate the success of such training. There is really no way to estimate how much more injury pesticides would have done in the absence of safety training. In any event, an intuitive grasp of the importance of such training has caused certain professional associations, government agencies, and interested chemical companies to spend millions of dollars on this work. The companies seldom receive just credit for the clear, uncompromising warnings that some of them issue in the form of (*a*) leaflets distributed with each package of the hazardous material, (*b*) posters to be put up in workplaces, (*c*) popular lectures, and (*c*) talks to workers. Warnings and precautions regarding the use of parathion have been especially noteworthy in this regard.

If any chemical produces injury, even infrequently, it is evidence of a need for additional or improved training.

9.4.1.1 Training of Workers. Because of the great variety of work situations, there is no possibility of setting down here specific instructions for workers. It must be emphasized that each worker should be told clearly and honestly, without depreciation or exaggeration, the dangers he is asked to face. Failure to do this is probably the most common mistake made in attempts to train workers in safety. The failure is probably made in the mistaken notion that men will not undertake work if they are acquainted with a particular danger or that they will demand extra pay or other consideration for the hazard. For generally accepted wages, men construct tall buildings, work in mines, or permit themselves to be shot into space. The physical dangers involved in these and many other jobs are obvious. The dangers involved in the use of chemicals may not be obvious, yet it is only by knowing them that the worker can grasp the reason for necessary precautions and begin to look for an even safer way to carry out each operation.

It is important to realize that real progress in safety is possible through education. Smith and Wiseman (1971) reported that the number of cases in poisoning by pesticides in the lower Rio Grande Valley dropped from 118 to 1968 to only 15 in 1969. Although the improvement depended on more than one factor, the author attributed part of it to the institution and enforcement of better safety habits in the aerial application industry.

9.4.1.2 Training of the Public.

Training of the public may have the limited aim of reducing misuse of dangerous materials and thus minimizing the injury done by them. Considerable progress already has been made along this line, and there is reason to think further progress can be made through poison control centers, and perhaps through expansion of safety messages in elementary schools.

Training of the young might have a far broader aim, namely, some public recognition and understanding of toxicology. Little progress has been made on this so far, but its importance justifies a vigorous effort.

Poison Control Centers. Poison control centers have become very popular. The first was established in Chicago in 1953 (Press, 1956). The Poison Control Center Directory (US Public Health Service, 1971) lists 644 centers for 49 stages, including 48 state coordinators' offices. Poison control centers in the Canal Zone, the District of Columbia, Guam, Puerto Rico, and the Virgin Islands also are listed. In addition, there are now poison control centers in Great Britain (Goulding, 1964), Australia (Johnson, 1963), Denmark (Myschetzky, 1964), Sweden (Karlsson, 1962), Belgium (Hilfman, 1968), and a number of other countries. The centers in the United States of America enjoy a variety of services from the National Clearing House for Poison Control Centers, including statistical assistance and the publication of comprehensive progress reports (Cann *et al.,* 1958). Regardless of their location, the centers maintain records of antidotes and lists of the ingredients of trade name products. Probably much more important is the safety education which some of the centers have money and staff to carry out (Jacobziner and Raybin, 1957). This education, carried out best by visiting nurses of the health department, promises to be very important in accelerating the improvement in the safety record of poisons.

Information on morbidity and mortality gathered by poison control centers in the United States of America is discussed in Section 7.1.1.2. One point is worth emphasis here. Most deaths and probably most nonfatal accidents caused by pesticides are nonoccupational. However, since an even greater problem of accidental poisoning is associated with drugs and household chemicals, and since the majority of victims of these accidents are children, it would seem best to focus on the problem rather than on any one class of chemicals. This is just what is being done by the poison control centers.

Safety Messages in Elementary Schools. In spite of the importance of present efforts and the fact that the victims of poisoning usually are of preschool age, it seems likely that chemicals would be used more wisely if children routinely received some training on the matter in school. If a child were taught the importance of dosage, he might learn why it is safe for him to have oil paints or a chemistry set, but important to use them and store them out of the reach of his baby brother.

The simplest and most generally useful message is: "Read the label." It cannot be emphasized too often that a good labeling program is the most important factor in safe use of pesticides. People need to be educated to use the information on the label, which is the product of so much study and care.

A Suggestion for the Future. In spite of the importance of indoctrination in safety, training really ought to be much broader. A reasonable coverage of toxicology should be a part of every textbook of biology, zoology, hygiene, and general science from the elementary grades through college (Hayes, 1971; Murphy and Hayes, 1972). Since we live in a chemical age, it is difficult to explain why our textbooks fail to state the basic principles of toxicology and even fail to identify the discipline that permits us to use chemicals safely. To be sure, some books, particularly the elementary ones, do express value judgments about certain specific compounds or classes of compounds. As often as not, however, these judgments are controversial. Certainly, they fail to offer the student any scientific basis for reaching his own conclusions. They do not even inform him that such a scientific basis exists.

The fact that texts make no mention of toxicology must depend on custom and lack of understanding of the science and its application. Correction of the neglect is overdue.

If toxicology is to be introduced into textbooks of biology and general science, where should emphasis be placed? Certainly it must be on natural phenomena, particularly those that do not involve man exclusively. The chemical age for living creatures began with the origin of life, not with the chemical aspects of the industrial revolution. Emphasis must be placed on the universality of the problems organisms face in adapting to chemicals. Prominence must be given to the dosage-response relationship and to modern ways of studying it. Undoubtedly, an example ought to be given of one of the forms of poisoning in which the biochemical lesion has been identified. Perhaps the case of cyanide would be suitable, since cyanide compounds occur in nature as well as in man-made situations.

If the material to be included in texts is well prepared and is confined to information and principles about which there is agreement, then we may hope that within a quarter of a century people generally will be able to exercise improved judgment regarding toxicology. Under these circumstances, it would be easier to justify a rational program of research on the one hand, and to avoid panic as a result of some isolated discovery on the other. Finally, general information on toxicology would offer a basis for recruiting the physicians, pharmacologists, chemists, veterinarians, and others who eventually specialize in one or another aspect of the discipline.

9.4.2 Community Relations

As pointed out in Section 1.6.2.2, pesticide problems have been solved promptly when they could be evaluated accurately in economic terms. Even when such evaluation is difficult or impossible, a genuine effort of the interested parties to understand one another's point of view can be rewarding.

From the community standpoint, there are mature and immature approaches to the use of agricultural chemicals or, in fact, chemicals of any kind. Maturity may be measured by the degree to which citizens are aware of the different factors influencing the community and the degree to which they cooperate for the mutual good. In the mature, basically agricultural community, the necessity for using agricultural chemicals is accepted, as is the potential danger some of these materials bring to those who use them. Partly because this problem of hazard to the worker has been met forthrightly, the safety record is often good. Each grower takes direct, personal responsibility for the chemicals to be used and the amount, method, and timing of their application. Neighbors are advised when pesticides are to be applied and recognize the necessity for their use.

Poor community relations have been observed in situations in which (a) suburbs encroached on farms, (b) the use of pesticides was frankly careless, or (c) some special interest group was attempting to promote their concepts without regard to the needs or views of others.

Although no specific directions can be given for improving community relations once they have deteriorated, the solution clearly lies in obtaining all relevant facts and in establishing communication leading eventually to mutual understanding and respect. Examples of reassurance of a community through a study of circumstances that had led to the concern of one or more people have been reported (Sumerford et al., 1953; Fowler, 1953; Quinby et al., 1958). For several years, the natural tendency to blame certain illnesses on pesticides has been aggravated by articles in magazines and newspapers, which have failed to recognize the fact that, in large populations, poisoning can be expected to appear most quickly, most frequently, most diversely, and most severely in those persons most extensively exposed to these compounds. The factory workers and farmers who come in contact with chemicals constitute large populations, and it is significant that the cases of poisoning that have occurred were almost all acute and were all the result of substantial exposure.

The varied claims of injury from incidental exposure to agricultural chemicals present a problem that can be met chiefly by correct diagnosis of each case. The fact that the studies made so far have failed to reveal injury from incidental exposure to these chemicals does not relieve the physician from examining the possibility in each new instance of suspicion. However, considerable reassurance of the community as a whole and of persons with incidental exposure to pesticides may be expected if they can be made to understand that their danger is less than that of workers whose exposure is direct and often substantial.

The special contribution of the occupational health physician is discussed in Section 9.3.1.8.

No matter what the initial state of community relations, it is important that those responsible for agricultural production, forest protection, or vector control gain the support of the local mass media. This may best be done through group action involving farm organizations, agroindustrial councils, and the like. Maintenance of support is relatively easy where benefits are constantly apparent. Maintenance of active support may be difficult where the benefit consists only of prevention of injury. The benefits of agriculture remain obvious in a community that depends economically on agriculture. On the other hand, the benefits of malaria control may be forgotten in a community that has been spared its ravages for a generation.

9.4.2.1 Interdepartmental Committees and Bilateral Agreements.

Federal Committees. The exigencies of war and the rapid technical advances in pest control led to the establishment at the federal level in the United States of America of an Inderdepartmental Committee on Pest Control (ICPC), which met for the first time in March, 1946. Members were named by the Departments of Agriculture; Defense; Health, Education, and Welfare; and Interior, and liaison members were drawn from the Armed Forces Pest Control Board, and later from the Tennessee Valley Authority. For a time the Committee was responsible for establishing the common or generic names of pesticides. The Committee also issued a number of statements on thermal vaporizers about which the members had reached agreement. However, the most important function of the Committee was always that of keeping the members aware of one another's programs so that they could communicate promptly and directly in the event some problem arose involving two or more departments.

According to a presidential announcement of September 6, 1961, the Secretaries of Agriculture; Defense; Interior; and Health, Education, and Welfare established a Federal Pest Control Review Board to review federal pest control programs and advise the various departments and agencies concerning problems in the use of pesticides and other chemicals, especially in cases involving interdepartmental interests and responsibilities. Each secretary appointed two members to the Board. In comparison with members of the ICPC, they were persons of greater administrative and lesser scientific responsibility. An early draft of the functions and procedures of the Board mentioned their future reliance of the Interdepartmental Committee on Pest Control for factual data and expert opinion, but there was little communication between the two groups.

In early April of 1964 an interdepartmental agreement was entered into between the Departments of Agriculture; Interior; and Health, Education, and Welfare, to coordinate the activities of the three departments pertaining to pesticides. This agreement outlined the responsibilities of the respective departments which related to the registration of pesticides and the setting of tolerances for pesticide residues. The agreement further provided that each department would undertake to keep each of the other departments fully

informed of developments in knowledge on this subject from research or other sources that might come into its possession. The agreement also outlined the procedures to implement these interdepartmental coordination procedures. The agreement stated that the Federal Pest Control Review Board might be asked from time to time to consider broad questions on policies relating to pesticides involving the interrelationship of control programs, research, registration, tolerances, and general departmental recommendations to the public. This agreement established no committee but did establish a review of registration. Applications for registration that might involve food were reviewed by FDA; those that might involve wildlife were reviewed by the Department of the Interior; and all application were received by the Public Health Service (PHS). Legal responsibility for registration remained with the Department of Agriculture.

In midsummer of 1964, the Federal Pest Control Review Board was replaced by the Federal Committee on Pest Control (Fed. Reg. 29:12945–12946, 1964). The ICPC was terminated also, its last meeting being on 18 June 1964. However, as individuals, many members of ICPC became members of the FCPC Subcommittee on Research. The new Committee consisted of not more than two members and two alternates each from the Departments of Agriculture; Interior; Defense; and Health, Education, and Welfare. However, for the first time, the interdepartmental cooperation was facilitated by a professional and clerical staff under the direction of an executive secretary. Specified functions of the Committee consisted of review of programs of federal agencies involving (a) control of pests, (b) monitoring of pesticides in man and the environment, (c) research in pest control, and (d) education concerned with pest control.

In 1969 the Federal Committee on Pest Control was replaced by a Subcommittee on Pesticides of the Cabinet Committee on Environment. In less than a year the Cabinet Committee on Environment was discontinued following formation by the Congress of the Council on Environmental Quality (42 USC 4321 *et seq.*). The Subcommittee on Pesticides then became the Working Group on Pest Control, responsible to the New Council on Environmental Quality, but with no change in function or membership.

Although some unification of approach was obtained through action of the various committees, their assigned functions could not be construed as limiting any of the statutory mandates of the departments. The political pressures relating to pesticides and to a more unified federal approach to pest control continued to mount and culminated in the establishment of the Environmental Protection Agency (EPA). This Agency was initiated by the President's Reorganization Plan No. 3 transmitted to Congress on July 9, 1970. The agency now combines under a single administration pesticide regulatory programs that formerly were in the Departments of Agriculture; Interior; and Health, Education, and Welfare—including FDA and PHS. (Some research laboratories, notably those of FDA and PHS, were transferred to EPA, but the Department of Interior retained a laboratory that was concerned primarily with pesticides.) It remains to be seen how this further unification of federal regulation of pesticides will serve the varied interests of the country.

Even with authority for registration vested in EPA, there is a continuing need for coordinating this activity with the activities of other departments regarding federal use of pesticides and research concerning their efficacy and usefulness. This coordination is achieved through broadening the base of the Working Group on Pest Control to become a Federal Working Group on Pest Management. This Group, like its predecessor, is responsible to the Council on Environmental Quality, although its secretariat, composed largely of the same persons who discharged this function under FCPC, is furnished by EPA. The membership has been extended to include Departments of State, Commerce, and Transportation, with liaison representation from the Department of Labor and the Office of Science and Technology (Fed. Reg. 36:23741–23742, 1971).

State Committees. At about the same time that the Federal Committee on Pest Control was formed, the idea of interdepartmental committees was taken up by some of the states. An especially active one of these committees is that in New York. Its organization and objectives have been described by Wills (1967), its first executive secretary.

Local Committees. Apparently no committees representing groups responsible for the use and limitation of pesticides in connection with agriculture, health, and wildlife have been formed at the local level. It cannot be said that imposing a committee of this sort on a community would correct poor community relations associated with the use of pesticides. It does seem likely that groups that established sufficient communication to form a committee voluntarily already would have solved their major problem.

Bilateral Agreements. Interdepartmental committees might be an extension of working agreements between only two departments. In some instances, however, bilateral agreements were set up to solve limited problems brought to light by committees involving several departments. An example was the early agreement between the US Department of Agriculture and the US Public Health Service by which the latter was consulted regarding the safety of any new unusual chemical pesticidal treatment (Fed. Reg. 24:7602–7605, 1959; 27:1878–1880, 1962).

9.5 Alternative Methods of Pest Control

Logically, the surest way to avoid poisoning is to stop using poisons. From a practical standpoint, this choice is not open. It appears likely that the use of chemicals, including pesticides, will increase. Of course, it is possible to seek alternative methods for pest control. Although a desire to improve safety has led to the development of effective chemicals of low toxicity, improved control of pests has been the main driving force leading to study of alternative methods. Furthermore, some alternative methods present potential hazards of their own. Physical methods, such as the use of light, or biological methods, such as the introduction of parasites, offer no hazard in the toxicological sense. However, the proposed use of microbial toxins would merely substitute less known compounds for better known ones, and the proposed use of living microorganisms for pest control would open a Pandora's box of unknown hazards.

The Sixteenth and Twentieth Reports of the WHO Expert Committee on Insecticides (WHO, 1967; 1973) commented on the safety of alternative methods of control. It was pointed out that, contrary to the popular belief that "natural" substances are harmless, the most poisonous materials known are of natural origin. The Committee noted that microbial toxins could—and should—be subjected to conventional through, pharmacological, and toxicological study, but a precise assessment of their hazard would require knowledge to their mode of action.

The Committe called attention to the special hazard of toxic fungi. They recommended that WHO ensure that the safety of any biological agent proposed for use in pest control should be assayed in a laboratory with the specialized knowledge appropriate for studying the particular agent in question. However, in view of the present state of research on the carcinogenic viruses, one may ask: What qualified laboratory would guarantee that any virus—even a live vaccine—is safe except in a limited context?

Alternative methods may be subject to problems not involving toxicity to a nontarget species. For example, resistance in a strain of the flour beetle to a synthetic juvenile hormone has been reported (Dyte, 1972).

REFERENCES

Advisory Committee on Official Water Standards (1925). Report of the committee. Public Health Rep., 40:693–722.

Advisory Committee on Pesticides and Other Toxic Chemicals (1967). *Review of the Present Safety Arrangements for the Use of Toxic Chemicals in Agriculture and Food Storage.* H.M.S.O., London.

American Conference of Governmental Industrial Hygienists (1963). *Respiratory Protective Devices Manual.* ACGIH, Braun and Brumfield, Inc., Ann Arbor.

American Conference of Governmental Industrial Hygienists (1968). Industrial Ventilation—A Manual of Recommended Practice, Ed. 10. ACGIH, Cincinnati.

American Conference of Governmental Industrial Hygienists (1971). *Documentation of the Threshold Limit Values for Substances in Workroom Air,* Ed. 3. ACGIH, Cincinnati.

American Conference of Governmental Industrial Hygienists (1973). *TLVs: Threshold Limit Values for Chemical Substances and Physical Agents in the Workroom Environment with Intended Changes for 1972.* ACGIH, Cincinnati.

Anonymous (1968). Deep well injection is effective for waste disposal. Environ. Sci. Technol., 2:406–410.

Anonymous (1969). Study group proposes revising regulation of hazardous cargo. News Report, National Academy of Sciences, 19(8): 4.

Association of American Pesticide Control Officials Incorporated (1973–1974). Suggested State Pesticide Control Act (pp. 20–39). Suggested State Pesticide Use and Application Act (pp. 40–58). In: *Official Publication,* 1973-1974. State Board of Agriculture, Topeka, Kansas.

Barnes, J. M. (1967). Food and health—the safe use of pesticides. In: *Proceedings of the 2nd British Pest Control Conference,* pp. 9–13. Industrial Pest Control Association, London.

Best's Safety Directory, Safety-Security-Pollution Control (1973). Ed. 14. A. M. Best Co., Morristown, NJ.

Bruggink, G. M., Barnes, A. C., Jr., and Gregg, L. W. (1964). Clinical problems in aviation medicine. Injury reduction trends in agricultural aviation. Aerosp. Med., 35:472–475.

Cann, H. M., Neyman, D. S., and Verhulst, H. L. (1958). Control of accidental poisoning—a progress report. J. A. M. A., 168:717–724.

Council of Europe (1968). Dangerous chemical substances and proposals concerning their labeling. Ed. 2. Strasbourg.

Chemical Specialties Manufacturers Association (1967). CSMA: Economic Poisons (Pesticides) Laws, Washington, DC.

Deichman, W. B., Brown, P., and Downing, C. (1952). Unusual protective action of a new emulsifier for the handling of organic phosphates. Science, 116:221.

Druckrey, H. (1967). Quantitative aspects in chemical carcinogenesis. In: *Potential Carcinogenic Hazards from Drugs: Evaluation of Risk,* edited by R. Truhaut. U.I.C.C. Monograph Serv. Vol. 7, Springer-Verlag, New York.

Duggan, R. E. (1968). Residues in food and feed. Pesticide residue levels in foods in the United States from July 1, 1963 to June 30, 1967. Pestic. Monit. J. 2:2–46.

Duggan, R. E., and Cook, H. R. (1971). National food and feed monitoring program. Pestic. Monit. J., 5:37–43.

Dutkiewicz, T., and Piotrowski, J. (1961). Experimental investigations on the quantitative estimation of aniline absorption in man. In: *Proceedings of the International Symposium on Maximum Allowable Concentration of Toxic Substances in Industry.* International Union of Pure and Applied Chemistry, pp. 319–323. Butterworths, London.

Dyte, C. E. (1972). Resistance to synthetic juvenile hormone in a strain of the flour beetle, *Tribolium castaneum.* Nature, 238:48–49.

Edson, E. F. (1958). Occupational health aspects of pesticides in Britain. Trans. Assoc. Ind. Med. Officers, 8(1):24–29.

Elkins, H. B. (1961). Maximum acceptable concentrations. A comparison in Russia and the United States. Arch. Environ. Health, 2:45–49.

Ettinger, M. B. (1960). A proposed toxicological screening procedure for use in the water works. J. Am. Water Works Assoc., 52:689–694.

FAO/WHO (1962). *Principles Governing Consumer Safety in Relation to Pesticide Residues.* WHO Tech. Rep. Ser. No. 240.

FAO/WHO (1964). *Evaluation of the Toxicity of Pesticide Residues in Food.* WHO/Food Add./23.

FAO/WHO (1965a). *Evaluation of the Toxicity of Pesticide Residues in Food.* WHO/Food Add./26.65.

FAO/WHO (1965b). *Evaluation of the Toxicity of Pesticide Residues in Food.* WHO/Food Add./27.65.

FAO/WHO (1965c). *Evaluation of the Hazards to Consumers Resulting From the Use of Fumigants in the Protection of Food.* WHO/Food Add./28.65.

FAO/WHO (1969a). *Guidelines for Legislation Concerning the Registration for Sale and Marketing of Pesticides.* FAO, Rome.

FAO/WHO (1969b). *1968 Evaluations of Some Pesticide Residues in Food.* WHO/Food Add./69.35.

FAO/WHO (1970a). *Pesticide Residues in Food.* WHO Tech. Rep. Ser. No. 458.

FAO/WHO (1970b). *1969 Evaluations of Some Pesticides in Food.* WHO/Food Add./70.38.

FAO/WHO (1971a). *Pesticide Residues in Food.* Report of the 1970 joint FAO/WHO meeting. WHO Tech. Rep. Ser. No. 474.

FAO/WHO (1971b). *1970 Evaluations of Some Pesticide Residues in Food.* WHO/Food Add./71.42.

FAO/WHO (1972a). *Pesticide Residues in Food.* Report of the 1971 joint FAO/WHO meeting. WHO Tech. Rep. Ser. No. 502.

FAO/WHO (1972b). *1971 Evaluations of Some Pesticide Residues in Food.* WHO Pestic. Resid. Ser. No. 1.

FAO/WHO (1973a). *Pesticide Residues in Food.* Report of the 1972 joint FAO/WHO meeting. WHO Tech. Rep. Ser. No. 525.

FAO/WHO (1973b). *1972 Evaluations of Some Pesticide Residues in Food.* WHO Pestic. Resid. Ser. No. 2.

FAO/WHO (1974). *Pesticide Residues in Food.* Report of the 1973 joint FAO/WHO meeting. WHO Tech. Rep. Ser. 545.

Farner, L. M., Yaffe, C. D., Scott, N., and Adley, F. E. (1949). The hazards associated with the use of lead arsenate in apple orchards. J. In. Hyg. Toxicol., 31:162–168.

Fawcett, H. H., and Wood, W. S. (1965). *Safety and Accident Prevention in Chemical Operation.* Interscience Publishers, Inc., New York.

Field, J. A. (1964). Pesticide development costs. Farm Chem., May issue: 28–31.

Fowler, R. E. L. (1953). Insecticide toxicology. Manifestations of cottonfield insecticides in the Mississippi Delta. J. Agric. Food Chem., 1:469–473.

Frawley, J. P. (1967). Scientific evidence and common sense as a basis for food-packaging regulations. Food Cosmet. Toxicol., 5:293–308.

Fulton, R. A., Konecky, M. S., and Smith, F. F. (1951). Determining the efficiency of respiratory cartridges and gas mask cannisters against dust and sprays. U. S. Bur. Entomol. Plant. Q., E830:1–8.

Fulton, R. A., and McClellan, W. D. (1957). Respiratory protective devices for agricultural pesticides. Phytopathology, 47:56–57.

Fulton, R. A., and Smith, F. F. (1958). Respiratory protective devices. Methods for testing them against pesticides. J. Agric. Chem., 13(8):30–32; 13(9):22–24.

Fulton, R. A., Smith, F. F., and Bushey, R. L. (1962). Respiratory devices for protection against certain pesticides. USDA, ARS-33-76.

Fulton, R. A., Smith, F. F., and Bushey, R. L. (1963). Respiratory devices for protection against certain pesticides. USDA, ARS-33-76, Supplement 1.

Fulton, R. A., Smith, F. F., and Bushey, R. L. (1964). Respiratory devices for protection against certain pesticides. USDA, ARS-33-76-1, Revised.

Fulton, R. A., Smith, F. F., and Gelardo, R. P. (1955) Respiratory protective devices for agricultural use. J. Econ. Entomol., 48:457–459.

Gaddum, J. H., (1956). The estimation of the safe dose. Br. J. Pharmacol., 11:156–160.

Gleason, M. N., Gosselin, R. E., Hodge, H. C., and Smith, R. P (1969). *Clinical Toxicology of Commercial Products*, Ed. 3. The Williams & Wilkins Co., Baltimore.

Golz, H. H. (1963). Problems in manufacturing and marketing pesticides. Am. J. Public Health, 53:1426–1427.

Goulding, R. (1964). The National Poisons Information Service. Med. Leg. J., 32:60–72.

Gray, W. H., Trevan, J. W., Bainbridge, H. W., and Attwood, A. P. (1931). The ureides of p-aminophenylstibinic acid. Proc. R. Soc. Lond. [Biol.], 108:54–83.

Great Britain (1952). Agriculture (Poisonous Substances) Act, H. M. S. O., London.

Hartwell, W. V., and Hayes, G. R., Jr. (1965). Respiratory exposure to organic phosphorus insecticides. Arch. Environ. Health, 11:564–568.

Hatch, T. F. (1972). The role of permissible limits for hazardous airborne substances in the working environment in the prevention of occupational disease. Bull. WHO, 47:151–159.

Hayes, W. J., Jr. (1971). Editorial. Toxicol. Appl. Pharmacol.,19:i–ii.

Hayes, W. J., Jr. and Pearce, G. W. (1953). Pesticides formulation. Relation to safety in use. J. Agric. Food Chem., 1:466–469.

Hilfman, M. H. (1968). Ervaringen van het Belgisch Toxicologisch Informatiecentrum. Ned. Tijdschr. Geneeskd., 112:413.

Hunter, C. G. (1968). Allowable body burdens of organochlorine pesticides. In: *Proceedings of the Fifth International Congress of Hygiene and Preventive Medicine*, pp. 1–10. Rome.

ILO/WHO (1969). Committee on Occupational Health: permissible levels of occupational exposure to airborne toxic substances. Sixth Report WHO Tech. Rep. Ser. 415: 5–16.

Jacobziner, H. (1966). Causes, control, and prevention of accidental poisonings. Public Health Rep., 81:31–42.

Jacobziner, H., and Raybin, H. (1957). A new approach to the control of chemical poisonings. N. Y. State J. Med., 57:209–215.

Johnson, A. (1963). The Commonwealth Poisons Register. Med. J. Aust. 2:659–660.

Karlsson, B. (1962). Poison Information Center at the Paediatric Clinic, Karolinska Sjukhuset. Sven. Läk.-Tidn., 59:263–270.

Lehman, A. J., and Fitzhugh, O. G. (1954). 100-Fold margin of safety. Assoc. Food Drug Officials Q. Bull., 18:33–35.

Mail, G. A., Hartwell, W. V., Hayes, G. R., Jr., and Funckes, A. J. (1960). Study of hazards in disposing of insecticide containers at a city landfill. Public Works Mag., 91:110–111.

Miller, E. J. (1965). The pesticides safety precautions scheme. Residue Rev., 11:100–118.

Monfore, K. E. (1965). The pesticide program of the Food

and Drug Administration. In: *Pesticides, People and Problems,* pp. 143–153. Proceedings Idaho Annual Health Conference.

Murphy, S. D., and Hayes, W. J., Jr. (1972). Toxicology—a neglected science? J. Coll. Sci. Teaching, 2(2):18–20.

Myschetzky, A. (1964). The Poison Center in Copenhagen. Proc. R. Soc. Med., 57:811–812.

National Academy of Sciences (1969). *Guidelines for Estimating Toxicologically Insignificant Levels of Chemicals in Food.* NAS-NRC, Washington, DC.

National Agricultural Chemicals Association (1967). *Law Guide,* NACA, Washington, D.C.

Papworth, D. S. (1965). Legislation and control of pesticides. J. Forensic Sci. Soc., 5:66–72.

Patty, F. A. (ed.) (1958). *Industrial Hygiene and Toxicology.* Ed. 2, Vol. I. Interscience Publishers, Inc. New York.

Perry, D. P. (1948). Explanation of the principal features of the federal insecticide, fungicide, and rodenticide act. Assoc. Food Drug Officials, US, Q. Bull., 12:64–68.

Press, E. (1956). Poison Control Centers: a new national movement. A.M.A. Arch. Ind. Health, 13:305–307.

Quinby, G. E., Walker, K. C., and Durham, W. F. (1958). Public health hazards involved in the use of organic phosphorus insecticides in cotton culture in the Delta Area of Mississippi. J. Econ. Entomol., 51:831–838.

Rohrman, D. F. (1968). Pesticide laws and legal implications of pesticide use. Food Drug. Cosmet. Law J., 23:142–163; 172–184.

Rollins, R. Z. (1965). Personal communication.

Rusnak, B. S., Gontovaya, N. A., and Dumitrash, I. P. (1968). Practical experience in controlling and application of agricultural poisons in the Moldavian SSR. Hyg. Sanit., 33:424–427.

Smith, D. A., and Wiseman, J. S. (1971). Pesticide poisoning. Epidemiology of pesticide poisoning in the Lower Rio Grande Valley in 1969. Tex. Med., 67:56–59.

Smith, I. (1969). Decontaminating accidental spills of pesticides. NAC News Pestic. Rev., 28:8–9.

Stokinger, H. E. (1969). Current problems of setting occupational exposure standards. Arch. Environ. Health, 19:277–281.

Stracener, C. E., Scherz, R. G., and Crone, R. I. (1967). Results of testing a child-resistant medicine container. Pediatrics, 40:286–288.

Sumerford, W. T., Hayes, W. J., Jr., Johnston, J. M., Walker, K., and Spillane, J. (1953). Cholinesterase response and symptomatology from exposure to organic phosphorus insecticides. Arch. Ind. Hyg. Occup. Med., 7:383–398.

Trasko, V. M. (1970). *Occupational Health and Safety Legislation: A Compilation of State Laws and Regulations.* U.S.D.H.E.W./P.H.S., Cincinnati.

Treasury Department (1914). Bacteriological standard for drinking water. Public Health Rep., 29:2959–2966.

Turner, S. A. (1967–1968). Trends in pesticide usage liability. In: *Offical Publication of the Association of American Pesticide Control Officials Incorporated,* pp. 73–77.

United Nations Industrial Development Organization (1972). *Industrial Production and Formulation of Pesticides in Developing Countries.* Vol. 1, United Nations, New York.

US Department of Agriculture (1964a). *The Federal Insecticide Fungicide, and Rodenticide Act.* Agricultural Research Service, Pesticides Regulation Division.

US Department of Agriculture (1964b). *Regulations for the Enforcement of the Federal Insecticide, Fungicide, and Rodenticide Act.* Agricultural Research Service, Pesticides Regulation Division.

US Department of Agriculture (1965). *Interpretations of the Regulations for the Enforcement of the Federal Insecticide, Fungicide, and Rodenticide Act.* Agricultural Research Service, Pesticides Regulation Division.

US Public Health Service (1962). *Public Health Service Drinking Water Standards.* PHS Publ. No. 956, Washington, DC.

US Public Health Service (1969). *Manual for Evaluating Public Drinking Water Supplies.* PHS Publ. No. 1820, Washington, DC.

US Public Health Service (1971). *Directory of Poison Control Centers.* PHS Publ. No. 1278, Washington, DC.

von Rümker, R., Guest, H. R., and Upholt, W. M. (1970). The search for safer, more selective, and less persistent pesticides. A questionnaire survey of pesticide manufacturers. Bioscience 20:1004–1007.

Ward, J. C. (1965). The functions of the Federal Insecticide, Fungicide, and Rodenticide Act. Am. J. Public Health, 55(7 Suppl. Part II): 27–31.

Weil, C. S. (1972). Statistics vs. safety factors and scientific judgment in the evaluation of safety for man. Toxicol. Appl. Pharmacol., 21:454–463.

Wills, J. H. (1967). Pesticides—a balanced view. Health News, 44(4):16–19.

Wolfe, H. R., Durham, W. F., Walker, K. C., and Armstrong, J. F. (1961). Health hazards of discarded pesticide containers. Arch. Environ. Health, 3:531–537.

Wolfe, H. R., Walker, K. C., Elliot, J. W., and Durham, W. F. (1959). Evaluation of the health hazards involved in house-spraying with DDT. Bull. WHO, 20:1–14.

World Health Organization (1967). *Safe Use of Pesticides in Public Health.* WHO Tech. Rep. Ser. No. 356.

World Health Organization (1970). *The Control of Pesticides.* WHO Chron., 24:516–520.

World Health Organization (1973). *Safe Use of Pesticides.* WHO Tech. Rep. Ser. No. 513.

World Health Organization (1972). *Modern Trends in the Prevention of Pesticide Intoxications.* World Health Organization, Copenhagen.

Yeomans, A. H., Fulton, R. A., Smith, F. F., and Bushey, R. L. (1966). Respiratory devices for protection against certain pesticides. USDA ARS 33–76–2, Revised.

10

EFFECTS ON DOMESTIC ANIMALS

This chapter outlines the epidemiology of the effects of pesticides on domestic animals and discusses some of the implications. The chapter is not concerned with diagnosis and treatment of poisoned animals. Radeleff (1970), Clarke and Clarke (1967), and Buck *et al*. (1973) have written excellent books on the clinical aspects of veterinary toxicology; these books are recommended to those concerned with animal care.

There is a marked similarity between the exposure of people to pesticides and the exposure of domestic animals and birds to these compounds. The similarity extends to the effects.

Laws regulating registration, transportation, use, and residues serve to protect domestic animals as well as man. In fact, some regulations primarily protect animals raised for meat and dairy products and protect man only secondarily. Domestic mammals and birds resemble man in having a limited number of short food chains, all subject to relatively complete control.

In all of these things, man and his domestic animals stand in contrast to wildlife. Except for certain precautionary labeling, the regulation of pesticides benefits wildlife only tangentially at best. Furthermore, the food chains of wildlife are innumerable and often complex.

It is not astonishing to find that the problems of domestic animals associated with pesticides are similar to those of people and different from those of some wildlife.

10.1 Incidence of Poisoning

10.1.1 Poisoning Generally

Since there is no systematic reporting of unintentional mortality among animals, it is impossible to prepare summaries comparable to those in Tables 7-1, 7-3, and 7-5 for human mortality. However, certain broad generalizations can be made. Since animals usually do not have access to alcohol and tobacco, they experience acute poisoning from them infrequently, and they almost never experience the long-term or indirect injuries these materials commonly produce in man. In general, animals have less contact than people with industrial chemicals, but in special instances, such as the contamination of pastures with fluorine wastes, animals have far greater exposure and suffer greater injury. Grazing animals are far more likely than people to ingest significant amounts of toxic plants. Finally, dermal applications are applied to animals more frequently and often in higher dosages and on relatively larger areas.

Most populations of domestic animals, except pets, differ sharply from human populations in both mortality and morbidity. Most cattle, sheep, and poultry are killed for food as juveniles or young adults. Some are killed in middle age. Only a very few reach old age. Therefore, to a large degree, domestic animals are spared the degenerative diseases. Well kept populations are protected from infections and deficiency diseases with an efficiency often better than that achieved in the most favored human populations. Thus, in comparison with man, the mortality of domestic animals is regulated and artificial.

In spite of the absence of exact statistics, it seems certain that poisoning is responsible for a higher proportion of the unintentional mortality of domestic animals than of people. This is true partly because animals have greater exposure to poisons, and partly because they are less liable to other causes of death.

In the absence of truly representative statistics, one might hope that the reports of diagnostic clinics and laboratories might offer some idea of the relative importance of different materials as causes of poisoning in the area served. Unfortunately, even this kind of information generally is lacking. In relation to activities of the Veterinary Diagnostic Laboratory of Iowa State University, it was reported that lead is still one of the most common causes of poisoning in livestock in the United States (Buck, 1970b), and that inorganic arsenic poisoning is second only to lead poisoning among all toxicoses detected in that Laboratory (Buck, 1970a). The arsenic usually was intended as a pesticide, but the lead usually was obtained from spent oil and grease from farm machinery or from old paint or batteries. The author also mentioned organic pesticides as sources of poisoning in cattle, but in the same context mentioned organic arsenic feed additives as toxicants in swine and poultry; and urea, nitrates, cyanide, mineral imbalance, mycotoxins, and low residue diets as sources of illness in one or more kinds of farm animals. No clue as to the relative importance of most of these toxicants seems to be available.

10.1.2 Poisoning by Pesticides

It was estimated that in 1948 pesticides caused the loss of about 0.2% of livestock in the United States of America. In recent years this loss has been reduced to 0.1% and it is considered unlikely that the loss can be reduced below 0.05%. In an $18,000 million industry, even 0.1% represents $18 million per year, or enough food for 200,000 people (Radeleff, 1969).

The possibility that occasional animals will be injured as the result of intentional application of pesticides to them is greater than the possibility of the corresponding human injury because treatment of animals is far more common and aggressive and because there can be no real cooperation on the part of animals. To achieve efficient treatment of uncooperative beasts, it may be necessary to use methods such as plunge dipping that involve a certain physical danger to the animals even if no pesticide were used.

Compounds for application to animals are selected on the basis of broad toxicological information, and the particular preparations to be used are tested carefully before their sale is permitted. Because of this care, only a few preparations prove unsatisfactory. Extensive experience has been reported for some preparations intended for direct application to animals, and these reports confirm their high degree of safety. For example, during the 4-year period 1964–1968, officials of the Tick Quarantine Area of New South Wales found, in connection with plunge dipping of more than a million cattle per compound, that the mortality due to poisoning was 0.00061% for coumaphos, 0.00342% for dioxathion, and 0.00349% for ethion. Experience with carbaryl, carbophenothion, diazinon, and Dursban® was more limited. The overall mortality rate among more than 17.5 million cattle dipped was 0.00322% (Roe, 1969).

10.1.2.1 Endemic Mortality and Morbidity. Undoubtedly the greatest cause of poisoning has been carelessness of the individual farmer. The occasional injury of one or a few animals on a single farm or this kind of injury on widely scattered farms clearly is an endemic situation. If the same kind of carelessness leads to injury of a large number of animals even on a single farm, the episode constitutes an epidemic. However, as illustrated in Section 10.1.2.2, some epidemics are distinguished more by the unusual circumstances that surround them than by the large number of animals involved.

The danger that pets will be poisoned is similar in many ways to the danger that children will suffer the same fate. Thus, the poisoning of dogs, cats, and other household pets is largely endemic in character. A number of case reports have been published, but few throw much light on circumstances that lead to poisoning. Many of the same reports do give valuable information on clinical and pathological findings and on the problem of differential diagnosis.

10.1.2.2 Epidemics of Poisoning by Pesticides. The following brief accounts of epidemics of poisoning among domestic animals are chosen and presented to illustrate some of the ways in which these misfortunes occur. No attempt has been made to list all episodes or to evaluate the hazard of different compounds. A discussion of factors that contribute to poisoning, whether endemic or epidemic, constitutes Section 10.4.

Improper Dosage. At about 5:30 o'clock one morning, a worker sprayed 54 milk cows with dichlorvos at a dosage 45 times greater than he intended. The proper dosage, which had been in use for some time, had proved entirely safe and had given good fly control leading to improved milk production. The grossly excessive dose produced severe poisoning in a few minutes. Fortunately, all the cows recovered in a few hours, although, judging from the presence of convulsions, some cows were in very grave danger for a time. After the excitement was over, it was found that the worker had taken dichlorvos from the wrong container, which, however, was of the same size and color as the one he had used before. The early morning light had been dim, and the worker may have been sleepy when he prepared the spray (Knapp and Graden, 1964).

The addition of an unmeasured amount of 57% malathion to a dipping solution that had been diluted by rain led to the poisoning of 24 dogs treated for ticks. Of the 24, 16 died or had to be killed. The final concentration of the dip was not determined but could have been as high as 15% malathion as compared to 0.25 to 0.5% commonly used for the purpose (McCurnin, 1969).

Use of Improper Compounds or Formulations. Although the extreme susceptibility of dairy calves to benzene hexachloride was revealed by early experiments (Radeleff *et al.*, 1955), this information did not prevent the application of a formulation containing DDT and lindane to a barn containing 21 young Sahiwal and Jersey calves. Symptoms occurred within 3 hours after spraying; four deaths followed within a short time, and others at longer intervals through the 3rd day. Only six calves survived (Singh *et al.*, 1969).

Of 19 cattle, 17 were poisoned and five died following spraying with a 0.25% emulsion of parathion (Lang and Nass, 1970).

Demeton taken from an unlabeled bag assumed to contain DDT killed 18 of 30 cattle sprayed with the material (Watson *et al.*, 1971).

Three cows suffered convulsions and one of them died after a rotenone formulation that actually contained approximately 30% endrin was applied to them (Moubry *et al.*, 1968).

Use of Treated Seed Grain as Feed. Apparently the largest outbreak of poisoning among animals following misuse of treated seed grain occurred on two collective farms in Saratov Province north of the Caspian Sea. Poisoning of swine followed the feeding of barley treated with ethyl mercury chloride for 23 days or

more. Poisoning described as acute was recorded in 481 of 858 animals, and apparently all those affected died or were destroyed. In subsequent months, further losses occurred, and the remaining pigs showed signs of chronic mercury intoxication (Alekseeva, 1969).

The inadvertent feeding of grain treated with methyl mercury dicyandiamide to a flock of 1,400 chickens undoubtedly killed part of about 45 that died within a month and a half after feeding began. However, the nature of the difficulty was determined not by clinical diagnosis but by chemical analysis of eggs and meat, which were withheld from the market until the residues were below 0.1 ppm (Howell, 1969).

Drift and Other Residues. Of 40 heifers, 11 were poisoned moderately by paraquat that had been sprayed on grass along a ditch beside which they walked on their way to and from pasture (.Piskac and Jordan, 1970).

Eighty bullocks died when 275 of them were allowed to graze along a road, the edge of which had been sprayed with sodium arsenite (Moxham and Coup, 1968).

Severe illness of cattle following respiratory exposure to drift has been documented in at least two instances (Quinby and Doornik, 1965). In one of them, dust containing 1% tepp was applied by aircraft at the rate of 0.56 kg of active ingredient per hectare to 18.6 ha of hops in a way that had been customary for 16 years. There was a thermal inversion and the air was unusually quiet so that the dust drifted very little beyond the crop and a farmhouse and barn about 210 m away, and it remained there about 2 hours. Fifteen cows showed typical signs of anticholinesterase poisoning and two heifers died. Persons trying to help the cattle experienced coughing and shortness of breath but were able to continue work. Chickens, geese, and a cat at the farmer's home 15 m away were not visibly affected.

Improper Storage. In a barn lot, three horses knocked off the lid of a machine for distributing poisoned grain, and among them consumed about 0.68 kg of oats containing 0.025% strychnine alkaloid. One horse died before treatment could be started, one recovered after treatment, and one was only mildly sick (Meek and Keatts, 1971).

Bags of 20% aldrin granules were used to form a temporary wall to hold corn cobs stored in a warehouse. In scooping up the cobs with a tractor, the operator inadvertently broke some of the bags and released aldrin granules into the cobs. When the latter were delivered to a farmer and used to feed 95 cattle, 36 were fatally poisoned. To make matters worse, the 36 carcasses were processed into tankage for animal feeds, and the surviving cattle (which undoubtedly still contained dieldrin residues) were slaughtered several months later for human food (Buck, 1970b).

Improper Disposal of Containers. Four heifers were found dead and another showed typical anticholinesterase poisoning after 20 of them were returned to the pasture from which they earlier had escaped. The cause of poisoning almost certainly was a partially empty bag of phorate that had been discarded not far from the pasture (Kitto, 1970; Bowen, 1970).

In another instance, seven cows were killed by disulfoton they obtained mainly from chewing bags that had blown into their pasture from an adjacent, sprayed potato field. The possibility could not be excluded that some disulfoton had contaminated irrigation water entering the pasture watering pond (Watson *et al.*, 1971).

Eight cattle died after they gained access to an old building and ate lead arsenate from bags that had been abandoned there (Rybolt, 1970).

The death of two heifers and a cow was traced to a drum discarded 4 years earlier that still contained a layer of paraquat overlaid by rainwater (Thomas and Amor, 1968).

10.2 Incidence of Storage and Excretion

Studies of storage and excretion have been carried out in domestic animals used either as experimental animals in the general sense, or in exploration of their special role in agricultural production. In the first instance, the results, whether obtained in dogs or cats or, more rarely, in livestock, are discussed along with results in rats, mice, and other laboratory animals in Chapter 3.

In the second instance, the results are of tremendous importance in determining the safety for man of agricultural procedures that might lead to residues in meat or dairy products; however, once a procedure has been found safe, the results of tests under necessarily experimental conditions are of little interest unless they happen to throw new light on some fundamental problem in qualitative or quantitative metabolism. Of far greater interest in connection with agricultural production are the results of monitoring meat and dairy products ready for human consumption. These results are discussed in Sections 6.1.1 and 6.1.5.

Factors (see Section 2.4) that lead to poisoning also may contribute to excessive residues in milk. In addition, the raising of hay on land previously treated with a chlorinated hydrocarbon insecticide for the control of soil insects affecting another crop has led to excessive residues in milk (Moubry *et al.*, 1968).

10.3 Other Possible Effects of Pesticides

Problems other than mortality, morbidity, and storage might be expected to follow the same pattern in connection with domestic animals as they have in relation to man, and in a sense this is true. For example, although it apparently has not been reported, some compounds applied to domestic animals must certainly induce liver microsomal enzymes in one or more species. The dosages involved in some instances certainly are as great as those that have produced this effect in man (see Section 7.3).

Of course, there have been instances of obvious illness that an author considered might represent poisoning and placed on record in the event his colleagues might observe the same kind of thing, even though the fact of poisoning could not be established. A good example of such alert, honest reporting is an account of possible poisoning of horses by a mixture of 2,4-D and 2,4,5-T that had been used to destroy nettles around the edge of a pasture (Pinsent and Lane, 1970). Of six horses, four became ill, one died, and one had to be killed. Some important findings did not correspond with those in livestock intentionally poisoned by large doses of the compounds, and it is difficult to conceive how the horses could have received a dosage nearly as large as livestock have withstood without any sign of injury (Radeleff, 1970). Thus, it is doubtful the illness in the horses represented poisoning, but circumstantial evidence strongly suggested this possibility, and no other cause of the small epidemic was found. Objective reporting of such episodes is a scientific necessity. It is only in this way that we can learn the peculiar combinations of circumstances (for example, mixtures of compounds and interactions between species) that may lead to poisoning. It is a pity that such reports lend themselves to misinterpretation and misuse.

Fortunately, the lunatic fringe has had little to say about the possibility that modern pesticides now determine the occurrence of diseases of animals that have been recognized for years but whose causes remain obscure. Perhaps this is only because the degenerative diseases are of less importance in livestock than in man.

10.4 Factors in Poisoning

The basic considerations regarding the relative importance of different factors in toxicology are the same for domestic animals as for other species. As explained in Section 2.4, dosage is the most important factor and compound the next most important one. Factors such as species, strain, age, sex, and others generally are far less important but may be critical in individual instances. In fact, certain classical examples of species difference involve domestic animals. The use of diazinon for fly control around duck pens on Long Island in 1954 led to the death of an estimated 15,653 of the birds (Dougherty, 1957). The same compound has been used for years around chicken pens without causing any difficulty. Another example that was recognized early is the high sensitivity of bees to carbaryl. Proper warnings prevented the occurrence of any catastrophic loss.

The unusual susceptibility of Dorset Down sheep to diazinon was observed in a flock composed of three varieties and a few animals of mixed breed (Smith, 1970).

Whether domestic animals will have unintentional access to pesticides is determined by the care with which people use and store the compounds. In almost all instances, the circumstances that led to poisoning of animals were similar to those that have produced human tragedy (see Section 7.1.4). The epidemics among domestic animals recounted in Section 10.1.2.2 are arranged under headings indicating the kinds of mistakes that have led to trouble. Briefly, pesticides mistaken for mineral supplements or some other wholesome material have been mixed directly into feed. Often the poison had been stored near the animals' proper feed. Unlabeled containers have been a frequent cause of trouble. The spraying of animals with the wrong compound has as a parallel the shampooing of children's heads with parathion. Usually, use of the wrong compound has been the result of ignorance and failure to read labels. In a few instances, use of the wrong compound was the result of mislabeling by the formulator. Fortunately, this particular kind of mistake is rare and promptly compensated.

REFERENCES

Alekseeva, A. A. (1969). Mercury retention in the muscles and internal organs of swine following Granosan poisoning. Veterinariya, 5:58–60.

Bowen, P. D. G. (1970). Deaths through careless disposal of an insecticide. Vet. Rec., 87:788.

Buck, W. B. (1970a). Diagnosis of feed-related toxicoses. J. Am. Vet. Med. Assoc., 156:1434–1443.

Buck, W. B. (1970b). Lead and organic pesticide poisonings in cattle. J. Am. Vet. Med. Assoc., 156:1468–1472.

Buck, W. B., Osweiler, G. D., and Van Gelder, G. A. (1973). Clinical and Diagnostic Veterinary Toxicology. Kendall Hunt Publishing Co., Dubuque, Iowa.

Clarke, E. G. C., and Clarke, M. L. (1967). Garner's Veterinary Toxicology, Ed. 3. Baillière, Tindall & Cassell, Ltd., London.

Dougherty, E., III (1957). Thiophosphate poisoning in white pekin ducks. Avian Dis., 1:127–130.

Howell, J. (1969). Mercury residues in chicken eggs and tissues from a flock exposed to methylmercury dicyandiamide. Can. Vet. J., 10:212–213.

Kitto, H. W. (1970). Deaths through careless disposal of a herbicide. Vet. Rec., 87:731–732.

Knapp, F. W., and Graden, A. P. (1964). Accidental exposure of dairy cows to excessive amount of dichlorvos. J. Econ. Entomol., 57:790–791.

Lang, E., and Nass, H. (1970). E 605 poisoning in a herd of Berlin cattle. Tieraerztl. Umsch., 25:128–131.

McCurnin, D. M. (1969). Malathion intoxication in military scout dogs. J. Am. Vet. Med. Assoc., 155:1359–1363.

Meek, D. G., and Keatts, W. H. (1971). Strychnine poisoning in horses. J. Am. Vet. Med. Assoc., 158:491.

Moxham, J. W., and Coup, M. R. (1968). Arsenic poisoning of cattle and other domestic animals. NZ Vet. J., 16:161–165.

Moubry, R. J., Myrdal, G. R., and Sturges, A. (1968). Residues in food and feed: rate of chlorinated hydrocarbon pesticides in dairy milk. Pestic. Monit. J., 2:72–79.

Pinsent, P. J. N., and Lane, J. G. (1970). A case of possible 2,4-D and 2,4,5-T poisoning in the horse. Vet. Rec., 87:247.

Piskac, A., and Jordan, V. (1970). Otrava skotu herbicidnim pripravkem "Gramoxone." Veterinarstvi, 20:471–473.

Quinby, G. E., and Doornink, G. M. (1965). Tetraethyl pyrophosphate poisoning following airplane dusting. J. A. M. A., 191:1–6.

Radeleff, R. D. (1969). Personal communication, June 20.

Radeleff, R. D. (1970). Veterinary Toxicology, Ed. 2. Lea & Febiger, Philadelphia.

Radeleff, R. D., Woodard, G. T., Nickerson, W. J., and Bushland, R. C. (1955). The acute toxicity of chlorinated hydrocarbon and organic phosphorus insecticides to livestock. USDA Technical Bulletin 1122, US Government Printing Office, Washington, DC.

Roe, R. T. (1969). The toxicity to cattle of some acaricides in use in plunge dips in New South Wales. Aust. Vet. J., 45:332–333.

Rybolt, D. (1970). Lead arsenate toxicosis—a case report. Iowa State Univ. Vet., 32:4–5.

Singh, H., Kunar, A., Singh, R., Bahga, H. S., and Sahu, S. (1969). Organochlorine insecticide poisoning in dairy calves, clinical report. Indian Vet. J., 46:910–912.

Smith, I. D. (1970). An unusual sequel to the shower dipping of sheep with diazinon. Vet. Rec., 86:284–286.

Thomas, P., and Amor, O. F. (1968). A case of diquat poisoning in cattle. Vet. Rec., 83:674–676.

Watson, M., Benson, W. W., and Gabica, J. (1971). Accidental organophosphate poisoning in cattle, two case histories. Arch. Environ. Health, 22:582–583.

11

EFFECTS ON WILDLIFE

This book is concerned primarily with the underlying principles of toxicology and with the real and potential injury that pesticides may produce in man. However, it is appropriate to outline the effects of pesticides on wildlife, partly because these effects constitute one aspect of the toxicology of pesticides, and partly because such consideration may increase understanding in two ways. First, certain ecological principles important in various degrees in all pest control operations are best understood and best illustrated in connection with wildlife (Moore, 1967). Second, the basic toxicological principle of dosage-response relationships, which often has been neglected in connection with study of wildlife, helps to explain the serious effects pesticides occasionally have. Application of this principle and appreciation of other factors in toxicity discussed in previous chapters may help to reconcile observations that, at first glance, appear entirely contradictory.

11.1 Toxicology

11.1.1 Inherent Susceptibility of Wildlife to Pesticides

A review of the inherent susceptibility of wildlife to pesticides is beyond the scope of this volume. It must be emphasized, however, that the range of species considered either as wildlife or at least as food for wildlife is almost limitless and certainly far more exten-

sive than the array of domesticated forms on which man depends directly. Therefore, the phenomenon of species variation in toxicity (Section 2.4.7) and in storage (Section 3.2.3.3) is of tremendous importance and complexity.

On the other hand, the susceptibility of wildlife to each compound at the level of the susceptible tissue, while showing some species differences, often is of the same order of magnitude as that of laboratory animals (see Section 3.2.3.4). The tremendous practical differences that exist depend mainly on differences in ability to concentrate, absorb, and eliminate the compounds in question.

In addition to many reports of individual investigations, there are several valuable reviews or tabular compendia concerning the toxicity of pesticides to wildlife. These include papers by Tucker and Crabtree (1970), Heath et al. (1972a), and Schafer (1972).

11.1.2 Storage of Pesticides in Wildlife

The storage of pesticides in wildlife obeys the rules governing the storage of chemicals in organisms generally, a subject discussed in Section 3.2.3. The measurement of storage in wildlife is of special importance because it offers the best and, frequently, only index of exposure of different species and of different populations of the same species. This approach is necessary because the exposure of wildlife to pesticides usually is unintentional and frequently indirect.

11.1.2.1 Compounds Found in Wildlife.
Biologists have placed greatest emphasis on DDT and its derivatives, and these compounds have been used by way of illustration in connection with most points discussed below.

A compound may be found in wildlife that is found rarely if ever in people. The occurrence of residues of mirex in terrestrial invertebrates, in birds, and in fish (Baetcke et al., 1972) might have been predicted because the compound was applied widely, often by aircraft, to open fields and brushland for control of the imported fire ant (Solenopsis saevissima). Undoubtedly the compound has been applied directly to water and also entered it indirectly by washing from the soil surface. In a similar way, a wide range of aquatic and marshland species associated with a waterway contaminated with methyl mercury store substantial amounts of mercury (Dustman et al., 1972).

A valuable review of chlorinated hydrocarbon residues in wildlife is that of Stickle (1973).

11.1.2.2 Monitoring of Pesticides. In order to obtain quantitative information systematically, an elaborate monitoring program has been established for certain chlorinated hydrocarbons and heavy metals (Johnson et al., 1967; Dustman et al., 1971). Species to be sampled were chosen on the basis of wide distribution, reasonable abundance and availability, food habits, and, no doubt, special interest. The species selected include the starling (Sternus vulgaris), mallard duck (Anas platyrhynchos), black duck (Anas rubripes), and the bald eagle (Haliaeetus leucocephalus). The black duck is substituted for the mallard in states where suitable numbers of mallards cannot be obtained. Birds are chosen rather than mammals chiefly because mammals that are sufficiently abundant and available (a) sample too small an area (because of their restricted home ranges), and (b) usually have only trivial residues (because they are herbivores). The omnivorous starling serves to monitor the terrestrial environment. Samples are collected for that purpose. Ducks serve as an index of contamination of the aquatic environment. Duck wings contributed by hunters constitute the samples for analysis, it having been shown (Dindal and Peterle, 1968) that there are highly significant correlations between residues in wings and in a wide range of tissues from the same birds. Eagles are at the top of a long food chain involving estuaries, where contamination with a variety of chemicals is considered especially critical. Because eagles are now scarce and protected by law, the only ones available for analysis are those found dead or incapacitated beyond recovery.

Early results of monitoring have been published for the starling (Martin, 1969; Martin and Nickerson, 1972), ducks (Heath, 1969), and the bald eagle (Reichel et al., 1969b; Mulhern et al., 1970; Belisle et al., 1972).

In addition to the few species that are being monitored systematically, a great range of species from worms to whales has been the subject of individual studies. Many of the results have been tabulated in an excellent review by Edwards (1970). Storage in eagles was reported by Belisle et al. (1972). The studies establish without doubt the widespread distribution of some of the chlorinated hydrocarbon insecticides, polychlorinated biphenyls, and heavy metals in organisms that live in areas where these materials are used or whose food chains can be traced to these areas or to drainage from them.

11.1.2.3 Geographical Distribution of Pesticides. Even wildlife in the most remote areas has been reported to contain DDT and related compounds, if not other chlorinated hydrocarbon insecticides. Thus, Sladen et al. (1966) reported concentrations of DDT-related compounds as high as 0.152 ppm in the fat of Adelie penguins (Pygoscelis adeliae) and lower concentrations in crabeater seals (Lobodon carcinophagus) from Antarctica. The analytical method was capable of measuring other chlorinated hydrocarbon insecticides but failed to detect any. The concentration of DDT and its metabolites in penguins corresponded in a predictable way with their physiological state. For example, the highest concentration was found in a penguin that had lost weight during molting. Whereas some doubt is involved in the measurement of small traces by gas chromatography (see Section 6.2.2.2), it must be pointed out that samples of fat from an emperor penguin (Aptenodytes fosteri), which had remained frozen since it was killed over 30 years before the extensive use of DDT, contained no detectable amount of that compound or its metabolites. Failure to find DDT in Antarctic ice argued against distribution of the compound by air currents. The authors discussed other possible sources of DDT in Antarctica, including direct contamination of the samples (unlikely in view of the precautions taken), waste disposal in the area, transfer by ocean currents, and transfer into local food chains by vast hordes of migrating scavengers and carnivores that move back and forth between the south polar regions and regions where pesticides are abundant.

Later, a concentration of 0.00004 ppm of DDT in water melted from Antarctic snow was reported (Peterle, 1969). This value is only a little less than that reported for rain and surface water in the United Kingdom and the USA (see Section 6.1.3.1).

The results on Antarctic wildlife were confirmed in connection with samples taken in the same general area. DDT only was found in 4 of 16 Weddell seals (*Leptonychotes weddelli*), and both DDT and DDE were found in most skuas (*Catharacta skua maccormicki*) examined. No pesticides were found in water or snow or in most invertebrates or fish on which penguins and other birds feed. Curiously enough, no pesticide was found in an emperor penguin (George and Frear, 1966).

A third study (Tatton and Ruzicka, 1967) was carried out on samples from Antarctica, but collected on Signy Island, some 4,500 km from the sites of the two earlier collections. The findings regarding DDT and its metabolites were confirmatory, but, in addition, traces of α-BHC, β-BHC, γ-BHC, heptachlor epoxide, and dieldrin were found in penguins and other birds restricted to the area. One other finding of special interest was high residues (0.73 ppm of heptachlor epoxide, 26 ppm of *p,p'*-DDE, and 2.5 ppm of *p,p'*-DDT) in the fat of a brown skua, a scavenger and predator known to migrate as far as the tropics. Most of the residues in other species were within the range of 0.001 to 0.010 ppm, but a few samples contained almost 0.050 ppm, usually of DDE. Another finding of great interest was the occurrence in krill (*Euphausia* sp.) of essentially the same pesticides as were found in birds restricted to the area. The concentrations in the krill were lower than those in the birds. Thus, migrant birds clearly constitute one way of transporting pesticides to the Antarctic, and krill clearly constitute one link in the food chain through which the material is passed.

Apparently the highest value reported in crude fish oils was 369 ppm of total DDT-related compounds in one species taken off Catalina Island, California, a very highly contaminated area (Burnett, 1971). Values from other areas of the United States of America or from other countries have been substantially less and sometimes undetectable. For example, consistently low levels were found in fish in the Caribbean Sea (Giam *et al.*, 1972).

DDT, its metabolites, and, to a much lesser extent, some other chlorinated hydrocarbon insecticides have been found in fish in remote parts of the world. A total of 14.4 ppm of DDT-related materials was found in the body oil of mackerel from the Pacific (Ribicoff and Larrick, 1964). Although it has been claimed that DDT or its metabolites may be found in species of fish that live their entire lives in the open ocean without coming near land, proof of the assertion apparently is poorly documented. The absolute extent of the area occasionally visited by the fish is incompletely known. Furthermore, little attention has been given to the food chains that might transfer materials from coastal waters to areas distant from any island or continental shelf.

11.2 Ecological Factors in Pest Control

11.2.1 Pests and Their Natural Control

11.2.1.1 The Nature of Pests. A pest is any organism that interferes with the convenience or well-being of man or another species he favors. Thus, pests may adversely affect not only man and his domestic animals and plants, but also desirable wildlife.

It is sometimes suggested that all pest situations depend on some kind of ecological imbalance. It is true, as pointed out in the following section, that pest problems may be increased by biotic simplification. However, it is inaccurate to suggest that all pest problems have this origin. It is even more misleading to suggest that all pest problems are somehow the result of human intervention, except in the purely semantic sense that if man were not involved at all, the definition of pest would never be applied. A number of vector-borne diseases including malaria, trypanosomiasis, sylvan yellow fever, plague, tularemia, several virus encephalitides, murine typhus, scrub typhus, and rickettsialpox are known to occur in animals that serve as reservoirs. There is reason to believe that these diseases antedate man, much less any recorded culture. Expeditions to the tundra are plagued by mosquitoes. The presence of these insects in tremendous numbers is entirely normal, but they are pests in spite of being a part of the regional ecological balance.

Abundance is not a prerequisite for a pest. A single infected malaria mosquito in a home carries a serious threat. It takes only a small number of tsetse flies to maintain sleeping sickness in parts of Africa to the extent that human life is imperiled and the introduction of cattle is impossible. Even the density of savannah species such as *Glossina morsitans* necessary to maintain human epidemics is only about 50 flies per hectare averaged over many square kilometers of bush. The riverine species such as *G. palpalis* and *G. fuscipes* may live in a small colony of a few hundred flies around a watering place and maintain transmission there. Transmission can occur wherever tsetse flies exist. Cattle trypanosomiasis is transmitted by densities below one fly to every 25 ha (ie, $<4/km^2$).

Thus, the seriousness of a pest must be judged more by the number of people it affects and the degree and nature of its injury rather than by its absolute abundance. A farmer can tolerate more plant lice than body lice.

11.2.1.2 Natural Control.

Control exercised over a "pest" species in the absence of man is no different from the control to which any other species is subject. This must be true because, in the absence of man, there can be no interference with man or his interests and, therefore, no pests.

Of course, the factors that keep natural populations in check vary somewhat from one species to another. However, ecologists agree that, in most instances, limitation of food and shelter is of more importance, and reduction of numbers by predators or parasites (including microorganisms causing disease) usually is of lesser importance. This generalization applies to both animals and plants. Among some but not all rodents, physiological changes conditioned by social relationships are of great significance in regulating populations (see Section 2.4.12.2). It is not known just how important this factor is in other animals, but it appears to be distinctly less important than in certain rodents. Unfortunately, populations of several rodent species may become excessive before limitation through any ecological mechanism reaches an important level.

Species-specific predators or parasites almost never reduce a prey population below a minimal level, much less exterminate it. Several models that have been proposed for predator-prey systems determine a stable limit cycle and provide a satisfying mathematical explanation for those communities in which populations are observed to oscillate in a rather reproducible, periodic manner (May, 1972; Gilpin and Rosenzweig, 1972). Thus, predators may increase in numbers in response to an increase in their prey and eventually lead to a precipitous decrease in the number of the latter. Predation may wipe out limited populations of prey. Cycles with high peaks and low nadirs in the populations of both predator and prey can occur, but such cycles are less common than was supposed formerly. In the long run, the predator depends on its prey as surely as herbivores depend on plants. The usual situation is for the predator to seize more of the young, the sick, and the old than of normal adults, with the result that influence on the breeding population is minimal. The prey is gathered almost as a crop that is harvested but also perpetuated. In the same way, a successful parasite does not destroy the host population although it may destroy certain individuals.

It follows from what has been said that the best pest control is that which limits food supply or harborage. Thus filling, draining, clearing, purposeful fluctuation of water level, and the like have been used with notable success for mosquito control. Rodent-proof construction and the proper collection and disposal of solid wastes contribute greatly to rat control. These and other environmental measures, if maintained, provide control that is effective, stable, and permanent. However, the practicality of any particular environmental measure will vary greatly according to circumstance. It may be practical to drain a malarious swamp but impractical to drain a malarious rice paddy. It may be practical to prevent urban rats from reaching their food but impractical to stop boll weevils from reaching theirs.

Since predators usually harvest their prey like a well kept crop, natural predators will offer satisfactory control of a pest only when substantial numbers of the pests can be tolerated. This does not mean that everything possible should not be done to foster desirable predators. It may even be feasible to develop predators as a commercial product so that, through human intervention, abundance of the predator does not depend on the survival of the pest it is meant to control.

11.2.2 Biotic Simplification, a Cause of Pest Problems.

Ecologists speak of the animals and plants that occupy a particular area as constituting a community. When the number of different species is great, the relationships among them are necessarily complex and constitute a system of checks and balances. When the number of kinds of organisms is small, their relationships are relatively simple and usually less stable.

In general, the number of species of plants and animals per unit area is greatest in the tropics and becomes progressively smaller at greater latitudes, being extremely small at the poles. The number of organisms that can survive an extremely cold climate is small. In a similar way, lack of heat and oxygen limits the number of species that can survive at the tops of very high mountains. Lack of water limits the number of species that can survive in deserts.

The inherent instability of simple communities is illustrated by the occasional overproduction of lemmings in Scandinavia. Lemming outbreaks have been recorded for centuries; they are not dependent on human activity. Another illustration involves the periodic increase of locusts in various semiarid parts of the world. Plagues of locusts are mentioned in the Bible. There is every reason to believe that the general behavior of lemmings and locusts was much the same before the advent of man as it has been during recorded history.

The relatively simple ecological community with which most people are familiar is that produced by agriculture. Agricultural ecology is not so simple as that of arctic or desert, partly because many native species thrive in woodlands and along roadways and hedgerows, but chiefly because the number of species of microorganisms in the soil remains very great. Nevertheless, land clearing and plowing inevitably lead to great biotic simplification. Agriculture is the necessary basis of essentially all civilization, including the most ancient cultures whose history has come down to us. Although biotic simplification is essential to agriculture, it is also a source of some pest problems.

During the last hundred years or so, there have been a number of important changes in agricultural practice. These changes involve: (a) introduction of power machinery; (b) introduction of chemical fertilizers; (c) introduction of pesticides; and (d) the extension of monoculture. All of these changes lead directly or indirectly to further biotic simplification. Another important change in agricultural practice, that is (e) the development of improved varieties of plants and animals, introduces little or no increase in simplification of the community, and, insofar as the varieties are more resistant to pests, this change actually stabilizes the community.

Various changes in agricultural practice are interrelated (see Section 1.4.2.4). For example, it seems doubtful that fertilizers or pesticides would be used so extensively in the absence of power equipment. Monoculture, the practice of raising a single crop in a very large area, has been greatly advanced by the availability of power equipment, although some degree of regional specialization in crops has existed for a very long time. Another example of the interrelation of agricultural practices is the fact that it is uneconomical to use fertilizer on a crop unless its destruction by pests can be limited.

The following sections consider specific ways in which biotic simplification can lead to pest problems.

11.2.2.1 Faunal Imbalance.
Any significant decrease in the number of individuals of a particular species in an area produces a state of faunal imbalance that is bound to influence some other species in the same community. For example, if a pest population is severely reduced, there will be a corresponding reduction in the populations of its predators and parasites. The degree of this secondary reduction will depend on the ability of the predators and parasites to find and use alternative sources of food. Although vertebrate predators usually prefer to eat animals of one or only a few species, they promptly attack other species when the favored ones are not plentiful. The alternative prey constitute what are called "buffer species" because they permit the predators to survive when their normal prey is scarce or even absent. Unlike vertebrate predators, insect predators are relatively specific in their choice of food; therefore, to a large degree, the control of insect pests brings simultaneous control of their natural enemies. If the means of control is a chemical, it often happens that the predators and parasites are also susceptible to the poison. Thus, many of them are killed directly rather than being killed secondarily through starvation.

No matter what the cause leading to the limitation of predators and parasites, the reduction in their numbers favors the recovery of the pest population. Thus, it may happen that the pest, no longer effectively limited by its enemies, may recover rapidly and the population may eventually exceed the level that originally was considered to require control measures.

In a somewhat similar way, the use of monoculture in connection with a given crop favors greater density and more uniform distribution of pests particularly adapted to that crop. At the same time, monoculture and various practices associated with it tend to discourage parasites and predators, especially those relatively nonspecific ones that find alternative hosts in native plants or in other crops.

Although it is common to think of grains, grapes, citrus, and many other crops as being grown on vast continuous areas, it must not be supposed that all monocultures are determined by man. Many forests in the subarctic are made up almost entirely of one species. Monoculture favors the spruce budworm no less than the corn borer. On the contrary, a solid stand is not a prerequisite for destruction. The American chestnut was exterminated by a blight even though it typically grew among other trees in the forest.

11.2.2.2 Emergent Pests.
A special case of faunal imbalance involves what has been called "emergent pests." These are species

that become pests only by virtue of some change in their environment. An example is found in the increased importance of mites following the use of DDT for the control of the codling moth. The mites were present before DDT was introduced, but not in sufficient numbers to cause appreciable harm. However, the use of DDT so affected the natural enemies of mites that the latter increased to a point of being serious pests, and other chemicals, notably parathion, had to be used for their control.

As discussed below, a reduction or elimination of enemies also may follow the transfer of a species to a completely new environment. However, the environmental change that causes a pest to "emerge" may involve its food rather than its enemies. The Colorado potato beetle became a pest when people brought the potato to it. Formerly it had fed on plants of no economic importance. Given an opportunity to eat potato plants, it rapidly spread eastward across the United States of America and on to Europe, rivaling the potato blight in its devastation.

Introduced Species.   Many important pests are not native to the area in which they do greatest damage. This fact is usually attributed to the introduced species' relative immunity from predation and parasitism in the simple community into which it is introduced. Undoubtedly, it often happens that introduced species fail to become established. However, if the ecological community is sufficiently simple, the relative absence of predators and parasites may favor an exceptional increase of the invader. Apparently, there is no example in which the use of pesticides favored the introduction of a pest. However, if a pest were already resistant to the pesticides in use, the possibility of its successful introduction might be increased by the artificially conditioned sparsity of enemies.

11.2.2.3 Evaluation of Biotic Simplification as a Cause of Pest Problems.

There can be no doubt that biotic simplification can increase the importance of certain species as pests, even to the point of making a species a pest when it was not one before. This tends to be especially true in agriculture and less true in public health. However, contrary to what is sometimes implied, making a biotic situation more complex does not always reduce the total pest problem. The introduction of irrigation may bring a threat of schistosomiasis as well as a more complex picture in agriculture and associated wildlife.

11.2.3 Food Chains

It was stated in Biblical times that all flesh is grass. One may question whether Isaiah had in mind an ecological principle or merely the ephemeral nature of the individual. In any event, the term "food chain" indicates the sequence of steps by which any particular animal derives its food from plants, whether they be grass or diatom.

Although man undoubtedly eats more kinds of food than any other animal, the major portion of his food chain is simple. Most human food comes from crops raised by man for the purpose, or from domestic animals that have been fed on crops raised for their use. Thus, man exercises considerable control over the major sources of his food and, consequently, over any chemicals used in the production of that food. To be sure, some people eat seafood and wildlife, over which there is little control. In primitive societies, an even wider range of wild food may be consumed. Available evidence indicates that the contribution of wild food to human intake of pesticide residues is small, either because the amount of such food eaten is small, or because the residues present are small, or usually for both reasons. The situation may be entirely different for other animals, as discussed in the following sections.

11.2.3.1 Secondary Poisoning.

Secondary poisoning is injury, fatal or otherwise, of one animal through contact with another that has been poisoned, intentionally or otherwise. Exposure usually takes the form of eating a disabled or dead animal. The major source of chemical in secondary poisoning may be the tissues of the animal consumed, but it usually is unabsorbed compound remaining in the gastrointestinal tract of the animal that is eaten.

The poisoning of young animals through contaminated milk, or the poisoning of parasites that feed on a systemically treated host could be considered forms of secondary poisoning, but they usually are not classified in this way.

In clearly documented instances of secondary poisoning, injury is the prompt result of one or more doses obtained by eating one or more poisoned animals. The possibility of delayed toxicity as a result of secondary poisoning cannot be denied, but its existence is speculative.

The victims of secondary poisoning are always carrion feeders or predators, including insectivores. Thus, commensal and wild rodents poisoned by sodium fluoroacetate, thallium, warfarin, and, no doubt, other compounds, have led to the death of dogs, cats, pigs, foxes, coyotes, birds of prey, buzzards, and the like. Of course, the hazard is relatively great with sodium fluoroacetate and quite small with warfarin. The death of chickens has been traced to the eating of roaches and other insects in houses sprayed with any of several compounds. In a similar way the death of fish, amphibians, and reptiles has been attributed to eating of aquatic insects killed by DDT, and many wild birds are thought to have been killed by eating insects disabled by DDT or other insecticides.

It also has been claimed that insect predators have been killed by eating insects poisoned by systemic compounds. However, since the compounds were applied to the surfaces of plants in some instances, and are contact poisons as well as systemics, it is difficult to see how the possibility of contact poisoning of the predators was excluded.

Resistance of vertebrates to pesticides is discussed in Section 3.1.3.2. It is of interest in connection with secondary poisoning that a single resistant mosquito fish (*Gambusia affinis*) may be treated with endrin in such a way that it survives but is able to release enough of the compound into 10 liters of clean water to kill five normally susceptible fish of the same species in 38.5 hours after they are placed in the water (Ferguson *et al.*, 1966). Individual resistant mosquito fish that had survived 2 ppm of endrin in the water for 7 days were force fed to 11 species of vertebrates (three other species of fish, frogs, turtles, three species of snakes, and three species of birds), including some that normally feed on mosquito fish. Mean survival time after ingestion of a single fish was less than 24 hours in most instances, even though the average weight of some of the species of predators exceeds that of the treated fish by over 700 times (Rosato and Ferguson, 1968). Thus, apparently some populations of mosquito fish can control their predators with endrin just as, through evolution, some other species can control their enemies with poisons they themselves elaborate. In fact, endrin-resistant mosquito fish collected in nature have been found lethal to susceptible sunfish (Finley *et al.*, 1970). For a discussion of allelochemics, see Section 1.2.1.6.

11.2.3.2 Biological Magnification.

Biological magnification is the phenomenon by which the concentration of a chemical is increased in successive steps of a food chain, with the danger that some species, especially the ones highest in the series, will be injured by the compound. There are several examples that illustrate the phenomenon. A classical example discussed below is the injury of fish-eating birds at Clear Lake, California, following the control of gnats in the lake. Another example is the injury of robins following efforts to control Dutch elm disease in a number of towns in the East and Midwest of the United States of America. A somewhat different kind of example involves the reproductive failure of certain populations of falcons and fish-eating birds associated with the widespread occurrence of DDE and perhaps other foreign compounds in the birds and their eggs. In this instance, no single usage of DDT or any other compound can be cited as the cause of trouble, although the sources of contamination may be less diffuse than some suppose.

Because each individual requires time to accumulate a substantial concentration of a chemical, and because a particular food chain may involve several species, there may be a delay in the onset of injury associated with biological magnification. However, "delayed toxicity" of this origin is no different from the effect of the same compound in the same species when the same rate of dosage is determined by some other mechanism. Once poisoning has occurred, the injury may be enzootic or epizootic. Outbreaks may occur because of significant new introductions of chemical into the ecosystem, or because of a seasonal increase in susceptibility associated with starvation or some other stress.

Whereas the term, biological magnification, has come to connote a steady increase in the concentration of a contaminant in the succeeding species of a long food chain, no two examples are exactly alike. Some of the chains really are short, and a high final concentration may depend more on unusual cumulation in a single species than on moderate cumulation in several. Certainly a few species are remarkable in their ability to concentrate one or more chemicals from their environment. Furthermore, the cumulation may not result from ingestion of the next lowest species in a food chain but from some other mechanism. Fish are able to take up DDT rapidly, directly from water. Absorption occurs mainly through the gills and does not depend on food, although fish can absorb DDT from that source also (Holden, 1962).

Two factors involved in direct uptake from water are adsorption and lipid partitioning. Both factors are involved in the behavior of DDT. It adsorbs not only on surfaces of gills, living algae, and particles of dead organisms, but on surfaces generally, including those of silt. No doubt this adsorption is conditioned in part by the marked insolubility of the compound in water. As soon as DDT comes in contact with a living membrane its absorption is favored by its relatively high solubility in lipids (see Section 3.2.2). High lipid solubility also favors storage in fat and, therefore, a relatively low degree of availability for metabolism and excretion (see Section 3.2.3.3).

Because of subtle differences in the relation of aquatic and terrestrial organisms to their environments, adsorption of fat-soluble pesticides plays an inordinately important role in the absorption of pesticides by aquatic organisms, and this explains to a large degree why the toxicity of pesticides to wildlife is predominantly an aquatic problem.

Cumulation associated with filtering has been spoken of as "biological concentration," in contrast to "trophic concentration" associated with ingestion (Herman *et al.*, 1969), but the different processes may overlap in different ways. Some fish obtain chemicals from their environment both by direct absorption from water and ingestion of food; other organisms obtain chemicals from particulate material they ingest as food after filtering it from their environment.

Oysters can tolerate concentrations of DDT that, depending on water temperature and duration of exposure, can lead to concentrations in the oysters as much as 700,000 times greater than that in the surrounding water (Butler, 1966). It was formerly supposed that this concentration was made possible by the ingestion of contaminated algae and other particulate matter the oysters filtered from the surrounding water. Although this may be true under natural conditions, some recent experiments suggest that oysters also absorb DDT by way of their gills (Brodtman, 1970).

Regardless of the exact mechanism by which concentration occurs, a single species with outstanding ability of this sort can have a striking effect on its predators.

In addition to the examples outlined below, many other naturally occurring episodes thought to illustrate biological magnification may be found in the reviews and proceedings listed at the beginning of Section 11.3.

The Clear Lake Gnat and Grebes. Clear Lake is a good fishing lake about 18,600 ha in size, located about 161 km north of San Francisco. The lake would be even more attractive to fishermen and other tourists if it were not for insects, especially a gnat (*Chaoporus astictopus*), the larvae of which develop in the lake bottom. Although the adults do not suck blood, they constitute a serious pest during the warm months because of their extremely high numbers. Efforts to control the gnat had been made for years but without significant effect. Eventually it was found that DDD, applied at a nominal rate of 0.0143 ppm, was capable of controlling the gnat larvae without injury to fish. Treatment at this rate applied in September, 1949, gave what was estimated to be 99% control. The results were so good

that, in spite of gradual increase in the gnat population, no further application of DDD was made until 1954. This application, at a slightly higher rate of 0.0200 ppm, was also considered 99% effective. The second recovery of the gnat population was more rapid. The third application of DDD made in September, 1957, was somewhat less effective, but adverse weather conditions may have been responsible. From 1949 through 1957 a total of 54,800 kg of DDD was put directly into the lake. Some other DDT-related material undoubtedly had found its way into the lake from the surrounding watershed (Rudd, 1964; Herman *et al.*, 1969).

It was not until several months after the third application of DDD to the lake that injury to grebes (*Aechmorphorus occidentalis*) was attributed to the chemical. It had been noted during the summer following the first application that the breeding colony of over 1,000 pairs of Western grebes did not return to the lake. Grebes did continue to visit the lake during each winter. Injury to these birds was not noted until December, 1954, when more than 100 were known to have died. Additional deaths occurred in March, 1955. No disease or other cause could be found in spite of search. Following the third application of DDD in September, 1957, a number of other grebes died in December. Analysis of fat from these birds revealed concentrations of DDD as high as 1,600 ppm. Analysis of a wide variety of samples then revealed not only that DDD was present in essentially all of them, but that the concentration increased in the order: plankton < small fish < big fish and grebes. The average concentration in plankton was 5.3 ppm, that in the edible flesh of various plankton-eating or plant-eating fish was 5 to 80 ppm, while that of predaceous fish was 1 to 196 ppm. Old fish contained 2 to 5 times as much DDD as young of the same species. Concentrations in the fat of all fish were much higher than those in their flesh, ranging from 40 to 2,500 ppm. It appeared that although the grebes and large, predaceous fish lived on small fish, the birds acquired somewhat less insecticide but were very much more susceptible to it. Fish in the lake apparently were not greatly affected. The way in which the samples were taken and analyzed does not permit any numerical estimate of the degree of increase in concentration of DDD in the successive steps of the food chain. However, it is inescapable that large increases did occur.

There were a number of other features of the Clear Lake episode that are not fully understood. It is said that the populations of egrets and herons decreased, but whether this was related to the use of DDD was not established. Although the death of grebes during winter and spring was apparently the uncomplicated effect of DDD poisoning, the reason so few birds came to the lake during the summer is not understood. Apparently there were no breeding birds at the lake from 1950 through 1957. Beginning in 1958 there were 15 to 20 pairs of birds, but no young were produced until 1962, and then only one. In 1967, 165 grebe nests in Clear Lake were marked and studied. More than 450 eggs were laid. Of these 89 were taken for incubation and analysis. It was estimated that a least 40 (11%) of the eggs left in the nests developed to full-sized grebes; one (6%) of the incubated eggs survived. The concentration of DDD in 17 eggs collected for analysis ranged from about 69.2 to 1,007 ppm on a lipid basis. Failure of the birds to raise young successfully was presumably caused by DDD, but the reason for birds to avoid the lake as a breeding place is entirely unknown.

A high degree of storage of DDD in one kind of fish (*Gambusia affinis*) under standardized laboratory conditions has been reported; and the ratio of DDD in these fish and in the water they inhabit is essentially the same as that of DDT and greater than that of DDE (Metcalf *et al.*, 1971a). On the contrary, higher vertebrates that have been studied degrade DDD efficiently, and other instances of persistence of the compound in the environment have not come to light. Thus, the demonstrated persistence of DDD in Clear Lake and its cumulation in grebes indicate a need for experimental study.

By 1969, the concentration of DDD in 28 eggs ranged from 32.1 to 257 ppm on a lipid basis. By 1970, reproduction of grebes at Clear Lake was essentially normal. The very rapid reduction in the concentration of DDD and also DDE in grebes and their eggs between 1967 and 1969 was attributed to the introduction of a small Atherinid fish to the lake in 1967 (Rudd and Herman, 1972). This kind of fish may be less efficient than others in concentrating DDD from water, or they may be more efficient than others in the biotransformation and excretion of DDT-related compounds.

No investigation of these possibilities has been reported.

Lake Trout. In 1955, young fish from all of more than 347,000 eggs collected from lake trout in Lake George and reared in the Lake George fish hatchery died. Detectable illness began when the fry had absorbed the yolk sac and were about ready to feed. The same thing happened in 1956, when eggs from Lake George fish were reared at the Lake George hatchery, and in 1957 even though they were reared at other hatcheries. In 1958, there was only negligible survival (0.9 and 1.4%) in two hatcheries. Crosses of females from Lake George with males from other waters failed to survive, but survival was normal when the opposite cross was made. The dead fry showed no pathology indicating a disease. DDT was suspected because of the large amount of it used in the watershed.

Study revealed that trout in some but not all other New York lakes were subject to the same difficulty. It was not possible fully to account for the difference between lakes by a history of the amount of DDT used in their watersheds. The only dependable figures for use were those for state and local agencies. Private use could be estimated only. There was some indication that application by aircraft or by blocks that released DDT directly into water for blackfly control led to more trouble than did fogging carried out by towns and villages. The watershed of Lake George was the only one studied where DDT had been used for control of the gypsy moth. Likewise, the concentration of DDT in trout did not correlate well enough with reproductive success to permit prediction. However, in both 1961 and 1962 it was found that the concentration of DDT could be linked to survival of the young when the compound in eggs was expressed in terms of the weight of fry at the onset of illness. When the DDT concentration was 2.93 ppm or more, the fry showed the characteristic syndrome and died, but when the concentration was 2.67 ppm or less, the fry remained healthy (Burdick *et al.*, 1964).

Although the failure of very young fish from Lake George and some other lakes to survive has been spoken of as reproductive failure, it is more precisely an example of simple poisoning of the fry associated with redistribution of DDT when it is released from the yolk lipids.

More recent studies have shown that many fish from Lake George contain slightly over 1 ppm of mercury. However, this probably was not the source of trouble, since fish of similar size taken from the lake about 1900 and made part of the collection of the Philadelphia Academy of Natural Sciences had similar levels (Harris *et al.*, 1972). Even more recently, substantial concentrations of polychlorinated biphenyls have been found in fish from the lake. In the meantime, there has been no appreciable decline in the concentration of DDT in the fish since 1964, but hatching and survival of a limited number of eggs taken from Lake George lake trout in 1971 were surprisingly good (Colson, 1973; Harris, 1973).

Dutch Elm Disease and Robins. The fungus that causes Dutch elm disease is transmitted from one tree to another by various bark beetles (May and Baker, 1952). The disease was first found to be in the United States of America in the late 1920's. Since that time the disease has spread from New York and Ohio to nearly half of the states in the Union and it has undoubtedly killed millions of trees. Unfortunately, the susceptible tree (*Ulmus americana*) has always been a favorite shade tree, and many streets in New England and the Midwest contain no other species. In most rural areas, the elms were scattered among other species of trees and, therefore, their death was less conspicuous. However, in certain areas of Iowa and perhaps elsewhere, there originally were few native trees except along streams. Most of the trees planted by farmers were elms, and death of these trees left the area almost denuded. Although DDT is relatively effective in preventing the spread of Dutch elm disease and of phloem necrosis (another disease of elms spread by leafhoppers), extremely heavy applications, ranging from 0.68 to 1.36 kg per individual tree, are required. Because of the extremely high dosage, direct injury to birds could have been predicted on the basis of studies already finished before trouble became severe.

Although direct kills of birds by the heavy doses of DDT required for the control of Dutch elm disease were observed early (Benton, 1951), and indirect kills by way of the food chain were suspected by 1950, a tentative explanation of the indirect kills was not published until much later (Barker, 1958). Briefly, it was found that soon after spraying, leaves contained residues of 174 to 273 ppm. After the leaves had dropped in the autumn, they still contained 20 to 28 ppm. Undoubtedly, a rather large amount of DDT fell on the soil immediately under the trees at the time of spraying. This pesticide, together with the residues on fallen leaves, combined to produce high residues in the very top layer of soil, including the leaf mold. Concentrations of DDT in earthworms taken from the soil beneath elm trees ranged from 33 to 164 ppm. Since earthworms form a very important element in the diet of robins (*Turdus migratorius*), it is not astonishing that many of the birds were killed from this source.

Although a high proportion of robins in many towns died soon after spraying and some 80 other species were affected (Wallace *et al.,* 1961), the same species remained unaffected in the neighboring countryside. Robins and many other birds are strictly territorial during the nesting season. Because of the expense involved, it was never practical to attempt to protect trees except those growing in towns and cities.

It is of interest that residues of chlorinated hydrocarbon insecticides in earthworms averaged 9 times those in agricultural soils from which they were collected, although the exact factor depends on the way in which the results were expressed. Insecticide levels were 11.5 times less in snails (analyzed with their shells) than in earthworms. However, residues in beetle larvae were 3.3 times, and residues in slugs were 3.7 times those in forms from the same sites. With very few exceptions, the concentrations of insecticides in the worms varied directly with the concentrations in the soils (Gish, 1970). Concentrations of DDT in earthworms living in forest soils tend to vary directly with the residues in those soils also. However, the persistence of the compound in forest soils, at least in a very cold climate, is longer than would be predicted from study of warm, agricultural soils (Dimond *et al.,* 1970).

11.2.3.3 Bases for Population Declines among Certain Falcons and Fish-Eating Birds.

The marked decline of populations of some falcons and fish-eating birds is viewed as a classical example of the effects of biological magnification. Comparison of the concentrations of certain pesticides and other compounds in these birds and their eggs with concentrations of the same compounds in their prey shows that such magnification has occurred in many instances and indicates high dosage levels for the predators. However, the relation of the chemicals to the decline of populations is sufficiently complex that it requires separate discussion. The matter is complicated by the fact that some of the endangered species were already in decline before the chemicals they now cumulate were invented. A comprehensive review of the matter as it involves eggshell thinning is that of Cooke (1973).

The frequency of eggshell thinning seen recently in susceptible species both in nature and experimentally is of an entirely different order of magnitude from the frequency of thinning seen earlier. It is worth noting that, whereas shock can cause poultry to lay soft-shelled eggs, these eggs are laid prematurely and lack the outer layers (Cooke, 1973), thus differing from the soft eggs laid by affected brown pelicans (*Pelicanus occidentalis*), which, in spite of their thinness, have the outermost layer present (Erben and Krampitz, 1971). Regardless of its cause, thinning of sufficient degree can lead to egg breakage, egg eating, or simply the disappearance of eggs from nests.

According to references cited by Potts (1968), egg breaking was recorded in several species before the chlorinated insecticides were introduced. Egg breaking can be caused not only by thinning but by a variety of stresses, including polygamy, confinement, crowding, and disturbance, as well as toxic substances, and egg eating is not rare among captive birds. However, such destruction or loss, of whatever cause, has been more frequent recently among species susceptible to eggshell thinning than was true before.

Recent Historical Background. Ratcliffe (1958) reported an apparent increase in egg breaking and egg eating among peregrine falcons (*Falco peregrinus*). His own first observation of breakage and disappearance of eggs was in 1951, but he cited a few earlier (1932, 1937, 1938) reports. Five years later, the same author (Ratcliffe, 1963) attributed the marked decline of peregrines to "agricultural toxic chemicals" obtained by the hawks from their contaminated prey. It was speculated that sublethal doses of chlorinated hydrocarbons cause first reduction in hatching success of eggs and then sterility of adult birds. It was emphasized that the actual decline in the number of falcons was preceded by a reduction in their breeding success and by their failure to attempt breeding. At least by 1963, and largely on the basis of personal communications, it was known that populations of peregrine falcons had declined seriously in France, Germany, Finland, Sweden, and the eastern United States of America, as well as in the United Kingdom (Ratcliffe, 1963).

At a conference held in Madison, Wisconsin, 29 August to 1 September 1965 (Hickey, 1969), the decline or "crash" of some peregrine populations in the United States of America and in other parts of the world was reported and discussed. Disease, predation, shooting, and other direct and indirect injury by man and his chemicals (including the DDT complex, dieldrin, mercury, and lead) were discussed at the conference as possible factors in population decline. However, the conference summary and conclusions (obviously completed during the final stages of editing the proceeding some years after the conference was held) contained a section on postconference research and, while judging that "the peregrine falcon population crash almost certainly resulted from a complex of environmental factors . . . ," placed predominant emphasis on dieldrin in Britain, DDE in the United States of America, and mercury in Sweden. Thus, the conference focused attention on the fate of the falcons, and the conclusion prepared later by Hickey and Roelle (1969) focused

attention on environmental pollution as the cause of trouble.

In addition to peregrine falcons, the conference considered ospreys (*Pandion haliaelus*) and some other birds of prey, and the research and discussion that followed the conference involved these birds, plus pelicans and gulls.

The next step in developing the current hypothesis (Ratcliffe, 1967) was to demonstrate thinning of eggshells of the peregrine falcon and the English sparrow hawk (*Accipiter nisus*) and to attribute the reproductive difficulty of these birds to this thinning. Further emphasis was placed on the probable importance of chemicals as causes of reproductive failure in susceptible species. Polychlorinated biphenyls and organic mercury were mentioned, as well as several chlorinated hydrocarbon insecticides. It was noted that DDT was used in 1945–1946, about the time thinning of eggshells began, whereas aldrin and dieldrin were not introduced until about 10 years later.

It was pointed out that 90% of the shells, as measured, consisted of calcium carbonate. Thus, the stage was set for the hypothesis that the inherent difficulty was one of calcium metabolism. It was noted, however, that there was no reason to suppose that there had been any significant change in the calcium intake of the birds.

In a crucial paper, Hickey and Anderson (1968) concluded that (a) many of the then recent crashes of raptor populations in the United States of America and western Europe had a common physiological basis, (b) eggshell breakage had been widespread but largely overlooked in North America, (c) significant decreases in shell thickness and shell weight were characteristic of the reproductive failures of raptor populations in certain parts of the United States of America, as had been shown earlier for some other populations, (d) the onset of the change was 1 year after the introduction of chlorinated hydrocarbons (actually DDT) into general usage and was not a random circumstance, and (e) these persisting compounds were having a serious, insidious effect on certain species of birds at the tops of contaminated ecosystems. Specifically, the authors showed that the eggshells of California peregrine falcons collected from 1947 and 1952 weighed 18.8% less than those collected from 1891 to 1939. Changes of the same order of magnitude were found in one or more declining populations of bald eagles, ospreys, and peregrine falcons from the eastern United States of America. Only minor changes (either increases or decreases) were found in the weight of eggshells of normally reproducing populations of peregrine falcons, ospreys, red-tailed hawks (*Buteo jamaicensis*), golden eagles (*Aquila chrysaetos*), and great horned owls (*Bubo virginianus*).

Measurements of museum specimens and of eggs collected more recently prove that there has been a decrease in the average thickness of the eggs of one or more populations of at least 22 species (Anderson and Hickey, 1972). Nearly always, the change was after 1945.

Correlation of Eggshell Thinning with Insecticide Content. As mentioned above, probable connection between eggshell thinning and various chlorinated compounds, especially DDT, was first pointed out by Ratcliffe (1967). A high degree of inverse correlation ($r = -0.9863$) and (what is the same thing expressed in a different way) an inverse linear relationship were found between the thickness of the shells of eggs laid by herring gulls (*Larus argentatus*) in 1967 and the DDE content of the same eggs. Polychlorinated biphenyls were not analyzed. Reproduction of the colonies of gulls from which the eggs were taken was normal with one possible exception. Although the authors spoke generally about chlorinated hydrocarbons, all evidence they presented or reviewed involved DDE (Hickey and Anderson, 1968). The general relationship reported by Hickey and Anderson (1968) and expressed either as inverse correlations or as inverse linear relationships between the thickness of eggshells and the concentrations of DDE in the same eggs was reported for populations of peregrine falcons (Ratcliffe, 1970), prairie falcons (*Falco mexicanus*) (Fyfe et al., 1969; Enderson and Berger, 1970), brown pelicans (Keith *et al.* 1970; Risebrough *et al.*, 1970; Blus *et al.*, 1971), white pelicans (*Pelecanus erythrorhynchos*) (Anderson *et al.*, 1969), cormorants (*Phalacrocorax auritus*) (Anderson *et al.*, 1969), the great blue heron (*Ardea herodias*) (Vermeer and Reynolds, 1970; Keith and Gruchy, 1972; Faber and Hickey, 1973), and the gannet (*Sula bassana*) (Keith and Gruchy, 1972).

In a study of residues of DDE, DDD, DDT, dieldrin, polychlorinated biphenyls (PCB's), and mercury, it was found by stepwise regression that, with only one exception, DDE was the only residue that accounted for a significant amount of variability in the weight and thickness of the eggshells of the brown pelican (Blus *et al.*, 1971). However, when a wider range of species was considered, dieldrin and PCB's as well as DDE appeared important for one species or another (Faber and Hickey, 1973).

The range of concentration of DDE reported was not great in any one of the papers just mentioned. However, when a wider range of concentrations was considered, the true inverse, straight-line relationship was found to involve thickness of shell and the logarithm of the concentration of DDE in the same eggs of peregrine falcons (Cade *et al.*, 1971) and brown pelicans (Blus *et al.*, 1972). The same relationship probably applied to other data on pelicans (Jehl, 1973) but it was not presented in this form. A linear relationship between shell thickness and the logarithm of the dietary concentration of a foreign chemical apparently was first demonstrated by Scott *et al.* (1944) in chickens fed sulfanilamide.

The estimated no-effect level appeared to be about 2.0 ppm of DDE in the eggs of falcons and 0.5 ppm for pelicans. The importance of species difference was emphasized. In brown pelicans, 15% thinning of shells appeared to be associated with DDE residues between 4 and 5 ppm in the eggs, whereas in cormorants 15% thinning was seen with average residues of 20 ppm, and in herring gulls only 11% thinning seemed to be associated with about 80 ppm. The mathematical relationship seemed to be similar in different species, but to operate in them at different levels (Blus *et al.*, 1972; Keith and Gruchy, 1972). There may be strain differences, for Kury (1969) found no effect among cormorants in Maine whose eggs contained DDE at average concentrations as high as 13.6 ppm.

On the other hand, Koeman *et al.* (1972) found no correlation between the concentration of DDE or any compound in the eggs of the European sparrow hawk and the shell index or thickness of the same eggs. This was true even though (*a*) the shells were thinner than normal, (*b*) the range of DDE concentrations was wide (6.2 to 69 ppm with means of 24 to 26 ppm in different years), and (*c*) a decline in reproduction was attributed to DDE. In a similar way, Wiemeyer *et al.* (1972) found a poor correlation between eggshell thickness (or the degree of thinning as compared with pre-1946 norms) and the concentration of DDE in the eggs of bald eagles (*Haliaeetus leucocephalus*) from different parts of North America. Correlation between reproductive success and DDE content was somewhat greater but still poor (Krantz *et al.*, 1970). However, some of the bald eagle eggs contained concentrations of dieldrin considered sufficiently high to interfere with reproduction (Weimeyer *et al.*, 1972).

A different kind of example of meaningful residues of other compounds involves eggs of brown pelicans on Anacapa Island in April, 1969. These eggs not only contained 40 to 135 ppm of *p,p'*-DDE, but also 0.6 to 4.6 ppm of *p,p'*-DDT (Lamont *et al.*, 1970), indicating a recent and perhaps continuing intake of DDT by the birds.

Some species, including the chicken, have proved immune to eggshell thinning by DDE. On the contrary, other compounds are capable of thinning the shells of other species. One polychlorinated biphenyl causes shell thinning in the chicken but not in the mallard duck (*Anas platyrhyncos*) or the bobwhite quail (*Colinus virginianus*) (Heath et al., 1972b).

The fact that DDT actually thickens the eggshells of the Bengalese finch (*Lonchura striate*) and the hen (Jefferies, 1969) does not alter the fact that certain chemicals including DDT thin the shells of some other species.

A valuable review and tabulation of residues in eggs is that of Stickel (1973).

Experimental Production of Eggshell Thinning. That DDE and other chlorinated hydrocarbons may have been the cause of eggshell thinning observed in nature is supported by a series of experiments indicating that these compounds can cause this effect in some species under controlled conditions. In the first of these studies, captive American sparrow hawks (*Falco sparverius*) were given diets containing on a dry weight basis: 1 ppm dieldrin and 5 ppm *p,p'*-DDT (low dosage), and 3 ppm dieldrin and 15 ppm *p,p'*-DDT (high dosage). Eggs laid by the original group of birds in 1967 and 1968 and by first generation young in 1968 were from 8 to 17% thinner than comparable eggs laid by the controls. In general, the number of unhatched eggs that showed no embryonic development and the number containing dead embryos were not greater for the treated birds. However, a significantly higher number of eggs disappeared from the nests of treated birds; it was assumed that this disappearance was due to breaking of thin-shelled eggs, and to eating of eggs or newly hatched young by parent birds. The higher dosage produced no greater effect of any kind than the lower dosage (Porter and Wiemeyer, 1969).

Nearly 1 year of feeding of *p,p'*-DDE at a dietary level of 10 ppm (dry weight basis), which was said to be equivalent to residue levels commonly found in the food of hawks in the wild, led to an average concentration of 32.4 ppm in the eggs and to a 9.7% thinning of their shells. The concentrations of DDT, DDD, dieldrin, and polychlorinated biphenyls were less than 0.3 ppm (Wiemeyer and Porter, 1970). Each female was killed for residue study as soon as she laid the first egg; therefore, reproductive success of the treated birds could not be followed.

Mallard ducks fed *p,p'*-DDE at dietary levels of 10 and 40 ppm (dry weight basis) laid eggs that were 13% thinner than normal, and 25% of them showed detectable cracks. Eggs with hairline cracks hatched at about half the rate of whole eggs, and those with definitie fractures did not hatch. As few as 21% as many ducklings per hen were hatched from ducks treated with DDE as from their controls. The higher dosage produced no more effect than the lower dosage, although the onset of its effect was more prompt. Successfully hatched ducklings from treated hens survived as well as those from controls. DDD at dietary levels of 10 and 40 ppm did not thin shells, but it did reduce the number of ducklings hatched per hen as compared to their own controls. *p,p'*-DDT at a dietary level of 25 ppm caused thinning of eggshells and a reduction of ducklings hatched per hen. These effects presumably were due to the metabolite, DDE. *p,p'*-DDT at dietary levels of 2.5 and 10 ppm did not cause eggshell thinning or measurable effects on reproduction. None of the treatments caused crippling among hatchlings (Heath et al., 1969).

The effects of feeding *p,p'*-DDE at dietary levels of 10 and 30 ppm (dry weight basis) to black ducks (*Anus rubripes*) were essentially the same as those observed with similar dietary levels in mallards. There was, however, a higher percentage of cracking at the higher dosage level, and it was found that the degree of thinning was greater at the apex and the caps than at the equator, the only place where measurements usually are made. The average DDE residues in eggs were 46 and 144 ppm following dietary levels of 10 and 30 ppm, respectively (Longcore et al., 1971).

Concentrations of DDE in the eggs of wild black ducks collected in 10 states ranged from 0.1 to 12.1 ppm, the average value for different states ranging from 0.4 to 5.5 ppm (Reichel and Addy, 1968).

Dieldrin at a dietary level of 1.6 ppm (dry weight basis) caused a 3.8% decrease in the thickness of eggshells of mallard ducks. Decreases little or no greater were caused by dietary levels of 4 and 10 ppm (Lehner and Egbert, 1969).

Feeding of DDE at a dietary level of 10 ppm (dry weight basis) produced a 12% thinning of the eggs of screech owls (*Otus asio*), compared to eggs laid earlier by the same bird (McLane and Hall, 1972).

In a study in which both the dietary concentrations of DDT and calcium were varied, it was found that reduction of the calcium level from 3.0 to 1.0% caused slightly more thinning of the eggshells of bobwhite quail and mallard ducks than did the feeding of 30 ppm of DDT to birds receiving 3.0% calcium. The combination of 30 ppm DDT with the low calcium diet had little additive effect. In no instance did the thinning exceed 10% (Tucker and Haegele, 1970). As a part of the same study the authors produced a greater thinning by a single large dose of DDT; but starvation of the birds after dosing makes interpretation of this part of the work difficult, because starvation is a recognized cause of eggshell thinning.

Japanese quail (*Coturnix coturnix*) fed either *p,p'*-DDT or *o,p'*-DDT at a concentration of 100 ppm in a diet containing 0.56% calcium laid eggs with thinner shells and lower shell calcium levels than those of controls fed the same low level of calcium (Bitman *et al.*, 1969). The same dosages of *p,p'*-DDT and *p,p'*-DDE produced from 16 to 19% reduction of carbonic anhydrase in the shell glands of Japanese quail, and it was claimed that this degree of inhibition is sufficient to explain the observed 10 to 15% decrease in eggshell thickness (Bitman *et al.*, 1970). In another study, somewhat lesser thinning of the eggs of Japanese quail with normal calcium intake was found at lower dietary rates (2.5 to 25 ppm of *p,p'*-DDT). The highest level fed was found to result in the death of some birds with typical DDT poisoning when they were under the stress of molting (Stickel and Rhodes, 1970).

Ring doves (*Streptopelia risoria*) fed *p,p'*-DDE at a dietary level of 40 ppm dry weight took an average of 2.5 times longer than controls to re-nest, produced 13.5% fewer eggs per clutch, had 10% thinner eggs, and experienced 3 times as great mortality of the young (Haegele and Hudson, 1973).

Relation of Eggshell Thinning to Shell Breakage, Reproductive Failure, and Population Decline. The exact relation of thinning to breakage varies with circumstances. Eggs thinned to the same degree undergo breakage somewhat more when incubated naturally than when incubated artificially with special care. Thinning of 2 to 5% may cause some damage, but it is difficult to distinguish this damage from normal loss. Thinning of 10% leads to some cracking and to increased embryonic mortality. Thinning of 20 to 25% leads to the breakage of many eggs, and in nature this degree of thinning is associated with reproductive failure and population decline. The most dramatic example is that involving brown pelicans on Anacapa Island in 1969.

Some species seem essentially immune to eggshell thinning by DDE. In others, such as the Japanese quail and the mallard duck, the maximal thinning ever observed has never reached a level associated with enough breakage to produce serious reproductive failure. It seems likely that there is some variation from one species to another in the exact degree of damage, even when all the species considered are susceptible and the degree of thinning is identical.

When eggshell thinning is of an intermediate degree, its effect on population dynamics may be obscured by other factors. For example, Anderson and Hickey (1970) concluded that the eggshells of three subspecies of brown pelican collected after 1949 were 15 to 26% lighter than normal. The relation of this limited observation to reproduction of the birds was unclear, for the authors noted that the fragmentary records "suggested possible fluctuations in number over the years"—a conclusion reached ealier by Bond (1942).

In a similar way it was reported that the shells of pelican eggs collected along the Atlantic coast of Florida and South Carolina and the Gulf coast of Florida in 1969 were 12 to 16% lighter than ones collected in the same areas before 1947 (Blus, 1970), but evidence for decline of the populations was not clearly established.

Although association does not constitute proof of cause and effect, it is a fact that the recent declines of some populations of peregrine falcons (Prestt, 1965), prairie falcons (Fyfe *et al.*, 1969), English sparrow hawks (Prestt, 1965; Ratcliffe, 1970), brown pelicans (Jehl, 1973), and white pelicans (Anderson *et al.*, 1969; Gress *et al.*, 1973) have been associated in nature with both eggshell thinning and failure of reproduction.

On the other hand, equal or even greater failure of reproduction has been recorded in some species even though there was no correlation between shell thickness and DDE content of the same eggs, and there was no more DDE in cracked eggs than in intact ones. For example, the wet weight concentration of DDE in the eggs of one colony of the common term (*Sterna hirundo*) ranged from 0.64 to 104.0 ppm, with a mean of 7.57 ppm, and was associated with a hatching success of only 24% and a fledgling success of only 5%; but the chemical findings were not statistically related to shell thinning or to shell cracking (Switzer *et al.*, 1971).

Species Differences. Thinning of eggshells has not been found in all species, including some reported to be decreasing in numbers. For example, Kreitzer (1971) reported that eggshell thickness in mourning dove (*Zenaidura macroura*) populations in 1969 and 1970 was normal compared to 1861–1935, even though it is claimed the species underwent a small but steady decline during 1960–1970.

In a similar way, Anderson and Kreitzer (1971) found that eggs of the whooping crane (*Grus americana*) laid in 1967–1969 were just as thick (0.612 mm) as those laid prior to 1910 (0.604 mm), when the species was considerably more numerous (Bent, 1926) and certainly not exposed to modern pesticides. The levels of insecticides in the birds themselves also were low (Lamont and Reichel, 1970).

Several British birds, the eggs of which have not shown thinning, were listed by Ratcliffe (1967).

Not even all species of predaceous birds are declining in population. Perhaps the clearest single set of data demonstrating this fact are those for resident populations of birds, based on mortality rates, recruitment rates (reproductive success), and ages at sexual maturity. Populations of great horned owls, barn owls, and red-tailed hawks were found to be stable in several areas. The same was true for the osprey in Florida, but not in Maryland or Connecticut. Evidence of lowered recruitment rates was found for the osprey, Cooper's hawk, red-shoulder hawk, and sparrow hawk, as well as for the brown pelican (Henny, 1972).

The annual Hawk Mountain count of migrating raptors has been made systematically since 1934, with the exception of 3 years during World War II. Like most long-term studies, it has changed somewhat over the years; specifically, counts were not made in August before 1947. A comparison of absolute numbers of counts from year to year may not always be valid. However, there is no reason to question the trend of each species compared to others. The numbers of observations per year vary from about 30 for some species to about 3,000 for others. Whereas the numbers of sharp-shinned (*Accipiter striatus*) and Cooper's (*A. Cooperii*) hawks have continued the decline evident before 1942, the number of red-tailed hawks, golden eagles, and peregrine falcons have remained steady since 1948 or earlier; and the numbers of red-shouldered hawks (*Buteo lineatus*), sparrow hawks, marsh hawks (*Circus cyaneus*), and ospreys have increased both in comparison to prewar years and progressively since 1948. The number of bald eagles was unusually high around 1950 but by 1962 returned to levels similar to those before 1940 (Spofford, 1969).

The two sets of data are in agreement regarding the decrease in Cooper's hawk and the steady state of the red-tailed hawk. The sets differ regarding the sparrow hawk, the red-shouldered hawk, and the osprey. The differences probably relate to the areas represented. Many of the birds seen at Hawk Mountain come from the Arctic where local pollution and persecution are minimal, but some populations do acquire high concentrations of pesticides during migration to South America.

Biochemical Basis of Reproductive Failure. Ringdoves (*Streptopelia risoria*) fed *p,p'*-DDT at a dietary level of 10 ppm for 3 weeks prior to mating showed a decrease of estradiol in the blood early in the breeding cycle and egg laying was delayed. There also was a marked decrease in deposition of medullary bone calcium and some decrease in eggshell weight. Intraperitoneal injection of *p,p'*-DDE (150 mg/kg) caused reduction of eggshell weight and inhibition of carbonic anhydrase in the oviduct by 59%, but injection of dieldrin (30 mg/kg) had no effect. It was considered that late breeding and failure to lay eggs to replace lost ones could be explained by reduced estrogen secondary to enzyme induction, whereas thinning and breakage of eggs could be explained by inibition of carbonic anhydrase, preventing the transfer of an essentialy normal supply of calcium from the body to the eggshell (Peakall, 1970a). It is of interest that the eggshell is laid down in about 20 hours just prior to laying. Therefore, any explanation of defective shells need involve only this brief period (Peakall, 1970b).

There has been no lack of effort to explain the phenomenon of eggshell thinning by chlorinated hydrocarbons. In fact, the multiplicity of explanations may have done as much to confuse as to convince. On the basis of experiments, the shell-thinning action of chlorinated hydrocarbons has been attributed to: (*a*) direct estrogenic action of DDT or its analogs (Bitman *et al.*, 1968); (*b*) inhibition of carbonic anhydrase (Bitman *et al.*, 1970; Peakall, 1970a); and (*c*) an effect on the thyroid (Jefferies and French, 1969). In addition, the possibility of (*d*) inhibition of the parathyroid gland and other derangements of calcium metabolism (Bitman *et al.*, 1969); and (*e*) inhibition of active transport of calcium through suppression of ATPase (Risebrough *et al.*, 1970) have been mentioned but not demonstrated experimentally. Delayed breeding has been attributed to (*f*) excessive degradation of natural estrogens due to induction of liver microsomal enzymes (Peakall, 1970a). The real importance of these factors or some combination of them in causing the effects observed in nature is in question. In fact, most of the biochemical reasoning has been concerned with DDT and dieldrin, although it is DDE that is most closely associated from an ecological point of view. Even for DDE, some hypotheses lack confirmation.

Work leading to reports that DDE inhibits carbonic anhydrase in the shell gland of ring-doves and Japanese quail (Peakall, 1970a; Bitman et al., 1970) was based on a claim by Keller (1952) that DDT inhibits this enzyme in bovine erythrocytes. However, the work of Keller could not be confirmed by Dvorchik et al. (1971). They point out that the reported reduction in enzyme activity in the gland usually was not enough to interfere with physiological function and that the method of investigation was unsatisfactory. The enzyme in red cells is as sensitive as that in any other tissue that has been studied properly. The results with shell glands require confirmation; if the study is repeated, it would seem best to use a species highly susceptible to eggshell thinning.

The biochemical relationships that have been studied as possible explanations of egg-shell thinning are as much subject to species differences as is thinning itself, but not necessarily in a parallel fashion. For example, dieldrin at a dietary level of 5 ppm increases the microsomal enzyme, aldrin epoxidase, in Japanese quail but does not affect cytochrome P–450 or NADPH-neotetrazolium reductase. On the other hand, concentrations of DDT up to 100 ppm not only fail to induce enzymes but actually depress epoxidase activity in this species. DDT also appears inactive as an inducer in pheasant (Phasianus colchicus) (Gillett et al., 1970). Species differences in the induction of enzymes occur in mammals also (see Section 3.1.3.1).

Not only is there some question whether the biochemical changes demonstrated in vitro are effective in vivo under field conditions, but there is doubt what chemicals are present in sufficient dosage in some wild populations to cause the observed changes. Eggshell thinning, loss of reproductive ability, or both have been attributed not only to DDE but to poly-chlorinated biphenyls (Risebrough et al., 1968) and to mercury compounds (Stoewsand et al., 1971; Spann et al., 1972). Some eggs may contain several compounds. For example, DDE, dieldrin, PCB's, and mercury were found in each of 23 bald eagle eggs analyzed for these compounds; both DDE and dieldrin were considered to be at a critical concentration in some of them (Wiemeyer et al., 1972).

The review by Cooke (1973) of possible mechanisms for the formation of thin egg-shells gives more detail about this matter in relation to wildlife than can be offered here. In addition, Cooke gave information on (a) the anatomy of the reproductive system of female birds, (b) anatomy of the eggshell, and (c) the results of studies in chickens. He pointed out that the chicken has been studied far more in this regard than any other species, but knowledge of shell formation in it is very incomplete. Furthermore, the chicken is a poor model because it is relatively resistant to shell thinning by organic chlorine compounds. Cooke considered that pesticides may cause thin shells through several (probably interrelated) mechanisms and that various factors such as species and environmental conditions might affect which mechanisms are dominant in any given situation. He went further and stated that shell thinning may be due to an unrecognized factor.

Dosage-Response Relationships. One cannot dismiss entirely the possibility that direct poisoning has contributed to the decline observed in some populations. Lethal levels of DDT or dieldrin have been reported in the brains of a few peregrine falcons (Risebrough et al., 1968) and eagles (Reichel et al., 1969a, 1969b; Mulhern et al., 1970; Belisle et al., 1972). Lethal levels of DDE were found in the brains of pelicans during a period of high mortality a year prior to the greatest eggshell thinning (Keith et al., 1970). At least in some instances (Mulhern et al., 1970), analyses were made simultaneously for polychlorinated biphenyls so that the possibility of confusing biphenyls and insecticides (Bagley et al., 1970) was excluded. Of the 153 bald eagles analyzed during 1964–1970, 15 possibly died of dieldrin poisoning (Belisle et al., 1972). Analysis of tissues other than the brain is a less satisfactory way of relating chemical effects of chlorinated insecticides to their residues. However, Robinson (1969) reviewed data on dieldrin (chiefly in liver) suggesting strongly that a few kestrels (Falco tinnunculus) and peregrine falcons had been poisoned by it in Holland and Britain. He concluded that about 5 to 20% of peregrine falcons found dead in Britain actually died from poisoning by dieldrin.

Although some persons have intimated or even stated that very low dietary residues of pesticides in general and of DDE in particular are a hazard to wildlife, egg or tissue residues clearly associated with significant eggshell thinning reflect substantial dosage. The conclusion that dosages of chlorinated hydrocarbon insecticides suspected of interfering with reproduction are almost at the lethal level is reinforced by the experimental finding that when DDE was fed at a dietary level of 2.8 ppm (wet weight basis) in order to study its effect on eggshell thickness, 2 of 14 male sparrow hawks died of DDE poisoning. Death occurred at a time of seasonal weight loss associated with molting. The relationship to DDE was supported by autopsy findings and the presence of DDE in the brains of the two birds at concentrations of 213 and 301 ppm, respectively (Porter and Wiemeyer, 1972). Similar findings were reported for Japanese quail (Stickel and Rhodes, 1970).

That substantial dosage is required to produce injury also is indicated by reports of increased thickness of eggshells and/or improved reproduction associated with reduction of egg or tissue residues. Such reports involve certain populations of peregrine falcons in Britain (Ratcliffe, 1969, 1972; Robinson, 1969), kestrels in Britain (Prestt, 1965), golden eagles in Scotland (Ratcliffe, 1970), pelicans on Anacapa Island (Gress *et al.*, 1973) and on Los Coronados (Jehl, 1973; Gress *et al.*, 1973), and herring gulls in Wisconsin (Keith, 1966; Hickey and Anderson, 1968).

Other Factors in Population Declines. Not all population problems are reproductive in origin, although a population that is hard pressed in some other way may reproduce poorly. Traditionally, farmers in the United States of America have considered large birds of prey as enemies, and many persons regard them as appropriate targets. This point of view has sometimes been given the force of law through the granting of bounties (Kalmbach *et al.*, 1964). As late as 1960–1965 and even later, trauma, primarily by shooting, was the greatest cause of mortality among bald eagles examined in the laboratory of the Patuxent Wildlife Research Center, Bureau of Sport Fisheries and Wildlife (Coon *et al.*, 1970; Belisle *et al.*, 1972).

Some consideration must be given to disturbance as well as to the more obvious forms of persecution. Dawson (1923) was so impressed by how much his own visit to Anacapa Island disturbed the pelicans there that he urged that such visits not be repeated. In some instances routine surveys recently have been made by low-flying aircraft. What would Dawson have thought of that?

Although no effort seems to have been made to measure the disturbance of populations, either indirectly through effects on the populations or in any other way, it is difficult to escape the conclusion that the importance of disturbance generally is increasing. In discussing declining populations of pelicans on Los Coronados and other islands along the California coast, Jehl (1973) mentions not only visits by tourists, but the shooting of birds from fishing boats and the buzzing of colonies by small planes.

Evaluation of the Data. Populations of several kinds of falcons and fish-eating birds have undergone marked decline in many areas. In spite of variations and shifts of local populations, no significant decrease in some of these species (eg, pelicans) was proved before chlorinated hydrocarbon insecticides were widely distributed in the environment. In other instances (eg, peregrine falcons), the recent change is clearly an acceleration of a long-standing decline. The fact that populations of some species of hawks have not declined has no bearing on the matter. According to the hypothesis under discussion, the difference is largely predictable from and explained by differences in food habits—fish-eating and bird-eating hawks being in greater danger than mammal-eating ones. Furthermore, species differences are the rule in toxicology, not the exception.

The primary importance of reproduction in maintaining populations must be recognized. The fact that an astonishing number of adults of some of the species with reproductive difficulties are killed by shooting detracts in no way from the critical importance of their reproductive problems. The same interpretation can be applied to other disturbances of populations by man.

The hypothesis that the reproductive failure of some populations of certain raptors and fish-eating birds is the result of chlorinated hydrocarbons is supported by (*a*) a correlation between the degree of eggshell thinning and the concentration of chlorinated compounds—mainly DDE—in birds, or in the defective eggs themselves; (*b*) some correlation between reproductive failure and eggshell thinning; (*c*) experimental proof that some degree of eggshell thinning and reproductive failure can be produced by chlorinated compounds—mainly DDE—in some species, including one of the genus *Falco*, several species of which have suffered decline; and finally, (*d*) a few instances of apparent increase in shell thickness and decrease in reproductive difficulty associated with reduction of residues of DDE in eggs. Not only is the correlation between shell thinning and concentration of DDE striking, but there now is no other explanation. No other compound is known to have become generally available about the time when eggshell thinning first occurred, soon after 1945. Polychlorinated biphenyls did not come on suddenly at that time and dieldrin was not available. The combined evidence is most impressive, but responsible wildlife toxicologists are the last to suggest that the evidence excludes other possibilities especially in view of certain considerations discussed later in this section.

From his exhaustive review, Cooke (1973) concluded that (*a*) residues of *p,p'*-DDE or other compounds or metabolites of the DDT group were responsible for eggshell thinning of certain species in North America and Great Britain since the Second World War; (b) in North America polychlorinated biphenyls and cyclodiene insecticides have played no more than minor roles, although in Britain cyclodienes have probably made a significant contribution; (c) mercury compounds apparently have not been associated with shell thinning under field conditions [although they have been associated with poisoning of wildlife in Sweden (Borg et al., 1966)]; and (d) in North America shell thinning often has been associated with population decreases, but to a lesser degree in Britain, where population declines of peregrines are considered due to deliberate breakage of eggs by sublethally poisoned parents and to adult mortality, rather than to accidental breakage of the thin shells.

In some instances, the thinning of eggshells may be less important as a cause of fragility than as an indication of residues in the egg leading to other injury. According to Cooke, foreign chemicals may cause the death of embryos or young chicks in three ways: (a) accidental breakage of thin-shelled eggs; (b) destruction of eggs or young by adults whose behavior has been rendered abnormal by poisoning; and (c) poisoning of embryos or young as the mobilization of chemical from the yolk reaches a critical stage. Each of these three separate causes of death may take the form of disappearance of eggs or young from the nest, even though destruction by the adult is primary in (b) only.

Because the hypothesis is impressive that chlorinated hydrocarbons have caused the reproductive failure observed in some populations of certain raptors and fish-eating birds, there is a danger that remaining questions will be ignored. Where the concentration of DDE is correlated with shell thinning and reproductive failure, these questions involve dosage, timing, and the possible importance of nonchemical factors. Where shell thinning is lacking or not correlated with the DDE present, the questions are more complex.

It is not certain that substantial dosages of chlorinated hydrocarbon insecticides always were available to susceptible populations when thinning of their eggshells began in nature. It has been pointed out that thinning of the eggshells of the peregrine falcon in the United Kingdom started quite suddenly in 1946 and that DDT was used there in 1945–1946 (Ratcliffe, 1967). Although this is true and although thinning occurs by the 3rd day of experimental dosage (Stickel and Rhodes, 1970), it is difficult to see how these birds got a substantial dosage at that time. The supply of DDT then depended very largely on production in the United States of America, and this production was put to military rather than agricultural use until 1945. Even in the USA, DDT was not available commercially until 1946. In that year, production reached 20,000 metric tons, a marked increase from the 4,366 metric tons produced in 1944, but a small amount compared with the world production of 200,000 to 250,000 metric tons annually reached considerably later. In the United Kingdom, it was not until 1948 that a reduction of the price of DDT permitted its general and increasing use in agriculture. One must question whether there was enough DDT available in 1946 in the remote areas inhabited by falcons and, if so, whether there was enough time for this chemical to be metabolized to DDE, and for that to work its way through the food chain to produce the thinning of eggshells of peregrine falcons already clearly evident in the United Kingdom in the spring of 1946. Finally, Ratcliffe (1970) speculated that DDT could have been used during the War to dust homing pigeons on which the peregrines fed. If one accepts, for point of argument, that there was enough DDE available to the hawks of the United Kingdom in 1946 to explain the observed change in eggshell thickness, then it becomes difficult to explain why there was no progression of thinning after 1948, when use of DDT began in earnest, or how the slight recovery of the population beginning in 1964 could occur; the amount of DDT certainly had increased by that time.

In other instances, what seemed an adequate dosage failed to produce the expected effect. The view that DDE is the culprit was accepted generally when Enderson and Berger (1968) noted with some astonishment that the eggs of peregrine falcons in Canada had about twice the levels of DDT, DDE, DDD, dieldrin, and heptachlor epoxide found in the stricken British peregrine population, yet reported that the birds "appear to be reproducing normally." The average levels observed in viable eggs in Canada were: 2.9 ppm of DDT, 17.8 ppm of DDE, 2.1 ppm of DDD, 0.8 ppm of dieldrin, and 0.4 ppm of heptachlor epoxide; the corresponding levels in the fat of breeding birds were: 37.3 for DDT, 284.0 for DDE, 39.5 for DDD, 3.3 for dieldrin, and 4.4 for heptachlor epoxide. Later evidence (Cade and Fyfe, 1970) indicated that Canadian populations of peregrines (presumably including the population studied by Enderson and Berger) had undergone marked decline by 1970. However, this later result does not negate or explain the earlier observation.

Timing as well as dosage presents some

problems. Following World War II, when they were persecuted severely, British populations of peregrines increased rapidly for several years, beginning in 1945. This recovery occurred even though the thinning of the eggs of these birds was clearly noticeable in 1946 and was essentially maximal by 1948 (Ratcliffe, 1967). Thus, the onset of reproductive difficulty really did not correspond with eggshell thinning. Cooke (1973) concluded that, whereas in North America shell thinning often has been associated with population decreases, in Britain declines in shell thickness are not thought responsible for the decrease observed in populations of certain raptor species, which are attributed instead to direct toxicity from cyclodiene insecticides. When population decline did come, it began in the south and spread northward like an epidemic, as was true in North America also.

A somewhat similar problem is posed by the injury to pelicans on Anacapa Island. It was stated by Banks (1966) that their reproduction was normal in 1963-1964. Although this judgment may not have been based on exact counts, the fact remains that later study (Anderson and Hickey, 1970) showed that eggs collected from the island in 1962 were 26% thinner than normal, and disastrous thinning leading to failure of reproduction in this population in 1969 was reported (Jehl, 1969; Keith et al., 1970; Risebrough et al., 1971). Some recovery of reproduction of pelicans on Anacapa Island in 1971 and especially in 1972 was reported (Gress et al., 1973). The factory that is said to be the source of local pollution began operation in 1947. Although industrial discharge of DDT was curtailed in April, 1970, the relatively rapid beginning of a possible resolution of the problem seems to be inconsistent with other evidence indicating that pelicans are unusually susceptible to DDT and its metabolites. Furthermore, a similar apparent increase in the breeding success of pelicans on Los Coronados in 1970 and 1971 was reported by Jehl (1973); it is difficult to see how a change in DDT release near Anacapa Island so rapidly would influence the breeding success of pelicans on Los Coronados about 200 km to the south.

Anderson and Hickey (1972) commented that when eggshell thinning is in the range of 15 to 20% for a period of years, the population in question seems to be generally in trouble. It is not clear why a period of years may be required. What further change is accomplished in those years, and why does population decline sometimes not occur?

All examples of eggshell thinning involve a reduction of average thickness or weight. In most instances, reduction of the average is associated with lowering of the entire range. However, for the bald eagle in Florida, reduction of average eggshell weight in 1947 involved little or no reduction of the lower part of the range—only a great reduction of the upper part. By the same token there were numerous "lightweight" eggs during the 1930's, 1920's, and even earlier (Anderson and Hickey, 1972). This situation raises a question of when thinning really occurred or, alternatively, whether lightweight eggs after 1947 were any more pathological than those laid decades earlier. The bald eagle is not the only species in which the change seen after 1945 was one of degree. Some breakage and disappearance of falcon eggs was reported prior to the introduction of DDT (Ratcliffe, 1967). This situation could indicate the introduction of a second adverse factor (ie, DDE) soon after 1945, but it could also represent accentuation of some unrecognized factor already present. To be sure, if such a factor does exist, there can be no assurance that it is chemical or, if chemical, what its nature may be.

Serious consideration of the existence of an unknown factor is required, especially in those situations where marked failure of reproduction is present, but the concentration of DDE (or any other recognized compound) in the eggs is not correlated with their thinning or breaking. In such instances, the presence of DDE in the eggs is merely evidence of its widespread occurrence. In the absence of correlation, any further interpretation is unwarranted.

The phenomenon of population decline and even extinction is not new. It is estimated that some 160 species or subspecies of birds have become extinct since 1600, most of them before 1900 (Vincent, 1966). On the contrary, some species have increased tremendously in recent years, in spite of whatever handicaps the "chemical age" may impose. Robinson (1969) has reviewed the exponential increase in the collared dove (Streptopelia decaoto) in Britain from 1955 to 1964.

Whereas the extinction of a few species seems adequately understood, the extinction of others remains a mystery. The great destruction of passenger pigeons (Ectopistes migratorius) is explained fully by their ruthless slaughter for meat (Bent, 1932), but their disappearance after they become too rare to be hunted profitably is a mystery. Some birds never become common yet survive without difficulty. There is more mystery about the decline of the peregrine falcon than may appear. In southeastern Canada and the eastern United States of America the decline began long before DDT was manufactured. Beebe (1969) speculated that it may have begun with the decline and extinction of the passenger pigeon, which was the natural and principal food of these hawks in these areas. Certainly peregrines suffered from reproductive problems before the advent of DDT, as reported by Hickey (1942) and by a number of others who participated in the 1965 conference (Hickey, 1969). Before DDT, the eastern North American peregrine population was considered in need of protection (Hickey, 1942). After 1947 the decline of this population continued at a rate "too rapid to have been caused by reproductive failure alone" (Hickey, 1970).

In a similar way, very thorough study of osprey populations in Cape May County, New Jersey, between 1939 and 1963 revealed a marked decline. However, the author (Schmid, 1966) cited papers published in 1890 and 1901 reporting earlier reductions in the same general area and concluded that "As in New England, the decline in the osprey population in Cape May County apparently began long ago, at least in some areas." He cited other published papers and his own observations suggesting that lack of available food supply could be a contributing cause. He also mentioned frequency of disturbance and persecution as possible causes. Before DDT was made in the United States of America, a 70% decline of osprey in one area was attributed to "pole-trapping, etc." around fish hatcheries (Hickey, 1943).

There is danger that fascination with the correlation between thickness of eggshells and concentration of DDE, or with any other single relationship, will exclude attention to other parameters of possible importance.

Need for Future Research. It would be desirable but difficult meaningfully to consider the possibility of genetic differences among populations of the same species. Resistance emerging under the influence of selection would explain the reports of apparent, slight recovery of some populations mentioned above. If resistance has developed, it would not be the first instance (see Section 3.1.3.2). Conversely, genetic drift may be considered as a cause of decline in rare species.

At the very least, more attention ought to be given to determining exactly when eggshell thinning and/or reproductive failure began in each species and in each area. A detail of special interest concerns shell thinning and reproduction of raptors in Switzerland, for DDT was used there for a few years before it became available elsewhere.

Inasmuch as highly responsible investigators (Bent, 1932; Hickey, 1942, 1969) reported the failure of some bird populations to reproduce before chlorinated hydrocarbon insecticides were invented, the possibility that this effect may occur spontanteously in populations reduced to a sufficient degree by other causes or be caused by naturally occurring chemicals or other factors must be kept in mind, and every clue must be investigated.

Mathematical modeling (Henny, 1972) has proved a keen tool for distinguishing premature mortality from reproductive failure as elements in the population dynamics of birds. If data could be developed regarding different factors contributing to this failure, there is no doubt that mathematical techniques could be developed for their evaluation.

Finally, a careful re-examination of the biochemical basis of reproduction in birds might help us to understand observed differences among species and apparent differences among populations of the same species.

11.2.3.4 Evaluation of Biological Magnification. It has been speculated that it is cumulation of effect that makes DDT dangerous to some wildlife, but repeated doses of several other compounds such as warfarin and mirex, which have not led to ecological complications, actually produce more cumulative effects in experimental animals (see Section 2.2.2).

The importance of biological magnification is tremendous in a few situations. However, some ecologists seem to view it as a necessary property of food chains. If this were true, it seems likely that more injury would be evident and that, with a model available, the cause could be traced easily. Actually, the phenomenon may be little more than a rare curiosity requiring a whole series of species that are inefficient at degrading and excreting the compound in question. Since food chains are of finite length, it is only necessary that one or at most a few species in a series be really effective in eliminating the compound, or that several species be moderately effective in eliminating it, in order to limit accumulation to a point that nothing really happens. Furthermore, even in susceptible food chains, biological magnification may be expected in connection with only a few compounds. Most pesticides are degraded readily by living organisms.

Some persistence of a compound in organisms and in the environment is necessary for biological magnification to occur. However, there has been a tendency in the literature to confuse the two and to assign an inordinate importance to environmental persistence. The heavy metals, which have absolute environmental persistence, generally have shorter biological halflives, exhibit less biological magnification than DDT and especially DDE, and have produced less injury to wildlife.

Because biological magnification clearly has been demonstrated in certain instances, there has been a tendency to view all high residues found in nontarget organisms as examples of it. Often more careful study has revealed that high residues were the result of high dosage, sometimes for an unexpected source. For example, the presence of DDT and related compounds in pelicans on Anacapa Island just offshore from Los Angeles has been viewed as an example of worldwide contamination. However, by analyzing a kind of crab (*Emerita analoga*) that lives by filtering detritus from sea water, Burnett (1971) showed that water near Los Angeles contained 45 times as much DDT-related material as water near the outflow of rivers draining extensive agricultural areas of the same state; the source of DDT at Los Angeles was said to be a single factory. In a similar way, differences in the concentrations of DDT-related compounds in Alaskan populations of peregrine falcons are explained largely by differences in their migration. Those with the highest residues migrate each winter as far south as Argentina, and therefore across parts of North and Central America where pesticides are used extensively (Cade *et al.*, 1971). Again, robins have been the victims of biological magnification of DDT through earthworms only in connection with the massive application rates of that compound required for control of Dutch elm disease.

Model Ecosystem. Fortunately an ingenious, simple, dependable test involving a model ecosystem has been developed to measure the tendency of a compound or its metabolites to undergo biological magnification (Metcalf *et al.*, 1971a, 1971b). This test now permits toxicologists to learn about any compound in a few months what it took ecologists 20 years to learn about DDT.

A series of experimental and control aquaria are maintained in a chamber providing carefully regulated temperature and light. Each aquarium contains a pool of water at one end and a gradually rising bank of sand at the other. Algae are grown in the water and sorghum on the land. Animals include plankton, snails, water fleas, mosquitoes, and fish in the water, and salt-marsh caterpillars on the land. Radioactive pesticide is applied to the sorghum, and its fate in the ecosystem is followed over an extended period.

Other Relevant Tests. More recently, it has been suggested that susceptibility of a compound to photooxidation offers an indication of its susceptibility to degradation by this and by other means also and, therefore, might be made the basis of a test (Crosby, 1972). The practical value of such a test involving photooxidation remains to be explored.

One difficulty in defining a pesticide that is subject to biological magnification lies in the fact that this property obviously constitutes a spectrum, and yet the dividing line between safety and danger in this spectrum is not known. It seems likely that measurements of the chronicity index (see Section 2.2.2) and concentration index (see Section 3.2.3.2) of compounds that have injured wildlife and of other compounds that have proved safe not only would define the limit of safety but would result in a relatively simple test of high predictive value. It might be that such tests would have to be made in selected, representative species. However, in spite of real variation between species, there is often considerable similarity in the general level of ability of different ones to metabolize a particular compound. It seems possible, therefore, that much could be learned by measuring the chronicity index and the concentration index of different compounds, even if the measurements were restricted to rats.

11.2.4 The Nature of Pest Control

Ecologists sometimes view each instance of pest control as an effort to rectify an imbalance of nature. Although this definition sometimes applies (Section 11.2.2), a far more general definition is that pest control is an effort to establish a new balance favorable to man, his crops, or desirable wildlife. The control of weeds in a crop is a purposeful effort to extend the imbalance produced by plowing and planting. The control of human parasites is an effort to avoid the vermin-ridden state in which man existed in the past, and still exists in primitive societies.

11.3 Injury to Wildlife

The potential of DDT for the control of malaria was realized within a few months after the first sample was brought to the United States of America in 1942. At first, of course, there was no way to predict the overwhelming predominance indoor house spraying with DDT would achieve in connection with malaria control. The possibility of using the compound as a larvicide was investigated during the early months of study. Those responsible for the work were thoroughly familiar with the effect of other pesticides, such as oil and Paris green, on aquatic insects and fish. A thorough study of the effects of DDT on these organisms was begun early and was essentially complete by the end of World War II.

Somewhat later, and as a supply of DDT became available, the potential of the compound for the control of forest insects was realized. Again, there was full awareness of the possibility of injury, and several quantitative studies were made of wildlife under practical conditions of forest insect control. These papers should be consulted not only by those interested in the detailed results, but also by those interested in a history of the relationship between pesticides and wildlife.

The early literature regarding the effect of pesticides on wildlife, under both practical and experimental conditions, was reviewed by Rudd and Genelly (1956). Later reviews or collections of papers including information on the ecological effects of DDT and, in some instances, other compounds are those of Hayes (1959), Rudd (1964), Tarzwell (1965), Moore (1966a), Miller and Berg (1969), Pimentel (1971), and Cope (1971).

11.3.1 Injury in Relation to Kind of Treatment

As might be predicted, injury to wildlife has varied tremendously, depending not only on the different compounds and dosages involved, but also on the circumstances of application. In general, it has been found that greatest damage has been done to aquatic organisms either by moderate to heavy dosages directly to water or by very extensive applications to non-agricultural land. Heavy, continuing or intermittent exposures to industrial discharges have been important sources of severe difficulty. With occasional exceptions, injury has been caused by heavy metals and by some, but not all, chlorinated hydrocarbon insecticides. In general, insecticides pose a greater threat to fish and other wildlife than herbicides and fungicides do. However, most insecticides when properly applied have caused little or no serious damage to wildlife. Of course, the safety of insecticides under practical conditions reflects careful study by wildlife experts to detect danger, and it also reflects general observance of the restrictions on use that finally are set down in labeling. The important fact remains that the majority of pesticides have not caused significant injury to wildlife.

11.3.1.1 Application to Water. During the latter part of the Second World War, DDT was applied to water for the control of malaria and mosquitoes. Since that time, the compound as well as several other chlorinated hydrocarbon insecticides and several organic phosphorus insecticides, including parathion and malathion, have been applied directly to water for the control of the aquatic larvae of other disease vectors or for the control of pest mosquitoes and blackflies.

Pentachlorophenol and some other molluscicides are added to water for the control of snails necessary for the complete life cycle of human blood flukes. 3-Bromo-4-nitrophenol and 3-trifluoromethyl-4-nitrophenol have been used for the control of lampreys, which are serious pests leading to the destruction of fish.

Insecticides are usually sprayed directly on water by means of hand equipment or by power equipment mounted on trucks, boats, or aircraft. Molluscicides may be sprayed or they may be metered into streams at rates determined by the rates of flow.

In recent times, almost all difficulty from the application of pesticides to water has been associated with some, but not all, chlorinated hydrocarbon insecticides.

Reviews regarding the presence and effects of pesticides in water are those of Hayes (1959) and Butler and Springer (1963).

Organisms Serving as Fish Food. The most important conclusion drawn repeatedly from careful observations under the conditions of malaria control is that anopheline mosquitoes may be controlled by DDT without undue injury to organisms considered important as fish food (Metcalf *et al.,* 1945; Hess and Keener, 1947; Tarzwell, 1947; 1948; 1950). This is true even though certain forms such as Diptera, Hemiptera, Coleoptera, Ephemeroptera, and amphipod crustacea are highly susceptible, and some of them such as surface Hemiptera were almost entirely eliminated by a complete season of applications.

A review (Hayes, 1959) showed that it frequently proved necessary to use higher application rates for the control of pest mosquitoes generally, and of salt-marsh mosquitoes in particular. Extensive mortality of the commercially important blue crab (*Callinectes sapidus*) has been reported in connection with the spraying of salt marshes. Fiddler crabs (*Uca crenulata*) on exposed beaches may suffer severe mortality, but crabs in water about two meters deep have remained uninjured when DDT was applied to the surface at very high rates.

Fish. The effect of DDT on fish is very similar to its effect on aquatic insects. The dosage of 11.2 mg/m² necessary for malaria control is not injurious as judged by the total number of fish, their weight, condition, species composition, and the abundance of very young fish (Hess and Keener, 1947). However, in routine malaria control operations, the rate of application sometimes exceeded the one recommended; thus Herald (1949) reported the loss of young milk fish in commercial ponds following the application of DDT by aircraft at a rate thought to be greater than twice that necessary for malaria control. As might be expected, even higher rates of application have led to heavy loss of fish, particularly when they were in shallow water from which they could not escape into deeper water or into unsprayed areas.

Birds and Mammals. The direct application of DDT to water has produced essentially no immediate mortality of birds or mammals. This has been true even in situations where gulls and herons were seen to enter the sprayed area to feed on dead arthropods. Rails successfully reared young in areas treated at the rate of 112 mg/m², and songbirds were unaffected and reared young successfully (Springer and Webster, 1949; 1951).

A completely different situation arose in connection with the locally massive applications required to control Dutch elm disease and as a delayed result of the repeated use of DDD for the control of the Clear Lake gnat, as described in Section 11.2.3.2.

11.3.1.2 Application to Non-agricultural Land. Applications to uncultivated land usually have been made for the control of a single dominant species of disease-bearing or destructive arthropod such as *Culex tarsalis* (the vector of one form of human encephalitis), the spruce budworm, the gypsy moth (*Porthetria dispar*), the white-fringed beetle, or the fire ant. Such treatments frequently were made by aircraft and might affect not only land animals in the treated area, but also animals living in streams passing through it. As discussed in Section 6.3.2.2, the possibility that a particular pesticide will be washed from the land and carried into streams in sufficient concentration to cause injury varies greatly from one compound to another.

Not only have different compounds been used for different purposes, but the same compound has been applied at very different rates. For example, oil solutions of DDT at the rate of 112 mg/m² are adequate for the control of many forest insects. However, dust and especially granular formulations have been applied at rates as high as 2,800 mg/m² for control of soil-infesting grubs such as the white-fringed beetle.

Aquatic Invertebrates. The application of 112 mg or more of DDT per square meter, which is required for the control of forest insects, constitutes a real threat to many

organisms in streams passing through forested areas. This application practically exterminates the surface insects and those breathing at the surface, and severely reduces free-swimming and crawling insects. Bottom forms are not so severely affected. The application of DDT to streams at the rate of 112 mg/m² can kill as much as 90% of the insect population and locally exterminate one-third of the species present.

Hoffman *et al.* (1946) observed that streams carry lethal amounts of DDT for only short distances and, therefore, concluded that the damage was done by insecticide deposited directly on the streams' surfaces and not by insecticide washed into the streams. However, dust formulations of DDT, as well as various formulations of some other pesticides, are carried more easily by runoff. Under certain conditions, even DDT in oil may be transported downstream as much as 48 km with lethal effect (Elson, 1967).

The effect of control programs extending over very large areas has not been remarkable in connection with aquatic invertebrates. Hoffman and Surber (1949) studied an area of 21,044 ha treated under practical conditions at a rate of 112 mg/m² for control of the gypsy moth. Although 70 to 80% of the stream insects were killed within 3 days, and although fish were killed in one stream over a period of 1 month, the loss of fish was small in comparison to the total population.

Terrestrial Invertebrates. Earthworms usually are not affected by insecticides. Their reaction to DDT is described in Section 11.2.3.2.

Insects are by far the most important land invertebrates, and as a group they are highly susceptible to insecticides. Their survival following an application of insecticide to a forest depends largely on their opportunity for exposure as determined by their ecology and life history. Species living in burrows or leaf mold, beneath bark, or in other protected situations may escape unharmed. Furthermore, invertebrates living below a cover may receive only a small dose. In a forest with a close canopy, only 2.5% of the DDT applied as an oil spray was recovered at ground level, although 30% was recovered in open areas (Hoffman and Merkel, 1948). In another study, the recovery under a forest canopy varied from less than 1 to 10%, and averaged 2.5%. When there was an additional cover of weeds, grass, or shrubs, the maximum recovery was 3% and the average recovery was 0.4% (Stewart *et al.*, 1946; Stickel, 1946). In a more open forest, the recovery of DDT averaged 4.6% (Goodrum *et al.*, 1949). Protection of animal life by low vegetation has been observed frequently.

The application of DDT as an oil spray at the usual rate for forest application (112 mg/m²) causes an almost immediate and pronounced effect on many species of insects inhabiting different kinds of forest. Mortality of exposed forms, as determined by carefully controlled population studies, frequently reaches 90%, and some species appear to be eliminated temporarily in the treated area. The residual effect of such an application lasted about a week. Applications at twice that rate lasted about 2 weeks, the effect of applications at 5 times that rate was severe after 6 weeks, and there was little recovery until 3 months after application (Hoffman and Merkel, 1948; Hoffman et al., 1949). Recovery from high dosage levels may be accompanied by inordinate reproduction of aphids and mites (Hoffman and Merkel, 1948; Hoffman et al., 1949).

Fish. Under practical conditions of forest treatment, even with dosages at twice the usual rate, the effect of DDT on fish populations may be slight, although some individuals are killed (Linduska and Surber, 1948; Adams et al., 1949). Thus, in general, fish have fared much better than fish food organisms (Hoffman and Surber, 1948; Surber and Friddle, 1949). However, recent studies have revealed higher initial mortality of fish and, perhaps much more important, mortality delayed 4 to 6 months after the early mortality had stopped. The delayed deaths were associated with spawning, the onset of winter, or other stresses (Graham, 1959; Elson, 1967).

Amphibians and Reptiles. The application of DDT at a rate suitable for the control of forest insects usually has little effect on frogs, salamanders, snakes, or turtles, although occasional ones are killed. A few striking exceptions have been reported. For example, apparently all wood frogs (*Rana sylvatica*) in two woodland pools were killed when the area was sprayed with DDT at the rate of 112 mg/m² for control of tent caterpillars. Many healthy frogs were present 1 day after spraying, but all were dead 2.5 days after application, presumably because they had eaten the larvae that fell into the water. The stomachs of 34 of the dead frogs contained an average of five caterpillars each.

Birds. The rate of application of DDT necessary for the control of Dutch elm disease is in the range of 6,000 to 13,000 mg/m². As described in Section 11.2.3.2, such a high rate of application of DDT regularly leads to immediate poisoning of various birds as well as to a delayed poisoning of robins by way of their food chain. Even a dosage of 448 mg/m² frequently leads to poisoning, so that birds showing clearcut signs of intoxication may be captured, and these birds almost invariably die (Hotchkiss and Pough, 1946; Linduska and Surber, 1948; Robbins and Stewart, 1949; George and Stickel, 1949; Speirs, 1949; Adams et al., 1949). On the contrary, the use of DDT at the rate of 112 mg/m² usually used for the control of forest insects produces little or no immediate effect on bird populations, the hatchability of eggs, the mortality of young, or the abandonment of nests (Hotchkiss and Pough, 1946; Kendeigh, 1947; Linduska and Surber, 1948).

The delayed effects of DDE, dieldrin, and alkyl mercury on susceptible birds are discussed in Section 11.2.3.2.

Mammals. Wild mammals seems to be somewhat less susceptible than wild birds to DDT. The difference probably is related more to food habits and other behavior than to inherent susceptibility. No serious injury to mammals has been produced by the application of DDT to non-agricultural lands, although applications at the rate of 560 mg/m² or higher have caused transient effects in some individuals (Linduska and Surber, 1948; Adams et al., 1949).

Although injury was not revealed, a study by Dimond and Sherburne (1959) did reveal how long DDT can persist in forest mammals following one or more applications to the forest at the rate of 1.1 kg/ha. Each application had covered 10^5 to 10^6 ha; the separate applications had been made 0 to 9 years earlier; and some areas had received only one treatment while others had received as many as three. An average concentration of 0.03 ppm of total DDT-related material was found in the whole bodies of vegetarian mice and voles, but 0.30 ppm was found in carnivorous shrews trapped in areas never known to have been treated. These residues presumably were the result of drift from considerable but unknown distances. Soon after a single treatment, the average residues in vegetarians and small carnivores were 1.06 and 15.58 ppm, respectively. Residues in mice and voles approached the level found in untreated areas 9 years after a single treatment but still averaged 1.18 in shrews (almost 4 times baseline values) after the same interval. It was estimated that, at the observed rates of decrease, residues in shrews would reach baseline in something over 15 years. Following three applications, residues were about twice as great as those after a single application when the interval from last treatment was the same. Dimond has shown about equal duration of residue persistence in other species.

11.3.1.3 Application to Agricultural Land.
Fish and Other Aquatic Organisms. There
has been virtually no study of aquatic insects
in connection with the ordinary application of
pesticides to agricultural lands. The traces of
pesticides ordinarily found in water (Section
6.1.3) would not be expected to influence these
organisms, and they have continued to thrive
in the streams of agricultural areas. In fact,
because of the great ability of fish to concentrate chlorinated hydrocarbon insecticides
from water, the finding of small residues in
some species serves to confirm their low rate
of exposure. Thus, Morris and Johnson (1971)
found dieldrin in the edible part of bottom
feeding fish in rivers draining areas where
aldrin had been used on row crops, mainly
maize. Far less dieldrin was found in pan and
predator game fish from the same rivers.
Rivers that do not drain row crops do not
produce elevated pesticide levels even in bottom feeding fish. The important point, however, is that the highest concentration of dieldrin was in large fish that obviously had
survived a long time. The very highest residue
found was only 1.6 ppm. Daily consumption of
fish with this highest residue would give an
intake harmless to people (see Table 7-24).

The fact that the concentration of pesticides
in water is generally extremely low does not
exclude the possibility that much higher concentrations will occur following heavy rains,
especially when all the land surrounding a
small stream has been treated recently with a
pesticide at a high rate. As discussed in Section 6.3.2.2, some compounds are relatively
easily transferred by water, while others rapidly become so firmly adsorbed to soil particles
that, even if the soil is washed into the
streams, the resulting suspension has little or
no toxicity to aquatic forms. DDT is firmly
attached to soil and apparently fish kills resulting from the agricultural use of this compound alone have not been reported. Fish kills
in small streams draining cultivated fields
have been attributed to toxaphene or endrin.

Terrestrial Wildlife. There is very little
information on what effect, if any, agricultural uses of pesticides have on terrestrial
wildlife. In the first place, desirable wild animals on farms are not primarily inhabitants
of highly cultivated land. Such animals may
live along fences, ditches, or unkept roadways
bordering fields, or they may live in orchards,
meadows, or woodlands from which they may
enter cultivated land to obtain a part of their
food. An unusually thorough study (Robel *et
al.*, 1972) found no statistically significant
effect on populations of rodents in fields

treated with aldrin, endrin, heptachlor, diazinon, parathion, and methyl parathion.

Some species, particularly birds, may be
injured in connection with crops such as fruit
and cotton that require large and frequent
applications of pesticides. However, the fact
that relatively few serious disruptions of farm
wildlife have been noted during the many
years in which pesticides have been used
extensively indicates that the effects of these
compounds usually are negligible. The most
striking exceptions have involved mortality of
birds associated with the use of aldrin and
other cyclodiene insecticides for treating seed
both in the United Kingdom (Murton and
Vizoso, 1963; Turtle *et al.*, 1963) and in Texas
(Flickinger and King, 1972). Not only seed-
eating birds but also some birds that feed on
invertebrates or on other birds were killed.
Difficulty was noted in the United Kingdom
beginning in 1956. In that and the following
years, increasingly large numbers of seed-
eating birds were found dead in cereal-grow-
ing areas in the spring. In each year, starting
in 1960, the Royal Society for the Protection of
Birds, in conjunction with the British Trust
for Ornithology, issued reports on such instances, and the occurrences received wide
publicity. Investigation showed that aldrin,
dieldrin, and heptachlor, which had not come
into general use in Britain until 1955 and
which were used to dress cereals sown in
spring, were almost certainly responsible for
the death among birds and probably also for
some secondary poisoning of mammals. The
concentrations of dieldrin, heptachlor epoxide,
and lindane in the tissues of poisoned birds
were similar to those in the tissues of birds
poisoned experimentally with the same compounds or their precursors. It was therefore
agreed in the summer of 1961 that these
dressings should not be used on spring-sown
cereals, and that in autumn they should be
restricted to cereals in districts where a specific need was demonstrable. The voluntary
agreement negotiated with manufacturers
and distributors of pesticides under the Pesticides Safety Precaution Scheme was well observed and there was no evidence of recurrence of the incidence after 1961 (Advisory
Committee on Poisonous Substances used in
Agriculture and Food Storage, 1964; Robinson, 1969).

11.3.1.4 Accidental Contamination. The
spilling or dumping of pesticides on land has
led to no serious injury to wildlife, although it
may well be that most desirable forms in the
immediate area are eliminated.

Gross contamination of water leads to an entirely different situation. There is no practical way to remove accidental spillage from water. Furthermore, unlike the situation on land, the poison spreads beyond the immediate area of contamination. If the spillage occurs in a stream, the poison is swept along with the water and it may kill all susceptible forms in its path for long distances. If the spillage occurs in a pond or a lake, the spread of the contaminant will be slower. However, it will certainly kill susceptible forms in the vicinity of spillage and if the material is not rapidly degraded, it may enter one or more food chains within the body of water and produce a delayed and perhaps unexpected effect. Although some fish kills have been the result of the intentional application of pesticides, the most extensive and serious injuries associated with foreign chemicals have followed accidental contamination of water, frequently through the inadvertent escape of industrial waste.

11.3.2 Overall Evaluation of Injury

One way of predicting future effects of pesticides is to consider trends found by monitoring the compounds in water (see Section 6.1.3), air (see Section 6.2.1), and soil (see Section 6.3.1). Although pesticides have been found in remote places, the trend is toward establishment of steady states, even when the same compound remains in use over a period of years. In some instances, residues of a particular compound in the environment have decreased as use of the material became more limited. Under these circumstances one can expect no increases and, in some instances, can expect decreased injury to wildlife by pesticides.

There has never been an overall evaluation of the injury to wildlife resulting from the use of pesticides. There have been, to be sure, very meticulous population studies of the effects of specific control programs. A few of these (especially ones concerned with the use of DDT for the control of malaria vectors or forest pests) have been cited in previous sections. Although some control programs, for example those directed against the spruce budworm, have involved vast areas and many years of experience, even these programs represent a relatively small fraction of the land area subjected to direct treatment with pesticides, and they do not account for most of the tonnage of the compounds that have been used.

Unfortunately, the majority of reports on the effects of pesticides on wildlife are, at best, similar to hospital bulletins, and, at worst, similar to accounts in tabloid newspapers. Hospital bulletins always reflect human misfortune, often with an unhappy ending. Even when accurate, such bulletins are not a valid source of information on community health. Isolated reports of injury to wildlife may reflect accidents and other misfortunes accurately, but they throw no light on the health of wildlife populations.

One notable attempt at a general evaluation of the condition of wildlife is that of the Advisory Committee on Poisonous Substances Used in Agriculture and Food Storage (1964). After concluding that the use of aldrin, dieldrin, and heptachlor as seed dressings had led to the death of seed-eating birds and perhaps a few predators, the report also concluded that limitation of the use of persistent pesticides would be wise in situations in which that degree of persistence was not required. However, in spite of recommending limitations to correct observed and even potential hazards, the report noted that "DDT and BHC have been in wide and extensive use in Great Britain for nearly twenty years," and concluded that it was unnecessary to place any restrictions at that time on either DDT or BHC (including γ-BHC). Indeed, the Committee considered that continued availability of these compounds was essential if their proposals for the limitation of aldrin and dieldrin were accepted.

Another way to learn the effects of pesticides on wildlife in general is to examine its effects on fur-bearing and game animals. In some instances, reports are required of hunters. The number of animals killed is a much more reliable and conservative record of populations than are counts based on sightings by a number of persons. Of course, a record could be misleading if the harvest in a given area has been excessive, but such an error would become evident through reduced harvests in succeeding years. The consistency of the values from year to year attests to the reliability of the figures.

Game animals in particular sometimes are spoken of as zoological "weeds" because their vigor and adaptability are said to be similar to that of plants that compete with our crops. Although the existence of a good growth of weeds is not evidence that the field is adapted for orchids, it is evidence of good soil and generally healthful conditions. By the same token, continuing high production of fur-bearing and game animals does not exclude the possibility of injury to some highly specialized species, but it does indicate a generally healthful environment.

As recorded in annual reports entitled *Fur*

Catch of the United States (US Department of the Interior), the harvest of some wild fur-bearers such as mink has decreased during the period in which modern pesticides have been in active use. However, the harvest of beaver, muskrat, racoon, and otter has remained essentially stable, while that of nutria has increased more than 4 times from 1954 to 1970.

Annual reports entitled *Big Game Inventory* (US Department of the Interior) show that big game has fared even better than fur-bearers. The harvest of black bear and Barbary sheep has remained about stable, but populations of peccary, wild boar, mountain goat, big horn sheep, antelope, moose, elk, mule deer, white-tailed deer, and black-tailed deer have increased from 1.5- to 20-fold.

Many states fail to report their harvest of small game, and apparently no national survey is attempted. Some states do record this kind of information. The record for Florida may be taken as typical. In that state, the harvest of squirrels more than doubled from 1950 to 1956 and then remained about the same through 1967, the last year of record. The harvests of duck, dove, quail, and wild turkey increased fairly steadily during the same period by overall factors of 2- to 6-fold (Florida Game and Fresh Water Fish Commission, 1968).

The maintenance or even increase of game is due largely to improved management. The state fish and game commissions deserve greatest credit, but farmers, ranchers, and foresters deserve credit, too. The difficulties have been great, and they remain so. The total area subject to complete habitat management is limited. Each year, more land is claimed for cities and highways. In general, game is produced on the poorest land. And yet, the fact of improved production is real. Of course, some years are better than others, but the trend is unmistakable, and it generally is consistent from state to state. An unusually dramatic example of increase involves white-tailed deer in Florida, where the recorded harvest of about 33,000 in 1967 exceeded the estimated total population of about 27,000 in 1942. This particular change was promoted not only by game management but by the eradication of the screw worm fly that attacked cattle as well as deer (Florida Game and Fresh Water Fish Commission, 1968).

The recognized and even the alleged harm to wildlife from pesticides tends to be localized both as regards geographical and species distribution. Sometimes only species that have very specialized habitat requirements are injured, and physical changes in the environment may, in themselves, be sufficient to cause the observed difficulty.

11.4 Control of Wildlife

Efforts to control wildlife have been made for centuries by individual farmers or groups of them intent on protecting their crops or herds. More or less recently, four major changes have occurred: (*a*) the means of control have become more diverse; (*b*) control has become the responsibility of government agencies as well as individuals; (*c*) the concept of control has extended to some forms of wildlife considered unfavorable to other forms of wildlife; and (*d*) there has been increasing disagreement as to whether one species or another should be controlled at all.

Considerable dependence is still placed on firearms for the control of large predatory birds and mammals. However, even for these species, and certainly for smaller forms, control is often by chemical means. As long as the effort is by individuals, it is unlikely to attract widespread criticism. When the control effort becomes official, it automatically becomes a target for persons with different economic or other interests or for persons of different political views.

In general, efforts to control enemies of game or other wildlife have attracted little public attention and most of that has been favorable. Examples include weed control in the feeding grounds of ducks, lamprey control in the Great Lakes, and the control of carp and other rough fish in ponds later restocked with sport fish.

It sometimes happens that ecologists, who are highly critical of pesticides and of other peoples' use of them, advocate some special use to which they themselves have contributed. An example is the sound, ecological use of herbicides for control of vegetation in right-of-ways and along roadsides and for naturalistic landscaping (Niering, 1968).

Efforts to control wildlife unfavorable to agriculture or forestry have been subject to more publicity and more severe criticism than is received by control programs to protect wildlife. The control of deer and similar animals, whether by hunting or other means, is almost always under the control of game managers. It is seldom criticized, but some groups even oppose hunting of managed herds. On the contrary, the control of mice in orchards and forests, the control of prairie dogs on open range, and especially the control of predatory birds and mammals commonly have led to debate about methods and even objectives. Some ecologists think coyotes (*Canis latrans*) maintain the balance of nature, but ranchers prefer that the particular balance not be maintained at the expense of their livestock. The case for ecology in the control of certain wildlife on marginal agricultural land has been described by Rudd (1964).

Ecological methods are unlikely to be used widely in agriculture until their effectiveness has been so thoroughly established and their methodology has become so perfected that farmers can be instructed in their use by county agricultural agents or by wildlife specialists.

Compounds that have been used in connection with wildlife include herbicides such as 2,4-D and 2,4,5-T; rodenticides such as sodium fluoroacetate and strychnine; fumigants such as cyanide; fish poisons such as rotenone and antimycin; and lampricides such as 3-bromo-4-nitrophenol and 3-trifluoromethyl-4-nitrophenol.

11.5 Limitations of Injury to Wildlife

11.5.1 Ecological Methods

It has been known for a long time that biotic simplification in agriculture increases the probability of injury from pests at the same time that it tends to increase crop yields. In some instances, it is practical to increase the diversity of a crop without reducing the yield. This is especially true in connection with pastures, ranges, and forests. A pasture composed of several species of grasses and broad-leaved plants, all wholesome for livestock, is less subject to destruction by pests than a pasture composed of one kind of grass. A mixed pasture is also better because the different plants mature at different times and may be used for a greater part of the year.

It is now possible to make paper from hardwoods as well as pine. It therefore becomes possible for the paper industry to plant and harvest a greater variety of trees.

The use of mixed stands in pastures or forests may make pest control unnecessary in these places. In connection with some other pests, especially commensal rodents, the limitation of food and shelter will reduce if not eliminate the need for chemical control (see Section 11.2.1.2).

11.5.2 Modified Use of Pesticides

When strictly ecological methods of control prove inadequate and the use of lethal chemicals is required, there is still much that can be done to shield wildlife. Protective measures include: (a) proper choice of pesticide; (b) limitation of dosage; (c) limitation of area of application; and (d) proper timing of application. Finally, (e) certain alternative methods that are either nonchemical or nonlethal, or both, may offer a possibility of pest control without significant injury to wildlife.

11.5.2.1 Choice of Compound.

Persistency. There seems to be general agreement that, of all pesticides, the persistent ones pose the major threat to wildlife (Rudd, 1964; Moore, 1966b). Some ecologists go so far as to suggest that if this problem were eliminated, no serious problem would remain. They cite the remarkable ability of populations to recover, provided the area from which the species has been eliminated is small or the survivors in a wider area are completely healthy and unimpeded. Early recognition serves to limit injury that is both immediate and spectacular, because efforts almost always are made to avoid a recurrence. Unfortunately, delayed effects of slowly increasing importance may be associated with persistent compounds.

Definition of the term "persistent pesticide" is not as easy as one might think. As discussed in Section 11.2.3.4, persistence has been confused with a tendency to cause biological magnification. The major offenders have been DDT, aldrin, dieldrin, heptachlor, mirex, and various alkyl mercury compounds. DDD was a problem at least in Clear Lake. All of these materials are degraded or dissipated slowly in air, water, and soil. Thus, they persist in the environment so that some species tend to receive a continuing intake. Once absorbed, they persist in the organism. Although strictly organic compounds are metabolized directly or indirectly to less toxic compounds, compounds of metals, whether organic or not, can only be metabolized to other toxic combinations.

The compounds now considered most injurious to wildlife are not known to produce damage disproportionate to their actual chemical accumulation in various species. This is true even of compounds that are metabolized and excreted promptly; if dosage is sufficient to produce injury, then the compound or a toxic metabolite can be demonstrated in the critical tissue during illness or at death. The possibility of injury to wildlife from compounds such as paralytic organic phosphorus compounds that produce chronic effects in the absence of chemical cumulation cannot be dismissed entirely. However, because of the very real danger of such compounds to man, their use is prohibited or severely limited. It seems unlikely that a compound of this kind would ever receive sufficiently widespread use to constitute a danger to wildlife.

Some uses of pesticides require persistency. Soil treatments for control of termites are useless unless they are long lasting. Indoor spraying for malaria control is doomed to failure unless each treatment persists for a month and preferably much longer. These particular uses have little or no effect on wildlife. On the contrary, it is clear that no real advantage is taken of the persistency of certain compounds known to injure wildlife when they are applied to cotton and other crops at intervals of a week or less. Thus, the uses that really require greatest persistency produce little or no injury to wildlife, simply because only relatively small quantities are involved and the compounds tend to remain where they are applied. The applications that make little or no real use of persistency are the ones that involve large tonnages, widespread application, and maximal availability to wildlife.

There would be great gain and little loss if use of highly persistent pesticides were restricted to those applications that require a high degree of persistence.

Specificity. All threat to wildlife would be eliminated and many problems of pest control would be solved if control could be specific. In spite of the use of broad spectrum pesticides, this goal is essentially reached in a few instances (eg, control of ectoparasites or indoor mosquitoes). However, the goal of specificity is far from accomplishment in connection with most agricultural and forest pests.

Some degree of specificity may be achieved by proper selection of conventional pesticides. For example, many organic phosphorus insecticides are less destructive to wild bees than carbaryl, which, however, produces a minimum of injury to other wildlife. Much greater specificity may be achieved in connection with some alternative methods of control discussed in Section 11.5.3.

Aid in Selection. The label is the most important aid in selecting compounds and specific formulations that will achieve control and yet minimize injury to wildlife. In the United States of America, the labels of all formulations likely to be used in such a way that they will contact wildlife are reviewed and if necessary revised by authorities in the Environmental Protection Agency, who have access to information developed by the Bureau of Sport Fisheries and Wildlife of the Department of the Interior. Thus, labels carry directions and warnings, which, if observed, not

only will protect man and domestic animals, but will help to protect wildlife. Unfortunately, there are no known solutions for some agricultural problems that are fully safe for wildlife. Such problems include widespread infestations with subterranean larvae of beetles and the need to prevent destruction of tree seed following their distribution for reforestation.

11.5.2.2 Limitations of Dosage. Since the toxic effects of compounds are dosage related, it follows that injury to wildlife may be minimized by using the smallest amount of pesticide necessary for control. The law of diminishing return places a limit on the rate at which pesticides may be applied profitably. However, there is a certain margin between the level that is barely effective and the highest profitable level. During recent years, increasing attention has been given to determining what the minimal effective level is. The problem is not an easy one and even an outline of it is beyond the scope of this chapter. Headley and Lewis (1967) have discussed the matter in their book, *The Pesticide Problem: An Economic Approach to Public Policy;* the different factors reviewed in their book must be considered realistically if application rates are to be reduced.

11.5.2.3 Limitation of Area of Application.

Extent of Area. Almost by definition, ecological effects are conditioned more by the duration and geographical extent of the injury than by its intensity. A flash flood that literally washes the fish out of a clear mountain stream will have little lasting effect compared to the gradual silting and warming that follow extensive destruction of forest on a large watershed. By the same token, serious injury to wildlife in a small area is often corrected much more quickly than perhaps less intense injury spread over whole states or continents. Not only does the difference have a scientific basis but its interpretation has a social basis. As soon as pest control extends to public lands or is carried out by a public agency it may become a target for public criticism and political attack. Clearly, public pest control must be carried out with more restraint and greater safeguards than is required in the private sector.

Character of Area. Even when the general extent of the area of application is fixed, considerable good can be done by excluding specific habitats. It is especially important to avoid direct application of pesticides to streams and lakes because of the unusual susceptibility of aquatic organisms. By the same token, mixing of formulations and disposal of used containers and waste pesticide should be done in such a way that contamination of water will not occur.

11.5.2.4 Timing of Application. It is sometimes possible to protect wildlife from a pesticide by adjusting the time of its application. Thus, injury to bees can be minimized by trying to avoid applications to cover crops while they are in bloom. If an insecticide is absolutely required during the blooming season, it may be applied at night or just after dawn, before the bees have left the hive. In a similar way, it may be possible to withhold application until bird nesting is past or until migratory birds have passed through.

11.5.3 Alternative Methods

What was said in Section 9.5 about the limited possibility of avoiding hazard to man through substitution of alternative methods for pest control also concerns hazards to wildlife. In fact, some alternative methods of control may be dangerous to wildlife although safe for man, just as is true of some chemicals. For example, the use of light to attract and control large sphinx moths that attack tobacco offers no danger to people but its harmlessness for other moths and even useful insects living in the same area remains to be proved. Thus, every new method of control, whether chemical, physical, or biological, must be studied individually to determine its effect on wildlife.

On the positive side, it must be said that methods will tend to be safe for wildlife to the extent that they are specific for the pest under attack. The use of male screwworm flies sterilized by radiation to eradicate this species in the eastern United States of America is not only one of the few examples of species eradication, but it is unique as an example of species specificity. The absolute specificity depended on the fact that the flies were reared and sterilized under essentially laboratory conditions. Unfortunately, the method must be adapted separately to each new use and this may be possible for few species of pests.

Finally, even specificity cannot exclude all complications. The use of myxoma virus in Britain affected directly only the rabbits it was meant to control; however, the ecological effects of myxomatosis were extremely complicated and involved many species of plants and animals (Moore, 1967).

The use of attractants seems to offer the most general promise of specificity. The attractants now known are compounds of striking specificity and low inherent toxicity.

When used in combination with poisons, it may be possible to use bait stations that prevent access of desirable species to the poison. Even when the combination of attractant and poison was exposed without any protection, as was done in the control of the oriental fruit fly (*Dacus dorsalis*), no detectable injury was done to wildlife because so little poison was required and most species had no contact with it.

REFERENCES

Adams, L., Hanavan, M. G., Hosley, N. W., and Johnston, D. W. (1949). The effects on fish, birds, and mammals of DDT used in the control of forest insects in Idaho and Wyoming. J. Wildl. Manage., 13:245–254.

Advisory Committee on Poisonous Substances Used in Agriculture and Food Storage (1964). *Review of the Persistent Organochlorine Pesticides.* H.M.S.O., London.

Anderson, D. W., and Hickey, J. J. (1970). Oological data on egg and breeding characteristics of brown pelicans. Wilson Bull., 82:14–28.

Anderson, D. W., and Hickey, J. J. (1972). Eggshell changes in certain North American birds. In: *Proceedings of the 15th International Ornithological Congress*, pp. 514–540. E. J. Brill, Leiden.

Anderson, D. W., Hickey, J. J., Risebrough, R. W., Hughes, D. F., and Christensen, R. E. (1969). Significance of chlorinated hydrocarbon residues to breeding pelicans and cormorants. Can. Field Nat., 83:91–112.

Anderson, D. W., and Kreitzer, J. F. (1971). Thickness of 1967–69 whooping crane eggshells compared to that of pre-1910 specimens. Auk, 88:433–434.

Baetke, K. P., Cain, J. D., and Poe, W. E. (1972). Residues in fish, wildlife, and estuaries: mirex and DDT residues in wildlife and miscellaneous samples in Mississippi— 1970. Pestic. Monit. J., 6:14–22.

Bagley, G. E., Reichel, W. L., and Cromartie, E. (1970). Identification of polychlorinated biphenyls in two bald eagles by combined gas-liquid chromatography-mass spectrometry. J. Assoc. Off. Anal. Chem., 53:251–261.

Banks, R. C. (1966). Terrestrial vertebrates of Anacapa Island, California. Trans. San Diego Soc. Nat. Hist., 14:173–188.

Barker, R. J. (1958). Notes of some ecological effects of DDT sprayed on elms. J. Wildl. Manage., 22:269–274.

Beebe, F. L. (1969). Passenger pigeons and peregrine ecology. In: *Peregrine Falcon Populations*, edited by J. J. Hickey, pp. 399–402. University of Wisconsin Press, Madison.

Belisle, A. A., Reichel, W. L., Locke, L. N., Lamont, T. G., Mulhern, B. M., Prouty, R. M., DeWolf, R. B., and Cromartie, E. (1972). Residues of organochlorine pesticides, polychlorinated biphenyls, and mercury and autopsy data for bald eagles, 1969 and 1970. Pestic. Monit. J., 6:133–138.

Bent, A. C. (1926). *Life Histories of North American Marsh Birds.* United States National Museum, Bulletin 135, US Government Printing Office, Washington, DC.

Bent, A. C. (1932). *Life Histories of North American Gallinaceous Birds.* United States National Museum, Bulletin 162, US Government Printing Office, Washington, DC.

Benton, A. H. (1951). Effects on wildlife of DDT used for control of Dutch elm disease. J. Wildl. Manage., 15:20–27.

Bitman, J., Cecil, H. C., Fries, G. F. (1970). DDT-induced inhibition of avian shell gland carbonic anhydrase: a mechanism for thin eggshells. Science, 168:594–596.

Bitman, J., Cecil, H. C., Harris, S. J., and Fries, G. F.

(1968). Estrogenic activity of *o, p'*-DDT in the mammalian uterus and avian oviduct. Science, 162:371–372.

Bitman, J., Cecil, H. C., Harris, S. J., and Fries, G. F. (1969). DDT induces a decrease in eggshell calcium. Nature, 224:44–46.

Blus, L. J. (1970). Measurements of brown pelican eggshells from Florida and South Carolina. Bioscience, 20:867–869.

Blus, L. J., Gish, C. D., Belisle, A. A., and Prouty, R. M. (1972). Logarithmic relationship of DDE residues to eggshell thinning. Nature, 235:376–377.

Blus, L. J., Heath, R. G., Gish, C. D., Belisle, A. A., and Prouty, R. M. (1971). Eggshell thinning in the brown pelican: implication of DDE. Bioscience, 21:1213–1215.

Bond, R. M. (1942). Banding records of California brown pelicans. Condor, 44:116–121.

Borg, K., Wanntorp, H., Erne, K., and Hanko, E. (1966). Mercury poisoning in Swedish wildlife. J. Appl. Ecol., 3:171–172.

Brodtman, N. V., Jr. (1970). Studies on the assimilation of 1,1,1-trichloro-2,2-bis-(*p*-chlorophenyl) ethane (DDT) by *Crassostrea virginica* Gmelin. Bull. Environ. Contam. Toxicol., 5:455–462.

Burdick, G. E., Harris, E. J., Dean, H. J., Walker, T. M., Skea, J., and Colby, D. (1964). The accumulation of DDT in lake trout and the effect on reproduction. Trans. Am. Fish. Soc., 93:127–136.

Burnett, R. (1971). DDT residues: distribution of concentrations in *Emerita analoga* (Stimpson) along coastal California. Science, 174:606–608.

Butler, P. A. (1966). Pesticides in the marine environment. J. Appl. Ecol., 3(Suppl.):253–259.

Butler, P. A., and Springer, P. F. (1963). Pesticides—a new factor in coastal environments. Transactions 28th North American Wildlife and Natural Resources Conference, pp. 378–390.

Cade, T. J., and Fyfe, R. (1970). The North American peregrine survey, 1970. Can. Field Nat., 84:231–245.

Cade, T. J., Lincer, J. L., White, C. M., Roseneau, D. G., and Swartz, L. G. (1971). DDE residues and eggshell changes in Alaskan falcons and hawks. Science, 173:955–957.

Colson, R. B. (1973). Personal communication.

Cooke, A. S. (1973). Shell thinning in avian eggs by environmental pollutants. Environ. Pollut., 4:85–152.

Coon, N. C., Locke, L. N., Cromartie, E., and Reichel, W. L. (1970). Causes of bald eagle mortality, 1960–1965. J. Wildl. Dis., 6:72–76.

Cope, O. B. (1971). Interaction between pesticides and wildlife. Annu. Rev. Entomol., 16:325–364.

Crosby, D. G. (1972). Environmental photooxidation of pesticides. In: *Degradation of Synthetic Organic Molecules in the Biosphere,* pp. 260–278. National Academy of Sciences, Washington, DC.

Dawson, W. L. (1923). *The Birds of California.* Vol. 4, pp. 1970–1982, South Moulton Co., Los Angeles.

Dimond, J. B., Belyea, G. Y., Kaduce, R. E., Getchell, A. S., and Blease, J. A. (1970). DDT residues in robins and earthworms associated with contaminated forest soils. Can. Entomol., 102:1122–1130.

Dimond, J. B., and Sherburne, J. A. (1969). Persistence of DDT in wild populations of small mammals. Nature, 221:486–487.

Dindal, D. L., and Peterle, T. J. (1968). Wing and body tissue relationships of DDT and metabolite residues in mallard and lesser scaup ducks. Bull. Environ. Contamin. Toxicol., 3:37–48.

Dustman, E. H., Martin, W. E., Heath, R. G., and Reichel, W. L. (1971). Monitoring pesticides in wildlife. Pestic. Monit. J., 5:50–52.

Dustman, E. H., Stickel, L. F., and Elder, J. B. (1972). Mercury in wild animals, Lake St. Clair, 1970. In *Environmental Mercury Contamination,* edited by R. Hartung and B. D. Dinman, pp. 46–52. Ann Arbor

Science Publishers, Ann Arbor, Mich.

Dvorchik, B. H., Istin, M., and Maren, T. H. (1971). Does DDT inhibit carbonic anhydrase? Science, 172:728–729.

Edwards, C. A. (1970). Persistent pesticides in the environment. In: *Critical Reviews in Environmental Control,* Vol. 1, Issue 1, pp. 1–67. Chemical Rubber Publishing Company, Cincinatti.

Elson, P. F. (1967). Effects on wild young salmon of spraying DDT over New Brunswick forests. J. Fish. Res. Board Can., 24:731–767.

Enderson, J. H., and Berger, D. D. (1968). Chlorinated hydrocarbon residues in peregrines and their prey species from Northern Canada. Condor, 70:149–153.

Enderson, J. H., and Berger, D. D. (1970). Pesticides: eggshell thinning and lowered production of young in prairie falcons. Bioscience, 20:355–356.

Erben, H. K., and Krampitz, G. (1971). Eischalen DDT-verseuchter Vögel: Ultrastruktur and organische Substanz. Abh. math-naturw. Klin. Akad. Wiss. Mainz, 1971 (2):31–64.

Faber, R. A., and Hickey, J. J. (1973). Eggshell thinning, chlorinated hydrocarbons, and mercury in inland aquatic bird eggs, 1969 and 1970. Pestic. Monit. J., 7:27–36.

Ferguson, D. E., Ludke, J. L., and Murphy, G. G. (1966). Dynamics of endrin uptake and release by resistant and susceptible strains of mosquitofish. Trans. Am. Fish. Soc., 95:335–344, 1966.

Finley, M. T., Ferguson, D. E., Ludke, J. L. (1970). Possible selective mechanisms in the development of insecticide-resistant fish. Pestic. Monit. J., 4:212–218.

Flickinger, E. L., and King, K. A. (1972). Some effects of aldrin-treated rice on Gulf Coast wildlife. J. Wildl. Manage., 36:706–727.

Florida Game and Fresh Water Fish Commission (1968). *A Quarter Century of Progress.* Publications-Printing Department, Florida Wildlife Magazine.

Fyfe, R. W., Campbell, B., Hayson, B., and Hodson, K. (1969). Regional population declines and organochlorine insecticides in Canadian prairie falcons. Can. Field Nat., 83:190–200.

George, J. L., and Frear, D. E. H. (1966). Pesticides in the Antarctic. J. Appl. Ecol., 3:(Suppl.)155–167.

George, J. L., and Stickel, W. H. (1949). Wildlife effects of DDT dust used for tick control on a Texas prairie. Am. Midl. Nat., 42:228–237.

Giam, C. S., Hanks, A. R., Richardson, R. L., Sackett, W. M., and Wong, M. K. (1972). DDT, DDE, and polychlorinated biphenyls in biota from the Gulf of Mexico and Caribbean Sea—1971. Pestic. Monit. J., 6:139–159.

Gillett, J. W., Porter, R. D., Wiemeyer, S. N., Gram, T. H., Schroeder, D. H., and Gillett, J. R. (1970). Induction of liver microsomal activities in Japanese quail. With supplemental information on: the induction of microsomal ethylmorphine demethylase activity in sparrow hawk livers by diets containing DDT and dieldrin or DDE. In: *The Biological Impact of Pesticides in the Environment.* Proceedings of Symposium held August 18–20, 1969, Environ. Health Sci. Ser. No. 1, edited by J. W. Gillett, pp. 59–64. Oregon State University, Corvallis.

Gilpin, M. E., and Rosenzweig, M. L. (1972). Enriched predator-prey systems: Theoretical stability. Science, 177:902–904.

Gish, C. D. (1970). Organochlorine insecticide residues in soils and soil invertebrates. Pestic. Monit. J., 3:241–252.

Goodrum, P., Baldwin, W. P., and Aldrich, J. W. (1949). Effect of DDT on animal life of Bull's Island, South Carolina. J. Wildl. Manage., 13:1–10.

Graham, R. J. (1959). Effects of forest insect spraying on trout and aquatic insects in some Montana streams. In: *Biological Problems in Water Pollution, Transactions of the 1959 Seminar.* US Department of Health, Education, and Welfare, Washington, DC.

Gress, F., Risebrough, R. W., Anderson, D. W., Kiff, L. F., and Jehl, T. R. (1973). Reproductive failures of double-crested cormorants in Southern California and Baja California. Wilson Bull., 85:197–208.

Haegele, M. A., and Hudson, R. H. (1973). DDE effects on reproduction of ring doves. Environ. Pollut., 4:53–57.

Harris, E. J. (1973). Personal communication.

Harris, E. J., and Karcher, R. W., Jr. (1972). Mercury: its historical presence in New York State fishes. Chemist, May.

Hayes, W. J., Jr. (1959). Pharmacology and toxicology of DDT. In: DDT, the Insecticide Dichloro-diphenyltrichloroethane and Its Significance, edited by P. Muller. Vol. 2, pp. 9–247. Birkhauser Verlag, Basel.

Headley, J. C., and Lewis, J. N. (1967). The Pesticide Problem: An Economic Approach to Public Policy. The Johns Hopkins Press, Baltimore.

Heath, R. G. (1969). Nationwide residues of organochlorine pesticides in wings of mallards and black ducks. Pestic. Monit. J., 3:115–123.

Heath, R. G., Spann, J. W., and Kreitzer, J. F. (1969). Marked DDE impairment of mallard reproduction in controlled studies. Nature, 224:47–48.

Heath, R. G., Spann, J. W., Hill, E. F., and Kreitzer, J. F. (1972a). Comparative dietary toxicities of pesticides to birds. Special Science Report No. 152, US Fish and Wildlife Service, Washington, DC.

Heath, R. G., Spann, J. W., Kreitzer, J. F., and Vance, C. (1972b). Effects of polychlorinated biphenyls on birds. In: Proceedings of the XVth International Ornithological Congress, edited by K. H. Voous, pp. 475–485. E. J. Brill, Leiden.

Henny, C. J. (1972). An Analysis of the Population Dynamics of Selected Avian Species. With Special Reference to Changes During the Modern Pesticide Era. Bureau of Sport Fisheries and Wildlife, Washington, DC.

Herald, E. S. (1949). Notes on the effects of aircraft-distributed DDT-oil spray upon certain Philippine fishes. J. Wildl. Manage., 13:316–318.

Herman, S, G., Garrett, R. L., and Rudd, R. L. (1969). Pesticides and the western grebe. In: Chemical Fallout, edited by M. W. Miller and G. G. Berg, pp. 24–53. Charles C Thomas, Springfield, Ill.

Hess, A. D., and Keener, G. G., Jr. (1947). Effect of airplane-distributed DDT thermal aerosols on fish and fish food organisms. J. Wildl. Manage., 11:1–10.

Hickey, J. J. (1942). Eastern population of the duck hawk. Auk, 59:176–204.

Hickey, J. J. (1943). A Guide to Bird Watching. Oxford University Press, London.

Hickey, J. J. (ed.) (1969). Peregrine Falcon Populations: Their Biology and Decline. The University of Wisconsin Press, Madison.

Hickey, J. J. (1970). Peregrine falcons, pollutants, and propoganda. Can. Field Nat., 84:207–208.

Hickey, J. J., and Anderson, D. W. (1968). Chlorinated hydrocarbons and eggshell changes in raptorial and fish-eating birds. Science, 162:271–273.

Hickey, J. J., and Roelle, J. E. (1969). Conference summary and conclusions. In: Peregrine Falcon Populations, edited by J. J. Hickey, pp. 553–567. The University of Wisconsin Press, Madison.

Hoffman, C. H., and Merkel, E. P. (1948). Fluctuations in insect populations associated with aerial applications of DDT to forests. J. Econ. Entomol., 41:464–473.

Hoffman, C. H., and Surber, E. W. (1948). Effects of an aerial application of wettable DDT on fish and fish-food organisms in Back Creek, West Virginia. Trans. Am. Fish. Soc., 75:48–58.

Hoffman, C. H., and Surber, E. W. (1949). Effects of an aerial application of DDT on fish and fish-food organisms in two Pennsylvania watersheds. Prog. Fish-Cult., 11:203–211.

Hoffman, C. H., Townes, H. K., Sailer, R. I., and Swift, H.

H. (1946). Field Studies on the Effect of DDT on Aquatic Insects. US Dept. Agriculture, Washington, DC.

Hoffman, C. H., Townes, H. K., Swift, H. H., and Sailer, R. I. (1949). Field studies on the effects of airplane applications of DDT on forest invertebrates. Ecol. Monogr., 19:1–46.

Holden, A. V. (1962). A study of the absorption of ^{14}C-labeled DDT from water by fish. Ann. Appl. Biol., 50:467–477.

Hotchkiss, N., and Pough, R. H. (1946). Effects on forest birds of DDT used for gypsy moth control in Pennsylvania. J. Wildl. Manage., 10:202–207.

Jefferies, D. J. (1969). Induction of apparent hyperthyroidism in birds fed DDT. Nature, 222: 578–579.

Jefferies, D. J., and French, M. C. (1969). Avian thyroid: effect of p,p'-DDT on size and activity. Science 166:1278–1280.

Jehl, J. R., Jr. (1969). The brown pelican, a vanishing American. Environ. Southwest, June:4.

Jehl, J. R., Jr. (1973). Studies of a declining population of brown pelicans in northwestern Baja California. Condor, 75: 69–79.

Johnson, R. E., Carver, T. C., and Dustman, E. H. (1967). Residues in fish, wildlife, and estuaries. Pestic. Monit. J., 1:7–13.

Kalmbach, E. R., Imler, R. H., and Arnold, L. W. (1964). The American Eagles and their Economic Status, 1964. US Department of the Interior, Washington, DC.

Keith, J. A. (1966). Reproduction in a population of herring gulls (Larus argentatus) contaminated by DDT. J. Appl. Ecol., 3:57–70.

Keith, J. A., and Gruchy, I. M. (1972). Residue levels of chemical pollutants in North American birdlife. In: Proceedings of the XVth International Ornithological Congress, edited by K. H. Voous, pp. 450–451. E. J. Brill, Leiden.

Keith, J. O., Woods, L. A., Hunt, E. G., (1970). Reproductive failure in brown pelicans on the Pacific coast. In: Transactions of the Thirty-Fifth North American Wildlife and Natural Resources Conference, pp. 56–64. The Wildlife Management Institute, Washington, DC.

Keller, H. (1952). Die Bestimmung Kleinster Mengen DDT und enzymanalytischem sege. Naturwissenschaften, 39:109.

Kendeigh, S. C. (1947). Bird population studies in the coniferous Forest Biome during a spruce budworm outbreak. Canada, Department of Lands and Forests, Div. Res. Biol. Bull., 1:1–100.

Koeman, J. H., vanBeusekom, C. F., and de Goeij, J. J. M. (1972). Eggshell and population changes in the sparrow-hawk (Accipter nisus). TNO-Nieuws, 27: 542–550.

Krantz, W. C., Mulhern, B. M., Bagley, G. E., Sprunt, A., IV, Ligas, F. J., and Robertson, W. B., Jr. (1970). Organochlorine and heavy metal residues in bald eagle eggs. Pestic. Monit. J., 4:136–140.

Kreitzer, J. F. (1971). Eggshell thickness in mourning dove populations. J. Wildl. Manage., 35:563–564.

Kury, C. R. (1969). Pesticide residues in a marine population of double-crested cormorants. J. Wildl. Manage., 33:91–95.

Lamont, T. G., Bagley, G. E., and Reichel, W. L. (1970). Residues of o,p'-DDD and o,p'-DDT in brown pelican eggs and mallard ducks. Bull. Environ. Contam. Toxicol., 5:231–236.

Lamont, T., and Reichel, W. (1970). Organochlorine pesticide residues in whooping cranes and everglade kits. Auk, 87:158–159.

Lehner, P. N., and Egbert, A. (1969). Dieldrin and eggshell thickness in ducks. Nature, 224:1218–1219.

Linduska, J. P., and Surber, E. W. (1948). Effects of DDT and other insecticides on fish and wildlife. Summary of investigations during 1947. US Fish and Wildlife Service Circ., 15:1–19.

Longcore, J. R., Samson, R. B., and Whittendale, T. W., Jr.

(1971). DDE thins eggshells and lowers reproductive success of captive black ducks. Bull. Environ. Contam. Toxicol., 6:485–490.

Martin, W. E. (1969). Organochlorine insecticide residues in starlings. Pestic. Monit. J., 3:102–114.

Martin, W. E., and Nickerson, P. R. (1972). Organochlorine residues in starlings—1970. Pestic. Monit. J., 6:33–40.

May, R. M. (1972). Limit cycles in predator-prey communities. Science, 177:900–902.

May, C., and Baker, W. L. (1952). Forests, trees, and pests. In: Insects. The Yearbook of Agriculture, 1952, pp. 677–682. US Government Printing Office, Washington, DC.

McLane, M. A. R., and Hall, L. C. (1972). DDE thins screech owl eggshells. Bull. Environ. Contam. Toxicol., 8:65–68.

Metcalf, R. L., Hess, A. D., Smith, G. E., Jeffrey, G. M., and Ludwig, G. L. (1945). Observations on the use of DDT for the control of Anopheles quadrimaculatus. Public Health Rep., 60:753–774.

Metcalf, R. L., Kapoor, I. P., and Hirwe, A. S. (1971a). Biodegradable analogues of DDT. Bull. WHO, 44:363–374.

Metcalf, R. L., Sangha, G. K., and Kapoor, I. P. (1971b). Model ecosystem for the evaluation of pesticides biodegradability and ecological magnification. Environ. Sci. Technol., 5:709–713.

Miller, M. W., and Berg, G. G. (eds.) (1969). Chemical Fallout. Charles C Thomas, Springfield, Ill.

Moore, N. W. (ed.) (1966a). Pesticides in the Environment and Their Effects on Wildlife. Supplement to Vol. 3 of J. Appl. Ecol.,pp. xii and 311. Blackwell Scientific Publications, Oxford.

Moore, N. W. (ed.) (1966b). An assessment of the discussions. In: Pesticides in the Environment and Their Effects on Wildlife. Supplement to Vol. 3 of J. Appl. Ecol., pp. 291–295. Blackwell Scientific Publications, Oxford.

Moore, N. W. (1967). Effects of pesticides on wildlife. Proc. R. Soc. B, 167:128–133.

Morris, R. L., and Johnson, L. G. (1971). Dieldrin levels in fish from Iowa streams. Pestic. Monit. J., 5:12–16.

Mulhern, B. M., Reichel, W. L., Locke, L. N., Lamont, T. G., Belisle, A., Cromartie, E., Bagley, G. E., and Prouty, R. M. (1970). Organochlorine residues and autopsy data from bald eagles 1966–68. Pestic. Monit. J., 4:141–144.

Murton, R. L., and Vizoso, M. (1963). Dressed cereal seed as a hazard to wood-pigeons. Ann. Appl. Biol., 52: 503–517.

Niering, W. A. (1968). The effects of pesticides. Bioscience, 18:869–875.

Peakall, D. B. (1970a). p,p'-DDT: Effects on calcium metabolism and concentrations of estradiol in the blood. Science, 168:592–594.

Peakall, D. B. (1970b). Pesticides and the reproduction of birds. Sci. Am., 222:72–78.

Peterle, T. J. (1969). DDT in Antarctic snow. Nature, 224:620.

Pimentel, D. (1971). Ecological Effects of Pesticides on Non-Target Species. Executive Office of the President Office of Science and Technology. US Government Printing Office, Washington, DC.

Porter, R. D., and Wiemeyer, S. N. (1969). Dieldrin and DDT: effects on sparrow hawk eggshells and reproduction. Science, 165:199–200.

Porter, R. D., and Wiemeyer, S. N. (1972). DDE at low dietary levels, kills captive American Kestrels. Bull. Environ. Contam. Toxicol., 8:193–199.

Potts, G. R. (1968). Success of eggs of the shag on the Farne Islands, Northumberland, in relation to their content of dieldrin and p,p'-DDE. Nature, 217:1282–1284.

Prestt, I. (1965). An inquiry into the recent breeding status of some of the smaller birds of prey and crows in Britain. Bird Study, 12:196–221.

Ratcliffe, D. A. (1958). Broken eggs in peregrine eyries. Br. Birds, 51:23–26.

Ratcliffe, D. A. (1963). The status of the peregrine in Great Britain. Bird Study, 10:56–90.

Ratcliffe, D. A. (1967). Decrease in eggshell weight in certain birds of prey. Nature, 215:208–210.

Ratcliffe, D. A. (1969). Population trends of the peregrine falcon in Great Britain. In: Peregrine Falcon Populations, edited by J. J. Hickey, pp. 239–269. University of Wisconsin Press, Madison.

Ratcliffe, D. A. (1970). Changes attributable to pesticides in egg breakage frequency and eggshell thickness in some British birds. J. Appl. Ecol., 7:67–115.

Ratcliffe, D. A. (1972). The peregrine population of Great Britain in 1971. Bird Study, 19: 117–156.

Reichel, W. L., and Addy, C. E. (1968). A survey of chlorinated pesticide residues in black duck eggs. Bull. Environ. Contam. Toxicol., 3:174–179.

Reichel, W. L., Cromartie, E., Lamont, T. G., Mulhern, B. M., and Prouty, R. M. (1969b). Pesticide residues in eagles. Pestic. Monit. J., 3:142–144.

Reichel, W. L., Lamont, T. G., Cromartie, E., and Locke, L. N. (1969a). Residues in two bald eagles suspected of pesticide poisoning. Bull. Environ. Contam. Toxicol., 4:24–30.

Ribicoff, A., and Larrick, G. P. (1964). Presence of DDT in fish oils. In: Intragency Coordination in Environmental hazards (Pesticides), Part I. Hearings before the Subcommittee on Reorganization and International Organizations of the Committee on Government Operations, United States Senate, Eighty-eighth Congress, First Session, May 16, 22, 23: June 4, 25, 1963. US Government Printing Office, Washington, DC.

Risebrough, R. W., David J., and Anderson, D. W. (1970). Effects of various chlorinated hydrocarbons. In: The Biological Impact of Pesticides in the Environment. Proceedings of Symposium held August 18–20, 1969, Environ. Health Sci. Ser. No. 1, edited by J. W. Gillett, pp. 40–53. Oregon State University, Corvallis.

Risebrough, R. W., Reiche, P., Peakall, D. B. Herman, S. G., and Kirven, M. N. (1968). Polychlorinated biphenyls in the global ecosystem. Nature, 220:1098–1102.

Risebrough, R. W., Sibley, F. C. and Kirven, M. N. (1971). Reproductive failure of the brown pelican on Anacapa Island in 1969. Am. Birds, 25:8–9.

Robbins, C. S., and Stewart, R. E. (1949). Effects of DDT on bird populations of scrub forest. J. Wildl. Manage., 13:11–16.

Robel, R. J., Stalling, C. D., Westfahl, M. E., and Kadoum, A. M. (1972). Effects of insecticides on populations of rodents in Kansas—1965–69. Pestic. Monit. J., 6:115–121.

Robinson, J. (1969). Organochlorine insecticides and bird populations in Britain. In: Chemical Fallout, edited by M. W. Miller and G. G. Berg. pp. 113–173. Charles C Thomas, Springfield, Ill.

Rosato, P., and Ferguson, D. E. (1968). The toxicity of endrin-resistant mosquitofish to eleven species of vertebrates. Bioscience, 18:783–784.

Rudd, R. L. (1964). Pesticides and the Living Landscape. University of Wisconsin Press, Madison.

Rudd, R. L., and Genelly, R. E. (1956). Pesticides: Their Use and Toxicity in Relation to Wildlife. State of California Department of Fish and Game, Game Bull. No. 7.

Rudd, R. L., and Herman, S. G. (1972). Ecosystemic transferal of pesticides residues in an aquatic environment. In: Environmental Toxicology of Pesticides, Part VII: Toxic Effect of Pesticide Residues on Wildlife, edited by F. Matsumura, G. M. Boush, and T. Misato, pp. 471–485. Academic Press, New York.

Schafer, E. W. (1972). The acute oral toxicity of 369 pesticidal, pharmaceutical and other chemicals to wild birds. Toxicol. Appl. Pharmacol., 21: 315–330.

Schmid, F. C. (1966). The status of the osprey in Cape May County, New Jersey between 1939 and 1963. Chesapeake Sci., 7:220–223.

Scott, H. M., Jungherr, E., and Matterson, L. D. (1944). The effect of feeding sulphanimide to the laying fowl. Poult. Sci., 23:446–453.

Sladen, W. J. L., Menzie, C. M., and Reichel, W. L. (1966). DDT residues in Adelie penguins and a crabeater seal from Antarctica. Nature, 210: 670–673.

Spann, J. W., Heath, R. G. Kreitzer, J. F., and Locke, L. N. (1972). Ethyl mercury p-toluene sulfonanilide: lethal and reproductive effects on pheasants. Science, 175: 328-331.

Speirs, J. M. (1949). The relation of DDT spraying to the vertebrate life of the forest, 1946. Canada, Department of Lands and Forests, Div. Res. Biol. Bull., 2:1–141.

Spofford, W. R. (1969). Hawk mountain counts as population indices in Northeastern America. In: Peregrine Falcon Populations, edited by J. J. Hickey, pp. 323–332. The University of Wisconsin Press, Madison.

Springer, P. F., and Webster, J. R. (1949). Effects of DDT on saltmarsh wildlife: 1949. US Fish and Wildlife Service, Special Sci. Rep., 10: 1–25.

Springer, P. F., and Webster, J. R. (1951). Biological effects of DDT applications on tidal salt marshes. Mosquito News, 11:67–74.

Stewart, R. E., Cope, J. B., Robbins, C. S., and Brainerd, J. W. (1946). Effects of DDT on birds at the Patuxent Research Refuge. J. Wildl. Manage., 10:195–201.

Stickel, L. F. (1946). Field Studies of a Peromyscus population in an area treated with DDT. J. Wildl. Manage., 10:216–218.

Stickel, L. F. (1973). Pesticide residues in birds and mammals. In: Environmental Pollution by Pesticides, edited by C. A. Edwards, pp. 254–312. Plenum Press, London.

Stickel, L. F., and Rhodes, L. I. (1970). The thin eggshell problem. In: The Biological Impact of Pesticides in the Environment. Proceedings of Symposium held August 18–20, 1969, Environ. Health Sci. Ser. No. 1, edited by J. W. Gillett, pp. 31–35. Oregon State University, Corvallis.

Stoewsand, G. S., Anderson, J. L., Gutenmann, W. H., Bache, C. A., and Lisk, D. J. (1971). Eggshell thinning in Japanese quail fed mercuric chloride. Science, 173:1030–1031.

Surber, E. W., and Friddle, D. D. (1949). Relative toxicity of suspension and oil formulations of DDT to native fishes in Back Creek, West Virginia. Trans. Am. Fish. Soc., 76:315–321.

Switzer, B., Lewin, V., and Wolfe, F. H. (1971). Shell thickness DDE levels in eggs, and reproductive success in common terns (Sterna hirundo) in Alberta. Can. J. Zool., 49:69–73.

Tarzwell, C. M. (1947). Effects of DDT mosquito larvicid-

ing on wildlife. I. The effects on surface organisms of the routine hand application of DDT larvicides for mosquito control. Public Health Rep., 62:525–554.

Tarzwell, C. M. (1948). Effects of routine DDT mosquito larviciding on wildlife. J. Natl. Malar. Soc., 7:199–206.

Tarzwell, C. M. (1950). Effects of DDT mosquito larviciding on wildlife. V. Effects on fishes of the routine manual and airplane application of DDT and other mosquito larvicides. Public Health Rep., 65:231–255.

Tarzwell, C. M. (1965). The toxicity of synthetic pesticides to aquatic organisms and suggestions for meeting the problem. In: Ecology and the Industrial Society. Fifth Symposium of the British Ecological Society. Blackwell Scientific Publications, Oxford.

Tatton, J. O'G., and Ruzicka, J. H. A. (1967). Organochlorine pesticides in Antarctica. Nature, 215:346–348.

Tucker, R. K., and Crabtree, D. G. (1970). Handbook of Toxicity of Pesticides to Wildlife. Bureau of Sport Fisheries and Wildlife, Resource Publ. No. 84. US Government Printing Office, Washington, DC.

Tucker, R. K., and Haegele, H. A. (1970). Eggshell thinning as influenced by method of DDT exposure. Bull Environ. Contam. Toxicol., 5:191–194.

Turtle, E. E., Taylor, A., Wright, E. N., Thearle, R. J. P., Egan, H., Evans, W. H., and Soutar, N. M. (1963). The effects on birds of certain chlorinated insecticides used as seed dressings. J. Sci. Food Agric., 14:567–577.

US Department of the Interior (for specific years). Fur Catch of the United States. Compiled from individual state records by the Division of Wildlife Research, Fish and Wildlife Service. Wildlife Leaflets Nos., 380, 388, 398, 424, 436, 444, 452, 460, 471, 474, 478, 482, 488, 493, 499.

Vermeer, K., and Reynolds, L. M. (1970). Organochlorine residues in aquatic birds in the Canadian prairie provinces. Can. Field Nat., 84:117–130.

Vincent, J. (1966). Red Data Book. Vol. 2. Aves. International Union for Conservation of Nature and Resources, Lausanne.

Wallace, G. J., Nickell, W. P., and Bernard, R. F. (1961). Bird mortality in the Dutch elm disease program in Michigan. Cranbrook Inst. Sci. Bull. 41:1–44.

Wiemeyer, S. N., Mulhern, B. M., Ligas, F. J., Hensel, R. J., Mathisen, J. E., Robards, F. C., and Postupalsky, S. (1972). Residues of organochlorine pesticides, polychlorinated biphenyls, and mercury in bald eagle eggs and changes in shell thickness—1969 and 1970. Pestic. Monit. J., 6:50–55.

Wiemeyer, S. N., and Porter, R. D. (1970). DDE thins eggshells of captive American kestrels. Nature, 227:737–738.

Chemical Names and CAS Registry Numbers of Compounds
Mentioned in This Volume Arranged by Group[a, b]

Nonproprietary name[b]		Chemical name	CAS No.
Inorganic and Organometal Pesticides			
arsenic		arsenic	
arsenic trioxide; 1810		arsenic trioxide	1327-53-3
cacodylic acid	WSA	dimethyl arsinic acid	75-60-5
calcium arsenate; 1907		tricalcium arsenate	**7778-44-1**
lead arsenate; 1892		lead arsenate	7645-25-2
MSMA; 1964	WSA	monosodium acid methanearsonate	2163-80
Paris green; 1867		copper acetoarsenite	12770-31-9
zinc arsenite; 1912 [ZMA]		zinc arsenite	10326-24-6
barium		barium	
barium carbonate		barium carbonate	513-77-9
chlorine			
sodium chlorate		sodium chlorate	7775-09-9
copper			
copper sulfate			7758-98-7
oxine-copper; 1942	ISO	copper 8-hydroxyquinolinolate	10380-28-6
fluorine			
cryolite; 1924		sodium aluminofluoride	15096-52-3
sodium fluoride		sodium fluoride	7681-49-4
lead		lead	
lead arsenate; 1892		lead arsenate	7645-25-2
mercury			
ethyl mercury compounds		ethyl mercury compounds	
mercuric **chloride**		mercuric chloride	7487-94-7
methyl mercury compounds		methyl mercury compounds	
phenyl mercuric acetate; 1945		phenyl mercuric acetate	62-38-4

Nonproprietary name	Chemical name	CAS No.

Inorganic and Organometal Pesticides (cont'd)

phosphorus	phosphorus	7723-14-0
sulfur	sulfur	
lime-sulfur; 1880	sulfur, water, and lime	
thallium	thallium	
thallium sulfate	thallium sulfate	7446-18-6
tin		
fentin acetate	triphenyltin	900-95-8
tricyclohexyltin hydroxide [Plictran®]	tricyclohexyltin hydroxide	13121-70-5

Pesticides Derived from Plants and Other Organisms

anabasine	L-3-(2'-piperidyl)pyridine	494-52-0
chlorotetracycline; 1955	7-chloro-4-dimethylamino-1, 4, 4a, 5, 5a, 6, 11, 12a-pentahydroxy-6-methyl-1, 11-dioxo-2-naphthacene-carboximide	57-62-5
cube; 1924	a vegetable preparation used as an insecticide and as a source of rotenone	
derris	a vegetable preparation used as an insecticide and as a source of rotenone	
gibberellic acid; 1960	gibberellic acid	77-06-5
nicotine; 1909	3-(1-methyl-2-pyrrolidyl)pyridine	54-11-5

pyrethrum and related compounds

allethrin; 1950	ESA, ISO	2, 2-dimethyl-3-(2-methylpropenyl) cyclopropanecarboxylic acid ester with 2-allyl-4-hydroxy-3-methyl-2-cyclo-penten-1-one	584-79-2
barthrin	ESA	6-chloropiperonyl 2, 2-dimethyl-3-(2-methylpropenyl)cyclopropanecarboxylate	70-43-9
pyrethrin I		2, 2-dimethyl-3-(2-methylpropenyl)cyclo-propanecarboxylic acid ester with 4-hydroxy-3-methyl-2-(2, 4-pentadienyl)-2-cyclopenten-1-one; pyretholone ester of chrysanthemum-monocarboxylic acid	121-21-1
pyrethrum; 1880		dried flower heads of Chrysanthemum cinariaefolium	8003-34-7
tetramethrin; 1971	ISO	2, 2-dimethyl-3-(2-methylpropenyl)cyclo-propanecarboxylic acid esters with N-(hydroxymethyl)-1-cyclohexene-1, 2-diacarboximide	7696-12-0

Nonproprietary name	Chemical name	CAS No.

Pesticides Derived from Plants and Other Organisms (cont'd.)

rotenone	1, 2, 12, 12a tetrahydro-2-isopropenyl-8, 9-dimethyoxy-[1]benzopyrano-[3, 4, 6] furo[2, 3-6][1]benzopyran-6(6aH)-one	83-79-4
sabadilla	sabadilla	8028-57-7
streptomycin; 1955 ISO	2, 4-diguanidino-3, 5, 6-trihydroxycyclo-hexyl-5-deoxy-2-0-(2-deoxy-2-methyl-amino-α-glycopyranosyl)-3-formyl pentofuranoside	57-92-1
strychnine	strychnine	57-24-9

Synergists

piperonyl butoxide; 1948	α[2-(2-n-butoxyethoxy)-ethoxy]-4, 5-methylenedioxy-2-propyl-toluene	51-03-6
piperonyl sulfoxide	1, 2-methylenedioxy-4-[2-(octylsulfinyl) propyl]-benzene	23715-11-9
n-propylisome	dipropyl-5, 6, 7, 8-tetrahydro-7-methyl-naphtho[2, 3-d]-1, 3-dioxole-5, 6-dicarboxylate	83-59-0
safrole	safrole	94-59-7
sesame oil	sesame oil	8008-74-0
sesamex	2-(2-ethoxyethoxy)ethyl-3, 4-(methylene-dioxy)phenyl acetal of acetaldehyde	51-14-9

Solvents, Propellants, and Oil Insecticides

dichlorodifluoromethane [Freon-12®]	dichlorodifluoromethane	75-71-8
kerosene	kerosene	8008-20-6
Tetralin®	1, 2, 3, 4-tetrahydronaphthalene	119-64-2
xylene	xylene	1330-20-7

Fumigants and Nematocides

acrylonitrile; 1953	propenenitrile	107-13-1
carbon disulfide; 1949	carbon disulfide	75-15-0
carbon tetrachloride; 1948	carbon tetrachloride	56-23-5
chloroform	trichloromethane	67-66-3
chloropicrin; 1949	trichloronitromethane	76-06-2
cyanide and related compounds	cyanide	57-12-5
calcium cyanide; 1922	calcium cyanide	592-01-8
calcium cyanamide; 1953	calcium cyanamide	156-62-7
hydrogen cyanide; 1877 [HCN]	hydrogen cyanide	74-90-8

Nonproprietary name	Chemical name	CAS No.

Fumigants and Nematocides (cont'd.)

Nonproprietary name	Chemical name	CAS No.
1, 2-dibromoethane; 1948	1, 2-dibromoethane	106-93-4
o-dichlorobenzene	o-dichlorobenzene	95-50-1
p-dichlorobenzene	p-dichlorobenzene	106-46-7
1, 1-dichloroethane	1, 1-dichloroethane	75-34-3
1, 2-dichloroethane; 1927	1, 2-dichloroethane	107-06-2
dichloroethyl ether	dichloroethyl ether	111-44-4
1, 2-dichloropropane; 1949	1, 2-dichloropropane	78-87-5
1, 2-dichloropropene; 1949	1, 2-dichloropropene	563-54-2
diphenatrile WSA	diphenatrile	86-29-3
1, 2-epoxyethane	1, 2-epoxyethane	75-21-8
1, 2-epoxypropane	1, 2-epoxypropane	75-56-9
hexachlorocyclopentadiene	hexachlorocyclopentadiene	77-47-4
methyl bromide; 1932	methyl bromide	74-83-9
methyl chloride	methyl chloride	74-87-3
methylene chloride	methylene chloride	75-09-2
naphthalene	naphthalene	91-20-3
Nemagon®; 1963	1, 2-dibromo-3-chloropropane	96-12-8
phosphides		
aluminum phosphide [Phostoxin®]	aluminum phosphide	20859-73-8
hydrogen phosphide [phosphine]	hydrogen phosphide	7803-51-2
zinc phosphide	zinc phosphide	
propargyl bromide; 1961	propargyl bromide	106-96-7
sulfur dioxide	sulfur dioxide	7446-09-5
sulfuryl fluoride; 1959	sulfuryl fluoride	2699-79-8
tetrachloroethylene	tetrachloroethylene	127-18-4
thiocyanates		
isobornyl thiocyanoacetate; 1938 [Thanite®]	isobornyl thiocyanoacetate	115-31-1
Lethane 384®; 1932	(2-[2-butoxyethoxy]ethyl thiocyanate)	112-56-1
1, 1, 1-trichloroethane	1, 1, 1-trichloroethane	71-55-6

Nonproprietary name		Chemical name	CAS No.

Fumigants and Nematocides (cont'd.)

trichloroethene		trichloroethene	79-01-6

Chlorinated Hydrocarbon Insecticides

BHC isomers; 1941	ISO	1, 2, 3, 4, 5, 6-hexachlorocyclohexane	
lindane	ESA, ICPC, ISO	gamma isomer of 1, 2, 3, 4, 5, 6-hexachlorocyclohexane	58-89-9

DDT and related compounds [c/]

bis(p-chlorophenoxy)methane; 1948		bis(p-chlorophenoxy)methane	555-89-5
Bulan® (see also dilan)		2-nitro-1, 1-bis(p-chlorophenyl)butane	117-26-0
chlorobenzilate; 1954	ISO	ethyl 4, 4'-dichlorobenzilate	510-15-6
chloropropylate; 1966	ISO	isopropyl 4, 4'-dichlorobenzilate	5836-10-2
DDA		bis(chlorophenyl)acetic acid	83-05-6
DDE		1, 1-bis(p-chlorophenyl)-2, 2-dichloroethylene	72-55-9
DDT; 1947		1, 1-bis(p-chlorophenyl)-2, 2, 2-trichloroethane	115-32-2
dicofol; 1956 [Kelthane®]	ESA, ISO	1, 1-bis(p-chlorophenyl)-2, 2, 2-trichloroethanol	115-32-2
dilan; 1951		mixture of [2-nitro-1, 1-bis(p-chlorophenyl)butane] and [2-nitro-1, 1-bis(p-chlorophenyl)propane]	8027-00-7
DMC		1, 1-bis(p-chlorophenyl) ethanol	80-06-8
methoxychlor; 1948	ISO	1, 1-bis(p-methoxyphenyl)2, 2, 2-trichloroethane	72-43-5
Perthane®; 1955		1, 1-bis(p-ethylphenyl)2, 2-dichloroethane	72-56-0
Prolan® (see also dilan)		2-nitro-1, 1-bis(p-chlorophenyl) propane	117-27-1
TDE [DDD]	ISO, ESA	1, 1-bis(p-chlorophenyl)-2, 2-dichloroethane	72-54-8

cyclodienes and related compounds

aldrin; 1950	ISO	1, 2, 3, 4, 10, 10-hexachloro-1, 4, 4a, 5,8, 8a-hexahydro-1, 4-endo-exo-5, 8-dimethanonaphthalene	309-00-2
chlordane; 1945	ICPC, ISO	1, 2, 3, 4, 5, 6, 7, 8, 8-octachloro-2, 3, 3a, 4, 7, 7a-hexahydro-4, 7-methanoindene	57-74-9
chlordecone; 1958 [Kepone®]	ISO	decachlorooctahydro-1, 3, 4-metheno-2H-cyclobuta[cd]pentalen-2-one	143-50-0
dieldrin; 1951 [HEOD]	ESA, ICPC, ISO	1, 2, 3, 4, 10, 10-hexachloro-6,7-epoxy-1, 4, 4a, 5, 6, 7, 8, 8a-octahydro-1, 4-endo-exo-5, 8-dimethanonaphthalene	60-57-1

Nonproprietary name		Chemical name	CAS No.

Chlorinated Hydrocarbon Insecticides (cont'd.)

cyclodienes and related compounds (cont'd.)

endosulfan; 1960 [Thiodan®]	ANSI, ISO	6, 7, 8, 9, 10, 10-hexachloro-1, 5, 5a, 6, 9, 9a-hexahydro-6, 9-methano-2, 4, 3-benzodioxathiepin-3-oxide	115-29-7
endrin; 1952	ICPC, ISO	1, 2, 3, 4, 10, 10-hexachloro-6, 7-epoxy-1, 4, 4a, 5, 6, 7, 8, 8a-octahydro-1, 4-endo-endo-5, 8-dimethanonaphthalene	72-20-8
heptachlor; 1952	ISO	1, 4, 5, 6, 7, 8, 8-heptachloro-3a, 4, 7, 7a-tetrahydro-4, 7-endo-methanoindene	76-44-8
heptachlor epoxide		1, 4, 5, 6, 7, 8, 8-heptachloro-2, 3-epoxy-3a, 4, 7, 7a-tetrahydro-4, 7, 7a-tetrahydro-4, 7, methanoindan	4067-30-5
isobenzan [Telodrin®]	ESA, ISO	1, 3, 4, 5, 6, 7, 8, 8-octachloro-1, 3, 3a, 4, 7, 7a-hexahydro-4, 7-methanoiso-benzofuran	297-78-9
isodrin	ICPC	1, 2, 3, 4, 10, 10-hexachloro-1, 4, 4a, 5, 8, 8a-hexahydro-1, 4-endo, endo-5, 8-dimethano-naphthalene	465-73-6
mirex; 1962	ESA	dodecachlorooctahydro-1, 3, 4-metheno-2H-cyclobuta[cd]pentalene	2385-85-5
terpene polychlorinates; 1955 [Strobane ®]		terpene polychlorinates	8001-50-1
toxaphene; 1945	ESA, ICPC	chlorinated camphene	8001-35-2

Organic Phosphorus Insecticides

dimethoxy compounds

azinphosmethyl; 1956 [Guthion®]	ESA, ISO	O, O-dimethyl S[4-oxo-1, 2, 3-benzo-triazin-3(4H)ylmethyl]phosphorodithioate	86-50-0
Azodrin®; 1965		dimethyl phosphate of 3-hydroxy-N-methyl-cis-crofonamide	6923-22-4
Bomyl®; 1964		dimethyl 3-hydroxyglutaconate dimethyl phosphate	122-10-1
bromophos	ESA, ISO	O, O-dimethyl-O-2, 5-dichloro-4-bromophenylthionophosphate	2104-96-3
Chlorthion®; 1954		O, O-dimethyl O-(4-chloro-3-nitrophenyl)phosphorothioate	500-28-7
Ciodrin®; 1961		1-methylbenzyl 3-(dimethoxyphosphinyl-oxy)-cis-crotonate	7700-17-6
cythioate; 1967 [Proban®]	ESA	O, O-dimethyl O-p-sulfamoylphenyl phosphorothioate	115-93-5
demeton-O-methyl [Metasystox®]	ISO	O, O-dimethyl-O-2(ethylthio) ethyl phosphorodithioate	867-27-6

Nonproprietary name		Chemical name	CAS No.

Organic Phosphorus Insecticides (cont'd.)

dimethoxy compounds (cont'd.)

Nonproprietary name		Chemical name	CAS No.
demeton-S-methyl [Metasystox®]	ISO	O, O-dimethyl-S-2(ethylthio) ethyl phosphorodithioate	640-15-3
dicapthon; 1958	ANSI, ESA	O, O-dimethyl O-(2-chloro-4-nitrophenyl)	2463-84-5
dichlorvos; 1960 [DDVP, Vapona®]	ESA, ISO	O, O-dimethyl 2, 2-dichlorovinyl phosphate	62-73-7
dicrotophos; 1963 [Bidrin®]	ISO	O, O-dimethyl cis-2-dimethylcarbonyl -1-methylvinyl phosphate	141-66-2
difenphos; 1965 [Abate®]		O, O, O', O'-tetramethyl O, O'-thiodi-p-phenylene phosphorothioate	3383-96-8
dimethoate; 1962	ANSI, ESA, ISO	O, O -dimethyl S(N-methylcarbamoyl-methyl)phosphorodithioate	60-51-5
endothion	ANSI, ISO	O, O-dimethyl S-[(5-methoxy-4-oxo 4H-pyran-2-yl)methyl] phosphorothioate	2778-04-3
famphur; 1969	ESA	O, O-dimethyl, O-p-(dimethyl sulfamoyl) phenyl phosphorothioate	52-85-7
fenitrothion [Folithion®, Sumithion®]	ISO	O, O-dimethyl O-(4-nitro-m-tolyl) phosphorodithioate	122-14-5
fenthion	ESA	O, O-dimethyl O[4-(methylthio)-m-tolyl] phosphorothioate	55-38-9
malathion; 1952	ESA, ISO	O, O-dimethyl-S-[1, 2-bis(ethoxycarbonyl) ethyl] phosphorodithioate	121-75-5
maloxon		O, O-methyl-S[1, 2-bis(ethoxy-carbonyl) ethyl] phosphorodithioate	1634-78-2
menazon	ESA, ISO	S-[(4, 6-diamino-s-triazine-2-yl)methyl] O, O-dimethyl phosphorodithioate	78-57-9
methidathion	ISO	O, O-dimethyl-S-(2, 3-dihydro-5-methoxy-2-oxo-1, 3, 4-thiadozol-3-yl-methyl)phosphorodithioate	950-37-8
mevinphos; 1957 [Phosdrin®]	ESA, ISO	O, O-dimethyl-1-carbomethoxy-1-propen-2yl phosphate	7786-34-7
monocrotophos	ISO	O, O-dimethyl-S-cis-1-methyl-2-(methylcarbamoyl) vinyl phosphate	6923-22-4
naled; 1959 [Dibrom®]	ANSI, ESA, ISO	O, O-dimethyl 1, 2-dibromo-2, 2-dichloroethyl phosphate	300-76-5
omethoate	BSI, ISO	O, O-dimethyl-S-(N-methyl-carbomyl-methyl)phosphorothioate	1113-02-6
oxydemeton-methyl; 1961 [oxydemetonmethyl] [Meta-Systox-R®]	ISO ANSI, ESA	O, O-dimethyl S-[2-(ethylsulfinyl)ethyl] phosphorothioate	2674-91-1

Nonproprietary name		Chemical name	CAS No.

Organic Phosphorus Insecticides (cont'd.)

dimethoxy compounds (cont'd.)

parathion-methyl	ISO	O, O-dimethyl O-p-nitrophenyl phosphorothioate	298-00-0
phosphamidon; 1960	ESA, ISO	O, O-dimethyl 1-chloro-diethyl-carbamoyl-1-propen-2yl phosphate	13171-21-6
ronnel; 1957 [fenchlorphos]	ANSI, ESA ISO	O, O-dimethyl 2, 4, 5-trichlorophenyl phosphorothioate	299-84-3
thiometon	ISO	O, O-dimethyl S-[2-(ethylthio)ethyl] phosphorothioate	640-15-3
trichlorfon; 1956 [Chlorophos®] [Dipterex®]	ESA, ISO	O, O-dimethyl (1-hydroxy-2, 2, 2-trichlorethyl) phosphorate	52-68-6

diethoxy compounds

Akton®; 1968		O-[2-chloro-1-(2, 5-dichlorophenyl) vinyl] O, O-diethyl phosphorothioate	1757-18-2
bromophos-ethyl	ESA, ISO	O, O-diethyl-O-2, 5-dichloro-4-bromo-phenylthiono phosphate	4824-78-6
carbophenothion [Trithion®]	ANSI, ESA, ISO	O, O-diethyl-S[(p-chlorphenylthio)-methyl] phosphorodithioate	786-19-6
chlorofenvinphos	ISO	O, O-diethyl-2-chloro-1-(2, 4-dichloro-phenyl) vinyl phosphate	470-90-6
chlorpyrifos [Dursban®]	ANSI	O, O-diethyl O-(3, 5, 6-trichloro-2-pyridyl) phosphorothioate	2921-88-2
coumaphos [Co-Ral®]	ESA, ISO	O, O-diethyl O-3-chloro-4-methyl-1-oxo-2H-1-benzopyran-7-yl phosphorothioate	56-72-4
demeton-O; 1952 [Systox® is a mixture of the O- and S- isomers]	ESA, ISO	O, O-diethyl O-2-(ethylthio)ethyl phosphorothioate	298-03-3
demeton-S; 1952	ESA, ISO	O, O-diethyl S-2-(ethylthio)ethyl phosphorothioate	126-75-0
diazinon; 1954	ESA, ISO	O, O-diethyl O-(2-isopropyl 4-methyl-6-pyrimidyl) phosphorothionate	333-41-5
dioxathion; 1956 [Delnav®]	ANSI, ESA, ISO	2, 3-p-dioxane S, S-bis(O, O-diethyl-phosphorodithioate)	78-34-2
disulfoton; 1958	ESA, ISO	O, O-diethyl S-2(ethylthio)ethyl phosphorodithioate	298-04-4
ethion; 1960 [Nialate®]	ANSI, ESA, ISO	O, O', O'-tetraethyl S, S'-methylene bisphosphorodithioate	563-12-2
fensulfothion; 1965 [Dasanit®]	ISO	O, O-diethyl O-[p-(methyl sulfinyl) phenyl] phosphorothioate	115-90-2

Nonproprietary name		Chemical name	CAS No.

Organic Phosphorus Insecticides (cont'd.)

diethoxy compounds (cont'd.)

HETP		hexaethyl tetraphosphate	107-49-3
paraoxon		O, O-diethyl O-p-nitrophenyl phosphate	311-45-5
parathion; 1946 [Folidol®]	ANSI, ESA, ISO	O, O-diethyl-O-p-nitrophenyl phosphoro-thioate	56-38-2
phorate; 1956	ANSI, ESA, ISO	O, O-diethyl S-(ethylthio)methyl phosphorodithioate	298-02-2
phosalone	ANSI, ISO	O, O-diethyl-S-(6-chloro-2-oxobenzoxa-lin-3-yl)methyl phosphorodithioate	2310-17-0
tepp; 1946	ESA, ISO	tetraethylpyrophosphate	107-49-3
thionazin; 1962		O, O-diethyl O-2-pyrazinyl phosphoro-thioate	297-97-2

other organic phosphorus compounds

crufomate [Ruelene®]	pINN, ANSI	4-tert-butyl-2-chlorophenylmethyl N-methylphosphoramidate	299-86-5
DFP		diisopropyl phosphorofluoridate	55-91-4
dimefox	ESA, ISO	bis(dimethyl-amino)phosphoryl fluoride	115-26-4
EPN; 1950	ESA	O-ethyl-o-p-nitrophenyl phenylphos-phorothioate	2104-64-5
Gardona®; 1966		2-chloro-1-(2, 4, 5-trichlorophenyl) vinyl dimethyl	961-11-5
Hinosan®		O-ethyl-S, S-diphenyl phosphorodithioate	17109-49-8
mipafox	ISO	n, n'-diisopropyldiamidosphoryl fluoride	371-86-8
Narlene® [Dowco 109]		O-(4-tert-butyl-2-chlorophenyl)O-methyl phosphoroamidothionate	5902-52-3
Phostex®		bis(dialkylphosphinothioyl) disulfides	
schradan; 1952 [OMPA]	ISO	octamethylpyrophosphoramide	152-16-9

Carbamates and Related Pesticides

N-methyl carbamates and related compounds

aldicarb; 1970 [Temik®]	ESA, ANSI, ISO	2-methyl-3-(methylthio)propionaldehyde O-(methylcarbamoyl)oxime	116-06-3
Banol®		3-chloro-4, 5-dimethyl phenyl N-methyl-carbamate	671-04-5
4-benzothienyl-N-methyl carbamate [Mobam®]		N-methyl-2, 3-substituted phenyl carbamate	1079-33-0

Nonproprietary name		Chemical name	CAS No.

Carbamates and Related Pesticides (cont'd.)

N-methyl carbamates and related compounds (cont'd.)

Nonproprietary name		Chemical name	CAS No.
BUX®; 1966		m-(1-ethylpropyl)phenyl methylcarbamate mixture	8065-36-9
carbaryl; 1958 [Sevin®]	ANSI, ESA, ISO	1-naphthyl N-methylcarbamate	63-25-2
carbofuran; 1969	ANSI, ESA	2,3-dihydro-2,2-dimethyl benzofuranyl-N-methylcarbamate	1563-66-2
isolan	ANSI, ISO	dimethyl 5-(1-isopropyl-3-methyl-pyrazolyl) carbamate	119-38-0
2-isopropylphenyl N-methylcarbamate		2-isopropylphenyl N-methylcarbamate	2631-40-5
3-isopropylphenyl N-methylcarbamate		3-isopropylphenyl N-methylcarbamate	64-00-6
methomyl; 1968	ESA, ANSI	S-methyl N-[(methyl-carbamoyl)oxy] thioacetimidate	16752-77-5
propoxur [Baygon®, aprocarb]	ISO	2-isopropoxyphenyl N-methylcarbamate	114-26-1
Zectran®; 1961		4-dimethylamino-3,5-xylyl N-methyl-carbamate	315-18-4

other carbamates and thiocarbamates

chlorpropham [CIPC]	ISO WSA	isopropyl N-(3-chlorophenyl carbamate	101-21-3
di-allate	ISO, WSA	S-2,3-dichloroally N,N-diisopropyl-thiocarbamate	2303-16-4
pebulate [PEBC]	ISO, WSA	S-propylbutyl-ethylthiocarbamate	1114-71-2
propham [IPC]	ISO	isopropyl N-phenyl carbamate	122-42-9

dithiocarbamates

copper dimethyldithiocarbamate [Wolfen® (German)]		copper dimethyldithiocarbamate	137-29-1
Dithane® M-45; 1961		manganese ethylenebisdithiocarbamate and zinc ion	12427-38-2
ferbam; 1948	ICPC, ISO	ferric dimethyldithiocarbamate	14484-64-1
mancozeb	ISO	complex of zinc and maneb containing 20% manganese and 2.5% zinc	8065-67-6
maneb; 1952	ISO	manganese ethylenebisdithiocarbamate	12427-38-2
nabam; 1945 [Dithane®]	ISO	disodium ethylene bisdithiocarbamate	142-59-6
thiram; 1931 [TMTD]	ICPC, ISO	tetramethylthiuramdisulfide	137-26-8

Nonproprietary name		Chemical name	CAS No.
Carbamates and Related Pesticides (cont'd.)			
dithiocarbamates (cont'd.)			
zineb; 1943	ICPC, ISO	zinc ethylene bisdithiocarbamate	12122-67-7
ziram; 1943 [Milbam®]	ICPC, ISO	zinc dimethyldithiocarbamate	137-30-4
Phenolic and Nitrophenolic Pesticides			
binapacryl	ISO	2-sec-butyl-4,6-dinitrophenyl 3,3-dimethylacrylate	485-31-4
2-chloro-4-phenylphenol; 1953		2-chloro-4-phenylphenol	92-04-6
dinitrocyclohexylphenol dicyclohexylamine salt; 1948	ESA	dicyclohexylammonium dinitro-o-cyclohexylphenate	317-83-9
2,4-dinitrophenol	ISO	2,4-dinitrophenol	51-28-5
2,4-dinitrophenol thiocyanoacetate; 1942		2,4-dinitro-1-thiocyanobenzene	1594-56-5
dinobuton	ISO	2-sec-butyl-4,6-dinitrophenyl isopropyl carbonate	973-21-7
dinocap; 1951	ESA, ISO	2-(1-methyl-n-heptyl)-4,6-dinitrophenol crotonate	6119-92-2
dinoseb; 1947	ESA, ANSI, ISO, WSA	dinitrobutylphenol	88-85-7
DNOC	ISO	4,6-dinitro-o-cresol	534-52-1
hexachlorophene		2,2-methylene-bis(3,4,6-trichlorophenol)	70-30-4
pentachlorophenol; 1936 [PCP]	ESA	pentachlorophenol and its sodium salt	87-86-5
o-phenylphenol; 1948		o-phenylphenol	90-43-7
p-phenylphenol		p-phenylphenol	92-69-3
2,3,4,6-tetrachlorophenol; 1948		2,3,4,6-tetrachlorophenol	58-90-2
2,2-thiobis(4,6-dichlorophenol) [TBP]		2,2-thiobis(4,6-dichlorophenol)	97-18-2
2,4,5-trichlorophenol; 1950		2,4,5-trichlorophenol	95-95-4
2,4,5-trichlorophenol, zinc salt; 1948		2,4,5-trichlorophenol, zinc salt	136-24-3
2,4,6-trichlorophenol; 1954		2,4,6-trichlorophenol	88-06-2
Miscellaneous Pesticides			
Aramite®; 1951		(2[p-tert-butylphenoxy]-1-methyl-ethyl 2-chloroethyl sulfite)	140-57-8
chlorbenside	ANSI, ESA, ISO	p-chlorobenzyl p-chlorophenyl sulfide	103-17-3
chlordimeform	ANSI	N'-(4-chloro-o-tolyl)-N,N-dimethylformamidine	6164-98-3

Nonproprietary name		Chemical name	CAS No.

Miscellaneous Pesticides (cont'd.)

chlorfenson; 1951 [ovex]	ISO ANSI	p-chlorophenyl p-chlorobenzene-sulfonate	80-33-1
Galecron®;1969		N,N-dimethyl-N'-(2-methyl-4-chloro-phenyl) formanidine	6164-98-3
Genite®; 1949		2,4-dichlorophenyl ester of benzene-sulfonic acid	97-16-5
phenothiazine		thiodiphenylamine	92-84-2
Sulphenone®; 1951		p-chlorophenyl phenyl sulfone	80-00-2
tetradifon [TCDS]	ANSI, ISO	p-chlorophenyl 2,4,5-trichlorophenyl sulfone	116-29-0
xanthone; 1939		9-oxoxanthone	90-47-1

Synthetic Organic Rodenticides

antu	ISO	1-(1-naphthyl)-2-thiourea	86-88-4
coumafuryl; 1955 [Fumasol®; Fumarin®]	ISO	3-(1-furyl-2-acetylethyl)4-hydroxy-coumarin	117-52-2
dicoumarol		3,3'-methylenebis(4-hydroxy coumarin)	66-76-2
ethylene thiourea		ethylene thiourea	96-45-7
fluoroacetamide		2-fluoroacetamide	640-19-7
norbormide	ANSI, ISO	5-(α-hydroxy-α-2-pyridyl-benzyl)-7-(α-2-pyridyl-benzylidene)norborn-5-ene-2,3-dicarboximide	991-42-4
sodium fluoroacetate [1080®]		sodium monofluoroacetate	62-74-8
warfarin	ICPC, ISO	3-(d-acetonylbenzyl)-4-hydroxy-coumarin	81-81-2

Molluscicides

metaldehyde		metacetaldehyde	9002-91-9

Herbicides and Related Compounds

acrolein	WSA	acrylaldehyde	107-02-8
ametryn [ametryne; 1964]	ISO WSA	2-ethylamino-4-isopropylamino-6-methylmercapto-s-triazine	834-12-8
amitrole; 1956	ANSI, ISO, WSA	3-amino-1,2,4-triazole	61-82-5
amitrole-T; 1960		3-amino-1,2,4-triazole and ammonium thiocyanate herbicide	8004-05-5
AMS; 1948	WSA	ammonium sulfamate	7773-06-0

Nonproprietary name		Chemical name	CAS No.
Herbicides and Related Compounds (cont'd.)			
atrazine; 1959	ANSI, ISO, WSA	2-chloro-4-ethylamino-6-isopropyl-amino-s-triazine	1912-24-9
benefin	WSA	N-butyl-N-ethyl-1,1,1-trifluoro-2,6-dinitro-p-toluidine	1861-40-1
Bladex®; 1971		2-(4-chloro-6-ethylamino-S-triazin-2-ylamino)2-methylpropionitrile	21725-46-2
bromacil; 1961	ANSI, ISO, WSA	5-bromo-3-sec-butyl-6-methyl-uracil	314-40-9
bromoxynil; 1965	ANSI, ISO, WSA	3,5-dibromo-4-hydroxybenzonitrile	1689-84-5
chloroacetic acid		chloroacetic acid	79-11-8
chloramben; 1960 [Amiben]	ANSI, ISO WSA	3-amino-2,5-dichlorobenzoic acid	133-90-4
chlormequat; 1962	INN, ISO	(2-chloroethyl)-trimethylammonium salts [of which the chloride is	999-81-5]
chlorbromuron; 1969	ISO, ANSI	3-(4-bromo-3-chlorophenyl)-1-methoxy-1-methylurea	13360-45-7
2-(4-chlorophenoxy)propionic acid; 1963 [4-CPP]		2-(4-chlorophenoxy) propionic acid	3307-39-9
chloroxuron; 1965	ANSI, ISO, WSA	N'-(4-chlorophenoxy)phenyl N,N-dimethylurea	1982-47-4
2,4-D; 1947	ISO, WSA	2,4-dichlorophenoxyacetic acid	94-75-7
2,4-DB; 1958	WSA	4-(2,4-dichlorophenoxy)butyric acid	94-82-5
dalapon; 1954	ANSI, WSA	2,2-dichloropropionic acid Na salt	127-20-8
dehydroacetic acid [DHC]		3-acetyl-6-methyl-2,4-pyrandione	520-45-6
dicamba; 1962	ANSI, ISO, WSA	2-methoxy-3,6-dichlorobenzoic acid	1918-00-9
dichlorprop; 1962 [2,4-DP]	ISO, WSA	2-(2,4-dichlorophenoxy)propionic acid	120-36-5
dicryl	ANSI, WSA	3'-4'-dichloro-2-methacrylanilide	2164-09-2
diphenamid; 1962	ANSI, ISO, WSA	N,N-dimethyl-2,2-diphenylacetamide	957-51-7
diquat; 1961	ANSI, ISO, WSA	1,1'-ethylene-2,2'-dipyridinium salts [of which the dibromide is	85-00-7]
diuron; 1954 [Karmex®]	ANSI, ISO, WSA	3-(3,4-dichlorophenyl)-1,1-dimethylurea	330-54-1
DSMA; 1964		disodium methanearsonate	144-21-8
erbon; 1955	ANSI, ISO, WSA	2-(2,4,5-trichlorophenoxy)ethyl-2,2-dichloropropionate	136-25-4
ethephon; 1971	ANSI, WSA	2-chloroethyl phosphonic acid	16672-87-0

Nonproprietary name		Chemical name	CAS No.

Herbicides and Related Compounds (cont'd.)

Nonproprietary name		Chemical name	CAS No.
ethoxyquin	ISO	1, 2-dihydro-6-ethoxy-2, 2, 4-trimethyl-quinone	91-53-2
fenac; 1960	WSA	2, 3, 6-trichlorophenylacetic acid	85-34-7
fenuron TCA; 1959	WSA, ISO	3-phenyl-1, 1-dimethylurea trichloroacetate	101-42-8
fluometuron; 1965	ANSI, ISO, WSA	3-(m-trifluoromethylphenyl)-1, 1-dimethylurea	2164-17-2
HCA; 1954	WSA	1, 1, 1, 3, 3, 3-hexachloro-2-propanone	116-16-5
2-hydroxyethyl hydrazine [BOH]		2-hydroxyethyl hydrazine	109-84-2
indoleacetic acid		indoleacetic acid	87-51-4
Kerb®; 1971		3, 5-dichloro-N-(1, 1-dimethyl-2-propynyl) benzamide	23950-58-5
linuron; 1961	ANSI, ISO, WSA	3-(3, 4-dichlorophenyl)-1-methoxy-1-methylurea	330-55-2
maleic hydrazide [MH]		maleic hydrazide	123-33-1
MCPA; 1952 [Methoxone®]	ISO, WSA	2-methyl-4-chlorophenoxyacetic acid	94-74-6
metobromuron; 1966	ANSI, ISO	3-(p-bromophenyl)-1-methyl-1-methoxyurea	3060-89-7
monuron; 1951 [Telvar®]	ANSI, ISO, WSA	3-(p-chlorophenyl)-1, 1-dimethylurea	150-68-5
monuron TCA; 1956	WSA	3-(p-chlorophenyl)-1, 1-dimethylurea trichloroacetate	140-41-0
morfamquat	ISO	1, 1'-bis[(3, 5-dimethylmorpholino) carbonylmethyl]4, 4'-bipyridinium	
naphthaleneacetamide; 1960		naphthaleneacetamide	86-86-2
naptalam; 1960 [NPA]	ISO WSA	N-1-naphthalenephthalamic acid	132-66-1
neburon; 1959	WSA, ISO	3-(3, 4-dichlorophenyl)-1-methyl-1-n-butylurea	555-37-3
noruron; 1965 [norea] [Herban®]	ISO ANSI, WSA	3-(hexahydro-4, 7-methanoidan-5-yl)-1 dimethylurea	2163-79-3
paraquat; 1964	ISO, ANSI	1, 1-dimethyl-4, 4'-bipyridilium	4685-14-7
picloram; 1963	ISO, ANSI, WSA	4-amino-3, 5, 6-trichloropicolinic acid	1918-02-1
piperalin; 1966		3(2-methylpiperidino)propyl-3, 4-dichlorobenzoate	3478-94-2
Planavin®; 1966		4-(methylsulfonyl)-2, 6-dinitro-N, N-dipropylaniline	4726-14-1

Nonproprietary name		Chemical name	CAS No.

Herbicides and Related Compounds (cont'd.)

Nonproprietary name		Chemical name	CAS No.
potassium cyanate; 1948		potassium cyanate	590-28-3
prometon; 1959 [prometone]	ISO WSA	2, 4-bis-(isopropylamino)-6-methoxy-s-triazine	1610-18-0
prometryn; 1964 [prometryne]	ISO WSA	2, 4-bis-(isopropylamino)-6-methyl-mercapto-s-triazine	7287-19-6
propanil; 1962	ISO, WSA	3, 4-dichloropropionanilide	709-98-8
propazine; 1961 [Gesamil®]	ISO, WSA	2-chloro-4, 6-bis(isopropylamine)-s-triazine	139-40-2
sesone; 1960	WSA	sodium 2-(2, 4-dichlorophenoxy)ethyl sulfate	136-78-7
siduron; 1964	ANSI, ISO, WSA	1-(2-methyl-cyclohexyl)-3-phenylurea	1982-49-6
silvex; 1954 [fenoprop]	ANSI ISO	2-(2, 4, 5-trichlorophenoxy)propionic acid	93-72-1
simazine; 1958	ANSI, ISO, WSA	2-chloro-4, 6-bis(ethylamino)-s-triazine	122-34-9
2, 4, 5-T; 1948	ISO, WSA	2, 4, 5-trichlorophenoxyacetic acid	93-76-5
2, 3, 6-TBA; 1958	ISO	2, 3, 6-trichlorobenzoic acid	50-31-7
TBA, DMA salt		2, 3, 6-trichlorobenzoic acid, dimethyl-amine salt	3426-62-8
TCA; 1949	ISO, WSA	trichloroacetic acid	76-03-9
terbacil; 1966	WSA, ANSI	3-tert-butyl-5-chloro-6-methyluracil	5902-51-2
terbutol; 1964 [Azak®]	WSA	2, 6-di-tert-butyl-p-tolylmethylcarbamate	1918-11-2
TOK® E-25; 1966		2, 4-dichlorophenyl 4-nitrophenyl ether	1836-75-5
S, S, S-tributyl phosphorothioate; 1960 [DEF®]		S, S, S-tributyl phosphorothioate	78-48-8
tributyl phosphorotrithioite; 1965 [Folex®]		S, S, S-tributyl phosphorotrithioite	150-50-5
trifluralin; 1961	ANSI, ISO, WSA	1, 1, 1-trifluoro-2, 6-dinitro-N, N-di-n-propyl-p-toluidine	1582-09-8
2, 3, 6-triiodobenzoic acid [TIBA]		2, 3, 6-triiodobenzoic acid	88-82-4

Fungicides and Related Compounds

Nonproprietary name		Chemical name	CAS No.
anthraquinone		9, 10-anthraquinone	84-65-1
azobenzene		azobenzene	103-33-3
Bordeaux mixture		cupric sulfate, basic	8011-63-0
captafol [Difolatan®]	ISO	N-(1, 1, 2-2-tetrachloro-ethyl-sulfenyl)-cis-Δ-4-cyclohexene-1, 2-dicarboximide	2425-06-1

Nonproprietary name		Chemical name	CAS No.

Fungicides and Related Compounds (cont'd.)

captan; 1949	ICPC, ISO	N-trichloromethylthio-4-cyclohexene-1,2-dicarboximide	133-06-2
chinomethionate	ISO	6-methyl-2-oxo-1,3-dithio(4,5-6) quinoxaline	2539-01-2
chloramphenicol		d(-)-thero-2,2-dichloro-N[β-hydroxy-α-(hydroxy-methyl)-p-nitrophenethyl] acetamide	56-75-7
chloranil	ICPC	tetrachloro-p-benzoquinone	118-75-2
chloroneb; 1967	ANSI, ISO	1,4-dichloro-2,5-dimethoxybenzene	2675-77-6
dichlone; 1943	ICPC, ISO, WSA	2,3-dichloro-1,4-naphthoquinone	117-80-6
dichloran	CSA	2,6-dichloro-4-nitroaniline	99-30-9
diphenyl		phenylbenzene	92-52-4
dodine; 1956	ANSI, ISO	n-dodecylguanidine acetate	2439-10-3
Dyrene®; 1958		2,4-dichloro-6-(o-chloroanilino)-s-triazine	101-05-3
folpet; 1958	ANSI	n-trichloromethylthiophthalimide	133-07-3
glyodin; 1946	ICPC, ISO	2-heptadecyl-2-imidazoline, monocitrate	556-22-9
griseofulvin	ISO	7-chloro-4,6-dimethoxycoumarin-3-one-2-spiro-1'-(2'-methoxy-6'-methyl-cyclohex-2'-en-4'-one	126-07-8
hexachlorobenzene [HCB]		hexachlorobenzene	118-74-1
Parnon®; 1967		bis-(p-chlorophenyl)-3-pyridinemethanol	177 81-31-6
8-quinolinol		8-hydroxyquinoline	148-24-3
quintozene	ISO	pentachloronitrobenzene	82-68-8
sodium azide		sodium azide	26628-22-8
thiabendazole	ISO	2-(4-thiazolyl)benzimidazole	148-79-8
1,2,3-trichloro-4,6-dinitrobenzene		1,2,3-trichloro-4,6-dinitrobenzene	6379-46-0

Chemosterilants

apholate		2,2,4,4,6,6-hexa hydro-2,2,4,4,6,6-hexakis (1-aziridinyl)-1,3,5,2,4,6-triazatriphosphorine	52-46-0
busulfan [Myleran®]		1,4-butanediol dimethanesulfonate	55-98-1
metepa	ESA	tris[1-(2-methylaziridinyl)]phosphin oxide	57-39-6
tepa		tris(1-aziridinyl)phosphine oxide	545-55-1
tretamine		s-triazine-2,4,6-tris(1-aziridinyl)-	51-18-3

APPENDIX I

Nonproprietary name		Chemical name	CAS No.
Repellants and Attractants			
butoxy polypropylene glycol; 1948		butoxy polypropylene glycol	
chloralose		glucochloralose	14798-36-8
deet; 1956	ESA	N, N-diethyl-$\underline{m}$-toluamide	134-62-3
diphenylamine; 1962 [DFA]		diphenylamine	122-39-4
ethyl hexanediol; 1947	ESA	2-ethyl-1, 3-hexanediol	94-96-2

a.   Where known, the approval status of nonproprietary names set by various agencies in the United States of America and by The International Organization for Standardization is given (see Section 1.7.1).

b.   Certain proprietary names and code names have come to be used almost as common names, and some of these are listed, usually in brackets.

c.   The $\underline{p}, \underline{p}'$- isomer is named in each instance, but others (notable the $\underline{o}, \underline{p}'$- isomer) occur.

APPENDIX II

Some Units of Measure Used in this Book

Concept	Description of unit	Abbreviation
dosage of animals or people	milligrams of compound per kilo-gram of body weight	mg/kg
storage in tissue, residue in food, or concentration in water	parts of compound per million parts of tissue, food, or water by weight	ppm
concentration in air	milligrams of compound per cubic meter of air	mg/m^3
concentration in formulation	parts of compound per hundred parts of formulation (weight/volume)	percent or %
rate of application to surfaces	milligrams of compound per square meter of area	mg/m^2

Conversion Table for the Units of Measure Frequently Used in Connection with the Toxicology of Pesticides. The Five Divisions of the Table Correspond to the Five Divisions in Appendix II.

1 ppm (by weight)	1	mg/kg
1 μg/100 g (μg%)	0.01	ppm
1 μg/g	1	ppm
1 μg/100 mg	10	ppm
1 mg/100 g (mg%)	10	ppm
1 grain/pound	142.9	ppm
1 mg/g	1,000	ppm
1 g/ pound	2,204.6	ppm
1 % (concentration)	10,000	ppm
1 μg/l	1	mg/m^3
1 g/1,000 cu. ft.	35.315	mg/m^3
1 ppm(of compound in air by volume) [a]/........		
1 pound/gallon	119.8	g/l
1 pound/gallon	12.0	% w/v
1 pound/acre	10.4	mg/sq. ft.
1 pound/acre	112.1	mg/m^2
1 pound/acre	1.121	kg/ha
1 mg/square foot	10.8	mg/m^2

a. This is an expression for concentration frequently used in industrial hygiene. It is based on the assumption that the material in question exists as a gas or vapor and expresses the number of volumes of compound per million volumes of air. The value may be calculated by the formula:

$$ppm = \frac{\text{observed concentration (mg/l) x 24,450}}{\text{molecular weight of compound}}$$

The figure, 24,450 ml, is the gram molecular volume of a gas at a pressure of 760 mm of mercury and a temperature of 25°C.

APPENDIX IV

Approximate Dosages (mg/kg/day) of a Compound for Certain
Animals on Diets Containing it at Different Concentrations that
do not Influence Food Intake[a]

Animal	Sex	Concentration (ppm) in the total diet excluding water						
		1	2	5	10	25	50	100
baby chicks	M -F	0.161	0.322	0.805	1.61	4.03	8.05	16.1
hens	F	0.058	0.116	0.290	0.58	1.45	2.90	5.8
adult mice	M	0.124	0.248	0.620	1.24	3.10	6.20	12.4
	F	0.133	0.266	0.665	1.33	3.33	6.66	13.3
weanling rats	M	0.100	0.200	0.500	1.00	2.50	5.00	10.0
	F	0.095	0.190	0.475	0.95	2.37	4.75	9.5
mature rats	M[b]	0.045	0.090	0.220	0.45	1.12	2.25	4.5
	F[b]	0.053	0.106	0.260	0.53	1.31	2.62	5.3
adult rhesus	M	0.016	0.032	0.080	0.16	0.40	0.80	1.6
	F	0.023	0.046	0.115	0.23	0.57	1.15	2.3
adult dog	M	0.019	0.038	0.095	0.19	0.47	0.94	1.9
	F	0.023	0.046	0.115	0.23	0.57	1.15	2.3
adult man	M - F	0.010	0.020	0.050	0.10	0.25	0.50	1.0

a. Whether a given concentration of a particular compound does change food intake must be learned by measurement. Dosage (mg/kg/day) =

$$\frac{dosage(mg/day)}{body\ weight\ (kg)} = \frac{dietary\ concentration\ (ppm)\ x\ food\ intake\ (kg/day)}{body\ weight\ (kg)}$$

b. The same values apply to 500 g guinea pigs.

INDEX

The chemical name of each pesticide considered in this book and indexed below is given in Appendix I but not repeated in this Index. Appendix I also lists the Chemical Abstracts Service registry number and other information, including, in some instances, the date of introduction of the compound.

A

Abano, Pietro d', 2
Abate ® (see Difenphos)
Abortion, effect of pesticides on, 364
Absorbent pads for measurement of exposure, 251–253
Absorption
  by plants, from soil, 268, 272
  dermal, 133–134, 140–150, 353–356
  dosage as factor in, 355
  eye, 150
  gastrointestinal, 135
  injection, in studies of, 117, 134, 150
  measurement of
    direct, 134–135, 256–257, 353, 355–356
    indirect, 134
  rate of, 143
  relative importance of different routes of, 71, 117
  respiratory, 136–140
  units for expressing skin permeability, 144
  unusual routes of, 150
Acceptable daily intake (ADI), 278, 442
Accipter niccus (English sparrow hawk), 493
Accuracy of statistical measurement, 53
Acetanilide, biotransformation of, 112, 115
Acetone, as solvent for
  collecting airborne compounds, 250
  dermal absorption tests, 144
Acetylcholine, 185
Acetylcholinesterase (see also Cholinesterase)
  inhibition of, 185, 413–414
  normal values for, 387
  reactivation of, by oximes, 411–412
N-Acetylcystyl, 108
Acetylsalicylic acid (see Aspirin)
Acids
  as therapeutic agents, 408
  corrosive action of, 183
Aconite, 3
Acrolein, 528
  poisoning in man, 317
  standards for, 451

Acrylonitrile, 519
  standards for, 449
Actinomycin-D
  action against porphyria, 90
  inhibition of RNA synthesis by, 90, 108
  toxicity of, to embryos, 200
Action levels for regulatory intervention, 446
Acute illness (see also specific illnesses), 38
Acute toxicity test, 217
Adaptation
  of liver, features distinguishing from injury, 117
  to pesticide exposure, in man, 362–363
Adhesive plaster, in dermal toxicity tests, 211–212
ADI (see Acceptable daily intake)
Adipose tissue (see Fat)
Adrenals
  characteristics of, 152
  storage of pesticides in, 348–350
Aechmorphorous occidentalis (grebe), 490–491
Aerosols, pesticide
  inhalation of, 138–140
  particle size of, 136–137
  workers' exposure to, 291–294
Aflatoxin, 6, 65, 69, 82
Africa, storage of DDT in human fat in, 343
Age, as factor in
  excretion and storage, 163, 358
  toxicity and poisoning, 81–82, 336–337
Aggression, 85–89
"Aging" of enzyme-inhibitor complex, 414
Agranulocytosis
  death rates in USA from, 364
  produced by aminopyrine, 389
Agricola, Georgius, 2
Agricultural Chemicals Approval Scheme in Great
    Britain, 432
Agricultural
  lands
    application of pesticides to, 507
    area of, 16–17
  pest control operators, 437

Agriculture
  benefits to, from pesticides, 17–18
  changes in practices of, 17–18, 487
  ecological community produced by, 487
  losses to, caused by pests, 15–16
Agriculture Poisonous Substances Act in Great Britain, 432, 437
Air
  ambient, measurement of chemicals in, as indication of exposure, 250–252
  exhaled
    analysis of volatile compound in, as measure of absorption, 142
    excretion in, 353
  monitoring, 462–463
  movement, as factor in residues, 286, 301
  pollution, 282–283, 285–288
  removal of poisoned persons to, 399
  residues in, 282–294
  sources of, for the worker, 464–468
Air-blast spraying of pesticides, 289–291
Aircraft, accident rates for applicators in, 364
Air-line respirator, 466
Air-purifying respirators, 466–467
Airway, maintenance of, in treatment of poisoning, 399–401
Akton ®, 524
δ-ALA (see δ-Aminolevulinic acid)
Alaska, pesticide residues in natives' food, 282
Albumen, as therapeutic agent, 403
Alcohol(s)
  as cause of mortality, 312
  as solvents in dermal toxicity tests, 212
  excretion of, in human milk, 339
  potentiation of action of other compounds by, 74–75
  relation to porphyria, 90
Aldicarb, 525
  poisoning by, in man, 317
  toxicity of, 68, 204
  use of, as systemic insecticide, 271
Aldrin, 521
  absorption of, through plant roots, 272
  as tumorigen, 191
  balance study of, 171–172
  disappearance of, from soil, 300
  epoxidation of, 109, 112
  excretion of, 168, 170, 351, 386
  interaction with other compounds, 73
  microsomal enzyme induction by, 121
  persistence of, in relation to wildlife, 510
  poisoning by, in man, 317, 319, 333, 370
  protein binding by, 132
  residues of, 268, 274, 278, 279, 282, 446
  standards for residues of, 443, 447, 450, 452
  storage of, as dieldrin
    in man, 157, 162–163, 342–343, 347, 384–385
  studies of, in volunteers, 231
  susceptibility of different species to, 77
  susceptibility of, to light, 88
  time-dosage relationships in soil, 299
  toxicity of
    to cells, 204
    to wildlife, 508
  use, 25
Alfalfa, residues in, 270
Aliesterase, liver, inhibition of, 75

"Alimentary aleukia," 320
Alkalis
  as therapeutic agents, 408
  corrosive action of, 183
Alkaloids, dermal absorption of, 149
Alkyl mercury fungicides
  epidemics caused by, 325–326
  treatment of grain with, 323
Alkyl phosphates, urinary metabolites of OP compounds, 353–355
Alkylating agents, as causes of dominant lethals and sterility, 188–189, 198
Allelochemics, usage of word, 7
Allergy
  dosage-response relationships in, 65–66
  tests for, 213–214, 390–391
Allethrin, 518
Alloxan, as cause of diabetes in rats, 5
Alphacellulose respirator pads, 251, 253
Alpha-fetoprotein, 194
Alternative methods for pest control, 474, 512
Altitude, as factor influencing toxicity, 88
Aluminum foil, use in dermal toxicity tests, 210–212
Aluminum phosphide (Phostoxin ®), 520
  poisoning by, in man, 317
Alveoli, 138
American Academy of Clinical Toxicology, 5, 9
American Chemical Society, 8
American College of Veterinary Toxicology, 9
American Conference of Governmental Industrial Hygienists, 9, 448
American Industrial Hygiene Association, 9
American Medical Association, 8
American National Standards Institute, Inc. (ANSI), 31
American Society for Experimental Pathology, 9
American Society for Pharmacology and Experimental Therapeutics, 8
American Standards Association (ASA) (see American National Standards Institute, Inc.)
Ametryn, 528
Amiben (see Chloramben)
4-Aminoantipyrine, product of aminopyrene, 112
p-Aminobenzoic acid, product of biotransformation, 112
δ-Aminolevulinic acid
  formation of, 94
  induction of synthetase of, 90–91
  structure of, 92
  urinary excretion of, 392
Aminoparathion, reduction of parathion to, 110
o-Aminophenol, conjugation of, 112
Aminopterin, as teratogen, 201
Aminopyrine
  and microsomal enzyme induction, 120, 122, 124
  as cause of agranulocytosis, 389
  biotransformation of, 112, 115
Amitrole, 528
Amitrole-T, 528
  as tumorigen, 192
Ammonium sulfamate (AMS), 528
  standards for, 451
Amphetamine
  deamination of, 112
  toxicity of, 134
Amphibians, effects of pesticides on, 506

Amphipod crustacea, susceptibility of to pesticides, 504
Amyl nitrite, as therapeutic agent, 422
Amyloidosis
  effect of, on pesticide storage, 359
  production by chemicals, 195
Anabasine, 518
  poisoning by, in man, 317
Anacapa Island, DDT in pelicans on, 499, 501
Analeptics, 405
Analgesics
  dermal absorption of, 149
  excretion of, in human milk, 339
Anaphylaxis and anaphylactic shock, 65, 404
Anas platyrhynchos (mallard duck), 495
Androgens, dermal absorption of, 149
Anemia
  aplastic
    chloramphenicol as cause of, 389
    deaths from, in USA, 367
  hemolytic, 127, 363
  pernicious, effect on porphyrin metabolism, 90
  sickle cell, 198
  treatment of, 403
Anesthetics
  action of, 186
  pesticides used as, 227
Aniline
  and microsomal enzyme induction, 120
  as product of biotransformation, 112
  differential protection technique in measurement of exposure to, 256
  exposure of workers to, 133, 463
  skin penetration by, 145
Animal repellants, poisoning by, in man, 315, 317
Animal(s)
  behavior of, in toxicity testing, 214–215
  domestic (see Domestic animals and specific names)
  preparation of, for dermal toxicity tests, 208–214
  products, residues in, 266–267
Anorexia, 83
Anoxia, relation to teratogenesis, 198
ANSI (see American National Standards Institute)
Antabuse, effect of, on excretion of trichloroacetic acid, 171
Antagonism, 73–75
Antarctic, residues in wildlife of, 484–485
Anthelmintics, pesticides used as, 224
Anthraquinone, 531
  as tumorigen, 193
Antibiotics
  as contrasted to probiotics, 86
  as therapeutic agents, 406
  excretion of, in human milk, 339
  pesticides used as, 227
Anticholinesterases, action of, 185, 240, 362
Anticoagulant drugs, pesticides used as, 227
Anticonvulsants
  as pharmacological antidotes, 410
  excretion of, in human milk, 339
Antidotes
  description or classification of, 72–74, 407
  detoxifying, 407–409
  pharmacological, 409–410
  specific, 410–423

Antiemetics, 405–406
Antihistamines
  dermal absorption of, 149
  excretion of, in human milk, 339
Antihormones, excretion of, in human milk, 339
Antimony potassium tartrate, use of, as emetic, 227, 458
Antimycin, use of in relation to wildlife, 510
Antipyrine, in tests for microsomal enzyme changes, 116, 120, 121
Antitoxin, usage of word, 7
α_1-Antitrypsin, inherited deficiency of, cause of chronic obstructive bronchopulmonary disease, 128
Antu, 528
  age as factor in toxicity of, 69
  as tumorigen, 192
  standards for, 451
  tolerance to, in rodents, 125
Apholate, 532
  toxicity of, 47
Apomorphine hydrochloride, as emetic, 395
Apples, pesticide residues on, 275
Application of pesticides
  area of, limitation of, 511–512
  directly to soil, 297–298
  improper, as cause of epidemics, 324–325
  methods of
    as factor influencing exposure of workers, 292
    as factor influencing residues in food, 269–271, 273–274
    as factor influencing residues in soil, 298–301
    equipment, formulations, and techniques, 26–27
    regulation of, 436–437
    timing of, 512
    to agricultural land, 507
    to non-agricultural land, 505–506
    to water, effect of on wildlife, 504–505
    ultra-low volume, 26–27
Applicators
  aircraft accidents of, 364
  storage of pesticides in, 344
Approved names of pesticides, 29
Aprocarb (see Propoxur)
Apronal
  and porphyria, 90
  as cause of thrombocytopenic purpura, 390
Aprons, for protection, 469
Aptenodytes fosteri (emperor penguin), storage of pesticides in, 484
Aquatic factors in toxicity, 97–98
Aquila chrysaetos (golden eagle), 494
Arabidopsis thaliana, for genetic studies, 204
Aramite ®, 527
  as tumorigen, 192
Argentina, storage of pesticides in people in, 342, 345
Arizona, moratorium on DDT in, 297
Armed Forces Act, permitting tests in man, 236
Arndt-Schulz rule, 57
Arsenic and arsenicals, 517
  adsorption of, by charcoal, 308
  beneficial effects of small dosages of, 57, 58
  excretion of, 354
  in dermal toxicity tests, 210
  inhibition of SH-enzymes by, 185
  mitochondrial swelling and axonal dystrophy in

Arsenic and arsenicals—*Continued*
  poisoning by, 197
  poisoning in animals, 479, 480
  poisoning in man, 314, 317, 318, 319, 333
  residues
    in foods, 267, 279
    in soil, 296
    in total diet, 278
  sale of, in USA, 436
  standards for, 449
  storage of, in man, 354, 385
  susceptibility of different species to, 80
  tolerance to, 125
  toxicity of, 38, 68
  treatment of poisoning by, 418–420
  use as drug, 227
  use as insecticide, 20, 22
Arteriosclerosis, insecticides as possible cause of, 359
Artificial respiration, 4, 399, 401
ASA (see American National Standards Institute)
Asia, storage or excretion of insecticides by people in, 343, 344, 346, 351
Aspergillus, genetic studies of, 204
Aspirin
  as common name, 30
  effect of, on HeLa cells, 204
  ingestion of, 316
  microsomal enzyme induction by, 124
  storage of, 162
  toxicity of, 68
Association of American Pesticide Control Officials, 31, 432
Asthma, effect of exposure to pesticides on, 327–328
Ataxia, in behavioral tests, 215
Atrazine, 529
  as tumorigen, 192
Atropine
  as pharmacological antidote, 409–410
  interaction of oximes with, 412–413
  tolerance to, as evidence of poisoning by organic phosphorus compounds, 379
  toxicity of, 47
Audiogenic seizures, 85
Australia
  accidental poisoning in, 333
  poison control centers in, 471
  storage of pesticides in people in, 343, 346, 351
"Automatic flagman," 470
Autoradiography, for studying dermal absorption, 141
Avoidance, conditioned and passive, in behavior tests, 214
Axon
  dystrophy of, in poisoning, 196
  potassium and sodium ions in, 186
Azak ® (see Terbutol)
Azinphosethyl, occupational disease caused by, 321
Azinphosmethyl, 522
  and microsomal enzymes, 75, 119, 122–123
  antagonism of, 75
  desulfuration of, 112
  exposure of workers to, 290
  poisoning by, in man, 317
  potentiation of, 74
  standards for, 443–450
  studies of, in workers, 229

susceptibility of different species to, 77
  toxicity of, 47
Azobenzene, 531
  as tumorigen, 193
  reduction of, 112
Azo compounds, 112
Azodrin ®, 522

B

Baby foods, pesticide residues in, 281
Backflow preventers, 470
Bacteremic shock, 404
Bacteria
  biotransformation of compounds by, 107, 302–303
  use of, in mutagenesis tests, 204–205
Bacterial toxins, 6–8
Baking soda, contraindicated as neutralizing antidote, 408
BAL (see Dimercaprol)
Balance study, 171–172
Banol®, 525
  and microsomal enzymes, 124
  toxicity of, in relation to protein deprivation, 83
Barbados, pesticide residues in air of, 285
Barbiturates
  and porphyria, 90
  as causes of mortality, 314
  as pharmacological antidotes, 410
Barium, 517
  storage of, in bone, 340
Barium carbonate, 517
  poisoning by, in man, 317, 323
Barley
  contamination of,
    by ethyl mercury chloride, 480
    by parathion, 323
  in genetic studies, 204
Barthrin (see also Pyrethrum and pyrethrins), 518
  studies of, in volunteers, 231
Basophil tests, 390
Baygon ® (see Propoxur)
Bean plants, in genetic studies, 204
Beetle, Colorado potato, 488
Behavior, tests of, 214–215
Belgium
  concentration of DDT in human milk in, 351
  participation of, in Council of Europe, 433
  poison control centers in, 471
  storage of pesticides in people in, 342
Benefin, 529
Benefits
  economic, from control of malaria, 13–15
  from disease control, 10–15
  from pesticides, 9–15
Bengalese finch, 495
1,2-Benzanthracene, and mechanism of photosensitization, 89
Benzene
  as solvent for dermal absorption tests in animals, 141
  inherent toxicity of, 456
Benzene hexachloride (see BHC)
4-Benzothienyl-*N*-methyl carbamate (Mobam®), 525
  poisoning by, in man, 317
  studies of, in workers, 229

Benzpyrene, 68
3,4-Benzpyrene, 57
  carcinogenicity of, 65
  enzyme induction by, 75
Benzylpenicillin, toxocity of, 47
Bernard, Claude, 3, 5, 182, 187
Bertrand's Law, 57–58
Beverages, pesticide residues in, 269
BHC, 520
  absorption of, through plant roots, 268
  as cause of blood dyscrasias, 363–364
  as tumorigen, 191
  disappearance of, from soil, 299
  excretion of, in man, 351, 352, 386
  exposure of workers to, 289
  microsomal enzyme induction by, 113, 120–122
  poisoning by
    in domestic animals, 480
    in man, 317, 319, 323
  porphyria production by, 90
  production of, USA, 22, 23
  residues of
    in air, 282
    in Antarctic birds, 485
    in food, 266, 268
    in soil, 296
    in total diet, 278, 279
    in water, 274
    removal of, from water, 276
    standards for, 443, 447, 450
  species differences in susceptibility to, 77–78, 480
  storage
    in man, 343, 345–346, 347, 349, 350, 384, 385
    of separate isomers, 161–162, 346
    relation to dosage, 157
  studies of
    in volunteers, 232, 233
    in workers, 229
  toxicity of, effect of protein on, 82–83
  use for treating dermatitis, 227, 232
  vaporizers, restriction of, 436
  vapor pressure of, 287
BHT, storage of, in man, 339
Bidrin® (see Dicrotophos)
Bile
  excretion of pesticides into, 168–169
  rate of flow, as factor in excretion, 169
Bilharziasis, treatment of, by pesticides, 227, 234
Binapacryl, 527
  exposure of workers to, 291
  standards for, 443
Biochemical lesion, 3, 132, 182, 184, 407, 410
Biochemical studies, in relation to toxicology, 172, 203
Biochemistry, in training of toxicologists, 8
Biodegradability, 302–303, 306
"Biological concentration" of pesticides by wildlife, 490
Biological index, 451–452
Biological magnification, 27, 46, 167–168, 489–492, 502–503
Biophysical tests in toxicology, 203
Biotic simplification
  as cause of pest problems, 486–488
  emergent pests, 487–488
  faunal imbalance, 487

Biotransformation (see also Metabolism), usage of word, 107
Birds, effects of pesticides on, 166–167, 490–491, 492–502, 505, 506, 507
Bis(p-chlorophenoxy)methane, 521
Bishydroxycoumarin, in tests for microsomal enzyme changes, 73–74, 116
Bladder, weight of, 152
Bladex®, 529
Blastula, teratogenesis in, 199
Blindness, in dogs, dithizon as a cause of, 197
Blood
  absorption of compounds into, 134–135
  as therapeutic agent, 403
  distribution of compounds by, 151–154
  dyscrasias (see Anemia; Agranulocytosis; Purpura)
  flow of, 151–152
  pressure, in supportive tests, 392
  storage of pesticides in, 346–349, 361, 385
  tests, in supportive treatment, 392
  vessels, toxic effects on, 194
Blood-brain barrier, 153–154, 414
Bluejay, effect of DDT on, 167
Bobwhite, effect of DDT on, 167
Body, human
  "standard" weight and height, 255
  surface area of, 255
  weight of organs of, 152
BOH (see 2-Hydroxyethyl-hydrazine)
Bomyl®, 522
Bone
  marrow
    porphyria and, 90
    storage of insecticides in, 348
    weight of, 152
  storage of elements in, 340
  weight of, 152
Bone-seekers, 161
Books, presentation of toxicology in, 471–472
Boots
  contamination within, 210
  for protection, 469
Bordeaux mixture, 531
Boric acid
  as cause of mortality, 319
  use to treat dermatitis, 227
Botfly larvae, control of, 76
Botulinum toxin A, toxicity of, 68
Brain
  biotransformation in, 115–116
  critical level of DDT in, 167
  distribution of compounds to, 151–154
  gold thioglucose as cause of injury to, 194
  hydrocephalus of, 196
  lipid concentration in, 361
  microcephaly of, in rats, 196
  storage of pesticides in, 166–167, 348, 350, 361
  susceptibility of, to teratogenesis, 200
  tumors, incidence of, effect of pesticides on, 367
  weight of, 152
Brazil, occupational poisoning by parathion in, 326
Breath analysis, 249, 389
Breeding (see Reproduction)
British Standards Institution (BSI), 31
Bromacil, 529

Bromide
  excretion of, 170
  residues of, in total diet, 278
  standards for, 443
Bromine, beneficial effect of small dosage of, 57
Bromobenzene, toxicity of, 62, 129
3-Bromo-4-nitrophenol, for lamprey control, 504, 510
Bromophos, 522
  standards for, 443
  studies of, in workers, 229
Bromophos-ethyl, 524
  standards for, 443
Bromoxynil, 529
Bromsulfalein, in supportive tests, 392
Bronchi and bronchioles, 138
Bronchopulmonary disease, assocatiated with deficiency of serum α_1-antitrypsin, 128
BSI (see British Standards Institution)
Bubo virginianus (great horned owl), 494
"Buffer species," as alternative prey, 487
Bulan® (see also Dilan), 521
  toxicity of, 402
Burial of pesticides for disposal, 462
Burning of pesticides, 462
Busulfan, 532
  as cause of sterility in male mammals, 189
  as teratogen, 201
Buteo jamaicensis (red-tailed hawk), 494
Butoxy propylene glycol, 533
Butter, pesticide residues in, 266
Butter yellow, 69
Buttermilk, pesticide residues in, 266
N,N'-di-n-Butylphosphorodiamine fluoride, toxicity of, 68
BUX®, 526
  toxicity of, to man, 317

C

Cacodylic acid, 517
  as tumorigen, 191
Cadmium, interaction of zinc with, 201
Caffeine
  excretion of in human milk, 339
  mutagenicity of, 207
  toxicity of, 47
Cage, for rat restraint, 211
Calcium
  as specific antidote, 423
  dermal absorption of, 149
  storage of, 164
Calcium arsenate, 517
  production and use of in USA, 23, 25
  standards for, 449
Calcium carbonate, in eggshells of birds, 493, 497–498
Calcium cyanamide, 519
  as tumorigen, 191
Calcium cyanide, 519
  use of, for rodent control, 430
Calcium disodium edetate
  as therapeutic agent, 418–421
  derivatives of, 419
Calcium gluconate, as specific antidote, 423
Calcium pantothenate, dermal absorption of, 149
Calcium polysulfide, as cause of mortality, 319

California
  regulation of pesticides in, 337, 437
  reports of occupational disease in, 321–322, 337, 339
  use of pesticides in, 26
Camphor, as cause of mortality, 319
Canada
  epidemic of poisoning in, 323
  excretion of pesticides by people in, 351
  levels of pesticides in birds' eggs in, 500
  pesticide residues in food in, 281
  storage of pesticides by people in, 342, 345
Canadian Association for Research in Toxicology, 9
Cannisters for respirators, 467
Capes, as protective clothing, 469
Capillaries, 130, 145
Captafol (Difolatan®), 531
  standards for, 445
Captan, 532
  as tumorigen, 193
  standards for, 445
  toxicity of, effect of protein on, 83
Carbamate insecticides
  as tumorigens, 192
  depression of cholinesterase by, 184, 386
  excretion of, 331, 332
  occupational disease caused by, 321
  poisoning by, in man, 317
  residues of
    in fruits, 269
    in total diet, 278
  safety for vector control, 330–333
  studies of
    in volunteers, 234
    in workers, 229
  toxicity to isolated cells, 204
Carbaryl (Sevin®), 526
  as tumorigen, 192
  death of cattle caused by, 479
  dermal absorption of, 141, 147
  excretion of, in man, 340
  exposure of workers to, 291
  for parasite control, 227
  inhibition of soil fungi by, 302
  metabolism of, 109
  microsomal enzyme induction by, 124
  poisoning by, in man, 317
  residues of, in total diet, 278, 279
  standards for, 444, 451
  storage of, in man, 340
  studies of
    in volunteers, 234
    in workers, 229
  testing of, for vector control, 331
  toxicity of
    effect of protein deficiency on, 83
    to isolated cells, 204
Carbofuran, 526
  poisoning by, in man, 317
  standards for, 451
Carbon dioxide
  as metabolite of carbon tetrachloride, 108
  combining power of blood in supportive tests, 392
  dermal absorption of, 149
Carbon disulfide, 519
  precautionary label for, 434

standards for, 449
Carbon monoxide
  as cause of accidental poisoning, 312, 382
  as metabolite of methylene chloride, 108
  hemoglobin and, 185–186
  oxygen as specific antidote against, 422
Carbon tetrachloride, 519
  as cause of poisoning, in man, 317
  excretion of, 108
  microsomal enzyme inhibition by, 120
  penetration of skin by, 142
  studies of, in volunteers, 231
  toxicity of
    effect of protein deficiency on, 82
    potentiation by alcohol, 74
  vapor pressure of, 287
Carbonic anhydrase, inhibition of, by DDT, 497–498
Carbophenothion (Trithion®), 73, 524
  exposure of workers to, 290
  microsomal enzyme substrate, 123
  mortality to cattle caused by, 479
  poisoning by, in man, 317, 323
  residues of, 278
  standards for, 443, 444
Carboxide gas, as cause of mortality, 319
Carboxyhemoglobin, 185
Carcinogenesis
  as cause of
    chronic illness, 37–38
    mortality, 312
  as possible result of probiosis, 86–87
  avoidance of, 439
  by asbestos, 139
  chemical, 64, 86–87, 190–194, 207, 439
  cocarcinogenesis, 190
  delay in onset of, 48–49
  dosage-response relationships, 64
  pesticides as cause of, 191–193
  radiation as cause of, 89
  study of, in man, 238–239
  tests for, 207
Carcinoma
  adrenal, treatment with DDD, 232
  effect of, on pesticide storage, 359–360
Cardinal, fatal level of DDT in brain of, 167
Cardiogenic shock, 404
Cardiovascular system,
  specific toxic effects on, 194
  tests of, 392
Carrageenin, as cause of hypersensitivity to cold, 194
Carrots
  residues of pesticides in, 272
  soils for raising, residues in, 297
Cases of poisoning (see Poisoning)
CAS registry numbers for pesticides, 31 and Appendix I
Casein, as test compound in study of microsomal enzyme induction, 122–124
Castor oil, as therapeutic agent, 397
Cat
  dermal absorption rate in, 143
  in war gas experiments, 51
Cataract, production, by chemicals, 197
Catatoxic steroids, to prevent poisoning, 406
Catecholamines, 84–85

Catharacta skua maccormicki (skua), storage of pesticides in, 485
Cathartics
  excretion of, in human milk, 339
  pesticides used as, 227
  saline, as therapeutic agents, 397–398
Cattle (see Livestock)
Ceiling value for TLV, 448
Cells
  injury to
    carcinogenesis, 190–194
    mutagenesis, 188–190
    spindle poisoning, 187–188
  isolated, toxicological studies on, 203–204
Central nervous system (CNS) (see Nervous system)
Centrifugal filter-blowers, 465
Centrifugation, differential, to separate cellular constituents, 113
Cereals, pesticide residues in, 267–268
Ceylon, malaria in, 11, 13–14
Challenge dose, in tests of sensitivity, 214, 389
Chaoporus astictopus (gnat), relation to biological magnification, 490–491
Charcoal, activated
  as therapeutic agent, 407–408
  in removing residues from water, 276
  similarity to chelating agent, 75
  to fix residues in soil, 272–273
Chard, contamination of, by toxaphene, 324
Cheese, pesticide residues in, 266
Chelating agent(s)
  and metals they bind, 418–419
  as causes of injury, 75, 197
  as specific antidotes, 417–421
  to diagnose lead poisoning, 385–386
Chemical
  basis of thresholds, in dosage-response relationships, 61–62
  burns, 183, 187, 321,
  carcinogenesis, 64, 86–87, 190–194, 207, 439
  potential of compounds, 183–184
  reactions, in metabolism of pesticides and other compounds, 107–111
Chemical Abstracts Services (CAS), 31
Chemical epidemiology, as aid to diagnosis, 379–382
Chemicals
  alteration of membrane properties by, 186–187
  dangerous, classes of, 433–435
  household, dermal absorption of, 133
  industrial, safety factors regarding, 439
  predictability of toxic effects of, 382–383
  production of pathological changes by, 5
  teratogenic action of, 197–201
  tolerance to, limitation of, 380
  transfer of, in body, 129–130
Chemistry, in training of toxicologists, 8–9
Chemosterilants
  as mutagens, 65
  chronicity index of, 45–46
  toxicity testing of, 43
Chevallier, J. B. A., 3
Chickens
  neurotoxicity in, 240–241
  poisoning of, by methyl mercury dicyanamide, 480

Children
  "keep out of reach of," on labels, 431
  reported cases of poisoning in, 314–316
  susceptibility of, to pesticides, 81–82, 336–337
Chinomethionate, 532
  exposure of workers to, 291
Chlamydomonas, resistance of, to colchicine, 187
Chloracetone, 51
Chloral hydrate, microsomal enzyme induction by, 73, 124
Chloralose, 533
  as cause of poisoning in man, 317
  as tumorigen, 193
Chloramben (Amiben), 529
Chloramphenicol, 532
  as cause of aplastic anemia, 65, 389
  microsomal enzyme induction by, 124
  use of, as drug, 227
Chloranil, 532
  as tumorigen, 193
Chlorates, danger of storage of, 460
Chlorbenside, 527
  residues of, 278
  standards for, 445
Chlorbromuron, 529
Chlorcyclizine, and microsomal enzyme induction, 123
Chlordane, 521
  disappearance of, from soil, 299
  excretion of, 386
  microsomal enzyme induction by, 120, 121, 122
  poisoning by, in man, 317, 319, 336
  porphyria production by, 90
  residues of
    in air, 282, 284
    in food, 278
  standards for, 443, 447, 450
  storage of, by people, 353, 384, 385
  studies of, in workers, 229
  susceptibility of different species to, 77–78
  toxicity of
    in relation to protein deprivation, 83
    to isolated cells, 204
Chlordecone (Kepone®), 521
Chlordiazepoxide hydrochloride, as test compound for microsomal enzyme induction, 121
Chlordimeform, 527
Chlorfenson (Ovex), 528
  as tumorigen, 192
  poisoning by, in man, 317
  toxicity of, to isolated cells, 204
Chlorfenvinphos, as test compound for microsomal enzyme induction, 122
Chlorinated hydrocarbon insecticides
  affinity of, for adipose tissue, 151–154
  as tumorigens, 191–192
  dermal absorption of, 134
  effect of, on reproduction, 217, 492–502
  excretion of, in man, 349–353
  in malaria eradication, 10–15
  in studies of interaction of compounds, 73
  in wildlife, monitoring of, 484
  poisoning by, in man, 317, 319, 323–324
  porphyria production by, 90–91
  residues of

  in air, 282–283
  in food, 266–269, 276–282
  in soil, 295–298
  in water, 274
  resistance to, 125–126
  safety of, 367–370
  storage of, in man, 339–349
  studies of
    in volunteers, 231–233
    in workers, 229
  toxicity of, to isolated cells, 204
  use of, as drugs, 227
  volatilization of, 273, 283, 286–288, 301, 302
Chlorine, 51, 517
Chlormequat, 529
  standards for, 445
Chloroacetic acid, 529
  as tumorigen, 192
Chlorobenzilate, 521
  as tumorigen, 191
  standards for, 443
  susceptibility of different species to, 77
p -Chlorobenzoic acid, production by soil organisms, 302
2-Chloroethyl-trimethyl ammonium chloride, as tumorigen, 192
Chlorofenvinphos, 524
  standards for, 443
Chloroform, 519
  as solvent, 146
  standards for, 449
  use of, as anaesthetic, 227
Chloroleukemia, in rats, 207
Chloroneb, 532
2-Chloro-4-phenylphenol, 527
2-(4-Chlorophenoxy) propionic acid, 529
Chlorophos® (see Trichlorfon)
Chloropicrin, 519
  as cause of poisoning, in man, 317
  standards for, 449
Chloropropylate, 521
Chlorotetracycline, 518
Chloroxuron, 529
Chlorpromazine
  as antiemetic, 406
  as microsomal enzyme substrate, 122
  as test substance for interaction with
    crowding, 85
    temperature, 88
  hydrochloride, 406
  sulfoxidation of, 112
Chlorpropham (CIPC), 526
  as tumorigen, 192
  effect of protein on toxicity of, 83
  residues of, in potatoes, 268
Chlorpyrifos (Dursban®), 524
Chlorthion®, 522
  exposure of workers to, 290
  susceptibility of different species to, 77
Cholinesterase
  as parameter in studies of pesticides in volunteers, 233–234, 240
  atypical, genetic factors in, 127–128
  inhibition of, 185, 362, 413–414
    in dermal absorption studies, 142

545 INDEX

normal values for, 387
reactivation of, by oximes, 411–412
Chromatography, gas, 172, 344, 352
Chromic acid, beneficial effect of small dosages, 57
Chromosome aberrations
in teratogenesis, 189, 201
in tests of mutagenesis, 205
usage of term, 188
Chronic diseases
in man, 359–360
usage of term, 38
Chronic poisoning, 38, 311–312
Chronic toxicity
tests for, 202, 204–207, 215–218
usage of term, 37
Chronicity index, 45–46, 159
Chronicity of injury, factors influencing, 37–38
Cigarette smoking, as cause of mortality, 312
Cigarettes, as means of oral exposure to pesticides, 294
Ciliary action, movement of particles by, 139
Ciodrin®, 522
CIPC (see Chlorpropham)
Circadian rhythms, as factor in toxicity, 91–97
Circus cyanius (marsh hawk), 497
Cirrhosis, of liver, effect of, on pesticide storage, 359
City soil, pesticide residues in, 297
Classes of poisons (A and B, I etc.), 431–432, 433, 435, 453–454
Clear Lake, in relation to biological magnification, 490–491
Clinical findings
in animals, 202
in man, as aid to diagnosis, 282–283
Clinical research (see Studies in man)
Clinical toxicology, 5
Clothing
contamination of, as source of poisoning, 223, 234
protective, 254–255, 468–469
Coal tar, use of, to control parasites, 227
Cobalt, dermal absorption of, 149
Cocarcinogenesis (see also Carcinogenesis), 190
Codeine, biotransformation of, 112
Codes of practice, for studies in man, 235–236
Codistillation, as a factor in pesticide volatilization, 287
"Cohort," in epidemiological study, 381
Coined names of pesticides, 29–30
Colchicine, as cause of spindle poisoning, 187–188
Cold, hypersensitivity to, 194
Coleoptera, susceptibility of, to pesticides, 504
Colinus virginianus (bobwhite quail), 495
Collards, contamination of by toxaphene, 324
Color, as warning, 432, 458
Colorimetric method, for determining storage of DDT, 340, 344
Columbia, epidemic of poisoning in, 323
Committees, for coordinating activities regarding pesticides, 433, 473–474
Common names of pesticides, 29–30
Community air standards, 447
Community relations, 472–474
Community studies, 329–330
Compatibility of pesticides in storage, 460
Competency, as factor in poisoning, 336–337

Complete differential protection technique for measuring absorption, 256–257, 355–356
Compound(s) (see also Residues)
antagonism of, 73
as factor in
absorption, 148–150
chronicity of poisoning, 37
protection of wildlife, 510–511
residues, 270–271, 278–280, 286, 300
storage and excretion, 161–163, 356
toxicity, 68–69, 334–335, 482
beneficial effects of, 57–62
biotransformation of, 107–118, 303
choice of, in prevention of injury, 455–456, 510–511
classes of, known to be absorbed, 148–150
competition for binding sites by, 132
cumulation of, effect of, 37–39
chronicity index of, 45–46
cumulation of storage, 154–161
concentration index of, 159–160
dangerous, classes of, 431–432, 433, 435, 453–454
derived, 69
interaction of, as factor in
excretion and storage, 162–163, 356
poisoning, 72, 336
residues, 271
kinds of, 72–75
methods of measurement, 72–73
persistency of, in relation to wildlife, 510–511
pharmacological action of, 207–208
potentiation of, 74–75
poisoning by, in man, 316–317
primary, 68–69
storage of, 161–166, 339–349, 355–362
Compound 1080 (see Monosodium fluoroacetate)
Concentration gradient, as factor in passage of compounds through membranes, 133
Concentration index, 159
Conditioning, in behavioral tests, 214
Confidence limits, 41–42
Congenital malformations, incidence of, 201
Congenital porphyria, 89–91
Coniine, 3
Conium maculatum, 3
Conjugation, of chemical compounds
enzymatic basis of, 116
importance of, in detoxification of cyanide, 108
usage of term and characteristic reactions, 108
Consent
of subjects, in testing, 235, 239
of workers, in testing, 243
proof of, 247
Container for poison
cleaning of, 460–461
disposal of, 460
improper, effect of on domestic animals, 481
labeling and location of, as factors in poisoning, 338
safe storage of, 459–460
Contamination, accidental
of clothing, 323, 324
of feed, 480–481
of food, 323–326, 434–436
of skin, 140–150
of soil, 507
of water, 508

Contamination—*Continued*
  removal of, 458–459
Control
  of pests, ecological methods for, 486
  of population, 84–86, 486
  of wildlife, 509–510
Controls in tests (see Statistics)
Convulsions
  monosodium fluoracetate as cause of, 196
  relation to behavioral tests, 215
Cooking of food, effect of, on residues, 275–276
Copper, 517
  and porphyrins, 90–91
  known in ancient Egypt, 3
  treatment of poisoning by, 421
Copper dimethyldithiocarbamate (Wolfen®), 526
  as tumorigen, 192
Copper 8-hydroxy quinoline, as tumorigen, 193
Copper oleate, mixed with tetrahydronaphthalene, as
    cause of mortality, 319
Copper sulfate, 517
  a dangerous emetic, 227, 394
Coproporphyrin, 94, 115
Coproporphyrinogen, 94
Co-Ral® (see Coumaphos)
Cormorants, eggshell thinness in, 494
Corn, in genetic studies, 204
Corn leaf blight, 18
Corn oil, as solvent for dermal absorption tests, 141
Cornea of eye, tests based on thickness of, 214
Corrosive action, of poisons, 183
Corrosive substances, graphic warning labels for, 433,
    434
Corticoid reduction, use of DDD for, 227
Cortisol, in tests for microsomal enzyme changes, 116,
    121
Cortisone
  as factor in teratogenesis, 198, 201
  dermal absorption of,
Cost, of
  developing a pesticide, 453–455
  imports and exports, 24
  pesticides, 23–24
  regulating pesticides, 453–455
Cost-benefit ratio, 27
Cotton, soil residues related to, 295
Cotton seed oil
  effect of, on dermal absorption of Bidrin®, 149
  residues of toxaphene in, 269
Coturnix coturnix (Japanese quail), 496
Coumafuryl (Fumarin®, Fumasol®,), 528
  poisoning by, in man, 317
Coumaphos, 524
  microsomal enzyme induction by, 123
  mortality to cattle caused by, 479
  species difference in susceptibility to, 76
  standards for, 444
  use of, as drug, 227
Coumarin
  as cause of mortality, 319
  species variations in susceptibility to, 126
Court action, involving tests in man, 238–239
Cover crops, as factor in soil residues, 301
Cow, storage of DDT in, 160
Cowbird, fatal level of DDT in brain of, 167

Cow's milk, excretion of pesticides in, 349
4-CPP (see 2-(4-Chlorophenoxy)propionic acid)
Crab
  injury to, 504
  studies of pesticide residues in, 503
"Crash," in avian populations, 493
Creams, prophylactic, 469–470
Cretinism, chemicals as causes of, 197
Criteria for safety, 367–370, 439–442
Critical molecules, inactivation of as mode of action of
    poisons, 185–186
Crop(s)
  cover, retardation of loss of pesticides from soil by,
    301
  production, 17
  type of, as factor in soil residues, 297
Cropworkers, poisoning of, 321, 326
Croton oil, 74
Crowding, effect of
  on avian reproduction, 493
  on toxicity, 84–85
Crufomate (Ruelene®), 525
  biotransformation of, 110
  species differences in toxicity of, 76
  standards for, 444, 550
  use of, as drug, 227
Cryolite, 517
Cube, 518
Cultivation of soil, as factor in residues, 301
Cumulation of effects
  chronicity index, 45–46
  general considerations, 37–39
  relation to storage, 166–167
  schedule of dosage in relation to, 70
Cupric chloride, 91
Cupric sulfate, a dangerous emetic, 395
Cuprizone
  as cause of hydrocephalus, 196
  effect of, on mitochondria, 195
Curve
  cumulative lognormal, 41
  logprobit, 41, 58–61
  logtime-logdosage, 48–52
Cushing's syndrome, 231
Creeping eruption, 233
"Custom applicator," use of term, 437
"Cutoff," in toxicity of homologous series, 184
C-value, 448
Cyanide and related compounds, 519
  as cause of acute illness, 38
  biotransformation of, 111
  dosage-response relationship of, 61
  inhibition of cytochrome oxidase by, 75, 185, 421
  mitochondrial swelling and axonal dystrophy in
    poisoning by, 197
  poisoning by, 51, 317, 319, 333
    treatment of, 421–423
  standards for, 443, 449
  toxicity of, in relation to storage, 166
Cyclophosphamide, 124
Cyclopropanoid fatty acids, safety evaluation of, 6
Cyclizine, and microsomal enzyme induction, 123
Cysteine, conjugation with, 108, 111
Cythioate (Proban®), 522
Cytochrome oxidase

inhibition of, by cyanide ion, 185, 203
release from inhibition, 75, 421–422
Cytogenetic study, relation to mutation, 205
Cytomegalic-inclusion disease, cause of teratogenesis, 201
Czechoslovakia
excretion of pesticides by people in, 351
storage of pesticides by people in, 342

D

2,4-D, 529
absorption and excretion of, 131, 135
as tumorigen, 192
poisoning by, in man, 317, 319, 333
production of in USA, 25
residues of
in air, 282
in soil, 296
in total diet, 278, 279
standards for, 445, 447, 451
studies of
in volunteers, 235
in workers, 229
susceptibility of different species to, 80
toxicity of, as influenced by other compounds, 73
4-DAB, logtime-logdosage curve, 49
Dairy products, pesticide residues in, 266
Dalapon, 529
poisoning by, in man, 317
DAM, use of, as therapeutic agent, 412
Daphnia magna, toxicity of sodium chloride to, 51–52
Dasanit ® (see Fensulfothion)
2,4-DB, 529
DCNB, residues of, 278
DCPA, residues of, 278
DDA, 521
excretion of, 168, 352, 353, 357, 386
production by soil organisms, 302
DDD (TDE), 521
as tumorigen, 191
excretion of, in man, 339, 351–353
for control of gnat larvae, 490–491
microsomal enzyme induction by, 121, 122
persistence of, 490–491, 510–511
production by soil organisms, 302
residues of
in fish, 267
in total diet, 278, 279
in water, 274
standards for, 143
storage of
in eggs of wild birds, 491, 494
in man, 341, 342–343, 344, 346, 347, 348, 350
studies of, in workers, 231
susceptibility to light, 88
toxicity to isolated cells, 204
use of, as drug, 227
DDE, 521
biotransformation from DDT, 107, 111, 118, 122, 302
effect of
on abortion, 364
on peregrine falcon population, 492–502
excretion of, in man, 351, 352, 386

microsomal enzyme induction by, 122
persistence of, 502–503
residues of
in air, 282, 285
in Antarctic birds, 485
in food, 266, 269
in total diet, 277, 278, 279
in water, 274
in wildlife, 484–485, 494
standards for, 443
storage of, in man, 305, 341, 342–343, 344, 346, 347, 348, 350, 361, 384, 385
toxicity of, to isolated cells, 204
DDMS, as product of hydrogenation of DDMU, 110
DDMU, reduction of, 110
DDNU, 110
DDOH, 110
DDT, 521
abortion, effect on, 364
absorption after
intravenous administration, 150
dermal exposure, 141
application of, to water, 504–505
as tumorigen, 191
biotransformation of, 107, 110, 111, 118
control of malaria by, 12, 303–304
critical level of, in brain, 167
disease, in relation to, 10, 86–87, 336–337
distribution in body, 153, 165, 166
dosage-response, in man, 369
enzyme induction by, 113, 120–123, 362
excretion of
in man, 339, 349–353
in milk, 166–167, 349–352
in volunteers, 232–233
in workers, 229
exposure of workers to, 289
metabolism of, 110, 113, 115–116, 118, 302–303
mode of action, 186–187
persistence of, in relation to wildlife, 510–511
poisoning by, 317, 319, 323
production of, in USA, 21–23
regulation of, 334–335
residues of
factors influencing, 267, 269–274, 280, 285–288, 291–294, 298–303
in air, 282–294
in eggs of wild birds, 492–502
in food, 265–282
in regular and special diets, 277, 278, 279, 280
in soil, 294–304
in water, 274–276
removal from various media, 275–276
standards for, 443, 446–447, 450
safety record of, 332–335, 367, 371, 456
storage of
in animals, 66, 77, 153, 157, 167, 168
in man, 162, 340–344, 345–349, 351–355, 361, 384–385
in wildlife, 484–485
susceptibility of different species to, 77–80
susceptibility of, to light, 88
toxicity
as influenced by other compounds, 73
effect of protein on, 83

DDT, toxicity—*Continued*
 in animals, 40, 47, 68, 78, 82, 83
 in relation to storage, 166, 167
 to isolated cells, 204
 to wildlife, 491–510
 use of
  as drug, 227
  in USA, 24, 25
 vapor pressure of, 287
 volatilization from water, 286–288
DDVP (see Dichlorvos)
Dealkylation, 109, 112
Deamination, 110, 112
Deaminomethyl Ruelene ®, as product of deamination
  of Ruelene ®, 110
Death (see Poisoning)
Decamethonium, 413
Decarboxylation, 115
Dechlorination, 110
Decontamination
 of vehicles, 461
 personal, 398, 399, 458–459
Deesterification, 112
Deet, 533
 poisoning by, in man, 317
DEF ® (see S,S,S-tributyl phosphorothioate)
Deferoxamine, as chelating agent, 418
Degradation of poisons in nature, 306
Dehydroacetic acid (DHC), 529
 as tumorigen, 193
Dehydrochlorinase, increase in activity of, by lindane
  and DDT, 113
Dehydrohalogenation, 111
Delille, R., 2
Delnav ® (see Dioxathion)
Demethylation, 113, 115
Demeton (Sytox ®)
 biotransformation of, 109, 112
 exposure to, relation of, to toxic dose, 294
 oxidation of, simple, 109
 poisoning by
  in cattle, 480
  in man, 317, 319
 standards for, 444, 450
 studies of
  in volunteers, 233
  in workers, 229
 sulfoxidation of, 109, 112
 susceptibility of different species to, 79
 use of, as systemic insecticide, 271
Demeton-O, 522, 524
Demeton-O-methyl (Metasystox ®), 522
Demeton-S, 523, 524
Demeton-S-methyl (Metasystox ®), 523
Demeton sulfone, as product of sulfoxidation of demeton, 109, 112
Demeton sulfoxide, as product of sulfoxidation of
  demeton, 109, 112
Denmark
 poison control centers in, 471
 storage of pesticides in people in, 342, 345
Depilatory, use of thallium acetate as, 227
Dermal absorption (see Absorption, dermal)
Dermal exposure
 measurement of, 252–255

 of workers, 288–294, 356
 relation to toxic dose, 293–294
Dermal toxicity
 in man, 327, 336
 of highly toxic compounds, 430–431
 tests for, 208–214
Dermatitis, use of pesticides to treat, 227, 231–234
Dermis, layer of skin, 145
Derris, 518
 studies of, in volunteers, 231
Design of studies in man, 240–248
Desulfuration, 75, 109, 112
Detergent, use of, for removal of pesticides, 399–459
Detoxication
 conjugation in, 108
 direct, by oximes, 412
 usage of word, 129
Detoxifying antidotes (see also Pharmacological and
  Specific antidotes), 407–409
Deuterium, dermal absorption of, 149
Dextrose injection, in supportive treatment, 402
DFA (see Diphenylamine)
DFP, 525
 studies of, in volunteers, 233
DHC (see Dehydroacetic acid)
Diabetes mellitus, chemicals as cause of, 5, 197, 412
Diacetylmonoxime, use of, as therapeutic agent, 412
Diagnosis of poisoning, 379–391
Diagnostic studies, in man, 228, 230
Di-allate, 526
 as tumorigen, 192
Dialysis, 409
Diazinon, 524
 biotransformation of, 123
 exposure of workers to, 290
 mortality to cattle caused by, 479
 poisoning by, in man, 317, 319, 323, 336
 residues of
  in total diet, 278, 279
  standards for, 444, 450
 studies of, in volunteers, 233
 susceptibility of different species to, 77–78
 toxicity of, effect of protein on, 83
Diazoxide, competition for binding sites by, 132
Dibenzanthracene
 mutations caused by, 188
 threshold for, 57
 toxicity of, 68
Dibrom ® (see Naled)
1,2-Dibromoethane, 520
 interaction with food to form toxic product, 274
 poisoning by, in man,
 standards for, 449
Dibucaine, 128
Dicamba, 529
 poisoning by, in man, 317
Dicapthon, 523
Dichlone, 532
 as tumorigen, 193
Dichloran, 532
 as tumorigen, 193
 studies of, in workers, 229
m-Dichlorobenzene, enzyme induction by, 115
o-Dichlorobenzene, 520
 in conjugation reactions, 111

standards for, 449
p-Dichlorobenzene, 520
  excretion of, in man, 340
  poisoning by, in man, 317
  standards for, 449
  studies of, in workers, 229
  vapor pressure of, 287
p,p'-Dichlorobenzophenone, 302
Dichlorodifluoromethane (Freon-12 ®), 519
  poisoning by, in man, 317
p,p'-Dichlorodiphenylmethane, 302
1,1-Dichloroethane, 520
1,2-Dichloroethane, 520
  interaction with food to form toxic product, 274
  poisoning by, in man, 317
  standards for, 449
Dichloroethyl ether, 520
  as tumorigen, 191
2,5-Dichlorophenol, conjugation of, 111
2,5-Dichlorophenyl glucuronic acid, 111
3,4-Dichlorophenylmercapturic acid, 111
1,2-Dichloropropane, 520
  standards for, 449
1,2-Dichloropropene, 520
Dichlorprop (2,4-DP), 529
  as tumorigen, 193
  poisoning by, in man, 317
Dichlorvos (DDVP, Vapona ®), 523
  detoxication of, by liver, 117
  for parasite control, 227
  poisoning by
    in domestic animals, 480
    in man, 317
  standards for, 443, 450
  studies of
    in volunteers, 233
    in workers, 229
  susceptibility of different species to, 78-79
  toxicity
    route of absorption, as factor in, 117
    to animals, 47, 210
  vapor pressure of, 287
Dicofol (Kelthane ®), 521
  exposure of workers to, 287
  metabolism by soil organisms, 302
  residues of, in total diet, 278, 279
  standards for, 443
  toxicity to isolated cells, 204
Dicoumarol, 528
  and microsomal enzymes, 122, 124
Dicrotophos (Bidrin ®), 523
  poisoning by, in man, 317
  toxicity of, in different solvents, 149
Dicryl, 529
  as tumorigen, 193
Dieldrin (HEOD), 521
  adaptation of the liver to, 117-118
  and duck hepatitis virus, 86
  as tumorigen, 191
  as product of epoxidation of aldrin, 109, 112
  defects of, for malaria control, 330
  dermal absorption of, 141
  disappearance of, from soil, 299
  distribution of, in body, 152-153
  dosage-response

curve, 42
  in man, 370
  effect of, on bird breeding, 493, 494, 498, 500
  excretion of
    in animals, 168, 170
    in man, 339-340, 352, 586
  exposure of workers to, 287
  microsomal enzyme induction by, 120, 122
  persistence of, in relation to wildlife, 510-511
  photochemical change of, 271
  poisoning by, in man, 317, 319, 323 327, 410
  protein binding of, 132
  residues of
    in air, 282, 285
    in Antarctic birds, 485
    in food, 266
    in soil, 296
    in total diet, 278, 279
    in water, 274
    removal from water, 276
    standards for, 443, 447, 450
  storage of
    age as factor in, 358
    dosage as factor in, 157
    in blood, 347, 384, 385
    in eggs of wild birds, 494, 497
    in fetus, 350
    in man, 162, 342-343, 345-348, 351, 352, 355, 357,
      361, 384
    race as factor in, 357
    sex as factor in, 358
  studies of
    in volunteers, 232
    in workers, 229
  susceptibility
    of different species to, 77, 78
    in relation to age, 81
    to light, 88
  testing of, 330
  tolerance to, 125
  toxicity of
    in relation to protein deprivation, 83
    in seed dressings, 507, 508
    to animals, 47
    to isolated cells, 204
  vapor pressure of, 287
Diet
  as factor in pesticide storage and excretion, 358
  geographical distribution of residues in, 280-281
  pesticides found in, 276-282
Diethylphosphate, excretion of, 354, 355
Diethylsuccinate, 115
Difenphos (Abate ®), 523
  standards for, 450
  studies of, in volunteers, 233
  toxicity of, 68
Differential protection technique for measurement of
      exposure by two routes, 256-257, 356
Diffusion, as form of passive transfer, 133
Diffusion coefficient, 286
Difolatan ® (see Captafol)
Digitalis, effect of altitude on toxicity of, 88
Dilan, 521
  disappearance of, from soil, 299
  exposure of workers to, 287

Dimefox, 525
    studies of, in volunteers, 233
    susceptibility of different species to, 79
Dimercaprol (BAL)
    effect of temperature on toxicity of, 87–88
    to combat arsenic, 418–420
Dimethoate, 523
    and microsomal enzyme induction, 119, 123
    beneficial effects of small dosages of, 58
    hydrolysis of, 110
    poisoning by, in man, 317
    standards for, 443
    studies of in volunteers, 233
    susceptibility of different species to, 77
    toxicity, to isolated cells, 204
Dimethoxon, and microsomal induction, 119
9,10-Dimethyl-1,2-benzanthracene, dosage-response
        relationship of, 74
O-O-Dimethyl-S-carboxyl-methyl   phosphorodithio-
        ate, biotransformation of, 110
Dimethylacetamid, solvent in dermal toxicity tests,
        212
Dimethyldithiophosphate, excretion of, 354–355
Dimethylformamide, solvent in dermal toxicity tests,
        212
Dimethylnitrosamine, carcinogenic dosage of, 69
Dimethylphthalate, solvent in dermal toxicity tests,
        212
Dimethylsulfoxide
    effect of, on dermal absorption of dicrotophos, 149
    solvent in dermal toxicity tests, 212
Dinitro compounds, toxicity of to isolated cells, 204
Dinitrobutylphenol
    poisoning by, in man, 317
    storage of, in human blood, 385
Dinitrocyclohexylphenol, 527
    toxicity to isolated cells, 204
2,4-Dinitrophenol, 527
    effect of temperature on toxicity of, 87
    poisoning by, in man, 317
    use of, as drug, 227
2,4-Dinitrophenol thiocyanoacetate, 527
Dinitrotoluene, dermal absorption of, 149
Dinobuton, 527
    exposure of workers to, 291
Dinocap, 527
    poisoning by, in man, 192, 317
    toxicity to isolated cells, 204
Dinoseb, 527
    exposure of workers to, 291
Dioxathion, 524
    and microsomal enzymes, 123
    mortality of cattle due to, 479
    standards for, 444
    studies of, in volunteers, 233
    susceptibility of different species to, 77, 79
Diphenamid, 529
    N-dealkylation of, 112
Diphenatrile, 520
    ᐧ as tumorigen, 191
Diphenyl, 532
    as tumorigen, 193
    poisoning by, in man, 317
    standards for, 445, 451
Diphenylacetamide, as product of diphenamid N-

    dealkylation, 112
Diphenylamine, 533
    standards for, 445, 451
Diphenylhydantoin (DPH)
    effect of, on storage of DDT, 356
    enzyme induction by, 121, 124
    incidence of anomalies produced by, 64
Diphenylthiocarbazone (see Dithizone)
Diptera
    in mutagenesis testing, 204–205
    susceptibility of to pesticides, 504
Dipterex ® (see Trichlorfon)
Diquat, 529
    poisoning by, in man, 317
    standards for, 445
Disease
    and probiosis, 86
    as speculative effect of pesticides, 327, 333, 366–367
    chemicals as causes of, 5, 182–218
    dosage in relation to, 380
    influence of, on toxicity, 85–87
    kinds of causes of, 380
    light as cause of, 88
    malaria, control by pesticides, 10–15
    plant, losses caused by, 15–16
    relation of pesticide storage in man to, 359–360,
        361–362
Disposal of pesticides and empty containers, 460–462
Dissociation constant, in ionization, 130
Distribution of compounds
    after absorption, 151–154
    as influenced by various factors, 130–133, 138–140,
        153–154
    dynamics of, 150–151
Disulfoton, 524
    and microsomal enzymes, 123
    beneficial effects of small dosages of, 58
    standards for, 450
    toxicity to isolated cells, 204
Di-Syston ® (see Disulfoton)
Dithane ® (see Nabam), 526
Dithane ® M-45, 526
Dithiocarbamate fungicides
    potentiation of alcohol by, 74
    residues of, in total diet, 278
    standards for, 451
Dithizone
    as chelating agent, 421
    toxicity of, 197
Diuron (Karmex ®), 529
    and microsomal enzymes, 124
    as tumorigen, 193
DMC, 521
    poisoning by, in man, 317
DNA
    in mutagenesis, 189, 206
    in relation to induction of enzymes, 108
    suspensions of, 90
DNOC, 527
    biotransformation of, 111
    exposure of workers to, 291
    poisoning by, in man, 317
    standards for, 451
    studies of,
        in volunteers, 234

in workers, 229
Doctor's First Report of Work Injury, in occupational disease, 321
Dodine, 532
  as tumorigen, 193
Dog
  poisoning of, by malathion, 480
  storage of pesticides in, 161, 359
  susceptibility of to chemicals, 77
Domestic animals
  importance to, of residues in different media, 305
  poisoning of, 478–482
  possible effect of pesticides on, 481
  storage of pesticides in, 481
Dominant lethal mutations and tests for them, 188, 206, 207
Dosage, 536
  as basis of safety standards, 440–442
  as factor in
    chronicity of injury, 37
    excretion, 157, 355
    poisoning, 335, 380, 480, 482
    residues, 269–270, 286, 298–300
    storage, 157, 355, 361–362
    testing in man, 241
    toxicity, 34, 64, 69–71, 335
  at tissue level, 53, 166–167
  choice of, for tests, 55, 241
  duration of, 37, 70–71
  limitation of, for wildlife protection, 511
  measurement of, in relation to human exposure, 249–257
  safe, calculation of, 440–442
  schedule of, as factor in toxicity, 69–70, 217
  selection of levels for tests, 55, 241
  small
    beneficial effects of, 57–58
    lowest effect level, 55
    model for effect of, 58–61
    no significant effect level, 55–56
    threshold
      chemical basis of, 61–62
      reality of, 56–57
  "supralethal," 48
  use of word, 39
Dosage-response relationship
  chemical basis of dosage-response relationships, 45
  chemical basis of thresholds in dosage-response relationships, 61–62
  importance of, 39, 69, 98–99
  in allergy, 65–66
  in carcinogenesis, 64–65
  in chemical control of ecological processes, 8
  in criteria of safety, 367
  in dermal absorption studies, 140–150
  in eggshell thinning and other injury to birds 494–495, 498–499
  in enzyme induction, 66–67
  in hypersensitivity, 65–66
  in metabolism, 66
  in mutagenesis, 65
  in neurotoxicity, 64
  in storage, 66
  in teratogenesis, 64
  in toxicity (sensu stricto), 64

in various phenomena, 45
  measurement of, 39
  to DDT, in man, 369
Dose
  toxic, relation of exposure to, 293–294
  usage of word, 39
Double blind studies, 246
Doves
  delayed breeding of, 497
  increase of, 501
Dowco 109 (see Narlene ®)
2,4-DP (see Dichlorprop)
DPH (see Diphenylhydantoin)
Draize test of eye irritation, 214
Drift, of pesticides in air
  effect of, on domestic animals, 480
  local, 283–284, 286
  worldwide, 284–285
Drosophila melanogaster (fruit fly), in study of mutation, 205
Drug addiction, as cause of mortality, 311
Drug Amendments Act of 1962, 228
Drugs (see Pesticides, Compounds, and names of specific compounds and groups of compounds)
Drums, to hold pesticides, cleaning of, 460–461
DSMA, 529
Duck
  eggshell thinning in, 495
  hepatitis virus and probiosis in, 86
  storage of pesticides in, 484
  susceptibility to certain compounds, 76, 482
Duration of dosage
  of toxicant, 46–47, 70–71
  relation to chronicity index, 45–46
Dursban ® (see Chlorpyrifos)
Dusts, pesticide
  collection of, 250–254, 285
  in dermal toxicity tests, 213
  relation to respiratory absorption, 136–140
  safety of, 457–458
  size of particles in, 137
  standards for, 448–452
  workers' exposure to, 288–294
Dutch elm disease, effect of its control on birds, 492
Dyrene ®, 532

E

Eagle
  bald
    effect on DDT on, 167
    eggshell thinning in, 494, 501
    storage of pesticides in, 484
    trauma as cause of mortality in, 499
  golden, egg weight of, 494
Earthworms, DDT in, 492
EC 50, 53
Ecological community, 486
Ecological factors in
  pest control, 485–503, 510
  protection of wildlife, 492–502, 511–512
Ecological toxicology, relation to environmental toxicology and to toxicology in general, 7–8

Ecology
  agricultural, 487
  monoculture, 17
Economic approach to solutions of pesticide problems, 28
Economic value
  of malaria control, 13–15
  of pesticides, 23
Ecosystem
  model, 27, 503
  storage of pesticides in relation to, 167–168
Ecothiopate, 185
Ectopistes migratourius (passenger pigeon), 501
Ecuador, occupational poisoning by dieldrin in, 327
ED 1, 41
ED 50
  as measure of teratogenicity, 64
  1-dose, 39–43
  90-dose, determination of, 43–45
ED 99, 41
Eddy diffusion, 284
Edema, 209
EDTA (see Ethylenediaminetetraacetic acid)
Education
  for prevention of injury, 464, 470–471
  poison control centers, role in, 471
Eggs
  destruction of, 492–493
  pesticide residues in, 267, 494
Eggshell thinning, 492–502
Egg white, as therapeutic agent, 408
Egypt, epidemics of poisoning in, 323
Electrocardiogram, as supportive test, 392
Electroencephalogram, as supportive test, 391
Electrolytes
  dermal absorption of, 148
  injection of, as therapeutic procedure, 402–403
Electromyography (EMG), in measure of pharmacological effects of pesticides, 365–366
Electro-osmosis, 148
Electrophoresis, effect of, on dermal absorption, 148
Ellenbog, Ulrich, 2
Embryo, injury to (see Teratogenesis)
Embryology, experimental, 217
Embryonic development, stage of, as factor in teratogenesis, 199–200
Emerita analoga (a crab), 503
Emesis, 185, 393–395
Emetics
  pesticides used as, 227
  use of as protective additive, 458
  use in therapy, 393–395
Emetime, 395
EMG (see Electromyography)
Emphysema, 128
Endocrine glands
  effect of isolation or crowding on, 84–88
  effect of light on, 89–96
  effect of, on toxicity, 80
  injury to, 197
Endoplasmic reticulum
  as source of microsomal enzymes, 113
  increase of, as an adaptation, 117
Endosulfan (Thiodan®), 522
  as tumorigen, 192

exposure of workers to, 287
poisoning by, in man, 317
residues of
  in soil, 297
  in total diet, 278, 279
  standards for, 443, 450
toxicity of, effect of protein on, 83
Endothion, 523
  poisoning by, in man, 317
Endrin, 522
  contamination of flour by, 323–324
  cumulation of, 295
  disappearance of, from soil, 299
  excretion of
    in animals, 168, 170
    in man, 386
  exposure of workers to, 287
  microsomal enzyme induction by, 120
  poisoning by, in man, 317, 319, 323
  residues of
    in air, 282
    in soil, 273, 295, 296, 297, 299
    in total diet, 278, 279
    in water, 274
    removal of, from water, 276
    standards for, 443, 447, 450
  resistance of fish to, 489
  storage of
    in animals, 157
    in man, 340, 348, 349, 384, 385
  susceptibility of
    different species to, 77, 78
    to light, 88
  tolerance to, among pine mice, 125
  toxicity of, 68
England (see also United Kingdom)
  excretion of pesticides by people in 351
  pesticide residues in food in, 281
  poisoning associated with pesticides in, 333
  storage of pesticides by people in, 342, 345, 359
Ensilage, reduction of residues by, 274
Enterohepatic circulation, 168
Entomological Society of American (ESA), 31
Environment (see Residues and Wildlife)
Environmental chemicals, effect of
  on metabolism, 75
  on storage, 344
Environmental Mutagen Scoiety, 9
Environmental pharmacology, 6–8
Environmental Protection Agency (EPA), 438, 474
Environmental Quality, Council on, 473
Environmental surveillance of pesticides for safety, 462–463
Environmental toxicology, relation to toxicology in general, 6–8
Enzymes
  anticholinesterases, 185
  as basis of
    biotransformation, 108–117
    conjugation, 108, 116
    interaction of compounds, 75
  biochemical lesions and, 184–185
  induction of
    dosage-response relationships in, 66–67, 108–117
    effect of, on nuclear RNA, 108

non-microsomal, 115
usage of term, 108
inhibition of, as mode of action of some poisons, 75, 184–185, 362
microsomal, induction of
by food or normal metabolites, 108, 116, 120, 122
in liver, 108–117
dosage-response relationships of, 66
factors influencing, 114
in man, 362–363
origin of, 113
pesticides in relation to, 118–124
relation of induction and inhibition, 118
tests for, 114–116
in other organs, 115–116
non-microsomal, induction of, 115
reactivation of, 75, 410–417, 421–422
relation of, totoxicity, 117–118
Eosin, 89
EPA (see Environmental Protection Agency)
Ephemeroptera, susceptibility of, to pesticides, 504
Epidemic
of posoning by pesticides, 322–327, 479–481
of teratogenesis, 5, 201
usage of word, 379
Epidemiology, chemical
in relation to pesticide storage, 362
of effects of pesticides on domestic animals, 478–482
usage of term and methods of study, 379–382
Epidermis
in dermal absorption, 140–150
structure of, 145
Epilepsy, interaction of DDT and drugs used in treatment of, 356–357
Epinephrine hydrochloride
as therapeutic agent, 404
delay of absorption by, 150
Epoxydation, 109, 112
1,2-Epoxyethane, 520
standards for, 449
1,2-Epoxypropane, 520
EPN, 525
and microsomal enzymes, 119–121, 123–124
as substrate in hydrolysis reaction, 115
poisoning by, in man, 317
potentiation of malathion by, 74, 75
standards for, 451
studies of, in volunteers, 233
toxicity of, 47
Epsom salts, use of, as cathartic, 398
Equipment, for handling pesticides, maintenance of, 458
Erbon, 529
Ergot, as cause of poisoning, 4
Erosion, of soil, as cause of migration of pesticides, 297
Erythropoietic protoporphyria, 90
ESA (see Entomological Society of America)
Escherichia coli, endotoxin of, induction of amyloid by, 195
Estradiol, and microsomal enzymes, 120, 122
Estrogens
dermal absorption of, 149
effect of DDT on, 497
Estrone, microsomal enzyme induction by, 122

Estuaries, residues in, 275
ET 50, 47–48
Ethacrynic acid, competition for binding sites by, 132
Ethanol
dermal absorption of, 149
solvent in dermal toxicity tests, 212
Ethephon, 529
Ether, often unsatisfactory for collecting airborne compounds for testing, 250
Ether cleavage (see *O*-dealkylation)
Ether/water partition coefficient, in dermal absorption, 146
Ethereal sulfates, formed by conjugation, 108
Ethics, codes of, in tests in man, 235–238
Ethion (Nialate®), 524
and microsomal enzymes, 123
exposure of workers to, 290
mortality of cattle caused by, 479
occupational disease caused by, 321
residues of, in total diet, 278, 279
standards for, 444
Ethionine, effects of, on cell metabolism, 108
Ethnic group, as factor in poisoning, 336
Ethoxyquin, 530
Ethygutoxin
and microsomal enzyme induction, 119
standards for, 445
Ethyl alcohol (see Ethanol)
Ethyl biscoumacetate, in tests for microsomal enzyme activity, 116
Ethylguthione, and microsomal enzyme induction, 116
Ethyl hexanediol, 533
Ethyl mercury compounds (see Mercury and its compounds)
O-Ethyl-methyl-*S*-phosphorylthiocholine iodide, toxicity of, 68
Ethylbromoacetate, 51
Ethylenediaminetetraacetic acid (EDTA), 51, 419–420
Ethylene dibromide, poisoning by, in man, 319
Ethylene dichloride
poisoning by, in man, 317
studies of, in workers, 229
Ethylesterenol, a catatoxic steroid, 406
Ethylene thiourea, 528
as tumorigen, 192
Euphausia sp. (krill), storage of pesticides in, 485
Europe
excretion of pesticides by people in, 351
storage of pesticides by people in, 342, 344, 345, 346, 351
European Association of Poison Control Centres, 9
European Society of Drug Toxicity, 8, 9
Evaluation of safety, relation to toxicology, 5–6
Evaporation, of pesticides, 273, 283, 286–288, 301, 302
Excretion
as measure of absorption, 135
biliary, 168–169
effect of, on storage, 164–165
factors influencing, 170–171, 355–362
fecal, 168–169, 352–353
in domestic animals, 481
in man, 349–354
in milk, 170, 349–352

Excretion—*Continued*
  respiratory, 168, 353
  study of, in volunteers, 231–235
  urinary, 169, 352–353
Experimental pathology (see Pathology)
Explosive substances, graphic warning labels for, 433–434
Export of pesticides
  cost of, 24
  kinds involved, 22–24
Exposure chambers, 208
Exposure to pesticides
  avoidance of, for safety, 458
  dermal, measurement of, 252–255
  effect of, on metabolism, 362
  history of, as aid to diagnosis, 382
  importance of residues in different media, 304–308
  incidental, in man, 328
  industrial, routes of, 133–134
  measurement of, 249–257
    differential protection technique for, 256–257, 356
    Symth technique for, 256, 356
  occupational, dermal and respiratory, 288–294, 368–370
  of wildlife, 335, 483–485
  oral, measurement of, 255–256
  relation of, to toxic dose, 293–294
  respiratory, measurement of, 249–252
  route of, effect on excretion, storage, and toxicity, 71, 335–336, 355–356
  standards for, 446–452
  via air, 282–294
  via food, 265–282
  via soil, 294–304
  via special diet, 281–282
  via total diet, 276–281
  via water, 274
Eye
  absorption by, 150
  injury to, 197, 321
  susceptibility of, to teratogenesis, 200
  tests for injury to, 214, 241
  washing of, in treatment, 398
  weight of, 152

F

Face, human, surface area of, 255
Factors influencing (see also Pesticides),
  absorption, 147–150
  distribution of chemicals in body, 129–133
  exposure, respiratory and dermal, 291–292
  maintenance of food supply, 17–18
  metabolism, 118–128
  pesticide residues
    in air, 285–288
    in animal products, 267
    in plants, 269–274
    in soil, 298–303
  poisoning, 334–339, 480–482
  population decline among birds, 492–502
  storage, 66, 151, 164, 355–362
  teratogenesis, 198, 201
  toxicity, 37, 67–99, 117–118, 166–167, 198–201
Falco peregrinus (falcon), 493

Falco sparverius (American sparrow hawk), 495
Falco tinnunculus (kestrel), 498
Fallout of pesticides, 283–284
Famphur, 523
  dermal absorption of, 141
Farm laborers, occupational disease among, 321
Farm land, utilization of, 16–17
Farmer, benefits of pesticides to, 15–18
Fat
  biopsy, technique for, 388–389
  blood flow to, 152
  distribution of compounds to, 151–154
  metabolism, 107
  storage of pesticides in, 340–346, 348, 350, 361, 384
    effect of starvation on, 86, 165–166
  vegetable, pesticide residues in, 269
Faunal imbalance, 487
FDA (see United States Food and Drug Administration)
Fecal excretion, 168, 352–353
Fechner's law, 62–63
Federal Aviation Agency, 437
Federal Committee on Pest Control, 473
Federal Environmental Pesticide Control Act, 9, 432
Federal Food, Drug, and Cosmetic Act, 442
Federal Insecticide, Fungicide, and Rodenticide Act (FIFRA), 20, 430–432, 442
Federal Pest Control Review Board, 473
Federal Working Group on Pest Management, 474
Feed additives, 58
Fenac, 530
Fenchlorphos (see Ronnel)
Fenitrothion (Folithion®, Sumithion®), 523
  standards for, 444
  studies of, in workers, 229
Fenoprop (see Silvex)
Fensulfothion (Dasanit®), 524
  poisoning by, in man, 317
  standards for, 444
Fenthion, 523
  for control of mosquito larvae, 274
  poisoning by, in man, 317
  studies of, in workers, 229
  testing of, 332
Fentin acetate, 518
  as tumorigen, 191
  standards for, 443
Fenuron TCA, 530
Ferbam, 526
  as tumorigen, 192
  standards for, 444, 451
Ferguson's principle, 183–184
Ferrous sulfate, use of, as drug, 227
Fertility index, in tests of reproduction, 215
Fertilizers, chemical, effect of, on agriculture, 19, 487
Fetal toxicity, 197–198, 201
Fetus
  human, storage of pesticides in, 163, 349–350
  injury to, 198
  microsomal enzymes in, 114
Fiber, loss and protection of, 15, 19
Fibrosis of lungs, by paraquat, 194–195
Fick's law for membrane penetration, 144
FIFRA (see Federal Insecticide, Fungicide, and Rodenticide Act)

Filtration, as form of passive transfer, 133
Finland
  decline of peregrine falcon population in, 493
  poisoning by parathion in, 327
Fire, caused by pesticides, prevention of, 460
First order kinetics, 157, 160, 298–299
Fish
  absorption of DDT and DDD by, 489–491
  effect of pesticides on, 490–491. 504–505, 506, 507, 508
  food, effect of pesticides on, 504, 505
  pesticide residues in, 267
Fish eating birds, population decline of, 492–502
Flagman, automatic, 470
Flammable substances, graphic warning labels for, 433–434
Fleas, control of, 76
Flies
  in tests of mutagenesis, 204–205
  tsetse, 485–486
Florida
  storage of pesticides in people in, 341, 345
    race as factor in, 357
    sex as factor in, 357–358
  Structural Pest Control Act, 438
Flour, contamination of, by pesticides, 323–324
Fluid balance, maintenance of, in therapy, 402–403
Fluometuron, 530
Fluorides, 517
  poisoning by, in man, 318, 319
  storage of, in bone, 340
Fluoroacetamide, 528
  poisoning by, in man, 317
Fluoroacetic acid, 129
Fluorocitrate, toxicity of, 196
5-Fluorouracil, absorption from gastrointestinal tract, 135–136
Fogs, pesticide, 136–138
Folex® (see Tributyl phosphorothioate)
Folidol® (see Parathion)
Folithion® (see Fenitrothion)
Folpet, 532
  as tumorigen, 193
  standards for, 445
Fontana, Felice, 2
Food
  additives, regulation of, 439, 442
  antinutritive substances in, 6
  contamination of, 323–326
  for babies, residues in, 281
  home grown, residues in, 281–282
  of Alaskan natives, residues in, 282
  pesticide residues in, 265–282, 294, 304
    removal of, 275–276
  safety, evaluation of, 5–6
  supply, maintenance of, 15–18
Food and Drug Administration (FDA), 30, 265, 445
Food chains
  biological magnification in, 167–168, 335, 488–492, 502–503
  usage of term, 488
Food poisoning, 312
Forearms, human, surface area of, 255
Forensic medicine (see Medicine, legal),
Forestry, benefits to, from pesticides, 15

Formaldehyde, as cause of mortality, 319
Formic acid, beneficial effect of small dosages of, 57
Formulation(s)
  as factor in
    exposure, 292
    interaction of compounds, 75
    residues, 271, 300
    safety, 456–458
    testing, 212–213
    toxicity, 75, 141
  dusts and powders, 26, 137, 457
  gases, 136–138
  granules, 137, 457
  liquids and pastes, 136–138, 456–457
  physical form at time of application, 136–138
Formulators, effect of exposure on storage in, 344
France
  decline of peregrine falcon populations in, 493
  legal attitude on tests in man in, 237
  participation of, in Council of Europe, 433
  storage of pesticides, by people in, 342, 344, 346
  use of war gases by, 51
Freon-12® (see Dichlorodifluoromethane)
Fruits, pesticide residues in, 269
Fumarin® (see Coumafuryl)
Fumasol® (see Coumafuryl)
Fumigants
  excretion of, 168
  for post-harvest pest control, 273–274
  physical characteristics of, 136–138
  poisoning by, in man, 317, 338
  studies of
    in volunteers, 231
    in workers, 229
  use of
    as drugs, 227
    in relation to wildlife, 510
Fungal toxins
  poisoning by, 322–323
  safety evaluation of, 6–7
Fungicides (see also separate compounds; groups of compounds; and Pesticides)
  ingestion of, 315
  poisoning by, in man, 38, 315, 316, 317, 321, 323, 324, 335
  studies of, in workers, 223
  treatment of foods with, 273
  years of introduction of, 20–21
Fungus, use of, in genetic studies, 204
Furocoumarin compounds, as causes of photosensitization, 89

G

Gaddum, 41, 440
Gagging to induce emesis, 394
Galecron®, 528
Gametogenesis, in tests of reproduction, 215
Ganglion cells, 197
Gangrene, ergot as cause of, 4
Gardens, home, use of pesticides in, 281–282
Gardona®, 525
Gas chromatography
  comparison with colorimetric method, 340, 344
  use of, 161, 172, 246, 352

Gas warfare, Haber's lecture on, 51
Gases
    dermal absorption of, 149
    pesticide, poisoning by, seasonal differences in, 338
Gastric lavage, 395–397
Gastrointestinal absorption, 135
Gastrointestinal system
    amyloid deposits in, 195
    liver, injury by cuprizone, 195
"Gaussian" curves, 41
"Gates," in nerve axons, 186–187
Generic names of pesticides, 29–30
Genetic factors
    and resistance, 125–128
    in relation to,
        mutagenesis, 189, 205
        susceptibility to poisoning, 80
    in teratogenesis, 199
    in tests of reproduction, 215
Genite®, 528
    as tumorigen, 192
Geographical location, as factor in
    distribution of residues in food, 280–281
    poisoning 337
    storage and excretion, 360, 484–485
Geometric mean, 62–63
Germany
    decline of peregrine falcon population in, 493
    poisoning by parathion in, 327
    use of war gases by, 51
Germany, East, storage of pesticides by people in, 342, 346
Germany, West
    participation of, in Council of Europe, 433
    storage of pesticides by people in, 342
Gesamil® (see Propazine)
Gestation index, in tests of reproduction, 215
G.I. tract (see Gastrointestinal system)
Gibberellic acid, 518
    as tumorigen, 191
Giddiness, resulting from acetylcholine excess, 185
Glauber's salt, use of, as cathartic, 398
Glaucoma, treatment of with DFP, 233
Gossina fuscipes, G. morsitans, and G. palpalis (tsetse flies), 485
Gloves
    contamination within, 210
    for protection, 468–469
Glucocorticoids, as therapeutic agents, 406
Glucose-6-phosphate dehydrogenase
    genetic basis of deficiency of, 127
    relation to forms of vitamin K, 423
    susceptibility of people with defect in, 363
Glucosides, 108
Glucuronic acid, 108, 111, 112
Glucuronide, formation by conjugation, 108
Glucuronyl transferase, increase in activity of, by lindane and DDT, 113
Glutamine, 108
Glutathione (GSH), liver, relation of to bromobenzene toxicity, 62
Glycine
    dependence, in tests for mutagenesis, 205
    in conjugation of foreign compounds, 108
    in synthesis of heme and other porphyrins, 94

Glyodin, 532
Glyoxylate, toxicity of, 61
Gnat, Clear Lake, 490–491
Gold thioglucose, as cause of hyperphagia and obesity, 194
Gonad, storage of chlorinated hydrocarbon insecticides in, 348, 349
Gout, treatment of, by colchicine, 187
Government, affiliation of toxicologists with, 9
Graded response, measurement of, 53
Grain
    pesticide residues in, 267–268
    seed, misuse as food or feed, 323, 480
Granules, pesticide
    residues from, 271
    safety of, 457–458
Graphic warning labels, 433–434
Great Britain (see also England; United Kingdom)
    labeling of pesticides in, 432–433
    poison control centers in, 471
Grebes, 490–491
Greece, malaria eradication in, 13
Griseofulvin, 532
    and microsomal enzymes, 124
    as cause of photosensitization, 89
    use of, as drug, 227
Grus americana (whooping crane), 497
GSH (see Glutathione)
Guatemala
    epidemic of poisoning by organic mercury in, 323
    pesticides in human milk in, 352
Guinea pig
    sensitivity tests in, 213–214
    skin permeability of, relative to other species, 147, 210
    susceptibility of, relative to other species, 77
Guthion® (see Azinphosmethyl)
Gutoxin, and microsomal enzymes, 119

H

Haber's rule, 51–52
Hair follicles
    in dermal absorption, 141, 145, 147
    structure of, 145
Half masks, as protective devices, 466
Halflife of compounds, 158
Haliaeetus leucocephalus (bald eagle), 494
Halogens, corrosive action of, 183
Hands, human, surface area of, 255
Harmful substances, graphic warning labels for, 433–434
Harvest, method of, as factor in residues in food, 273
Hats, for protection, 469
Hawaii, storage of pesticides by people in, 341, 345
Hawks, 494, 495, 497
Hay fever, insecticides suggested as cause of, 328
Hazardous materials, federal regulation of, 431
HCA, 530
HCB (see Hexachlorobenzene)
HCN (hydrogen cyanide) (see Cyanide),
Headache, from acetylcholine excess, 185
Health
    as factor in excretion and storage, 359
    benefit, to from pesticides, 10–15

occupational, toxicological aspects of, 4–5
pesticide residues in relation to, 278
"Health" foods, pesticide residues in, 281
Heart
storage of pesticides in, 349, 350
susceptibility of, to teratogenesis, 200
weight of, 152
Heart disease, insecticides suggested as causes of, 328
Heinz body, 127
HeLa cells, exposure of, to compounds, 204
Helium, dermal absorption of, 149
Hellebore, 3
Helminthiasis
susceptibility of parasites and hosts to chemicals, 76
treatment of with pesticides, 231, 233, 234
Hematocrit, in supportive tests, 392
Heme, regulation of δ-ALA synthetase by, 90–91
Hemiptera, susceptibility of, to pesticides, 504
Hemlock, 3
Hemodialysis, 409
Hemoglobin
inactivation of, by carbon monoxide, 185–186
in supportive tests, 382
P-450 Hemoprotein, increase in, as adaptive measure, 117
Hempa (see Hexamethyl phosphoric triamide)
Henderson-Hasselbach equation, 130
HEOD (see Dieldrin)
Heparin, susceptibility to, in warfarin resistance, 126
Hepatic microsomal enzyme induction, 108, 112–115, 119–124
Hepatic portal absorption
contrast of effect with that of absorption by a systemic vein, 117
measurement of, 134
Hepatitis
danger of, in blood transfusions, 403
DDT as cause of, 366
porphyrin metabolism and, 90
Heptabarbital, and microsomal enzymes, 122, 124
Heptachlor, and its epoxide, 522
absorption of, through plant roots, 273
disappearance of, from soil, 299
excretion of
in animals, 170
in man, 351, 352, 386
microsomal enzyme induction by, 122, 124
persistence of, in relation to other pesticides, 510–511
residues of
in air, 282, 284
in Antarctic birds, 485
in food, 267
in soil, 297, 298
in total diet, 278, 279
standards for, 443, 447, 450
storage of
in animals, 162
in man, 339, 345–346, 347, 348, 350, 384, 385
susceptibility of different species to, 77
toxicity of
in seed dressings, 507, 508
to isolated cells, 204
Herban® (see Noruron)

Herbicides (see also separate compounds, groups of compounds, and Pesticides)
as tumorigens, 192–193
ingestion of, 315
poisoning by, in man, 315, 317, 335
residues of
in air, 282
in food and other crops, 267
in soil, 296
in total diet, 278–279
standards for, 445, 447, 451
studies of
in volunteers, 235
in workers, 229
use of, in relation to wildlife, 510
years of introduction of, 20–22
Hernia, contraindication to vomiting, 394
Herons, eggshell thinning of, 494
Herring gulls, eggshell thickness of, 494
HETP, 525
studies of, in volunteers, 233
Hexachlorobenzene (HCB), 532
and porphyria, 90
poisoning by, in man, 317, 323
standards for, 445
storage and excretion of, 354, 384
storage of, in man, 342–343, 384
Hexachlorocyclopentadiene, 520
Hexachlorophene, 527
as cause of photosensitization, 89
concentration of, in blood, 339, 385
for parasite control, 227
storage and excretion of, 339, 354
Hexamethyl phosphoric triamide (hempa), toxicity testing of, 43
Hexane, as solvent, 146
Hexobarbital sleeping time, as measure of microsomal enzyme activity, 114, 119, 122–124
Hinosan®, 525
and microsomal enzymes, 123
poisoning by, 317
HIOMT (see Hydroxyindole O-methyltransferase)
Hippuric acids, formed by conjugation, 108
Histidine, dependence, in tests for mutagenesis, 204
Histochemical techniques, for studying dermal absorption, 141
History of exposure, as aid to diagnosis, 382
"Hit and run" poisons, 38
Hodgkin's disease, death rate in USA from, 367
Hog
contamination of meat from, 325–326
storage of pesticides in, 163
Homicide, 312, 320, 327
Hoods, as protective devices, 465–466
Hormesis, use of word, 58
Hormoligant, use of word, 58
Hormoligosis, use of word, 58
Hormone(s)
effect of, on storage, 163
excretion of, in human milk, 339
induction of enzymes by, 113
usage of word, 7
Hose mask, 466
Host-mediated tests, for mutagenesis, 205
Houses, pesticides in mud walls of, 303–304

Hueppe's rule, 57
Humidity, relative, as factor in
    teratogenesis in birds, 199
    toxicity, 97
Hungary
    concentration of DDT in milk in, 351
    storage of pesticides by people in, 342, 346
Hydrocephalus, in mice, 196
Hydrochloric acid, corrosive action of, 183
Hydrocortisone
    dermal absorption of, 147
    use of, in therapy, 406
Hydrogen phosphide, 520
    toxicity of, in man, 317
Hydrolysis, metabolic, 110, 112, 113, 115
o-Hydroxyacetanilide, 112
17-Hydroxycorticosteroids, as parameter in studies of
        pesticides in volunteers, 232
2-Hydroxyethyl hydrazine (BOH), 530
    as tumorigen, 193
Hydroxyindole O-methyl transferase (HIOMT), 96
Hydroxyl amine, relation to oximes, 412
4-Hydroxyl-1-naphthyl N-methyl carbamate, 109
Hydroxylation, of ring or side chain, 109, 112
6-Hydroxyzoxazolamine, 112
Hyperbilirubinemia, unconjugated, treatment of,
        with DDT, 362–363
Hyperemia, effect of, on dermal absorption, 148, 213
Hyperglycemia, 197
Hyperphagia, 194
Hyperpyrexia, 85
Hypersensitivity
    dosage-response relationships in, 65–66
    induced by light, 89
    limitations of tests for, 389–391
    to cold, carrageenin as cause of, 194
Hypertension, effect of, on pesticide storage, 359
Hyperthermia, as effect of nitrophenol poisoning, 407
Hypocalcemia, 423
Hypocyames, 3
Hypoglycemia, 197
Hypovolemic shock, 406
Hypoxanthine dependence, in tests for mutagenesis,
        205
Hypoxia of tissues, from carbon monoxide poisoning,
        185–186

                                I

ICPC (see Interdepartmental Committee on Pest
        Control)
Icterus index, in supportive tests, 392
Idaho, storage of pesticides by people in, 341, 345, 347,
        358
Illinois, race as factor in pesticide storage in, 357
Illiteracy of workers, as obstacle to use of labeling, 430
Immunity to infectious diseases, contrast with poison-
        ing, 380
Importation of pesticides
    cost of, 24
    kinds involved, 22–23
    regulation of, 436
Inborn errors of metabolism, 90, 198
Incineration of pesticides, 462

Index(es)
    chronicity, 45–46
    concentration, 159–160
    of reproduction (fertility, gestation, lactation, sur-
        vival, and viability), 215–216
    tests in man, 240
India
    epidemic of poisoning by parathion in, 323
    malaria in, 11–14
    occupational poisoning by dieldrin in, 327
    pesticide residues in food in, 268
    storage of pesticides in people in, 343, 344, 346, 359
Individual differences, as factors in
    metabolism, 118
    storage and excretion, 357
    toxicity, 78
Indoleacetic acid, 530
    as tumorigen, 193
Indonesia, occupational poisoning by dieldrin in, 327
Induction of enzymes (see Enzymes)
Industrial exposure
    equipment for protection from, 464
    measurement of, 249–257
    routes of, 133
    tests of, in workers, 243
Industry, affiliation of toxicologists with, 9
Infant
    mortality, from sodium chloride, 69
    susceptibility of, to pesticides, 81, 349–352
Infection
    epidemiology of, 380
    injury to embryo by, 198, 201
Information on pesticides, sources of, 29–31
Infusions, in treatment of poisoning, 402–403
Ingestion of pesticides, in USA, 315
Inhalation toxicity (see Respiratory toxicity)
Inheritance in man, relation to mutation, 189–190
Injury (see Poisoning; Toxicity)
Inorganic pesticides
    as tumorigens, 191
    poisoning by, in man, 317, 319
    studies of, in volunteers, 231
    used as drugs, 227
Inositol, dependence in tests for mutagenesis, 205
Insanity, insecticides suggested as cause of, 328
Insect repellants, poisoning by, in man, 315
Insecticides (see also specific compounds, groups of
        compounds, and Pesticides)
    ingestion of, 315
    poisoning by, in man, 315, 317, 334, 335
    production of, USA, 20–24
    years of introduction of, 20, 22
Inspection, relation to regulations, 438–439
Insurance, for tests in man, 247
Interaction of compounds (see also Compounds; Po-
        tentiation; Antagonism)
    antidotal oximes with atropine, 415
    as factor in
        residues on crops, 271
        storage and excretion, 135–136, 356–357
        toxicity, 72–75, 336
    importance of environmental chemicals in, 75
    kinds and measurement of, 72–73
    mechanisms of, 75, 131–132
Interdepartmental Committee on Pest Control

(ICPC), 31, 473
International regulation of pesticides, 433, 436
International Maritime Consultive Organization, 436
International Organization for Standardization
    (ISO), 31
International Society of Toxinology, 9
Intestine
    absorption from, 134–135
    biotransformation in, 116
Intoxication, epidemiology of, 379–381
Intravenous
    injection, in studies of absorption, 141–142
    toxicity, in comparison of dosage-response by two
        routes, 117
Invertebrates, effects of pesticides on, 504, 505–506
Investigator, legal protection of, 247–248
Iodine
    beneficial effect of small dosage of, 57
    corrosive action of, 183
    deficiency of, as factor in teratogenesis, 201
    tincture of, as neutralizing antidote, 409
Ion-exchange resins, 75
Ionization
    as factor influencing interaction of compounds, 75
    as factor limiting compound transfer, 130–131
    as influenced by dissociation constant, 130
Ionizing radiation, 89
Ionosphere, pesticide vapors in, 284
Iowa, death of elm trees in, 492
IPC (see Propham)
Ipecac, syrup of, use of, as emetic, 394–395
Iran, epidemics of poisoning by pesticides in, 323–324
Iraq, epidemic of poisoning by organic mercury in, 323
Irradiation, as factor in teratogenesis, 198, 201
Irritant gases and vapors, safety limits for, 453
Irritation and tests for it, 197, 208, 213, 214
ISO (see International Organization for Standardiza-
    tion)
Isobenzan (Telodrin®), 522
    as tumorigen, 192
    poisoning by, in man, 317
Isobole, 72
Isobornyl thiocyanoacetate (Thanite®), 520
    as cause of mortality, 319
    studies of, in volunteers, 231
Isodrin, 522
    disappearance of, from soil, 299
    storage of, 157
Isolan, 526
    as tumorigen, 192
    poisoning by, in man, 317
    route of absorption of, as factor in toxicity, 117
    toxicity of, 71
Isolation, effects of, on toxicity, 84–85
Isomers, variation in metabolism and storage of,
    161–162
Isomerization, 111
Isoprenaline (see Isoproterenol)
Isopropanol
    as solvent in dermal toxicity tests, 212
    effect of, on dermal absorption of dicrotophos, 149
2-Isopropyl-4-pentenoyl urea, porphyria production
    by, 90
o-Isopropylphenyl-N-methylcarbamate, 526
    studies of, in workers, 229

3-Isopropylphenyl-N-methylcarbamate, 526
    poisoning by, in man, 317
    studies of, in workers, 229
    testing of, for vector control, 332
Isoproterenol, 84, 88
Isotopes, for tagging compounds, 171
Israel
    epidemic of poisoning in, 323
    poisoning by pesticides in, 333, 336
    storage of pesticides by people in, 343, 359
Italy
    concentration of DDT in milk in, 351
    participation of, in Council of Europe, 433
    storage of pesticides by people in, 342, 346

                                J

"Jake leg" paralysis, 64
Japan
    parathion poisoning in, 327, 334
    pesticide residues in food in, 281
    storage of pesticides by people in, 343, 346
Johnson Wheeled Sprinkler, 21

                                K

Karmex® (see Diuron)
Kelthane® (see Dicofol)
Kepone® (see Chlordecone)
Kerb®, 530
Kerosene, 519
    contraindication to vomiting, 394
    emetic action of, 405
    poisoning by, in man, 317
Kestrels, mortality of, caused by dieldrin, 498
Kidney
    blood flow to, 152
    function of, effect on storage, 161–166
    in biotransformation, 115
    injury to, by chemicals, 195–196, 365
    lipid concentration in, 361
    storage of pesticides in, 348, 349, 350, 361
    weight of, 152
Kinetics, use of, in pesticide monitoring, 298–300
Kobert, Edward Rudolph, 3
Korea, epidemic of poisoning by warfarin in, 323
Krill, storage of pesticides in, 485
Kuru, an infection mistaken for poisoning, 380

                                L

Labeling of pesticides
    graphic, 433–434
    importance of, 471
    in Great Britain, 432–433
    international proposals for, 433
    in USA, 430–432
    limitation of sale through, 430
    relation to poisoning, 325, 338
Laboratory findings, as aid to diagnosis, 383–391
Laboratory staff, as volunteers in studies in man, 242
Lactation index, in tests of reproduction, 216
Lake trout, 491
Lambs, susceptibility of, to pesticides, 81
Lampreys, control of, 504, 509, 510

Land
  application of pesticides to, 505–507
  utilization of, for farming, 16–18
Larus argentatus, herring gull, 494
Lavage, gastric, for treatment of poisoning, 395–397
Law (or principle or rule)
  Agriculture Poisonous Substances Act, 432, 437
  Armed Forces Act of 1956, 236
  Arndt-Schulz law, 57
  Bertrand's, 57
  California Agricultural Code, 432, 437
  Drug Amendments Act of 1962, 228
  Fechner's, 62
  Federal Aviation Act of 1958, 438
  Federal Environmental Pesticide Control Act of
     1972, 9, 432, 437, 438, 439, 459
  Federal Food, Drug, and Cosmetic Act of 1938, 442
  Federal Insecticide Act of 1910, 430
  Federal Insecticide, Fungicide, and Rodenticide
     Act of 1947, 430, 438, 442
  Federal Seed Act, 458
  Ferguson's, 183–184
  Fick's, 144
  Florida Structural Pest Control Act, 438
  Food Additives Amendment of 1958, 442
  Haber's, 51–52
  Hueppe's, 57
  in relation to
    labeling, 430, 434
    liability, 455
    medicine, 2–4
    samples of pesticides as legal evidence, 388
    studies in man, 235–240
    surveillance of workers, 463
    tests of effectiveness of drugs, 228
    toxicity criteria, 431
    transport of formulations, 434–436
    working conditions, 438
  Karnofsky's, 198
  Miller Amendment of 1954, 442
  Occupational Safety and Health Act of 1970, 438,
     452
  of geometric mean, 63
  permitting or requiring tests in man, 236–238
  Poison Prevention Packaging Act of 1970, 459
  State Pesticide Use and Application Act, 432, 437
LC 50, 53
LD 1, 41
LD 50
  1-dose, 29–42
  90-dose, 43–45
  history of term, 40
  in relation to teratogenicity, 64, 199
  litter, 199
  maternal, 199
  test using small number of animals, 42
LD 99, 41
Leaching of soil, effect on residues, 301
Lead, 517
  blood concentrations of, 339, 385
  corrosive action of, 183
  diagnostic test for, 385–386
  early reference to, 3
  effect of on porphyrin metabolism, 90–91
  poisoning
    in domestic animals, 479, 481
  in man, 2, 317, 318
    treatment of, 418, 420–421
  storage and excretion of, 160–161, 162, 321, 339,
     340, 354
Lead arsenate, 517
  as cause of poisoning, in man, 317, 333
  production and use, 23, 25
  residues of, 275
  standards for, 449
Leafy vegetables, pesticide residues in, 268
Legal medicine (see also both Medicine and Law), 2–4
Legumes, pesticide residues in, 268
Lehmann, Karl Bernhard, 3
Lemmings, in Scandinavia, 486–487
Leptonychotes wenddelli (Wenddell seal), storage of
     pesticides in, 485
Lethal synthesis, 69, 129, 300
Lethane 384®, 520
  poisoning by, in man, 317
Leukemia, deaths from, in USA 366–367
Levarterenol bitartrate, use of, as therapeutic agent,
     404
Lewin, Louis, 3
Liability, a deterent to misuse, 455
Lice, use of parathion in treatment of, 322, 324
Licensing
  of drugs, for sale, 237
  of operators, 437–438
Light (see also Radiation), effects of on toxicity, 88–89
Lime-sulfur, 518
Lindane (see BHC)
Linuron, 530
Lipid
  in organs, relation to pesticide storage, 361
  in membranes, 130, 132–133
  solubility in, as factor in
    absorption by aquatic organisms, 489
    gastrointestinal absorption, 135
Lipid-partitioning and lipid/water coefficient, 133,
     489–490
Liquid pesticide formulations,
  in dermal toxicity tests, 212–213
  in relation to safety, 456–457
Literacy, as factor in poisoning, 338
Litter LD 50, 199
Liver
  adaptation of, 117–118
  amyloid in, 195
  carcinoma of, 361
  changes in function of, by pesticides, 365
  effect of on storage, 161–166
  enzymes, induction of, 115–116, 362
  injury to, 117–118, 195
  lipid concentration of, 361
  mitochondria of, 195
  net effect on biotransformation, 117
  storage of pesticides in, 348, 349, 350, 361
  weight of, 152
Liverstock, poisoning of, by pesticides, 478–482
"Loading dose," 157
Lobodon carcinophagus (crabeater seal), storage of
     pesticides in, 484
Locusts, plagues of, 487
Logprobit
  conversion and the lognormal model, 41
  model, relation to small dosage, 58

phenomena obeying model, 45
relation to other models, 60–61
Logtime-logdosage curve
development of the concept, 48–49
form of the complete curve, 49–50
relation to Haber's rule, 52
use of, for prediction, 51
Lonchura striata (Bengalese finch), 495
Losses caused by
malaria, 11–12
pests, to agriculture and forestry, 15–16
LT 50, 47–48
Lumbar puncture, in supportive tests, 392
Lung
carcinoma of, in man, 311, 312
fate of inhaled materials in, 139–140
fetal, pesticide concentrations in, 350
fibrosis of, 194–195
storage of pesticides in, 348
ventilation of, in athletes, 251
weight of, 152
Luxembourg, participation of, in Council of Europe, 433
Lymph
absorption of compounds into, 135
nodes, storage of pesticides in, 348
vessels, injury to by chemicals, 194
Lymphoblastic transformation test, 391
Lymphocyte cultures for demonstrating chromosome aberrations, 188
Lymphoid tissue, weight of, 152

M

MAC (see Maximal allowable concentration)
Machinery, effect of, on agricultural production, 17, 487
Mackerel, pesticide residues in, 485
Macrophages, in respiratory system, 139
Magendie, Francois, 2
Magnesium salts, as cathartics, 398
Malaria
economic benefits of control of, 13–15
eradication attempted by pesticides, 11–12, 330–333
history of, 11
in Greece, 13–14
in Panama, 11
military importance of, 10–11
potentiation of some drugs, in treatment of, 73
protection from, 12–13
Malathion, 523
absorption of, dermal, 142–144
and microsomal enzymes, 123
beneficial effect of small dosages of, 58
excretion of, in man, 355
exposure to, occupational, 290
for parasite control, 227
measurement of intake of, 354, 355
poisoning by
in animals, 480
in man, 319, 333
postharvest application, 273
potentiation of, by some other compounds, 73–75
residues of
in air, 282
in grain, 267

in total diet, 278, 279
standards for, 444, 450
species differences in susceptibility to, 77–80
studies of
in volunteers, 233
in workers, 229
testing of, for vector control, 330–331
toxicity of, 68
effect of temperature on, 87
to isolated cells, 204
ultra-low-volume application of, 26–27
Malaya, epidemic of poisoning by parathion in, 323
Maleic hydrazide (MH), 530
as tumorigen, 193
Malidixic acid, competition for binding sites by, 132
Mallard duck, storage of pesticides in, 484
Malnutrition (see also Nutrition)
insecticides suggested as cause of, 328
in tests of reproduction, 215
protein, influence of on susceptibility to chemicals, 82–83
Maloxon, 523
as substrate in decarboxylation reaction, 115
studies of, in volunteers, 234
toxicity of, to isolated cells, 204
Malpractice, relation to tests in man, 238
Mammals
circadian rhythms in, 96–97
mutagenesis in, as indicated by sterility, 189, 206
wildlife, effects of pesticides on, 505, 506
Man
dermal absorption rates in, 143
effects of pesticides in, 311–371
inheritance in, relation to mutation, 189–190
relative importance, of residues in different media to 304–305
skin permeability of, relative to other species, 147, 210
storage of pesticides in, 339–350, 354, 355
studies in, 225–264
teratogenesis in, 201
Mancozeb, 526
standards for, 444
Maneb, 526
as tumorigen, 192
poisoning by, in man, 317
standards for, 444
"Market Basket" and related studies of pesticides in food, 276–282, 445
Masks, as protective devices (see also Respirator), 466
Mass spectography, 172
Maternal LD 50, 199
Mathematics
as basis for safety factors, 440–441
of storage, 151–153, 157–161
Mating index, in tests of reproduction, 215
Maximal allowable concentration (MAC), 447
"Maximum tolerated dose," 440
MCPA (Methoxone®), 530
poisoning by, in man, 317
residues of
in meat, 267
in total diet, 278
Measurement of exposure of people to chemicals, 249–257
Meat, pesticide residues in, 267, 280, 325

Median lethal dose, 40
Medical surveillance of workers for safety, 463–464
Medical use of pesticides, 10–15, 226–227, 330–333
Medicine
  clinical, toxicological aspects of, 5
  legal
    books on, 31
    toxicological aspects of, 2–4
  occupational
    books on, 31
    toxicological aspects of, 4, 243
  training of toxicologists in, 8–9
  veterinary, toxicological aspects of, 5
Medicolegal importance of samples, 388
Mefenamic acid, competition for binding sites by, 132
Melatonin, endogenous, 96
Membranes
  as sites of toxic action, 186
  properties of, 130
  transfer of chemicals across, 129–130
Menazon, 523
  and microsomal enzymes, 123
Mendelian patterns of inheritance, 201
Mental
  derangement, as result of poisoning, 363
  incompetence, as factor in poisoning, 336–337
Meprobamate, microsomal enzyme induction by, 121
Mercapturic acids, formed by conjugation, 108
Mercury, and its compounds, 517
  adsorption of, by charcoal, 408
  alkyl mercury compounds, 323, 325–326
  as tumorigens, 191
  beneficial effects of small dosages of, 57
  dermal toxicity, as influenced by volatility, 211
  effect of, on bird population, 493, 498, 500
  ethyl mercury compounds, 323, 480
  human tolerance for, 69
  in red blood cells of people, 190
  in treatment of syphilis, 1, 133
  methyl mercury compounds, 201, 323, 480
  organic, poisoning by, in man, 317, 323–326
  phenyl mercuric acetate, as tumorigen, 191
  poisoning by, 317, 318, 319, 323–326, 333, 480
  rate of absorption of, 143
  standards for, 449
  storage and excretion of, 190, 339, 354, 385
  toxicity of, 201
  treatment of poisoning by, with BAL, 419–420
  use as cathartic, 227
Mesenteric fat, storage of pesticides in, 348
Metabolic pool technique, 172
Metabolism (see also Absorption; Distribution; Stor-
    age; Excretion)
  balance studies in, 171
  biotransformation, including specific chemical
    reactions in, 107–118
  concentration index, 159
  conjugation in, 108, 111, 112, 116
  definition of, 107
  dosage-response relationships in, 66
  enzymes in, 108–133
  "external," 107
  extrahepatic, 115–116
  factor(s) in, 108, 117–118, 127–128
  fat, 107
  measurement of, 172–173

  nonmicrosomal, 115
  protein, 107
  qualitative, 107–129
  quantitative, 129–172
  relation to
    adaptation and injury, 117–118
    resistance, 118–126
    tolerance, 118–125
    toxicity, 117–118, 129
Metabolites, of pesticides
  excretion of, 352, 354–356
  qualitative aspects, 107–128
  toxicity of, 129
Metaldehyde, 528
  poisoning by, in man, 317
Metals
  monitoring of, 294–297, 484
  persistence of residues of, in soil, 300
Metaphase, effect of colchicine on, 188
Metaraminol bitartrate, use of, as therapeutic agent,
    405
Meta-Systox® (see Oxydemetonmethyl)
Metepa, 532
  as tumorigen, 193
  toxicity of, 47
Methanol, dermal absorption of, 149
Methemaglobin, in supportive tests, 392
Methidathion, 523
  standards for, 444
Methionine sulfoximine, mitochondrial swelling and
    axonal dystrophy in poisoning by, 197
Methods (see Techniques)
Methomyl, 526
Methoxone® (see MCPA)
Methoxychlor, 521
  and microsomal enzymes, 121
  excretion of, 168, 170
  poisoning by, in man, 317
  residues of,
    in soil, 296
    in total diet, 278, 279
    standards for, 443, 447, 450
  storage of, 157, 163, 342–343
  studies of, in volunteers, 232
  susceptibility of different species to, 77, 79
  toxicity to isolated cells, 204
5-Methoxypsoralem, as cause of photosensitization,
    89
Methyl amine, 110
Methyl bromide, 520
  poisoning by, in man, 317, 319
  standards for, 449
  vapor pressure of, 287
Methyl chloride, 520
Methyl demeton
  occupational poisoning by, in Brazil, 326
  poisoning by, in man, 317
  standards for, 450
  studies of
    in volunteers, 234
    in workers, 229
Methyl mercury compounds (see Mercury and its
    compounds)
Methyl paraoxon, and microsomal enzymes, 119
Methyl parathion, 524
  and microsomal enzymes, 119, 123

circadian rhythms as factor in toxicity of, 96
exposure of workers to, 290
metabolism, 109
occupational poisoning by, in Brazil, 326
poisoning by, 317, 319
residues of
    in air, 282
    in soil, 296
    in total diet, 278
    standards for, 444
studies of, in volunteers, 234
susceptibility of different species to, 77, 79, 97
Methyl salicylate
    effect of, on dermal absorption of dicrotophos, 149
    solvent in dermal toxicity tests, 212
N-Methylaniline, oxidation of, 112
Methylazoxymethanol, as cause of microcephaly, 196
Methylchloroformate, 51
Methylcholanthrene
    as photosensitizer, 89
    carcinogenicity, 57, 60, 65
    microsomal enzyme induction by, 75, 122, 123
    mutations in mice caused by, 188
    toxicity of, 65, 68
Methylene blue
    as photosensitizing agent, 89
    in measurement of oral ingestion, 255
Methylene chloride, 520
    metabolism of, 108
    penetration of skin by, 142
    poisoning by, in man, 317
    standards for, 449
    studies of, in volunteers, 231
Methyprylon, and microsomal enzymes, 121
Metobromuron, 530
Mevinphos, 523
    and microsomal enzymes, 123
    poisoning by, in man, 317, 319, 323, 336
    standards for, 444, 450
    susceptibility of different species to, 77
Mexico, epidemics of poisoning by parathion in, 323, 326
MH (see Maleic hydrazide)
Microcephaly, in rats, 198
Micronutrients, influence of, on pesticide absorption by plants, 273
Microorganisms, biotransformation of compounds by, 107, 302–303, 487
Microscopy, fluorescent, for studying dermal absorption, 141
Microsomal enzymes (see Enzymes, microsomal)
Microsomal fraction, 113
Microsomal protein, increase of, as adaptive measure, 117
Milbam® (see Ziram)
Military
    importance of malaria, 10–11
    personnel, as volunteers in testing, 242
Milk
    as neutralizing antidote, 408
    excretion of compounds in, 170, 339, 349–352
    lactation index, 216
    pesticide residues in, 266–267
Milk of magnesia, use of
    as cathartic, 398
    as neutralizing antidote, 408

MINA, use of, as therapeutic agent, 412
Mineral(s)
    excretion of, in human milk, 339
    requirement for, 58
    supplement, ferrous sulfate as, 227
Mint, aldicarb residues in, 271
Miosis, resulting from acetylcholine excess, 185
Mipafox, 525
    poisoning by, in man, 317
Mirex, 522
    as tumorigen, 192
    effect on wildlife, 484, 510
    residues of, in soil, 269
    toxicity of, 47
Mississippi River, pesticide residues in, 275
Mists, pesticide, 136–137
Mites, as pests, 488
Mitochondria of liver, kidney, and nerve, 195–196
Mitomycin C, teratogenesis of, as related to schedule of dosing, 217
Mobam® (see 4-Benzothienyl-N-methyl carbamate)
Mode of action
    general considerations, 182
    nonspecific, 183–184
    of eggshell thinning in birds, 497–498
    relation to
        biochemical lesion, 184
        critical molecules, 185–186
        enzymes, 184–185
        Ferguson's principle, 183–184
        membranes, 186–187
        reversibility, 38–39
        "supralethal" dosage, 48
    specific, 184–187
Model(s)
    cumulative lognormal, of toxicity, 41
    of dynamics of storage, 155–156
    of ecosystem, 27, 503
Moisture, as factor in residues in soil, 301
Mold, slime, in genetic studies, 204–205
Molecular weight, effect on dermal penetration, 144
Molecules, critical, usage of term, 185
Molluscicides
    application of, to water, 504
    poisoning by, in man, 317
    to control schistosomiasis, 10
Molybdenum, 75, 83
Monetary model for pesticide storage, 155
Mongolism, 189
Monitoring, for pesticides
    in food, 445–446
    is soil, 295–297
    in wildlife, 484
    in workers, 462–464
Monkey
    in toxicity testing, 76
    storage of DDT in, 77, 163
Monocrotophos, 523
    poisoning by, 317
    standards for, 444
Monoculture, 17, 487
Monoisonitrosoacetone, use of, as therapeutic agent, 412
Monolayer, of hexadecanol to limit evaporation of water, 288

Monosodium fluoracetate (compound 1080)
  as cause of convulsions, 196
  history of name, 29
  poisoning by, 317, 488
Monosodium L-glutamate, damage to retina by, 197
Monuron (Telvar®), 530
  as tumorigen, 193
  toxicity of, effect of protein on, 83
Monuron TCA, 530
Morbidity (see also Poisoning)
  chemical carcinogenesis as cause of, 194
  endemic
    in animals, 479
    in man, 313-316, 320-322
  malaria as cause, 11
Morfamquat dichloride, 530
  toxic effects of, 195-196
Morphine
  as product of codeine O-dealkylation, 112
  tolerance to, 380
Mortality (see Poisoning)
Mosquito
  anopheline, in malaria transmission, 11
  resistance of, to insecticides, 13
Mosquito fish, pesticide resistance in, 126
Moth balls, poisoning by, in man, 314, 315
Motivation of volunteers, 248
Mourning dove, eggshell thickness in, 496
Mouse, susceptibility of, compared to other species, 77
mppcf (million particles per cubic foot), 448
MSMA, 517
Mucor alternans, pesticide degrading capability of, 303
Mud walls of homes, distribution of residues in, 303-304
Murder (see Homicide)
Muscle
  fasciculation, 140
  weight of, 152
Mustard, dry, powdered, use of, as emetic, 394
Mustard greens, contamination of, 324-325
Mutagenesis
  dosage-response relations of, 65, 206-207
  general considerations, 188-190
  pesticides as cause of, 189
  tests for, 204-207
Myasthenia gravis, treatment of, with pesticides, 233-234
Myleran® (see Busulfan)
Myocardium, blood flow to, 151
Myxomatosis, 512

N

Nabam, 523
  as tumorigen, 192
  standards for, 444
Naled (Dibrom®)
  poisoning by, in man, 317
  studies of
    in volunteers, 234
    in workers, 229
Names (see Nomenclature)
Naphthalene, 520
  poisoning by, in man, 317

standards for, 450
1-Naphthaleneacetamide, 530
  as tumorigen, 193
Naptalam (NPA), 530
  as tumorigen, 193
1-Napthol, toxicity to isolated cells, 204
1-Napthyl-N-hydroxyl-methyl carbamate, 112
Narcosis, in behavioral tests, 215
Narlene® (DOWCO 109), 525
National Association of Coroners, 9
National differences in epidemiology of poisoning, 338
National Institute for Occupational Safety and Health (NIOSH), 452
National soil monitoring, 295-296
Nausea, resulting from acetylcholine excess, 185
Neburon, 530
Neck, human, surface area of, 255
Necrosis, of retinal ganglion cells, 197
Nemagon®, 520
  poisoning by, in man, 317
Nematocides
  poisoning by, in man, 317
  studies of
    in volunteers, 231
    in workers, 229
Nematodes, 76
Neoplasia (see Carcinogenesis)
Neostigmine, and acetylcholinesterase, 411
Nephrosis, 131
Nerves, damage to, 186-187
Nervous system
  axons of, sodium and potassium ions in, 186
  central
    blood flow to, 151
    effect of acetylcholine excess on, 185
    specific toxic action on, 85, 196-197
  peripheral, injury to, by anticholinesterases, 185
  stimulation of, by analeptics, 405
  tests on, 392
Nervousness, resulting from acetylcholine excess, 185
Netherlands
  participation of, in Council of Europe, 433
  storage of pesticides by people in, 342, 346
Neurogenic shock, 404
Neuromuscular junction, depolarization of, by oximes, 413
Neurospora crassa, in study of mutation, 204
Neurotoxicity
  a distinct kind of injury, 37
  dosage-response relationships in, 64
  to be avoided in tests in man, 240
New York Academy of Sciences, 8
New Zealand, storage of pesticides in people in, 343, 346
Nialate® (see Ethion)
Nickel, dermal absorption of, 149
Nicotine, 518
  adsorption of, by charcoal, 408
  dermal absorption of, 149
  detoxication of, 117
  excretion of, in human milk, 339
  poisoning by, in man, 317, 319, 324, 333, 335
  standards for, 449
  tolerance for, 125
  toxicity of, 68, 117
  vapor pressure of, 287

Nigeria
    occupational poisoning by dieldrin in, 327
    storage of pesticides in people in, 343
Nikethamide, use of, in therapy, 405
NIOSH (see National Institute for Occupational
        Safety and Health)
Nitrites, and sodium thiosulfate in treatment of
        cyanide poisoning, 75, 421–422
p-Nitroanisole, in relation to biotransformation, 120,
        121, 124
Nitrobenzene, dermal absorption of, 149
p-Nitrobenzoic acid
    and microsomal enzymes, 120
    reduction of, 112, 115
Nitrogen, dermal absorption of, 149
Nitrophenolic pesticides
    hyperthermia in poisoning, 407
    metabolism of, 112
    poisoning by, in man, 317
    studies of
        in volunteers, 234
        in workers, 229
    use of, as drugs, 227
No effect level (see also Dosage), 39, 55-57, 440
Nomenclature
    for drugs, 30
    for particle sizes, 136
    for pesticides
        CAS Registry Number, 31
        proprietary, nonproprietary, approved, coined,
            common, generic, and official names, 29–30
        sources of information on, 31
Non-agricultural land, application of pesticides to,
        505-506
Nonproprietary names (see Nomenclature)
Nonspecific action, 183–184
Norbolethane, a catatoxic steroid, 406
Norbormide, 528
    species differences in toxicity, 76
    tolerance to, in rodents, 125
Norea (see Noruron)
Norepinephrin, 404
Norpipanone, effect of temperature on toxicity of, 88
North America
    epidemics of poisoning by pesticides in, 323–324
    storage of pesticides by people in, 341, 342–345
Noruron (Herban®, norea), 530
    and microsomal enzymes, 124
    as tumorigen, 193
Nose, aerodynamics of, 138, 250, 251–252
"No significant effect level," 55–56, 440
NPA (see Naptalam)
NPN (nonprotein nitrogen of blood), in supportive
        tests, 392
Nuclear fallout, 285
"Nuisance dusts," 448
Numerical safety factor, 440–441
Nuremberg Military Tribunal, 235
Nursing care, in treatment of patients, 406–407
Nutrition
    anorexia, 88
    influence of, on
        excretion, 358
        pesticide penetration of plants, 273
        storage, 165, 358
        teratogenicity, 198, 201

    toxicity, 82–83
    protein, 82–83
    starvation, 82–83
    studies of, in man, 240
    trace elements, 83

                            O

Obesity, 194
Obidoxime chloride, as therapeutic agent, 412,
        416–417
Occupation, as factor in poisoning by pesticides, 339
Occupational disease, including poisoning,
    reports of, in USA, 321–322, 324, 326
    silicosis, 139
Occupational exposure (see Exposure to pesticides,
        occupational
Occupational health, 4–5, 136
Occupational Safety and Health Act of 1970, 164, 438,
        452
Occupational Safety and Health Administration
        (OSHA), 452
Occupational safety, regulations for ensuring, 436–439
Oceania, storage of pesticides by people in, 343, 346
n-Octanol, as solvent in dermal toxicity tests, 212
Official names of pesticides, 29–30
Oils
    dietary, as cause of chloroleukemia, 207
    vegetable, pesticide residues in, 269
Olive oil/water partition coefficient, 146
Omethoate, 523
OMPA (See Schradan)
Onion plants, in genetic studies, 204
Operant conditioning, in behavior tests, 214
Operators, pesticide, licensing of, 437–438
Opium, 3
Oral absorption, 133
Oral dosing
    required by regulations, 431
    techniques for, 217
Oral exposure
    of workers, 294
    measurement of, under practical conditions,
        255–256
Orfila, M. J. B., father of toxicology, 2, 3
Organ, function tests of, effect on storage, 164–165,
        207–218
Organic mercury (see Mercury and its compounds)
Organic phosphorus compounds
    absorption, dermal, 133
    acetylcholinesterase, 185
    additon to water, 274
    excretion of, 353–355
    inhibition of enzymes by, 362
    mental alertness in relation to, 363–364
    metabolism, extrahepatic, 116
    neurotoxicity caused by, 64
    poisoning by
        in animals, 479–481
        in man, 317, 319, 321, 323–327
        treatment of, 409–417
    potentiation of toxicity of, 73
    residues of
        in air, 282
        in food, 267, 269
        in total diet, 276–280

Organic phosphorus compounds, residues of—*Continued*
    standards for, 443–444, 447, 450
    study of
        in volunteers, 233–234
        in workers, 229
    toxicity of
        cumulative, 46
        dermal, measurement of, 140
        to isolated cells, 204
    use of, as drugs, 227
Organometal pesticides (see separate elements)
Organs, storage of pesticides in, 349
Ornithines, 108
Orotic acid, 108
OSHA (see Occupational Safety and Health Administration)
Osprey, 493
Ouabain, mitochondrial swelling and axonal dystrophy in poisoning by, 197
Ovex (see Chlorfenson)
Owl, great horned, 494
Oxidation, chemical, in metabolism, 109, 112
Oxidation of nitrogen, 112
Oxidative phosphorylation, inhibition of, 184
Oxidizing substances, graphic warning labels for, 433–434
Oximes, as specific antidotes, 410–417
Oxine-copper, 517
    as tumorigen, 193
Oxydemetonmethyl (Meta-Systox ®), 523
    susceptibility of different species to, 77
Oxygen
    as antidote, 401–402, 422–423
    dermal absorption of, 149
    in photodynamic processes, 89
Oxythioguinox, as photosensitizer, 89
Oysters, absorption of DDT by, 490
Ozone, in reduction of pesticide residues in water, 276

P

p (Permeability constant), 144
Palate, susceptibility of, to teratogenesis, 200
2-PAM
    as diagnostic agent, 379
    restoration of enzymes by, 75, 415–416
Panama Canal, malaria control at, 11
Pancreas
    concentration of pests in, 350
    injury to beta cells of, by dithizon, 197
    weight of, 152
Pandion haliaelus, osprey, 493
Panniculus fat, storage of pesticides in, 348
Pants, contamination of, by mevinphos, 323–324
Paracelsus, 1–2
Paramecium, 89
Parameters
    for studies of pesticides in man, 231–235, 240–241
    of storage, 156
Paranitrophenol, toxicity to isolated cells, 204
Paraoxon, 525
    absorption of, dermal, 140, 142, 143
    and microsomal enzymes, 119, 123
    conversion of parathion to, 88, 112, 326
    metabolism of, by skin, 116, 141, 144–145

relative solubility of, 146
    studies of, in volunteers, 234
    toxicity to isolated cells, 204
Paraquat, 530
    effect of, on lungs, 136, 194–195
    poisoning by
        in animals, 480–481
        in man, 317
    standards for, 445, 451
    toxicity of, 47, 136
Parasite-host differences in susceptibility, 75–76
Parasympathetic system, excessive activity of, 185
Parathion (Folidol®), 525
    absorption of, dermal, 140, 141, 143, 356
    adsorption of, by charcoal, 408
    and microsomal enzymes, 119, 123
    as substrate in desulfuration reaction, 115
    conversion to paraoxon, 69, 88, 112, 326
    excretion of, in man, 340
    exposure of workers to, 290, 356
    metabolism of, by microorganisms, 302
    poisoning by, in man, 317, 319, 323, 324, 334, 336
    reduction of, species differences in, 110
    regulation of importation of, 436
    residues of
        in air, 282
        in soil, 294
        in total diet, 278, 279
        removal of, from water, 276
        standards for, 444, 450
    studies of
        in volunteers, 234
        in workers, 229, 356
    susceptibility to, in different species, 77, 78, 79
    toxicity of
        effect of protein binding on, 69, 83
        effect of temperature on, 87
        in animals, 47, 68
        to isolated cells, 204
    toxification of, by liver, 117
    vapor pressure of, 287
Parathion-methyl (see Methyl-parathion)
Paris Green, 517
    effect of, on fish, 503–504
Parnon®, 532
    microsomal enzyme induction by, 124
Particle size
    as determinant of inhalation, 138–140
    of pesticidal dusts and sprays, 136–138
Partition coefficient, between water and oil, 141, 184
Passenger pigeon, extinction of, 501
Passive transfer across membranes, 132–133
Paste, formulations of pesticides, safety of, 456–457
Patch test, 214
Pathology, experimental, relation of toxicity to, 2–5
Patients
    as volunteers in studies in man, 242
    nursing of, 406–407
    storage and excretion of pesticides by, 384–386
PCB's (see Polychlorinated biphenyls)
PCP (see Pentachlorophenol)
Peanuts, residues in soils for raising, 297
Pea plants, in genetic studies, 204
PEBC (see Pebulate)
Pebulate (PEBC), 526
    as tumorigen, 192

biotransformation of, 110
Pediatric disease, studies of, 240
Pediculosis, treatment of, with pesticides, 227, 232, 234
Pelicanus erythrorhynchos (white pelican), 494
Pelicanus occidentalis (brown pelican), 492
Pellagra, effect on porphyrin metabolism, 90
Penacillamine, and metals bound by it, 418, 421
Penguins, storage of pesticides in, 484, 485
Pentachlorophenol (PCP), 527
  application of, to water, 504
  as tumorigen, 192
  excretion of, in man, 339, 354, 386
  poisoning by, in man, 317, 324, 380, 382
  residues of, in total diet, 278
  standards for, 451
  storage of, in man, 339, 354, 385
  studies of, in workers, 229
Pentobarbital
  microsomal enzyme substrate, 121
  use of, as pharmacological antidote, 410
"Percent-per-day," rate of storage loss, 156
Perchlormethyl mercaptan, 51
Percutaneous absorption (see Absorption, dermal)
Pericarditis, acute, piscofuranine as cause of, 196
Peripheral nervous system, specific toxic actions on, 185, 186, 197
Perirenal fat, storage of pesticides in, 348
Permeability
  constant, and units for expressing, 144
  dermal in different species, 210
Permissible level of residue, 442
"Persistent pesticides," effect of, on wildlife, 510–511
Perthane®, 521
  as cause of fire, 460
  as tumorigen, 191
  excretion of, 168
  exposure of workers to, 287
  residues of, in total diet, 278, 279
  studies of, in volunteers, 232
  toxicity to isolated cells, 204
Pest control
  alternative methods of, 474, 512
  natural, 486
  nature of, 503
Pest control operators
  licensing of, 437–438
  occupational disease in, 321
Pesticides (see also Factors influencing; Poisoning; Toxicity), 317–333
  absorption, rates of, 141–148
  application of
    methods for, 21, 26–27
    to land and water, 504–507
  as anthelmentics, 227
  benefits from, 9–20, 57
  chemical reactions in metabolism of, 107–129
  cost of, 23–24, 453–455
  definition of, 9
  disposal of, 461–462
    container for, 460–461
  effects of, on man
    marginal, 363–366
    observed, 311–363
    speculative, 366–367
  evaporation of, 273, 283, 286–288, 301, 302

excretion of, in man, 349–362
exports of, 22–23, 24
formulations of, as factor in
  respiratory absorption, 136–138
  safety, 456–458
geographical location as factor in residues in
  food, 280–281
  people, 360
  wildlife, 283–284, 484–485
imports, 22–23, 24, 436
induction of microsomal enzymes by, 118–124, 362–363
information on, 31
inhibition of blood cholinesterase by, 362
introduction of, dates of, 20–21
losses of livestock caused by, 479–481
methods of application
  as factor in
    exposure of people, 291–294, 304–305
    residues in food, 281–282
    residues in soil, 298–301
  general considerations, 21, 26–27
modified use to limit injury to wildlife, 510–512
monitoring for, 295–297, 484
mutagenic action of, 189
nomenclature of, 29–30, 33
persistence of, 510–511
physical characteristics of, at time of application, 136–137
poisoning by
  in domestic animals, 478–482
  in man, 311–339, 391–423
post-harvest application of, 273–274
problems, related to, 27–29
production of, 20–27
proprietary and non-proprietary names, 29–30
regulation of, legal, 429–455
residues of
  in air, 282–294
  in food, 265–282
  in soil, 294–304
  in total diet, 276–282
  in water, 274–276
specificity of, 511
storage of
  in domestic animals, 481
  in man, 339–349, 355–362
  in wildlife, 483–485
studies of
  in volunteers, 231–235
  in workers, 229–230
units of measure, 33, 144–145, 534, 535
use
  as drugs, 227
  number of compounds and products involved, 24–26
  regulation of, 436–439
  tonnage of, 24–25
Pesticides Safety Precautions Scheme, in Great Britain, 38, 432, 507
Pests
  as factors in disease, 10
  control of, by natural and alternate means, 486, 512
  definition of, 9
  "emergent," 487–488
  losses caused by, 13, 14, 15–16

Pests—*Continued*
  nature of, 485–486
  problems, biotic simplification, as cause of, 486–488
Peters, Rudolph A., 3, 69, 129, 184
Petrolatum emulsion, liquid, as cathartic, 397
pH
  as factor influencing toxicity, 97, 130–131
  effect of, on adsorption of chemicals by charcoal, 408
Phagocytosis, in respiratory system, 139
Phalacrocorax aurilius (cormorant), 494
Pharmacogenetics, 127
Pharmacological antidotes (see also Detoxicating and Specific antidotes), 409–410
Pharmacological effects
  in tests in man, 241
  relation of tissue levels to, 53
  tests for, 207, 386
Pharmacology, relation to toxicology, 2, 8, 9
Pharynx, 138–140
Phasianus colchicus (pheasant), 498
Phenobarbital
  carcinogenicity in man and mouse, 194
  effect of, on pesticide toxicity, 118
  effect of, on storage of DDT, 356–357
  microsomal enzyme induction by, 120–124, 410
  storage of, 162
  use of, as pharmacological antidote, 410
Phenols and related compounds
  corrosive action of, 183
  dermal absorption of, 149
  occupational disease caused by, 321
  poisoning by, in man, 317, 324
  studies of
    in volunteers, 234
    in workers, 229
  use of, as drugs, 227
Phenosulfophthalein, in supportive tests, 392
Phenothiazines, 528
  as cause of photosensitization, 89
  as tumorigens, 192
  use of, as antiemetics, 406
Phenoxyacetic acid herbicides, poisoning by, 333
Phenyl mercuric acetate (see Mercury and its compounds)
Phenylacetone, as product of amphetamine deamination, 112
Phenylbutazone
  and microsomal enzymes, 116, 122
  as cause of thrombocytopenic purpura, 389
  protein binding of, 132
o-Phenylphenol, 527
  as tumorigen, 192
p-Phenylphenol, 527
  as tumorigen, 192
Phenyramidol, and microsomal enzymes, 124
Pheochromocytoma, removal of, as cause of shock, 404
Pheromone
  threshold concentration of, 57
  usage of word, 7
Phloem necrosis, a disease of elms, 492
Phorate, 525
  and microsomal enzymes, 123
  metabolism of, by microorganisms, 302
  poisoning by, in man, 317
  standards for, 450

Phosalone, 525
  standards for, 444
Phosdrin® (see Mevinphos)
Phosgene, 51
Phosphamidon, 524
  N-dealkylation of, 109
  poisoning by, in man, 317
  standards for, 444
  susceptibility of different species to, 77
Phosphine (see Hydrogen phosphide)
Phosphorus, 518
  adsorption of, by charcoal, 408
  poisoning by, in man, 317, 319
  restriction of sale of, 436
  standards for, 449
Phostex®, 525
  poisoning by, in man, 317
Phostoxin® (see Aluminum phosphide)
Photochemical change, 89, 271, 284
Photodieldrin, 271
Photodynamic processes, 89
Photoperiodicity, 89, 96
Photosensitization, 89–91
Physical action of compounds, 183–184
Physician, role of, in education of workers, 464
Physiological studies in man, 230–235
Physostigmine, acetylcholinesterase inhibition by, 411
Phytonadione, as specific antidote, 423
Picloram, 530
  standards for, 451
Picrotoxin, effect of temperature on toxicity of, 87
Pig, skin permeability of, 210
Pineal gland, 96
pINN (see Nomenclature, nonproprietary names)
Pinocytosis, 133
Piperalin, 530
Piperonyl butoxide, 519
  as tumorigen, 191
  effect of, on microsomal enzymes, 118, 119
  interaction with other compounds, 73
  standards for, 443
  studies of, in volunteers, 231
Piperonyl sulfoxide, 519
  as tumorigen, 191
Piscofuranine, as cause of pericarditis, 196
Pk$_a$ values, 130
Placebos, use of, in tests in man, 238, 246
Plague, 10
Planavin®, 530
Plants
  enzymes of, biotransformation by, 107
  losses of, caused by pests, 15–16
  poisonous, relation to toxinology, 7
  residues in, 267–269
    factors influencing, 269–274
  "systemic" pesticides in, 76
  temperature of leaves, 273
Plasma, as therapeutic agent, 403
Plasma cholinesterase
  atypical
    as cause of intolerance to succinylcholine, 127
    genetic basis of, 128
  inhibition of, 362
  normal values for, 387
Platelet count, in supportive tests, 392
Plictran® (see Tricyclohexyltin hydroxide)

Pneumonitis, insecticides suggested as cause of, 328
Point mutation, 188
Poison(s)
  arrow, 2
  classes of, definitions of, 433, 435, 441–442, 453–454
  place of, in world history, 3
  regulation of, 429–455
  spindle, 187–188
"Posion," marking on labels, 431
Poison control centers
  information from, 314–316, 321
  organization of, 471
Poison oak, illness caused by, 321
Poison Prevention Packaging Act of 1970, 459
Poisoning
  accidental, in animals
    by pesticides, 478–482, 490–502, 504–509
    evaluation of injury
      to domestic animals, 478–479
      to wildlife, 508–509
    factors contributing to, 480–482, 504
    importance of residues in different media, 305–306
    limitation of, 510–512
    secondary, 488–489
  accidental, in man
    cases, as sources of information, 226
    diagnosis of, 379–391
    epidemics due to pesticides, 322–327
    epidemiology of, as aid to diagnosis, 379
    experience of special groups, 327–333
    factors contributing to, 322–327, 334–339
    history of, as aid to diagnosis, 382
    importance, relative to other causes of death, 311–312
    in different countries, 333–334, 338
    information from poison control centers, 314–316, 321
    morbidity
      from all compounds, 313–316
      from pesticides, 320–322
    mortality, endemic
      from all compounds, 311–313
      from pesticides, 316–320
    occupational, 321–322, 326–327, 339
    pesticides that have caused, 316–317
    prevention of, 429–475
    regional differences in, 337–338
    secondary, 325–326, 380
    treatment of, 391–423
  intentional, 320–327
  possible, 363–367, 481
Poisonous plants, relation to toxinology, 6–7
Poland
  concentration of DDT in milk in, 351
  storage of DDT by people in, 342
Poliomyelitis
  effect of DDT on susceptibility to, 366
  effect on porphyrin metabolism, 90
  insecticides suggested as cause of, 328
Pollution (see also Contamination), 6, 70, 447
Polychlorinated biphenyls (PCB's)
  and duck hepatitis virus, 86
  effect of, on bird breeding, 493, 494, 498, 500
  residues of, in fish, 267
  storage of, 339, 484
Polyethylene screen, for collecting surface microlayers.

  of water, 287
Polyethylene sheet, in dermal toxicity tests, 212
Poncho, as protective clothing, 460
Population control, 85, 486
Population decline, in some birds, 492–502
Pork, contamination of, by alkyl mercury, 324, 325–326
Porphin, 90, 92
Porphobilinogen, 92, 94
Porphyria
  general discussion, 89–91, 92–95
  in relation to chemical epidemiology, 380
Porphyrins, in supportive tests, 94–95, 392
Post-harvest application of pesticides, as factor in residues, 273–274
Potassium antimony tartrate, use as emetic, 394
Potassium cyanate (see also Cyanide and related compounds), 531
Potassium cyanide (see also Cyanide and related compounds)
  cumulative effect of, 43
  production of acute illness by, 38
  toxicity of, 47
Potassium gate, derangement of, 186–187
Potassium ions, in nervous system, 186–187
Potassium permangenate, as neutralizing antidote, 409
Potassium sodium tartrate, use of as cathartic, 398
Potatoes
  pesticide residues in, 268, 446
  residues in soils for raising, 297
Potentiation
  cocarcinogenesis as form of, 190
  in interaction of compounds, 74–75
  relation of to storage, 158–159
Poultry, pesticide residues in, 267
"Practical residue limit," 447
Pralidoxime chloride, 412, 415–416
Predator-prey systems, stable populations in, 486
Predators, 486, 487, 488–489
Pregnancy
  as factor
    influencing toxicity, 80–81
    in pesticide storage, 358
  contraindication to emesis in, 394
Pressure, atmospheric, as factor influencing toxicity, 88
Prevention of injury, by
  choice of compound or formulation, 455–458, 510–511
  protective devices, 464–470
  protective practices, 458–464, 510–512
  regulations, 429–455
Primaquine, as cause of hemolytic anemia, 127
Principle(s) (see Law)
Prisoners
  as volunteers, in testing, 242–243
  of war, in testing, 236
Private institutes, affiliation of toxicologists with, 9
Proban® (see Cythioate)
Probiosis and probiotics, 86
Probit, 41, 440
Procaine, de-esterification of, 112
Production of pesticides, 20–23
Products, stored, protection of, 19
Prolan®, 521
  toxicity to isolated cells, 204

Proline dependence, in tests for mutagenesis, 205
Prometon (Prometone), 531
Prometryn (Prometryne), 531
Propanil, 531
Propargyl bromide, 520
Propazine (Gesamil®), 531
  as tumorigen, 193
  poisoning by, in man, 317
Propham (IPC), 192, 526
  as tumorigen, 192
  metabolism of, 109
Propoxur (Baygon®, aprocarb), 526
  poisoning by, in man, 317
  standards for, 451
  studies of
    in volunteers, 234
    in workers, 229
  testing of for vector control, 331–332
Proprietary names (see Nomenclature)
Propylene glycol, in dermal toxicity tests, 212
n-Propylisome, as tumorigen, 191
Prospective study in epidemiology, 381–382
Prostate, weight of, 152
Protection of
  crops, 17
  investigators, from law suits, 247–248
  people, from malaria, 12–13
  stored products, 19–20
  volunteers, from injury, 246–247
Protective equipment and devices, 464–470
Protective practices, 458–464
Protein
  as neutralizing antidote, 408
  binding, as factor in chemical interaction, 75,
    131–132
  dietary deficiency of, influence of, on toxicity, 82–83
  from plasma, use in therapy, 403
  induction of amyloid by, 195
  in membrane structure, 130
  metabolism of, 107
  microsomal, increase in, 117
Prothrombin
  depletion of, 423
  effect of vitamin K on formation of, 423
  time, in supportive tests, 392
Protocol, in studies in man, 243–246
Protocoproporphyria, 94
Protoporphyrin III, 92
Psychiatric disease, studies of, 240
Psychological factors affecting toxicity, 85
Pulmonary edema, counteracted by oxygen, 401
Puromycin
  action against porphyria, 90
  effects of, on cell metabolism, 108
Purpura
  death rate in USA from, 364
  thrombocytopenic, caused by drugs, 389
Pygoscelis adelinae (adeline-penguins), storage of
    pesticides in, 484
Pyrethrum and pyrethrins, 518
  for protection of staple food, 273
  interaction with other compounds in vivo, 73
  persistence of, 273
  poisoning by, in man, 317, 319
  standards for, 443, 449
  studies of, in volunteers, 231

toxicity of, 68
use as drug, 227
Pyridine-2-aldoxime, use of, as therapeutic agent, 412
Pyridoxine, dermal absorption of, 149
Pyrimethamine, 73
Pyrroloporphyria, 94

Q

Qatar, epidemic of poisoning by endrin in, 323
Quail, eggshell thinning in, 495–496
Qualitative aspects
  of biotransformation, 113, 129
  of metabolism, 107–129
Quantitative aspects of metabolism, 129–172
Quinidine, as cause of thrombocytopenic purpura, 389
Quinine
  as cause of thrombocytopenic purpura, 389
  excretion of, 131
Quinolin, as tumorigen, 193
8-Quinolinol, 532
  as tumorigen, 193
  standards for, 445
Quintozene, 532
  as tumorigen, 193

R

Rabbit
  eye irritation tests in, 214
  skin permeability of, 147, 210
  susceptibility of, compared to other species, 77
Race, as factor in
  exposure, 305
  poisoning, 336
  storage and excretion, 357
Radiation
  as factor in toxicity, 88
  as cause of
    aggressiveness, 89
    carcinogenesis, 190
    injury to embryo, 198, 201
    sex ratio reversal, 89
    sterilization of screw-worm flies, 89
  ionizing, 89
  sensitization to, 89–91
  ultraviolet, 89
  visible, 89
Radioactive substances, graphic warning labels for,
    433–434
Radioactive tracers
  in balance studies, 172
  in dermal absorption studies, 140–143
  in measuring metabolism, 172
  in metabolic pool technique, 172
Radium, its interference with its excretion, 159, 160
Radon, dermal absorption of, 149
Rain, effect of, on residues, 273, 301–302
Rainwater, pesticide residues in, 274, 284–285
Ramazzini, Bernardino, 2
Randomization of subjects, 55
Rat
  dermal absorption by, 141, 147
  in toxicity testing, 43–44
  resistance of, to warfarin, 126
  skin permeability of, compared to other species,
    147, 210

storage of DDT in, 81, 167
Rational Monitoring Program, 445
recINN (see Nomenclature, nonproprietary names)
Red squill, effect of altitude on toxicity of, 88
Reduction, chemical, in metabolism, 108, 110, 112, 115
Reentry poisoning, 321, 326
References, scientific and legal, 33
Regional differences in poisoning, 337
Regulation (see also Law)
    cost of, 453–455
    of pesticides, 429–455
    of surveillance of workers, 463
    of use, 436–437
    of working conditions, 438
    relation to liability, 455
Relative humidity, as factor in toxicity, 97
Remainder analysis, 134, 140–141
Removal of residues from food and water, 275–276
Renal collecting ducts, specific injury to, 195–196
Repellents
    ingestion of, 315
    poisoning by, in man, 315, 317
Reproducibility of results of tests, 63–64
Reproduction
    failure of, in birds, 490–491, 492–502
        possible biochemical basis of, 497–498
    tests of, 215–217
Reproductive system, injury to, 197
Reptiles, effects of pesticides on, 506
Research, clinical, regulation of, 235–240
Reserpine, effect of temperature on toxicity of, 88
Residues of pesticides
    drift in air, 283–285
    effect on domestic animals, 480
    exposure of general population, 276–283
    exposure of workers
        dermal and respiratory, 288–294
        oral, 294
    factors influencing
        in air, 285–288
        in animal products, 267
        in plants, 269–274
        in soil, 298–303
    importance
        to man, 304–305
        to other organisms, 305–306, 502–503
    in air, 282–294
    in food, 265–282
    in mud walls of homes, 303–304
    in soil, 294–304
        following application to crops, 295–297
        following application to soil, 297–298
    in special diets, 281–282
    in total diet, 276–282
    in water, 274–275, 446
    in wildlife, 483–484
    permissible level of, 442
    qualitative and quantitative, changes in, 298
    regulation of, 439–453
    removal from food and water, 275–276
    standard for, 446–452
    volatilization of, 273, 286–288, 302
Resistance
    to compounds,
        as factor in secondary poisoning, 489

    in mammals, 126–128
    in mosquitoes, 13, 330
    metabolism as source of, 125–126
    to disease, reduction of, by chemicals, 86
    usage of word, 118, 125–126
Respiration, inhibition of, by cyanide ion, 184, 421–422
Respirator(s)
    kinds and maintenance of, 464–468
    modified, for measuring respiratory exposure, 251–252
Respiratory absorption (see Absorption, respiratory)
Respiratory excretion, 168, 353
Respiratory exposure
    measurement of, under practical conditions, 249–252
    of workers, 288–294
    protection from, 464–468
Respiratory system
    absorption from, 136–138
    clearance, 139–140
    excretion, 168
    fibrosis of lung, paraquat as cause of, 194–195
    injury to, 194–195, 321
        measurement of, 208–209
    macrophages, injury to, 140
    penetration of, by particles, 138
    phagocytosis, in clearance of, 139–140
    structure of, 139
Respiratory toxicity
    degree of, determining classification for regulatory purposes, 431
    tests of, 208–209
Responses
    conditioned, in behavioral tests, 214
    graded, measurement of, 53
Reticulocytes, count, in supportive treatment, 392
Retina, necrosis of ganglion cells of, 197
Retrospective study in epidemiology, 381
Reversibility of toxic effects, 38–39, 207
Riboflavin, dermal absorption of, 149
Ribosomes, relation of, to microsomal enzymes, 113
Rickets, use of white phosphorus in treatment of, 227
Ringdoves, delayed egg production in, 497
RNA
    effect of inducers on, 108
    messenger, in microsomes, 108
    synthesis, 90–91
Robins, effect of DDT on, 167, 492
Rochelle salt, use of, as cathartic, 398
Rodenticides
    as tumorigens, 192
    poisoning by, in man, 314, 315, 317, 334–335
    use of
        in disease control, 10
        in relation to wildlife, 510
Ronnel (Fenchlorphos), 524
    and microsomal enzymes, 123
    residues of, in air, 284
    species differences in, toxicity of, 76
    standards for, 444, 450
    use of, as drug, 227
Root vegetables, pesticide residues in, 268, 271, 272
Rotenone, 519
    as cause of spindle poisoning, 188
    as tumorigen, 191

Rotenone—*Continued*
  as photosensitizer, 271
  inhibition of oxidative phosphorylation by, 184
  interaction of, with dieldrin, 271
  poisoning by, in man, 317, 319
  standards for, 449
  use of, in relation to wildlife, 510
Romania, storage of DDT by people in, 342
Route(s) of exposure
  as factor in storage and excretion, 355–356
  as factor in toxicity, 71, 335–336
  methods of measuring absorption by, 256–257
Rubber sheet, in dermal toxicity tests, 212
Rubella, as factor in teratogenesis, 201
Ruelene® (see Crufomate)
Rule (see Law)
Rural areas, USA
  atmospheric levels of pesticides in, 282–283
  deaths from pesticides in, 337

S

Sabadilla, 519
  poisoning by, in man, 317
"Safe concentration zone," 451
Safe dosage, calculation of, 439–442
Safety
  closures, 459
  community relations, in relation to, 472–474
  criteria and evaluation of, 5–8, 214–215, 248–249,
      367–371, 439–442
  dosage in relation to, 69, 440–442
  education for, 470–472
  factors (including 100-fold margin), 440–442
  pretesting for, 5
  regulations regarding, 429–455
Safrole, 519
  and microsomal enzymes, 119, 120
Sale of pesticides, limitation of, 430, 436
Salicylates, teratogenicity of, 198
Salicylic acid
  beneficial effect of small dosages, 57
  dermal absorption of, 149
Salivary gland, weight of, 152
Salmonella typhimurium, in tests of mutagenesis, 204
Salt (see Sodium chloride)
Samplers, for measurement of dermal exposure,
      253–254
Samples
  medicolegal importance of, 388
  primary, collection of, 226
  selection, collection, labeling, and shipment of,
      386–388
Sanarelli-Schwartzman phenomenon, 194
Sandwiches, as means of oral exposure to pesticides,
      255–256, 294
Sarin
  absorption of, rate in cat, 143
  detoxification of, by oximes, 412
  inactivation of, by skin enzymes, 145
Saudi Arabia, epidemic of poisoning by endrin in, 323
Scabies
  improper treatment with parathion, 324, 327
  proper treatment with some other pesticides, 232
Schecter-Haller colorimetric method for DDT analy-
      sis, 340–344
Schedule of dosage, as factor in toxicity, 69–70

Schistosomiasis, control of, by molluscicides, 10, 504
Schools, teaching of safety in, 471–472
Schradan (OMPA), 525
  and microsomal enzymes, 123
  oxidation of N of, 112
  species differences in toxicity of, 79
  studies of, in volunteers, 79
Screens to collect dust, 250–251, 285
Schulz rule, 57
Scillicoside, and microsomal enzymes, 120
Scotland, pesticide residues in air of, 284–285
Scrotum, cancer of, 190
Seals, storage of pesticides in, 484–485
Seasonal differences, as factors in,
  poisoning in man, 338
  storage and excretion, 360
  toxicity, 97
Sebaceous glands, in dermal absorption, 145, 146
Secondary poisoning, 380, 488–489
Sedatives
  excretion of, in human milk, 339
  use of, as pharmacological antidotes, 403–404, 410
Sediment, residues in, 274–275
Seed-grain, treated, as source of poisoning, 323, 325,
      507
Selenium
  relation of beneficial and toxic dosages of, 59
  uniformity of concentrations of, in blood, 280–281
Sensitization, tests of, 213–214, 389–391
Sequestration (see also Chelation), of colloidal mate-
      rial injected intravenously, 134, 150
Sesame oil, 191, 519
Sesamex, 519
Sesone, 531
Sesoxame, and microsomal enzymes, 119
Sevin® (see Carbaryl)
Sewage, addition of pesticides to, 462
Sex
  as factor in
    poisoning, in man, 336
    storage and excretion, 163, 357–358
    toxicity, 80–81
  differences in microsomal enzymes, 114
SGOT, in supportive tests, 392
SGPT, in supportive tests, 392
SH-enzymes, inhibition of, by arsenic, 185
Sheets, contamination of, by parathion, 323, 324
Shellfish (see Fish)
Shock, definition and treatment of, 402–405
Siduron, 531
Sigmoid curve, 40–41
Silica
  contraindicated in pesticide formulations, 136
  dosages of, as factor in silicosis, 335
  respiratory exposure to, significance of, 133, 136,
      252
Silicosis, 85–86, 139, 457, 463
Silver, dermal absorption of, 62, 147
Silvex (Fenoprop), 531
  as tumorigen, 193
Simazine, 531
  as tumorigen, 193
  poisoning by, in man, 317
Singapore, epidemic of poisoning in, 324
Sinusitis, insecticides suggested as cause of, 328
Skeleton, axial, relative susceptibility to teratogenesis
      of, 200

SKF 525A, enzyme inhibition by, 75, 118, 123
Skin
  absorption from, 130–134, 140–150, 355–356
  cancer of, 89
  excised, in absorption tests, 144
  exposure of workers, 288–294
  "farmer's," 89
  fatigue, 209
  injury to, 89
    occupational, 321
    tests of, 208–214
  permeability of, 140–145, 210, 256
  sensitization, tests of, 209–210, 213–214
  structure of, 145–146
  washing of, to remove poison, 399
  weight of, 152
Skua, storage of pesticides in, 485
Sleeping time, as indicator of microsomal enzyme
    activity, 114, 119–124, 215
Smoke, retention of chemical in, 138
Smyth technique, for measuring exposure by two
    routes, 256, 356
Soap, provision for washing, 459
Social factors, affecting toxicity, 85
Sociedad Venezolana de Toxicologia, 9
Societies related to toxicology, 8–9, 31
Society of Toxicology, 8, 9
Sodium, dermal absorption of, 149
Sodium arsenate, poisoning by, in man, 317
Sodium azide, poisoning by, in man, 317, 532
Sodium calcium edetate, 418, 420–421
Sodium chlorate, poisoning by, in man, 317, 319, 517
Sodium chloride
  as emetic, 394
  chronicity index of, 46
  poisoning by, in man, 69
  teratogenicity of, 198
  toxicity of
    to animals, 47, 51, 68
    to isolated cells, 204
Sodium cyanide, restriction of, as rodenticide, 430
Sodium fluoride, 517
  poisoning by, in man, 317, 323
Sodium fluoroacetate (1080®), 528
  addition of nigrosine black to, 458
  poisoning by, in man, 317
  restriction of use of, 430, 456
  rodent tolerance to, 125
  standards for, 451
  use of, in relation to wildlife, 510
Sodium gate, derangement of, 186–187
Sodium nitrite, as therapeutic agent, 422
Sodium pentabarbital, 97
Sodium phosphate, use of, as cathartic, 398
Sodium sulfate, use of, as cathartic, 398
Sodium thiosulfate and nitrites, action of, 75, 421–422
Soil
  of cities, residues in, 297
  residues in and factors influencing them, 272,
    294–304
  progressive binding of residues in, 297
  specific gravity of, 295
  temperature of surface, 301
Solubility of compounds, in determining absorption,
    146–150
Solvents
  excretion of, 162

for use in dermal toxicity tests, 212
in partition coefficient determination, 141
safety of, 456
standards for, 449–450
studies of
  in volunteers, 231
  in workers, 299
used as drugs, 227
South Africa
  race as factor in pesticide storage in, 357
  sex as factor in pesticide storage in, 358
South African porphyria, 95
South America, storage of pesticides by people in,
    342, 345
Spain, storage of DDT by people in, 342
Sparrow, effect of DDT on, 167
Sparrow hawks (American and English), 493, 495
Specialized transport across membranes, 132–133
Species
  choice of, in toxicity testing, 210, 214, 240
  differences
    as factor in clinical research, 225
    in eggshell thinning in birds, 496–497
    in metabolism, 114, 118, 482, 498
    in mutagenesis testing, 206–207
    in storage, 163–164
    in toxicity, 75, 77–79, 118–128, 482
    "introduced," 488
Specific action, 184–187
Specific antidotes (see also Detoxifying and Pharma-
    cological antidotes), 410–423
Specific gravity, of soils, 295
Specific-locus test for mutagenesis, 205
"Specific pesticides," 511
Spinal cord
  pesticide concentrations in, 350
  weight of, 152
Spindle poisoning, 187–188
Spironolactone, a catatoxic steroid, 406
Spleen
  storage of pesticides in, 348, 350
  weight of, 152
Spraymen, as subjects of studies, 228–229, 289–291,
    353, 356
Sprays, size of particles in, 136–138
Staphylococcus epidermidis, 86
Starling, storage of pesticides in, 484
Starvation, effect of, on storage and toxicity, 82, 165,
    358–359
State committees, 474
Statistics
  abnormal values in controls, 64
  as element of toxicology, 2
  books on, 53
  geometric mean, 62–63
  grouping of subjects, 55
  "no significant effect level," 55–56
  number of subjects, 53–55
  randomization of subjects, 55
  reproducibility of results, 63–64
  selection of dosages, 55
  sigmoid curve, 40–41
  small dosages, effects of, 55–62
  vital, 312–313, 318–320
Sterility, in mammals, 188–189, 206
Sternus vulgaris (starling), storage of pesticides in,
    484

Steroids
  as therapeutic agents, 406
  endogenous, induction of enzymes by, 108
Stimulants
  behavioral tests of, 215
  use of, as therapeutic agents, 404–405
Stomach (see also Gastrointestinal tract),
      absorption of compounds by, 135
"Stomach tube," in oral dosing, 217
Storage
  as factor in chronicity of injury, 37–38
  as indicator of absorption, 134–135
  concentration index of, 159–160
  cumulative, 38
  dosage-response of, 66, 157, 355
  dynamics of, 150–168
  factors influencing, in man and animals, 66,
      151–164, 355–362
  loss following last dose, 154–161
  mathematical treatment of
    after dosing stops, 151–153, 160–161
    cumulative stage, 157–158
    equilibrium state, 158–159
  models of, 155–156
  of food, effect on pesticide residues, 274
  of pesticides
    for safety, 436, 459–460
    improper, as cause of poisoning, 323–325, 480–481
    in blood, 346–349
    in domestic animals, 266–267, 481
    in ecosystem, 167
    in fat, 340–346
    in fetus, 349–350
    in man, 339–362
    in organs, 348–349
    regulation of, 436
    study of, in volunteers, 231–235
  parameters of, 156
  relation to toxicity, 166–167
Strain differences
  in metabolism, 118–125
  in toxicity, 75–78, 482
Stratum conjunctum, 145, 146
Stratum corneum, 145
Stratum germanativum, 145
Stratum granulosum, 145
Stratum lucidum, 145–148
Stratum spinosum, 145
Streptomycin, 519
  use of, as antibiotic, 227
Streptopelia decapto (collared dove), 501
Streptopelia risoria (ringdove), 496
Strobane® (see Terpene polychlorinates), as tumori-
      gen, 192
Strontium
  dermal absorption of, 149
  storage of, in bone, 164, 340
Strychnine, 519
  adsorption of, by charcoal, 408
  cancellation of use of, for predator control, 430
  dermal absorption of, 149
  poisoning by, in man, 314, 317, 318, 319, 333
  rodent tolerance to, 125
  standards for, 449
  toxicity of
    effect of altitude on, 88

    effect of temperature on, 87–88
  use of
    as drug, 227
    in relation to wildlife, 510
Students, medical, as volunteers, in studies in man,
      242
Studies, in man
  closing ceremony in, 246
  conclusion regarding, 248–249
  consent of persons involved, 239–240, 247
  contribution of, to criteria of safety, 367–371
  design of, 240–248
  diagnostic and therapeutic, 228–230
  dosage selection in, 241
  double blind, 246
  initiation of, 245–246
  laws permitting or requiring, 236–238
  legal considerations, 235–240
  malpractice in relation to, 238
  measurement of exposure of subjects, 249, 257
  physiological, 230
  protection of investigators and volunteers, 246–248
  protocol for, 243–246
  tests applicable to, 114–115, 141–144, 213–214
  volunteers
    choice of, 241–243
    motivation of, 248
    protection of, 246–247
    workers as, 229–230, 243
Subacute toxicity tests, 43, 202
"Sufficient challenge," 58
Sugar, pesticide residues in, 269, 323
Suicide, 312, 320, 327
Suits, as protective devices, 469
Sulfate ions, 108, 111
Sulfides, 108
Sulfonamids and derivatives, as causes of photosen-
      sitization, 89
Sulfonethylmethane, porphyria production by, 90
Sulfoxidation, 109, 112
Sulfur, 518
  occupational diseases caused by, 321
Sulfur dioxide, 520
  poisoning by, in man, 319
  relation to aerosols, 139
  standards for, 450
Sulfuryl fluoride, 520
  poisoning by, in man, 317
Sulphadiazine, 73
Sulphenone®, 528
Sumithion® (see Fenitrothion)
Sunburn, 89
Superficial barrier, in dermal absorption, 145, 147
Supplied-air respirators, 466
Supportive test, 391
"Supralethal dosage," 48
Surveillance (see Monitoring)
Survival index, in tests of reproduction, 216
Susceptibility (see Toxicity)
Swamper, 470
Sweat glands, in dermal absorption, 145
Sweating, resulting from acetylcholine excess, 185
Sweden
  concentration of DDT in milk in, 351
  poison control centers in, 471
  poisoning of children in, 336

regulation of tests in man in, 238
Swedish porphyria, 94
Switzerland, poisoning in, 334, 336
Sympathomimetic effects of oximes, 413
Synergists, as tumorigens, 191
Synthesis of compounds (see Conjugation)
Synthetic organic pesticides, production data on, 22
Synthetic organic rodenticides
    posioning by, in man, 317
    studies of, in volunteers, 231
    use of as drugs, 227
Syphilis
    as teratogen, 201
    mercury in treatment of, 1, 133
Syrup of ipecac, 394–395
Systemic insecticides, 271
Systemics, for mammals, 76
Systox® (see Demeton)
Systox sulfoxide, as product of systox oxidation, 109

T

2,4,5-T, 531
    absorption of, 135
    as tumorigen, 193
    poisoning by, in man, 317
    residues of
        in air, drift of, 284
        removal of, from water, 276
        standards for, 447, 451
    storage of, 384, 385
    studies of, in workers, 229
    use of
        in relation to wildlife, 510
        tonnage, 25
Tannic acid, as neutralizing antidote, 408
Tapetum ludicum, of the eye, destruction of, 197
TBA, DMA salt, 531
2,3,6-TBA, 531
TCA, 531
    poisoning by, in man, 317
TBP (see 2,2-Thiobis(4,6-dichlorophenol)
TCDS (see Tetradifon)
TDE (see DDD)
Techniques
    chromatography, 172
    covering of animals for dermal testing, 210–212
    formulation, selection of for testing, 212–213
    mass spectrography, 172
    metabolic pool, 172–173
    of adjusting urine samples, 388
    of dermal dosing, 210–214
    of fat biopsy, 165–166, 388–389
    of gastric lavage, 396–397
    of measuring
        dermal absorption, 140–145
        dermal toxicity, 208–214
        respiratory toxicity, 208
    of oral dosing, 217
    of respiratory dosing, 208
    of studies in man, 225–257
    species, choice of, 210, 214, 240
    volume of dose, 213, 218
Teeth, weight of, 152
Telodrin® (see Isobenzan)
Telvar® (see Monuron)
Temik® (see Aldicarb)

Temperature
    as factor in residues, 301
    as factor in teratogenesis in birds, 199
    as factor in toxicity, 87–88
    coefficient, in poisoning, 186–187
    control of, in care of poisoned patient, 407
    effect of, on dermal absorption, 146–148
    of plant leaves, 273
    of soil surface, 301
1080® (see Sodium fluoroacetate)
Tepa, 532
    as cause of sterility in mice, 189
Tepp (tetraethylpyrophosphate), 525
    and microsomal enzymes, 123
    dermal absorption of, 140, 149
    dust, application of, 292
    exposure to, 289–291, 293–294
    poisoning by, in man, 317
    species differences in, susceptibility to, 78
    studies of
        in volunteers, 234
        in workers, 229
    toxicity of, 68
Teratogenesis
    dosage-response in, 64, 198
    factors in, 198, 201
    general discussion, 197–201
    in man, 201
    in tests of reproduction, 215
    measurement of, 217
    relation to general toxicity, 198–199
Teratogenic zone, 199
Teratogens
    classes of, 198
    interaction of, 74
Teratology, 5, 217
Terbacil, 531
Terbutol (Azak ®), 531
Termites, control of concentration and availability of poison, 297–298
Terpene polychlorinates (see also Strobane ®), 522
    as tumorigens, 192
Testis
    injury to, 197
    weight of, 152
Testosterone, and microsomal enzymes, 123
Test(s) (see also Techniques)
    acute toxicity, 202
    basophil, 390–391
    biochemical and biophysical, 203
    breath analysis, 389
    chronic toxicity, 202
    cost of, 454–455
    diagnostic, 383–391
    dosage for, choice of, 55, 241
    for hypersensitivity, limitations of, 389–391
    formulation as factor in, 212–213
    for pharmacological effects, 386
    for toxicants or metabolites, 383–386
    in man (see also Studies in man), 225–249
    index, 240
    legal requirement for, 237
    of behavior, 214–215
    of biological magnification, 503
    of carcinogenesis, 207
    of dermal toxicity, 208–214
    of eye irritation, 214

Test(s)—*Continued*
  of isolated cells, 203–204
  of microsomal enzyme activity, 115, 116
  of mutagenesis, 204–207
  of oral toxicity, 217–218
  of primary irritation, 208, 213
  of reproduction, 215–217
  of respiratory toxicity, 208
  of sensitization
    other tissues, 389–391
    skin, 213–214
  of teratogenesis, 217
  patch, 213–214
  pharmacological, 207–208
  preparation of animals for, 210–212
  relation to toxicology, 201–203
  subacute toxicity, 202
  supportive, 391
  using chelating agents, to mobilize lead, 385–386
  using small numbers of subjects, 42
  volume of dose, as factor in, 213, 218
Tetrachlorethylene, 520
  penetration of skin by, 142
  poisoning by, in man, 317
  storage loss of, 161
  standards for, 480
  studies of, in volunteers, 231
  use of, as drug, 227
2,3,4,6-Tetrachlorophenol, 527
Tetradifon (TCDS), 528
  as tumorigen, 192
  exposure of workers to, 291
  residues of, in total diet, 278
Tetraethylpyrophosphate (see tepp)
Tetralin ®, 317, 519
  toxicity of, to man, 317
Tetramethrin (see also Pyrethrum and pyrethrins), 518
Thalidomide, as teratogen, 5, 201, 217
Thallium and its compounds, 518
  as cause of chronic illness, 38
  dithizon in treatment of poisoning by, 421
  poisoning by, in man, 317, 319, 323
  restriction of use of, 436
  secondary poisoning by, 488
  standards for, 449
  studies of, in volunteers, 231
  use of, as depilatory, 227
Thanite ® (see Isobornyl thiocyanoacetate)
Therapeutic studies in man, 228, 230–235
Theriaca, remedy, 4
Thermodynamic activity, 183–184
Thiabendazole, 532
  poisoning by, in man, 317
  standards for, 445
Thiamine
  deficiency of, 184
  dermal absorption of, 149
2,2-Thiobis (4,6-dichlorophenol) (TBP), 527
  as tumorigen, 192
Thiocyanate, conversion of cyanide to, 111, 421, 422, 520
Thiodan ® (see Endosulfan)
Thiometon, 524
  poisoning by, in man, 317
  studies of, in workers, 229

Thionazin, 525
Thiopental, importance of blood flow in distribution of, 151
Thiouracil, toxic effects of, 197
Thiourea
  dermal absorption of, 149
  safety factor of, 440
Thiram (TMTD), 526
  as tumorigen, 192
  poisoning by, in man, 317
  standards for, 444, 451
Thorium, dermal absorption of, 149
Three generation test of reproduction, 215–217
Threshold
  biological reality of, 56–57
  chemical basis of, 61–62
  effect, 440
Threshold limit values (TLV's), 133, 446–452
Thrombocytopenic purpura, some chemicals producing, 389
Thromboembolic disease, treatment of with warfarin, 235
Thumb, absorption of compounds through, 142
Thymidine dependence, in tests for mutagenesis, 205
Thymus, weight of, 152
Thyroid
  autoimmunization of, as factor in teratogenesis, 201
  injury to, by chemicals, 183, 197, 497
  weight of, 152
Thyroxine, protein binding of, 131
TIBA (see 2,3,6-Triiodobenzoic acid)
Time (see also Season), from application to harvest, 270
Time-dosage relationships
  ET 50 and LT 50, 47–48
  Haber's rule, 51–52
  logtime-logdosage curve, 48–52
    use to predict proper dosage for long-term tests, 51
  of residues
    in soil, 298–300
    in vegetable foods, 270
  of storage, 150–168
  of toxicity, 46–47
Tin and its compounds, 518
  standards for, 449
Tissue
  as factor in storage and excretion, 153–154, 163–164, 360–361
  connective, weight of, 152
  dosage in, 39, 53, 167
  supportive, injury to, 196
TKT (see Tyrosine alpha-ketoglutarate transaminase)
TLV's (see Threshold limit values)
TMTD (see Thiram)
Tobacco, cigarettes, poisoning by, in man, 311–312
TOCP, potentiation of malathion by, 75
TOK ®, 531
Tolbutamide
  and microsomal enzyme induction by, 116, 122
  as teratogen, 201
Tolerance
  legal for residues, 442–446
  to chemicals including nicotine, 125, 380
  usage of word, 118, 125, 442

Tort claims act, for protection by medical investigators, 247–248
Toxaphene, 522
  disappearance of, from soil, 299
  dosage-response curve, 42
  excretion of, in man, 386
  microsomal enzyme induction by, 120, 122
  poisoning by, in man, 317, 319, 324
  residues of
    in air, 282
    in cotton seed oil, 269
    in soil, 296
    in total diet, 278, 279
    standards for, 447, 450
  storage of, in people, 384, 385
  studies of, in volunteers, 232
  toxicity of, effect of protein on, 83
  use of, in USA, 25
Toxaplasmosis, as teratogen, 202
Toxicant
  concentration of, effect on toxicity, 53
  dispersed, measurement of, 52–53
  removal of, by washing, 141, 211, 253–254, 398–399
  tests for, 383–386
  usage of word, 7
Toxication, usage of word, 129
Toxicity (see also Compound, Dosage, Exposure)
  acute, 37, 202
  as influenced by
    accessibility of poison, 437–438
    adaptation, 117–118
    age (including embryo), 81–82, 199–200, 336–337
    aggregation, 84–85
    altitude, 88
    circadian rhythms, 91–96
    competence of people, 336–337
    compound, 37, 68–69, 146–147, 149–150, 199, 334–335
    containers for poison, 338
    crowding, 84–85
    disease, 85–87
    dosage, 37, 64–67, 69–70, 199, 335
      duration of, 37, 70–71
      schedule of, 69–70
    ecological factors, 488–492, 502–503, 504–508
    enzymes, 117–118, 125–129
    formulation, 75, 212–213
    genetic factors, 127–128
    individual differences, 78–80
    interaction of compounds, 72–75, 336
    isolation, 84–85
    light and other radiation, 88–91
    nutrition, 82–84
    occupation, 339
    organ susceptibility, 194–197, 200
    pH, 97
    photosensitization, 89
    pregnancy, 80–81
    pressure, atmospheric, 88
    psychological factors, 85
    race, 326
    relative humidity, 97
    route of exposure, 71, 335, 336
    season, 97, 338
    sex, 80–81, 336
    skin area, 142–145, 213
    skin covering, 210–212
    skin integrity, 145–148
    social factors, 85
    species, 75–79, 118, 194
    stage of development, 199–200
    storage in tissues, 37, 166–167
    storage of formulations, 322–325
    strain, 75–76, 199
    temperature, 87–88, 148
    water hardness, 97–98
  chronic, 37, 202
  chronicity of, 37–39
  corrosive action in, 183
  dosage-response relationships, 64–67
  duration of injury, 37–39
  expression of, 37, 39
  intravenous, 134
  kinds of, 37, 64–67, 182–218
  nonspecific action in, 183–184
  of metabolites, 129
  ratings or classes, 431–432, 433, 435, 453–454
  specific action in, 184–187
  subacute, 202
  tests for (see Tests)
  to cells, 187–194
  to chromosomes, 188–190
  to embryo and fetus, 197–201
  to organ systems, 194–197
  to wildlife, 483–512
Toxic dose, percentage per hour, 293–294
Toxicologically insignificant levels, 441–442
Toxicologists, affiliations and training of, 8, 9
Toxicology
  definition of, 1
  information on, sources of, 31–33
  landmarks of, 2–3
  societies, 8–9
  subdivisions of, 2–8
  training in, 8, 470–472
Toxic substances graphic warning labels for, 433–434
Toxin
  bacterial, 6
  fungal, 6, 320
  usage of word, 7
Toxinology, relation to toxicology, 6–7
Toxogonin (see Obidoxime chloride)
Trace elements, 57, 83–84, 215
Tracers, 141, 142, 171, 172
Tracheostomy, in treatment of poisoning, 400
Training, 8, 470–472
Tranquilizers
  behavioral tests in relation to, 215
  excretion of, in human milk, 339
  population control in relation to, 85
Transfusions, in treatment of poisoning, 402–403
Translocation of pesticides in plants, 271, 272
Transport of chemicals in blood, 134–135, 150–151
Transport of pesticides
  regulation of, 434–436
  spillage during, as cause of epidemics of poisoning, 323–325
Treatment of poisoning, 3–4, 391–423
Tretamine, 532
  as tumorigen, 193
Trevan, 40, 440

S,S,S-Tributyl phosphorothioate (DEF ®), 531
  atmospheric levels of, 282
Tributyl phosphorothioite (Folex ®), 531
Tributyrin, for test of microsomal enzymes, 115
Trichinella spiralis and trichinosis, 86
Trichlorfon (Chlorophos ®, Dipterex ®), 524
  effect of, on oxime concentrations in brain, 414
  in treatment of helminthiasis, 76
  poisoning by, in man, 317
  species differences in toxicity of, 76
  standards for, 444
  studies of, in volunteers, 234
  toxicity to isolated cells, 204
  use of, as drug, 227
1,2,3-Trichloro-4,6-dinitrobenzene, 532
1,1,1-Trichloroethane
  penetration of skin by, 142
  poisoning by, in man, 317
  standards for, 450
  studies of, in volunteers, 231
  rate of absorption of, by man, 143
Trichloroethene (see Trichloroethylene)
Trichloroethylene (Trichloroethene), 521
  excretion of, 169, 171
  penetration of skin by, 142
  persistence of residues of, in grain, 274
  poisoning by, in man, 317, 333
  standards for, 450
  studies of,
    in volunteers, 231
    in workers, 229
Trichlorodinitrobenzene, residues of in potatoes, 268
2,4,5-Trichlorophenol, 527
2,4,5-Trichlorophenol, zinc salt, 527
2,4,6-Trichlorophenol, 527
  as tumorigen, 192
Tricyanoaminopropene, toxic effects of, 197
Tricyclohexyltin hydroxide, 443, 449, 518
Triethylenemelamine, as cause of sterility, 206
Triethyl tin, inhibition of oxidative phosphorylation
  by, 184
3-Trifluoromethyl-4-nitrophenol, for lamprey control,
  504, 510
Trifluralin, 531
2,3,6-Triiodobenzoic acid (TIBA), 531
Trimedoxime, use of, as therapeutic agent, 412
Trimethylamine, *N*-oxidation of, 112
1,1'-Trimethylene bis (4-formyl pyridinium), use of,
  as therapeutic agent, 412
Triorthocresyl phosphate
  as cause of chronic paralysis, 38, 64, 380
  potentiation of malathion by, 74
  susceptibility to, in man and hens, 76
Tri-*p*-ethylphenyl phosphate, neurotoxicity of, to
  chickens, 240
2,4,6-Trisethyleneimino-1,3,5-triazine, as cause of
  sterility in dogs, 206
2,4,6-tri-*tert*-butylphenol, 62
Trithion ® (see Carbophenothion)
Tritium, dermal absorption of, 149
"Trophic concentration," of pesticides by wildlife, 490
Tuberculosis, 85
Tumorigenicity of various compounds, 64–65, 191–193
Tumors, adrenal, treatment of, with DDD, 232
Turdus migratorius (robin), 492
Turkey (bird), storage of DDT in, 66

Turkey (country), poisoning by hexachlorobenzene in,
  323
Turnip greens, effect of, on benzpyrene hydroxylase,
  116
Typhus, controlled by DDT, 10
Tyrosine alpha-ketoglutarate transaminase (TKT),
  96

U

Ulmus americana (elm), 492
Ultra-low volume technique, of pesticide application,
  26–27
Ultraviolet radiation
  action on pesticides, 107, 284, 306, 503
  conversion of 7-dehydrocholesterol, 89
  injuries caused by, 89
  photosensitization by, 89
Unconsciousness
  as contraindication to emesis, 394
  care of people in, 407
Union of Soviet Socialist Republics
  concentration of DDT in milk in, 351
  epidemics of poisoning in, 320, 323, 480
  industrial exposure in, 448, 451, 453
United Kingdom
  effects of pesticides on birds in, 493, 496, 498–501,
    507
  labeling of pesticides in, 432–433
  participation of, in Council of Europe, 433
  poisoning of people in, 333, 336
  requirements for tests in man in, 237–238
United States Adopted Name Council, 30
United States Department of Agriculture (USDA), 31
United States Department of Transportation, 436
United States Food and Drug Administration (FDA),
  30
United States of America (USA) (see also specific
    states)
  concentration of DDT in human milk in, 349–351
  effects of pesticides on birds in, 490–491, 492–502,
    505, 506, 507
  epidemics of poisoning by pesticides in, 323–324
  excretion of pesticides by people in, 349–355
  geographical distribution of residues in food in,
    280–281
  labeling of pesticides in, 430–432
  legal requirements for tests in man in, 237
  mortality rate for accidental poisoning in, 311–313
  regulation of transport in, 434–436
  reports of occupational disease in, 321–322
  residues of pesticides in air of, 280, 282–283
  storage of pesticides by people in, 339–351
United States Tariff Commission, 21
Units, of measure, used in toxicology, 33, 141–145,
  448, 534, 535
"Universal antidote," 408
Universities, affiliation of toxicologists with, 9
Urban-rural distribution of poisoning, 337
Urea
  dermal absorption of, 149
  metabolite of carbon tetrachloride, 108
  movement of, across membranes, 130
Urinalysis, as supportive test, 392
Urinary pH, effect of, on dynamics of storage, 161

Urine
  adjustment of samples of, 388
  analysis of compound in, as measure of absorption, 142
  excretion via, 169, 352–255, 386
Urogenital organs
  injury to, by chemicals, 195–196
  susceptibility of, to teratogenesis, 200
Uroporphyrin, 93, 94, 95
Uroporphyrinogen, 94
USAN Council (see United States Adopted Name Council)
USDA (see United States Department of Agriculture)
Use experience, as source of information on safety, 226, 228
Use of pesticides
  economic benefits from, 13–15, 18–19
  methods of application, 21, 26–27
  modified, for protection of wildlife, 510–512
  number of compounds and products, 24–26
  regulation of, 436–439
  tonnage, 24, 25

V

Valinomycin, effect of, on conductance in membranes, 186
Vapor pressure, of pesticides, 286–287
Vasoconstrictors, effect of, on dermal absorption, 148
Vasopressor drugs, use of, as therapeutic agents, 404–405
Vector control
  and dermal exposure, 293
  WHO testing of compounds for, 330–333
Vegetables, pesticide residues in, 267–274
Veils, as protective clothing, 469
Venenum, Latin root of venom, 7
Venezuela
  occupational poisoning by dieldrin in, 327
  storage of pesticides by people in, 242, 345
Venom, 7
Vertebrates
  resistance to chemicals in, 126, 489
  species differences in, 76–78
Veterinary medicine, in training of toxicologists, 9
Veterinary Products Safety Precautions Scheme in Great Britain, 432
Veterinary toxicology, 5
Viability index, in test of reproduction, 216
Viruses, bacterial for genetic studies, 204
Visible radiation, effects of, 89
Vitamin A
  dermal absorption of, 149
  teratogenicity of, 198, 215
  threshold dosage for action of, 56–57
Vitamin C, dermal absorption of, 149
Vitamin D
  dermal absorption of, 149
  formation of, in irradiated skin, 89
  threshold dosage for action of, 56–57
Vitamin K
  as specific antidote, 423
  dermal absorption of, 149
  in relation to warfarin resistance, 126

Volatilization, of pesticides, 273, 283, 286–288, 301, 302
Volume of dose, for oral or dermal administration, 42–43, 213, 218
Volunteers (see Studies in man)
Vomiting (see Emesis)

W

Wales, poisoning by pesticides in, 323, 333
Warfarin, 528
  chronicity index of, 46
  competition for binding sites by, 132
  cumulative effect of, 46, 160
  in tests for microsomal enzyme activity, 116, 124
  poisoning by, in man, 317, 319, 323
  replacement for dangerous rodenticides, 456
  resistance to, in rats and man, 126
  secondary poisoning by, 488
  standards for, 451
  studies of, in volunteers, 235
  susceptibility of different species to, 80
  toxicity of, 43–44, 47, 48, 50, 87
  use of, as drug, 227
Warning
  graphic, 433–434
  marking on labels, 432
Washing
  in measurement of dermal exposure, 253–254
  in prevention of poisoning, 458–459
  in treatment of poisoning, 398–399
Water
  as toxicant, 69
  effect of, on dermal absorption of dicrotophos, 149
  effects on wildlife of, pesticides in, 504–505, 506, 507, 508
  hardness of, as factor in toxicity, 97–98
  pesticide residues in, 274–275, 276
  provision of, for washing, 459
  rate of absorption, in man, 143
  standards for residues in, 446–447
Water-electrolyte balance, restoration of, 402–403
Water-wettable powders, 26
  in dermal toxicity tests, 213
  safety of, 457
  size of particles in, 137
Weather, as factor in residues in food, 273
Weed(s), losses caused by, 16
Weed Society of America (WSA), 9, 31
Weight
  loss of,
    effect on storage and toxicity, 82, 166–167, 358–359
    influence on toxicity, 82
  pesticides used in reduction of, 227
West Pakistan, epidemic of poisoning in, 323
Wheat, contamination of, by parathion, 323
Wheat plants, in genetic studies, 204
White blood cells, 86–87, 390–391
White phosphorus, use of, as drug, 227
WHO (World Health Organization)
  pesticides testing program, 330–333
  responsibility for nonproprietary names of drugs, 30
Whooping crane, 497
Wick evaporation, 286

Wildlife (see also specific forms)
    alternative methods of pest control, 512
    control of, 509–510
    effects of pesticides on, 483–512
    exposure of, to pesticides in different media, 306
    geographical distribution by pesticides in, 484–485
    importance to, of residues, 306
    inherent susceptibility of, to pesticides, 483
    injury to, 503–509
    limitation of injury to, 510–512
    storage of pesticides in, 283, 284, 483–484
Wilson's disease, use of penicillamine in treatment of,
        421
Wind
    as factor in exposure of workers, 292
    in relation to residues in air, 286
Wisconsin, pesticides in soils in, 296–297
Wolfen ® (see Copper dimethyldithiocarbamates)
Women, storage of pesticides in, 357–358
Workers
    advantages as subjects for studies, 243
    "buddy system" among, 459
    exposure of, to pesticides, 288–294, 368
    marginal effects of pesticides, rare in, 363–366
    measurement of exposure of, 249–257
    medical surveillance of, 463–464
    occupational disease in, 321–322
    storage of pesticides in, 384–385
    studies of pesticides in, 229–230
    training of, 470–471
    urinary excretion of pesticides by, 386
Working conditions, regulation of, 438
Working in pairs for safety, 459
World Health Organization (see WHO)
World Wars, malaria in, 10–11
WSA (see Weed Society of America)

                            X

Xanthone, 528

X-radiation
    carcinogenic action of, 190
    teratogenic action of, 64, 198
X-ray of chest, as supportive test, 392
Xylene, 519
    effect of, on dermal absorption of dicrotophos, 149
    in dermal toxicity tests, 212–213
    poisoning by, in man, 317, 324
Xylylbromide, 51

                            Y

Yeast, in genetic studies, 204
Yellow fever, urban, control by DDT, 10

                            Z

Zectran ®, 526
    as tumorigen, 192
    poisoning by, in man, 317
Zenaidura macroura (mourning dove), 496
Zinc
    effect of deficiency of, on eye, 197
    effect on metabolism of molybdenum, 75, 83
Zinc arsenite (ZMA), 517
Zinc phosphide, 520
    poisoning by, in man, 317
    rodent tolerance to, 125
Zinc sulfate, use of, as emetic, 394
Zineb, 527
    as tumorigen, 192
    poisoning by, in man, 317
    standards for, 444
Ziram (Milbam ®), 527
    as tumorigen, 192
    poisoning by, in man, 127, 317
    standards for, 444
ZMA (see Zinc arsenite)
Zoxyzolamine, and microsomal enzymes, 122
Zygote, teratogenesis in, 199